SYNOPSIS OF
SURGERY

SYNOPSIS OF
SURGERY

RICHARD D. LIECHTY, M.D.

Professor of Surgery and Associate Dean, Graduate Medical Education,
University of Colorado College of Medicine,
Denver, Colorado

ROBERT T. SOPER, M.D.

Professor of Surgery, Director, Pediatric Surgical Services,
University of Iowa College of Medicine,
Iowa City, Iowa

FIFTH EDITION

with **811** illustrations

The C. V. Mosby Company

ST. LOUIS • TORONTO • PRINCETON   1985

MOSBY

A TRADITION OF PUBLISHING EXCELLENCE

Editor-in-chief: Karen Berger
Assistant editor: Sandra L. Gilfillan
Manuscript editor: Carl Masthay
Book design: Jeanne Genz
Cover design: Suzanne Oberholtzer
Production: Barbara Merritt, Ginny Douglas

FIFTH EDITION

The C.V. Mosby Company
11830 Westline Industrial Drive, St. Louis, Missouri 63146

Library of Congress Cataloging in Publication Data

Liechty, Richard D., 1925–
  Synopsis of surgery.

  Bibliography: p.
  Includes index.
  1. Surgery—Handbooks, manuals, etc. I. Soper,
Robert T., 1925–   . II. Title. [DNLM: 1. Surgery,
Operative. WO 500 L718s]
RD37.L53   1985   617   84-25465
ISBN 0-8016-3099-1

T/VH/VH   9 8 7 6 5 4 3 2 1   01/C/041

Contributors

WILLIAM H. BAKER, M.D.

Professor and Chief, Section of Peripheral Vascular Service, Stritch School of Medicine, Loyola University of Chicago, Chicago, Illinois

EDWARD BARTLE, M.D.

Assistant Professor, University of Colorado School of Medicine, Denver, Colorado.

GEORGE E. BLOCK, M.D.

Professor of Surgery, Pritzker School of Medicine, University of Chicago, Chicago, Illinois

JEFFREY R. CLARK, M.D., Col.

Chief of Surgery, Fitzsimmons Army Hospital, Aurora, Colorado

DANIEL L. CLARKE-PEARSON, M.D.

Associate Professor, Division of Gynecologic Oncology, Department of Obstetrics and Gynecology, University of Illinois at Chicago, Chicago, Illinois

REGINALD R. COOPER, M.D.

Professor and Chairman, Department of Orthopaedics, University of Iowa College of Medicine, Iowa City, Iowa

ROBERT J. CORRY, M.D.

Professor and Head, Department of Surgery, University of Iowa College of Medicine, Iowa City, Iowa

ALBERT E. CRAM, M.D.

Associate Professor, Department of Surgery, University of Iowa College of Medicine, Iowa City, Iowa

MERRIL T. DAYTON, M.D.

Assistant Professor, Department of Surgery, University of Iowa College of Medicine, Iowa City, Iowa

DONALD B. DOTY, M.D.

Clinical Professor of Surgery, Staff Surgeon, LDS Hospital and Children's Medical Center, Salt Lake City, Utah

BEN EISEMAN, M.D.

Professor of Surgery, University of Colorado Medical Center, Denver, Colorado

ADRIAN E. FLATT, M.D., M.Chir., F.R.C.S.

Chairman, Department of Surgery, Norwalk Hospital, Norwalk, Connecticut; Clinical Professor of Orthopaedic Surgery, Yale University, New Haven, Connecticut

DAVID W. FURNAS, M.D.

Professor of Surgery and Chief of Plastic Surgery, University of California, Irvine, California

JONATHAN C. GOLDSMITH, M.D.

Associate Professor, Department of Internal Medicine, University of Nebraska Medical Center, Omaha, Nebraska

HOWARD P. GREISLER, M.D.

Assistant Professor, Section of Peripheral Vascular Surgery, Stritch School of Medicine, Loyola University of Chicago, Chicago; Attending Surgeon, Hines Veterans Administration Hospital, Chicago, Illinois

NELSON J. GURLL, M.D.

Professor, Department of Surgery, University of Iowa College of Medicine, Iowa City, Iowa

JOHN F. HANSBROUGH, M.D.

Assistant Professor of Surgery and Director of Emergency Services, University of Colorado Medical Center, Denver, Colorado

CHARLES E. HARTFORD, M.D.

Director, Burn Treatment Center, Crozer-Chester Medical Center, Chester, Pennsylvania

CHARLES J. KRAUSE, M.D.

Professor and Chairman, Otolaryngology—Head and Neck Surgery, University of Michigan, Ann Arbor, Michigan

WADE C. LAMBERTH, Jr., M.D.

Assistant Professor, Thoracic and Cardiovascular Surgery, Department of Surgery, University of Iowa College of Medicine, Iowa City, Iowa

RICHARD D. LIECHTY, M.D.

Professor of Surgery and Associate Dean, Graduate Medical Education, University of Colorado College of Medicine, Denver, Colorado

EDWARD E. MASON, M.D., Ph.D.

Professor of Surgery, University of Iowa College of Medicine, Iowa City, Iowa

BRIAN F. McCABE, M.D.

Professor and Head, Department of Otolaryngology—Head and Neck Surgery, University of Iowa College of Medicine, Iowa City, Iowa

J. SCOTT MILLIKAN, M.D.

Instructor in Surgery, University of Colorado School of Medicine, Denver, Colorado

GEORGE E. MOORE, M.D.

Professor of Surgery, Denver General Hospital, Director, Surgical Oncology, Denver, Colorado

HIRO NISHIOKA, M.D., F.A.C.S.

Assistant Clinical Professor of Neurosurgery, Medical College of Wisconsin, Milwaukee, Wisconsin

ISRAEL PENN, M.D.

Chief of Surgery, Veterans Administration Medical Center, Cincinnati, Ohio

JACK R. PICKLEMAN, M.D.

Professor of Surgery, Chief, Division of General Surgery, Stritch School of Medicine, Loyola University of Chicago, Chicago, Illinois

SAMUEL D. PORTER, M.D.

Clinical Associate Professor of Surgery, University of Iowa College of Medicine, Iowa City, Iowa

KEVIN C. PRINGLE, M.D., Ch.B.

Associate Professor, Department of Surgery, University of Iowa College of Medicine, Iowa City, Iowa

NICHOLAS P. ROSSI, M.D.

Professor, Thoracic and Cardiovascular Surgery, Department of Surgery, University of Iowa College of Medicine, Iowa City, Iowa

JOSEPH D. SCHMIDT, M.D.

Professor of Surgery/Urology, Head, Division of Urology, School of Medicine, University of California, San Diego, California

JAMES A. SCHULAK, M.D.

Assistant Professor, Department of Surgery, University of Iowa College of Medicine, Iowa City, Iowa

SIROOS S. SHIRAZI, M.D., F.A.C.S.

Professor and Director of Gastrointestinal Surgery, Department of Surgery, University of Iowa College of Medicine, Iowa City, Iowa

RAYMOND SILVA, M.D.

Instructor, University of Colorado School of Medicine, Denver, Colorado

JOHN T. SOPER, M.D.

Assistant Professor, Division of Gynecologic Oncology, Department of Obstetrics and Gynecology, Duke University Medical Center, Durham, North Carolina

NATHANIEL J. SOPER, M.D.

Senior Surgical Resident, University of Utah Medical Center, Salt Lake City, Utah

ROBERT T. SOPER, M.D.

Professor of Surgery, Director, Pediatric Surgical Services, University of Iowa College of Medicine, Iowa City, Iowa

GREG VAN STIEGMANN, M.D.

Assistant Professor of Surgery, University of Colorado School of Medicine, Denver, Colorado

NEIL R. THOMFORD, M.D.

Professor and Chairman, Department of Surgery, Medical College of Ohio, Toledo, Ohio

TIMOTHY A. THOMSEN, M.D.

Clinical Assistant Professor of Surgery, University of Iowa College of Medicine, Iowa City, Iowa

JOHN H. TINKER, M.D.

Professor and Head, Department of Anesthesia, University of Iowa College of Medicine, Iowa City, Iowa

IVAN M. TURPIN

Assistant Professor of Surgery, University of California Medical School at Irvine, Irvine, California

RICHARD WEIL, III, M.D.

Professor of Surgery, University of Colorado School of Medicine, Denver, Colorado

To
Valerie and Hélène

Preface

Almost twenty years ago, we began outlining the first edition of *Synopsis of Surgery*. At that time we adopted the philosophy of writing for those medical students just beginning their clinical studies. Our coauthors have readily accepted this concept of "... the textbook carefully designed for a particular audience, the student, whether still in school or fifteen years out of school..." (*J.A.M.A.* **197:**133, 1966). In this editorial, the author cautions medical writers to avoid the temptation to combine textbooks with "... reference books which discuss specific topics in substantial detail. Whoever tries to mix these two types is, at the present complex level of medicine, performing only a disservice."

Although we have resisted the constant pressures to include more data, to make this a textbook for all readers, *Synopsis of Surgery* has inevitably grown since the first edition. We hope, nevertheless, that this fifth edition will continue to give the students a broad understanding of surgical principles yet allow them some occasional extra moments with a Bach, a Dostoevski, or perhaps a Tom Landry, to leaven their data-gorged existence. As Hamlet reminds us, students and teachers alike: "There are more things in heaven and earth, Horatio, than are dreamt of in our philosophy."

Richard D. Liechty
Robert T. Soper

Contents

SYNOPSIS OF
SURGERY

1
Origin of Surgical Disease

Richard D. Liechty
Robert T. Soper

Each day of the year our medical school libraries add the equivalent of three new *volumes* of medical literature to their already extensive collections. As in other scientific fields, the medical profession, and especially the medical student, face an "information crisis." The volume and scope of medical literature dramatically emphasize the diversity of specialization. However, common bonds do exist across the specialty fields. Obstruction is still obstruction whether in the lacrimal duct, ureter, or spinal canal. We would like to begin by emphasizing some of these common concepts that link one specialty to another.

All somatic diseases, regardless of the specialty fields treating them, have their origins in the following six basic pathological processes:

1. Congenital defects
2. Inflammations
3. Neoplasms
4. Trauma
5. Metabolic defects and degeneration
6. Collagen defects

Four phenomena that result from these fundamental pathological processes are responsible for almost all surgical diseases and for many nonsurgical diseases as well. These phenomena are (1) obstruction, (2) perforation, (3) erosion, and (4) tumors (or masses).

OBSTRUCTION

Cerebrovascular disease (strokes) and coronary heart disease (coronaries) are two of the leading causes of death in the United States. Both result from obstruction of vital arteries carrying blood to the brain or to the heart muscle. Glaucoma, one of the two leading causes of blindness in our country, also results from obstruction, in this case obstruction to the outflow of fluid from the anterior chamber of the eye.

Free flow of blood, urine, cerebrospinal fluid, lymph, and other fluids, as well as air, is essential for health. Table 1-1 shows the wide variety of diseases that result from obstruction.

Table 1-1. Diseases resulting from obstruction

System	Disease	Nature of obstruction
C.N.S.	Hydrocephalus	Congenital obstruction of cerebrospinal fluid
E.N.T.	Middle ear infection	Eustachian tube obstruction
Eye	Glaucoma	Obstruction of aqueous humor
Lung	Atelectasis	Mucus plug in bronchus
Biliary tract	Cholecystitis	Cystic duct stone
G.I.	Appendicitis	Fecalith, appendix
G.U.	Prostatism	Prostatic hypertrophy
Extremity	Intermittent claudication	Arteriosclerosis

Table 1-2. Examples of perforation

System	Disease	Nature of perforation
C.N.S.	Cerebral hemorrhage	Rupture of central nervous system artery
E.N.T.	Perforation of tympanic membrane	Infection with pressure
Lung	Spontaneous pneumothorax	Rupture of bleb
Biliary tract	Rupture of gallbladder	Obstruction, distension, necrosis
G.I.	Duodenal ulcer	Perforation of ulcer
G.U.	Ruptured bladder	Obstruction and distension
Vascular	Aortic aneurysm	Rupture of aneurysm

Table 1-3. Examples of erosion

System	Disease	Nature of erosion
C.N.S.	Meningitis	Erosion of abscess wall; mastoiditis
E.N.T.	Pharyngeal carcinoma	Bleeding; erosion into blood vessels
Lung	Tuberculosis	Bleeding; granulomatous erosion into blood vessels
G.I.	Duodenal ulcer	Bleeding; ulcer erosion into blood vessels
G.U.	Bladder stone	Bleeding; erosion of bladder wall
Extremity	Raynaud's phenomenon	Digital ulceration; ischemic erosion of skin

PERFORATION

Perforation, similarly, is the direct cause of many surgical diseases. Perforation is often such an intensely dramatic event that few medical students will forget the "boardlike" abdomen of the patient with a ruptured peptic ulcer or the shock that overwhelms the patient with a ruptured aortic aneurysm. Examples are given in Table 1-2.

EROSION

Erosion is a "partial perforation," a slower process of ulceration (i.e., a break in the continuity of a tissue surface). Examples of erosion are given in Table 1-3.

TUMORS

The most subtle of these four phenomena is a tumor or a mass. This explains in large measure why cancer is so often detected only after it induces one of the previous three processes; e.g., we occasionally see tumors of the breast that have grown to astonishingly large size. Because no vital flow is obstructed and perforation or erosion of the skin occurs very late, symptoms and consequently diagnosis are delayed, often tragically.

These four phenomena, *obstruction, perforation, erosion,* and *tumors,* are the underlying direct causes of most surgical diseases. Like the theme of a symphonic work, they recur in many different forms. Sometimes they appear unmistakably loud and clear; at other times soft, muted, and elusive. The able physician will learn to recognize and understand them. Such recognition and understanding are the chief concern of this book.

2
Wounds, Wound Healing, and Drains

David W. Furnas
Richard D. Liechty

Although the healing of wounds is a vital part of surgery, it also plays an important role in other medical fields. For example, the fibrous healing of myocardial infarcts often leads to life-threatening arrhythmias or ventricular aneurysms, and fibrous vegetations threaten embolization from rheumatic valvular disease. In posthepatitic patients scar tissue infiltrates the liver and in some cases fatally encases the regenerating liver cells or produces portal venous hypertension. In these examples fibrous tissue healing in its exuberant, sometimes misdirected, growth may eventually prove fatal. Wound healing, the surgeon's constant concern, is of more than casual interest to other physicians as well.

Healing by regeneration in man is limited to simple tissues, such as epithelium, and one compound organ, the liver. All other organs (skin, bowel, heart, brain) heal by merely sealing or patching of the wound. Paraplegia, for example, results from transection of the upper spinal cord. Scar tissue joins the severed cord ends but blocks all nerve impulses; the distal neurons, separated from their cell nuclei, degenerate and die. Unfortunately man has, in his evolutionary past, virtually lost the ability to regenerate compound tissues. There remains, however, this remarkable process of sealing or patching that man depends on to survive his hostile environment.

Tissues heal by three main processes: *epithelialization, fibrous tissue synthesis,* and the powerful force of *contraction*. Many surgical decisions depend on a clear knowledge of these extraordinary phenomena. When to remove sutures, where to make incisions, when to release a postoperative patient for normal activities, when to splint a wound, when to primarily close a wound, and when to leave it open are practical applications that the student should keep in mind as he studies the fundamental aspects of wound healing.

We first discuss the healing of *incised wounds, avulsed wounds,* and *contaminated wounds.* Pathological wound healing, wound complications, placement of incisions, suture materials, wound drainage, and drainage tubes complete this chapter.

INCISED WOUNDS AND SUPERFICIAL WOUNDS

A simple *clean incised wound* heals by *primary intention* after accurate surgical closure (*primary closure*). Within the first few hours of injury the cut edges of the wound are coapted by a fibrinous coagulum, which serves as a scaffold for granulation tissue to form. During the first day, leukocytes, mast cells, and mascrophages enter the area to dispose of local debris and bacteria. The *epithelial cells* of the neighboring epidermis dedifferentiate, flatten out, multiply, migrate into and across the wound, and redifferentiate. Within 24 hours the epidermal surface is intact in an incised and sutured wound. This same sequence of fibrin deposition, granulation tissue, and epithelialization serves to replace and heal the surface of broader wounds, such as second-degree burns or light abrasions, within a few days or weeks.

During the first few days that an incision is healing, the *inflammatory phase,* almost no tensile strength is gained. Meanwhile, *capillary buds* begin to sprout from the wound edges and differentiate into functioning networks, and *fibroblasts* migrate into the wound area, probably from nearby loose connective tissue. These fibroblasts form *collagen,* the material that knits the wounded dermis and deeper structures and gives strength to the wound. First the fibroblasts secrete *tropocollagen,* which aggregates into large *procollagen* fibers. These herald the *collagen phase,* the earliest evidence of tensile strength. Procollagen, through polymerization and cross linkages, becomes collagen, and from the fifth through the fifteenth days there is a rapid gain in tensile strength.

The young collagen fibers mature, link with one another, and orient along lines of stress. The wound reaches almost its full strength within 6 weeks. Although a slight gain continues over a number of months, the scar seldom, if ever, becomes stronger than the surrounding skin and fascia.

The *rate of healing* is accelerated by a rich blood supply and perhaps by warmth of the wounded part. Thus the face heals rapidly and sutures may be removed in a few days. In contrast, sutures must be left for 10 to 14 days in wounds of the lower leg because of its poorer blood supply.

As *wound maturity* progresses, the fibroblasts and capillaries greatly diminish in number, and the resultant scar is composed chiefly of collagen connective tissue, capped with epithelium. This progress is observed clinically as an initial red, raised, hard *immature scar* that molds into a flat, soft, and pale *mature scar* over a period of 3 to 12 months or more, as collagen molecules and cross links rearrange.

An excised wound or defect closes more slowly but in identical fashion, except that contraction of the wound edges plays the principal role. The edges of the defect advance into the defect probably from the action of contractile myofibroblasts. These recently described cells resemble *smooth muscle cells* and can be inhibited in experimental animals by smooth muscle antagonists. Wound contraction is a consistent, powerful force that all experienced surgeons respect (Figs. 2-3 and 2-4).

"EXCISED" OR AVULSIVE WOUNDS

If a wound cannot be primarily closed, it must heal by *secondary intention* by means of the mechanisms of contraction and epithelialization. Examples are wounds that are excessively contaminated, wounds in which treatment has been delayed, or burns and wounds that involve necrosis of large skin surfaces. In a few days the raw, exposed area becomes filled with *granulation tissue* ("proud flesh") (Fig. 2-1) composed of sprouting capillaries and fibroblasts. The wound edges creep toward each other by *contraction* and *epithelial migration.* If a mantle of necrotic skin clings to the surface of the defect, it is called an *eschar.* Formed of coagulated collagen and debris, it is much thicker and tougher than the scab of a superficial wound (Fig. 2-2). Tightly attached at first, it eventually separates from the underlying granulation tissue and falls away.

Healing is speeded by removal of dead tissue,

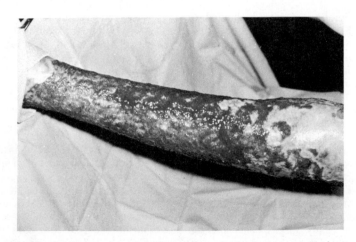

Fig. 2-1. Granulation tissue. Red, moist bed of fibroblasts and capillaries covering surface of leg that sustained full thickness burns 6 weeks before.

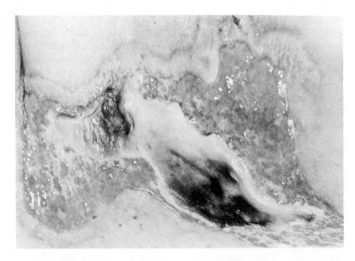

Fig. 2-2. Eschar. Deep burn coagulated full thickness of skin several weeks before. Eschar is in process of separating from underlying bed of granulation tissue. Copious exudate from local bacterial activity speeds process.

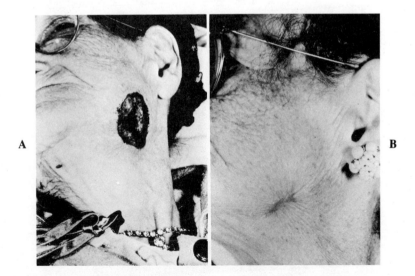

Fig. 2-3. Useful wound contraction. **A,** Wide removal of carcinoma of skin with electrocoagulation leaving open 3 × 4 cm. defect. **B,** Defect several months later after spontaneous closure by contraction and epithelialization. (Courtesy Department of Dermatology, University of Iowa Hospitals.)

debris, and secretions by surgical excision (débridement) and by application of intermittent dressings moistened with antibacterial solutions to the wound. The capillarity of the dressings drains away bacterial exudate. Dead tissue adherent to the dressings is removed when the dressings are changed. There soon emerges a clean granulating surface that resists reinfection. Wound closure can be hastened by *secondary closure* (if the wound edges can be apposed) undertaken a few days after injury. Sutures are used to appose the wound edges, usually after the granulation tissue is first excised. Larger wounds are closed with split skin grafts. If the defect is *too* large, an unstable scar may result.

In many instances healing by *secondary intention* is convenient and desirable (Fig. 2-3). However, when the wound is located on the face or over a joint (where mobility of the part favors excessive displacement), contracture is likely and it results in diminished motion and sometimes grotesque deformity (Fig. 2-4). This is prevented by early closure of the wound with skin grafts or pedicles before contraction occurs. In addition, splints and physical therapy may help prevent skin grafts from contracting.

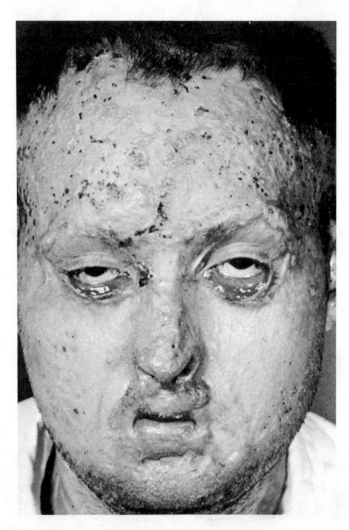

Fig. 2-4. Inimical wound contraction. Ectropion of eyelids and stenosis of mouth resulted from spontaneous closure of burn wounds of face by contraction and epithelialization.

CONTAMINATED WOUNDS

Wounds received outside of the operating room are contaminated wounds. They may be *grossly clean* or *dirty, neat,* or *ragged* and contused ("*tidy*" or "*untidy*" in British parlance).

A "golden period" of approximately *6 hours* was cited several decades ago as the optimum time to close a contaminated wound, after which the wound should be left open to prevent infection. This concept should not be entirely ignored, but more important is the answer to the question: Can this *contaminated wound* be converted into a surgically *clean wound,* or is this a *contaminated wound* in which bacterial activity is already so advanced that it *cannot* be converted?

We now have antibiotics and more refined surgical techniques so that, *with an excellent blood supply, we can take liberties with the golden period.* A 2-day-old wound of the foot that shows no sign of infection can be closed with appropriate preparation (not simply "putting in stitches") with small risk of infection. A grossly clean, neat wrist laceration, 12 hours old, can be repaired safely. However, a 3-hour-old wound of the lower leg received from a dirty barnyard source should probably be left open.

A contaminated wound is always converted to a *surgically clean wound* before early closure, by the following steps:

1. Take culture; start antibiotics if wound is large; tetanus prophylaxis
2. *Clean* all foreign material and loose debris by use of syringes, scrub brushes, and curets; avoid traumatic tattoos
3. *Hemostasis*
4. *Irrigate* with several liters of sterile solutions (saline, hydrogen peroxide, benzalkonium chloride) to dilute the number of bacteria remaining in the wound and to carry away microscopic debris
5. *Match* the landmarks of the wound so that a tentative plan for débridement, shifting of tissues, and closure can be made
6. *Débride,* i.e., excise with scalpel ragged wound edge, all dead or questionably viable tissue, and tissues that contain embedded foreign material
7. *Close* with sutures, grafts, or pedicle, *or* if heavy contamination or missing tissue:
8. Dress frequently with moist antibiotic dressings and carry out delayed closure several days later *or* dress and await secondary healing

PATHOLOGICAL WOUND HEALING

At times an excessively hard, raised, red, itching, unsightly *hypertrophied scar* (Fig. 2-5) may result from excessive tension on the wound, unfavorable site, inaccurate wound closure, or unknown factors. Exuberant hypertrophied scars sometimes result from partial thickness burns in children (Fig. 2-6). Improvement usually occurs with time; surgical excision and revision of the scar may be necessary. The patient must understand that *scar "removal" can never eradicate scarring but can only minimize it.*

Occasionally a massive overgrowth of scar tissue invades the normal surrounding skin and creates unsightly, gnarled protuberances called *keloids* (Fig. 2-7). Keloids occur only in susceptible individuals, most often in pigmented races. They have great propensity for *recurrence* when excised.

If a granulating wound defect is too large, closure by the process of contraction will be unsuc-

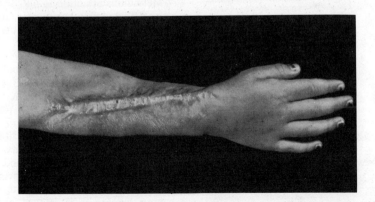

Fig. 2-5. Hypertrophied scar resulting from closure of forearm defect under tension.

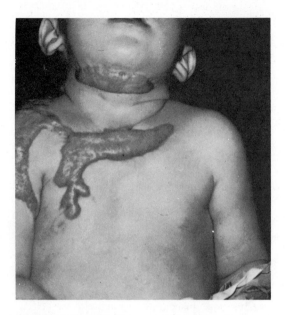

Fig. 2-6. Exuberant hypertrophied scar resulting from scalds (deep partial thickness burn).

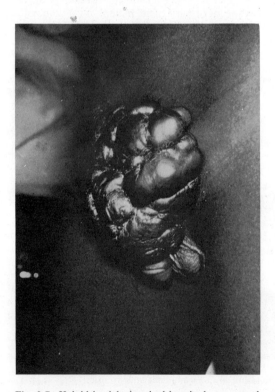

Fig. 2-7. Keloid in right inguinal hernioplasty wound.

cessful and will leave an open expanse of granulation tissue. In time the capillaries and fibroblasts diminish, and the granulation tissue is gradually transformed into avascular scar tissue. Epithelial migration yields only a thin, fragile mantle over the scar. The result is an *unstable scar* that is prone to reinjury and chronic ulceration. If recurring ulceration proceeds for several decades, metaplasia and finally squamous carcinoma *(Marjolin's ulcer)* may occur at the site of the injury. To prevent an unstable wound, the surgeon converts exposed granulation tissue into a closed wound by application of a split-thickness skin graft or pedicle.

WOUND COMPLICATIONS

Healing of wounds is retarded by the *protein deficiency* seen in severely depleted patients (particularly deficiency of the amino acid methionine), but healing is not greatly affected in patients who have moderate deficiencies. *Ascorbic acid deficiency* interferes with formation of collagen from collagen precursors, and the wounds develop little tensile strength. Because all collagen, and especially wound collagen, is continually being built up and destroyed, lack of vitamin C can cause a disruption in wounds that are years old. This explains the mystifying wound disruptions in scorbutic sailors, so well described in seafaring tales. Excessive *adrenocortical hormones* suppress fibroblastic activity. *Diabetes mellitus* sometimes engenders poor healing. *Infection, excessive motion, hematomas, seromas, edema, venous stasis, foreign material,* and *heavily traumatized tissue* in the wound area all impede satisfactory healing. *Reduced vascular supply* from any cause retards or prevents wound healing, e.g., *excessive tension* on the wound edges, *radiation changes, heavy scarring,* or *arteriosclerosis.*

Meticulous attention to nutrition, antisepsis, operative technique, hemostasis, and postoperative care will favor satisfactory wound healing.

PLACEMENT OF INCISIONS

Minimum scar formation and maximum camouflage are most likely to result when incisions are placed in the *wrinkle lines* of Kraissl and Conway (Fig. 2-8). These lines fall at right angles to the direction of pull of the underlying muscles. On the face they are most easily identified by having the patient grimace and perform exaggerated expressions. Elsewhere they are found by close inspection of the skin. Sometimes incisions may be hidden at or above the hairline, in the eyebrows, behind the ears, in the mouth, or along the areolar border of the nipple (Fig. 2-8, *A* and *B*). If an incision must cross the flexor surface of a joint, it is

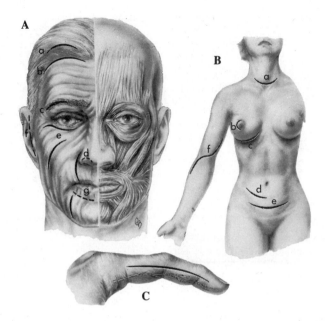

Fig. 2-8. A, Incisions camouflaged, *a,* in scalp, *b,* at scalp line, *c,* in eyebrow, *d,* in nostril, *e,* in wrinkle lines, *f,* in retroauricular area, and *g,* inside mouth. **B,** Incisions camouflaged in, *a,* neck creases, *b,* areolar border, *c,* submammary fold, *d,* skin creases of abdomen, *e,* wrinkle line and pubic hair of abdomen, and *f,* design of incision across the flexor surface of a joint to avoid contracture. **C,** Incision along neutral border of finger (where flexor skin creases meet extensor creases) to avoid contracture.

important that it curve or zigzag, nearly paralleling the transverse joint crease for part of its distance. Access to the flexor surface of the finger is made through the midlateral line or *neutral border* of the finger (Fig. 2-8, *C*). Straight longitudinal incisions across flexor surfaces of joints are notorious for the contractures they cause. On the abdomen, transverse (wrinkle line) incisions generally offer superior healing, though the need for extensive exposure sometimes dictates vertical incisions. Because the main muscular pull is transverse, transverse incisions paralleling these tensions have less tendency to disrupt. Transverse incisions are preferable on the chest also. Vertical incisions on the sternal region are noted for their tendency to hypertrophy.

SUTURE MATERIALS

Catgut and *chromic catgut* are made from intestinal submucosa of sheep. They are *absorbed* by the tissues, an advantage in contaminated wounds. They cause more inflammatory reaction, i.e., they are more *reactive* than other suture materials, and they are not so easy to manipulate as sutures of natural fiber. *Polyglycolic acid sutures* are also absorbed.

Natural-fiber sutures, silk, cotton, and linen, are *not absorbed,* are *much less reactive,* and have more tensile strength. They are the *easiest of all sutures to handle.* If buried in a contaminated wound, they act as a nidus for bacteria and tend to cause small draining sinuses that persist for many months until the sutures are finally expelled or removed.

Synthetic-fiber sutures, nylon, Dacron, polyster, polypropylene, etc., are *not absorbed.* They are *stronger* and *less reactive* than silk, with much less tendency to cause draining sinuses after closure of contaminated wounds, particularly if they are *mono*strand rather than *poly*strand. The monostrand sutures are *more difficult to handle* than natural-fiber sutures, but they have an advantage of minimum capillary action.

Wire sutures, stainless steel, silver, or tantalum, are *not absorbed,* have minimum capillarity and minimum reactivity, and are the *strongest* of sutures. They are *more difficult to handle* than the other materials and tend to cut through tissues.

Table 2-1. Surgical procedures commonly followed by drainage

Procedure	Material to be drained
Cholecystectomy	Bile from accessory bile ducts—from liver to gallbladder
Pancreatic resection	Pancreatic juice, from many tiny pancreatic ducts
Parotidectomy	Secretions from transected parotid gland
Thoracotomy	Air or serous fluid drained from intrapleural space; important to keep lung expanded
Splenectomy	Tail of pancreas is often very close to splenic hilum; drainage of pancreatic juice
Nephrectomy	Drainage of perinephric fat that is susceptible to infection
Incision and drainage of furuncles	Drain pus, allow wound to heal from bottom
Large flaps	Serum and blood prevented from collecting with suction catheters

WOUND DRAINAGE

Drains are placed in wounds only when *abnormal fluid collections* are present or expected. The purpose of drainage is to provide an exit for these fluids. Collections of body fluids can be harmful in the following ways:

1. Provide culture media for bacterial growth
2. Cause tissue irritation or necrosis, e.g., bile, pancreatic juice, pus, urine
3. Cause elevation of skin flaps with loss of vascularity and sloughing
4. Cause pressure on adjacent organs

In clean wounds, when no abnormal collection of fluids is expected, drainage is *unnecessary,* i.e., after a thyroidectomy or hernia repair. Bleeding should seldom, if ever, be used as an alibi for draining. Hemostasis should be attained at the time of operation. Blood clots may obstruct drains and entice the surgeon into a sense of security while bleeding proceeds in the wound.

Surgeons vary somewhat in their indications for drainage. Table 2-1 lists surgical procedures in which drains are commonly used.

Soft rubber or plastic drains are commonly used for wound drainage; when large amounts of drainage material are expected or when a "dry wound" is important, suction applied to hollow tube drains is effective.

Drains act as foreign bodies. Granulation tissue forms about them and walls them off rapidly. Thus the area in which drains are effective is soon limited by this "isolating effect" of healing tissue. Drains are usually removed slowly as the amount of drainage decreases over a period of days or rarely weeks.

T TUBES AND OTHER "FISTULA"-FORMING TUBES

Hollow drainage tubes are often used to form *fistulas* (hollow connections) from internal organs, either to drain a body fluid (bile) to the outside or to instill materials into body organs (feeding jejunostomy).

The short member of the T tube is placed in the common bile duct whereas the longer member leads outside the body, thus providing a bypass for the bile to the outside. It is also used to inject radiopaque dye for x-ray studies of the bile ducts. Granulation tissue soon forms a fibrous wall about the T tube, walling it off from the remainder of the peritoneal cavity—the rubber tube is a foreign body. After 9 to 10 days a T tube can be removed with no fear of internal bile leak. However, if a T tube is pulled out within 48 hours of its insertion, a bile leak invariably occurs into the peritoneal cavity with consequent bile peritonitis. This same walling-off process occurs around *gastrostomy, jejunostomy, cecostomy, cystostomy,* and other tubes. If these tubes become dislocated before the fibrous tract forms, extravasation will almost always result, often with serious or fatal consequences. Because of their important function, these tubes are stitched securely to the skin and should seldom be removed before 10 days after insertion.

Urinary catheters, nasogastric tubes, and rectal tubes pass through natural orifices that are lined by epithelium, and therefore they can be removed at any time with no heed to this important principle of fibrous sealing-off of the tube. *Thoracotomy tubes are discussed in Chapter 30.*

3
Fluids and Electrolytes

Edward E. Mason

The subject of fluids and electrolytes is sometimes neglected because of both its simplicity and its potential complexity. Probably 95% of surgical patients require only short-term, routine replacement of fluids. When patients resume oral intake, they regulate themselves. Furthermore, with short-term intravenous therapy, patients can withstand gross insults. Normal kidneys, by excreting excess fluids, readily compensate for most fluid overloads, and when fluid replacement is inadequate, the kidneys conserve fluids.

This chapter is dedicated to the presentation of a simple scheme for rational analysis of the daily fluid requirements for all patients whether the problem is simple or complex, but especially to the recognition, understanding, and logical analysis of requirements for the occasional difficult patient whose kidneys are not functioning well and whose life may depend on this portion of the treatment.

Three major questions must be answered in order to provide optimum parenteral fluids:
1. What metabolic fluids (urine and insensible loss) are needed?
2. What abnormal body fluids (vomiting, diarrhea) currently being lost must be replaced?
3. What fluids are needed to correct accumulated fluid and electrolyte imbalances?

The first two questions are commonplace. Serious, neglected illnesses and injudicious fluid therapy underlie the last question.

A clear comprehension of this chapter is best attained by an initial rapid reading, followed by methodical study with concentration on those areas each student finds most difficult.

COLLECTION OF INFORMATION

What information is required to answer these questions about a particular patient, and how is it obtained? Four major sources are used: (1) history (including accurately maintained records of intake and output), (2) physical examination, (3) laboratory analyses, and (4) diagnosis *ex juvantibus* (the response to treatment).

History

If the patient is seen by a physician for the first time, only an estimate may be available for the amounts of *fluid loss* such as vomitus, liquid stools, and urine. Similar rough estimates should be made for *fluid intake* in terms of containers familiar to the patient and relatives.

For the hospitalized patient with intake and output recorded, a table should be made of all the solutions that have been given to the patient, starting from the time the patient was last believed to be in balance. The total amounts of the following should be determined: (1) intravenous electrolytes and water, (2) urine excreted, and (3) electrolyte-containing fluids lost from the body by gastric suction or other routes. An estimate must also be made of the insensible loss by evaporation from skin and lungs. In the average adult at normal temperatures and humidity, this loss will total about 800 ml./day.

Physical examination

During the physical examination, an estimate should be made of the amount of subcutaneous extracellular fluid (ECF) present. This requires an awareness of the effect of varying amounts of subcutaneous fat and elastic tissue on skin turgor. One can evaluate skin turgor by pinching the skin into a fold and observing the rate of return to normal. In the very obese patient, severe depletion of extracellular fluid may be masked by fatty turgor of the skin. In the elderly and often poorly nourished patient with little fat and elastic tissue, poor skin turgor often suggests depletion of extracellular fluid even though the extracellular fluid volume is normal. In a young, lean, acutely ill adult, severe deficiency of extracellular fluid is characterized by skin that can be pinched up into a fold and remains in that position for several seconds.

Overexpansion of extracellular fluid is sometimes difficult to determine until the patient develops dependent edema along the back or buttocks or, if the patient has been in a standing or sitting position, pitting edema of the ankles. Sometimes, even though definite edema cannot be found, the jellylike movement of the tissues on percussion will be suggestive of waterlogged subcutaneous tissues. *Changes* in the findings are often much more helpful than the static findings at any single examination. These changes in *extracellular fluid* (skin turgor, edema, and ascites) are easier to detect than changes in total body water. *Rapid changes in total body water*, either overhydration or dehydration, do lead to mental confusion, coma, and convulsions (which may mimic the signs and symptoms of a poorly localized cerebrovascular accident). However, total body water abnormalities, in contrast to extracellular fluid changes, produce no detectable changes in skin turgor.

Physical examination not only reveals signs of gross abnormalities of total body water and extracellular fluid volumes but also may provide clues to abnormal *chemical composition* of body fluids. A patient with suspected potassium deficiency will often have weakness of the muscles and distension of the bowel with poor bowel sounds. A high serum potassium may cause rhythm disturbances of the heart as the potassium approaches a lethal level of 8 to 10 mEq./L. High serum calcium levels cause mental confusion, nausea and vomiting, and profound weakness. Low calcium levels are accompanied by muscle spasm and neuromuscular irritability, so that tapping over the facial nerve causes contraction of the facial muscles (Chvostek's sign).

Central nervous system diseases, such as encephalitis and cirrhosis, often result in comatose states. The consequent rapid ventilation causes "blowing off" of carbon dioxide, which results in *respiratory alkalosis.* This causes a decrease in ionized calcium and may be accompanied by the signs of calcium deficiency. Patients with metabolic acidosis breathe rapidly and deeply in an effort to blow off sufficient carbon dioxide to lower carbonic acid levels and, by virtue of this respiratory alkalosis, to compensate for the *metabolic acidosis.* The physician who is familiar with the patient's basic underlying disease is in an excellent position to recognize various physical signs of abnormal fluid and electrolyte balance. Reexamination of the patient is important. Changes in physical findings not initially evident are often recognized during repeated examinations. Changes in body weight, skin turgor, alertness, and breathing rate *during treatment* also contribute to the evaluation.

ANALYSIS OF DATA
Estimation of body fluid volumes in health

In the average healthy adult male who is well nourished but has a minimum of fat (fat contains almost no free water), about 60% of the body weight is made up of fluid components. Women have more fat than men. By finding out what an obese patient weighed before becoming obese (or, if necessary, by simply estimating what the patient should weigh after a satisfactory regimen of weight reduction), one can arrive at a rough idea of the patient's expected normal lean (nonfat) body mass. From *lean body mass,* estimates of the volume of fluids in the body compartments can be calculated easily.

The lean body weight is converted from pounds into kilograms by use of the factor 2.2 pounds/kg. The patient's extracellular fluid volume is estimated by multiplication of the lean body mass by 20%. This leaves, therefore, 40% of the lean body mass as intracellular fluid; 15% of the lean body mass as fluid between the cells, or interstitial fluid; and 5% as fluid in the circulating blood volume exclusive of the blood cells. A 70 kg. lean man should therefore possess about 3.5 liters (L.) of plasma; 7% to 8% of the lean body mass is the usual estimate of normal blood volume (plasma + cells).

VOLUME, TONICITY, AND BODY SOLUTES

Every solution has a characteristic solute curve, illustrated by Fig. 3-1, where the horizontal axis is the *volume,* the vertical axis is *concentration,* and the curving line represents a given amount of *solute.* Since the amount of solute is fixed, any volume increase causes a reciprocal decrease in concentration. Similarly, with decreasing volume the concentration rises.

The equation *Volume × Concentration = Total body solute* depicts this relationship mathematically. The body solutions share this same relationship, but obviously life depends on these three variables remaining within a limited physiological range.

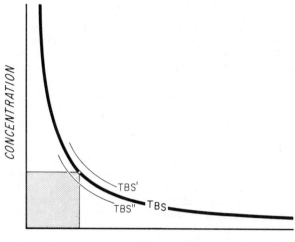

Fig. 3-1. Concentration-volume relationship. Concentration of electrolytes on vertical axis against fluid volume on horizontal axis. Because total body solutes *(TBS)* is a fixed amount of solutes, any point on the curving line equals any other point. Since concentration × volume = TBS, then if volume increases, concentration must decrease; if volume decreases, concentration must increase. *TBS'*, Increase in solutes (electrolyte overinfusion). *TBS''*, Decrease in solutes (from vomiting and diarrhea).

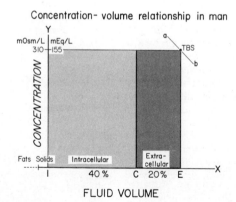

Fig. 3-2. Concentration of electrolytes on vertical axis against fluid volume on horizontal axis. Distribution of body fluids into, *I*, intracellular (40%) and, *E*, extracellular compartments (20%). Remaining 40% of body weight is composed of solids and normally distributed fat. Total body solutes, *TBS*, are depicted by a curving line, *a-b*, which is a *mathematical constant*. (Concentration × volume = total solutes in *any* solution.) This line naturally falls at the intersection of volume and concentration. Diagram depicts mathematical relationship of concentration × volume = total solutes. When one changes, another *must* also change. A clear understanding of these diagrams in health and in the disease states that follow is as fundamental to understanding fluid and electrolyte problems as are the multiplication tables to understanding mathematics.

Body solutions differ from simple, in vitro solutions because the body has two distinct fluid compartments (cellular and extracellular). Cells separate the body solutes by pumping sodium out and allowing potassium to replace the displaced sodium, but the concentration of solute in the cellular compartment *always equals* the concentration of solute in the extracellular compartment. This is the *law of osmotic equilibrium*. The concentration of intracellular cations (chiefly potassium) always equals the concentration of extracellular cations (chiefly sodium). Water diffusing freely between the two body compartments maintains this osmotic equality. Fig. 3-2 shows the concentration–volume–total solute relationship as it applies to man.

Although we depend on extracellular fluid (serum) samples for concentration measurements, we know they reflect intracellular concentrations as well. Despite the dual fluid compartments and the physiological segration of cations in the body, the *Concentration × Volume = Total body solute* relationship is equally valid in living organisms as in the test tube.

Sodium concentration, the dominant extracellular cation, holds the key to body tonicity and volume. Since sodium represents 92% of all extracellular cations, we can use it as if it were the only cation. The body zealously guards sodium concentration between 136 and 145 mEq./L. Despite wide individual variations in the intake of salt and water, control of thirst and antiduretic hormone stabilizes sodium concentration within this narrow range.

Sodium concentration is a measure of *tonicity* of body fluids: sodium concentrations below 136 mEq./L. denote *hypotonicity;* concentrations above 145 mEq./L. indicate *hypertonicity.*

We can estimate acute body volume changes by determining weight changes, skin turgor, pulse rate, dryness of tongue, hematocrit, hemoglobin,*

---

*Red blood cells and concentration defects: Another concentration measurement helpful in the diagnosis of extracellular fluid deficit is the concentration of the red blood cells. Plasma is part of the extracellular fluid. Plasma volume contracts along with the interstitial fluid volume. The result is an increase in the hemoglobin concentration and hematocrit. Often a hemoglobin or hematocrit has not been determined before the patient loses extracellular fluid. An estimate can still be helpful, however, if the patient has not had signs or symptoms of anemia or polycythemia. Under such circumstances a hematocrit of 60 or above or a hemoglobin of 19 gm./dl. allows a strong presumption that contraction of the extracellular fluid volume has occurred. The single measurement is interpreted as *a change in concentration caused by a change in compartment volume.*

etc. We can also accurately determine body tonicity (sodium concentration) in the laboratory. With the aid of these two measurements and clear understanding of the concentration–volume–total solute relationship, we can diagnose and treat most body fluid abnormalities. The six chief abnormalities are total body water loss, total body water gain, extracellular fluid loss, extracellular fluid gain, pure salt deficit, and malnutrition. I will discuss and illustrate these abnormalities in terms of the concentration–volume–total body solute diagrams.

BODY FLUID ABNORMALITIES
Total body water loss

An estimate is made of the total body water deficit incurred, by lack of oral intake and the duration of desiccation from loss of urine and continued evaporation from skin and lungs. This number of liters of water is subtracted in the diagram when the line *E* is moved appropriately closer to *I;* e.g., if a 70 kg. man has been unable to drink for 2½ days and during this time has continued to evaporate water, he has an estimated loss of 2 L. Also, if during this time he has excreted 1 L. of urine, his total body water deficit would amount to 3 L. (approximately 7% of his lean body weight). This is depicted by a 7% decrease in the distance between *I* and *E*. (See Fig. 3-3.)

The cells also participate in this loss depicted by a 7% decrease in the distance between *I* and *C*. Any change in total body water is a change in both the *cellular volume* and the *extracellular fluid*

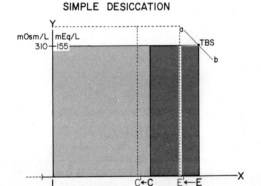

Fig. 3-3. In simple desiccation, volume decreases, concentration increases, and total body solutes (the product of volume × concentration) remain the same. Remember, the curving line, *a-b*, is a constant. (Any point on this line equals any other point.) Both extracellular and intracellular compartments share in water loss.

volume. Water moves freely across the cell membranes, equalizing the osmotic pressure *outside* the cell and *inside* the cell. Since no solutes are lost, the concentration rises.

Total body water gain

If the patient has retention of water without any change in total body salt, concentration of salt decreases; e.g., if the retention is 4 L. in a 70 kg. man (total body water is about 42 L.), this is a 10% increase in total body water, and the concentration of solutes (as depicted by sodium) can be expected to decrease by 10% (Fig. 3-4). This means that the sodium should now be 129 mEq./L. instead of 143.

Extracellular fluid loss

The extracellular fluid volume is altered when the patient loses electrolyte-containing fluids as in vomiting and diarrhea or after a severe burn. In major trauma (as after prolonged and extensive operations and after major hemorrhage), a decrease in extracellular fluid occurs. An effort should be made to estimate the actual number of liters of electrolyte-containing fluid lost—one depicts this by moving the line *E* to the left but with no change in the intracellular fluid volume *IC* (Fig. 3-5). Sometimes, when the diagnosis of extracellular fluid deficit can be made, the data necessary for quantitation are deficient. The degree of ECF contraction must then be estimated from physical findings plus response to treatment. A loss of one fourth to one third of the extracellular fluid volume is sufficient to cause signs of circulatory disturb-

ance such as a lowered blood pressure, especially with the patient in a sitting position. Urinary output is low. A patient who has vomiting and diarrhea and who has very poor skin turgor may therefore need as much as 3 to 4 L. of expansion of extracellular fluid before he begins to look well, to resume normal renal function, and to have a normal blood pressure and normal peripheral circulation.

Extracellular fluid gain

Patients with heart failure or with cirrhosis and increased aldosterone, or patients with decreased renal function who are given too much sodium-containing fluid, may develop edema, ascites, or pleural fluid. One can estimate this retention by knowing the increase in *total body weight,* and it should be depicted in Fig. 3-2 as an increase in extracellular fluid volume *EC* and a new *TBS* line, which is to the right of line *a-b*. Congestive heart failure and overtransfusion of blood and salt solutions are two common examples.

Pure salt deficit

The patient who loses extracellular fluid (containing electrolytes) and receives nonelectrolyte fluid may have a normal body weight and a normal total body water volume but a *decrease* in total body solute. This is depicted in Fig. 3-6 by *TBS'*. With simple loss of extracellular fluid (Fig. 3-5), the position of the cell membrane, *C*, does not change. However, in pure salt deficiency (with vomiting of electrolyte solution and replacement with water),

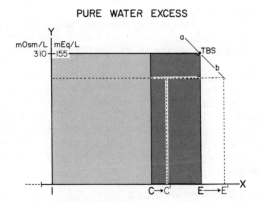

Fig. 3-4. In pure water excess (usually renal failure), fluid volume increases and concentration decreases. Total body solutes remain the same. Notice that this excess water is distributed throughout total body water.

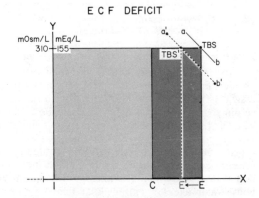

Fig. 3-5. Extracellular fluid deficit. Because body solutes are *lost* from body (vomiting, diarrhea, burns), *TBS* changes to *TBS'* (the new constant is parallel curving line *a'-b'*). Concentration stays the same, but volume of extracellular fluid decreases.

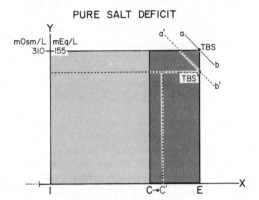

Fig. 3-6. Vomiting or diarrhea followed by drinking water is common cause of pure salt deficit. Volume stays the same; concentration decreases. Again, since body solutes have been lost, position of *TBS* changes to *TBS'*. The excess water distributes evenly between intracellular and extracellular compartments. Overall effect is shrinking of extracellular compartment. Hematocrit reflects this shrinkage by rising. Intracellular fluid volume is increased.

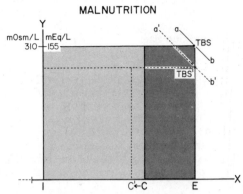

Fig. 3-7. Chronically malnourished patient has low concentration of serum sodium but total body sodium is increased. Deficit in body solute is in exchangeable potassium. There is movement of sodium into cells as well as expansion of extracellular fluid and total body water. Plasma volume is actually above normal and hematocrit is reduced. History and physical findings should distinguish this condition from pure water excess. Low hematocrit distinguishes malnutrition from pure salt deficiency.

an internal shift to *C'* (water goes into cells) occurs. Even though the patient's body weight is normal, the concentration of sodium is low and the hematocrit and hemoglobin are elevated. This paradoxical decrease in sodium concentration and rise in hematocrit and hemoglobin concentration strongly suggest a pure salt deficit. The white blood count is usually greatly elevated. This may be suggestive of infection, but the body temperature is usually below normal and when the salt is replaced, the white count falls toward normal along with the hematocrit.

Total body water excess versus pure salt deficiency

Sometimes the information from history and physical findings is insufficient to make a complete diagnosis in a patient with a *low* concentration of serum sodium, and the differential diagnosis must be made between total body water excess and pure salt deficiency. Examination of Figs. 3-4 and 3-6 reveals how this diagnosis can be settled. The lowered concentration of serum sodium indicates that if total body solute is normal (a simple total body water excess), extracellular fluid volume is increased (*E'* would now be opposite *b*). With the increase in extracellular fluid volume, intracellular fluid volume (including red blood cells) would be equally increased. The hematocrit would be normal. In contrast to this, if the problem is one of loss of electrolyte solution and replacement with non-

electrolyte solution (a pure salt deficiency), total body water and body weight are unchanged. There is, however, an internal shift of fluids into the cells depicted by an increase in *IC* and a decrease in *EC*, with *C'* the position of the cell membranes. Since the extracellular fluid volume is contracted, the hematocrit will be high. The rise in hematocrit with pure salt deficit distinguishes it from total body water excess in which the hematocrit is unchanged.

There is still another possibility for explaining a low concentration of serum sodium—protein malnutrition. Under such circumstances serum albumin is decreased and plasma volume tends therefore to be inadequate. Retention of sodium occurs and water retention also occurs to the extent that an effective plasma volume is established by increase in extracellular fluid and total body water. A simplified summary of these changes is shown in Fig. 3-7. Because of the decrease in cellular tissue and potassium, total body solute is decreased.

Assessing laboratory data

Two concepts must be mastered regarding the interpretation of serum sodium concentration. These are the rules of (1) *osmotic equilibrium,* which we have already discussed, and (2) *electrical neutrality.* The second rule states that *total anions must equal total cations* in an electrolyte solution.

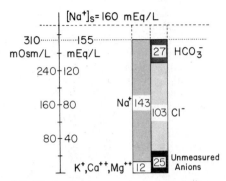

Fig. 3-8. Total anions must always equal total cations. Dilution or concentration of body electrolytes will affect both sides of Gamble diagram so that change in anion concentration is proportional to change in cation (sodium) concentration.

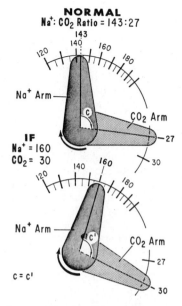

Fig. 3-9. Arms to circular slide rule are set as normal ratio of CO_2 to sodium. Arms with this fixed ratio are then moved to observed sodium, and expected CO_2 is read. Expected chloride for any observed sodium is determined in same fashion.

It implies that any change in concentration of sodium must be accompanied by an equal change in concentration of anions.

Once the use of sodium concentration as an index of tonicity of body fluids and the rule of electrical neutrality are accepted, the clinician may evaluate the accuracy of a set of laboratory data (Fig. 3-8). The internal consistency of a set of laboratory data should be carefully scrutinized. If the concentration of chloride plus CO_2 (as bicarbonate) approaches or exceeds the value given for sodium, obviously a laboratory error involves at least one of these ions. All three of the determinations must be repeated.

If the concentration of sodium is excessively high in comparison to the concentration of CO_2 plus chloride, this may be a laboratory error, but it may also indicate an abnormal accumulation of unmeasured anions as occurs in uremia, ketosis, severe infection, and circulatory insufficiency. If the patient has no disease or condition that would cause an elevation of unmeasured anions, laboratory error should be suspected.

Bedside proportions

A small circular slide rule was once helpful (Fig. 3-9) for these propoportions and for other calculations at the bedside. Today a wrist or pocket calculator is used, but the calculations remain the same. The ratio of normal concentration of chloride to sodium can be established (143 to 103), and then with this ratio maintained as a fixed angle, the sodium arm can be moved to the observed, abnormal value of, e.g., 160. For such a patient, with a relative deficiency in total body water (Figs. 3-3 and 3-9), the expected chloride should be 115. Changes in concentration of major anions should be proportional to changes in concentration of sodium unless an associated disturbance of electrolyte *composition* of the extracellular fluid exists.

The normal ratio of CO_2 content to sodium concentration is 27 to 143. This ratio (or fixed angle) is established on the arms of the slide rule (Fig. 3-9). As the sodium arm is moved over to 160, it is observed that the normal CO_2 content for the patient becomes 30. In this way the rule of electrical neutrality allows determination of the internal consistency of a set of data as well as determination of whether an observed chloride or CO_2 concentration is simply altered by virtue of the change in *total body water* or whether it is altered by a true change in the *composition* of the electrolytes in extracellular fluid.

A reciprocal relationship is also seen between CO_2 content (HCO_3 in Fig. 3-8) and chloride. A compositional change in which the concentration of one of the anions increases greatly cannot exist without a decrease in another of the anions, e.g., when a patient with a peptic ulcer vomits acid gastric juice containing high concentrations of chloride, the remaining fluid in the body has a deficit of chloride (hypochloremia). This is a deficit of chloride in the entire extracellular fluid. The bicarbonate anion will be above normal. When the CO_2 content (bicarbonate) is normal or decreased and the chloride is greatly decreased, some cause for elevation of the *unmeasured anions,* such as phosphate, ketone bodies, or organic acids, must be sought. One of the more common causes of this is renal insufficiency; the blood urea nitrogen and creatinine will be elevated.

The other ions exist in such low concentrations that they neither participate in the reciprocity with total body water, nor are influenced in a significant way by considerations of electrical neutrality. One trace cation is normally present in a concentration of 40 nm./L. This is the hydrogen ion, and in so-called *metabolic* disturbances of acid-base balance (diabetic acidosis, uremia) the serum CO_2 content in mEq./L. may permit a very good estimate of the severity of hydrogen ion increase (acidosis) or decrease (alkalosis). If the patient has been vomiting, the resultant hypochloremia and an increase in the bicarbonate (or CO_2) content indicate a *hypochloremic alkalosis.* In situations in which chloride or other anions are increased in concentration and bicarbonate is decreased, a diagnosis of *metabolic acidosis* is made. Whether this is primary metabolic acidosis or is compensatory to respiratory alkalosis is a question that is discussed in the section on acid-base balance (p. 21).

WRITING THE PRESCRIPTION

The physician at the bedside who understands the concentration volume relationships *and* the clinical status of his patient is well prepared to order replacement fluids. In order that nothing be left out of this order, he should consider THREE ITEMS: *metabolic fluid losses, current abnormal fluid losses,* and *accumulated imbalances.*

Replacing urine and insensible fluid loss

First the patient needs *metabolic fluids* for urine and insensible loss. This fluid is relatively low in electrolyte concentration and can be supplied by the use of 5% glucose. The average patient will produce about 1,000 ml. of urine in 24 hours and will require some 800 ml. of the same fluid for replacement of insensible loss from skin and lungs. This does *not* include sweat, which should be considered as an abnormal fluid and would require some replacement with salt. This may approach 2,000 or 3,000 ml. in hot weather or with fever. Accurate body weights are essential when losses that cannot be measured occur. They are indicated in all patients receiving intravenous fluids.

Replacing abnormal fluid losses

The second type of fluid required depends on *ongoing abnormal losses.* Usually the orders are written on morning rounds. At this time about 8 hours of the day have passed, and it is a simple calculation to determine the amount of fluid in the gastric suction or drainage from other parts of the gastrointestinal tract and simply to multiply the amount of fluid by 3 to estimate total 24-hour requirements. If the patient has no abnormal fluid losses, this item can be ignored. If the fluid being lost is acid gastric juice, as determined by a quick bedside determination with pH-sensitive paper, replacement should be with 0.9% saline. If the intestinal juices are quite alkaline, as is the case with a fresh ileostomy or leakage from a duodenal fistula, replacement should be with saline and one-sixth molar sodium lactate in the ratio of 2 parts and 1 part. If the patient is losing extracellular-like fluid with a normal body fluid pH, e.g., the removal of a large volume of pleural or peritoneal fluid, this should be replaced with a fluid that has the composition of normal extracellular fluid. This can be approximated by use of isotonic saline and one-sixth molar sodium lactate in the proportions of 4:1, which is the ratio of the major anions in extracellular fluid—chloride and bicarbonate, 103 and 27.

Restoring normal balance

The third and most complex item to be considered is the *correction fluids.* The concentration volume diagram is of great help in situations of imbalance. A few examples of the various abnormalities just discussed are given in the following paragraphs:

1. If the patient is deficient in *total body water* as is evidenced by a 10% increase in sodium concentration (and weight loss of 8 pounds), he will require a 10% increase in total body water, which can be supplied as 5% glucose. This means that to change a sodium concentration from 158 to 143 in a lean 70 kg. man, it would be necessary to provide 4 L. of 5% glucose. Remember, this is *in addition to* the fluids required for metabolic purposes (urine and insensible loss) and replacement of current abnormal losses.

2. If the patient has a *deficit of extracellular fluid* estimated to be approximately one fourth of his normal expected extracellular volume, this can be replaced with lactated Ringer's solution or with a mixture of saline and M/6 sodium lactate in the proportions of 4:1. For the hypothetical 70 kg. lean man, this would require 20% of 70, which is 14 L. times a one-fourth deficit, or 3.5 L. of extracellular fluid replacement.

3. For the patient who has a *pure salt deficiency* and a normal total body water (Fig. 3-6), corrective salt replacement is calculated as follows: Given a serum sodium concentration of 121 mEq./L., the deficiency is 143 mEq./L − 121 mEq./L. = 22 mEq./L. Since in this situation the "excess" water has shifted into cells (remember, water moves freely across cell membranes), the deficit in sodium (22 mEq./L.) must be multiplied by the *total body water* (42 L.) to give 924 mEq. This is the total deficit, which is the amount of salt contained in 6 L. of extracellular fluid.

This much salt should never be given as a single order. Initially a hypertonic salt solution can be used, but not more than 9 to 10 gm. of salt should be given without reevaluation of the patient. This is the amount of salt present in 200 ml. of 5% sodium chloride or 300 ml. of 3% sodium chloride. In such a severe extracellular fluid salt deficiency, this order may be repeated twice, but then the remainder of the deficit should be made up of isotonic electrolyte solution. Additional salt can thus be administered in the fluids needed for metabolic requirements for urine and insensible loss. Usually these are nonelectrolyte solutions, but in the patient with a salt deficit the entire intravenous fluid therapy can consist in giving electrolyte solution over a period of several days until the deficiency is corrected.

4. If the patient has a *hypochloremia*, the replacement solutions should be composed of 0.9% saline. *Saline is an acidifying solution* and will correct a metabolic alkalosis because saline has 155 mEq./L. of chloride in comparison with normal extracellular fluid, which has only 103 mEq./L. This means that in every liter of 0.9% saline approximately 50 mEq. of extra chloride is provided to increase the chloride concentration. The *extracellular fluid total chloride deficit* and the number of liters of 0.9% saline required to supply this amount of excess chloride can be calculated.

If the metabolic alkalosis is severe, hydrochloric acid may be infused by use of a 0.1 to 1 N solution administered through a central venous catheter by gravity drip at 1 mEq./min. until two thirds of the calculated dose has been given. Such treatment is indicated only when two of the following three criteria are met: pH 7.45 or above, base excess 7 mEq./L. or more, partial pressure of arterial carbon dioxide 50 torr or higher.

5. If the patient has a *metabolic acidosis* with a bicarbonate of 17 mEq./L. and one desires to increase this to 27, the deficit of 10 mEq./L is multiplied by the estimated liters of *extracellular fluid,* which in the 70 kg. person should be 14 L., for a total of 140 mEq. A molar solution of sodium lactate contains 1,000 mEq./L. of lactate. The lactate is metabolized, and the result is bicarbonate. One-sixth molar sodium lactate solution contains one-sixth as much bicarbonate as molar lactate, or 166 mEq./L. This means that some 850 ml. of one-sixth molar sodium lactate would supply the required 140 mEq. of bicarbonate.

Selecting and administering fluids

As the various requirements of fluid and electrolytes are added up, some of the electrolytes may be placed in metabolic fluids if necessary to avoid use of hypertonic electrolyte solutions. In a patient who has large current losses and an extensive past deficit (in addition to his metabolic needs), the administration of 8 to 9 L. of fluid in 24 hours may be required. If this is the case, the order should be written so that the nurse will run the fluids at a rate to approximate 9 L. in 24 hours. The size of drops varies, but the average is about 16 drops/ml.; 9 L. of fluid contain 144,000 drops. There are 60 minutes in the hour, and in 24 hours there are 1,440 minutes. A simple division reveals that the intravenous fluid should run at the rate of 100 drops/minute. Always specify the rate at which intravenous fluids should be infused.

Recording intake and output

The various bags of fluid ordered should be numbered. The nurse should write the numbers on the bags when they are prepared for the patient, so that they correspond with the physician's orders. When each bag is empty, it should be kept near the patient's bed—at any time the numbered bags can be reviewed to determine what fluids have been given and what fluids are yet to be given. At least once every 24 hours, usually at midnight, all the bags are gathered together and the total 24-hour urine volume is measured as well as the volume of gastrointestinal juices. This information must then be recorded accurately in the chart.

Bedside tests

Much of the information is now available for writing a new set of fluid orders for the next 24 hours. Either the nurse or the physician can obtain additional useful information at the bedside by measuring the specific gravity of the urine. With color-coded test tape, pH should be measured for the urine and all other fluids removed from the patient. A patient who is losing acid gastric juice will develop an alkalosis, and his urine will tend to become more alkaline. A patient who is losing alkaline juices in excess of what is replaced will gradually develop a metabolic acidosis, and his urine will become more acid. A patient who is not receiving enough water will develop a high specific gravity of the urine. A patient who is receiving gavage feedings with a high-protein, high-calorie feeding and an inadequate amount of water may have 1 L. of urine but the specific gravity may be 1.035, indicating that the water intake is inadequate for this solute load.

Bedside tests are available for estimation of the *urine chloride* (the Fantus test) or the *urine sodium* (the zinc uranyl acetate precipitation test). These tests show whether the urinary salt excretion is normal or high or low; e.g., if a patient with a low or normal serum sodium concentration has 8 to 9 gm. of salt in the urine continuously despite the fact that a seemingly adequate amount of salt is being given intravenously each day, either adrenal insufficiency or a salt-losing disease of the kidney should be suspected. Such a patient can be given 8 to 10 mg. of desoxycorticosterone acetate (Doca). If this causes an immediate reduction in the salt excretion, the patient has adrenal insufficiency and will need treatment with corticosteroids. If steroids are ineffective, a renal abnormality exists and the salt loss will have to be replaced as an abnormal loss in the same way that loss of electrolyte in gastrointestinal secretions is replaced.

Clinical reevaluation

When the fluids have been ordered, the physician should examine the patient again periodically to make sure that the diagnosis is correct and that the patient is responding to the fluid therapy as anticipated. A patient with severe metabolic acidosis who is receiving one-sixth molar sodium lactate should have a progressive decrease in the rate and depth of respiration. A patient with a severe extracellular fluid volume deficit who is receiving 3 to 4 L. of extracellular fluid should have an improvement in his skin turgor, pulse, blood pressure, and rate of urinary output. A patient with a total body water deficit should have improvement in his sensorium, an increase in output, and a decrease in specific gravity of the urine. If such a patient has an excessive amount of urine and seems to be losing urine as fast as 5% glucose is given, one should suspect diabetes insipidus and test for it by giving vasopressin (Pitressin). These are examples of *diagnosis ex juvantibus*. If the response to treatment is not as expected, the collection and analysis of information must be reviewed since the basis for the fluid orders may have been erroneous.

SPECIAL PROBLEMS

The healthy, young, thin patient with a surgical problem such as inguinal hernia or appendicitis receives parenteral fluids for a very short time and will tolerate gross errors of fluid therapy ranging from receiving no fluids to receiving only glucose solution or saline. Since the majority of patients do not require careful analysis, there is a real danger that a physician will become careless and fail to think through the logical analysis, which may be lifesaving in the critically ill patient. The general analysis has been presented, and after some experience in its use it actually requires only a few minutes to complete in the majority of patients. In addition to the preceding outline, the experienced physician will apply additional reasoning when he recognizes certain specific problems such as complicated acid-base imbalance, disturbances in potassium metabolism, acute trauma, and other problems, some of which will be discussed briefly.

Acid-base balance

The hydrogen-ion concentration in body fluids plays a critical role in enzyme systems and other physiological processes (conservation of base by the kidneys and the binding of oxygen by hemoglobin, for example). Remarkable *buffer systems* dampen or moderate any rapid changes in hydrogen-ion concentration. The main buffer system, the bicarbonate ion–carbonic acid buffer, is aided first by pulmonary regulation of excretion of volatile acid as CO_2 and second by renal excretion of nonvolatile acids such as those of phosphate and ammonium. The ratio of bicarbonate ion to carbonic acid in body fluids is normally 20:1. The Henderson-Hasselbalch equation expresses this important relationship of body pH, bicarbonate ion (nonvolatile), and carbonic acid (volatile) in mathematical terms:

$$pH = pK + \log \frac{BHCO_3}{H_2CO_3}$$

In clinical concepts, this may be expressed as:

$$\text{Acid-base balance} = \text{Constant} + \frac{\text{Kidney function}}{\text{Ventilation}}$$

Primary diseases in the kidneys, which cause ineffective excretion of nonvolatile acids, are compensated for by increased excretion of volatile (carbonic) acid by the lung. The converse is also true. In assessment of acid-base disturbances, CO_2 content, which measures volatile and nonvolatile acids, is of limited value in patients with complicated metabolic, renal, and pulmonary problems.

Two pieces of data and a diagram (Fig. 3-10) are necessary to analyze acid-base disturbances more completely. These are pH and P_{CO_2}. They are

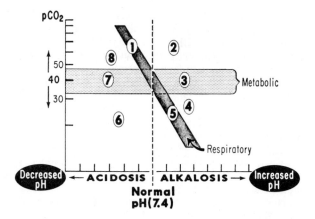

Fig. 3-10. All possible acid-base abnormalities in terms of P_{CO_2} and pH. (Modified from Siggaard-Andersen, O.: The acid-base status of the blood, Baltimore, 1964, The Williams & Wilkins Co.)

1. Respiratory acidosis
2. Mixed respiratory acidosis and metabolic alkalosis.
3. Metabolic alkalosis
4. Mixed metabolic and respiratory alkalosis
5. Respiratory alkalosis
6. Mixed metabolic acidosis and respiratory alkalosis
7. Metabolic acidosis
8. Mixed metabolic and respiratory acidosis

obtained rapidly and accurately from arterial blood samples.

Concept of pH

pH is the negative log of the hydrogen-ion concentration and is a convenient way of stating a very small number. The normal arterial pH is 7.4. With increasing hydrogen-ion concentration, the pH decreases, and this is referred to as a state of *acidosis*. Hydrogen-ion concentration decrease is associated with an increased pH and is called *alkalosis*.

Two types of pH disturbance are classified according to whether they are caused by a change in the body carbonic acid, *respiratory disturbances,* or whether they are caused by a change in concentration of nonvolatile, nonrespiratory substances, *metabolic disturbances*. Whenever fluids that are excreted, secreted, or lost from the body differ in their hydrogen-ion concentration from normal body fluids, an opposite change occurs in the hydrogen-ion concentration of the fluids remaining in the body; i.e., if a patient loses acid gastric juice, the body changes toward an alkalosis. If the patient excretes very alkaline urine, the body fluids change toward a state of acidosis. Acidosis and alkalosis (or basosis) are, for the clinician, terms signifying a deviation around a normal body pH of 7.4.

Concept of P_{CO_2}

The second important datum is the partial pressure of carbon dioxide (P_{CO_2}) in the body fluids and in the alveolar air, which is in equilibrium with these fluids.* A normal P_{CO_2} is usually about 40 mm. Hg. The rate of excretion of carbon dioxide by ventilation regulates the carbonic acid in the body. A P_{CO_2} above normal (hypercapnia, hypercarbia) indicates *respiratory acidosis*. If the ventilation is above normal so that the patient is blowing off excessive amounts of CO_2 (hypocapnia, hypocarbia), the P_{CO_2} will be below normal, *respiratory alkalosis*.

Types of acid-base imbalances

Acid-base deviations from normal can be classified as *primary, compensatory,* or *mixed;* e.g., a patient with a *primary metabolic acidosis* from retention of lactic acid (attributed to poor circulation or shock) will usually respond to the increased concentration of hydrogen ions by breathing more rapidly and increasing the rate of excretion of carbonic acid. This is *compensatory respiratory alkalosis. Primary respiratory alkalosis* may occur in a patient with portal hypertension and cirrhosis. Portacaval shunt may cause an increase in ammonia in the blood and, as a result of this, stimulation of the respiratory center. Increased ventilation results in "blowing off" carbonic acid,

---

*Usually the alveolar CO_2 concentration is about 5.6%. Partial pressures, measured in mm. Hg, vary with barometric pressure and vapor pressure.

which eventuates in primary respiratory alkalosis. Sometimes a patient develops two primary conditions, one of which is respiratory and the other metabolic, and yet neither of these is compensating. Both are the result of some disease process or its complication, and these are referred to as *mixed forms of acid-base imbalance;* i.e., a patient with emphysema may be unable to excrete carbon dioxide normally and develops an elevated P_{CO_2}, or a *primary respiratory acidosis,* from the retained carbonic acid. At the same time such a patient may have one of several different conditions that might also cause a *primary metabolic alkalosis,* such as an obstructing duodenal ulcer causing vomiting of acid gastric juice.

Graphic summary of acid-base abnormalities

The pH, P_{CO_2} diagram (Fig. 3-10) makes it possible to sumarize all primary, compensatory, and mixed acid-base abnormalities. Pure abnormalities of nonrespiratory, or metabolic, origin are depicted in areas 7 and 3, and pure deviations from normal (caused by decreased or increased excretion of carbonic acid or respiratory abnormalities) are shown in areas 1 and 5. Areas 2, 4, 6, and 8 are all mixed areas. Area 6 is a common location for patients who have a primary metabolic acidosis and a compensatory respiratory alkalosis. Area 2 includes patients with mixed primary problems but also *respiratory compensation for a metabolic alkalosis.* If a patient with a primary metabolic alkalosis moves into area 2, it may signify that he also has a primary abnormality in his pulmonary function, and one should look for airway obstruction, pneumonia, pulmonary embolism, or another cause of impaired gas exchange.

Importance of clinical correlation

The preceding examples illustrate that *understanding of the particular patient's acid-base problem requires more than just laboratory data.* The clinician must know what primary acid-base abnormalities might be present according to the disease process; i.e., increased ventilation may result because the lungs and the central nervous system function in a normal manner to compensate for a metabolic acidosis. If a patient has a high blood urea nitrogen and diseased kidneys fail to excrete excess organic acids, the retention of these acids will cause a metabolic acidosis. If the patient has severe ketosis, secondary to uncontrolled diabetes, and the lungs are clinically normal, then the excessive ventilation is compensatory, and the clinician knows, before he enlists the help of the laboratory, that the patient's P_{CO_2} and pH will converge somewhere in area 6.

With accurate clinical knowledge of the patient, measurement of P_{CO_2} and pH is often unnecessary. The CO_2 content of blood will provide a sufficiently accurate estimation of the abnormality in base excess. Normally the CO_2 content is 27 mEq./L. in such samples, and in the patient described the CO_2 content might be 17 or even 7. The difference from normal in CO_2 content is -10 or -20 and is the deficit in base; i.e., if the CO_2 content is only 7, this means a 20 mEq. deficit. A 70 kg. lean patient with 14 L. of extracellular fluid would need 20 times 14, or 280, mEq. of bicarbonate or lactate to bring the CO_2 content back to 27. This would require 1,687 ml. of M/6 sodium lactate since 166 mEq. are present in 1 L.

When pH and P_{CO_2} measurements are necessary

Situations arise in the seriously ill patient (often found in postoperative and intensive care areas) in which the patient probably has both metabolic and respiratory abnormalities. In these complex situations measurements of P_{CO_2} and pH are invaluable guides to determine whether the primary abnormality is metabolic, respiratory, or both.

From the examples given, simple calculations will determine the amount of one-sixth molar sodium lactate required for treatment of a metabolic acidosis or the amount of 0.9% saline, with its 50 mEq./L. chloride excess, required to treat a metabolic alkalosis (provided that it is not secondary to potassium deficiency). Primary respiratory abnormalities, of course, are best treated by measures to restore normal ventilation rather than by administration of any particular type of intravenous fluid. Alkaline solutions (one-sixth molar sodium lactate) may be necessary to correct a compensatory metabolic acidosis before sedation is given to correct the primary respiratory alkalosis (inappropriate overactivity of respiratory center).

Blood gas measurements

Arterial blood gas measurements may be needed frequently in patients who are seriously ill with abnormal cardiopulmonary function. Single samples can be obtained, or an indwelling arterial cannula may help to provide samples as needed. Allen's test consists in compression of the radial and ulnar arteries while the patient pumps blood out of the hand by fist-clenching. Releasing only one artery at a time demonstrates whether there is adequate collateral blood flow should the radial artery become occluded. If the blood supply of the hand is dependent on the radial artery, other vessels should be used to obtain arterial blood samples, especially if an indwelling cannula is to be considered.

Arterial blood samples are frequently analyzed not only for Pco_2 and pH but also for Po_2, and not just to determine acid-base balance but to evaluate the adequacy of ventilation and oxygenation. Respiratory failure may occur suddenly without prior signs and symptoms but will usually be preceded by a progressive fall in Pao_2. Pao_2 is normally 97 mm. Hg when a patient is breathing air. A decrease below 80 is abnormal and requires explanation and appropriate treatment. Oxygenation and ventilation are assessed separately by determination respectively of Pao_2 and $Paco_2$. Perfusion of areas of the lung that are not properly aerated causes a decrease in Pao_2 because of the venous admixture or so-called shunt. Frequently ventilation is appropriate to maintain a normal $Paco_2$ even though there is a decrease in Pao_2. A rising $Paco_2$ indicates ventilatory failure. The focus of management then should be on the restoration of a more normal ventilation and not just on the administration of oxygen or correction of acid-base imbalance.

Oxygen therapy will usually help a patient with hypoxia provided that ventilatory failure is not present. If $Paco_2$ is high and the respiratory drive is dependent on hypoxia, administration of oxygen alone will not help and may even result in a worsening of ventilatory failure. An endonasal endotracheal tube and ventilatory support may be urgently needed in addition to increased oxygen inhalation. The cause of CO_2 retention must be found and corrected. Blood gas analysis is the first step in recognition, evaluation, and determination of appropriate treatment of respiratory failure.

Potassium

Special thought must be given to potassium balance because potassium is the chief cation within cells (94% of total body potassium is in the cells). Young adult women have 2,000 to 3,000 mEq. total potassium and men have up to 5,000 mEq. The correlation in humans between total exchangeable potassium and energy consumption (in calories per day with moderate activity) is around 0.90. The total exchangeable body potassium can be measured by dilution with radioactive potassium, but this is not a practical clinical test. The clinician must rely on analyses of serum potassium. There are only about 70 mEq. of potassium in the extracellular fluid. The normal serum potassium ranges between 3.5 and 5 mEq./L. If as much as 70 mEq. of potassium moves out of its location in cells into extracellular fluid or if this much potassium is retained in extracellular fluid during intravenous potassium administration, the patient will probably die of cardiac arrest.

Recognition of potassium abnormalities

Like the recognition of sodium deficiency, recognition of body potassium deficiency is dependent to a great extent on the suspicion of the clinician. His suspicion is raised by knowledge of circumstances that cause potassium loss. Potassium is continually excreted in the urine. In contrast to sodium, despite cessation of potassium intake, the kidneys continue to excrete potassium (minimum rate, 10 to 20 mEq./day). It is also lost in gastrointestinal juices. If a patient has been losing large amounts of such fluids and the replacement solutions have contained no potassium, total body potassium deficiency will eventually occur, usually accompanied by a lowering of serum potassium concentration. The degree of lowering of serum potassium concentration, however, tells little about the magnitude of total body potassium deficiency.

Patients unable to take food by mouth or subjected to trauma, burns, and major operative procedures, or treated previously with steroids or diuretics are likely to have a potassium deficiency. The physical signs are nonspecific. Such patients have weakness (occasionally almost to paralysis), decreased deep tendon reflexes, and commonly ileus, abdominal distension, and a picture easily confused with chronic bowel obstruction. The electrocardiogram shows a flattening or even inversion of the T wave. These patients are quite sensitive to digitalis and may, if treated with digitalis, show signs of intoxication with nausea and abnormal rhythm.

Patients with high serum potassium also may have muscular paralysis and complain of paresthesias. The electrocardiogram shows elevated and peaked T waves and, with near lethal potassium levels, the electrocardiogram loses all of its normal components.

Potassium problems are divided into (1) those patients in whom the extracellular fluid potassium concentration is abnormal, but without any intracellular deficit, and (2) those patients who have a total body potassium deficiency. The extracellular fluid potassium is affected by the rate of potassium absorption or absence of intake, the rate of loss from the body in various fluids, and the maintenance of a normal cellular metabolism. Sodium is continuously pumped out of cells, allowing a high concentration (or gradient) of potassium within the cells compared with the concentration of potassium in extracellular fluid. If the patient becomes severely ill so that metabolism is impaired and the sodium pump begins to fail, then sodium tends to remain in cells and potassium tends to leak out; the extracellular fluid potassium will rapidly reach a level incompatible with life.

Potassium excess. If a heavy object crushes large masses of muscle, potassium leaks out into the extracellular fluid along with myoglobin. The kidneys may become damaged from the pigment and from impaired circulation, and such a patient will die of potassium poisoning within 18 to 24 hours after the crushing injury. Severe burns and major operative procedures are also followed by elevation of serum potassium because of tissue damage and impaired renal function.

In most instances all that is required relative to potassium balance is to restrict potassium during the first 24 hours after a major operation or during the first few days after a burn. The patient with crush syndrome has to have vigorous treatment with peritoneal dialysis or use of the artificial kidney, and the dialyses may have to be carried on almost continuously during the first few days while the large amounts of potassium are being lost from the crushed muscle. The patient in negative nitrogen balance who is burning his own cellular protein also loses potassium, and the amounts of potassium entering extracellular fluid can be reduced when 400 to 800 calories a day are supplied by the administration of glucose in the intravenous fluids so as to minimize protein catabolism.

Potassium- and hydrogen-ion concentration. The concentration of potassium in extracellular fluid is influenced by the hydrogen-ion concentration. Increasing concentrations of hydrogen ion in the extracellular fluid (acidosis) cause hydrogen to move into cells and potassium to move out of cells so that the serum potassium will rise. If the acidosis is treated with sodium bicarbonate or sodium lactate, the serum potassium concentration will fall as the patient becomes less acidotic. If a patient has an alkalosis, this will cause the serum potassium to fall. The patient with severe diabetic acidosis may on initial examination have a serum potassium that is high and then in the course of treatment (and in a matter of hours if the acidosis is rapidly corrected) the potassium may fall to a very subnormal level partly as a result of the change in acid-base balance and also because the patient may have a severe total body deficit of potassium.

Potassium deficit. Total body potassium deficit may arise in a variety of situations, but one of the classic examples is the patient who develops pyloric obstruction from a duodenal ulcer; vomiting produces a *hypochloremic alkalosis*. The physician prescribes an amount of saline that he believes should correct the hypochloremic alkalosis and, after treatment with this, finds that the patient still has a low chloride concentration and a high CO_2 content in blood. He may also observe that the patient has an acid urine, which seems inconsistent in a patient with alkalosis. In the days before the

flame photometer, this was sufficient to justify a diagnosis of potassium deficiency, but with potassium analysis it is possible to document this by finding a low serum potassium.

For every 3 mEq. of potassium lost from the cells, 2 mEq. of sodium and 1 mEq. of hydrogen ion enter the cells. The hydrogen, of course, is bound to protein and other buffers, but, as a result of this exchange, the cells become more acid. The cells lining the renal tubules participate in potassium deficiency and cellular acidosis so that the urine formed is acid (Fig. 3-11). Excretion of acid urine produces hypochloremic alkalosis in extracellular fluid. In the patient who has been vomiting acid gastric juice and also losing potassium, there are therefore two reasons for developing hypochloremic alkalosis. Both potassium and chloride are required to correct the potassium deficiency and the extracellular alkalosis.

Notice that two different problems related to potassium and hydrogen ion have been discussed. In the first situation a primary *extracellular acidosis* occurs and hydrogen ion moves into the cell forcing potassium out, causing an increase in concentration of serum potassium. In the other situation the primary abnormality is an *intracellular potassium deficiency* and an increase in cellular hydrogen-ion concentration along with movement of sodium into the cell, followed by the production of an extracellular alkalosis. In the first situation the acidosis begins in extracellular fluid and also involves intracellular fluid. In the second situation, an intracellular acidosis initiates and sustains extracellular alkalosis. As you might expect, some patients who develop an extracellular acidosis, as in diabetic ketosis or with diarrhea, also develop a depletion of cellular potassium.

Treating potassium imbalances

The best treatment is prevention; potassium imbalance, like other fluid and electrolyte problems, can be prevented by replacement of abnormal fluid losses as they occur and provision of adequate calories and metabolic fluids together with 40 mEq. of urinary loss potassium per day. The potassium requirements may be slightly higher if the patient is receiving steroids or diuretics. The requirements are nil if the patient is oliguric, is acidotic, or has recently undergone a major operation.

Gastrointestinal juice losses should be replaced in the same quantity and at the same rate as they are being lost. For each liter of intravenous electrolyte solution required, 40 mEq. of potassium chloride should be added. Potassium should almost always be diluted in intravenous fluids so that 40 mEq. is distributed in at least a liter of fluid. If,

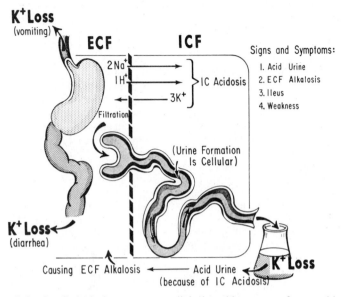

Fig. 3-11. Hypokalemic alkalosis is a common clinical problem seen after vomiting because of obstructing duodenal ulcer or pyloric stenosis with replacement of NaCl but *not* K^+. K^+ leaves cells. H^+ and Na^+ enter cells. Intracellular *acidosis* results from this exchange. Kidney cells are also acidotic and therefore secrete acid urine; ECF alkalosis is exaggerated. This situation is reversed only by correction of the K^+ deficit.

however, the serum potassium is below 3 mEq./L., as much as 80 mEq. can be placed in each liter of intravenous fluid. In some instances it will be necessary to give several hundred milliequivalents in a day, perhaps for a number of days, until the total body potassium deficit is repaired. This must be monitored with serum potassium analyses, and the treatment is tapered to maintenance levels as soon as the serum potassium reaches a normal range.

High potassium levels in patients who are greatly acidotic and who have adequate renal function will return to normal as the patient's acidosis is corrected. In oliguria or acute renal failure a serum potassium of 7 mEq./L. or above should be treated with emergency measures such as the administration of one-sixth molar sodium lactate to correct the acidosis, calcium to counteract the effect of potassium on myocardial irritability, and the administration of glucose and insulin to cause deposition of potassium along with phosphate and glycogen in the liver. If the patient can take sodium polystyrene sulfonate (an exchange resin) with sorbitol by mouth, this will remove potassium but should not be relied on in the emergency situation. The exchange resin can also be given as a retention enema. Peritoneal dialysis or hemodialysis is often

required to restore the potassium to normal in the patient with renal failure; delay is deadly.

Calcium and phosphate
Hypocalcemia

The administration of parenteral calcium or phosphate is infrequently required, but the circumstances in which it is required may be very dramatic. Tetany usually occurs within 2 days after parathyroidectomy or injury of the blood supply of the parathyroid glands during radical thyroidectomy. Recognition may be delayed for several weeks if the deficiency is mild. Hypocalcemia also occurs after removal of parathyroid adenomas or hyperplastic parathyroid glands and is to be expected if the patient has osteitis fibrosa cystica or other evidence of bone demineralization such as an elevated alkaline phosphatase.

Hypocalcemia is common in chronic acidosis and becomes manifest when the acidosis is treated. Acidosis tends to sustain a relatively high concentration of *ionized* calcium. When the acidosis is treated and the body fluids become more alkaline, rapid reduction in ionized calcium causes onset of symptoms. This is seen in patients with chronic renal insufficiency and occasionally in patients treated for acidosis from other causes such as diabetic ketosis or acidosis associated with chronic diarrhea. Patients with malabsorption and steatorrhea, such as that occurring after the removal of small bowel or sidetracking of small bowel for purposes of treating obesity, may lose calcium from bone but maintain normal serum calcium levels.

The symptoms of low serum calcium are tingling of the fingers and feet and paresthesias about the face and especially around the lips and tongue. Some patients have severe spasm of various muscles, more commonly the back muscles and the muscles of the hands and feet, so that the patient develops a characteristic flexion of the wrist and the metacarpophalangeal joint with extension of the distal phalangeal joints, referred to as carpopedal spasm. One can demonstrate the muscular irritability by tapping over the facial nerve and observing the contraction of the facial muscles, especially the orbicularis oris (Chvostek's sign). Production of carpopedal spasm by application of a tourniquet (Trousseau's sign) is less often demonstrable but is equally pathognomonic of hypocalcemia.

The muscle spasm and paresthesias cause anxiety, which commonly causes the patient to hyperventilate. The subsequent reduction in carbonic acid and respiratory alkalosis lead to a further decrease in the ionized calcium, which increases the symptoms and frightens the patient, causing further hyperventilation. This is similar to the hyperventilation syndrome with tetany occasionally seen in a patient who has a normal serum calcium, but it is much more likely to occur in a patient with hypoparathyroidism.

The suspected diagnosis is confirmed by a serum calcium below 8 mg./dl. and, probably of even more importance, a serum phosphorus that is above 4.5 mg./dl. If both calcium and phosphorus are below normal, there may be a problem of inadequate nutrition rather than hypoparathyroidism. Patients with uremia have retention of phosphate and a lowering of serum calcium so that the laboratory values may imitate primary hypoparathyroidism, and in the chronic forms of uremia, a compensatory hyperplasia of the parathyroid glands may result.

Treating hypocalcemia. Parathyroid tetany is safely and dramatically treated by the administration of 10 ml. of 10% calcium gluconate intravenously. This should be given slowly, and if the patient is not completely relieved of his symptoms, a second 10 ml. can be administered. This may have to be repeated several times in the first few days, and for the patient who has had hyperparathyroidism and depletion of his bone minerals, it may be necessary to add up to 80 ml. of 10% calcium gluconate to each liter of intravenous

fluids and to run the intravenous infusion of 5% glucose continuously at a rate sufficient to keep the patient from having tetany.

Vitamin D_2 (calciferol) is given in oral doses of 50,000 units/day along with oral calcium gluconate. This calcium salt is rather insoluble and must be given in a saturated solution or a suspension. Vitamin D has a slow action requiring at least a week for its full effect. If a patient still has hypocalcemia after several weeks, the dosage can be increased to 100,000 units. Occasional patients require as much as 200,000 units/day of vitamin D_2 to maintain a normal serum calcium. The patients are taught how to test their own urine with Sulkowitch reagent, and they are advised to report immediately if the urinary calcium precipitation is too dense to see newsprint through. The hypoparathyroidism that occurs after thyroidectomy may be temporary, and it is important to avoid vitamin D poisoning. These are toxic doses of vitamin D for a patient whose parathyroid function returns to normal. The urinary calcium test is not very accurate, and serum calcium determinations are also required until the patient is well regulated. Even then the serum calcium should be measured several times a year. The use of calcium in the intravenous fluids can be discontinued as soon as the patient is able to get along without the medication for several days without any signs or symptoms of tetany. Mild tetany is not dangerous. Prolonged hypocalcemia should not be tolerated, however, because such patients develop cataracts.

Hypercalcemia

Hypercalcemia causes many nonspecific symptoms that are related to the gastrointestinal tract, the kidneys, and the neuromuscular and skeletal tissues. These patients complain of anorexia, nausea, vomiting, constipation, diarrhea, abdominal pain, nocturia, polyuria, thirst, headache, backache, bone pain, aching thigh muscles, weakness, lethargy, loss of interest, exhaustion with mild physical effort, dizziness, fainting, and confusion, as well as symptoms of acute peptic ulcer, pancreatitis, renal stones, and kidney infection. Hyperparathyroidism has been referred to as "a disease of stones, bones, abdominal groans, and psychic moans with fatigue overtones." Despite all these symptoms the diagnosis was often not made for months or years, and many patients developed parathyroid crisis with serum calcium levels of 14 mg./dl. or above and serum phosphorus levels below 3 and often in the range of 1.5 mg./dl. We now almost routinely measure serum calcium and phosphorus levels in hospital patients. This practice detects hyperparathyroidism before severe complaints or serum chemical alterations have had time to develop. An elevation of parathyroid hormone confirms the diagnosis.

There are no typical physical signs. The patients are irritable, seclusive, distracted, and dull. They often have laxity of their joints, which makes them able to put their feet behind their head and also causes them to have a peculiar and unsteady gait. The diagnosis is made from the typical serum calcium elevation and extremely low serum phosphorus. Once these chemical abnormalities are found, a differential diagnosis arises that involves hyperparathyroidism, multiglandular adenomas, cancer of the breast and other cancers with bone metastases (or cancerous production of parathormone), sarcoidosis, and milk-alkali syndrome. The last condition is infrequent but results when a patient with peptic ulcer drinks several quarts of milk a day and ingests large amounts of alkaline powders in the treatment of the ulcer.

Treating hypercalcemia. Albright suggested in 1932 that sodium phosphate might be used in the treatment of hyperparathyroidism, since excessive excretion of phosphates by the kidney and a consistently low serum phosphorus were found in those patients who had not yet developed uremia. The retention of phosphorus is greatly in excess of the observed rise in serum phosphorus during the recovery of patients who have had hyperparathyroidism, and this has suggested that these patients probably have a great deficit of phosphate in extraskeletal tissues. Acute hypercalcemia has been treated successfully by isotonic disodium phosphate and monopotassium phosphate. This causes a prompt reduction in serum calcium levels from the dangerous areas above 14 mg./dl. to normal levels and is effective whether the hypercalcemia is caused by hyperparathyroidism or cancer. Improvement in stupor, nausea, renal function, and other symptoms and signs of hypercalcemia is usually rapid.

This treatment should not take the place of appropriate diagnostic measures and surgical treatment of the underlying cause of the hypercalcemia, but it does solve the emergency problem and allows the surgeon to perform a necessary operation under more optimum conditions. High serum calcium also causes renal damage. In animals even 24 hours of hypercalcemia will cause calcification in the kidney, with resultant decrease in glomerular filtration rate and elevation of blood urea nitrogen. Myocardial and brain damage may also occur during prolonged and severe hyperparathyroidism.

Magnesium
Magnesium deficiency

Magnesium deficiency is likely to be present in patients with delirium tremens, in patients with cirrhosis in whom fluid and salt retention require the use of diuretics, and in patients with ulcerative colitis and chronic diarrhea. The signs and symptoms of magnesium deficiency in such patients may be mimicked by other deficiencies likely to be present at the same time. Prolonged parenteral fluid therapy without magnesium supplement is a common precedent now to magnesium deficiency, just as in similar patients a few years ago prolonged parenteral fluid therapy without addition of potassium was a common antecedent to hypokalemia. Another similarity between potassium and magnesium deficiencies is their occurrence in those patients with chronic renal disease who have a high urine output, but without uremia. Magnesium deficiency may appear in the patient who has been operated on for severe hyperparathyroidism. The serum magnesium concentration tends to fall parallel to the decrease in calcium concentration during the early hypocalcemic phase of recovery from hyperparathyroidism. This is undoubtedly related to the repletion of magnesium in the bones. Magnesium is also localized in cells, particularly in the mitochondria. The intracellular fluid magnesium is around 28 mEq./L., whereas the serum levels normally range between 1.5 and 2.5 mEq./L.

Deficiency of magnesium causes central nervous system and neuromuscular hyperirritability with hallucinations, jerking, plucking at the bedclothes, and movements of the hand that simulate the so-called hepatic flap of liver failure. Convulsions may occur. The reflexes are usually hyperreactive, and the patient may develop nystagmus or a positive Babinski sign and other signs suggestive of central nervous system disease. This picture is easily confused with water intoxication, which can also cause convulsions and coma. Treatment is usually given intramuscularly with 50% magnesium sulfate in doses of 2 ml. at a time, repeated every 6 hours until the serum magnesium is again normal. One gram a day of magnesium sulfate is sufficient for maintenance, but in the majority of patients parenteral fluids are not required over a long enough period of time so that a significant magnesium depletion would occur.

Magnesium excess

Magnesium intoxication is difficult to separate from hyperkalemia and other associated abnormalities that occur in uremia. A patient with acute renal failure who is treated frequently with peritoneal or extracorporeal dialysis should not develop magnesium intoxication.

Extracellular fluid loss

Internal sequestration of sodium-containing fluids is a common circumstance in the surgeon's practice and is difficult to recognize or to treat quantitatively because the fluid is hidden. Extracellular fluid loss occurs in patients with burns, intestinal obstruction, peritonitis, serum sickness, and multiple soft-tissue injuries. This also occurs in connection with hemorrhage if the blood is not immediately replaced. Since bleeding is a part of major operations and extensive fractures, such patients require a mixed type of replacement with both blood and extracellularlike fluid. Physicochemical changes occur in the collagen in burned skin and cause it to swell by taking up extracellular fluid. Anyone who has seen an obstructed bowel with its severe edema or exudate of peritonitis involving large surface areas, including both visceral and parietal peritoneum, can readily understand the mechanism of sodium fluid sequestration.

Trauma and hemorrhage

If blood is lost by simple hemorrhage and is immediately replaced and if no tissue damage occurs either from the injury or from a period of shock, no electrolyte solution is required. If a few hours transpire during or after the hemorrhage before treatment, sodium-containing fluids become sequestered within the body. The resultant reduction in effective extracellular fluid volume requires both replacement of the blood and restoration of the effective extracellular fluid volume. In the average adult one should give as much as 2 L. of extracellular-like fluid while waiting for the blood to be cross matched. If more than 1,000 ml. of blood are required, some additional electrolyte solution may also be given.

During major prolonged operations, a reduction in effective extracellular fluid volume of 15% to 20% is often seen. Administration of this fluid during the operation will reduce the amount of blood required to maintain normal vital signs. This does not obviate the replacement of blood loss. The electrolyte fluid should be given in addition to blood.

In all of these patients with burns, trauma, hemorrhage, and operative procedures (lasting longer than 2½ hours), the extracellular-like fluid can be made up of 0.9% saline and one-sixth molar sodium lactate in the proportions of 4:1. In most hospitals lactated Ringer's solution is available and has the composition of extracellular fluid.

When extracellular fluid is sequestered as a result of a burn, trauma, or shock-induced tissue injury, and the patient receives appropriate electrolyte solutions to replace this fluid, a mobilization and excretion of such fluid must follow. If the kidneys do not function well and the fluid is retained, pulmonary edema may occur. After resuscitation, electrolyte-containing solutions should

be withheld and, if necessary, diuretics should be given until the fluid overload is corrected.

Patients should be prepared for major operative procedures by having blood volume and hemoglobin levels restored to normal before the operation. Severe depletion of body proteins should also be corrected by the administration of either plasma or human serum albumin. The normal patient has approximately 60% of his blood volume in veins, including the large veins leading into the right side of the heart; he may lose 1 to 1.5 L. of blood before he becomes hypotensive simply because of the constriction of these veins, thereby maintaining venous return.

The normal patient also has about 60% of his albumin in extravascular areas and can lose this much of his total body albumin before he begins to show the signs and symptoms of reduced plasma volume. If a patient with reduced blood volume and reduced body albumin is subjected to a major operation and does not have more than his operative blood loss replaced, he may in the postoperative period demonstrate a failing renal function, poor peripheral circulation (even with the appearance of arterial thromboses in major vessels), and an extremely high hematocrit. If the problem is not recognized and treated vigorously with electrolyte solution, plasma, and blood, such a patient will die. Deficiencies of albumin and whole blood should be repaired *before* the operation.

Replacement of gastrointestinal fluid loss

Much of the imbalance in fluid and electrolytes could be avoided if gastrointestinal fluids were properly replaced at the time of their loss. This implies, of course, accurate records of the type and volume of fluid lost. In the adult this is a loss of isotonic fluid and it is simply replaced with isotonic fluid, such as 0.9% saline or saline plus one-sixth molar sodium lactate. Since all the fluids lost and the two replacement solutions have the same concentration of electrolytes, the chief difference relates to the anion *composition and therefore the pH* (Table 3-1). The pH of the fluid being lost can be determined at the bedside with pH paper. If acid juice is lost from the stomach (and not all juice aspirated from the stomach is acid gastric juice), the fluids remaining in the body are more alkaline. Fluid lost from the upper small bowel (through a long intestinal tube or a duodenal fistula) is alkaline, resulting in an acidosis. If the loss is a balanced loss of gastric and intestinal juices having a pH of approximately 7.4, then the acid-base balance of the patient is unchanged.

If the juice being lost is acid with an excess of chloride, the replacement solution should be isotonic saline, which has an excess of 50 mEq./L. of

Table 3-1. Effects of treatment of acid-base disturbances

Type of fluid loss	Resultant acid-base disturbances	Intravenous fluid ratio (0.9% NaCl:M/6 Na lactate)		
		Neutral (4:1)	Acidifying (1:0)	Alkalinizing (2:1)
Balanced loss	None	Balance	Acidosis	Alkalosis
Acid juice loss	Alkalosis	Alkalosis	Balance	Severe alkalosis
Alkaline loss	Acidosis	Acidosis	Severe acidosis	Balance

chloride as compared with the chloride concentration in normal extracellular fluid. If the fluid being lost is alkaline, the replacement solution should be made up of only 2 parts of saline and 1 part of one-sixth molar sodium lactate. If the solution lost is approximately that of extracellular fluid, the proportions of isotonic saline and one-sixth molar sodium lactate should be 4:1, which is the proportion of bicarbonate to chloride in extracellular fluid.

A few physicians stubbornly maintain that the kidney will take care of any imbalance and that any electrolyte loss may be treated by the administration of 0.9% saline. If a patient loses alkaline intestinal juices and therefore has a metabolic acidosis and is then treated with saline solution, which causes its own hyperchloremic acidosis, even a normal kidney cannot correct this condition. The kidneys in a patient with severe acidosis do not function normally.

The patient with ulcerative colitis who has a total colectomy and ileostomy illustrates the need for continuous monitoring of the type of intestinal fluids lost. During the early postoperative period, the loss is primarily one of acid gastric juice from the stomach that tends to produce an alkalosis and requires treatment with saline. As the intestine begins to function several days after the operation and acid gastric suction fluid loss ceases and alkaline ileostomy fluid loss begins, a large loss of alkaline intestinal juices results in acidosis. At this time the treatment must suddenly be changed from the administration of the acidifying saline solution to an alkalinizing replacement solution containing 2 parts saline and 1 part one-sixth molar sodium lactate. In the replacement of all intestinal fluid loss, 20 to 40 mEq. of potassium should be added for each liter of fluid lost. Gastric juice potassium concentration is usually around 8 to 10 mEq./L. Intestinal juices may contain as high as 50 or 60 mEq./L. potassium.

Acute renal failure

Kidney shutdown is usually the result of a combination of several factors such as hypoten-sion, intravenous hemolysis (infusion of mismatched blood or distilled water), dehydration, extensive trauma, crushing of muscle, and release of myoglobin. *Ischemia* is the common denominator of most causes of acute renal failure.

All degrees of injury from mild tubular injury to complete renal cortical infarction are seen. In most patients there is a lysis of tubular cells with varying numbers of breaks in basement membranes. The latter results in permanent tubulovenous fistulas or obstructed nephrons. Tubulolysis is a reversible lesion, analogous to a burn, with remaining islands of viable cells from which regeneration occurs. Recovery of function requires a few days to as long as 3 weeks. During the period of regeneration, the patient remains oliguric. As the nephrons begin to retain the glomerular filtrate, polyuria develops. As the living cells mature and begin to show subcellular organelles such as mitochondria, normal concentrating function is restored and the diuretic phase of recovery is replaced by normal renal function.

Prevention of acute renal failure requires adequate and early replacement of blood and extracellular fluid, as discussed on pp. 15 and 27. A traumatized patient requiring four units of blood replacement may, in addition, need 3 or 4 L. of lactated Ringer's solution before the urine output is adequate.

Mannitol or furosemide may restore urine flow even though there is a persistent inadequacy of blood and extracellular fluid volume, but it will not correct, and may obscure, the circulatory insufficiency at fault.

Progressive decrease in urine volume to less than 500 ml./day or a rising blood urea nitrogen and creatinine with a greater volume of urine indicates probable acute renal failure. Persistent circulatory insufficiency must be ruled out, and a trial of blood or lactated Ringer's solution may be given to see if normal urine volume can be restored. Simple retention must be ruled out by catheterization or irrigation of an indwelling catheter. The urine is examined for blood cells and casts; tests for urea, creatinine, and electrolytes in the urine are not usually necessary. With renal failure, the urine approaches the chemical composition of the blood.

Acute renal failure causes a retention of any fluids that are administered to the patient; the dilution of total body solute depends on the magnitude of accumulated water, as illustrated in Fig. 3-4. The percent decrease in serum sodium concentration will be equal to the percent increase in lean body mass calculated from change in body weight. If acute renal failure is recognized early and if fluid is restricted adequately, serum sodium concentration remains normal.

Potassium and organic acids accumulate with a resultant progressive fall in CO_2 content. If the patient vomits or has loss of acid gastric juice by nasal gastric suction, the CO_2 may remain normal, with decrease in the serum chloride. This is ideal, since retained *organic acids* do not cause acidosis. A low serum chloride never requires treatment if the CO_2 content is normal. As phosphate is retained, the serum calcium falls. Death occurs after about 10 to 12 days from high potassium, from retained fluids and pulmonary edema, or from pneumonia. Death may occur in 24 hours with crushing injuries, as mentioned on p. 24. No patient should die from renal failure.

Emergency treatment of a high serum potassium requires (1) *glucose and insulin* to force potassium into glycogen stores, (2) *correction of the acidosis* to force potassium into cells, (3) *elevation of serum calcium* to counteract the effect of potassium on myocardial irritability, and (4) dialysis as soon as possible.

Patients without recent abdominal operations can be subjected to peritoneal dialysis within a very short time. Peritoneal dialysis or hemodialysis is required at intervals of every few days to maintain reasonably normal body chemistries while the kidneys are recovering. Peritoneal dialysis is less efficient than hemodialysis with an artificial kidney, and it must be used more frequently and for longer periods of time—but peritoneal dialysis can be used when an artificial kidney is not available.

In addition to the treatment of hyperkalemia, management of acute renal failure should include (1) replacement of only insensible and renal water losses, (2) weighing the patient daily—about 1 pound is the anticipated daily loss, (3) calories given in the form of sugar-sweetened butterballs for protein-sparing effect, and (4) oral administration of ion-exchange resins that bind potassium and increase its excretion in the stool.

SUMMARY

The surgeon is a physician who operates. He is responsible for the complete day-to-day care of his patients and should make a habit on rounds of asking himself what each patient needs for (1) metabolic fluids, (2) replacement of abnormal loss, and (3) restoration of any imbalance that exits. The latter should be defined on the basis of the data available from history, physical findings, intake and output records, and any laboratory analyses of abnormalities of (a) volume, (b) tonicity and chemical composition, and (c) acid-base balance. The diagrams—(1) volume versus concentration, (2) bar graph of extracellular fluid cations and anions, and (3) P_{CO_2}, pH—should be drawn in the patient's chart (progress notes) together with appropriate modifications from normal. One should adjudicate inconsistencies in the analyses by collecting additional data, repeating examinations of patient and laboratory tests, and reviewing the logic of the diagnostic analysis. Finally the needs for fluids, electrolytes, and nutrients should be totaled for the day and incorporated into a simple prescription that the nurse can supply, with prepared intravenous solutions.

4

Disorders of Hemostasis: Diagnosis and Treatment

Jonathan C. Goldsmith

Acquired or congenital hemostatic abnormalities may preclude or complicate surgical procedures. Hemorrhage and poor or delayed wound healing add to morbidity and may result in mortality. When disorders of hemostasis are diagnosed preoperatively, the defect can be corrected and hemorrhagic sequelae avoided.

NORMAL HEMOSTASIS

Arrest of hemorrhage is dependent on an interplay among blood vessels, humoral coagulation factors, platelets, and the fibrinolytic mechanism. Abnormalities in any of these elements can contribute to hemostatic failure. When a vessel is severed, the collagenous subendothelial components of the vessel wall are exposed. Platelets adhere to these exposed components. Hageman factor (factor XII) can also be activated by collagen with subsequent generation of thrombin (Fig. 4-1) and a fibrin clot. Tissue factor made available by trauma activates factor VII (proconvertin), which also generates thrombin. Thrombin, a serine esterase, is not only important in the production of a fibrin clot, but also aggregates platelets. Platelets adherent to subendothelium release ADP from their dense granules, which induces aggregation of other platelets. This interplay of platelets and fibrin results in a hemostatic plug and the primary arrest of bleeding. The normal clearance mechanism for restitution of blood flow is fibrinolysis. Plasminogen deposited in a clot at the time of fibrin formation is activated in an orderly fashion to plasmin, a serine protease, capable of digesting fibrin, which results in thrombus dissolution.

PREOPERATIVE SCREENING

The three essential components of preoperative screening for a bleeding disorder are (1) medical history, (2) physical examination, and (3) focused laboratory evaluation.

Medical history

The most important aspect of the preoperative evaluation is a thorough history. Duration of symptoms helps determine if the patient has a defect that is congenital (e.g., bled after circumcision) or acquired (e.g., underwent major surgery 10 years ago but had difficulty after a dental extraction last year). Superficial hemorrhage (cutaneous, gastrointestinal tract, genitourinary tract) is more suggestive of a platelet abnormality, whereas bleeding into deeper structures (joints, muscle, or soft tissue) is suggestive of a defect in humoral coagulation factors. Spontaneous hemorrhage is consistent with a severe defect, whereas bleeding only after surgery suggests a milder abnormality. Delayed wound healing with broad scars occurs in factor XIII deficiency and in milder deficiencies of the blood coagulation factors. A patient's family history is important in establishment of a diagnosis (e.g., X-linked recessive for hemophilia, autosomal dominant for von Willebrand's disease). A careful review of the patient's prescription and nonprescription medications should be performed because many substances, such as aspirin-containing drugs, induce qualitative platelet defects.

Physical examination

A general physical examination with emphasis on the skin, mucous membranes, and joints may confirm suspicions of a hemostatic defect. The presence of petechiae or purpura is suggestive of a platelet defect, whereas ecchymoses are more often a consequence of a deficiency of a humoral coagulation factor or excessive fibrinolysis. Laxity of skin occurs in connective-tissue disorders (e.g., Ehlers-Danlos syndrome). Poorly healed scars may be found in patients with abnormalities of connective tissue and in those with defects in coagulation factors. The increased fibrinolytic activity of mucous membranes such as that found in the oral cavity may make mild hemostatic defects clinically apparent. Few or disordered platelets or deficiencies of blood clotting factors can cause oral-cavity bleeding. Deformity of joints because of repeated intra-articular hemorrhage is consistent with a severe deficiency of factor VIII or factor IX.

Laboratory evaluation

Laboratory screening for hemostatic defects is directed by the medical history, physical examination, and the nature of the surgical procedure. Patients with a negative history and examination undergoing minor surgery in a nonvital area do not require laboratory testing. However, if surgery is major (thoracic, orthopedic, or abdominal) or in a vital area (ocular, ear-nose-throat, oral cavity,

or central nervous system), *laboratory testing is mandatory*.

Screening tests should include a platelet count, prothrombin time (PT), partial thromboplastin time (PTT), fibrinogen, thrombin-clotting time (TCT), bleeding time, factor XIII, and a test for excessive fibrinolysis such as the euglobulin lysis time. Abnormalities in the screening tests will determine appropriate subsequent determinations. A prolonged PTT suggests a defect in the intrinsic or common pathways of coagulation (Fig. 4-1). Based on the history, specific assays for factor VIII, factor IX, or factor XI may be indicated. Although deficiency of factor XII also prolongs the PTT, it is not associated with a hemorrhagic diathesis. An isolated prolongation of the PT is associated with factor VII deficiency. Prolongation of both the PT and PTT suggests a deficiency in the common pathway involving factor X (Stuart factor), factor V (proaccelerin), or factor II (prothrombin). A long TCT is found when there is a deficiency of clottable fibrinogen or the presence of fibrin (or fibrinogen) degradation products (FDP), heparin, or monoclonal immunoglobulins. Factor XIII deficiency is demonstrated by the dissolution of clots in urea or monochloroacetic acid. Rapid lysis of clots in the euglobulin lysis time (ELT) is suggestive of plas-

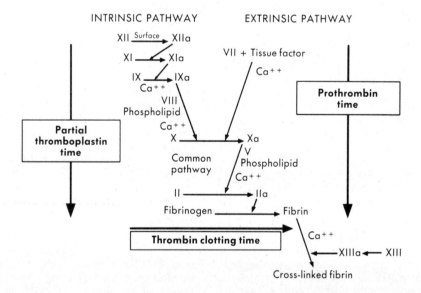

Fig. 4-1. Scheme of cascade hypothesis of blood coagulation. Partial thromboplastin time assesses intrinsic and common pathways. Prothrombin time allows evaluation of extrinsic and common pathways. Thrombin clotting time is affected by qualitative and quantitative abnormalities of fibrinogen and presence of inhibitors of fibrinogen conversion and fibrin polymerization. Specific assays are required to detect abnormalities of factor XIII. (From Goldsmith, J.C.: J. Iowa Med. Soc. **71:**291-297, 1981.)

minogen activation or a small clot secondary to fibrinogen deficiency, as occurs in disseminated intravascular coagulation.

CONGENITAL DISORDERS
Hemophilia

A deficiency of factor VIII (antihemophilic factor, AHF) or factor IX (plasma thromboplastin component, PTC) activity results in clinically indistinguishable bleeding disorders. Both deficiencies are inherited as X-linked recessive conditions characterized by soft-tissue and intra-articular hemorrhage. The clinical severity of the disorders correlates with the degree of deficiency of clotting-factor activity. Patients with less than 1% of the normal amount of factor VIII or IX activity have severe disease with lifelong, recurrent spontaneous bleeding. Patients with 1% to 5% of the normal amount of activity have moderate disease with rare spontaneous, but predictable posttraumatic or postsurgical hemorrhage. Patients with 5% to 50% of normal are mildly affected and bleed excessively only after trauma or surgical challenge.

Several therapeutic materials are available for correction of the clotting defect in hemophilia. Factor VIII is present in fresh whole blood, fresh frozen plasma (FFP), cryoprecipitate, and commercial lyophilized factor VIII concentrates (Table 4-1). Whole blood is a poor replacement source in view of the large volumes required and the rapid loss of factor VIII activity in storage. Fresh frozen plasma also has a high volume for a given amount of AHF activity but is stable for several weeks at −20° C. Cryoprecipitate is the residue of insoluble material remaining when fresh frozen plasma is thawed at 4° C. It is a highly concentrated source of AHF but requires special storage facilities. Factor VIII concentrate is stable at 4° C in lyophilized form for years and, after reconstitution, for hours at room temperature. The risk of hepatitis transmission is great with commercial materials prepared from nonvolunteer plasma. Risks are much less with fresh frozen plasma or cryoprecipitate obtained from volunteer donors.

Before major thoracic, abdominal, orthopedic, ophthalmologic, ear-nose-throat, or dental procedures, patients with classic hemophilia (AHF deficiency) should be replaced to a plasma factor VIII activity level of 80% to 100% of normal. Cryoprecipitate would be an appropriate blood product for mildly affected patients who will require few total lifetime transfusions. Factor VIII concentrate is appropriate for frequently transfused (weekly to monthly), severely affected patients. Dose calculation is based on patient weight. A bag of cryoprecipitate contains 80 to 100 units of factor VIII.

Units required for 100% correction: Weight (kg.) × 50

One half the priming dose should be given every 8 to 12 hours for 3 to 5 days postoperatively and then one fourth the priming dose every 12 hours for a total of 14 days of replacement. Postinfusion factor VIII levels should be 80% to 100% for the first few postoperative days and 30% to 50% subsequently. Factor VIII can also be administered continuously by infusion pump after an initial priming dose. The resultant factor VIII levels should be similar to intermittent infusions. Epsilon aminocaproic acid (EACA) is useful in a dose of 50 mg./kg. orally q.6h. for 7 to 10 days after oral surgery and decreases the need for factor replacement. However, EACA is of no benefit in other types of surgery in patients with hemophilia.

Therapy for factor IX–deficient patients may be accomplished with fresh frozen plasma or commercial factor IX (prothrombin complex) concentrates. Plasma exchange may be required to overcome volume constraints when fresh frozen plasma is used. Patients with hemophilia B should have their plasma level of factor IX activity raised to 50% to 60% of normal preoperatively.

Units required for 50% correction =
Weight (kg.) × 30 to 40

One fourth of the primary dose should be given every 12 hours for 3 to 5 days postoperatively and then every 24 hours for a total of 14 days of replacement. Postinfusion factor IX levels should be approximately 50% for the first few postoperative days and 20% to 30% subsequently. Factor IX levels greater than 60% or dosing more frequently than 8 hours may be associated with inappropriate arterial and venous thrombosis.

Table 4-1. Replacement materials

	Volume (ml.)	Units AHF/ml.	Units PTC/ml.
Fresh whole blood	500	0.5	0.5
Fresh frozen plasma	225	1.0	1.0
Cryoprecipitate	20	5.0	1.0
Factor VIII concentrate	20-50	~20.0	—
Factor IX concentrate	30-50	—	~20.0

Von Willebrand's disease

Von Willebrand's disease (vWD) is an autosomal dominant inherited disorder clinically manifested by surface and postoperative hemorrhage. In laboratory determinations, defects in factor VIII function are identifiable as well as a prolonged bleeding time. Replacement therapy should be in the form of plasma or cryoprecipitate. Lyophilized factor VIII concentrates often lack "von Willebrand factor" activity necessary for correction of the bleeding time and are therefore ineffective and inappropriate.

Goals are twofold in replacement therapy. The factor VIII level should be increased to a range of 80% to 100% and the bleeding time shortened to normal or near normal. In elective procedures eight to ten bags of cryoprecipitate should be given approximately 12 hours before surgery. This permits the production of additional factor VIII activity by the patient with von Willebrand's disease. A second infusion of eight to ten bags should be given preoperatively. If the factor VIII level is not 80% to 100% or the bleeding time not less than 13 minutes by a template method, additional cryoprecipitate should be infused. Six to eight bags of cryoprecipitate should be administered postoperatively and then four to six bags every 8 hours for 3 days. Four to six bags should then be given every 12 hours for an additional 7 to 10 days. Frequent dosing with cryoprecipitate is required postoperatively as correction of the bleeding time is transient even when factor VIII levels are normal.

1-Desamino-8-D-arginine vasopressin (DDAVP) will be licensed for intravenous use in the United States in 1984. Infusion of DDAVP raises factor VIII levels in patients with mild hemophilia and von Willebrand's disease. A dose of 0.3 to 0.5 μg./kg. before procedures and repeated postoperatively has permitted oral and abdominal surgery without the need for transfusion of blood products.

ACQUIRED DISORDERS
Platelet disorders

The most common cause of bleeding is thrombocytopenia. This may be the result of decreased production, an increased space of distribution (splenomegaly), or enhanced destruction. Possible causes for decreased production include bone marrow failure, drugs, alcohol, radiation, and nutritional deficiencies (folic acid, vitamin B_{12}). Shortened platelet survival may be attributable to disseminated intravascular coagulation, immune destruction (idiopathic thrombocytopenic purpura, ITP), or mechanical causes (e.g., cardiac prosthetic valve).

Qualitative platelet defects are manifested by a prolonged bleeding time when normal or near-normal numbers of platelets are circulating. There are rare congenital disorders with abnormal platelet function, but more commonly a prolonged bleeding time is secondary to drug ingestion (e.g., aspirin or nonsteroidal anti-inflammatory drugs) or administration (e.g., carbenicillin), uremia, or liver disease.

If a patient has not been previously sensitized to platelet antigens, the equivalent of 6 units of random donor platelets should be administered preoperatively. Although the goal is to reduce the bleeding time to near normal (less than 13 minutes), a platelet count in excess of 50,000/μl. is also desirable. Platelet counts in patients with thrombocytopenia secondary to enhanced destruction usually do not respond to platelet transfusion. Surgery in these patients carries great risk and should be performed only when no other approach has been satisfactory. One exception to this is the patient with ITP who has increased platelet destruction because of increased platelet-associated immunoglobulin G. These patients often have normal or near-normal bleeding times and are candidates for curative surgery, such as splenectomy, with very low platelet counts and no preoperative or postoperative platelet transfusions.

Perioperative hemorrhage

Intraoperative hemorrhage in a previously normal individual is caused by massive transfusion, thrombocytopenia, disseminated intravascular coagulation (DIC), or primary fibrinolysis. Rapid transfusion with greater than 5 units of banked blood may dilute out the normal coagulation factors to levels insufficient to support hemostasis. Platelet counts may fall secondary to utilization or loss on mechanical devices such as cardiopulmonary bypass pumps. Intraoperative DIC may be secondary to sepsis, malignancy, mismatched blood with hemolysis, or obstetric causes, such as amniotic fluid embolism. The fibrinolytic mechanism is normally activated intraoperatively. However, excessive activity may be generated during urologic surgery.

Postoperative hemorrhage may be attributable to anatomic bleeding sites or caused by intraoperative hemorrhage (see above). Anatomic bleeding is usually local and begins soon after surgery. Systemic coagulopathies result in hemorrhage away from the operative site and may be delayed in onset. Routine screening tests may clarify the type of defect. In cardiopulmonary bypass cases, a reptilase time should also be performed to determine if there is residual heparin effect.

Coagulopathy-related bleeding can often be terminated or slowed by the infusion of 2 or 3 units of fresh frozen plasma or 1 unit of fresh frozen plasma for each 3 or 4 units of transfused red cells. Platelet support may be indicated and can be supplied as the equivalent of 6 donor units. In occasional patients postoperative hemorrhage may not cease until fibrinogen (contained in 10 to 15 units of cryoprecipitate) has been infused. Rarely is it necessary to interrupt the fibrinolytic mechanism with EACA. Exceptions occur in oral surgery and occasionally after genitourinary surgery.

Disseminated intravascular coagulation (DIC)

The excessive generation of thrombin may lead to a clinically important bleeding and less often thrombotic disorder. DIC is manifested by consumption of blood clotting factors V and VIII and fibrinogen, consumption of platelets, and activation of fibrinolysis. Typically patients have long prothrombin times and PTT's, lowered platelet counts and fibrinogen, elevated fibrin(ogen) degradation products (FDP), and circulating fibrin monomer.

Therapy of DIC is directed at correction of the underlying disorder such as sepsis or malignancy. Infusion of FFP as a source of antithrombin III and cryoprecipitate as a source of fibrinogen may be needed for hemostasis in some patients pending treatment of the cause of DIC. Heparin in doses of 200 to 500 units/hour may be needed in rare patients with hemorrhagic DIC. EACA should not be given to patients with suspected or proved DIC because fibrinolysis is protective under these circumstances.

Vitamin K deficiency

Starvation or poor caloric intake after gut sterilization may lead to vitamin K deficiency. This can be avoided by the weekly parenteral administration of 10 mg of vitamin K_1 to postoperative patients who are not taking anything by mouth for prolonged periods. Vitamin K deficiency because of malabsorption can be corrected by the parenteral administration of 10 to 15 mg of vitamin K_1. Intravenously administered vitamin K may be attended by cardiac arrhythmias, which make the subcutaneous or intramuscular route preferable.

Patients on warfarin requiring long-term anticoagulation can have their clotting defect immediately but temporarily reversed by the infusion of 2 to 4 units of FFP. Parenteral vitamin K will also correct the clotting defect but only after 6 to 24 hours and will make subsequent anticoagulation with warfarin very difficult. If therapy with warfarin is not desired postoperatively, FFP and vitamin K are given concurrently, allowing immediate surgery.

Liver disease

The patient with hepatocellular disease presents a difficult problem for management. Eighty-five percent of these patients have coagulation abnormalities, wheras bleeding occurs in only 15%. The normal liver plays a central role in blood coagulation and fibrinolysis. Clotting factors, fibrinolysis factors, and enzyme inhibitors are primarily synthesized in the hepatocyte. Quantitative and qualitative defects in clotting factor synthesis, as well as inadequate production of inhibitors of clotting and fibrinolysis, can result from hepatocellular disease. In addition to its synthetic function, the liver clears activated clotting factors from the circulation. These hepatic clearance mechanisms may also be impaired in liver disease, permitting the circulation of activated factors, fibrinolytic activators, and degradation products of coagulation. Hepatic dysfunction also results in both qualitative and quantitative platelet defects.

It is often impossible to distinguish liver disease from DIC in a patient with hepatocellular damage. Correction of the coagulopathy is mandatory before any surgical procedure. Fresh frozen plasma contains both procoagulants and inhibitors of coagulation, making it the preferred replacement material. Platelet concentrates may also be indicated. Prothrombin complex concentrates (factor IX concentrates) are contraindicated; although these materials had an activity of factors II, VII, IX, and X activity, they lack antithrombin III and have caused thromboembolic complications and death when infused into patients with liver disease.

If DIC is suspected in the presence of liver disease, FFP should be given initially. If clinical hemorrhage continues, heparin may be useful at a rate of 200 to 500 units/hour. Heparin may worsen bleeding. If this happens, it should be discontinued.

A structural cause for gastrointestinal hemorrhage should be sought in the presence of liver disease. Vigorous efforts should be made to find an anatomic bleeding site. Local nonoperative measures such as gastric lavage with iced saline and norepinephrine, infusion of vasopressin, and use of a Sengstaken-Blakemore tube may prove effective.

5
Shock

Timothy A. Thomsen
Robert T. Soper

Shock may be defined as a condition of inadequate vascular perfusion to satisfy the minimal metabolic demands of the cells, or the inability of tissues to utilize oxygen and other nutrients. The clinical situation triggering shock produces a defect, or a combination of defects, that impedes cellular utilization of high-energy substrates.

Shock may result from many different causes, but all have the common effect of reducing vascular perfusion of body cells leading to tissue hypoxia, metabolic acidosis, and cellular death, if uncorrected. The absence of a single simple test to measure effective blood flow to the tissues accounts for much of the confusion about the diagnostic criteria of shock and for the widely divergent approaches to its classification and treatment. Lacking such a test, the physician must base his diagnosis of shock on signs, symptoms, and measurements that are suggestive of, but do not absolutely prove, the presence of shock. The two most important factors in restoring the shock patient to a normal, stable condition are to recognize the state of shock and to reverse the mechanisms that caused it.

Shock is the terminal event in all deaths. Trauma with attendant shock is said to be the most common primary factor causing death during the first four decades of life in the United States. Recent studies have provided new and intriguing concepts to the understanding of shock. We now recognize that shock, though usually associated with systemic hypotension, may occur with normal arterial pressures, as in patients with gram-negative septicemia. However, low arterial pressures do not necessarily signify shock.

NORMAL CELLULAR PERFUSION

Normal perfusion of body tissues begins with the heart, which pumps oxygenated blood and nutrients into the major arteries of the body in a pulsatile manner. Regulators of organ blood flow are concentrated in the precapillary sphincters of the metarterioles of the body. These regulators produce resistance to arterial flow to maintain blood pressure and convert the pulsatile circulating stream to an even flow (Fig. 5-1, *A*). A single precapillary sphincter regulates flow to several capillaries. Normally, only about 20% of the capillaries of the body are perfused at any one time (the other 80% are closed). If all the capillaries were open simultaneously, the circulating blood volume would have to be increased many times to fill all vascular channels of the body. The capillaries carrying blood at a given time are rotated, so that all cells are periodically perfused with oxygen and nutrients. This orderly rotation of perfused capillaries is probably assured by the following mechanism: as the cells of inactive capillaries become anoxic, there is released some vasoactive substance (histamine? lactic acid?) that dilates the capillary sphincters to allow perfusion through these channels, thus diverting flow from capillaries nourishing freshly oxygenated tissue.

The blood flow through the open capillaries is rapid, and the decrease in pH of the blood is small. End products of cellular metabolism are picked up on the venous end of the capillaries, and the blood is returned in the venous channels to the heart pump. Arterial blood not needed by its capillary branches at that moment is diverted directly back to the veins via arteriovenous shunts by contrac-

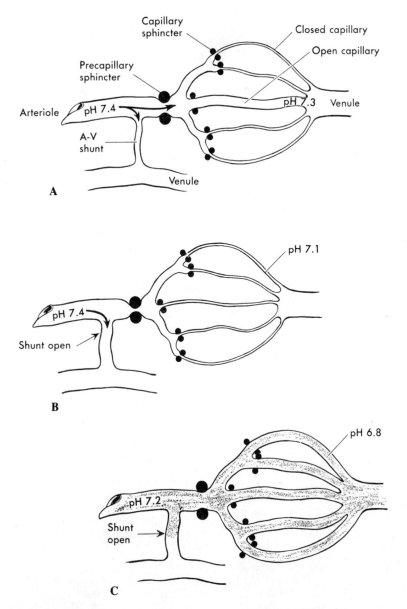

Fig. 5-1. A, Diagram of normal microcirculation. Precapillary sphincter is partially constricted, diverting some arterial blood directly to veins through the arteriovenous shunt. Blood entering capillary system is perfusing only about 20% (1 out of 5 capillaries in diagram) of cells nourished by this system at any given time. Intermittent opening and closing of capillary sphincters assure periodic perfusion of all tissue. Blood flow is rapid through the perfused capillary, and decrease in blood pH is small. **B,** Vasoconstriction phase of shock. Majority of blood in arteriole is diverted across arteriovenous shunt to venous side by constriction of precapillary sphincter. Capillary perfusion is reduced and blood flow slowed to produce greater drop in capillary blood pH. **C,** Vasodilatation phase of shock. Capillaries and venules dilate, blood volume is inadequate to fill large vascular bed, blood flow stagnates, pH drops, and thrombosis may occur.

tion of metarteriole sphincters. Maintenance of flow discourages clumping of cells and increased blood visosity to prevent intravascular clotting.

A derangement of one or more of these components of normal circulation may impair cellular perfusion and produce shock. The physician must pinpoint and correct these derangements to treat shock adequately.

PATHOPHYSIOLOGY OF SHOCK

In early shock, *hyperventilation* is always seen. The increased respiratory rate is usually associated with a decrease in tidal volume and a diminution of P_{CO_2} to 25 to 35 mm. Hg. The P_{O_2}, however, may remain normal as a result of this hyperventilation despite minor lung damage. This early hyperventilation may be caused by platelet aggregates that impede blood flow and may form microemboli producing pulmonary respiratory failure.

Most shock states are associated with *hypovolemia* and *hypotension*. These nonspecific stimuli stimulate the sympathetic alpha adrenergic receptors and result in pronounced compensatory vasoconstriction (Fig. 5-1, *B*). Constricted metarteriole sphincters divert more of the arterial blood across the arteriovenous shunts to increase venous return to the heart, reducing blood flow in the capillary system controlled by the metarteriole. The scanty blood that does enter the capillaries flows slowly and has more oxygen extracted and a lower pH than normal. The sympathetic discharge also constricts the venous (capacitance) bed providing compensation for as much as a 25% volume deficit.

In the presence of hypotension or hypovolemia, interstitial fluid tends to move into the intravascular space. This occurs, according to the Frank-Starling hypothesis, because the colloid osmotic pressure is normal and the filtration pressure is dramatically reduced at the arteriolar end of the capillaries. This accounts for as much as 1 liter of increased intravascular fluid.

Late in the shock state as cellular anoxia increases, lysosomal breakdown occurs with release of proteolytic enzymes, the most powerful being bradykinin. These potent vasodilators expand the vascular bed (Fig. 5-1, *C*). This increases the vascular bed volume to well above what could be filled by even a "normal" circulating blood volume. This phenomenon generally worsens the relative hypovolemia that already exists.

The inadequate perfusion of tissue that occurs during shock deprives the affected cells of oxygen and substrates essential to normal cell function. A series of complex chemical transformations are necessary for the synthesis of adenosine triphosphate (ATP), the ultimate source of energy for life

processes. In the absence of oxygen, ATP is inefficiently produced by anaerobic metabolism. Two moles of ATP are produced per mole of glucose. (Under normal aerobic conditions, pyruvate is converted to acetyl CoA and then enters the Kreb's cycle to produce 38 moles of ATP per mole of glucose.) Under anaerobic conditions, lactic and pyruvic acid accumulate in the tissues, helping to produce the metabolic acidosis of shock. Stored high-energy phosphate bonds decrease, and cellular enzyme systems become disorganized. Organ function then begins to deteriorate. Gastric erosions and hemorrhage are seen. Intestinal ischemia leads to bacteremia and diarrhea; pulmonary capillary leak leads to pulmonary edema and respiratory failure. Renal and hepatic injury results in failure of both of these organs, and cerebral dysfunction is manifest as confusion and obtundation. In the final stages of shock, there is intracellular edema, increasing capillary endothelial damage with leak of protein and fluid into the extravascular space. As metabolites and vasoactive substances increase, there is increasing capillary stagnation and a tendency to develop disseminated intravascular coagulopathy. Ultimately, these factors of *stagnation* of capillary flow, *acidemia*, and *capillary thrombosis* are a vicious cycle that leads to cellular death, organ failure, and the death of the patient.

CLASSIFICATION OF SHOCK

Shock may be classified in several ways. One of the simplest is on the basis of the cause of the shock and is outlined as follows:

1. *Hypovolemic shock:* hemorrhage, burns, trauma, intestinal obstruction, diarrhea, fractures, dehydration
2. *Septic shock:* septicemia, endotoxemia, exotoxemia
3. *Cardiogenic shock:* myocardial infarct, cardiac tamponade, cardiac arrhythmias
4. *Neurogenic shock:* spinal anesthesia or trauma, simple fainting, overdose of vasodilating agents
5. *Other* hypoglycemia, drug overdose

Hypovolemic shock

Hypovolemic shock occurs when there is a significant loss of circulating blood volume, extravascular fluid, or both. This is the most common type of shock seen in surgical practice and is characterized clinically by cold skin, tachycardia, lowered blood pressure, decreased central venous pressure, decreased urine flow, increased arterial blood lactate level, and decreased cardiac index. Whole blood loss may occur either externally by surface injury or internally into tissue planes as with crush injuries, pancreatitis, major fractures, and peritonitis. Bleeding into the lumen of the gastrointestinal tract is another major cause of hypovolemic shock in the surgical patient. External blood loss is easy to recognize, quantitate, and treat, whereas internal bleeding or third-space sequestration of fluid is frequently more difficult to recognize, quantitate, and manage.

When the arterial blood pressure falls from any cause, the compensatory response is mediated primarily through the sympathetic nervous system by increasing peripheral resistance (arteriolar constriction through alpha adrenergic receptors) and increasing cardiac output (through beta adrenergic receptors). In addition, venomotor tone is increased to deliver more blood from venous reservoirs into the circulation. The vessels of the heart and brain are not involved in arteriolar constriction and thus remain protected.

There are additional endocrine responses such as the release of antidiuretic hormone (ADH) and aldosterone, both of which act to retain salt and water. Renin is released from the juxtaglomerular apparatus in response to decreased pressure. This proteolytic enzyme forms angiotensin from plasma precursors, and after conversion to angiotensin II, it leads to increased production and release of aldosterone from the adrenal gland. When plasmalike fluid is the primary constituent of the blood that is sequestered in tissues injured by burns, cellulitis, or trauma, hemoconcentration occurs with a consequent increase in viscosity. Under these circumstances blood sludging occurs in the microcirculation, with the added risk of intravascular coagulation. When whole blood is lost, the additional deleterious effect on the tissue of sludging does not occur because of subsequent hemodilution.

Septic shock

Septic shock has two distinctly different mechanisms for producing shock: (1) *Hypodynamic septic shock* secondary to extensive cellulitis or diffuse infections of body cavities (peritonitis) whereby large amounts of plasmalike fluid sequester in the injured tissue to produce hypovolemia, and (2) *hyperdynamic septic shock* in which toxins produced by infecting organisms exert profound effects on the circulation and impair cellular metabolism.

Septic shock may be produced by either gram-negative or gram-positive organisms, but more commonly by gram-negative organisms. Peculiarly predisposed to septic shock are immunosuppressed organ-transplant patients and patients receiving chemotherapy. In contrast to hypovolemic shock, the patient with septic shock is usually warm and has pink extremities. Cardiac output is increased and peripheral vascular resistance is decreased. As in early hypovolemic shock, a moderate state of

alkylosis occurs secondary to hyperventilation. Circulating blood volume is usually normal or above normal, but oxygen utilization is maintained at a lower than normal level. This seems to indicate an inability of the cell to utilize oxygen in septic shock. Many mechanisms have been studied with respect to this particular cellular paralysis; of the systems studied, 2,3-diphosphoglycerate (DPG) is the most likely culprit responsible for the inefficient oxygen utilization by the cells.

Sepsis may produce profound shock with a high mortality (40% to 90%). Shock produced by gram-positive organisms tends to be less severe than that triggered by gram-negative organisms. Often septic and hypovolemic shock occur simultaneously to compound each other. However, it is clear that septic shock can occur alone, such as the shock occasionally provoked by instrumentation of the lower urinary tract with release of endotoxin from a small prostatic abscess or urinary tract infection.

Endotoxin will occasionally produce an abnormal acceleration of the clotting process known as disseminated intravascular coagulation (DIC). When massive DIC consumes large amounts of platelets and fibrin, diffuse hemorrhage occurs. Under these circumstances the patient may die of hypovolemic shock.

In recent years a special form of septic shock has been described, termed the *toxic shock syndrome*. This shock state is attributed to a toxin that is produced by *Staphylococcus aureus* bacteria. The syndrome is manifest by fever, headache, rash, vomiting, and significant hypotension. It was initially described in young menstruating females and may be related to tampon use. However, it also is seen in patients with postoperative surgical abscesses, wound infections, bursitis, the postpartum state, and a host of other clinical settings.

Cardiogenic shock

Cardiogenic shock occurs when there is inadequate cardiac output despite a normal blood volume. These patients have increased peripheral resistance, increased pulse rate, and decreased cardiac output. This results in cool, clammy skin.

The most common cause of cardiogenic shock is myocardial infarction. When infarction results in functional loss of more than 45% of myocardial tissue, there is profound decrease in cardiac output. Many other conditions result in diminished cardiac output. For example, the heart may not fill adequately because of pulmonary embolus, pericardial tamponade, tension pneumothorax, or venacaval obstruction. The heart may not pump the circulating volume efficiently because of ineffective emptying of the chambers (atrial and ventricular arrhythmias), sudden changes in myocardial conduction or contraction, or total cessation of heartbeat (cardiac arrest).

Cardiogenic shock continues to have a high mortality and is best managed through an aggressive combined approach that should include vasodilators to decrease the myocardial afterload and vasopressors to support the cardiac contractility. Occasionally the intra-aortic balloon pump is used for temporary support. Rarely, in specific instances, emergency cardiac surgery is necessary to correct the complication of coronary occlusion.

Neurogenic shock

Neurogenic shock occurs when there is blockage or damage to the sympathetic nervous system with subsequent vasodilatation, therefore rendering the "normal" blood volume totally inadequate to fill the expanded vascular space. This situation is observed in spinal and epidural anesthesia, antihypertensive or alpha blocking drug overdosage and in some spinal cord injuries. Simple fainting caused by emotion, pain, or fright might also be considered a form of neurogenic shock, but the degree of hypotension is minimal and the treatment is relatively simple. It is important to stress that head injury never produces hypotension except immediately before death. The usual hemodynamic response to head injury is compensatory hypertension to improve cerebral perfusion. Therefore a patient with hypotension and a head injury must be presumed to have other injuries producing hypovolemia to account for the shock.

Other forms of shock

Various other nonspecific forms of shock are observed. One is that seen with rapid release of histamine into the bloodstream, as with major antigen antibody reactions, severe cellular anoxia, and the terminal phases of hypovolemic shock. Other forms include hypoglycemic shock, shock observed with drug overdosage (particularly the barbituates in very high doses), acute adrenal insufficiency, and acute gastric dilatation.

DIAGNOSIS OF SHOCK

The early diagnosis of shock and the simple statement "This patient is in shock" does more to speed treatment and enhance care than any other factor. However, the most difficult aspect of shock management is its diagnosis. Although several specific types of shock have been listed, the clinical setting for each of these is very nonspecific. To recognize the presence of shock or its manifestations becomes critical. The classic signs of shock are metabolic acidosis, systolic pressure less than a range of 80 to 90 mm. Hg, oliguria, and poor tissue perfusion. However, if the diagnosis is delayed

until these signs are present, treatment will be too late in many cases. The early diagnosis of shock depends on a high level of clinical suspicion and careful observation of the patient's vital signs. Early in shock the pulse pressure (the difference between the systolic and diastolic pressures) will be reduced, indicating a decrease in stroke volume; the patient will also have tachycardia. Before major changes in urine volume are observed, urine concentration increases and the urine sodium decreases. When there is a major drop in blood pressure or renal blood flow, urine volume may decrease dramatically or stop. Another early sign of shock is tachypnea with associated respiratory alkylosis. Metabolic acidosis is a very late sign and reflects the severity of cellular damage and decreased metabolism. Changes in mental state and signs of poor peripheral perfusion (cold, clammy skin) are also helpful diagnostic signs.

The following priorities are assigned to organ systems relative to the order in which they are deprived of adequate blood flow in hypovolemic shock:

1. Skin and subcutaneous fat
2. Intestinal and skeletal muscle
3. Major viscera such as kidney and liver
4. Finally, in the terminal stages of shock, heart and brain

Clinical criteria and bedside tests roughly parallel the selective perfusion of tissues noted above. *Pale, cold,* and *clammy skin* and mucous membranes reflect the skin and subcutaneous vasoconstriction, *weakness* and *ileus* reflect reduction in blood flow to muscle and intestine, *oliguria* results from renal vasoconstriction and changes in distribution of renal blood flow, and alterations in the state of *consciousness* roughly reflect cerebral blood flow.

TREATMENT OF SHOCK
General principles

The goal of shock treatment is to restore normal cellular perfusion. *Shock must first be recognized,* and a quick clinical assessment made of its degree of severity. The patient is placed at rest in bed in the Trendelenburg position, airway and adequate respiratory exchange are assured, and baseline monitors of the vital signs are taken: temperature, pulse rate and volume, arterial blood pressure. A urethral catheter is inserted, and the hourly urine output is recorded. If the cause of the shock is readily apparent, one must then prevent its progression, if possible, by control of bleeding, splinting of fractures, nasogastric suction, etc. Life-threatening aspects of shock must be controlled before any strenuous manipulations are carried out to determine the more exact and complex cause of shock.

If the cause is not apparent, the functional derangements imposed by the shock are assessed, and steps are taken to treat them appropriately: the efficiency of the heart pump is restored if necessary, the volume of circulating blood and extracellular fluid is replenished, peripheral vasomotor activity is evaluated, and the pH and viscosity of blood are restored to normal. The patient is observed frequently and carefully by the same person to note the response to treatment. The goal of treatment is a patient who is alert and no longer complaining of thirst or air hunger, who has warm, pink, and dry skin with prompt capillary refill on compression of the nail beds, and who is excreting satisfactory amounts of urine.

Specific measures

The physician must first be certain that the patient's heart is beating. Cardiac arrest is the inevitable result of severe shock, and one must treat it by (1) establishing an adequate airway, (2) assisting respirations, and (3) beginning external cardiac massage. An emergency electrocardiogram distinguishes between ventricular fibrillation and asystole as the cause of the arrest, the former being treated by electrical shock to defibrillate. Sodium bicarbonate buffer is given to correct acidosis, and finally cardiac stimulants are introduced intravenously or directly into the heart, if the preceding measures are unsatisfactory.

If the heartbeat is present but the pumping action is inefficient and sluggish, inotropic agents are indicated. Distant heart tones with a large heart are suggestive of pericardial tamponade, which is treated by needle aspiration of the blood or fluids sequestered within the pericardial sac.

In less severe shock the first priority is attention to the patient's ventilatory status. All patients with shock should receive supplemental oxygen and must be critically and frequently observed to determine if ventilatory decompensation is beginning and if ventilatory assistance is needed.

Hypovolemia is next corrected by volume replacement, preferably of the volume and type of body fluids that have been lost. Prompt, aggressive fluid resuscitation is critical. Large-bore needles or catheters are placed into two veins. Ideally, a catheter is advanced into either the superior or inferior vena cava to allow monitoring of central venous pressure. A specimen of the patient's blood is removed for immediate type and cross match. Until blood becomes available, fluid is infused in the form of saline, bicarbonate, Ringer's solution, hetastarch, or albumin, depending on the needs of the patient and the fluids available. The immediate

effect of electrolyte solution in increasing blood volumes is as good as that of colloid, though colloid (plasmanate, hetastarch, or albumin) does remain in the vascular tree longer than electrolyte solution and smaller volumes are needed to achieve comparable volume expansion. When blood becomes available, it is given to the point of restoring the red blood cell count to normal. Fluids in excess of this are often needed, but they are better supplied by electrolyte solution than by additional blood.

If blood has been lost, a crude estimation of the amount of hemorrhage is helpful in estimation of the replacement need. Mild blood loss of 10% to 15% of blood volume does not produce clinical signs of shock unless it has been lost rapidly, and replacement is often optional. However, shock will be produced by a 10% blood loss in the elderly or otherwise debilitated patient, and replacement is wise. With moderate blood loss of 20% to 30% of blood volume, clinical signs of shock appear, and a corresponding amount is replaced. After replacement of lost blood, additional amounts of electrolyte solution should be given to replenish the extracellular fluid that earlier had been drawn into the vascular space to compensate for lost blood. Fluids in addition to these estimated losses are necessary if the vascular space has been abnormally enlarged in response to poor tissue perfusion. Even a "normal" blood volume is inadequate to fill this enormous vascular space, and additional electrolyte solution is necessary to maintain adequate central venous pressure and venous return to the heart. During the recovery phase of shock, fluid in excess of the "normal" blood volume is excreted by diuresis.

Attention should next be directed to the acid-base balance of the patient. Of course, if the patient has been well ventilated and well perfused through resuscitation, the acid-base situation should take care of itself. However, in periods of severe and prolonged shock it may be necessary to administer bicarbonate or perhaps tromethamine (THAM) to help overcome some of the problems of acidosis. After adequate volume expansion has occurred as assessed by Swan-Ganz or central venous pressure measurements, it may become necessary to administer various inotropic agents to achieve an acceptable blood flow or blood pressure. The first drug in the line of importance is dopamine HCl. When it is given in a dose of 2 to 5 μg./kg./min., renal blood flow and splenic blood flow is enhanced, whereas there is little change in cardiac output or blood pressure. At doses of 5 to 10 μg./kg./min. cardiac output increases, with some elevation in peripheral vascular resistance. At higher doses (greater than 10 μg./kg./min.) the affects become very similar to epinephrine, with severe peripheral vasoconstriction. Another drug that can be used with properties similar to dopamine HCl is dobutamine HCl. This drug increases cardiac contractility without dramatically increasing myocardial oxygen demands. The dose of this drug initially is 2.5 μg./kg./min. At high doses in excess of 15 μg./kg./min. tachycardia and severe vasodilatation may become a problem. Some physicians believe that epinephrine is the optimal drug for cardiac inotropic enhancement. However, the problems with peripheral constriction and dangerous arrhythmias are more common. If the unusual situation of bradycardia exists, atropine sulfate 1 mg. is the initial treatment. If the problem persists, the patient might be treated with isoproterenol at a dosage of 1 to 2 μg./kg./min. If the patient still demonstrates signs of excessive vasoconstriction after all therapeutic modalities have been attempted, vasodilators may be tried. Vasodilators should be used with great caution, since prompt vasodilatation may aggravate the clinical setting of shock. The drug of choice at the present time is sodium nitroprusside in the dosage of 0.5 to 3 μg./kg./min., and one should carefully adjust it on a continuous intravenous infusion pump.

Intravascular coagulation occurs in severe stages of shock because of stagnation of excessively viscid and acid blood within capillaries, to which is frequently added hypercoagulability associated with trauma, red cell hemolysis, and bacterial toxins. This tendency is reduced when the blood volume is expanded, the flow rates through capillaries and veins are increased, and the blood viscosity is reduced. Acidosis is corrected by administration of bicarbonate, tromethamine (THAM), or lactated Ringer's solution.

Septic shock is treated by replacement of body fluids that have sequestered in areas of cellulitis or peritonitis, if present. There is no drug to counteract the bacterial toxins, other than bactericidal antibiotics to remove the source of the toxins. Blood cultures are obtained, and broad-spectrum antibiotics are administered. It may be necessary to change these when the bacterial sensitivities are determined. Obviously, surgical drainage or removal of the septic source is of paramount concern, if feasible. Body temperature should be monitored carefully in septic shock, with cooling blankets often being necessary to reduce dangerous hyperthermia. The role of corticosteroids in septic shock is still debated, but probably should be considered after all the preceding derangements have been corrected. It is believed that steroids stabilize lysosomal membranes, improve microvascular flow, and decrease histamine release.

Steroids should be administered early, either methylprednisolone 30 mg./kg. per 12 hours or dexamethasone 3 mg./kg. per 12 hours.

In recent years attention has been directed to the beta endorphins. These endogenous opiates are produced by the pituitary and are increased in shock states. It is known that opiates may produce hypotension by virtue of expanding the venous capacitive system, and therefore the increase in beta endorphins may aggravate the shock state. It is believed that the administration of naloxone, an opiate blocking agent, might reverse the hypertensive effects of the beta endorphins.

MONITORS AND GUIDEPOSTS TO ADEQUATE TREATMENT

The *general appearance* of the patient is important in judging how appropriate and adequate shock treatment has been. The mental status of the patient offers a crude indication of cerebral perfusion, with the goal being an alert and communicative patient. The skin and mucous membranes should be pink and warm, and the skin should be dry and of a normal temperature. Capillary refill should be prompt, as evaluated by the speed with which the color returns to the nail beds after compression.

The *vital signs* (pulse, arterial blood pressure, and respiratory rate) are monitored frequently and preferably by the same techniques. A return toward normal of all these parameters indicates a favorable response to treatment. A stable patient should have normal vital signs: pulse rate less than 120/min., respirations less than 28/min., and systolic blood pressure greater than 90 mm. hg.

Urinary output is one of the most valuable monitors of shock treatment. Hourly measurements of urinary output are especially valuable in determination of the rate of fluid replacement. This monitor is important enough to justify passing a urethral catheter into each patient who is seriously shocked. Hourly urine output should be as follows:

10 ml./hour in an infant or child (1½ ml./kg./hr.)
30 ml./hour in a normal adult
20 ml./hour in the elderly

The urine specific gravity and pH are measured on each of the hourly specimens.

Venous pressure determinations are a useful guide to the rate of fluid volume replacement in shock. One can make a crude estimate of venous pressure by observing the filling of the neck and extremity veins at various elevations from the heart. Far more accurate than this is the central venous pressure (CVP), which is measured with a catheter in the superior or inferior vena cava, where no valve dampens the pressure between the end of the catheter and the heart. Normal central venous pressure varies from 5 to 15 cm. of water. It is elevated by positive pressure respiration and the Valsalva maneuver. Most patients in shock initially have a low central venous pressure, which rises to normal with adequate replacement of fluid volumes. High central pressure may indicate right heart failure, pulmonary venous obstruction (massive pulmonary embolus), left-side heart failure, pericardial tamponade, or excess fluid and blood administration. The correct cause must be determined and appropriate efforts made to bring the venous pressure back to normal. The central venous pressure is not infallible, and foolish reliance cannot be placed on it. Far more important than the absolute measurements obtained is the trend observed while therapy is administered (as a depleted fluid volume is expanded, the CVP should rise.) If the catheter migrates or becomes misplaced, or the end comes to lie against the vein wall, the recorded pressure is misleading. This is especially likely when massive amounts of blood have been given through the catheter, requiring checks of position and placement periodically.

Left atrial pressure measures preload, which in turn dependably reflects left ventricular filling (LVEDP), a vital factor in the response to shock. Measuring left atrial pressure is difficult to perform directly; however, pressure recorded from a flow-directed balloon catheter (Swan-Ganz) that is wedged in the pulmonary capillary bed correlates directly with simultaneously measured left atrial pressure, except when ventilation is being supported with high positive end-expiratory pressure

(PEEP). Many of these catheters also have a thermistor, which allows cardiac output to be estimated by the thermodilution technique. Therefore the percutaneously introduced Swan-Ganz catheter may be a valuable aid in the resuscitation and management of a patient in shock.

Arterial blood gas studies are helpful to determine the degree of acidosis and the efficiency of respiration. A low blood pH in a severely shocked patient justifies treatment with a buffer solution such as sodium bicarbonate. High P_{CO_2} or low P_{O_2} indicate that respiratory assistance is needed.

Serum electrolyte determinations often help one in the choice of repair solutions, especially when the shock results from major body fluid losses (Chapter 3).

Serial hematocrits are useful if the shock results from blood or body fluid loss. The hematocrit is normal immediately after blood loss and gradually decreases as extracellular fluid is drawn into the vascular space to replenish circulatory volume. The hematocrit of the bank blood is 35% to 37%, and with massive blood replacement the patient's hematocrit is limited to this level. Conversely, the hematocrit rises with plasma loss and falls back toward normal when extracellular fluid is drawn into the vascular tree or is administered in therapy.

All the preceding parameters are useful in allowing judgement of the degree of shock and the response to treatment. None of them is used alone, and total patient evaluation is most important in the evaluation of the response to therapy. *Restoring adequate tissue perfusion assures successful therapy.*

6
Surgical Infection

Merril T. Dayton

Serious infections remain an important cause of complications threatening surgical patients despite advances made in the understanding of preoperative nutrition, the development of more potent and broader spectrum antibiotics and improvements in surgical technique. In addition to being life threatening on occasion, surgical infections cause significant morbidity, result in enormous increases in hospital costs, which total billions of dollars per year, and cause a significant increase in the work load on surgical services. The pattern of complicating infections has changed in the last two decades from one dominated by gram-positive cocci to one of nosocomial infections that are gram-negative bacilli over half the time; nevertheless the attendant morbidity, mortality, and financial impact of serious infection has not changed and remain a formidable problem for the surgeon.

DEFINITION

Any definition of the term "surgical infection" must stress the unique relationship between a given infection and the primary etiological or therapeutic role of an operative procedure with regard to its outcome. "Medical infections" generally are associated with a single type of bacteria, have minimal local tissue reaction, manifest with constitutional symptoms, and, by definition, can usually be successfully treated with antibiotics alone. On the other hand, "surgical infections" are those that are either the direct result of an operative procedure (complication) or those that can be successfully treated only by surgical intervention. They are usually polymicrobial, are associated with a significant local tissue reaction such as erythema, fluctuation, and point tenderness, will not respond to antibiotics alone, and eventually require either incision and drainage or excision for resolution. Common examples are abscesses, necrotizing fasciitis, cholangitis, wound infections, empyema, gas gangrene, and appendicitis.

HOST DEFENSE MECHANISMS

Man is surrounded by a multitude of potentially pathogenic bacteria, fungi, and viruses, which remain harmless because of a delicate immunological balance between the host and these potential pathogens. Any perturbation of this balance such as a breakdown of host defenses or an increase in pathogen inoculum results in a potentially serious infection.

Because of their invasive nature, operative procedures often interrupt these defense barriers (skin, bowel wall, peritoneum) and render the host more liable to infection. Reports from the Communicable Disease Center underscore this liability to infection by demonstrating the highest infection rates among hospitalized patients on surgical services. Paradoxically, while operations sometimes predispose the patient to infection, in other circumstances the patient may recover from a serious infection (abscess, gas gangrene, necrotizing fasciitis) only after aggressive surgical treatment.

One irony of modern medical progress is the further compromise of host defenses related to implementation of new apparatuses, surgical techniques, and mechanical equipment such as endotracheal tubes, Foley catheters, and vascular cannulas used in monitoring and treating such patients.

Successful defense of the host against microbial invasion thus depends on properly functioning immune mechanisms. Intact skin and mucous membranes play an invaluable role in protecting the host; the high infection rates in burn patients confirm the importance of this tough, reliable protective layer. Normal cellular and humoral function are imperative in preventing serious infections; the neutropenic or agammaglobulinemic patient is easy prey for microbes that ordinarily are not pathogenic.

Upon penetrating the host's first line of defense, the pathogen triggers a complex array of humoral and cellular defense mechanisms (Fig. 6-1). Commonly the invasion is associated with tissue injury, which stimulates an inflammatory vascular response mediated by the kinin system and other vasoactive substances. The result is increased capillary permeability, vascular dilatation, and increased capillary sphincter tone. Consequently,

plasma proteins ooze into the interstitium along with neutrophils and monocytes by diapedesis.

Two general mechanisms now play complimentary roles in the defense process. Humoral factors, including antibody-antigen aggregates, activate the complement system promoting chemotaxis, increased adherence, and anaphylactoid substances. This results in amplified phagocyte function and eventual bacterial cell wall lysis. Similarly, cellular factors make critical contributions after opsoninization leads to phagocyte attachment to the bacterium, followed by engulfment and subsequent intracellular digestion of the bacterium. Although both neutrophils and lymphocytes are capable of phagocytosis, the neutrophil plays the most important role in early defense against invading pathogens.

PATHOGENESIS OF INFECTION

Any imbalance of the host defense system whether from *overloading, intrinsic abnormalities,* or *host defense interference* results in infection.

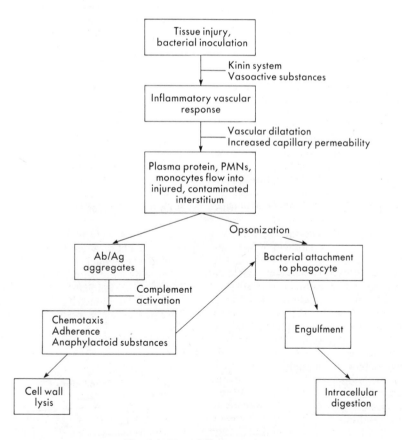

Fig. 6-1. Host defense system.

Table 6-1 Factors increasing incidence of surgical infections

Factors	X-fold increase in infection
Host intrinsic factors	
1. Malnutrition	3
2. Alcoholism	
3. Steroids	2
4. Diabetes	2
5. Poor tissue perfusion	
6. Anemia	
7. Obesity	2
8. Chronic renal failure	
9. Malignancy	
10. Immune suppression	
11. Hypoproteinemia	
12. Infection at nonrelated site	3
13. Age over 60 years	3
Local wound factors	
1. Contaminated wound	6
2. Foreign body	
3. Devitalized or necrotic tissue	
4. Preoperative hospitalization	4
5. Excessively tight sutures	
6. Emergency operation	3
7. Excessively long operation (over 3 hours)	2
8. Hematoma, seroma	
9. Electrocautery	2
10. Penrose drain use	2

In addition, the type of bacteria invading the host plays a role in whether an infection develops; some types inhibit phagocytosis because of cell surface structures, others produce potent exotoxins, and still others are toxic because of surface components.

Overloading occurs when the inoculum is large or continued; unresolved contamination simply overwhelms the host's defense capabilities. Intrinsic abnormalities relate to systemic conditions that suppress the humoral and cellular limbs of host defense. Examples include malnutrition, alcoholism, steroid administration, diabetes, poor tissue perfusion, anemia, obesity, chronic renal failure, malignancy, immune suppression, and hypoproteinemia. Host defense interference is usually caused by local factors in surgical patients. Devitalized or necrotic tissue, foreign bodies, excessively tight sutures interfering with blood supply, dead space with hematoma or seroma, and rough tissue handling resulting in injury are all known deterents of wound healing. Large clinical studies have clearly shown the correlation between the factors aforementioned and an increased risk of wound or surgical infection (Table 6-1).

INFECTION PREVENTION

Without question the most effective, least expensive, and most desirable method of dealing with infection is to prevent it from ever occurring. Systemic conditions that suppress normal host defense should be dealt with preoperatively. Malnourished patients should be appropriately alimented before surgery, steroid use should be minimized if possible, diabetes should be carefully controlled, anemia should be corrected, and weight loss for obese patients is highly desirable.

Bacterial contamination intraoperatively can be minimized by a careful antiseptic preparation of both the patient and surgical team members. Breaks in technique (e.g., glove tears) should immediately be rectified, devitalized tissue should be debrided, all foreign bodies should be removed or kept to a minimum (e.g., suture), and any time a contaminated organ is entered or transected, the remainder of the field should be carefully excluded. Careful hemostasis and wound closure without tension are of paramount importance in successful wound healing without infection. Other important factors include minimizing the length of the operative procedure and limiting the length of the preoperative and postoperative "in-hospital" stay.

Prophylactic antibiotics are another important weapon in the armamentarium of infection prevention. Whereas multiple studies have clearly demonstrated the efficacy of prophylactic antibiotics in high-risk surgical patients, other studies have shown that prophylaxis regimens need not be prolonged or expensive to be effective. Similarly, little benefit is derived when prophylactic antibiotics are used in low-risk patients; on the contrary, improper use results in increased patient cost, the development of drug-resistant bacteria, and serious complications such as pseudomembranous colitis. Determinants of surgical patients with high risk of wound infection have been previously described and surgical procedures have been classified according to degree of bacterial contamination, as follows:

1. Clean
   a. No hollow viscus entered
   b. Primary wound closure
   c. Elective procedure
   d. No breaks in septic technique
   e. No inflammation
   f. Infection incidence 2%

2. Clean-contaminated
   a. Hollow viscus entered but controlled
   b. Primary wound closure
   c. Mechanical drain used
   d. Minor break in aseptic technique
   e. No obvious inflammation
   f. Infection incidence 10%
3. Contaminated
   a. Uncontrolled spillage from hollow viscus
   b. Open, traumatic wound
   c. Major break in aseptic technique
   d. Inflammation apparent
   e. Infection incidence 20%
4. Dirty
   a. Uncontrolled, untreated spillage from hollow viscus
   b. Open, suppurative wound
   c. Pus present in operative field
   d. Severe inflammation, patient toxic
   e. Infection incidence 50%

The procedures requiring prophylactic antibiotics are as follows:

High infection rate or high risk
   Colon and rectum surgery
   Vaginal hysterectomy
   Vascular procedures involving prostheses
   Biliary procedures at risk (acute cholecystitis, cholangitis, common duct obstruction)
   Procedures for gastric obstruction, bleeding, cancer, or ulcer with achlorhydria
   Appendectomy (nonincidental)
   Major head and neck resections
   Urethra and bladder surgery in females
   Noncardiac thoracic surgery (lung and esophageal resections)
   Open-heart procedures

Presence of indwelling prosthesis
   Cardiac valve
   Arterial graft
   Artificial joint
   Ophthalmological implant
   Ventricular shunt
   Synthetic mesh

In summary, proper prophylaxis therapy is short term, inexpensive, properly timed (i.e., must be started before the incision is made), and used only in high-risk patients.

DIAGNOSIS OF SURGICAL INFECTIONS

Physical examination remains the most effective modality in diagnosing surgical infection. The majority of the latter are associated with local erythema, fluctuation, crepitus, calor, induration, or point tenderness. Radiological procedures may be helpful in the diagnosis of intra-abdominal infections; flat plate and upright films of the abdomen may show an elevated hemidiaphragm (subphrenic abscess), a soap-bubble pattern (lesser sac ab-

scess), obliterated psoas margin (appendiceal abscess), pneumoperitoneum (perforated ulcer), and air-fluid levels outside the bowel lumen (abscess secondary to gas-forming organism). Soft tissue roentgenograms often show subcutaneous air associated with clostridial infection. Ultrasound is particularly helpful in identification of large fluid collections or cystic spaces; it is limited when there is excessive bowel gas. Computed tomography scanning also helps identify pancreatic and other abdominal fluid collections even in the face of significant bowel gas. Labeled-leukocyte scans are becoming increasingly helpful in identification of occult infection and are replacing gallium scans for that specific indication.

GENERAL PRINCIPLES IN TREATING SURGICAL INFECTIONS

Incision and drainage are indicated in virtually all abscesses wherever encountered in the body (exceptions include amebic liver abscesses and lung abscesses). Because of altered local blood supply, inadequate antibiotic levels, closed spaces under pressure, and overwhelming inoculum, conservative therapy is normally doomed to failure. Adequate surgical therapy involves widely opening the abscess cavity, draining its contents, breaking up loculations, and leaving a drainage tube.

Excision of the diseased organ or source of infection is often definitive therapy and no further treatment including drainage or antibiotics may be necessary. Not infrequently antibiotics and excision are used concomitantly to provide optimal therapy.

Débridement is an important principle of surgical infection that is used when necrotic tissues are present or a virulent, advancing fasciitis or myositis threatens the patient's life.

Diversion of the fecal stream is often helpful in treatment of bowel perforation, fistulas, and severe perianal infections.

For small localized abscesses without attendant septicemia, incision and drainage may be all that is required for adequate treatment of the condition. However, when there is a large abscess with adjacent organs involved, bacteremia and obvious systemic manifestations such as hypotension, tachycardia, high fever, decreased urine output, and respiratory deterioration, antibiotics become a crucial ally of surgical therapy for optimal patient management. Selection of the appropriate antibiotic should initially be made after Gram stain of the pyogenous drainage or after detection of the diseased organ responsible for the contamination; further modification of the antibiotic regimen can be made after carefully collected aerobic and anaerobic speci-

Table 6-2. Preferred antibiotics for serious surgical infections

Organism	First choice	Second choice
Streptococcus viridans	Penicillin G	Cephalosporin
Streptococcus pyogenes	Penicillin G	Cephalosporin
Streptococcus sp., group B	Penicillin G	Cephalosporin
Streptococcus as enterococcus form	Ampicillin	Penicillin G or vancomycin
Staphylococcus aureus		
penicillinase (−)	Penicillin G	Cephalosporin
penicillinase (+)	Oxacillin, nafcillin	Cephalosporin
Peptostreptococcus	Penicillin G	Clindamycin
Streptococcus pneumoniae	Penicillin G	Erythromycin
Clostridium perfringens	Penicillin G	Chloramphenicol
Clostridium tetani	Penicillin G	Tetracycline
Clostridium difficile	Vancomycin	Metronidazole
Bacteroides, oral strains	Penicillin G	Clindamycin
Bacteroides, GI strains	Metronidazole	Clindamycin
Enterobacter	Gentamicin or tobramycin	Amikacin
Escherichia coli	Gentamicin or tobramycin	Amikacin, ampicillin
Klebsiella	Gentamicin or tobramycin	Amikacin
Proteus mirabilis	Ampicillin	Gentamicin
Proteus indole (+)	Gentamicin or tobramycin	Amikacin
Serratia	Gentamicin or amikacin	Cefotaxime
Pseudomonas aeruginosa	Gentamicin or tobramycin and carbenicillin or ticarcillin	Amikacin and carbenicillin
Providencia	Amikacin	Cefotaxime
Candida	Amphotericin B	—

mens are cultured and organism sensitivity to the various antibiotics is determined (Table 6-2).

SPECIFIC SURGICAL INFECTIONS
Cellulitis

Cellulitis is a nonsuppurative infection of soft tissue, which is often the earliest host response to bacterial invasion. Pathophysiologically it is characterized by bacterial invasion and multiplication with concomitant capillary dilatation, leukocyte infiltration, and increased capillary permeability and edema of the dermal and subcutaneous layers. It manifests clinically as a diffuse erythema that is palpably warm and often tender. There is usually a trauma or wound site, which is the portal of entry, and the patient often has a fever. Frank abscess rarely occurs, and the disease is mentioned here primarily because it may be confused with the true surgical infections that have attendant inflammation. It is most commonly caused by streptococci and should be treated by large doses of penicillin given intravenously, warm soaks, elevation, and immobilization of the involved area, if possible.

Lymphangitis

A previously established infection serves as a nidus for the disease process called lymphangitis, which results when bacterial invasion occurs into the lymphatic system draining a local infection. Clinically, one sees a tender, edematous extremity with linear erythematous streaks in the distribution of the lymphatic channels leading to the regional lymph nodes. In the prepenicillin era this condition was known as "blood poisoning" and was a harbinger of serious complications related to the infection. Treatment is identical to that for cellulitis because streptococcus is usually the offending organism.

Furuncle/carbuncle

In contrast to the spreading, diffuse nature of streptococcal infections, staphylococcal infections are usually localized and indurated and have a central cellulitic area that necroses and forms a cutaneous abscess. Furuncle is an example of a staphylococcal infection that starts most commonly when a sebaceous gland at the base of a hair follicle becomes obstructed and the normally colonized follicle develops a localized abscess. This may then enlarge, extend into subcutaneous tissues, and even rupture spontaneously. Clinically the patient will complain of a local, raised lesion that is tender, fluctuant, and inflamed. A carbuncle is a necrotizing infection of dermis and subcutaneous tissues originating as a cluster of furuncles. As the lesion progresses, multiple pus-draining sinuses develop, central suppuration occurs, and occasionally existing skin bridges slough. Treatment of an uncomplicated furuncle is incision and drainage; for more advanced furuncles with surrounding inflammation or multiple lesions, antibiotics with incision and drainage are required. The procedure involves opening the lesion widely, evacuating pus, breaking up loculations, and either packing the wound open or "saucerizing" it (removing a superficial ellipse of skin) to prevent superficial wound closure before deep tissues have healed. Treatment of carbuncles involves appropriate antibiotics given intravenously and aggressive surgical therapy consisting of incision, drainage, and even excision of sinus tracts on occasion. A penicillinase-resistant agent such as oxacillin or nafcillin should be used to treat this family of infections.

Postoperative wound infections

Postoperative wound infections occur in 3% to 10% of patients undergoing operative procedures. Their development is the result of a complex interaction between (1) surgical technique and wound care, (2) bacterial contamination during surgery, and (3) the relative efficacy of the host's immune system. Risk factors and high-risk patients for developing postoperative wound infections were previously discussed in this chapter. Importantly the two most common sources of bacterial contamination are the patient's skin and any colonized hollow organ of the patient entered during the operation (e.g., colon, trachea, gallbladder). Exogenous sources such as operating team members and operation room environment play a minor etiological role in postoperative infections. The most common pathogens isolated from postoperative wound infections remain *Staphylococcus aureus* and gram-negative rods. With the exception of *Clostridium* and β-hemolytic streptococcus wound infections, which may manifest within 24 hours postoperatively, the majority become evident some 5 to 7 days postoperatively. The clinical picture is one of low-grade fever, wound pain, erythema, local edema, and drainage. Treatment consists in widely opening the wound by removal of skin stitches or clips, evacuating pyogenous material, appropriately debriding, and loosely packing the wound open to heal by secondary intention. Antibiotics usually are not required but may be added if systemic symptoms are present.

Tetanus

Tetanus is a disease that manifests primarily with neurological symptoms directly related to a potent bacterial exotoxin called tetanospasmin. The etiological agent (*Clostridium tetani*) is a gram-positive, anaerobic, spore-forming rod, which is usually introduced into the injured area as a spore. Under conditions of warmth and low tissue-oxygen tension, the spores convert to the vegetative form, which produces the toxin. Wounds that are predisposed to develop tetanus include deep stab injuries, injuries with massive tissue necrosis, and farm injuries. The incubation period is 3 to 21 days, and when symptoms occur, they do so in one of three ways: (1) generalized tetanus with trismus, local spasm, lethargy, irritability, dysphagia, abdominal cramps, and laryngeal spasm; (2) local tetanus with persistent muscle rigidity near the injury site; and (3) cephalic tetanus, a rare condition characterized by involvement of cranial nerves. The most common form is generalized tetanus, which has a mortality of 50%.

The most important principle in treating tetanus is prevention by appropriate wound care and primary immunization. The latter consists of three sequential doses of tetanus toxoid followed by a booster dose 1 year after the third dose. Further booster doses should be repeated every 10 years. Wound care involves copious irrigation and aggressive débridement of skin injuries, usually with the skin being left open to heal by secondary intention. Determining adequate immunization in the recently injured patient may be difficult; treatment guidelines are indicated in Table 6-3. When the diagnosis of tetanus is made, treatment should include aggressive débridement of the surgical wound, high doses of intravenously administered penicillin, intramuscular doses of human tetanus immune globulin, and supportive care including sedation and use of paralytic agents. With the latter, endotracheal intubation and ventilatory support are necessary.

Clostridial infections

Clostridial organisms cause a wide spectrum of disease ranging from simple contamination to an aggressive, invasive myonecrosis. *Clostridium perfringens* is causal in 80% of cases. The organism is a gram-positive rod that requires a low redox potential and anaerobiosis for optimal growth. Trauma, ischemia, foreign body, or pyogenic infection cause conversion of spores to the vegetative forms, which produce the toxin responsible for the clinical manifestations. The toxins include fibrinolysin, lecithinase, collagenase, and hyaluronidase. Although not common, different diseases in the spectrum must be differentiated because their treatments are vastly different. Examples are clostridial cellulitis and clostridial myonecrosis.

Clostridial cellulitis is usually initiated by a puncture wound of an extremity. The first symptom

Table 6-3. Guidelines for tetanus prophylaxis in injured patients

| | Previously immunized | | | | Not previously immunized | |
| | Immunized more than 10 years ago | | Immunized less than 10 years ago | | | |
	Minor wound	Tetanus-prone wound	Minor wound	Tetanus-prone wound	Minor wound	Tetanus-prone wound
Wound	Wash, removal of foreign body	Débridement, Irrigation, Removal of foreign body	Wash, removal of foreign body	Débridement, Irrigation, Removal of foreign body	Wash, removal of foreign body	Removal of foreign body, Aggressive débridement, Removal of devitalized tissue, Copious irrigation
Tetanus toxoid	0.5 ml. of tetanus toxoid intramuscularly	0.5 ml. of tetanus toxoid intramuscularly	If no booster within 5 years, tetanus toxoid	If no booster within 1 year, tetanus toxoid	Basic immunization starting with 0.5 ml. of tetanus toxoid intramuscularly	0.5 ml. of tetanus toxoid intramuscularly; then continue immunization
Human tetanus immune globulin	No	250 units of tetanus immune globulin intramuscularly, contralateral side	No	No	No	250 units of tetanus immune globulin intramuscularly, contralateral side
Antibiotics	No	Penicillin intravenously	No	No	No	High dose of penicillin intravenously

occurs after 3 or 4 days and is usually pain. Thereafter, multiple blebs occur extruding foul-smelling, reddish brown fluid; frank necrosis of the skin and subcutaneous tissue then completes the cycle. The dissection develops immediately above the deep fascial planes and is often associated with skin discoloration. Crepitus is always a prominent feature, with gas being both extensive and easily demonstrable; muscle is not involved, however. The patient usually has few constitutional symptoms, a finding that helps distinguish this form from myonecrosis. Gram stain of aspirated, watery pus usually confirms the diagnosis. Therapy involves radical incision, drainage, débridement, high-dose intravenously administered penicillin, and wound packing. Later skin grafting may be necessary.

Clostridial myonecrosis or "gas gangrene" is the most severe form of clostridial infection and usually occurs after extensive lacerations or muscle devitalization, ischemia, gross soil contamination, or delayed wound treatment. Incubation is usually 3 days, and the disease onset is acute, with the initial symptoms being a sense of increasing weight and deep pain. Progression of the disease is rapid, and the patient becomes pale, diaphoretic, and often delirious. Tachycardia and hypotension follow and shock may develop at any point in the course. The wound has a profuse serosanguineous discharge that has a sweet, musky odor initially; overlying skin is white, shiny, and tense. Gas bubbles may be seen at the wound entrance, and exposed muscle is edematous and noncontractile; crepitus is often noticed when the disease is advanced. A Gram stain of the drainage confirms the diagnosis though the clinical picture is strongly suggestive. Roentgenograms also demonstrate subcutaneous air. Treatment includes radical débridement of nonviable muscle and opening of fascial compartments; if the disease is extensive and far advanced, amputation of the extremity may become necessary. Ancillary treatment includes high-dose intravenously administered penicillin and hyperbaric oxygenation; although the method is somewhat controversial, some also advocate the administration of clostridial antitoxins. Inadequately treated, clostridial myonecrosis invariably has a lethal outcome. Overall mortality is 20%.

Necrotizing fasciitis

Necrotizing fasciitis is one of the most common of the serious surgical infections. It may complicate either traumatic or surgical wounds, especially when an abdominal hollow viscus has been opened. The condition is a mixed infection caused by a synergistic combination of aerobic gram-negative rods and anaerobes plus microaerophilic streptococci or hemolytic staphylococci. The disease is a rapidly invasive infection of superficial fascia with associated thrombosis of penetrating vessels from the deep system to the skin. The latter results in skin necrosis along with impressive fascial dissection (Fig. 6-2).

Clinically one sees lymphedema extending in all directions associated with mottled, reddish purple skin. As the disease progresses, blebs filled with serosanguineous fluid form followed by skin necrosis in 30% of cases. The fascia is a grayish, nonviable color ("dishwater appearance") and easily separates from the subcutaneous layer without pain. The patient is most frequently profoundly toxic with fever, hypotension, tachycardia, tachypnea, and mental confusion. Aggressive fluid resuscitation is necessary before the patient is taken to the operating room; hypocalcemia and anemia may also occur and mandate correction before anesthetic induction.

Treatment involves radical excision of all nonviable fascia and skin back to healthy tissue. Where necrotic fascia undermines viable skin, long parallel incision may be made with removal of all nonliving fascia and preservation of overlying skin. Antibiotics are supplementary and should include an aminoglycoside and penicillin initially with appropriate adjustments made after culture and sensitivity tests are completed.

Serious streptococcal infections

Streptococcal hemolytic gangrene (necrotizing cellulitis) is produced by hemolytic streptococci usually after a minor skin wound. Clinically the patient develops a low-grade temperature along with edema, warmth, erythema, and pain in the skin region involved. Over a 2- to 3-day period, even with antibiotics, the skin becomes dusky and forms large, dark, serous blebs; in contrast to clostridial infections, the fluid in the blebs has no odor. The last stage in the disease is cutaneous necrosis and gangrene (Fig. 6-3). Treatment includes emergency incision and drainage beyond involved tissue longitudinally and deep to underlying fascia; undermining skin flaps is usually not necessary. The incision releases skin tension, prevents ischemia, and allows wound packing, elevation, and débridement of necrotic skin.

Streptococcal myositis is caused by anaerobic streptococci and is characterized as a massive infection of muscles with skin discoloration, edema, local pain, crepitation of muscle and generalized toxemia. In contrast with clostridial myositis, cutaneous erythema is more pronounced, involved muscle while edematous is still alive and contractile, the odor is distinctly different from that of *Clostridium*, and Gram stain shows no gram-positive bacilli. Management consists in inci-

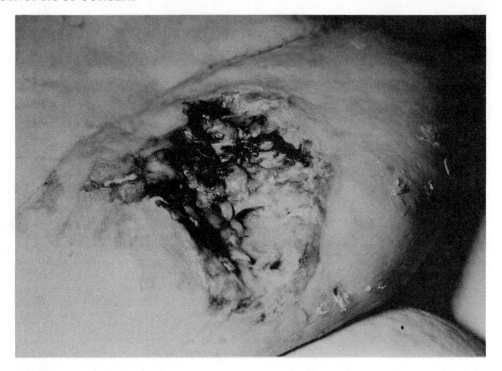

Fig. 6-2. Postoperative necrotizing fasciitis with obvious skin necrosis, mottling, and fascial dissection.

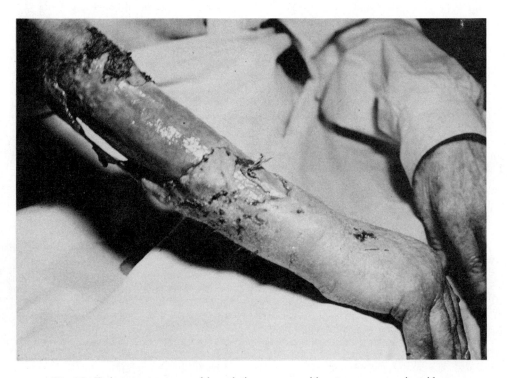

Fig. 6-3. End-stage streptococcal hemolytic gangrene with cutaneous necrosis evident.

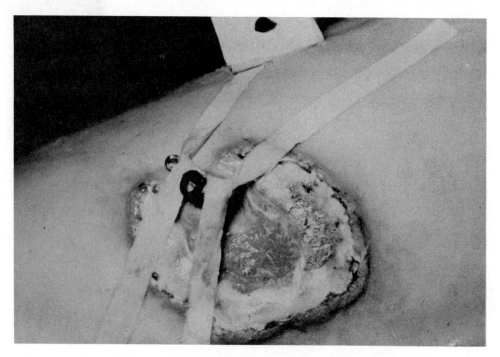

Fig. 6-4. Progressive bacterial synergistic gangrene with three characteristic zones: peripheral erythema, purplish skin in the middle, and central necrosis.

sion, drainage, and occasionally excision of necrotic muscle.

Progressive bacterial synergistic gangrene

Also known as Meleney's synergistic gangrene, this infection develops 2 weeks after an operative or skin wound and is caused by a nonhemolytic streptococcus and a hemolytic staphylococcus. The wound has a characteristic appearance typified by three zones: (1) peripherally, a wide area of edema and erythema, (2) adjacent to a zone of purplish, painful skin, and (3) a central zone of necrosis and ulceration (Fig. 6-4). Low-grade fever, anemia, and weakness are occasionally present; systemic manifestations may occur early and should be treated with fluids and intravenously administered antibiotics. Definitive treatment, however, is radical excision of all nonviable layers extending well into viable tissue. Skin grafting may become necessary later.

Nonclostridial gangrene

Gangrenous lesions with associated subcutaneous gas are usually classified as clostridial in origin. However, a host of gram-negative organisms can produce gas with extensive soft-tissue dissection; these are probably more common and less severe than "gas gangrene" from clostridial organisms. *Escherichia coli,* anaerobic streptococci, *Bacteroides* species, and *Enterobacter* species have all been associated with this infection. Commonly the infection occurs after wet gangrene of an extremity develops; crepitus is then detected on physical examination or roentgenogram. A lack of systemic toxicity with extensive air dissection is suggestive of the diagnosis. Therapy involves débridement and local wound care; the extensive gas dissection can generally be ignored.

Fungal infection

Actinomycosis is caused by a gram-positive fungus that branches into filamentous structures; it is anaerobic and is often part of the normal oral flora. Three major clinical types of the disease are described: cervicofacial (which is the most common), thoracic, and abdominal. It is characterized by firm, nodular granulomas that break down, suppurate, and discharge pus through multiple

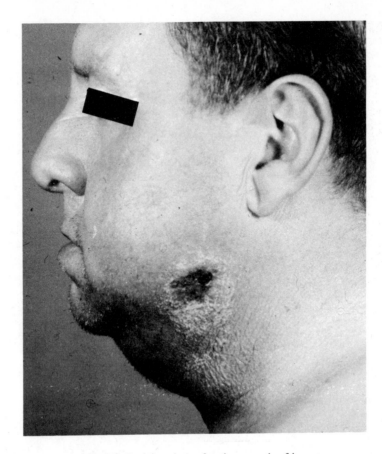

Fig. 6-5. Draining sinus of actinomycosis of jaw.

sinuses (Fig. 6-5). Gram stain reveals "sulfur granules" that are aggregates of mycelia. Long-term treatment with penicillin is necessary as well as occasional excision of the sinus tracts.

Nocardiosis is caused by *Nocardia*, a gram-positive aerobic fungus that has become an important complication of immune suppression or immunodeficiency. It presents as a chronic, suppurating, draining sinus tract similar to actinomycosis. It may also extensively involve the central nervous system or respiratory system and present with systemic manifestation of low-grade fever, lethargy, weakness, weight loss, and irritating cough. Primary treatment involves administering sulfonamides, but surgical therapy in the form of sinus tract excision and abscess drainage may be necessary.

7
Surgical Nutrition

Nathaniel J. Soper
Robert T. Soper

A well-balanced diet has long been recognized as necessary for good health. However, the fact that disease states, trauma, and operations increase nutritional requirements has been appreciated and documented only during the past half century. Further, the materials and delivery systems that have allowed these increased demands to be met in patients who, for one reason or another, are unable to eat ordinary diets have evolved only during the past 2 or 3 decades. The purpose of this chapter is to review current concepts of basic nutritional requirements, the manner in which they are affected by disease and operations, and different techniques by which these increased nutritional demands may be met.

BASIC METABOLIC CONSIDERATIONS
Energy requirements

Carbohydrate and protein (4 kcal./gm. each) and fat (9 kcal./gm.) supply dietary energy. The daily energy requirements can be calculated when the energy requirements for activity are added to those demands required for basal metabolic purposes. Basal energy demand varies with size and age. Thus an infant requires approximately 100 kcal./kg./24 hours to meet the enormous metabolic demands for growth and development, whereas a young adult male needs only 20 to 30 kcal./kg./24 hours to meet his basal energy requirements. Generally, 1 ml. of fluid is required for each calorie of energy that is expended. Fig. 7-1 graphically portrays a simple method of estimating maintenance body fluid and calorie requirements, based on body weight. Many other formulas for calculating basal

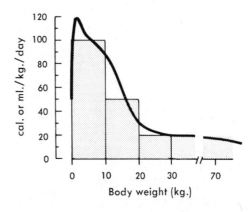

Fig. 7-1. Maintenance needs, caloric or fluid.

energy requirements are available, including the Harris-Benedict equation, which is presented later in this chapter.

Energy requirements are increased by a number of factors, including the following: (1) fever (7% per 1° F); (2) major long bone fractures, (3) severe burn injures, (4) body growth and development, (5) healing of wounds, (6) pregnancy, (7) hyperthyroidism, and (8) physical activity.

Protein requirements

Protein needs must be considered separately from caloric requirements. Protein cannot be stored except in functional tissue, as somatic and visceral protein. Normal daily protein requirements vary from 2 gm./kg. in infants to 40 to 60 gm. in adults. If inadequate calories are supplied, structural proteins will be "cannibalized" to produce energy, a process termed *gluconeogenesis*. This accelerated protein breakdown is reflected by increased urinary nitrogen excretion. Stressed or injured patients should receive twice the normal daily protein requirements. Such severe injuries as major thermal burns may increase the protein requirements to 300 gm./24 hours.

An important characteristic of the supplied diet is the calorie-to-nitrogen ratio. Energy is required to incorporate protein into tissue protoplasm. Dietary protein will be converted to glucose and used for energy rather than to form structural proteins if less than 150 nonprotein calories are supplied per gram of nitrogen. Depletion of body protein in surgical patients results in impaired wound and anastomotic healing, increased infection rate, anemia, edema, and weakness.

Carbohydrate and fat

These substances are the body's primary energy substrates. Certain tissues (brain, myocardium, erythrocytes, and phagocytes) require glucose as their principal energy source. Many of these tissues can, however, adapt during the course of starvation to use ketone bodies from the oxidation of fat. Thus, during the initial period of fasting, much protein will be catabolized to form glucose, whereas later the demand for gluconeogenesis decreases. The initial period of catabolism can be minimized by addition of as little as 100 gm. of carbohydrate per day to the patient's intake.

There are ample stores of energy in the body under normal circumstances in the form of body fat—100 to 150 kilocalories in an average adult. In sharp contrast, carbohydrate storage in the form of glycogen is minimal. Approximately 500 gm. (2,000 calories) of glycogen is available in liver and muscle, but it is quickly exhausted during stress.

A specific dietary requirement is that for essential fatty acids, so-called because they cannot be manufactured or stored in the body. For example, approximately 2% of the caloric intake must be linoleic acid to prevent deficiency states. Essential fatty acid deficiency may quickly become apparent in infants, but it is uncommon in adults; it can be prevented when intravenous fat emulsion (Intralipid or Liposyn) is supplied once or twice per week.

Requirements for vitamins, minerals, and trace elements

In order for the body to optimally utilize these nutrients, certain additives such as fat- and water-

Table 7-1. Metabolic response to stress in adults

Clinical status	Calorie requirements (kcal./kg./day)
Unstressed starvation	20
Basal metabolism	25-30
Elective surgery	35
Trauma	40
Severe infection	50
Major burns	50-70

soluble vitamins, minerals, and trace elements (zinc, copper, manganese, iodine, magnesium) are required. Commercial solutions of water-soluble vitamins and trace elements are available and should be routinely supplemented during prolonged nutritional therapy. Vitamin K (as indicated by clotting studies) and iron (given as intramuscular iron dextran or blood transfusion) may also be necessary during prolonged nutritional therapy.

Effects of stress and trauma

Stress and trauma activate the sympathoadrenal axis to release catecholamines, glucocorticoids, and glucagon. These hormones stimulate gluconeogenesis, glycogenolysis, and the release of free fatty acids, with the resulting hyperglycemia leading to the so-called "diabetes" of stress. This hypermetabolic pattern may greatly increase caloric requirements (Table 7-1).

Catecholamines trigger protein catabolism for gluconeogenesis, and explain why protein demands are so much greater during stress than with unstressed starvation. Great amounts of protein may be lost, particularly with coexistent trauma and infection. In excess of 30 gm. of urinary nitrogen may be excreted daily, which equates to the loss of 190 gm. of protein, or 1 kg. of wet muscle. Even when large quantities of protein and calories are provided, it may be difficult to reverse nitrogen-wasting. Therefore nutritional support should be instituted early after trauma and in adequate amounts to patients such as those with extensive burns, which are known to trigger a prolonged catabolic state.

Consequences of malnutrition

Recent studies have documented quite clearly why we need to be concerned about the nutritional status of our patients. These studies have shown that as many as 50% of hospitalized surgical patients suffer from protein-calorie malnutrition. In turn, malnutrition is associated with increased mortality and morbidity (primarily infectious), decreased healing rates, and depressed in vivo and in vitro parameters of immunity. Furthermore, optimal nutritional support has been shown to improve mortality and to lower the sepsis rate in surgical patients.

Measuring nutritional status

A thorough history and physical examination are the primary screening tests to determine which patient needs nutritional support. There are many clinically utilized tests by which nutritional status can be estimated, as follows: (1) anthropometrics (triceps skin fold, etc.), (2) biochemical tests (creatinine-height index, albumin, prealbumin, transferrin, nitrogen-balance determinations), and (3) tests of immune competence (total lymphocyte count, delayed hypersensitivity skin testing). The tests that we have found most useful to evaluate the adequacy of nutritional therapy are serial measurements of caloric intake and body weight, and frequent determinations of albumin/transferrin levels and nitrogen balance. Useful nutritional constants and equations follow:

Harris-Benedict equation to calculate basal energy expenditure (BEE):

BEE (men) = 66.47 + 13.75 × Weight (kg.) + 5.0 × Height (cm.) − 6.76 × Age
BEE (women) = 655.10 + 9.56 × Weight + 1.85 × Height − 4.68 × Age
BEE (infants) = 22.10 + 31.05 × Weight + 1.16 × Height

Nitrogen balance = [Administered protein (gm.) ÷ 6.25] − [Urinary urea nitrogen (UUN; 24-hour sample) + 3 gm. (stool losses, nonurea urinary nitrogen)]

Protein catabolized = UUN × 6.25
Muscle broken down = UUN × 30
(Muscle = 73% water, 23% protein)

DELIVERY OF NUTRITIONAL SUPPORT
Total parenteral nutrition

Total parenteral nutrition (TPN) is a technique whereby all the required proteins, calories, and essential minerals are delivered intravenously. TPN can be administered either into a small peripheral vein or into a large central vein. When given peripherally, the fluid can be only mildly hypertonic, thus requiring large volumes to satisfy nutritional needs; new venipunctures are required daily or more often. On the contrary, when infused centrally, the solution can be quite hypertonic, since it is delivered into a large vascular channel where blood flow is rapid. This dilutes the solution quickly to isotonic concentrations, before being disseminated throughout the body.

TPN is generally indicated for anyone who is unable to take enough nutrition by way of the gastrointestinal tract and who has no prospect for improvement for a predictable, but variable, time interval; 1 week of starvation is sufficient to render newborns malnourished, and 2 weeks of starvation will initiate the process in adults. TPN is especially indicated when there exist excessive caloric demands from illness or injury, as after major thermal injuries, in sepsis, or after multiple trauma.

TPN can provide the lengthy periods of gastrointestinal rest that is required by certain medical problems, such as prolonged diarrhea, disaccharidase deficiencies, protein-losing enteropathies, severe gastrointestinal allergies, or inflammatory bowel disease. However, the majority of diseases for which parenteral hyperalimentation is indicated fall within the surgical realm and include patients who have had massive bowel resection, prolonged or multiple intestinal obstructions, gastroenteric fistulas, prolonged paralytic ileus, or wound dehiscence, or who face lengthy and debilitating chemotherapy or x-ray therapy.

The TPN formula

Most hospitals stock a "standard" TPN solution, which consists of 25% dextrose, 3.5% to 4.5% amino acids, and appropriate electrolytes. This mixture results in a calorie-to-nitrogen ratio of 150:1 to 225:1. Water-soluble vitamins and trace elements are provided daily, and heparin may be added to each bottle to inhibit venous thrombosis. Emulsified fat solution should be administered twice weekly.

Meticulous attention to sterility must be maintained by the pharmacy when the TPN solutions are being made because the high glucose content is an excellent culture medium. The solutions should be prepared in a laminar airflow hood with appropriate quality-control precautions.

Special clinical situations may require one to alter the standard TPN formula. Patients who are in renal failure require a higher calorie-to-nitrogen ratio, either by the supplying of 35% dextrose or by exclusive delivery of essential amino acids (Nephramine solution). Carbon dioxide retention in patients with chronic lung disease may be lessened when an increased percentage of calories is supplied as fat, to lower the respiratory quotient. Recently there have been marketed branched–chain–enriched amino acid solutions, which are claimed to improve the clinical outcome in patients with hepatic failure or after major trauma.

The TPN delivery system

Because TPN formulas are hypertonic compared to serum, they must be delivered into a high-flow part of the vascular system for rapid dilution and to

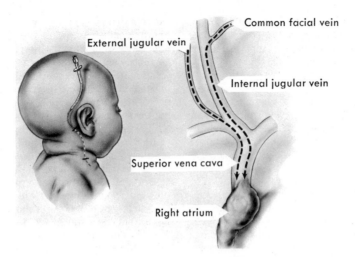

Fig. 7-2. Insertion of delivery-system catheter into external or internal jugular vein in infant.

minimize endothelial damage and thrombosis. The superior vena cava is admirably suited for this purpose. The inferior vena cava can be used, but the problems with sterility and immobilization of the catheter in the lower venous compartment make it less desirable.

In the school child and adult the catheter can be introduced percutaneously into the subclavian vein from just below the midpoint of the clavicle, the catheter being threaded easily into the superior vena cava. However, in the infant and younger child it is safer to insert the catheter by a surgical cutdown into either the external jugular vein or a branch of the internal jugular vein through which the tip is threaded into the superior vena cava (Fig. 7-2). The fact that the tip of the catheter has been accurately placed into the superior vena cava must be confirmed by fluoroscopy or x-ray examination, since malposition is common and dangerous.

For sterility purposes, it is best to separate the point where the catheter penetrates the skin as far as possible from the place where the catheter enters the vein. In the infant and young child the catheter can be tunneled subcutaneously to exit from the skin either over the flat portion of the mastoid bone behind the ear (Fig. 7-2) or alternatively it can be tunneled down the chest wall to exit at midsternum. The entire procedure is carried out in the operating room under strict aseptic technique.

We prefer an intravenous catheter that is constructed of Silastic (silicone rubber) that has been impregnated with silver to render the catheter radiopaque. Silastic is much softer than conventional plastic catheters. It is nonirritating and nonreactive and can lie in the venous system for years without provoking phlebitis. The catheter is anchored by a suture at the point where it penetrates the vein so as to discourage inadvertent removal. The Broviac and Hickman catheters have a Teflon felt cuff affixed to the subcutaneous part of the catheter, which has obviated the need for suture fixation at the point where the catheter exits from the skin. These catheters are commonly tunneled around the rib cage to exit over the midsternum. Granulation tissue "grows into" the Teflon felt cuff to anchor the catheters in place.

The entire system, including the intravenous tubing from the formula bottle to the Silastic catheter, is changed daily under aseptic conditions and must be maintained as a completely closed system. Under no circumstances should this venous line be violated for drawing blood, administering other intravenous fluids, or determining central venous pressure. A small sterile dressing (Op-site or Tagaderm) covers the Silastic catheter where it exits from the skin. This dressing is changed three times weekly by specially trained nurses. The skin is defatted with acetone and cleaned with an appropriate antiseptic, and povidone-iodine (Betadine) ointment is placed over the exit site.

The formula is usually administered at a constant hourly rate over each 24-hour period. A gravity drip will suffice if monitored closely by skilled personnel, but an infusion pump is generally preferable. Nurses especially trained in TPN techniques can teach catheter care and infusion techniques to either the patient or his family to allow the patient to be discharged home when lengthy periods of nutritional support are anticipated. Under these circumstances, it is often possible to limit the nutritional infusions to the nocturnal hours so as to allow the patient greater freedom and activity during the waking hours of the day. Some patients have been managed at home with TPN successfully for years provided that proper catheter care is maintained.

Special considerations of TPN

During the first few days of hyperosmolar intravenous feeding, amino acids and sugar are commonly lost in the urine to pose the threat of osmotic diuresis and dehydration. This threat is minimized by use of a half-strength TPN solution the first day, a three-fourths solution the second day, and then the full-strength TPN formula the third day. During this period of TPN initiation, frequent examinations of the urine for sugar may justify administration of exogenous insulin on a sliding scale to prevent serious hyperglycemia and glycosuria. After several days of parenteral hyperalimentation, endogenous insulin production increases so that blood and urine glucose levels are maintained within normal limits. By the same token, the hyperalimentation infusion must never be abruptly discontinued or hypoglycemia will ensue.

When TPN is first started, the body weight, fluid balance, serum electrolytes, and blood and urine glucose and serum osmolality are monitored daily. When the patient has stabilized on TPN, weekly checks of these parameters suffice for proper monitoring, except that urine glucose levels should be measured four times daily while therapy is initiated, and it is wise to make spot checks of urine glucose levels daily until therapy is discontinued. During TPN infusion the body is in an anabolic state, and potassium and phosphate requirements are often increased above maintenance needs. Potassium, like nitrogen, is incorporated intracellularly and usually given in direct ratio to the amount of administered nitrogen (10 to 15 mEq./gm. of nitrogen).

As the patient recovers, oral feedings are begun and gradually increased as tolerated. TPN administration is proportionately reduced in a stepwise manner. As the patient approaches normal oral feedings, the TPN solution is diluted in concentration and gradually diminished in volume before being terminated.

Complications of TPN

Thrombosis around the catheter is a common complication of lengthy TPN administration and may be minimized by use of Silastic catheters and the addition of dilute heparin to the formula. Catheter misplacement and occult pneumothorax are avoided by x-ray or fluoroscopic evaluations carried out along with catheter placement.

Septicemia is unquestionably the most serious complication of TPN. It ultimately will occur when any foreign body, such as the TPN catheter, dwells in the vascular system for lengthy periods of time, especially in debilitated patients who frequently have other sites of infection associated with their surgical problem. However, the rate of infection is directly proportional to the care that is exercised during the initial catheter placement, the length of the subcutaneous tunneling of the catheter, and the subsequent day-to-day care of the catheter. With careful attention to these points, infection can be minimized. We have frequently had a single catheter in place for a period of several months with no infection developing.

Ultimately, however, infection will occur with lengthy superior vena cava or inferior vena cava catheterization. Under these circumstances, sepsis often is caused by bizarre organisms such as fungi or yeast, or by skin bacteria that are usually not considered to be pathogenic.

At the first sign of infection (unexplained temperature elevation, leukocytosis, hyperglycemia, or simply an unexpected deterioration in the patient's general condition) serial blood cultures are drawn; if these return positive, the TPN catheter is withdrawn and cultured. The patient's general condition is carefully assessed for possible infection elsewhere and antibiotic therapy is directed by results of Gram stain and culture. After appropriate treatment of septicemia is underway, the catheter can be placed in another vein within 24 to 48 hours.

Metabolic complications, frequently seen during administration of TPN, necessitate changes in the formula or its rate of administration. These complications include azotemia, hypophosphatemia, trace-metal deficiency, and carbon dioxide retention. Hepatobiliary problems may also arise during TPN therapy. Fatty liver and cholestasis, manifested by elevated liver enzymes and serum bilirubin, may be corrected when one lowers the glucose content of the solution. Acalculous cholecystitis, presumably attributable to biliary stasis, has recently been recognized as a potential complication of long-term TPN administration in fasting patients.

Peripheral vein hyperalimentation

Recently, solutions have been formulated that are low enough in tonicity (less than 600 mOsm./L.) to allow their safe infusion into small peripheral veins without provoking phlebitis. Because of lower glucose concentration, large volumes must be given to satisfy nutritional needs. Alternatively, amino acids or amino acids and 5% dextrose may be given as "protein-sparing" therapy during periods of fasting that are predictably relatively short. The main advantage of peripheral hyperalimentation is to eliminate the major complications of thrombosis and sepsis of centrally placed catheters.

The basic solution used in peripheral hyperalimentation is 3% to 4.25% amino acids in a 10% dextrose solution. Fat emulsion is added to supply 50% to 60% of the nonprotein calories as fat.

Electrolytes and vitamins are added to satisfy daily requirements. Dilute heparin may be added to discourage phlebitis. Obviously, larger volumes of this fluid must be infused to satisfy nutritional needs than the more hypertonic fluid that is used in central infusion. Renal failure, cardiac failure, and overhydration are indications to shift to a central infusion. Because of the need for frequent venipunctures, peripheral vein hyperalimentation is limited to the hospitalized patient.

Enteral nutrition

If the patient's condition allows, enteral tube feeding is preferable to either peripheral or central nutrition for the following reasons: lower cost, fewer catheter-associated complications, hepatic and gastrointestinal "integrity" can be maintained better, and possibly the provision of greater resist-

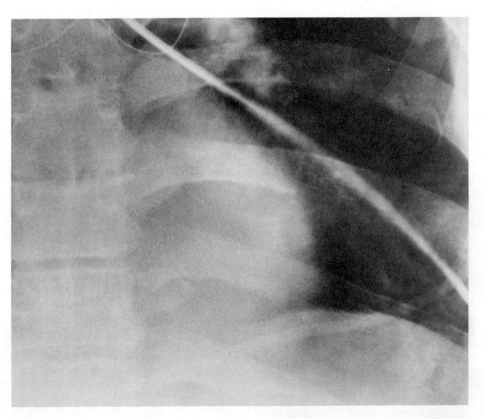

Fig. 7-3. Spot film taken to check placement of radiopaque feeding tube. Patient was asymptomatic, even though feeding tube traverses left lower lobe bronchus. Had feedings been given, a pulmonary disaster would have ensued.

ance to intra-abdominal infection. Enteral alimentation is indicated in patients who have an intact gastrointestinal tract but who are unable or unwilling to consume adequate nutrients; it is useful in patients with swallowing problems or who have psychiatric inanition, in patients suffering oropharyngeal or esophageal disturbances or diseases, and in patients with burns or multiple trauma. Tube feedings may be administered through nasoduodenal tubes, gastrostomy tubes, or tubes placed percutaneously into the jejunum.

Tube-feeding formulas

Commercial diets vary widely in calorie density, osmolality, protein source, and cost. Patients with normal gastrointestinal tracts can utilize meal-replacement formulas that consist of casein or soy protein isolates, oligosaccharides, and long-chain fatty acids. Examples of these diets include Ensure, Osmolite, and Isocal.

Patients with short bowel syndromes, selective malabsorption, or fistulas often require elemental diets. These contain crystalline amino acids or protein hydrolysates, glucose, oligosaccharides, and medium-chain triglycerides and therefore need

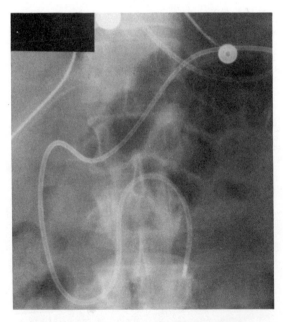

Fig. 7-4. Plain abdominal roentgenogram showing correct position of radiopaque feeding tube. Tube has a single loop in stomach and then traverses duodenal C-loop; mercury-weighted tip of tube lies in jejunum just beyond ligament of Treitz.

minimal digestion. Because of their rich carbohydrate content, these diets are generally higher in osmolality. Examples of elemental formulas include Vivonex and Vital.

Techniques of enteral feeding

Feedings administered through nasogastric tubes are often complicated by gastroesophageal reflux and aspiration. Silastic tubes of 7 to 9 Fr have recently been introduced bearing a mercury-weighted tip; these tubes can be passed transnasally into the distal duodenum for drip feeding into the small bowel. Passage of these flexible tubes into the stomach may be facilitated by a guidewire. With the patient positioned on his right side, gravity and peristalsis will then commonly propel the tube through the pylorus and around the duodenum. If the tube does not pass spontaneously, metoclopramide may be given to stimulate gastric emptying, or the tube can be manipulated through the pylorus and into the duodenum under fluoroscopic control.

If the need for enteral nutritional support is recognized at laparotomy, a standard or needle catheter jejunostomy may be inserted at that time. Feedings can generally be started within 48 to 72 hours postoperatively, after the injection of water-soluble contrast material has verified correct catheter placement.

It is mandatory to verify tube position every time a feeding tube is passed. Small tubes may be inadvertently passed into the bronchus without triggering respiratory symptoms (Fig. 7-3), and the simple auscultation of injected air may be misleading. Tube position can be verified by plain roentgenograms or fluoroscopy (Fig. 7-4), as well as by aspiration of gastric contents and bile.

Bolus feedings can be given directly into the stomach. However, when the feedings are administered into the duodenum or jejunum, continuous infusions controlled by pumps are desirable. Half-strength feedings are initiated at 50 ml./hour in adults, with 25 ml./hour increases every 8 hours until the volume goal is achieved. The solution strength is then gradually increased to meet caloric requirements.

Complications of enteral feedings

Metabolic complications of tube feedings are similar to those seen with TPN, and mandate intensive glucose, electrolyte, and metabolic screening, particularly early in therapy. Mechanical problems include nasopharyngeal irritation, tube displacement, and aspiration. Gastrointestinal disturbances that are related to tube feedings include cramping, distension, and diarrhea and are the most common complications of enteral nutrition. The strength or infusion rate of the solution should be decreased, and the possibility of lactose intolerance must be considered.

CONCLUSIONS

Parenteral hyperalimentation, whether infused into a peripheral or central vein, is a very useful and sometimes life-saving technique to prevent or treat serious malnutrition in patients whose medical or surgical illness precludes enteral feedings. Tube feeding can often be used in patients with intact gastrointestinal tracts but who are unable or unwilling to consume adequate nutrients. When adequate nutrients are provided by any of these modalities, the following objective evidence of nutritional improvement will occur: weight gain, prompt wound healing, closure of intestinal fistulas, reversal of severe inflammatory gastrointestinal disorders, improvement in serum albumin concentration, etc. Many patients enjoy a general feeling of well-being. It is no longer necessary for a patient to starve simply because he temporarily is unable to eat.

8
Preoperative Care

Edward Bartle

Judging precisely which patients will survive, or succumb to, any specific operations for a disease, or diseases, is impossible. The many obvious variables such as age, seriousness of the primary disease, and coexisting diseases, account for the intangible nature of risk in any operation. Healthy, good-risk patients have died after simple operations, and aged, poor-risk patients have eased through procedures of astonishing magnitude. Therefore estimation of surgical risk is at best an educated guess based on past experiences. When asked to guarantee an operation (and this happens not infrequently), the experienced surgeon refuses to guarantee anything but his professional concern and competence. Sound surgical judgment, nevertheless, requires an estimation of surgical risk, especially in difficult cases when surgical risk must be cautiously weighed against any expected benefit from the operation. Surgical risk involves three main elements—the patient, the disease, and the treatment. This risk is in the form of the following equation:

$$\text{The patient} + \text{The disease} + \text{The treatment} = \text{Surgical risk}$$

THE PATIENT
Age

Prematurity and extreme old age are associated with increased operative risk. Little difference is seen, however, in operative mortality in the third decade as compared to the eighth decade with *brief procedures* that disturb physiological functions minimally, such as thyroidectomy or hernia repair; with operations of greater magnitude, involving increased physiological stress, the mortality is substantially greater in older patients. The mortality of combined abdominoperineal resection, for example, rises strikingly with age.

Heart

"A man is as old as his arteries," according to an old adage. We could add, "especially his coronary and cerebral arteries." For example, more than half of the patients who survive major arterial reconstructions (femoroiliac, internal carotid) and who have diabetes or coronary disease will die within 5 years after these procedures. Most die from myocardial infarction.

In addition to recent myocardial infarction (less than 6 months) Goldman lists eight other factors that increase life-threatening cardiac complications in the postoperative period:

1. An S_3 gallop or distended jugular veins prior to operation
2. Myocardial infarction in the preceding 6 months
3. Rhythm other than sinus or premature atrial contractions on the preoperative electrocardiogram
4. More than five premature ventricular contractions per minute at any time before operation
5. An intraperitoneal, intrathoracic, or aortic operation
6. Age greater than 70 years
7. Important valvular aortic stenosis
8. An emergency operation
9. Poor general condition

The New York Heart Association ranks patients

with cardiac symptoms from Class I (no symptoms) to Class IV (symptoms at rest). More than half of the deaths in Goldman's series came from within Class IV.

When life-threatening diseases arise in a patient with serious cardiac disease, even a few hours of intensive cardiac care—to control hypertension, arrhythmias, or heart failure—can increase survival.

Venous thrombosis and pulmonary embolism, which are more common in patients with chronic heart disease, may be decreased by low-dose heparin (5,000 units subcutaneously every 12 hours). Many believe that this prophylactic therapy lowers mortality, especially in older persons.

Lungs

Pulmonary dysfunctions—inability to move air in and out of the lungs, to clear the bronchial tree by coughing, and to perfuse the lungs—often underlie postoperative pulmonary complications. Heavy cigarette smoking is often a precedent cause. We can anticipate pulmonary problems by asking simple clinical questions. How many flights of stairs can the patient climb? How many blocks can he walk without dyspnea? Can he comfortably carry out routine tasks? If normal exertion prompts shortness of breath, pulmonary ventilation tests (vital capacity, forced expiratory volume in 1 second) and arterial blood gases, before and during exercise, will help quantitate the deficit and indicate the urgency for postoperative respiratory support.

Kidneys

Chronic renal failure increases operative risk. A useful screening test for renal function is serum and urine creatinine levels. Urine creatinine concentrations should exceed by tenfold the normal serum levels (<1.6 mg./dl.). Meticulous attention to fluid and electrolyte replacement can prevent problems in patients with compromised renal function. Dialysis (peritoneal or hemodialysis) should precede all elective operations in patients with chronic renal disease and elevated BUN and creatinine levels.

Liver

Jaundice and ascites usually indicate severe liver disease. Unremitting, progressive jaundice signals a need for urgent remedial operation for the jaundice, if the jaundice is "surgical." A negative history for jaundice and normal serum bilirubin, proteins, alkaline phosphatase, transaminases, and prothrombin time usually indicate an adequate liver. Abnormalities in any of these tests should indicate the need for further investigation of liver functions. The type of liver disease will often influence the choice of anesthetic.

Blood

A diffuse organ, the blood and blood-forming tissues can be the limiting element in any surgical procedure. Anemia, with fewer red cells to carry oxygen, lowers oxygen delivery to tissues. Clinical and experimental studies show that a hematocrit of 30% will provide adequate oxygen transportation during surgical procedures. (However, it must fall to 7%, a level that barely sustains life, before wound healing is substantially impaired.) Platelet activity, essential for blood clotting, depends on platelet counts above 50,000/ml. (normal values are 150,000 to 300,000/ml.). Counts below this level require pre-operative or intraoperative platelet transfusions, or both.

White blood cells and macrophages defend against infections. Leukemia, Hodgkin's disease, diabetes, and immunosuppressive drugs will impair these first-line defenses. In addition, remember that general anesthetic agents and major operations interfere with the body's immune responses. Broad-spectrum antibiotics can help such patients withstand the additional stresses from surgical procedures.

Endocrine system

Endocrine factors are discussed in Chapters 7, 13, 14, and 15. *Diabetes* coexists with many surgical problems. Uncontrolled diabetes, a distinct hazard, must be treated vigorously before induction of anesthesia.

Preoperative treatment of diabetes

Carbohydrate (minimum of 200 gm.) and insulin must be given together to utilize the carbohydrate. In general, hypoglycemia (coma, convulsions) is more hazardous than hyperglycemia. Blood glucose levels of 200 to 250 mg.% are innocuous in the absence of ketoacidosis. For moderate diabetes, the usual regimen includes the following:

1. Giving half the patient's usual insulin (NPH or lente) dose subcutaneously at the beginning of the operative procedure along with 1,000 ml. of 10% glucose in water
2. Repeating the same dose at the end of the procedure while infusing 10% glucose solution (total 2,000 to 3,000 ml. in 24 hours)

For poorly controlled diabetes, start with 10 units of subcutaneous crystalline insulin every 6 hours and give 5 to 10 additional units for each 50 mg./dl. increase in blood glucose above 200 mg./dl. (or for each 3+ or 4+ urine glucose reaction).

Dehydration states

Varying states of simple desiccation, extracellular fluid loss, hemorrhage, or loss of specific electrolytes can appreciably affect operative risk. They are discussed at length in Chapter 3.

Nutritional status

Chronic disease and subsequent malnutrition impede wound healing. Surgeons now have the tools, given adequate time, to improve a patient's nutritional status before operation. Parenteral hyperalimentation can provide proteins, amino acids, calories (glucose), vitamins, minerals, and fats—in short, total nutritional needs. Infusing these hypertonic solutions into high-flow veins (superior vena cava) has made this lifesaving procedure possible.

Lacking time to reverse preoperative malnutrition in emergency situations, such as a perforated colon cancer, the surgeon begins hyperalimentation during the operation and continues it postoperatively. (See Chapter 7.)

Obesity is associated with renal disease, pulmonary problems, diabetes, hypertension, cerebrovascular diseases, and orthopedic problems. As a consequence, morbidly obese patients (100 pounds more than ideal weight) lose about 10 to 15 years of life expectancy. Because obesity increases operative time, this adds to the risk of septic, pulmonary, and vascular complications. Patients require brief operative procedures, intensive respiratory support, rapid mobilization, and sometimes antibiotics and heparin.

THE DISEASE

The variability of the physical status of patients parallels the wide range of diseases that may afflict them. The nature of the disease (malignant or benign, infected or sterile), the physiological disturbances it causes, the site, and the length of time the disease has been present are all important factors affecting surgical risk.

With critical disorders (cancers or diseases causing exsanguinating hemorrhage), consideration of surgical risk becomes a clear, hard question of life or death. When the alternative to operative treatment is so obvious, most surgeons (and patients) would choose an operation with even the slight probability of saving life as the hoped-for reward.

Malignant versus benign disease

Operations on specific organs are, by and large, more hazardous for malignant diseases than for benign diseases. A gastric operation for cancer, for example, carries a higher mortality than one for benign gastric ulcer. Operations for thyroid nodules are less hazardous than those for thyroid cancer.

Septic versus sterile disease

Septic diseases are more complicated, with a higher mortality, than sterile or relatively sterile diseases are. Perforated appendicitis has a higher mortality than early acute appendicitis. Septic cholecystitis is more often fatal than aseptic, uncomplicated cholecystitis.

Site of the disease

The site of the disease is an important determinant of surgical risk. Operative risk decreases in descending order in the following sites: heart, thoracic esophagus, brain, rectum, colon, stomach, and lung. The nature and extent of the disease is, of course, an important factor in each specific site.

Time element

The greater the length of time the patient has had the disease, the poorer the operative risk. For example, the complication rate from a septic source (e.g., a perforated appendix) varies directly with the time interval between perforation and treatment. Debilitating effects from cancer that has lurked undetected for long periods also increase surgical risk.

THE TREATMENT

Treatment strongly influences both the *patient* and the *disease*. This is the only one of the three factors of surgical risk over which the surgeon has much control. Knowledge of the patient's overall status and the disease that afflicts him keynotes successful management. After assessing the patient and the disease as completely as possible, the surgeon plans the operative treatment.

Magnitude of the operation

After restoring the ill patient to as near normal as possible, the extent of the operation must be considered. One thought should be clearly in mind: *surgical risk increases with the magnitude of the procedure.* Blood loss, trauma to the patient, and operating time are all cofactors. Replacement of an intracardiac valve is obviously more hazardous than the comparatively simple mitral valvulotomy. Cholecystostomy is a shorter, simpler, and safer procedure than cholecystectomy for acute cholecystitis. A wide variety of other examples illustrate the importance of surgical judgment. In choosing among the possible therapeutic options, the surgeon must weigh this critical factor of surgical magnitude carefully. In most instances decisions are relatively easy; in a few they are immensely difficult.

An additional important but largely unassessable factor is the skill of the surgeon and his team. What can be performed expeditiously with a well-trained team in a modern hospital may, unfortunately, become catastrophic under less favorable conditions.

Postoperative care

The quality of postoperative care is another important, yet variable, factor in operative risk. Experienced nursing personnel in intensive care units have reduced postoperative mortality more than any other factor. Their efficiency, skill, and dedication are more important than electronic monitors, suction and inhalation equipment, or any of the other mechanical devices that aid in the care of the postoperative patient. Their continued training is the responsibility of the surgeons who work with them.

• • •

Operative risk is an intangible yet invaluable and practical concept. The spectrum of variables inherent in the *patient,* the *disease,* and the *treatment* defies precise analysis. Eventually computers may help in assessing operative risk; at the present time valid statistical analyses of the many variables (to program a computer) exist only as research projects. Estimation of surgical risk must, as always, be based on experience, intuition, and a generous measure of common sense.

9
Anesthesia

John H. Tinker

Before the 1840s, "surgery" was limited to the "procedures" that could be accomplished in seconds or minutes in concert with screams of agony from the patient. The development of anesthesia changed all this and is variously credited to Crawford Long's use of ether in 1842, or Horace Wells' 1845 report of nitrous oxide rendering the patient pain-free but still moving on the table, or William Morton's use of ether in 1846 (under public scrutiny) to prevent both pain and movement. Diethyl ether gained early supremacy in the United States, whereas chloroform became popular in Europe. Anesthesia was "discovered" many years before hypodermic needles, electrocardiography, blood pressure measurement (in man), intravenous fluid therapy, etc. Regional anesthesia developed with usage of cocaine during the 1880s and procaine before 1910. Cyclopropane (1929) and thiopental (1935) were both in widespread usage before penicillin was. In the mid-1950s, halothane gained worldwide acceptance because of potency, ease of administration, and nonflammability. It was followed by several other nonflammable fluocarbon potent volatile agents, plus new potent narcotics and other injectables. Anesthetics are administered to over 20 million Americans yearly today.

The objectives of surgical anesthesia are fourfold, as follows: (1) to prevent perception of pain, (2) to obliterate awareness of surroundings (unless regional anesthesia is employed, (3) to provide muscle relaxation if needed, and (4) to obtund untoward autonomic reflexes. Clearly anesthesia satisfying these requirements is not "sleep"! The state we call anesthesia must be a subtle set of alterations of physiological function. It must be readily reversible, i.e., must not constitute significant physiological or pharmacological trespass. Xenon, a "noble" gas, which does not enter into conventional chemical reactions, is an anesthetic. Anesthesia thus does not necessarily have to be attributable to a drug binding to a specific receptor. Removal of pain, awareness, muscle tone, and many protective reflexes places squarely on the anesthetist the responsibility of maintaining safe circulation, respiration, metabolism, etc. Producing an anesthetic state in a patient is not difficult. Keeping that now-helpless patient safe while at the same time providing adequate conditions to permit effective and expeditious surgery is another matter.

There is a strange conundrum that because anesthesia is seldom if ever directly therapeutic, it must necessarily be inherently *safe*, and that any and all untoward outcomes must, of necessity, be caused by poor practice. Not so. Anesthetics and accompanying adjuvants are potent and dangerous drugs, with many actions and interactions neither explored nor explained. Why such safety should be demanded of these agents and techniques is a mystery, since all other drugs and procedures are accepted to have risk/benefit ratios. Patients who would not have been considered viable candidates just a few years ago today are presented for major operations. They are often taking a variety of other potent drugs and have complex fluid or electrolyte disturbances, metabolic derangements, and multiple organ failure. Some form of "anesthesia" can almost always be given to even the most moribund patient, but always there is a price.

PHYSIOLOGICAL AND TOXIC DERANGEMENTS DURING ANESTHESIA
Ventilatory and respiratory effects

Ventilation is gas exchange, whereas respiration is adequacy of oxygen delivery to tissues. The anesthetist must often take over, control, and monitor both. The *airway*, glibly mentioned as important in cardiopulmonary resuscitation courses, becomes crucial to the anesthetist. Beginners are amazed and dismayed at (1) how rapidly the patient loses ability to maintain his or her airway and (2) how difficult it can be to obtain and maintain an unobstructed safe airway. General anesthesia results in loss of muscle tone to produce nearly complete inspiratory obstruction (snoring is but a hint). Various maneuvers, such as tilting the head backward, lifting the mandible anteriorly, placing artificial oral and nasopharyngeal airways, adding positive pressure to inspired gases, and inserting an endotracheal tube are all airway maintenance and protection procedures. Securing the airway and providing adequate ventilation in a patient who has a bronchopleurocutaneous fistula, wherein positive pressure ventilation causes most of the gas to take the "least resistance path" out the fistula is an extreme example, but it does serve to point out the range of difficulties with the airway that can be encountered during anesthesia.

Just ventilating the lungs may indeed adequately remove carbon dioxide from the blood, but it does not necessarily assure adequate oxygenation of the blood, or tissue delivery thereof. During anesthesia, especially when muscle paralysis is added (with neuromuscular blocking agents), gradual increases often occur in regional pulmonary ventilation-perfusion mismatch, especially in patients with diseased lungs. This can result in decline, sometimes to alarmingly low levels, in arterial oxygen partial pressure, unless careful monitoring is performed. Precise mechanisms causing this problem are not known, but there often (not necessarily) is a gradual decrease in lung functional residual capacity (FRC), sometimes to the point wherein airway closure ("closing capacity") may occur during tidal breathing. Maintaining a clear airway is not all that is necessary to assure adequate tissue oxygen delivery during anesthesia.

Cardiovascular effects

With the exception of some narcotics, anesthetics are *all direct myocardial depressants*. This includes agents like ketamine and cyclopropane, which also excite the sympathetic nervous system (and may raise the blood pressure). An agent like ketamine, which usually results in sympathetic activation, may still produce myocardial depression in a patient whose cardiac muscle has been depleted of endogenous catecholamines (i.e., severe myocardial failure). Certain narcotics, notably fentanyl, are not direct myocardial depressants, though they are not complete anesthetics either. Other narcotics, such as meperidine *are* myocardial depressants. Is this direct myocardial depression necessarily harmful? Not always. Judicious myocardial depression may decrease cardiac oxygen demand and be protective if there is severe coronary artery disease. If myocardial depression and the peripheral vasodilatation that usually accompanies it are carried too far, the resultant hypotension may compromise pressure-dependent areas in myocardium or brain and produce infarction. Furthermore, peripheral vasodilatation may trigger undersirable reflex tachycardia—again compromising a diastolic time-dependent coronary artery–diseased heart.

Not only do anesthetics cause varying degrees of myocardial depression and arteriolar vasodilatation, but also there is often venodilatation and decreased venous return. All these effects may combine to produce hypotension. Dysrhythmias may occur from direct anesthetic-catecholamine interaction (usually seen with halothane), or from insufficient sympathoadrenal suppression.

Circulatory *hyperdynamism* may also occur, from anesthetic levels that are insufficient to counteract the effects of sudden or gradual surgical stimulation. The resultant hypertension or tachycardia may result in sufficient myocardial regional oxygen supply and demand imbalances to produce ischemia or infarction. Clearly, monitoring and control of hemodynamics play a major role in anesthetic management.

Central nervous system effects

Anesthesia itself implies suppression of at least some activity in the central nervous system (CNS), whether it is by blocking major nerve trunks, or spinal cord (via spinal or epidural anesthesia), or the entire CNS. The student should clearly understand that "anesthesia" is *not sleep* but just as clearly that it is *not coma*. Such selective depression of the CNS must preserve vital integrity, namely, basal (often medullary) functions. All modern potent anesthetics can be fatal in high enough concentrations just on the basis of massive CNS depression. Anesthetics in reasonable concentrations do spare vital CNS functions and yet suppress awareness (cortical function). The reverse corollary to this is that sympathetic stimulation during surgical maneuvers *will* often get through; i.e., the CNS is not sufficiently depressed to prevent some activation of the sympathetic system. This results often in "roller coaster" blood pressure, heart rate, and systemic vascular resistance during actual anesthesia and operation, and this effect is a continual problem for anesthetists. The student should realize that many of these major stimuli do "get through." Hypnosis studies have even shown that voices and other happenings in the operating room are getting through also, at least at a subconscious level. Actual conscious subsequent recall of events during anesthesia has concerned anesthetists who care for critically ill patients wherein high concentrations of anesthetics might prove too depressant to compromised cardiovascular systems. Another group of patients wherein "too-light" anesthesia may result in awareness are pregnant patients, in whom the clinical objective is to administer sufficient anesthesia to obliterate maternal awareness, without dangerously depressing the delivered infant. Awareness under anesthesia can be a problem, for example, during emergency cesarean sections.

Renal effects

If anesthesia decreases arterial blood pressure, renal blood flow will decrease, usually proportionally. The formerly used anesthetic methoxyflurane underwent approximately 50% metabolic degradation. The most frequent by-product of that agent, inorganic fluoride, occasionally caused nephrotoxicity, which resulted in a form of high-output renal failure. The only modern anesthetic metabolized into appreciable inorganic fluoride is enflurane. Careful studies in animals and in patients with mild to moderate renal failure have shown that fluoride levels do not increase sufficiently to produce nephrotoxicity with enflurane.

Another side of the renal effect question comes when the anesthetist tries to "protect" the kidney against postoperative acute renal failure. These situations often occur during major vascular surgery, whether aortic cross-clamping occurs above or below the renal arteries. Which anesthetic technique is best to optimize renal protection is not known. Whether to administer loop or osmotic diuretics before the expected renal insult is also controversial. Anesthetists often give a "prophylactic" dose of mannitol before aortic cross-clamp, but valid, controlled outcome studies are not available. Whether any particular rate of urine formation is any more protective against postoperative renal failure than any other is not known. Postoperative renal failure is a devastating, often fatal complication that has not yet achieved a satisfactory solution.

Hepatic effects

Chloroform, first used as an anesthetic in 1847, is clearly a hepatic toxin. When halothane was introduced in 1956, anesthesiologists were concerned that it might also be hepatotoxic because its chemical structure is similar, as shown below:

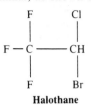

Halothane

Halothane is a potent, nonflammable, extremely clinically useful anesthetic. It became immensely popular and has been given to millions upon millions of patients throughout the world. Reports of rare but devastating postoperative fatal hepatic necrosis began to appear shortly after the introduction of halothane. This prompted the massive National Halothane Study in 1961. In that study, halothane was clearly the safest anesthesia then in use, but there *were* several unexplained cases of massive hepatic necrosis occurring after halothane anesthesia. Most experts today do believe there is a clinical entity called "halothane hepatitis." Unfortunately, today some internists (and lawyers) blame halothane for many (most?) postoperative hepatic difficulties despite the fact that there is absolutely no way in which "halothane hepatitis" can be distinguished pathologically from other causes of centrilobular hepatic necrosis. Indeed, numerous cases of "halothane hepatitis" have been "diagnosed" despite the record-proved fact that the patient in question did *not* receive halothane at all!

Can we make sense out of all this? There are animal models (rats) wherein postanesthetic hepatic centrilobular necrosis can be reproducibly obtained. With halothane as the anesthetic, this model requires all of the following together: (1) hepatic microsomal mixed function oxidase (cytochrome P_{450}) *induction*, with either barbiturates or polychlorinated biphenyl (PCB), (2) a *hypoxic* gas mixture of less than 14% oxygen, and (3) halothane in low doses, approximately 0.5%. The situation gets complicated, however, by the fact that both enflurane and isoflurane (the two other volatile anesthetics in use today) can be substituted for halothane in the above model and hepatic centrilobular necrosis still results. With the other two anesthetics, lower oxygen levels (about 10%), higher anesthetic dosages (1.5% to 2%), and *fasted* (24-hour) animals are required. Probably, postanesthetic hepatic necrosis is real and is related to a complex series of events, including diminution of oxygen delivery to the liver. It is likely that the halothane is somewhat more likely to be associated with this toxicity than either enflurane or isofluorane is, but the syndrome is rare. There *are* situations where halothane is a nearly ideal choice for reasons beyond the scope of this chapter. Halothane should not disappear from the anesthesiologists' armamentarium. Clearly, hepatic effects of general anesthetics are important, controversial, and interesting. Surgical stress itself affects liver function in many ways discussed in other chapters.

HOW IS ANESTHESIA PRODUCED?

General anesthesia is often (but not necessarily) *induced* with a rapidly acting intravenously administered drug, such as sodium thiopental, etomidate, diazepam, or sodium methohexital. The uptake and distribution characteristics of these drugs make them difficult to use, continuously or intermittently, to *maintain* lengthy anesthesia. A "sleep dose" of sodium thiopental, for example, may wear off in approximately 17 minutes. It is not metabolized or eliminated in that short of a time period. Instead, a *redistribution* of the agent away from the brain occurs. A significant percentage of the administered dose originally lodges in brain tissue simply because about 15% of the resting cardiac output goes to that organ. The fatty tissues elsewhere, though poorly perfused, constitute a vast reservoir into which these highly lipophilic drugs will eventually be redistributed. Thus the patient awakens after a "sleep dose" of thiopental because of redistribution. *Maintenance* of general anesthesia is readily achieved with gaseous or volatile agents because they are rapidly removable and changeable in their concentrations in blood and brain via the *lungs*.

Therefore much general anesthesia is *induced* with a rapidly acting intravenous agent and then *maintained* with a volatile or gaseous anesthetic. Today, "volatile" applies to a liquid that is vaporized. Halothane, enflurane, and isoflurane are the three such agents currently in use. "Gaseous" applies to nitrous oxide, in use since 1845. The latter is relatively impotent, requiring high concentrations. Consequently it is often if not almost always used as an adjunct, or supplement. If nitrous oxide is used as a supplement to volatile agent anesthesia, it is generally considered to be a volatile agent–based anesthetic. If, by contrast, nitrous oxide is used to supplement intravenous agents including narcotics such as morphine or fentanyl, or hypnotics such as diazepam or barbiturates, the anesthesia is said to be a *balanced* type.

During general anesthesia, *muscle relaxation* formerly was provided by administration of high concentrations of agents such as diethyl ether. These "deep" anesthetics carried risks of severe circulatory and respiratory depression. In other words, the advent of specific neuromuscular blocking drugs permitted much "lighter" anesthetics to be given, undoubtedly rendering them safer. Certainly not all general anesthetics require addition of muscle relaxants.

Regional anesthesia offers a wide range of choices. Many believe that regional anesthesia is "less" anesthesia and therefore inherently safer. There is little evidence that this is true. A major regional anesthetic might very well result in severe hypotension, for example. On the other hand, an axillary block of the upper extremity may be an ideal choice for a patient with a full stomach who requires emergency hand surgery. Spinal (intrathecal drug injection) or epidural (local anesthetic injected into the epidural space) are commonly chosen to try to lessen the amount of anesthetic drug absorbed by the fetus during labor or delivery. Herniorrhaphy is well performed under the near-cadaveric abdominal muscle relaxation that results from a spinal anesthetic.

Many times, a combination of regional and general anesthesia seems reasonable. For instance, for a cholecystectomy, it is possible to first perform bilateral intercostal nerve blocks at T6 through T12, administer a light general anesthetic with an intravenous induction, and then maintain it with nitrous oxide plus narcotic supplementation, with ventilation controlled through an endotracheal tube. There are as many potential nerve blocks as there are points at which nerves can be reasonably approached with local anesthetics.

Patient acceptance of regional anesthesia is not always enthusiastic. Patients who object to being "awake" often can be given a light general anesthetic in addition to the regional block. Patients who believe friends or relatives have been injured by regional anesthesia are not likely to be impressed with the mathematics of event psychology, i.e., the fact that random occurrences associated with (before or after) a significant event are anecdotally likely to be causally associated with it. Patients should never be coerced into either an anesthetist's or a surgeon's preconceived ideas about the ideal anesthetic for a particular procedure.

The idea that the sickest patients should get regional anesthesia is also not necessarily logical. General anesthesia may result in less hypotension, better oxygenation, carbon dioxide elimination, and airway control. On the other hand, a small dose of local anesthetic, deposited in the subarachnoid space, does provide a large area of superb surgical anesthesia, with little drug to be metabolized or excreted. Regional anesthesia has perhaps received best acceptance during labor and delivery because of the objective of avoiding fetal depression.

CLINICAL ANESTHESIA MANAGEMENT
Preoperative evaluation

Anesthesia is complex *medical* care. A thorough evaluation of the patient before anesthesia is mandatory. This must include detailed knowledge of the patient's medical history, including details of prior cardiac and cerebrovascular events, specific systemic disease, drug reactions, current drug therapies, difficulties with prior anesthetics, and all other relevant vital organ problems. Specific areas of further interest include potential for difficult airway management, problems with dentition, neck and jaw ranges of motion, and potential difficulties in obtaining vascular access.

In addition to a medical work-up, plus determining that the patient's ongoing medical diseases or problems are in optimal control, plus the specific anesthesia-related problems mentioned above, the preoperative visit serves the additional extremely useful purpose of allaying patient fear and uncertainty to a considerably greater degree than any pharmacological premedicant. Patient and family questions can be answered, and unknowns are replaced by expectancies. Media publicity about risks associated with anesthesia have increased public awareness to the point where careful explanations and achievement of trust are often demanded by the patient before permission is given to perform anesthesia and surgery.

Preoperative preparation includes a suitable nothing-by-mouth (NPO) period (not necessarily "NPO past midnight") to try to attain gastric emptying. Premedication may include a drying agent (atropine or scopolamine), an analgesic (morphine, meperidine, etc.), and a sedative (diazepam, lorazepam, barbiturate, etc.). The sedatives should be given by mouth with a sip of water whenever possible. Premedication is difficult at best. Heavy sedation, with airway and respiratory compromise resulting in hypercarbia may severely increase intracranial pressure in patients with space-occupying intracranial lesions. Too-light premedication plus anxiety may trigger an anginal episode indistinguishable (without work-up) from a beginning myocardial infarction. No combination or recipe works well all the time. Personal contact and trust is often most important.

Selection of monitoring

The anesthetist must plan carefully the degree to which the patient's physiological responses to anesthesia and surgery are to be monitored. Few patients today are or should be anesthetized without continuous monitoring of at least one lead of the electrocardiograph. Blood pressure is monitored by cuff, automated oscillometry, or invasive arterial catheter through a strain gauge transducer, depending on the degree to which major blood pressure fluctuations are expected *plus* a careful estimate as to whether such fluctuations will likely be dangerous to that particular patient.

Estimates of *right* ventricular preload by central venous pressures give some idea of dynamic blood volume status in patients with healthy hearts undergoing procedures wherein major ($\pm 15\%$) blood loss is expected or has occurred. Thermistor-equipped flow-directed pulmonary artery catheters permit measurement of cardiac output, calculation of systemic and pulmonary vascular resistances, and estimates (by use of pulmonary artery wedge pressures) of *left* ventricular preload. Such invasive and potentially hazardous monitoring equipment is reserved for *patients undergoing major surgery in whom there is known or suspected myocardial dysfunction.* The pulmonary artery catheter has been controversial because it is expensive, complex, and potentially hazardous. It is not proper to use it always for certain procedures and never for others, without taking into account the degree of the patient's myocardial dysfunction. It is extremely useful during anesthesia and well into the critical postoperative period.

The *brain* can be monitored by an electroencephalograph, computerized EEG analysis, somatosensory cortical evoked potentials, and verbal contact during regional anesthesia. EEG monitoring is often performed during carotid endarterectomy. Evoked potential monitoring may find use as a monitor of spinal-cord integrity during scoliosis repair and thoracic aortic aneurysmectomy.

Pulmonary function monitoring consists in constant observation for color changes, arterial and mixed venous blood gases, and various devices to guard against delivery of hypoxic gas mixtures or ventilator failure. Special pulmonary artery catheters with fiberoptic infrared sensors are available for detection of changes in mixed venous oxygen saturation. Transcutaneous noninvasive oxygen saturation monitors of several types are available.

Renal function monitoring usually consists in measuring urine output, but more sophistication can be lent by measurement of urinary electrolytes or osmolarity, or both. *Liver function* monitoring generally is not done during anesthesia. *Endocrine function* monitoring may be especially important in diabetics (serial blood glucoses). *Coagulation* monitoring during operation can range from simple activated coagulation times to all-out efforts by sophisticated coagulation laboratories. Electrolyte disturbances of all types can occur during anesthesia, and Na^+, K^+, ionized Ca^{++} plus serum osmolarity can all be easily measured.

Conduct of the anesthetic

The patient is generally not anesthetized outside the operating room, though "induction rooms" are used for regional anesthetics in some institutions. Once the patient is in the operating room, induction by inhalation, intravenous agents, or regional anesthesia is accomplished after planned monitors have been attached and validated. It is not always necessary to have an intravenous tube established for every minor short procedure in healthy patients (e.g., myringotomy in a healthy NPO 5-year-old child).

The decision to maintain the airway using a mask, mask and oral or nasal airway, endotracheal tube, or tracheostomy is complex and outside the scope of this chapter. Every "long" case does *not* necessarily mandate an endotracheal tube. Anesthesia, whether regional or general, *should not ever be performed without the presence of someone experienced in airway management*, someone who can obtain and maintain airway patency throughout the procedure. A deadly trap is to perform, for example, a local or regional anesthetic in a situation where airway maintenance is dubious or no one present is sufficiently skilled. Such a patient may well undergo collapse for various reasons and need immediate airway maintenance by someone highly skilled. The student's respect for airway maintenance difficulty will grow, no matter what field he or she chooses.

Special techniques

In addition to availability of special monitoring, several special techniques are available to facilitate anesthesia or surgery. *Deep hypothermia* with subsequent deliberate circulatory arrest during certain cardiac and cerebral operations requires forethought and skill. *Deliberate arterial hypotension*, achieved by direct vasodilatation or other ways may reduce blood loss, provide better exposure of tumor margins, reduce risk of transfusion hepatitis, etc. *Deliberate hypertension* is often employed during carotid endarterectomy. *Deliberate hyperthermia* for cancer treatment requires numerous anesthetic skills. *Autotransfusion* of shed blood, often after centrifugal "washing," is now commonplace. Endotracheal *jet ventilation* can facilitate laser excision of laryngeal lesions. *High-frequency ventilation* may be useful in surgery for bronchopleural fistulas. Intra-aortic *balloon counterpulsation, left ventricular assist devices*, and *optimal pacing* are all employed in cardiac surgery.

Subspecialty anesthesia

Cardiovascular, neurosurgical, pediatric, obstetric, orthopedic, and other surgical specialties have developed highly technical procedures. Anesthetists have also specialized in trying to provide optimal management of these specialized cases. Just a few examples should suffice. The coronary artery bypass operation is often relatively straightforward, but a difficult emergence from bypass in a patient with severe ventricular dysfunction requires skills best (perhaps only) developed with frequent and extensive experience. Neurosurgical sitting-position craniotomies pose severe air embolism hazards, requiring Doppler monitoring and special treatment techniques. Operations on tiny infants may pose severe size-related, metabolic or respiratory problems. The student should not be taken in by the "glamour" of these highly specialized situations. Anesthetic management of major abdominal surgery in a heavy smoker with cardiac disease may be a considerably greater challenge than a coronary artery bypass procedure!

Problems during anesthesia

Arterial hypotension can occur suddenly and to life-threatening levels during anesthesia. Possible causes include anesthetic overdose, hypoxemia, major blood loss, surgical positioning, retractor obstruction of venous return, myocardial ischemia or cardiac arrhythmias or both, various drug-to-drug interactions, anaphylaxis, and other drug or transfusion reactions. The anesthetist often does not have the luxury of an extensive work-up but must make rapid therapy decisions, objectively evaluate the ongoing results of those decisions, and be willing to alter therapy if subsequent events indicate.

Problems with *airway management* are common. Examples include inadvertent disconnection of the breathing circuit, secretions plugging the endotracheal tube, and endobronchial intubation and tube cuff overinflation. Again, diagnosis and therapy must be prompt, for these are potentially humbling and disastrous experiences.

In addition to problems with circulation and respiration, the anesthetist must try to prevent pressure injuries, electrocautery ground return plate burns, dental damage, peripheral nerve injuries from malpositioning of extremities, and injuries to the eyes, ears, and vocal cords.

"Vigilance" is an easy word to write in a chapter such as this, and is, with good reason, the official motto of the American Society of Anesthesiologists. It implies discipline and dedication. The minute-to-minute care during anesthesia and surgery is one of the few times any physicians personally render such continuous care. Improper drug administration, technical maneuvers, and incorrect therapies are often as immediately apparent as the results of poor surgical technique.

Postoperative and intensive care

The period during which patients recover from anesthesia is one of rapid fluctuations in vital signs and mental status and may therefore be quite hazardous. Recovery room nursing is a recognized subspecialty of that profession, with good reason. Rapid assessment of deteriorating neurological function in a postoperative neurosurgical patient may, for example, signal the need for immediate reoperation. Assessments of circulation, respiration, renal status, and neurological status are crucial. Outpatients who have undergone general or major regional anesthesia need informed critical evaluation to determine their ability to leave the hospital. In large hospitals, the recovery room is a fast-changing, sometimes chaotic-appearing place. Professionalism must reign if safe anesthesia and surgery are to be carried out.

Critically ill postoperative patients who will require extended care are often transferred directly to the surgical intensive care unit from the operating room. Here, all manner of difficult acute and chronic medical and surgical problems must be managed. Nursing personnel again bear the brunt of the front-line action. The morale and organization have much to do with the success, or lack of it, of such a unit. Jurisdictional disputes among various physician specialists must be solved with professionalism in the patient's best interest. It is important for all to remember that these are critically ill patients, outcomes are not always going to be rosy, and occasionally treatments will fail. Physicians facing such failures must *deal effectively with their own anxieties and insecurities* regarding these difficult patients. Those insecurities must not be defended by arrogance, dogmatism, or arbitrary and capricious behavior. Successful care of these patients really does require a dedicated, professional *team* approach.

Involvement of anesthesiologists in intensive care activities is natural because of their expertise in ventilatory and circulatory support, airway management, and respiratory care. Critical care specialists now come from anesthesiology, pulmonary and other areas of internal medicine, pediatrics, and surgery backgrounds. If these persons are to become truly critical care experts, they must not assume that any of their original backgrounds confers the requisite totality of expertise.

Pain management

Many patients have chronic pain syndrome of various sorts. Therapies such as repeated peripheral nerve blocks with local anesthetics, intrathecal or epidural steroids or narcotics, and even ablative therapy with nerve blockade using ethanol or phenol are sometimes successful. Many anesthesia departments have established or have participated in pain clinics. Sometimes these are multidisciplinary, with psychological, psychiatric, neurological and surgical support. These are difficult patients to help. They may be taking large dosages of numerous drugs, may be addicted, may have numerous secondary gains, and may be litigation prone. Nonetheless, many can be helped to return to gainful employment. Furthermore, in-hospital pain management services may provide better acute pain care. Pain therapy research is currently very active. Knowledge about these hitherto poorly understood disorders is burgeoning. Anesthesiologists have therapy to offer and are participating.

Overview

Anesthesia has been said to be "hours of boredom and moments of sheer terror." Not true. Competent anesthetists are in tune with their patient's physiology. When perturbations occur, decisive, logical, previously thought out steps are taken to obtain a diagnosis, administer treatment, objectively evaluate results, and alter therapy accordingly. Anesthesia is, in other words, the detailed, technical, and critical *practice of medicine*.

10
Postoperative Care

Richard D. Liechty
Raymond Silva

Complications may occur after almost any operation regardless of its magnitude. Even simple, routine diagnostic procedures (with catheters or needles, drugs, or various contrast media) may cause complications or even death.

In the study of surgical complications, *anticipation* and *early recognition* keynote successful treatment. The majority of all postoperative complications are signaled by two signs: *fever* or *shock* (cardiovascular collapse). Pain and tenderness, so important preoperatively, are often masked by operative pain or suppressed by sedation, especially in the first few hours after operation. Because sedation dulls the patient's responses, the surgeon must develop exceptional sensitivity to the *signs* of postoperative complications. In this chapter we outline a general overview of postoperative complications and refer the reader to other chapters that discuss specific problems in detail.

PATTERN OF SURGICAL COMPLICATIONS
Chain reaction

Fortunately, surgical complications usually appear singly, but all too often, especially in the older, debilitated patient, they occur as *chain reactions*—one complication begets another; e.g., a prolonged ileus requires gastrointestinal suction and intravenous feeding. The patient is shackled to his bed for prolonged periods by a tube in his nose and a needle in his arm. Thus the stage is set for thrombophlebitis (from inactivity) or pneumonitis (from irritation of the upper respiratory areas) with sepsis. These secondary and tertiary complications

are serious and occasionally fatal. Any number and variety of these chain reactions may arise, but they almost invariably begin with one complication. Anticipation and prevention of these initial complications can thwart the sinister chain reaction. Predisposing factors in surgical complications are discussed in Chapter 8.

RECOGNIZING SURGICAL COMPLICATIONS

Fever is the most common evidence of postoperative complications. *Cardiovascular collapse,* though less common, is more dramatic and emergent. Together these two signs forecast at least 90% of postoperative complications. Since early recognition is so important, we will discuss complications in association with these two signs that tell us something is wrong.

Fever

Mild transient fevers appear after most operations from tissue necrosis, hematoma, or cauterization. Higher sustained fevers arise with the following four most common postoperative complications:

1. Atelectasis
2. Wound infections
3. Urinary infections
4. Thrombophlebitis

These causes of fever occur frequently and should be committed to memory as the *Four W's:* "Wind, wound, water, and walk." When fever occurs, the student should think first of these four common sources.

Lung problems (wind) within the first 48 hours

Lung complications commonly occur after operations for the following reasons:

1. Endotracheal tubes; oxygen and ether irritate the respiratory tree, and increased secretion results.
2. Atropine causes inspissation of bronchial secretions.
3. The position of the patient cannot be changed on the operating table and secretions tend to fill the lung and thereby encourage the growth of organisms.
4. An anesthetized patient cannot cough to clear secretions.
5. In the immediate postoperative period the patient, because of sedation or pain, cannot move or cough to clear secretions adequately; an obstruction (from secretions) and atelectasis (collapse of portions of the lung) result.
6. Abdominal distension impairs diaphragmatic excursion.

Fever, tachypnea, and cyanosis (when large portions of the lung are affected) characterize atelectasis. Pneumonitis may result from sustained obstruction. Coughing, deep breathing, moving percussion of the chest wall, and humidified air help clear the respiratory tree of these secretions. If large areas of lung are involved by pneumonia, the patient becomes confused with few other signs and symptoms. Confusion means poor oxygenation of the brain and should prompt the physician to order a roentgenogram of the chest. In the older male with chronic disease of the lung or heart, gram-negative rod pneumonia is common. In certain outbreaks in hospitals *Staphylococcus aureus* is the prime cause of pneumonia in elderly postoperative patients. Bronchoscopy or tracheal catheterization with aspiration of mucus plugs can stimulate patients who have difficulty in coughing. These procedures themselves may introduce new bacteria into the lung, bypassing the usual host-resistance barriers.

Respiratory distress syndrome

Adult respiratory distress syndrome (ARDS, posttraumatic lung, shock lung) follows massive trauma, burns, sepsis, shock, or multiple blood transfusions. Representing a complex reaction to these many possible insults, the injured pulmonary capillary endothelial cells leak fluid and proteins into the lung interstitium, perivascular lymphatic spaces, and alveoli. The flooded alveoli collapse creating pulmonary shunts, which lower arterial Po_2—the hallmark of ARDS. Postmortem studies show grossly heavy lungs (three to six times normal), chiefly from edema fluid and some fibrosis.

The syndrome usually appears 1 or 2 days after correction of the circulatory problems. Restlessness and respiratory distress accompany the roentgenographic picture of increasing patchy opacification of the lung fields. The Pao_2 progressively decreases, and hyperventilation keeps the $Paco_2$ low. Pulmonary studies show falling lung compliance, decrease in functional residual capacity, and increase in respiratory work. The patchy lung lesions may become confluent. Without ventilatory support the patient succumbs.

Mechanical ventilation and positive end-expiratory pressure keynote the treatment. The added pressure increases functional capacity, opens collapsed alveoli, and prevents further collapse. The Swan-Ganz catheter, monitoring left atrial filling pressures and cardiac output, helps to guide therapy. Any source of sepsis should be treated concurrently. (See Chapter 29.)

Wound infections (wound) 5 to 7 days

Wound infections may occur after any operation. They are most common, however, after gallbladder or gastrointestinal operations and operations on the breast (Table 10-1). Drying of tissues by long exposure, operation on contaminated structures, gross obesity, or operations on the very young or very old are directly related to an increase in sepsis rate. Experiments on medical students by Elek show that the infection rate from inoculated staphylococci increases a thousandfold with a foreign body (suture).

Patients who harbor infections remote from the operative site are likely to have greater wound infection rates than those without such remote infections. Wound infection rates rise proportionately with the duration of operative procedures and

Table 10-1. The occurrence rate of wound infections

Operation	Septic wounds (%)
Gallbladder	21
Breast	15
Miscellaneous abdominal	13
Thorax	9
Hernia	7
Miscellaneous orthopedic	3
Meniscectomy	0
Overall average for England*	9.7
Overall average for U.S.A.†	7.5

*Public health laboratory source incidence of surgical wound infection in England and Wales, Lancet **2**:659, 1960.
†Howard, J. M., et al.: Ann. Surg. **160**(suppl.):1-192, 1964.

Table 10-2. Bacteria found in wound infections*

Staphylococcus aureus	60%
S. aureus and coliforms†	13
Coliforms alone	17
Other specified organisms	4
No pathogens	6

*Data from Public health laboratory source incidence of surgical wound infection in England and Wales, Lancet 2:659, 1960.
†*Escherichia coli, Klebsiella-Enterobacter, Proteus,* and paracolon.

with the length of prophylactic antibiotic administration. Any break in aseptic technique can contribute to wound infections during operations or with later dressing changes.

Heat, redness, and tenderness in a wound demand investigation and drainage. Wound infections involve staphylococcus alone in 60%, staphylococcus with enteric organisms in 13%, and enteric organisms alone in 17%. A prudent plan of treatment should proceed as follows: wound culture and sensitivities, antistaphylococcal penicillin (penicillinase-resistant) or cephalosporins (both are lipophilic agents), change in antibiotics according to the patient's response, and laboratory evidence of sensitivity (Table 10-2). (See Chapter 6.)

Abdominal wound dehiscence. Heralded by a serosanguineous discharge about 5 to 6 days postoperatively, the abdominal incision opens and viscera usually protrude through it. Hematomas, seromas, infection, excessive coughing, retching, distension, or poor nutrition (diabetes, uremia, starvation, immunosuppression) often underlie this catastrophe. Inadequate sutures or excessively tight closures—which compromise blood supply—are the chief technical offenders.

In most cases immediate operative closure with through-and-through wire or other strong materials solves the urgent problem. With infection or immunosuppression our transplant surgeons have reemphasized an invaluable technique: they pack these wounds open and let them heal secondarily, with surprising success.

For a discussion of other wound problems, see Chapter 2.

Urinary infection (water) 5 to 8 days

Postoperative patients often have difficulty voiding and sometimes require catheterization. Although urinary infections occur without catheterization, the usual initiating factor is the introduction of a catheter that mechanically carries organisms into the bladder. Single catheterizations are associated even under the best of circumstances with a 4% infection rate. Irrigation of the anterior urethra with bacitracin or neomycin, frequent catheter changes, and constant irrigation with 0.25% acetic acid or neomycin-bacitracin-polymyxin mixtures help prevent sepsis. A round pad of plastic foam about 2 inches in diameter and about 1 inch thick, threaded on a Foley catheter and pushed up to rest against the external urinary meatus, helps anchor the catheter. Subsequently the pad can be moistened with an antiseptic or with antibiotic solution or cream.*

Thrombophlebitis (walk) 7 to 14 days

We do not understand all the factors leading to spontaneous thrombosis in the deep leg and pelvic veins of certain postoperative patients. However, *stasis* and *increased coagulability* of blood are two important factors. Obesity, birth control medications, immobility, advanced age, cardiac problems, and abdominal malignancies are associated factors. Thrombophlebitis is characterized by fever, pain, tenderness, and redness along superficial veins. Pain and edema occur with thromboses in deep veins. The great hazard of blood clots in deep veins rests in the possibility of the clots moving to the lungs (pulmonary emboli). About 25% of patients who develop pulmonary emboli die from one or more of the following: arrhythmias, bronchoconstriction, pulmonary edema, or inadequate return of blood to the left side of the heart (which causes right ventricular failure). Early movement, ambulation, and wrapping of the legs help prevent stasis. Most thromboses respond to rest, elevation of the legs, and chemotherapy with heparin and fibrinolytic agents. Ligating or narrowing the lumen of the inferior vena cava can prevent subsequent emboli if patients develop emboli while on full heparin anticoagulation (Fig. 10-1). (See Chapters 30 and 33.)

Third day fever

The "third day surgical fever" comes from inflammation surrounding intravenous catheters. Removal and antibiotic therapy bring rapid relief.

---

*Experimental work with *Serratia marcescens* has shown that these organisms migrate into the bladder in the fluid (urine and exudate) that forms alongside the catheter. Thus these local procedures help prevent the upward migration of organisms. Patients with infection develop dysuria, frequency, urgency, hesitancy, and fever. Systemic antibiotics can control generalized sepsis but cannot control localized urinary infections as long as the catheter is in place. Recent experience shows that intermittent catheterization, under rigid aseptic precautions, carries less risk than continuous (Foley) catheterization.

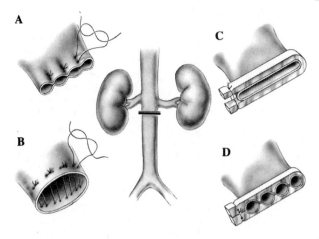

Fig. 10-1. Vena cava narrowing to prevent emboli. **A,** Multiple channel method. **B,** Suture sieve method. **C,** Slit Teflon clip. **D,** Serrated Teflon clip.

Table 10-3. Postoperative shock

Cause	Diagnosis	Treatment
Bleeding Usually in peritoneal or pleural cavities or retroperitoneal areas	Check wounds, drain sites, open wounds, or use diagnosis aspiration if necessary; central venous pressure is low	Blood and immediate ligation of bleeding vessel (see Chapters 3 and 5)
Cardiac shock Myocardial infarction or arrhythmias, arrest	Check for pulse irregularities, electrocardiogram, absence of pulse and cyanosis suggest cardiac arrest; SGOT aids diagnosis of infarction; central venous pressure is high	Dependent on diagnosis general measures, oxygen, sedation, cardiopulmonary resuscitation (see Chapters 5, 29, and 31)
Pulmonary embolus	No specific signs; chest pain, hemoptysis suggest diagnosis; angiography, ventilation, and perfusion scans can make diagnosis; obesity, previous cardiac difficulties, cancer and pelvic operations, immobility, and increased age are associated factors	Embolectomy; heparin, fibronlytic agents to dissolve clots are promising (see Chapters 29, 30, and 33)
Transfusion reaction (contaminated blood)	Smears of blood show gram-negative organisms; shock rapidly follows blood administration; usually fatal	Discontinue blood; corticosteriods; massive doses of antibiotics intravenously (see Chapter 4)
Sepsis	Culture of blood or suspicion of gram-negative bacterial source of septicemia; symptoms often subtle: tachycardia, hypotension, oliguria, fluid retention, respiratory failure—"silent signs of sepsis"	Massive intravenous antibiotics, fluids, corticosteroids (see Chapters 5 and 6)
Adrenal failure	Must be diagnosed by suspicion or history of steroid therapy, lack of other causes	Intravenous corticosteroids (100 to 300 mg. of hydrocortisone) (see Chapter 15)
Anaphylactic shock	Obscure clinical picture; history of drug sensitivities is vitally important; urticaria and edema may aid diagnosis	Epinephrine, antihistamines, corticosteroids
Fat embolism	Tachycardia, dyspnea, hypotension, increased central venous pressure; nodular pulmonary infiltrates	Ventilatory support, heparin, dextran, steroids, immobilization of fractures (see Chapters 30 and 38)

Cardiovascular collapse

The signs of cardiovascular collapse—a cold, clammy, pale patient, decreased blood pressure, and a rapid, thready pulse—usually occur with alarming suddenness in the postoperative patient. Table 10-3 is a helpful guide in the rapid detection and treatment of postoperative shock. The cited chapters discuss these causes of shock in detail. The student should think of bleeding and cardiac disease (myocardial infarction) as the two most common causes.

LESS COMMON COMPLICATIONS
Acute parotiditis

Acute parotiditis is a rare complication that occurs in older, debilitated patients. An acute, painful, tender swelling of the parotid gland is an unmistakable sign. Dehydration may cause inspissation and obstruction in the duct, with a secondary staphylococcus invasion. This is one of the few instances in which x-ray therapy is used for benign disease. It is effective in the early stages. Surgical incision and drainage may be necessary if x-ray therapy fails to halt suppuration.

Postoperative cholecystitis and pancreatitis

Postoperative cholecystitis and pancreatitis are rarely seen; consequently they are often overlooked. Dehydration may engender these conditions as in parotiditis. Treatment is conservative (fluids, gastrointestinal suction, atropine, and rest). Occasionally, cholecystostomy or cholecystectomy is required.

Fat emboli

See Chapter 38.

GASTROINTESTINAL COMPLICATIONS

A high percentage of anesthetized patients will be nauseated and vomit in the postoperative period. Such a common phenomenon cannot be considered a complication.

Aspiration of vomitus

Aspiration of vomitus is a serious complication that must be prevented by emptying of the stomach before anesthesia (with a nasogastric tube when necessary). Turning the patient on his side with the head lowered when vomiting occurs may prevent this complication.

Paralytic ileus

A temporary cessation of peristalsis of the gastrointestinal tract will occur after anesthesia, trauma, and abdominal operations. If it becomes sustained, electrolyte imbalance, wound infections, or some metabolic disturbance (myxedema or ad-

renal failure) may be the cause. Nasogastric suction and fluid replacement will correct most cases.

Acute gastric dilatation

Acute gastric dilatation is an uncommon complication that may follow abdominal, chest, spine, or central nervous system procedures. The precise cause is obscure. An astonishing amount (several liters) of gas and dark, foul material may collect in the stomach. Vomiting and distension are the main diagnostic points. The vomiting, which is seldom accompanied by retching, features an overflow type of regurgitation that, curiously, may not be attended with nausea.

The distension may rapidly progress to fatal cardiovascular collapse within hours. Immediate intubation of the stomach with aspiration of its contents and fluid and electrolyte replacement may be lifesaving. Aspiration of 2 liters or more of gas and liquid material virtually assures the diagnosis of acute gastric dilatation. Continuous decompression will usually relieve the gastric dilatation immediately and reverse the gastric atony within 48 hours. The surgeon can safely discontinue aspiration at that time if no mechanical obstruction coexists.

Hiccup

Hiccuping in the postoperative patient may indicate some potentially serious underlying problem; this is its chief significance. Most commonly hiccups are a short-lived nuisance and nothing more. Abscesses near the diaphragm, uremia, gastric dilatation, paralytic ileus, peritonitis, anxiety, and acidosis are the more common conditions that cause these spasms of the diaphragm. Rarely hiccups may persist for days or weeks and utterly exhaust the sufferer. Correcting the associated disease is the obvious and logical treatment. Vagal pressure, rebreathing air or carbon dioxide, sedation, or tranquilization may bring symptomatic relief.

OTHER URINARY COMPLICATIONS
Retention of urine

Anesthesia, narcotics, anticholinergic drugs (atropine), operative trauma, advanced age, and diseases of the urinary system (an enlarged prostate) contribute to urine retention. Having the patient sit or stand to void is helpful. Sterile catheterization of the bladder must be done to prevent overdistension of the bladder, if the patient cannot void.

Acute renal insufficiency

Acute renal insufficiency is a rare condition that may occur after operative procedures. The urine output decreases despite adequate intake. Precise replacement of fluids will often be sufficient therapy, and the patients will begin excreting urine within 7 to 10 days in most cases. (See Chapter 3.)

Lavaging the peritoneum with fluids designed to collect and remove nitrogenous wastes and potassium provides a "substitute kidney" in severe cases. Because peritoneal dialysis is relatively simple, it has largely replaced the more complicated renal dialysis with the artificial kidney for short-term therapy.

ANAPHYLACTIC REACTIONS AND SERUM SICKNESS

In addition to shock, anaphylactic reactions are characterized by urticaria, angioedema, rhinitis, conjunctival congestion, wheezing, dyspnea, or any combination of these manifestations. An injection of foreign material induces an antigen-antibody response; subsequent exposure triggers the reaction. In humans the cardiorespiratory system (nose, glottis, pulmonary artery, bronchioles, and right ventricle), the hepatic venules, and renal glomeruli are specific targets for these reactions. A generalized urticaria often covers many patients.

Almost any organic substance such as blood proteins, enzymes, horse serum, glues, and many foods (fish, chocolate, egg whites) may cause anaphylaxis. Penicillin, dextran, local anesthetics, contrast media, and dyes are proved offenders.

Serum sickness is a close relative of anaphylaxis but with onset 4 to 10 days after administration of the causative serum or drug. Adenopathy, arthralgia, fever, leukopenia, neuropathy, and rash characterize serum sickness.

When systemic anaphylactic symptoms appear, 0.25 ml. of 1:1,000 epinephrine is given immediately and repeated every 5 minutes until nervousness or tachycardia appears. Asthmatic symptoms may be relieved by intravenous aminophylline. Antihistamines and corticosteroids are slower acting but may curtail advancement of symptoms. Tracheostomy may be required to bypass obstructing glottic edema. Since serum sickness is much less violent than anaphylaxis, symptomatic treatment with aspirin or corticosteroids will prove adequate in most instances.

BEDSORES (DECUBITUS ULCERS)

Bedsores are caused by *pressure* over bony areas (sacrum, elbows, heels). Ischemia is induced by compression of the blood vessels that supply these areas. Since decubiti can form within hours in living tissues (but not in cadavers), some surgeons hypothesize a lytic factor arising from ischemic, compressed, viable tissue. Ischemia (arterio-sclerosis) and anesthesia (paraplegia) are precedent factors in most cases. The disease affects the older, debilitated patient or the younger patient who has a neurological disease; paraplegics are extremely susceptible to bedsores.

Protection and *frequent movement* are the key words in prevention of bedsores. The nurse plays the principal role in prevention.

POSTOPERATIVE NEUROSES AND PSYCHOSES

When a surgical procedure has been successful and nonmutilating, most patients react with mild euphoria. They feel an inner satisfaction in having overcome a hazardous experience. *Depressions* normally occur after loss of any important part of the body, whether it be functionally or cosmetically deforming. Anxiety for an uncertain future in the patient's new state adds to the depression. Most patients, fortunately, adapt to these changes and resume a reasonably normal life. Severe depression characterized by withdrawal, restlessness, insomnia, expressions of hopelessness, and the desire for death should arouse suspicion of suicidal intent. The surgeon's responsibility includes listening to his patient, reassuring him, and closely following a patient with symptoms of depression. Much aid can be given to the patient with a colostomy, for example. Introducing him to colostomy clubs can mean an abrupt change of attitude. When he sees others who have accepted their colostomies and lead successful, normal lives, his adjustment to his colostomy is rapid and gratifying. Similarly with amputees, early positive emphasis on physical therapy and rehabilitation is one of the most important factors in a successful recovery.

Major personality disturbances are fortunately uncommon in the postoperative period. The stress of the illness, the intensity of therapy, and previous emotional makeup are the important underlying factors. A sudden, acute onset of symptoms, especially when the patient seems to overreact to the stresses, often foretells a good prognosis. The immediate problem lies in physically restraining and sedating the patient. Psychiatric consultation should be obtained for these reactions as well as for severe depressions, suicidal tendencies, or any other aberrancies of behavior that may threaten a normal recovery.

Dehydration and other disturbances in fluid and electrolyte balance may cause severe personality changes. (The problems are discussed in Chapter 3.) Sepsis, uremia, alcoholism, barbiturates, and other drugs are also known offenders in producing aberrant behavior patterns. History, physical examination, or specific chemical tests can uncover most of these causes.

SPECIFIC COMPLICATIONS

The purpose of this chapter has been to discuss complications that may arise after any operative procedure. Specific complications that arise only in certain circumstances such as thyroid storm or hypoparathyroidism are discussed in later chapters.

Each of the many highly technical operative procedures has its own technical complications. In shunting procedures for hydrocephalus, for example, a variety of technical failures result from attempts to shunt excess cerebrospinal fluid from the brain through man-made conduits to other parts of the body. As new operative techniques evolve in whatever field, a new set of technical complications will follow. Of necessity, these complications must be managed by those trained to recognize and treat them.

11
Malignant Neoplasms

George E. Moore

IMPACT OF CANCER

Cancer is a group of diseases (about 150 recognized types) of varied causes arising from many different tissues. The term "cancer" includes all disease with uncontrolled growth of cells that leads to serious disability and often death of the host. One must understand that these different cancers vary tremendously both in biological characteristics and in their effects on the patient. Each kind of cancer should be considered separately.

Cancer is the second leading cause of death in the United States (Fig. 11-1). Unless some unforeseen and providential cancer prevention or treatment is discovered, one in four persons, or almost 52 million people living today, have or will develop cancer. In 1984 there were about 870,000 new cases of cancer plus about 45,000 cancers in situ of the cervix and 400,000 skin cancers. (Skin cancers are listed separately because of their high, 98$^+$%, curability.) Melanomas of the skin are quite deadly and are considered separately. About 450,000 patients will die of cancerous neoplasms or tumors—over 1,200 each day. In the last 10 years there have been over 4.5 million cancer deaths and medical costs exceeding $30 billion a year.

Much of this pain and suffering and expense could be avoided. In the past 30 years the 5-year "cure rate" (without evidence of disease 5 years after treatment) has improved from one in four to one in three persons. Improvement in detection and treatment as well as changes in the incidences of several major cancers influence this result. As the number of elderly persons increases, so does the total number of cancer patients.

In this chapter we discuss the chief features of this enormous medical, economic, and sociological problem. The management of specific types of cancer is outlined in following chapters.

EPIDEMIOLOGY— THE GLOBAL PERSPECTIVE

Cancer is a worldwide problem with poorly understood but intriguing racial, ethnic, sex, age, and geographical differences; e.g., carcinoma of the stomach has been rapidly decreasing in the United States. On the other hand, female breast cancer so common in the United States (one in 11) is rare in Japan.

Burkitt's lymphoma, a curious malignancy frequently affecting children in tropical Africa, may be caused in part by a DNA virus (Epstein-Barr virus, EBV) and perhaps impairment of the victim's resistance by malaria or other environmental factors. Another strange tumor—nasopharyngeal cancer—is frequent in China and localities in the Mideast and has a causative relationship with EBV.

There are many myths about special places that are cancer free. Usually there are no health facilities in such places and thus few authentic diagnoses, and also the inhabitants usually die at a young age. In brief, there are no multicellular animal species free of cancer. There are environmental and genetic factors that alter the development of various kinds of cancer, but unknown factors predominate.

Cancer of the lung, the leading cancer in men, is about five times more common in male than in female Americans. However, women (who started

Rank	Cause of Death	Number of Deaths	Death Rate per 100,000 Population	Percent of Total Deaths
	All Causes	**1,913,841**	**785.0**	**100.0**
1.	Heart Diseases	733,235	294.4	38.3
2.	Cancer	403,395	169.4	21.1
3.	Cerebrovascular Diseases	169,488	66.4	8.9
4.	Accidents	105,312	44.9	5.5
5.	Chronic Obstructive Lung Disease	49,933	20.5	2.6
6.	Pneumonia & Influenza	45,030	17.6	2.4
7.	Diabetes Mellitus	33,192	13.6	1.7
8.	Cirrhosis of Liver	29,720	13.1	1.6
9.	Arteriosclerosis	28,801	10.6	1.5
10.	Suicide	27,206	11.4	1.4
11.	Diseases of Infancy	23,448	12.2	1.2
12.	Homicide	22,550	9.4	1.2
13.	Nephritis	15,729	6.3	0.8
14.	Aortic Aneurysm	14,031	5.7	0.7
15.	Congenital Anomalies	13,526	6.8	0.7
	Other & Ill–defined	199,245	82.7	10.4

Source: Vital Statistics of the United States, 1979.

Fig. 11-1. Mortality for leading causes of death in the United States in 1979. (From Cancer Statistics, 1984, CA-A Cancer Journal for Clinicians **34**(1):7,1984; from Vital Statistics of the United States, 1979.)

Table 11-1. Selected human carcinogens

Carcinogens	Organ system
Chemical (occupational and social)	
Chimney soot	Scrotal skin
Asbestos (usually with smoking)	Mesothelioma, lung
Cigarette smoke	Lung, bladder, larynx
Aniline dyes	Bladder
Hydrocarbon compounds	
Benzene	Bone marrow
Coal tar and pitch, creosote	Skin, scrotum, lip
Mineral oils, other petroleum	Skin, scrotum
Halogenated hydrocarbons	Various tumors
Ethylene dibromide (EDB)	
DDT, DBDP, heptachlor, etc.	
Vinyl chloride	Liver (hemangiosarcoma)
Arsenic	Skin, lung, liver
Chromium, nickel, cadmium	Lung, nasal cavity
Physical	
Ionizing radiation	Many organs, bone
Particulate: Thorotrast, etc.	marrow, thyroid connective tissue
Ultraviolet radiation	Skin (basal and squamous cell carcinoma, possible melanoma)
Dietary	
Aflatoxins	Liver
Nitrosamines	Gastrointestinal tract
Toxic plants: cycad, bracken, safrole	Small and large bowel, liver
Alcohol	Oral cavity, esophagus, liver
Immunosuppressive agents and antineoplastic drugs	Reticulum cell sarcoma, epithelial malignancies of skin and viscera
Antilymphocyte serum	
Corticosteroids	
Anticancer agents (many)	
Hormones	
Estrogens (prenatal)	Vagina, cervix
Androgenic steroids	Liver
Hypohormone, e.g., thyroid	Thyroid
Biological	
Viruses	Over 300 malignancies, many species
Epstein-Barr virus	Burkitt's lymphoma (?), nasopharynx (?)
Unknown virus	Acquired immunodeficiency syndrome (AIDS), Kaposi's sarcoma
Oncogenes	Many tissues

smoking heavily about two decades after men) are beginning to catch up. Breast and uterine cancer are the most common female cancers, but lung cancer will soon be more frequent. Most of these excessive cancer deaths from tobacco use (affecting cells of the lung, mouth, throat, esophagus, bladder, and pancreas) could be prevented.

Despite the association of cancer and aging, malignancies can occur at any age. Malignancies are now a major cause of death in children. (See Chapter 28.) The development of cancers may take from 5 to 40 years, and the host's ability to destroy or restrain cancer cells may be lessened with aging.

ETIOLOGY

The causes of some of the 150 kinds of human cancer are known; causes of others are complex or unknown. Genetic factors and susceptibilities are associated with both precancerous and cancerous growths, as follows:

Hereditary neoplasia—examples
    Retinoblastoma
    Nevoid basal cell carcinoma
    Trichoepithelioma
    Multiple endocrine adenomatosis
    Chemodectomas
    Gardner's syndrome
Genetic factors—examples
    Polyposis coli
    Albinism or light skin and blue eyes
    Immune deficiencies
    Chromosome abnormalities

Cancers develop more frequently in patients with suppressed immunity after organ transplantation, a condition resembling some inherited immune deficiencies. Breast cancer is more frequent in daughters whose mothers or maternal grandmothers have had breast cancer, especially if it developed before menopause. Persons with red hair, blue eyes, and light skin are far more likely to develop skin cancers and malignant melanoma. Some known and suspected causes of cancers are listed in Table 11-1. There are also "promoting agents" that by themselves do not cause cancer but increase the carcinogenicity of causal factors by stimulating the growth of the cancerous cells.

Cancerous cells have permanent genetic changes and often both increased numbers of chromosomes and abnormal chromosomes. Cancer cells escape many but not all the normal restraints of the body.

COMMON SITES OF CANCER

Although cancers can originate in any organ, certain sites are more common than others (Fig. 11-2). With the exception of melanomas, skin cancer, the most common human cancer, is seldom

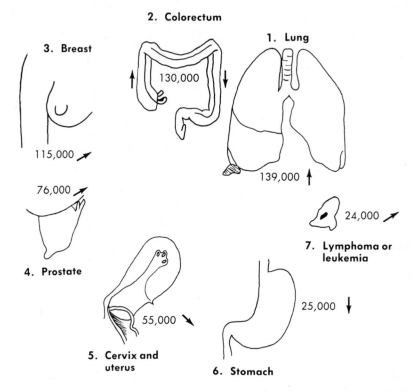

Fig. 11-2. Sites of cancer (in adults of both sexes) in frequency of occurrence, 1984. *Arrows,* Increase or decrease in incidence. (↑ , Increasing rapidly; ↓ , decreasing rapidly; ↗ , increasing slowly; ↘ , decreasing slowly.)

fatal. Table 11-2 lists the eight that are the most common killing cancers (Fig. 11-3). Together they account for about two thirds of all cancer fatalities.

SPONTANEOUS REGRESSION OF CANCER

The course of almost all cancers is relentlessly progressive, but rare instances of spontaneous regression are recorded. Spontaneous regression of cancer strongly suggests an immune response by the host or a change in hormone levels that the cancer cells required for growth. Some malignancies such as malignant melanoma may have high (5% to 10%) regression rates, whereas others such as gastric carcinoma have regressions less than 0.1%.

KNOWN IMMUNE FACTORS

Two examples of the enormous effects of immune factors upon the development of cancer are (1) the development of malignancies when the normal immune defenses are suppressed so that

Table 11-2. Most common cancers that kill

Site	Estimated new cancers (1984)
Lung	139,000
Colon and rectum	130,000
Breast	115,000
Prostate	76,000
Uterus	55,000
Pancreas	25,000
Stomach	25,000
Hematopoietic tissue	24,000

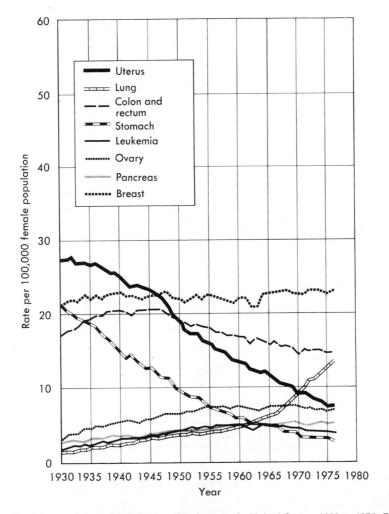

Fig. 11-3. Death rates, male and female, by site of cancer in United States, 1930 to 1976. Rates for male and female population standardized for age on 1940 United States population. (Data from U.S. National Center for Health Statistics and U.S. Bureau of the Census.) *Continued.*

kidney transplants will survive and (2) the use of topical immunotherapy to destroy superficial skin cancers. Patients with kidney transplants have a much higher risk of several kinds of cancer: cancers of the skin and hematopoietic tissues as well as epithelial and connective tissues. A foreign cancer accidently implanted with a donor kidney will regress if the immunosuppression is reversed.

The second example reflects the ability of lymphoid cells to recognize and destroy tumor cells after adhering to them.

SPREAD OF CANCER CELLS

A few malignancies consist of cells with a strong adherence for each other. Such cancers, e.g., basal cell carcinoma of the skin, may grow and invade immediate normal tissues but rarely spread or metastasize to distant organs. They can be cured by local treatments: excisional surgery, radiation therapy, or cautery.

Unfortunately a majority of malignancies have cells that can live and divide as single elements. They penetrate into lymphatic and blood vessels, grow along tissue planes, and colonize distant

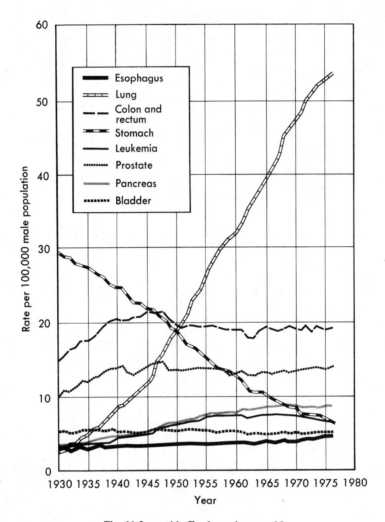

Fig. 11-3, cont'd. For legend see p. 85.

organs and body cavities. Clumps of malignant cells carried by the lymph and blood to distant organs embolize smaller vessels, penetrate into the tissues, and form enlarging metastases that interfere with vital organ functions.

In general, sarcomatous malignancies spread predominantly through the vascular system and epithelial carcinomas through the lymphatic vessels. Many cancers spread by both routes. Although some tissues are more receptive ("make better soil") to some kinds of cancer cells, anatomic considerations affect the predominant sites of metastases. Carcinomas of the colon are more likely to invade the blood vessels of the portal system; therefore liver metastases are common,

whereas cancers of the kidney more often invade systemic blood vessels leading to metastases of the lungs.

Isolated single metastases are rare. Usually, if the cancerous cells and clumps of cells have the biological capability of producing metastases, metastases will develop in more than one organ. However, even multiple metastases can sometimes be destroyed or controlled and the patient cured by a combination of therapies; e.g., the use of surgery, radiation, and chemotherapy to cure Hodgkin's disease.

The clinician must remember that metastases often represent selective growth of tumor cells that have mutated and may no longer have the same

Table 11-3. Cancers that mimic endocrine syndromes

Syndrome	Hormone	Source
Polycythemia	Erythropoietin	Kidney cancer
Ectopic Cushing's syndrome	ACTH-like	Lung cancer
Hyperglycemia	Glucagon-like	Sarcomas
Hypercalcemia	Parathyroid-like	Breast, lung cancer
Carcinoid syndrome	Serotonin	Carcinoid, bowel cancer
Inappropriate ADH	ADH	Lung cancer, others

responses to therapy as the primary tumor did. For example, a primary beast tumor may have progesterone receptors and be expected to respond to hormone antagonists, but one half of the metastases will not have the receptors and therefore must be treated by cytotoxic agents.

HORMONE RECEPTORS

Many tumor cells retain the normal receptor proteins for various hormones such as insulin, thyroxine, cortisone, estrogen, progesterone, and testosterone. In general more primitive cancer cells do not have hormone receptors and are independent of the need for hormones for growth. The detection of hormone receptors in breast cancers have importat prognostic significance and indicate whether hormones and hormone antagonists can be used to control tumor growth.

CANCER-ENDOCRINE SYNDROMES

Some cancers have the extraordinary ability to produce hormones and thus mimic endocrine syndromes. Oat cell lung cancer, a notable example, can secrete a number of hormones (or hormone-like substances), such as ACTH, parathyroid hormone, ADH, and TSH. These curious syndromes are listed in Table 11-3.

These interesting syndromes tell us much about the multipotentials of the living cell. All somatic cells have a complement of 46 chromosomes and have the potential to produce a wide variety of proteins, enzymes, and hormones. Many genes in these chromosomes are repressed ("turned off") during the process of normal differentiation and maturation, and so the expression of only a few specific genes is allowed in each cell. The neoplastic cell, by additions, deletions, and functional changes in the genes, escapes from these controls. By a process of derepression, some inactive genetic loci become activated. These loci direct the production of embryonic proteins, hormones, and enzymes that can sometimes be detected in cancer patients. For example, the appearance of carcinoembryonic antigen (CEA) in the blood is helpful in allowing detection of some early recurrent

tumors of the colon and pancreas. Removal of the tumor can reverse the endocrine abnormality, but usually these syndromes reflect an underlying, inoperable cancer.

DIAGNOSIS

The symptoms and signs of cancer are as diverse as the wide variety of cancer sites and the resultant functional disturbances. In some cases metastases may herald the existence of the cancer. The origin of the metastasis may sometimes be determined by (1) histological appearance, (2) electron microscopy, (3) cancer cell products or hormone receptors, and (4) the pattern of lymphatic spread. In some cases of diffuse carcinomatosis the precise origin of the cancer remains obscure. About 50% of all patients dying from cancer have predominant metastatic spread to lymph nodes, 36% have liver metastases, and 30% have pulmonary involvement; as previously mentioned, epithelial cancers usually spread through the lymphatics, and sarcomas spread through the bloodstream. The cancers that metastasize to the liver most frequently are those of the pancreas, stomach, esophagus, and colon, which invade the portal vein.

About 15% to 20% of patients with fatal cancers show skeletal metastases. Cancers frequently metastasize to the bones from the breast, prostate, lung, thyroid, kidney, and even malignant lymphomas and Hodgkin's disease. The bones most frequently involved include the vertebrae, ribs, skull, femur, pelvis, humerus, and sternum. The bones and areas of bones with cellular marrow trap the cancer cells from the blood. Distant spread to the brain occurs in about 5% of fatal cases of malignant neoplasm. Cancers of the breast, lung, and kidney, and melanoma contribute most of the metastatic growths in the brain. Curiously, primary cancers in the brain rarely metastasize to other parts of the body.

Some recent developments allow more specific and early localization of both primary and metastatic disease, e.g., brain and liver scans with radioisotopes, CT scans, ultrasound, angiography, and mammography—a very important special

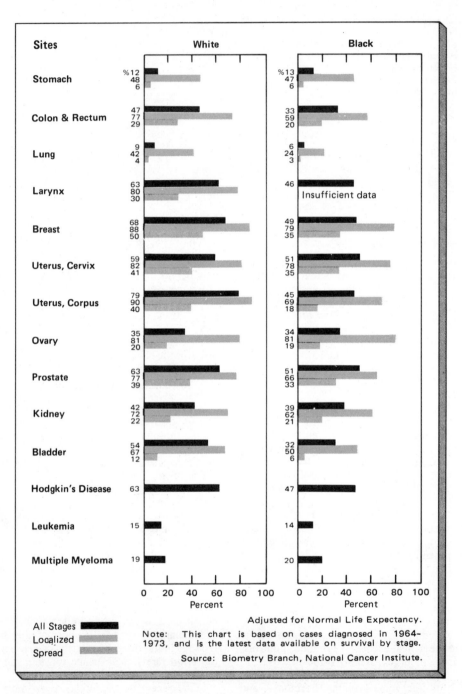

Fig. 11-4. Five-year cancer survival rates for selected sites by race, 1964 to 1973, and adjusted for normal life expectancy.

x-ray study of the breasts. Flexible bronchoscopes gastroscopes and colonoscopes have decreased the discomfort to the patient and greatly improved the diagnosis. Of particular value is the ability to biopsy suspected lesions through them.

Cytological samples of tumor tissue can be obtained for the pathologist by suction aspiration of cells through a fine needle. A core of tissue can be excised by larger needles with a cutting mechanism. Still larger specimens are obtained by surgical incision or excision of the suspected tumor. The presence of tumor cells in a pleural or peritoneal effusion is detected after the cells are concentrated by centrifugation and then they are fixed and stained on slides for microscopic examination.

A new method of tumor cell identification uses monoclonal antibodies against specific cell products or antigens. These can be applied to both cytological preparations and sections of tissue.

PROGNOSIS

The 5-year "cure" rate for all cancer is now about one in three patients. Fig. 11-4 gives the 5-year survival rates for some common neoplasms. The importance of lymph-node metastases in the prognosis of cancer is obvious from these examples.

TREATMENT

Three methods of treating cancers are widely used: surgery, irradiation, and chemotherapy. The mode of treatment depends on the type and extent of the tumor. Immunotherapy and chemoimmunotherapy are still chiefly experimental.

Surgery

The fundamental aim of surgery is to remove all of the tumor with the least disruption of the structures and functions of the host. In some cases of advanced cancers palliative procedures such as bypassing bile around a cancer of the pancreas may bring gratifying symptomatic relief. Resection of a colon cancer may prevent obstruction even though liver metastases are present. Occasionally resection of isolated metastases to lung, liver, brain, or other sites results in astonishingly long survivals and rarely even cures.

In early cancers without evidence of systemic invasion, surgical excision is often the preferred primary treatment used in an attempt to cure the patient. It may be extended to include the removal of regional lymph nodes. Excisional surgery may be supplemented with adjuvant radiation therapy and hormonal and chemotherapy.

Radiation therapy

Because ionizing radiation alters the reproductive process of cells, it can destroy cancer and inhibit its growth. Although it destroys both normal and neoplastic cells, normal cells have a greater capacity for repair and recovery. The degree of success depends on the difference in radioresponsiveness of the tumor compared to the surrounding normal tissues (Table 11-4). This response differential (therapeutic ratio) is extremely important, for it may enable us to control tumors whose cells have little sensitivity to radiation but are growing in tissues that will tolerate the high dose of radiation necessary for tumor control, e.g., soft-tissue sarcoma in an extremity. On the other hand, some radiosensitive tumors may be surrounded by tissues that will not withstand even the lowest effective tumor dose, e.g., lymphoma in the region of the kidneys.

The primary intent of radiation therapy is to cure; the secondary intent is to palliate. When evaluating a patient with cancer, the radiotherapist must first decide whether the tumor is likely to be susceptible to growth reduction by its sensitivity to radiation and by its overall size and site as well. He must localize the tumor precisely by radiographic studies, radioactive isotope scans, diagnostic ultrasound, and sometimes even surgical exploration. He must spare the surrounding normal tissues from unnecessary radiation. Computers play a valuable role in complex mathematical calculations needed to plan treatment.

Radiation functions either as a primary mode of treatment or in combination with surgical removal, chemotherapy or both. Radiotherapy may be used either preoperatively or postoperatively, depending on the type, location, and extent of the tumor.

Radiotherapy and surgery, in general, are not competitive treatments. Each has its area of greatest effectiveness, though many tumors respond equally to either modality. Factors such as cosmetic results, length of treatment cost and availability of facilities help the physician and patient choose the best treatment. Whatever method is selected, *the optimal time for cure is the first therapeutic attempt.*

Therefore the overall treatment of a patient is often planned by a conference of radiologist, surgeon, internist-oncologist, and pathologist before any treatment is started.

Palliation

The radiotherapist often treats painful or crippling metastases. Patients sometimes respond with gratifying relief of symptoms. New high-voltage generators and linear accelerators have greatly increased the effectiveness of radiotherapy. Interstitial needles, "threads," and other applicators of radioisotopes are available for intensive radiation of extensive tumors.

Table 11-4. Radiosensitivity classification of normal tissues and malignant tumors

Relative radiosensitivity	Normal tissues	Primary malignancies
High	Lymphoid Hematopoietic Spermatogenic cells (testis) Follicular epithelium (ovary) Optic lens	Leukemia Lymphoma Hodgkin's disease Medulloblastoma Seminoma Dysgerminoma Retinoblastoma Anaplastic carcinoma

Medium	Skin
	Epithelium (mucosal linings)
	Endothelium (vascular)
	Growing cartilage
	Growing bone
		Basal cell carcinoma
		Squamous cell carcinoma
		Adenocarcinoma
		  Uterus
		  Breast
		  Bowel
		  Prostate
		Liposarcoma
		Bronchogenic carcinoma
		Astrocytoma
		Rhabdomyosarcoma

Low	Connective tissue Muscle Fat Bone Nerve	Other adenocarcinomas Hypernephroma Teratoma Osteogenic tumors Melanoma Other sarcomas (differentiated)

Chemotherapy

The quest for a specific drug or drugs to destroy tumor cells selectively has brought some striking results, most notably a 70% (or higher) cure rate for choriocarcinomas with methotrexate. Many cures and extended periods of remission have been achieved in patients with leukemias, lymphomas, childhood sarcomas, and kidney malignancies. Chemotherapy can be used effectively in association with radiation therapy and surgical excision. Grossly and morphologically, cancers differ from normal tissues, but no known qualitative difference separates them on a chemical or molecular level. There are, however, a number of quantitative dissimilarities (enzymes and metabolites) and growth rates that permit selective chemotherapy. If a qualitative difference is discovered, a drug or drugs can be designed to exploit this difference. Of the hundreds of thousands of antitumor agents tested in the past, only a few have proved to be useful clinically.

The same therapeutic principles apply to cancer drugs as to surgery and irradiation. The drugs must destroy the tumor but must not irreparably injure the host. Unfortunately, the results of chemotherapy are often uncertain, unpredictable, and temporary. The drugs currently available have a very slight therapeutic advantage when compared to their toxicity on normal cells. Thus chemotherapy drugs are given in doses as high as possible before serious toxicity occurs. Just as radiation is fractionated so that the normal cells have a preferential chance of recovery, so too are chemotherapy drugs given in cycles. Most of the drugs interfere with RNA or DNA synthesis. Many cells of the body (especially those of the blood-forming organs, gastrointestinal tract, and hair follicles) divide rapidly and are therefore vulnerable to cytolytic agents.

Combinations of drugs attack cancer cells at several critical points of protein synthesis and DNA replication. Tumor masses often originate from a single cell but are unstable and mutate into related cells with differing susceptibility to chemotherapy; therefore combinations of drugs are desirable.

Agents in current use are classified as follows:

Alkylating agents: nitrogen mustard, cyclophosphamide, phenylalanine mustard, Thio-TEPA, nitrosoureas (BCNU, CCNU), glycarbylamide, dacarbazine (DTIC)

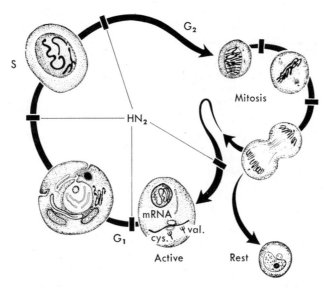

Fig. 11-5. Cell cycle and chemotherapy. Most cytolytic agents act on cell at some point in cell cycle. Nitrogen mustard (HN_2) can act at almost any position. Cells are usually most vulnerable during S, or synthetic, phase of DNA synthesis. *cys.*, Cysteine; *val.*, valine.

Antimetabolites: methotrexate, 6-mercaptopurine, 5-fluorouracil
Antibiotics: actinomycin D, doxorubicin (adriamycin), bleomycin
Alkaloids: vincristine, vinblastine
Hormones: estrogens, androgens, corticosteroids, thyroxine
Antihormones: antiestrogens, antiadrenaline, antiprolactin
Miscellaneous: urethan, *o,p'*-DDD, stilbestrol

Most of these drugs disrupt metabolic functions at certain phases of the cell cycle (Fig. 11-5). Nitrogen mustard, cyclophosphamide, and other alkylating agents can disrupt function at almost any point in the cycle, whereas other drugs are more specific. Alkylating agents are often termed "radiomimetic." They bind and disrupt the DNA strands and therefore have an effect somewhat like radiation therapy. The *Vinca rosea* alkaloids produce their antineoplastic effect during the mitotic phase of the cell cycle. Actinomycin D prevents the transcription of DNA to RNA during the G1 phase of the cycle. Many of the other drugs including 5-fluorouracil, 6-mercaptopurine, cytosine arabinoside, and methotrexate act during the S (synthetic) phase of the cell cycle. Drugs can modify the metabolic processes in the cell at either a molecular or an organelle level.

Some drugs attack specific cells, e.g., *o,p'*-DDD versus adrenocortical tumors; streptozotocin versus pancreatic islet cell tumors.

Some of the solid tumors that are palliated by cytotoxic agents are listed in Table 11-5.

Adjuvant chemotherapy supplements surgery (or radiation) with drugs. For example, a series of drugs and drug combinations have improved the life of breast cancer patients. The advent of hormone receptor assays will permit antihormone therapy in selected patients. Ovariectomy, adrenalectomy, and hypophysectomy may be considered either adjuvant surgery or adjuvant hormone therapy. Medical "adrenalectomy" can be achieved by the interruption of steroids from cholesterol by aminoglutethimide.

Thyroxine is frequently used as an adjuvant to the excision of thyroid cancer by reason of its inhibition of thyrotropic hormone release from the pituitary.

The thesis that adjuvant chemotherapy should produce cures or more effective palliation when the least number of tumor cells are present is logical, but, unfortunately, well-controlled studies have not confirmed the effectiveness of most available drugs.

Complications of chemotherapy

Since the therapeutic amount of these drugs approaches the toxic level, cancer chemotherapy carries a substantial morbidity. All normal, rapidly dividing cells within the organism are vulnerable to these cytolytic agents. The most serious complication of this type of therapy is bone marrow depres-

Table 11-5. Selected solid tumors palliated by cytotoxic agents.

Malignancy	Primary drug(s)	Secondary drug(s)
Hodgkin's disease and lymphomas	COPP: cyclophosphamide, vincristine sulfate (Oncovin), procarbazine, prednisone	Doxorubicin, chlorambucil
Wilms' tumor	Actinomycin + vincristine	Doxorubicin
Sarcomas	Doxorubicin, methotrexate + "rescue"	Vincristine, cyclophosphamide
Bladder	Doxorubicin, fluorouracil	Cyclophosphamide, *cis*-platinum
Breast		
Hormones	Fluoxymesterone, tamoxifen	Stilbestrol, testolactone
Cytotoxins	Fluorouracil, cyclophosphamide, methotrexate, doxorubicin	Melphalan
Lung	Doxorubicin + cyclophosphamide + vincristine	
Colon and rectum	Fluorouracil	Combinations
Stomach	Fluorouracil	Mitomycin, combinations
Melanoma	Dacarbazine	Combination
Liver and biliary tract	Fluorouracil, antiestrogens	Doxorubicin, cyclophosphamide
Ovary	Doxorubicin + cyclophosphamide	Melphalan
Uterus, endometrium	Melphalan + fluorouracil	Antihormones
	Doxorubicin + cytoxin	*cis*-Platinum

sion. Most drugs depress all elements of active bone marrow. An alkylating agent (cyclophosphamide) usually spares the thrombocytes, whereas actinomycin may attack them. Vincristine is more selectively neurotoxic than myelotoxic (marrow toxic). Doxorubicin (adriamycin) has unique and dangerous toxic effects on the cardiac cell.

The cells in the hair follicles divide rapidly and consequently are vulnerable to chemotherapy; temporary baldness may occur. The incidence of alopecia may be 30% with a single drug such as fluorouracil and 100% with doxorubicin (adriamycin) and with combinations. Hair regrows after cessation of therapy. Occasionally dermatitis may result from drug therapy, but it is usually limited to the period of drug administration.

The cells within the alimentary tract also have a rapid turnover rate. Cytotoxic agents cause varying degrees of mucosal damage and attendant symptoms—melena, cramps, diarrhea, dysphagia, and sepsis.

Maximum toxicity may not become manifest until 5 to 10 days or to as long as 3 weeks after discontinuance of therapy; thus multiple doses must be given with great care. A 2% to 4% mortality is associated with the use of potent cytolytic agents. Infection is the most common cause of death.

If a malignant lesion is sensitive to drug therapy, it usually responds early, completely, and for long intervals.

Tumors may develop resistance to the effect of chemotherapy after a period of 2 to 18 months. Usually this results from the overgrowth of mutant cancer cells insensitive to the drug. In such an instance other drugs should be given.

The dosage of toxic chemotherapeutic agents must be given accurately and with consideration of the patient's condition. The dosage is usually calculated from body surface or normal body weight. If a patient is obese, the dosage should be estimated from "ideal" weight.

The physician must be particularly careful to avoid serious toxic reactions, especially common with (1) multiple drugs, (2) malnutrition, (3) combinations of therapies, e.g., surgery and x-ray treatments, (4) infection, (5) diabetes, (6) obesity, (7) old age, and (8) passivity and inactivity.

Hyperalimentation and new antiemetic drugs such as metoclopramide have improved the ability of patients to tolerate high does of chemotherapy.

Regional administration of chemotherapeutic agents

Widely disseminated tumors require systemic chemotherapy, but localized tumors respond best to high concentrations of drugs. Infusion and perfusion increase drug concentration to the tumor yet spare other parts of the body.

Intra-arterial infusion. Since cells are most vulnerable during certain stages of mitosis, the anticancer drug must be present at this time. Often cancer cells are "mitotically" out of step; therefore the drug must be offered over a period of time. We inject the anticancer agent through a cannulated

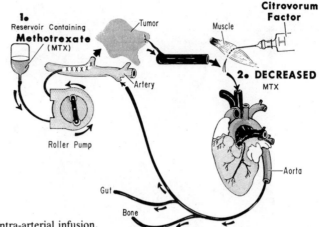

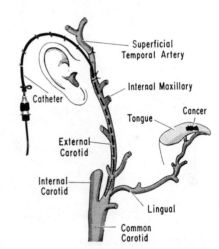

Fig. 11-6. Regional intra-arterial infusion.

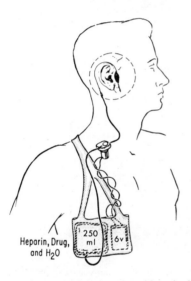

Fig. 11-7. Intra-arterial infusion. Portable unit allows full ambulation. Implantable units are available.

Fig. 11-8. Intra-arterial infusion. Notice precise placement of catheter orifice at takeoff of lingual artery to infuse cancer of tongue.

artery supplying the tumor. The tumor receives the full force of the drug continuously over a period of weeks or months. It can be diluted and antagonized in the peripheral circulation by the normal metabolite so that other areas of the body receive only minimal dosages of the agent (Fig. 11-6). Citrovorum factor is used with methotrexate to antagonize its action on normal cells. Head and neck tumors, advanced pelvic tumors, melanomas of the extremities, and hepatic metastases have been

controlled by this method (Figs. 11-7 and 11-8).

Perfusion. A portion of the body (usually an extremity) is isolated by tourniquet, and the isolated portion is made a part of an extracorporeal circuit by cannulation of both artery and vein. An anticancer drug (e.g., phenylalanine mustard, actinomycin D, or doxorubicin) in high concentration is then introduced. After perfusion, the therapist washes out the isolated area and restores vascular continuity. This technique can be repeated at inter-

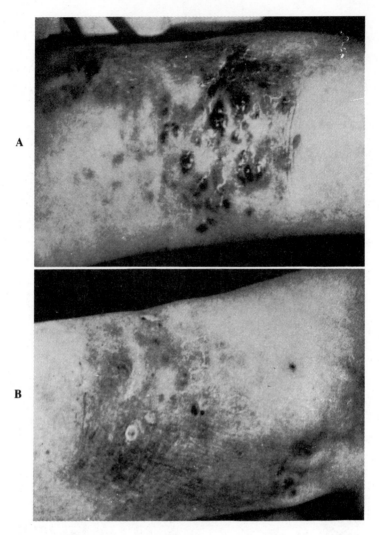

Fig. 11-9. Recurrent melanoma. **A,** Before perfusion. **B,** After perfusion (phenylalanine mustard). (From Stehlin, J.S., Jr., and others: Ann. Surg. **151:**605-619, 1960.)

vals necessary to control cancer growth. Perfusion (prophylactically) supplements primary resection of cancers, notably melanomas (Figs. 11-9 and 11-10). After wide excision of all gross tumor (primary melanoma), the incidence of local recurrence and in-transit metastases (metastases between the tumor and nearest lymph nodes) average 15% to 20%. These smaller aggregates of cells in lymphatic blood vessels and tissues are probably most vulnerable to prophylactic perfusion at the time of excision of the primary tumor and its metastases. Perfusion also helps palliate far-

advanced or recurrent malignant melanomas and sarcomas of the extremities. Implantable reservoirs connected to cannulated vessels are useful over many months (Gyres et al., 1984).

Combined therapy

Irradiation combined with infusion has successfully palliated far-advanced cancers in the head and neck region (Fig. 11-11).

Combinations of drugs systemically have improved results, e.g., methotrexate, chlorambucil, and actinomycin D in the treatment of embryonal

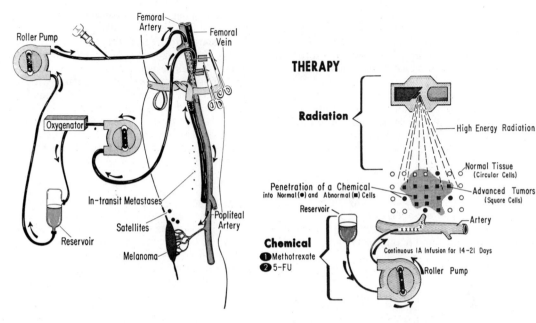

Fig. 11-10. Regional intra-arterial perfusion.

Fig. 11-11. Simultaneous radiation and chemotherapy.

cancer of the testicle. Some regimens include as many as five to seven drugs and may be combined with hyperthermia.

Nonspecific important treatment of cancer patient

A majority of patients will suffer from advanced cancer. The physician must combine his technical skill with a vitally important sensitivity and sympathy. He must sustain some degree of hope for the patient, yet not mislead him. The cancer patient often goes through phases of rage (Why me?) and rejection (I don't believe it.) and antagonism to those caring for him before progressing to an acceptance of his serious and possibly fatal disease. The physician must guide the patient through these emotionally grueling periods. The patient will sense that he is in the hands of an aggressive yet sympathetic therapist who is knowledgeable about new therapies. Optimal care and support of the patient require the skills of internist, radiologist, surgeon, physiotherapist, nurse, social worker, and, of great importance, the informed close relatives. In addition to this desirable team effort a patient should have a single physician to whom he can relate his hopes and fears.

Patients with cancer, even when far advanced, do not necessarily have severe pain. The discomfort is often a minimal physical stimulus (fatigue, loss of interest) with maximum overlay of anxiety and the loss of normal activity and work patterns. The loss of independence and an increasing dependence on others is frustrating. There are many methods of controlling pain without narcotics. Local or regional pain, can be controlled by peripheral nerve blocks with alcohol, epidural instillation of phenol, and other modifications of local and regional anesthesia. (See Chapter 40.) Early addiction of a cancer patient induces tolerance, which reduces the effectiveness of narcotics when tolerance is most needed. Combination of tranquilizers, sleep-inducing drugs, and programs of activities all aid in minimizing the use of narcotics. Oral forms of many drugs permit the competent patient to adjust his medications to meet his individual needs.

In addition to the psychological and painful aspects of malignant disease, other manifestations of distant and local involvement demand treatment. Effusions of the pleural and peritoneal cavities can be controlled by drainage, systemic chemotherapy, local instillation of drugs, sodium restriction, and diuretics. Pleural effusions are particularly distressful because they slowly suffocate patients. Patients who cannot tolerate cytolytic agents because of bone marrow depression may require quinacrine injections (50 mg. initially, and daily increments of up to 200 or 250 mg.). Peritoneal effusions may be shunted back into the venous system through catheters with one-way valves (the Denver shunt). Care must be exercised, since disseminated intravascular coagulation may occur.

Metastases to the central nervous system are common from lung and breast cancer and melanomas. Craniotomy may be worthwhile to remove a single mass that causes symptoms. Steroids and radiotherapy may also relieve increased intracranial pressure.

Metastasis can collapse vertebral bodies, with subsequent pressure on the spinal cord or spinal nerves. Epidural metastases may impinge on nerves without bony involvement. When symptoms of compression rapidly progress, emergency laminectomy and radiotherapy may prevent complete paralysis.

Bony metastases occasionally result in pathological fractures. The pain of bone metastasis can often be controlled with radiation therapy, and pathological fractures will often heal. Fractures of weight-bearing bones often require immobilization by the use of intramedullary devices followed by radiation therapy. If possible, these techniques should be applied before the fracture occurs.

The superior vena cava may be selectively obstructed in patients with lymphomas and lung cancer. Simultaneous chemotherapy and radiation therapy may be palliative for these patients.

The patient with bowel obstruction may benefit from a resection, intestinal bypass, gastrostomy, ileostomy, or colostomy. Cervical esophagostomy (which prevents accumulation of secretions in the pharynx and bronchial aspiration) can be palliative for patients with high esophageal obstruction. By supplying calories and other nutritional elements, hyperalimentation aids healing, extends palliation, and supports the patient during chemotherapy. (See Chapter 7.)

The prompt treatment of the cancer-endocrine syndromes, e.g., hypercalcemia in association with breast cancer, can prolong and improve vitality. Adrenocortical steroids, mithramycin, restriction of calcium, and increased fluid intake with diuretics may lower hypercalcemia. Adrenalectomy or o,p'-DDD may palliate ectopic Cushing's syndrome. Bromocriptine mesylate, aminoglutethimide, fluorouracil, and other newer drugs may inhibit hormone synthesis.

Several nonspecific antigens associated with tumors are useful clinically; their appearance in serum helps to detect underlying cancers and their recurrence. About 70% of patients with hepatomas show elevated serum levels of alpha fetoglobulin.

The hepatoma cells, reverting back to the embryonic forms that normally produce this antigen during early life, secrete it pathologically. Elevated serum levels indicate hepatoma or hepatocarcinoma. Carcinoembryonic antigen (CEA), another fetal antigen, increases in the serum with gastrointestinal cancers and some other cancers such as those of the lung and breast but with inflammatory diseases as well. CEA will detect most patients with recurrent colon cancers. CEA serum levels drop after successful resection and rise with recurrence.

IMMUNOLOGY AND CANCER

Investigators, long suspecting a link between cancer and the body's defense mechanisms, have cited the following evidence to support their suspicions: (1) some cancers have miraculously disappeared without explanation other than some "inherent defense mechanisms"; (2) pathologists have noticed that lymphoid cells tend to cluster about certain cancers, and these cancers seem to have a favorable course; (3) cytological studies have revealed convincing evidence that cancer cells flood the circulation, especially during surgical procedures, yet few grow into neoplasms; (4) some defense mechanisms even in patients with advanced cancers resist the development of additional tumors; (5) immunosuppression may enhance carcinogenesis and cell growth. Malignancies develop more frequently in patients with organ transplants and in those with AIDS (acquired immunodeficiency syndrome).

Immune response

The body, sensing foreign cells through memory-cell surveillance, responds immunologically in two ways to cancer: (1) a cell-mediated reaction and (2) with humoral antibodies. Lymphoid cells play a leading role. The T-cells, derived from the thymus, include subsets of "killer cells." They recognize the cancer cell as "foreign," attach to cell membranes, and lyse the cells. The B-cells (from bursal equivalent) produce tumor antibodies (Ab) that neutralize antigen or act in delayed sensitivity reactions and, with complement, can lyse cells. Although the cell-mediated response appears dominant, both mechanisms interact in their attempt to destroy tumors. (See Chapter 36.)

Immunotherapy

Because radiation and surgery are effective only against local and regional sites of primary and metastatic cancer, the oncologist must consider systemic therapy to kill or control disseminated cancer cells. Chemotherapy, hormones, hormone

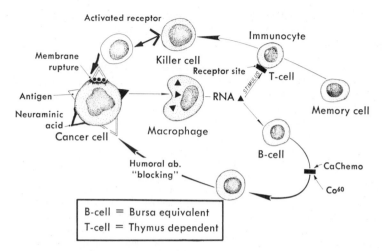

Fig. 11-12. Immunological surveillance: tumor-specific antigen or cancer cell processed by macrophage. Product (immune RNA?) sensitizes T-cells, which seek out and destroy cancer cell if it is not protected by "blocking" substance.

antagonists, and maturation agents are used for this purpose. Immunotherapy theoretically would attack only antigen-associated cancer cells, thus sparing normal cells. The ablative therapies reduce the main mass of tumor cells (called "debulking"), thus helping to override immunotherapy's chief weakness: the overwhelming of the body's immune responses by advanced cancers. Chemotherapy may also prevent formation of "blocking" substances that interfere with immunological defenses (Fig. 11-12). Antibodies to unique DNA sequences in tumor cells, such as oncogenes, may be useful for tumor localization but probably won't provide effective therapy in the near future. Monoclonal antibodies can be generated from hybrid cells expressing tumor antigens.

Agents that suppress the immunological responses to grafts are discussed in Chapter 36. Tumor immunologists seek just the opposite. They seek mechanisms that enhance the immunological response to cancer. The approaches to cancer immunotherapy are (1) active, (2) passive, (3) nonspecific and topical, and (4) adoptive.

Active immunotherapy

Researchers try to increase the antigenicity of tumor vaccines by coupling tumor cells with rabbit gamma globulin (a highly antigenic protein) and by using neuraminidase to "unmask" antigens (Fig. 11-12). Up to now, these attempts to fashion more potent cancer vaccines have been disappointing.

Passive immunotherapy

Antitumor antibodies, produced by patients cured of cancer, have failed to achieve clear-cut clinical results when given to patients with similar cancers. Although experiments utilizing homologous tumors in experimental animals have been encouraging, tests with autochthonous tumors usually fail. Antiserum therapy may neutralize blocking factors or stimulate macrophages and lymphocytes to lyse tumor cells, but the effects are inadequate.

Infusion of extracts from lymphocytes removed from patients with cancer or cured from cancer have produced some tumor regressions. RNA extracts or transfer factors provide informational molecules that transmit to host lymphocytes a specific sensitization to "unwanted" cells. The recipient's own immune reaction then fights the foreign cells, but the effects have been disappointing. Interferons have caused some tumor regression; perhaps new tumor-specific interferon will be more effective.

Nonspecific therapy

Some nontumor substances stimulate the general immune defenses. For several years interest centered on BCG, an attenuated, bovine tuberculous bacillus, and extracts from it, which provided some regressions of animal tumors. In a few patients some melanomas that were injected directly with BCG regressed, and in rare instances other lesions, apart from those injected, also regressed. In brief, the use of various immune stimulants systemically as an adjuvant therapy has been a failure.

Topical therapy

Dinitrochlorobenzene (DNCB) or fluorouracil incites a local delayed sensitivity reaction that destroys cancer cells when either one is applied to superficial, squamous, or basal cell cancers of the skin (topical immunity).

The mechanism of action probably involves the various lymphoid cells attracted to the inflamed area.

Adoptive immunity

Adoptive immunity consists in culturing the patient's lymphocytes and reinfusing them after they are exposed to tumor antigens. The limitations of this adoptive therapy include an inability to stimulate a majority of the cells to recognize and attack the tumor cells and the need to grow a large number of cells in a few weeks without exposure to foreign proteins.

Marrow transplants

Recently patients have been given chemotherapy to rid the bone marrow of malignant cells, and then bone marrow is removed and preserved by special freezing. If the patient's lymphoma or leukemia recurs, large—even lethal—doses of chemotherapy can be used and the bone marrow can be replenished with the preserved cells. This is another form of adoptive immunity, the replenishing of live lymphoid cells. It has been successful against acute leukemias but less so against other malignancies. Transplants of marrow from identical twins have been successful, but marrow transplants with minimal adverse histocompatibility have been less so.

12
The Skin

David W. Furnas
Ivan M. Turpin

The skin is the largest organ of the body and is the device that allowed our distant forebears to emerge from the sea without fear of desiccation or bacterial ambush. The skin is composed of several different structures, each giving rise to characteristic disease processes. Only the few that have surgical significance are considered here.

THE EPIDERMIS AND ITS ADNEXAL STRUCTURES

Hair follicles, sebaceous glands, and sweat glands (eccrine and apocrine) are formed by labile epithelial cells that can quickly regenerate to repair any superficial injury. (See discussion on skin grafts in Chapter 34.) Infections and tumors are common in these structures.

Infections

Furuncles, or "boils," are caused by *Staphylococcus aureus* infections of hair follicles; they respond to surgical incision, drainage, and antibiotics. *Carbuncles* are staphylococcal infections of the back or of the posterior part of the neck that burrow and branch into the deep dermis and subcutaneous tissue fat. Adequate drainage requires wide and deep incisions. *Hidradenitis suppurativa* is a chronic infection of apocrine sweat glands in the axilla or the perineum. If far advanced, this disease is treated by excision of the involved skin and repair of the resultant defect with skin grafts or pedicles. The surgical importance of *acne vulgaris*, a recurring pustular infection of the skin follicles of the face, arises from the need to improve resulting scars with excision, dermabrasion, or collagen injections.

Benign conditions

Rhinophyma is a grotesque hyperplasia of the nasal skin, treated simply by sculpting a more desirable shape with a scapel; it arises after years of the chronic inflammatory process *acne rosacea* (Fig. 12-1).

Epidermal cysts (sebaceous cysts, or wens) occur anywhere on the body but particularly on the face, neck, or scalp (Fig. 12-2). They may result from bits of epidermis implanted in the depths of the skin by sharp objects (see discussion on implantation cyst, Chapter 39), or possibly from a blocked hair follicle or sebaceous gland. They are lined by epidermis and are filled with epidermal debris. Rarely, a *true sebaceous cyst* is encountered that is lined by sebaceous cells and filled with sebum. The lining of *dermoid cysts* contains not only keratinizing epidermis but also adnexal structures. They presumably arise from primordial islands of skin that were displaced during embryonic development. They are common around the eyes (Fig. 12-3) and nose, and sometimes they extend into the cranial vault; therefore the surgeon undertaking their excision should be properly forearmed. *Seborrheic keratoses* are brownish, raised, "velvety-feeling" blotches, common in old patients. They have no potential for malignancy. Because of their superficial purchase on the skin, they can be shaved off with a knife, and the wound will epithelialize. Sometimes they are so numerous that excision is impractical. There are numerous types of *benign adenomas, papillomas,* and *polyps* of epidermal and adnexal origin for which excision (or dermatological removal) is performed to obtain a diagnosis and to improve appearance.

A   B

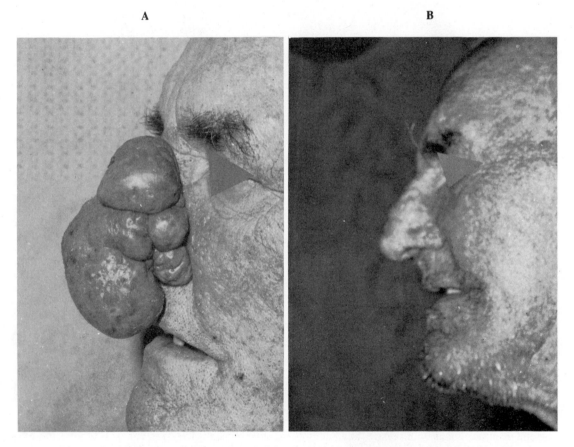

Fig. 12-1. Rhinophyma. **A,** Preoperative condition. **B,** Nasal bulk reduced by simple surgical paring.

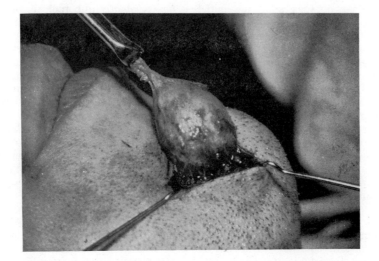

Fig. 12-2. Epidermal cyst of chin exposed at operation.

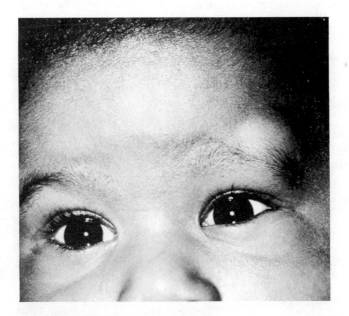

Fig. 12-3. Dermoid cyst of upper lateral part of left orbital rim. Cyst caused indentation in frontal bone.

Premalignant lesions

There are numerous premalignant lesions of the skin that develop into squamous cell carcinomas or basal cell carcinomas decades after the initial inciting insult (Fig. 12-4). *Senile* or *actinic keratoses* result from years of exposure to sunshine (e.g., in farmers and sailors). The solar radiation responsible for the malignant degeneration in skin is ultraviolet radiation with wavelength between 290 and 320 nm (UV). *Keratotic radiation changes* result from repeated small doses of ionizing radiation (e.g., hands of dentists) or from therapeutic doses of radiation received many years before (Fig. 12-5). Long-term treatment for syphilis or psoriasis with Fowler's solution or other arsenical drugs results in premalignant *arsenical keratoses*, which are found on palmar or plantar surfaces. Chronic contact with certain hydrocarbon compounds, accompanied by irritation or sunlight, may result in keratoses such as those that lead to the scrotal carcinoma of chimney sweeps. *Chronic unstable burn scars* or *chronic draining osteomyelitis* causes premalignant changes that lead to *Marjolin's ulcer*, which is a squamous carcinoma. The unfortunate children who inherit *xeroderma pigmentosum* through an incomplete sex-linked recessive gene have an exquisite sensitivity to ultraviolet radiation, causing keratoses and ultimately multiple squamous cell carcinomas, basal cell carcinomas, and even sarcomas and melanomas. They are doomed to die before adulthood. Patients with *lupus vulgaris* (tuberculosis of the skin) develop keratoses and frequent basal or squamous carcinomas (lupus carcinoma) in their later years. *Nevus sebaceus* is an ovoid, hairless, yellow-brown plaque with a verrucous surface that is present at birth or develops in childhood. Such nevi are associated with epilepsy, mental retardation, and secondary neoplasms such as basal cell carcinoma and syringocystadenoma.

Most of the skin cancers that arise from these predisposing lesions are prevented if one avoids exposure to the various inciting causes. Diagnosis is confirmed by histological examination of suspicious lesions. Either *excisional biopsy* (complete removal of suspicious lesions including margins of normal tissue on all sides) or *incisional biopsy* (removal of only a sample of the lesion) with a knife or punch is done. Premalignant lesions may be treated by excision, shaving, dermabrasion, electrodesiccation, application of chemotherapeutic agents, or careful observation.

Malignant lesions

Basal cell carcinomas and *squamous cell carcinomas* that arise in the epidermis (sometimes

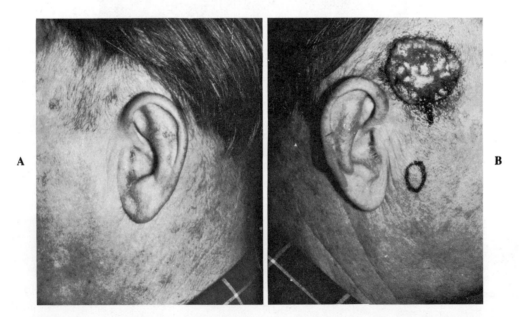

Fig. 12-4. Progress of precancerous change to cancer. **A,** Senile keratoses of left temple (just anterior to hairline) and scaphoid fossa of external ear. **B,** Frank squamous epidermoid carcinoma of right temple of same patient with metastasis to preauricular lymph nodes (*inked circle*).

called *epitheliomas*) are the *most common of all malignant tumors*. They arise from the epidermis because of the previously mentioned factors, or from no obvious cause. Of the predisposing factors, sunlight is by far the most important. Light-complexioned male outdoor workers in hot climates receive the most solar radiation and are therefore the most frequent victims. Hands, faces, and necks are the most common sites. The most superficial epitheliomas are *multicentric basal cell carcinoma, intraepidermal squamous cell carcinoma,* and *Bowen's disease.*

Basal cell carcinoma (basal cell epithelioma) (Fig. 12-6) of the skin is most common on the face, particularly the cheeks, eyelids, nose, and lips (nonvermilion surface). Northern European ancestry strongly predisposes to basal cell carcinoma. It

has a raised, pearly, translucent appearance and a delicate capillary network, frequently without ulceration. Ulceration develops as the lesion increases in size. It almost never metastasizes, but if inadequately treated, it relentlessly erodes through soft tissues, cartilage, and bone until death ensues from invasion of arteries, brain, or airway (hence the name *rodent ulcer*). If the patient is seen early and excision and histological study are carried out properly, the cure rate should approach 100%.

Squamous cell carcinoma (squamous cell epithelioma) (Figs. 12-4, *B*, and 39-28) of the skin has the power to metastasize to regional lymph nodes; however, it is a well-differentiated carcinoma, and metastases occur late. Antecedent trauma such as radiation injury (Fig. 12-5), chronic chemical exposure (hydrocarbons, arsenic), burns from plastic or

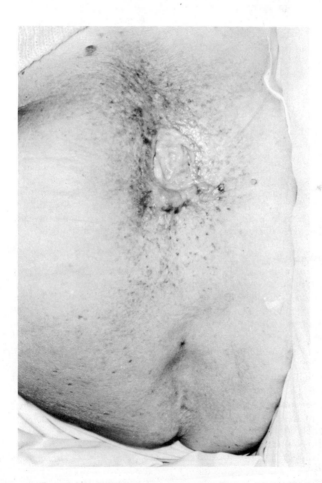

Fig. 12-5. Radiation changes in lumbar area caused by radiation received for "lumbago" 35 years previously. Central area of necrosis is surrounded by atrophic keratotic skin. Many basal cell and squamous cell carcinomas were found on microscopic examination.

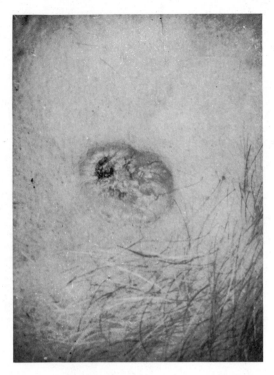

Fig. 12-6. Basal cell carcinoma. Translucency, mild lobulation, delicate vasculature, and slight ulcerations are seen.

hot metal, or unstable scars (as well as sunlight) predispose to squamous cell carcinomas. They are horny, crusted lesions and frequently show rolled margins surrounding an area of ulceration. The ears, temples, upper parts of the face, and dorsum of the hands are the most common sites. Squamous cell carcinoma is almost as common as basal cell carcinoma, but it affects an older group of patients. Wide excision or radiation of early lesions yields a 5-year survival rate of over 90%. The outlook is gloomier for patients with very large lesions and lymph node metastases. Regional lymphatic dissection is carried out when lymphatic metastases are suspected.

Keratoacanthoma (self-healing epithelioma, molluscum sebaceum) grows rapidly from a small papule to a sizable raised tumor with an umbilicated, necrotic center in 6 to 8 weeks and then subsides, leaving a scarcely visible mark. It has the microscopic picture of a well-differentiated squamous cell carcinoma. Rarely, it fails to regress, behaving like an invasive squamous carcinoma. The numerous types of neoplasms of the adnexal structures of the skin will not be discussed because of their rarity.

For certain spindle cell and poorly differentiated carcinomas of the skin, electron microscopy or immunoperoxidase procedures may be of help in making the diagnosis.

THE DERMIS

Excessive proliferation of dermal fibroblasts occurs in hypertrophied scars and keloids (see Chapter 2), as well as some rare lesions such as desmoids.

PIGMENT-PRODUCING CELLS

The surgically important pigmented lesions, nevi and melanomas, arise from pigment-producing cells of neuroectodermal origin (melanocytes, Schwann cells, or both). Freckles and lentigines are pigmented but are not composed of pigment-producing cells.

Pigmented nevi

Junctional nevi (Figs. 12-7 and 12-9), in which the nevus cells are clustered at the junction of the dermis and the epidermis, are flat and hairless and can give rise to malignant melanomas. *Intradermal nevi* (Figs. 12-8 and 12-9) are formed of nests of

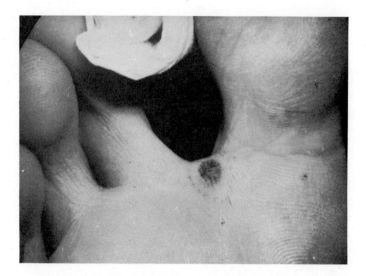

Fig. 12-7. Junctional nevus. Flat, hairless, brownish gross appearance (proposed incision line marked with ink).

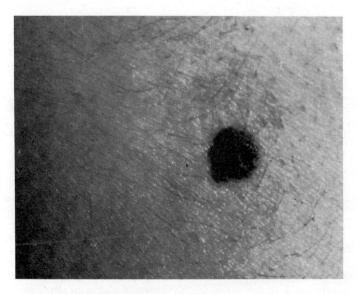

Fig. 12-8. Intradermal nevus. Notice elevated contour.

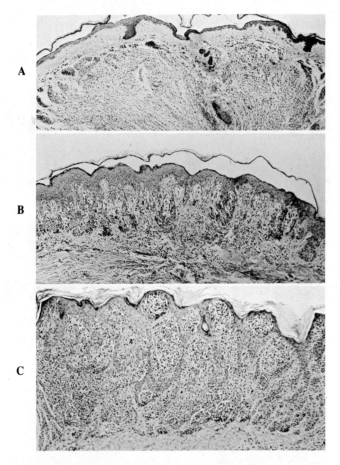

Fig. 12-9. Nevi. **A,** Intradermal nevus. Nevus cells are all well below dermo-epidermal junction and occupy the entire lower four fifths of pictured specimen. **B,** Junctional nevus. Nevus cells are found only in clusters at junction area between dermis and epidermis. **C,** Compound nevus. Nevus cells are seen in nests at dermo-epidermal junction and also throughout much of dermis. (Courtesy Dr. James H. Graham, Department of Dermatology, University of California, Irvine, Calif.)

Table 12-1. Description of nevi

Junctional nevus	Compound nevus	Intradermal nevus
Flat	⟵⟶	Raised
Hairless	⟵⟶	Often hairy
Often present below knee		Rarely present below knee
Present in most young children		80% of nevi in adults
70% of nevi in children under 15 years		Rarely present in young children
Nevus cells in clumps at dermoepidermal junction	Nevus cells at both sites	Nevus cells in nests within the dermis
Precursor to malignant melanoma	Same significance as junctional nevus	Not premalignant

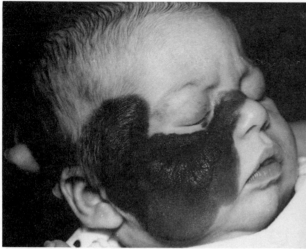
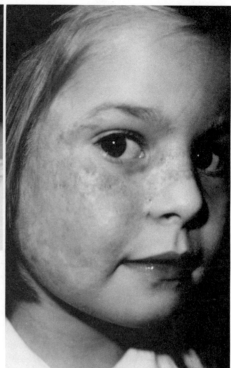

A

B

Fig. 12-10. A, Congenital hairy nevus. **B,** Five years after treatment by dermabrasion.

nevus cells buried in the dermis, deep to the dermoepidermal junction. They are usually raised, may be hairy, and do not become malignant. The *compound nevus* (Fig. 12-9) has both junctional and intradermal elements and has the same malignant potential as the junctional nevus. (See Table 12-1.)

Junctional nevi are much more common in children than in adults (70% of nevi in children under 15, but only 20% in adults), yet, paradoxically, malignant melanoma is almost unknown in children. (*Juvenile melanomas*, which microscopically resemble malignant melanomas, occur in children but are not malignant.) Curiously, almost all nevi below the knee in adults are junctional nevi.

There are so many nevi and such a minute percentage of them turn into malignant melanomas that it is impractical to excise every flat, hairless mole. However, nevi at points of constant irritation (foot, belt line, neck, bearded area) and nevi that show any sort of change, such as increase in size, deeper pigmentation, itching, or bleeding, should be excised and examined microscopically.

The uncommon *blue nevus* (benign dermal melanocytoma) derives its color (sometimes a striking deep blue) from intense pigmentation plus its loca-

tion deep within the dermis. Occasionally the regional lymph nodes become pigmented, but metastases are almost unknown.

The *giant hairy nevus* and *"bathing trunk" nevus* appear at birth and may cover half of the body surface. These sometimes give rise to true malignant melanomas in childhood. Removal by dermabrasion before 10 months of age has been promising (Fig. 12-10).

Malignant melanomas

Malignant melanomas (Fig. 12-11) are highly malignant pigmented skin lesions (rarely nonpigmented) found anywhere on the skin (and rarely on oral mucosa or anoderm). The most common sites are the head, neck, and lower limbs. They can metastasize through both the lymphatic system and the bloodstream and may spread to any organ of the body. Small islands of microlymphatic spread near the primary lesion are called *satellites*. Other foci of spread may outline the course of regional lymphatic vessels. About half the malignant melanomas arise from junctional or compound nevi, and half arise anew. They occur particularly in young adults and throughout the adult years. The blotchy *Hutchinson's spot* or *malignant lentigo*,

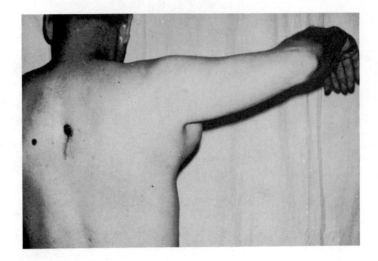

Fig. 12-11. Malignant melanoma. Malignant melanoma of back has metastasized to right axillary lymph nodes, causing large axillary mass.

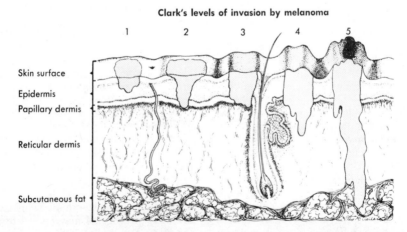

Fig. 12-12. Clark's five levels of invasion by melanoma.

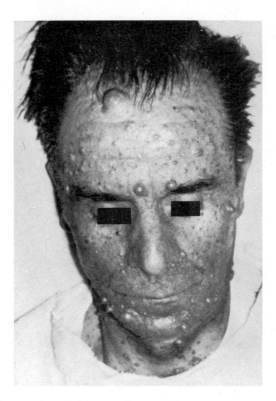

Fig. 12-13. Neurofibromatosis. Multiple neurofibromas of face in patient with von Recklinghausen's syndrome.

seen on the facial skin of elderly patients, is a relatively indolent melanoma and metastasizes only at a late date. It has a proclivity to local recurrence.

Malignant melanomas are radioresistant and must be treated by wide local excision, frequently combined with removal of the regional lymphatics. Chemotherapeutic or immunological agents are sometimes useful adjuncts. (See Chapter 11.) Prognosis depends on clinical type, level of invasion, and metastasis. *Lentigo malignant melanoma* commonly afflicts the aged and has the best prognosis. *Superficial spreading malignant melanoma* and *nodular malignant melanoma* arise in youth and middle age and carry an intermediate and poor prognosis, respectively. Clark classifies malignant melanomas in five levels (Fig. 12-12): (1) in situ, above basal lamina of epidermis; (2) extension through basal lamina into papillary layer; (3) tumor fills papillary level to the junction of the reticular dermal layer; (4) invasion into the reticular layer; and (5) invasion of subcutaneous fat. Breslow measures the thickness directly. Lesions less than 0.76 mm. thick rarely metastasize. Depending on type and level, the prognosis for localized malig-

nant melanomas ranges from 20% to 100% in 5-year survivals. Lymphatic spread reduces the expected survival to 15% or less, and bloodstream seeding cuts it to practically nil.

NERVE TISSUES

A *neuroma* (traumatic neurilemoma) is an outgrowth of Schwann cells and axons, mixed with scar tissue, located at the proximal cut end of a severed nerve. (See discussion on benign tumors of the hand, Chapter 39.) A *neurilemoma* is a discrete, encapsulated, benign tumor arising from the Schwann cells of peripheral nerves. It is usually solitary, but it may occur in neurofibromatosis. A *neurofibroma* (Fig. 12-13) is a benign, nonencapsulated, diffusely infiltrating benign tumor, usually found in multiple sites. At times neurofibromas cause strikingly grotesque deformities. They are usually associated with café-au-lait spots and are part of the hereditary disorder *von Recklinghausen's syndrome*. The multiplicity and permeation of the lesions can make a mockery of ablative surgery, though often the patient's appearance can be improved. Sarcomatous degeneration is a late complication.

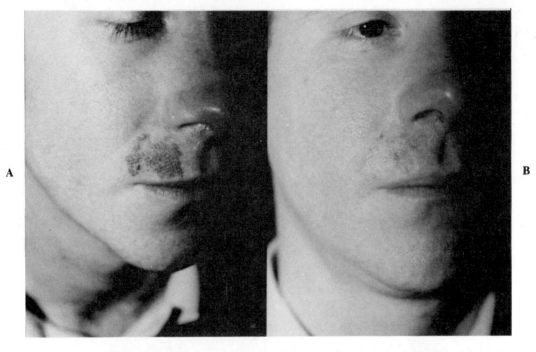

Fig. 12-14. A, Capillary hemangioma involving the right upper lip. **B,** Appearance after treatment with the argon laser. (Courtesy Dr. Bruce M. Achauer, University of California, Irvine Medical Center, Orange, Calif.)

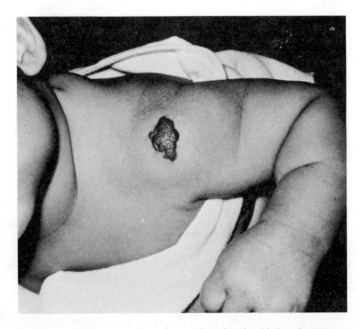

Fig. 12-15. Strawberry nevus. Lesion appeared several weeks after birth and spontaneously subsided before 2 years of age.

VASCULAR TISSUES
Capillary hemangioma

The port-wine stain, or nevus flammeus, commonly appears as a large, flat, purplish blotch on the face or neck with no disruption of normal contour. It is present at birth, does not regress, and is important only because of its appearance. It can be camouflaged with skillful makeup. The argon laser is now the treatment of choice (Fig. 12-14). "Stork bites" are purplish areas of delicate capillary dilatation on the nape of the neck, eyelids, or glabella of newborn babies, and they subside before the child reaches 1 or 2 years of age. Strawberry mark (or nevus vasculosus) (Fig. 12-15) is a highly cellular capillary hemangioma that appears as a raised, bright red lesion anywhere on the body. It regresses spontaneously.

Cavernous hemangiomas

Involuting cavernous hemangiomas appear shortly after birth as small, blue-red lesions, commonly on the face or neck, which rapidly grow into

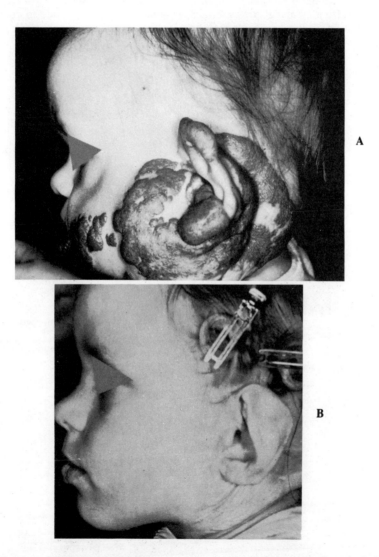

Fig. 12-16. Involuting cavernous hemangioma. **A,** Appearance at height of growth cycle during first year of life. **B,** Appearance several years after spontaneous involution. (Courtesy Dr. Richard Caplan, University of Iowa Hospitals, Iowa City, Iowa.)

large space-occupying masses that may cause grotesque disfigurement (Fig. 12-16). They usually involute before the age of 2 or 3 years, but they may leave in their wake distortion and displacement of facial features, which necessitates reconstructive surgery. Early excision may be needed to prevent amblyopia or airway obstruction. Pressure devices and steroid therapy may accelerate involution.

Ordinary cavernous hemangiomas may be of any size, shape, or location, may be multiple, and may be associated with arteriovenous fistulas, hemorrhage, or infection. Treatment is usually excision. At times location or size may make surgical attack impractical. Injection of sclerosing agents may be of help.

Malignant tumors of vessels are very rare and are highly malignant.

SUBCUTANEOUS FAT

Lipomas are soft, multilobulated, benign lumps of fat that have a color and texture different from that of immediately surrounding subcutaneous fat (Fig. 12-17). They are treated by excisional biopsy in order to differentiate them from malignant soft tissue tumors such as *liposarcoma, fibrosarcoma,* or *rhabdomyosarcoma.* If the mass is large, hard, and truly suspicious for malignancy, an incisional biopsy with study of permanent microscopic sections is the best prelude to definitive surgery.

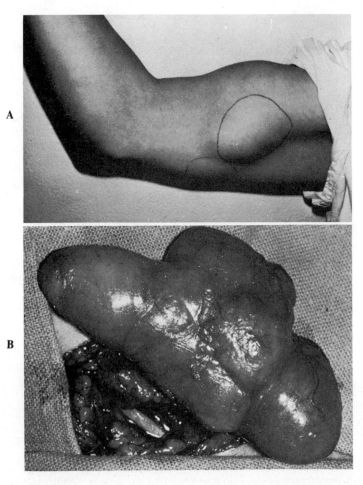

Fig. 12-17. Lipoma. **A,** Preoperative lumps on right arm, suspected to be lipomatous. **B,** Operative specimen showing fat lobulations of lipoma in contrast to pattern of adjacent subcutaneous fat.

13
The Thyroid Gland

Richard D. Liechty

The normal human thyroid gland weighs only 20 to 30 gm. As is true of other endocrine glands, the hormonal activity of the thyroid gland far overshadows its size.

Thyroid hormones have three vitally important functions in man: (1) they control metabolism within the cells, (2) they have a profound effect on growth and development, and (3) they strongly influence tissue differentiation.

The cellular actions of these hormones remain poorly understood, but the clinical consequences of excesses or deficits of thyroid hormones are well known and most important. The diseases of function and structure of the thyroid gland are the main concern of this chapter.

PHYSIOLOGY

The thyroid gland is the only tissue in the body with the ability to store significant amounts of iodine. It combines the trapped iodine with tyrosine to form two active hormones, thyroxine (tetraiodothyronine, T_4) and triiodothyronine (T_3). These hormones, stored in the thyroid as thyroglobulins, are released into the circulation and are immediately bound to thyroid-binding globulin. The concentration of serum T_4 is about 40 times that of T_3. But the more potent T_3 accounts for at least half the total metabolic effect. Some researchers believe that T_4 is converted to T_3 and that T_3 is the only active hormone intracellularly.

Hypothalamic-pituitary-thyroid triangle

The pituitary gland controls the thyroid gland through its thyroid-stimulating hormone, TSH (TSH is released by TRH, thyrotropin-releasing hormone from the hypothalamus), which incites thyroid cells to produce and release thyroid hormones. Without the TSH stimulus, the thyroid gland (the target gland) is absolutely powerless to function, and it consequently atrophies.

The thyroid hormones, as they increase in the blood in response to TSH, inhibit or cut off production of TSH. This negative-feedback control system monitors the amount of thyroid hormones at a steady level. This level is "set" in brain centers (probably the hypothalamus), and TRH conveys this message to the responsive thyrotropic cells in the anterior pituitary (Fig. 13-1).

Understanding this hypothalamic-pituitary-thyroid feedback relationship is vital to understanding thyroid disease; e.g., whenever functioning thyroid tissue is ablated, thyroid hormones decrease and TSH increases (the blocking action of

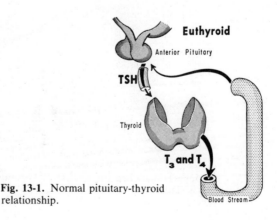

Fig. 13-1. Normal pituitary-thyroid relationship.

thyroid is removed). This increased TSH, in turn, will stimulate any remaining thyroid tissue to grow.

On the other hand, when thyroid hormones are added, they block TSH and place the thyroid gland at rest. This latter effect explains the action of thyroid hormones in suppressing growth of goiters, nodules, and even some cancer, all of which theoretically arise in response to increased TSH. Exogenous thyroid hormones, acting much like a cast on an extremity, "splint" and rest the thyroid gland.

THYROID MEDICATIONS

Probably no other common drug is more misunderstood or misused than desiccated thyroid. The active substances in *desiccated thyroid* are thyroxine (T_4) and lesser amounts of triiodothyronine (T_3), purified from animal thyroids. It has a long action (up to 2 months) with peak action in 10 to 14 days. The normal daily requirement in adults is 120 to 180 mg. Giving subnormal amounts for losing weight or "pepping up" patients is worthless; e.g., 30 mg. a day will suppress the production of TSH "30 mg. worth." The feedback system goes into action, TSH drops, thyroid production decreases, and the consequent level of thyroid hormones remains the same.

Synthetic thyroid substances offer more predictable physiological effects than desiccated thyroid does. Triiodothyronine (Cytomel in its sodium form, T_3) acts rapidly (within hours) and probably is cleared from the body within a week (25 μg. of T_3 is equal to 65 mg. of desiccated thyroid). L-Thyroxine (Synthroid, T_4) acts less rapidly than T_3. The usual daily dose is 100 to 200 μg.

Normal adults require full replacement doses of any thyroid drug. The only valid indication for smaller doses is in beginning treatment of myxedema. These patients are sensitive to thyroid hormones, and the dosages must be increased gradually, especially in those with cardiac disease and in the elderly.

DISEASES OF THE THYROID

Thyroid disease may be divided into two main types: functional diseases and anatomical or structural diseases.

Functional diseases
Hyperthyroidism (Graves' or Basedow's disease, thyrotoxicosis)

Hyperthyroidism is probably caused by an immunological process; an abnormal protein mimicking TSH releases excess T_3 and T_4 (Fig. 13-2). At the present time thyrotoxicosis is best thought of as a "runaway" thyroid gland. TSH is low. The onset may be preceded by sudden emotional shock, such as the death of a loved one. Thyrotoxicosis is four times more common in women than in men. Secondary hyperthyroidism attributed to increased pituitary TSH secretion is rare.

Clinical picture. The clinical picture of hyperthyroidism includes the following: nervousness, weight loss, fine moist skin, increased appetite, tremor, exophthalmos, goiter, rapid pulse, increased pulse pressure, exaggerated deep tendon reflexes, irritability, agitation, heat intolerance, and pretibial myxedema. Older patients show fewer signs and symptoms of hyperthyroidism; occasionally only refractory congestive heart failure or arrhythmias indicate thyrotoxicosis in older patients ("masked hyperthyroidism"). Severe hyper-

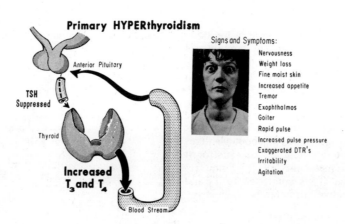

Fig. 13-2. Primary hyperthyroidism. Excess thyroid hormones released by overactive thyroid gland. TSH is suppressed.

thyroidism in time may also appear paradoxically as a decrease in activity and appetite ("apathetic hyperthyroidism"). Such a state must be aggressively treated even to forced feedings.

T_3 thyrotoxicosis appears rarely (1%) as a variant of thyrotoxicosis. The usual laboratory values remain low or normal, but elevated serum T_3 levels and failure to suppress (positive Werner's test) are diagnostic.

Laboratory tests. The most dependable thyroid function tests are the serum thyroxine level (T_4) test, T_3 uptake test, and ^{131}I uptake test (Table 13-1).

The *serum thyroxine test* (T_4 test) measures the total serum thyroxine (by displacement with radioactive T_4 or radioimmunoassay). Increased serum proteins (chiefly thyroid-binding globulin [TBG]) cause falsely elevated T_4 values. Preg-

Table 13-1. Important diagnostic thyroid tests

Test	Normal values	Theory	Comments
Serum thyroxine	4-11 µg./dl.	Measures total thyroxine in serum	Neither inorganic nor organic iodides interfere; increased serum proteins elevate values; decreased serum proteins depress values
T_3-resin uptake test (T_3RU)	25%-35%	Measures excess radioactive T_3 that becomes absorbed on resin; in toxic patients the protein molecules are "saturated"; thus radioactive T_3 will be absorbed on resins	Radioactive T_3 is incubated with patient's blood in vitro; can be used in pregnancy; not affected by I_2 or antithyroid drugs; thus can be used to check patients treated with these drugs; low-serum proteins cause falsely increased values; increased serum proteins cause falsely depressed values
Free thyroxine index	4.6-16	Multiplying $T_4 \times T_3$-resin uptake (and dividing by mean value of T_3RU) gives artificial number that corrects for increases or decreases in thyroid binding proteins.	Excellent screening test of thyroid function; especially useful in pregnancy or patients taking birth control medications
Radioactive iodine (^{131}I) uptake	15%-40% 4 and 24 hr.	Measures amount and rate that thyroid takes up ^{131}I in 4 and 24 hr.	A reliable test; not used during pregnancy; I_2 and antithyroid drugs will block this test
Serum T_3	96-172 ng./dl.	T_3 may be ultimate, active product of T_4	Valuable in diagnosing T_3 thyrotoxicosis; other tests usually normal
Scintiscan	Normal glands show an even distribution of ^{131}I throughout gland	^{131}I map of thyroid	Cysts, nodules, and cancer may be "cold"; little help in picking out malignant nodules; one definite asset is recording thyroid metastases to other areas (neck, bones, etc.)
Suppression test	4- and 24-hr. ^{131}I uptake is depressed by 50% (after suppression with 5-day course of T_3)	The pituitary-thyroid axis is tested by oral exogenous T_3 to suppress TSH; normal patients will suppress by 50%; toxic patients do not suppress	Very useful in determining the borderline hyperthyroid patients, when other laboratory values are equivocal
TSH	Values vary with laboratory	Elevated with any disease that depresses thyroid function; decreased with hyperthyroidism or exogenous thyroxine	Excellent method to check adequacy of thyroid suppression
TSH response to TRH	Values vary with laboratory	Tests hypothalmic-pituitary-thyroid triangle Exaggerated response in hypothyroidism Flat response in thyrotoxicosis Flat response, with normal or low TSH, points to pituitary failure	Completed in 2-3 hr. Gradually replacing suppression test

nancy and contraceptive agents are common causes of abnormally elevated serum proteins and consequently falsely increased levels of serum thyroxine.

The *T₃ uptake test* measures thyroid function based on the binding capacity of the patient's serum proteins for a known amount of radioactive triiodothyronine (T_3). The patient's serum is incubated with a measured amount of radioactive T_3. The patient's unbound proteins bind the T_3. The excess or unbound radioactive T_3 is taken up on a resin sponge, where it is measured by a radiation counter. A hyperthyroid patient, for example, will have fewer binding sites available on his TBG, thus the radioactive T_3 will be taken up in larger amounts by the resin sponge.

Conditions that cause increased serum proteins (pregnancy, contraceptive agents) will cause falsely depressed T_3 values. But these same conditions falsely elevate the T_4 test. Thus, by obtaining both T_4 and T_3 uptake tests and free thyroxine index, the physician can evaluate a patient's thyroid function despite abnormal serum proteins.

The *^{131}I uptake test* measures the amount of radioactive iodine taken up by the thyroid in 4 hours and 24 hours. A scintillation counter records the uptake in percentages of radioactivity given. In addition to measuring thyroid activity, the radioactive iodine within the thyroid gland can be mapped by a scintillation scanner to show the size and shape of the gland, *a thyroid scan.*

The *TSH test* measures plasma TSH. It is elevated with hypothyroidism, after total thyroidectomy, or with any disease that lowers T_4 or T_3. Conversely, hyperthyroidism or exogenous thyroid depresses TSH.

The *suppression test,* utilizing the thyroid-pituitary feedback relationship, can often distinguish the suspected thyrotoxic patient from the anxious patient (who may appear thyrotoxic) when other laboratory tests are equivocal.

^{131}I uptakes taken before and after a 5-day course of triiodothyronine (75 to 125 μg. each day) show no significant difference in the thyrotoxic patient (the TSH cannot be further depressed). Given the same test, the euthyroid patient shows a

Table 13-2. Antithyroid drugs—dosage and action

Drug	Dosage	Action
Thiocarbamides		
Propylthiouracil	100-300 mg. q.6-8h.	Blocks organic binding of iodine
Methimazole (Tapazole)	5-30 mg. q.6-8h.	
Potassium perchlorate	200-400 mg. q.6h.	Inhibits thyroid iodide transport mechanism
Iodine (Lugol's solution)	5-10 drops daily	Poorly understood
Propranolol	40-720 mg./day, divided doses	Beta-receptor blocking agent relieves toxic symptoms

Table 13-3. Comparison of three common methods of treatment of hyperthyroidism

Method	Action	Advantages	Disadvantages
I. Antithyroid drugs	Block thyroid hormone synthesis	1. Avoids surgery and irradiation	1. High incidence of drug reaction, blood dyscrasias, skin reaction 2. Frequent visits to physician necessary 3. Recurrence rate high when therapy discontinued
II. Surgery	Removal of functioning tissue	1. Most rapid method of permanent control 2. Avoids irradiation	Complications of surgery 1. Damage to recurrent laryngeal nerves 2. Damage to parathyroid glands (1%) 3. Wound complications 4. Permanent hypothyroidism (<10%) (leaving 10 gm. remnants of thyroid)
III. ^{131}I	Radioactive destruction of thyroid cells	1. Avoids surgery 2. Permanent control 3. Avoids drug reaction	1. Danger of irradiation 2. Hypothyroidism rate is high, 50% or more in 10 years; probably 100% in 20 years 3. Often treatment period is lengthy (up to 2 years) 4. Contraindicated in pregnancy and very young

50% depression in the ^{131}I uptakes after suppression with T_3. This test illustrates the important principle that thyrotoxic glands become autonomous; euthyroid glands remain under pituitary (TSH) control.

Treatment of thyrotoxicosis. Three methods for treatment of thyrotoxicosis are commonly employed: (1) antithyroid drugs, (2) surgery, and (3) radioactive iodine (^{131}I). Surgery and ^{131}I permanently *ablate* thyroid tissue; antithyroid drugs only *block* thyroid function (by blocking hormone synthesis by thyroid tissue) (Table 13-2). Unfortunately, thyrotoxicosis often recurs when drug therapy is discontinued. Therefore in most instances ablation of thyroid tissue is the preferred treatment. Many physicians do not favor using ^{131}I in young (or pregnant) women or children because of fear of irradiation. Before surgical removal of the thyroid gland, thyrotoxicosis *must* be controlled by antithyroid drugs to prevent *thyroid storm*. Thyroid storm is probably caused by massive release of thyroid hormones at operation or during other stress. A frighteningly rapid pulse, high fever, and rapid fluid loss can result in death. Fluids, steroids, antithyroid drugs, hypothermia, and adrenergic blocking agents, especially propranolol, headline the current therapy. Prevention by proper patient preparation is the best treatment. Advantages and disadvantages of the three treatment methods are summarized in Table 13-3.

Prognosis. The treatment of hyperthyroidism is most gratifying. All the signs and symptoms of thyrotoxicosis predictably diminish with treatment except for exophthalmos.

Exophthalmos. Occasionally exophthalmos may become more exaggerated after treatment. The unknown etiology of exophthalmos is rendered even more obscure by the fact that exophthalmos may occur in euthyroid persons. Some ascribe exophthalmos to long-acting thyroid-stimulating (LATS) hormones, but the origin and function of this substance are still obscure. No satisfactory treatment for severe or malignant exophthalmos exists. Tarsorrhaphy and, rarely, orbital decompression may be necessary to prevent optic nerve injury and blindness.

Hypothyroidism (myxedema)

Cause. The most common cause of myxedema is *spontaneous atrophy* of the thyroid gland (Fig. 13-3). An autoimmune mechanism (a sensitization to thyroxine) may play a role in this process. The second leading cause of myxedema, postirradiation myxedema, occurs after treatment of hyperthyroidism with ^{131}I. In some series the incidence approaches 50% of those patients treated in follow-up studies of 10 years or more. TSH serum levels are usually increased. Failure of TSH production (secondary myxedema) because of pituitary failure is rare. Hypothyroidism may vary from mild signs and symptoms to the full-blown picture of myxedema.

Clinical picture. The clinical picture of myxedema includes coarse thick hair, dry skin, puffy face, deep voice, yellow skin (carotenemia), sluggish reflexes, and constipation. In more severe cases ascites, pleural and pericardial effusions, paralytic ileus, hypothermia, and coma appear. The diagnosis is strongly suggested by a serum T_4 below 4 μg./dl., a T_3 uptake below 25%, a decreased ^{131}I uptake below 5% and 10% (4 hours and 24 hours), and elevated serum TSH levels.

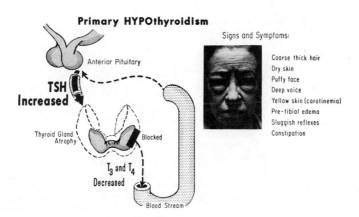

Fig. 13-3. Primary hypothyroidism. Most common cause is spontaneous atrophy. Thyroid hormones are diminished. TSH and TRH are increased.

Treatment. Perhaps no other disease responds to treatment more successfully than myxedema. Small doses of thyroid substances initially, increasing to full replacement doses (65 to 180 mg. of desiccated thyroid) restore normal function in almost all patients.

Anatomical or structural diseases
Goiters and nodules

A *goiter* is, by definition, an enlargement of the thyroid gland. A goiter may be diffusely enlarged (simple goiter) or nodular (nodular goiter). A nodule may occur in an otherwise normal gland; these are called solitary thyroid nodules.

The most common cause of goiter is a deficiency in iodine ingestion or metabolism (endemic goiter). The thyroid responds by increasing in size in an effort to produce the necessary thyroid hormones. Nodules and cysts may form as a consequence of thyroid enlargement.

Another cause of goiter is the ebb and tide of metabolic stress, e.g., menstrual cycles and pregnancy. This explains why women have more goiters and nodules (5:1) than men do.

Thyroiditis and malignancy also cause thyroid enlargement and will be discussed separately.

Solitary thyroid nodules (Fig. 13-4 and Table 13-4) are suggestive of malignancy because they arise in a gland otherwise normal to palpation. About 50% of these "solitary" growths are really dominant nodules in a multinodular goiter; the other nodules are too small to be palpated clinically. Some of them are "new growths"; thus all solitary nodules should be evaluated for malignancy by fine needle aspiration biopsy or large cutting needle biopsy. These tests yield cells for cytological study and tissue specimens for histological study. They are most accurate in the diagnosis of papillary cancer (psammoma bodies and "ground-glass" nuclei) and lymphocytic thyroiditis (lymphocytes and fibrous trabeculas). They

Table 13-4. Pathology of solitary nodules of thyroid (from composite studies)

Multinodular goiters	50%
Adenomas	20
Cancer	20
Thyroiditis	5
Cysts	5
TOTAL	100

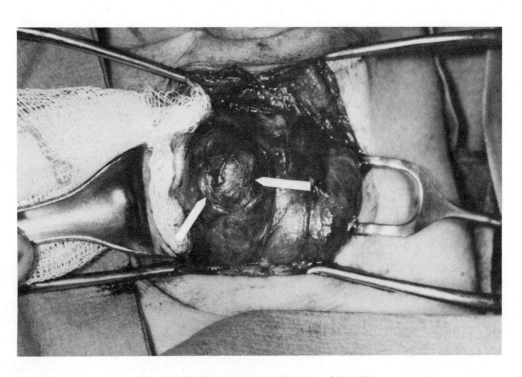

Fig. 13-4. Solitary nodule in right lobe of thyroid.

are least accurate in the diagnosis of follicular cancer. The most helpful of all preoperative tests, needle biopsies give more definitive information than scintiscans or ultrasound imaging. Scintiscans may show "cold" nodules, but these are usually cysts or benign adenomas rather than cancer. Similarly, ultrasound may differentiate cystic from solid lesions, but so will needle aspiration and at far less cost.

Treatment of goiters and nodules. As a useful rule, all *solitary nodules are considered malignant* until proved benign; all *multinodular goiters are considered benign* until some evidence is suggestive of malignancy. The incidence of malignancy in *clinically solitary* thyroid nodules is about 20% nationwide. No infallible tests short of microscopic diagnosis can detect the dangerous nodules. If needle biopsy specimens are abnormal or equivocal, the nodules should be excised with margins of surrounding normal tissue (lobectomy). Many soft nodules that occur in pregnancy will regress on giving suppressive doses of desiccated thyroid, or after the pregnancy is terminated; thus these nodules can be treated conservatively.

Diffuse and multinodular goiters are not removed routinely. Small, palpable nodular goiters are very common (5% to 10% of adults); thyroid cancer is uncommon. Thus operative mortality for routine thyroidectomy would likely exceed any saving of life from thyroid cancer. We operate only on suspicious goiters, i.e., a rapidly growing nodule, a hard or fixed lobe or nodule within the goiter, or evidence of cervical metastasis. Goiters are removed also for cosmetic reasons or for obstruction of the trachea or esophagus. Since nodules occurring in children carry a high risk of malignancy, all such nodules should be excised and examined.

Thyroiditis

Thyroiditis is a general term that describes the four types of inflammatory diseases of the thyroid gland. The lymphocytic type is by far the most common.

The four types of thyroiditis and the approximate relative incidence are as follows:

	Number of cases
Lymphocytic type (Hashimoto's struma, struma lymphomatosa)	100
Viral type (subacute, granulomatous, de Quervain's)	10
Riedel's (woody)	1
Suppurative (acute, bacterial)	<1

Clinical characteristics. Clinical characteristics of the lymphocytic, viral, Riedel's, and acute suppurative types of thyroiditis are discussed in the paragraphs that follow.

Lymphocytic type. Lymphocytic thyroiditis is probably caused by an autoimmune mechanism. Thyroid tissue becomes sensitized to its own hormones, resulting in an invasion of lymphocytes and fibrous tissue. A diffuse, rubbery, nontender goiter results. The thyroid antibody titer is usually elevated. Although chiefly afflicting woman 20 to 50 years of age, it is the most common cause of goiter in children. Many believe it eventually leads to myxedema. Biopsy and replacement of thyroid (T_3 or T_4) keynote the treatment.

Viral type. Viral thyroiditis causes a tender, diffuse enlargement or occasionally a tender nodule, mild fever, increased sedimentation rate, and general malaise. Bed rest, sedation, aspirin, and in extreme cases steroids (to reduce inflammation) are the usual methods of treatment. Biopsy diagnosis is rarely necessary for the skilled clinician.

Riedel's type. Riedel's type is very rare. Probably the fibrous end stage of lymphocytic thyroiditis, the gland atrophies and becomes woody hard. Because it mimics the firmness of cancer, it demands biopsy and treatment with replacement doses of T_3 or T_4.

Acute suppurative thyroiditis. Acute suppurative thyroiditis is a medical oddity. Having seen only one case, I mention this entity last to emphasize its rarity. The source of bacterial thyroiditis is most often from abscessed lower teeth. Treatment, as with any abscess, includes drainage and antibiotics.

Cancer

Cancer of the thyroid has an extremely wide range of behavior. It is rivaled in this respect only by breast cancer among the common malignancies. Most differentiated types grow slowly over years. The undifferentiated types grow rapidly and may be lethal within weeks or months. Since most undifferentiated types afflict older adults, advanced age often signals an ominous prognosis. Cancer of the thyroid may be classified as follows:

Differentiated 80%	Intermediate 5%	Undifferentiated 15%
Papillary	Medullary	Small cell
Follicular		Large cell
Mixed papillo-follicular		Sarcomas

Papillary cancer occurs in children and young adults of the third and fourth decade, often with a history of prior irradiation to the neck area. It is the most common thyroid malignancy. For small lesions (1.5 cm) with no metastases, lobectomy alone is often adequate treatment. With progression of the tumor, metastases usually appear in the neck and grow slowly. Total thyroidectomy and excision of regional metastases form the basic treatment. Total thyroidectomy accomplishes two objectives: (1) it removes thyroid tissue that competes (with tumor) for ^{131}I; (2) it removes possible multicentric foci of tumor. When cervical spread has occurred, most surgeons prefer conservative removal of only the involved tissues. The patient is allowed to become hypothyroid. If residual tumor is shown to take up iodine, ^{131}I is given in large therapeutic doses. TSH, or a thiouracil drug to increase the body's TSH, often increases the ^{131}I uptake in the metastases. Suppressive doses of thyroid are administered for the remainder of the patient's life.

Follicular cancer tends to metastasize distantly and occurs in a slightly older age group (fifth decade). Before ^{131}I treatment, total thyroidectomy prepares the patient by removing tumor and allowing any remaining metastases to pick up ^{131}I more effectively.

Mixed type is a commonly occurring composite of the preceding two types. A variant of papillary cancer, it is treated accordingly.

Medullary cancers contain varying amounts of amyloid and carry an intermediate prognosis. The 10-year survival rate exceeds 60% in operable patients. Medullary cancers tend to be familial and are associated with pheochromocytomas, hyperparathyroidism, and neurofibromatosis. Some medullary cancers produce calcitonin. Elevated levels of serum calcitonin have predicted medullary cancers, preoperatively, in family members who carry this trait.

Undifferentiated thyroid cancer is aggressively malignant. It occurs in older people and rarely takes up [131]I. Radical surgical excision and external irradiation are the only, and usually ineffective, treatment.

Sarcomas of various types are rare. Occasionally, wide excision will offer a favorable prognosis.

14
Parathyroid Glands

Richard D. Liechty

A multihormonal system regulates calcium, magnesium, and phosphate homeostasis in all vertebrates. The organs involved in this regulation are bone, kidney, and gut, and the major hormones are parathyroid hormone (parathormone, PTH), calcitonin (CT), and vitamin D. In general PTH and vitamin D act in concert with (but opposing) CT to maintain serum calcium between 8.5 and 10.5 mg./dl. Calcium regulates neuromuscular excitability, blood coagulation, membrane function, secretory processes, and many enzyme reactions; to maintain these vital functions, nature zealously keeps calcium within these narrow limits.

ANATOMY AND EMBRYOLOGY

Man normally has four parathyroid glands situated close to the posterior surface of the thyroid, one gland near each pole. Each gland should weigh no more than 70 mg. Their small weight and their location make the parathyroid glands liable to accidental removal or damage during thyroid surgery. The parathyroid glands, derived from the third and fourth branchial pouches, differentially migrate caudally so that the lower pair come from the third pouch and the upper pair from the fourth. About 10% of parathyroid glands are ectopically located within the thyroid, thymus, superior mediastinum, and even pericardium. Histologically, parathyroid glands contain cords of chief and oxyphilic cells. Chief cells, subdivided into water-clear and dark cells according to their content of secretory granules, secrete PTH. Most adenomas feature dark cells; hyperplastic parathyroid glands arise from either cell.

Calcitonin comes from "C-cells" (for calcitonin). Derived from the ultimobranchial body, these cells disperse into thyroid, thymus, and parathyroid tissues in man. They resemble adrenal medullary cells and pancreatic alpha cells, with which they probably share a common origin.

PHYSIOLOGY (Figs. 14-1 and 14-2)

PTH, a polypeptide hormone, elevates plasma calcium levels in three ways. First, it shifts calcium from bone to plasma, probably by stimulating osteoclasts. Second, it inhibits tubular reabsorption of phosphate, thus promoting phosphaturia, while enhancing calcium reabsorption. Third, it stimulates the conversion of 25-OH vitamin D_3 to 1,25-$(OH)_2$ vitamin D_3 (1,25-dihydroxycholecalciferol) in the kidney. In turn, 1,25-$(OH)_2$ vitamin D_3 incites the intestinal absorption of calcium and phosphorus. This potent metabolite of vitamin D_3 also helps shift calcium from bone to plasma, but only in the presence of PTH. Low phosphorus and high PTH levels turn on the kidney's 1-hydroxylation mechanism; high phosphorus and low PTH levels turn it off. This dual control provides the body with a constant supersaturated solution of calcium and phosphorus, ions vital to cell metabolism (cardiac conduction, ATP) and bone metabolism.

Calcitonin, by suppressing osteoclastic activity, will antagonize any sudden rise in calcium levels. Thus these three hormones, coupled with their classical feedback systems (PTH and calcium; PTH and vitamin D_3; calcitonin and calcium), maintain plasma calcium and phosphorus concen-

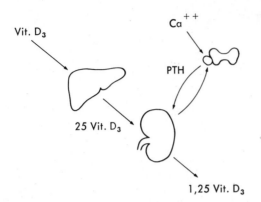

Fig. 14-1. Vitamin D_3, a hormone. Renal parenchymal cells convert vitamin D_3 to 1,25-$(OH)_2$ vitamin D_3 under influence of two stimuli: (1) elevated PTH or (2) lowered serum PO_4. PTH and 1,25-$(OH)_2$ vitamin D_3 form feedback control system. Kidney is endocrine organ and 1,25-$(OH)_2$ vitamin D_3 is hormone.

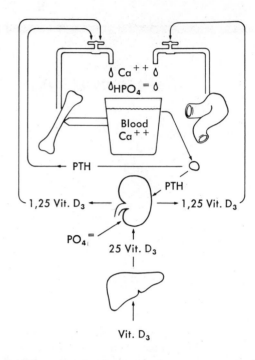

Fig. 14-2. PTH–vitamin D interaction. Vitamin D_3 is hydroxylated in liver to 25-OH vitamin D_3. Kidney adds another hydroxyl group to make 1,25-$(OH)_2$ vitamin D_3. This sterol stimulates intestinal absorption of Ca^{++}. It also releases calcium from bone but only when PTH is present. High PTH + low $PO_4^=$ levels turn on 1-hydroxylase mechanism.

trations at remarkably constant levels. They control these levels precisely despite widely varying intakes and bodily demands.

Calcium circulating in blood and extracellular fluid represents less than 1% of the total body content. About half is in an active or ionized form; the rest is protein bound or non-ionized and therefore biochemically inactive. Calcium binds chiefly to albumin; lesser amounts bind to globulins. To correct for variations in serum proteins, they should be measured along with serum calcium levels. About 0.9 mg. calcium is bound per gram of protein, allowing for a rough estimation of the ionized calcium level. The binding of calcium to albumin is enhanced by alkalosis (e.g., the tetany of hyperventilation) and decreased by acidosis.

HYPERPARATHYROIDISM
Primary hyperparathyroidism

Clinical features. About one case of primary hyperparathyroidism emerges from every 1,000 carefully screened hospital admissions. This disease results from the autonomous and increased secretion of PTH, usually from neoplastic transformation (Fig. 14-3). About 80% of patients with hyperparathyroidism have as the cause a single parathyroid adenoma; hyperplasia, multiple adenomas, or a mixture of the two (and rarely cancer) account for the rest. Most pathologists agree that distinguishing hyperplastic from adenomatous tissue, especially on frozen section, is unreliable, if not impossible.

Cancers of other organs commonly elevate serum calcium chiefly from osteolytic metastases, but some tumors (notably in the lung and kidney) secrete a PTH-like substance and thus mimic primary hyperparathyroidism.

The nonspecific symptoms of muscle weakness, fatigue, nausea, anorexia, constipation, mental changes, polyuria, polydipsia, and renal colic and infections characterize hypercalcemia. Between 60% and 75% of patients have detectable renal involvement including stones or gravel, repeated infections, hematuria, nephrocalcinosis, and azotemia. About 5% to 10% of all patients with renal stones will prove to have hyperparathyroidism. Clinical bone involvement caused by excessive resorption is found in about 20% of patients. Most often this is diffuse, resembling osteoporosis. Less frequently seen now are the classical lesions of osteitis fibrosa cystica. Fig. 14-4 shows subperiosteal resorption, which is diagnostic. This resorption usually involves the fingers and lateral third of the clavicles.

Hyperparathyroidism, usually featuring chief cell hyperplasia or adenomas, runs in some fam-

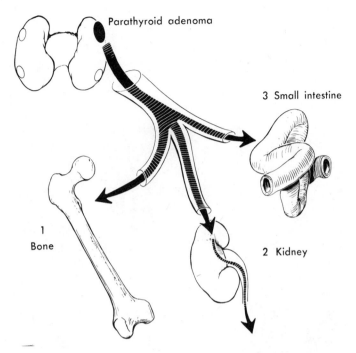

Fig. 14-3. Primary hyperparathyroidism. *1*, PTH releases calcium from bone while inhibiting new bone formation. *2*, PTH promotes renal reabsorption of calcium and inhibits tubular reabsorption of phosphate. *3*, PTH stimulates 1,25-(OH)$_2$ vitamin D$_3$ secretion, and this hormone increases intestinal absorption of calcium.

ilies. Pheochromocytomas, pancreatic adenomas, medullary thyroid carcinomas, and pituitary and thyroid tumors also characterize these syndromes of multiple endocrine adenomas. Peptic ulcer, pancreatitis, and hypertension increase in incidence with hyperparathyroidism and often defy therapy until the adenoma is removed. All patients with these diseases should have a serum calcium determination. Occasionally the serum calcium will become acutely and severely elevated, leading to a life-threatening aggravation of the symptoms listed above—a *parathyroid crisis*.

Diagnosis. The causes of hypercalcemia in hospitalized patients are as follows:

Bone metastases	55%
Hyperparathyroidism	20%
Ectopic PTH	15%
Other causes	10%
Thiazide ingestion	
Sarcoidosis	
Vitamin D poisoning	
Milk-alkali syndrome	
Thyrotoxicosis	
Adrenal failure	

Differential diagnosis. Asymptomatic patients with mild hypercalcemia for a year or more who deny excessive intake of milk products and vitamins and have no family history of endocrine disorders will virtually all have hyperparathyroidism. Elevated serum PTH levels (Fig. 14-5), depressed phosphorus levels, and a chloride-to-phosphorus ratio of more than 33 further confirm this diagnosis. In addition, elevated serum alkaline phosphotase indicates the degree of bone destruction. Hyperchloremia, mild metabolic acidosis, and hyperuricemia often coexist. Hypercalciuria is common, but the total calcium excretion is usually less than 400 mg./day because PTH promotes calcium reabsorption.

A long duration of hypercalcemia without weight loss eliminates malignant disease, both osteolytic and ectopic. The lack of familial hypercalcemia, of hypocalciuria, and of early onset (before age 10 years) rules out familial hypocalciuric hypercalcemia (FHH). The absence of symptoms and signs of the other causes of hypercalcemia effectively eliminates them from consideration. The tests used in the differential diagnosis of hyperparathyroidism (listed in order of importance) are as follows:

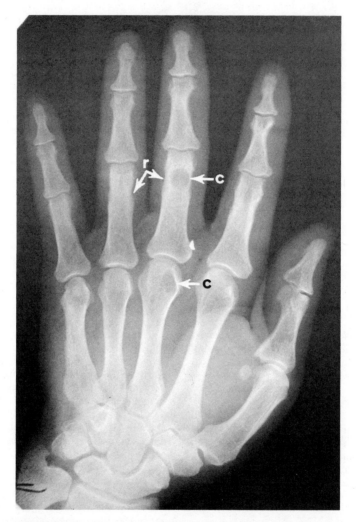

Fig. 14-4. Radiologically diagnostic lesions of subperiosteal resorption, *r*, and associated cysts, *c*. Such lesions are more likely demonstrable in patients with large adenomas.

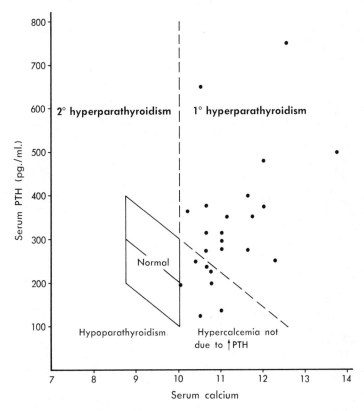

Fig. 14-5. PTH levels help differentiate causes of hypercalcemia. High levels of both calcium and PTH indicate primary hyperparathyroidism. Low levels of PTH with high levels of calcium point to some other cause. (See causes listed under "Differential diagnosis.")

Serum:
Calcium
PTH
Phosphate
Chloride
Alkaline phosphatase
Uric acid
Total protein/albumin
Hematocrit (HCT)
Sedimentation rate
pH
BUN (blood urea nitrogen)
Creatinine

Other tests:
Urinary calcium, urinalysis, chest roentgenogram, KUB (kidney-ureter-bladder) abdomen or intravenous pyelogram, hydrocortisone suppression test, urinary or nephrogenous cAMP

Selective venous catheterization, with subsequent determinations of PTH on venous blood samples, may help localize the adenoma. Arteriography can sometimes pinpoint the adenoma in unusual sites, such as the mediastinum. At the first operation, experienced surgeons can successfully cure hyperparathyroidism in 95% of all patients. Thus the cost of these procedures and the risks of arteriography (brain dysfunction in about 5% of all patients) outweigh their possible advantages in routine cases. They are usually reserved for the difficult, reoperative cases.

Therapy. Three problems complicate surgical treatment: (1) there may be more or less than the normal four glands, (2) 10% of glands arise ectopically (Fig. 14-6), and (3) frozen section diagnosis often fails to distinguish between hyperplasia and adenomas. Knowing that the initial operation allows him the golden chance to evaluate the parathyroid pathological condition, the surgeon must plan his operation methodically as follows. Because about 10% of parathyroid glands arise ectopically, he must attempt to identify all four glands, no matter how tedious and time consuming this may prove. He should remove the one enlarged gland if he finds three other normal or atrophic

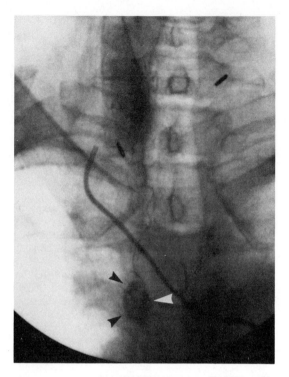

Fig. 14-6. Arteriogram showing ectopic parathyroid adenoma in mediastinum.

ones, and if he finds only three glands, he should resect the thyroid on the side of the missing gland. He should select subtotal parathyroidectomy (three and one-half glands removed) (1) for gross enlargement of more than one gland, (2) if all glands appear normal or minimally enlarged with no evidence of a fifth gland, (3) for familial parathyroid disease, or (4) for chronic, mild renal insufficiency. An alternative procedure involves removing all glands and transplanting a remnant (about 50 to 70 mg.) into neck or arm muscle. The remnant must be divided into 1 to 2 mm fragments that are dispersed into muscle pockets. Some surgeons use subcutaneous pockets. These plans offer the greatest chance for permanent cure with minimal risk of permanent hypoparathyroidism or recurrence.

Parathyroid crises (Ca^{++} 15 mg./dl. or higher) call for immediate action, including: (1) intravenous phosphates, (2) saline diuresis, and (3) mithramycin or calcitonin infusions. These measures aim at lowering the serum calcium before *urgent* exploration.

When operative removal is not feasible, chronic medical treatment with oral phosphate-phosphorus (2 to 5 gm./day) can normalize serum calcium

levels in most patients. Many physicians prefer mithramycin because they fear renal precipitation of calcium phosphates.

Secondary hyperparathyroidism

In chronic renal failure the kidney's 1-hydroxylation mechanism fails, causing 1,25-(OH)$_2$ vitamin D$_3$ levels to drop. To compensate, PTH increases and in time the stressed parathyroid glands become hyperplastic. The elevated levels of PTH, if sustained, produce renal osteodystrophy, a painful, often crippling bone disease. Because the diseased kidneys lose their ability to excrete phosphorus, plasma phosphorus levels increase. This elevation (1) further suppresses 1-hydroxylation and (2) favors ectopic calcifications. Although calcium levels tend to remain normal or even low, increased phosphate levels (exceeding the solubility coefficient) favor deposition of calcium phosphate salts. These deposits can obstruct vital arteries (coronary, renal). Thus *renal osteodystrophy* and *ectopic calcifications* characterize advanced renal failure with secondary hyperparathyroidism. PTH remains under feedback control but only by higher levels of calcium. The treatment of secondary hyperparathyroidism includes (1) treatment of the renal disease, (2) 1,25-(OH)$_2$ vitamin D$_3$ to bypass the defective 1-hydroxylation mechanism, and (3) low phosphate diet. In almost all instances this regimen, which on occasion includes renal transplantation, will control the secondary hyperparathyroidism.

Tertiary hyperparathyroidism

Occasionally, the normal feedback controls fail. Hyperplastic parathyroid glands become autonomous, causing calcium levels to rise to dangerous levels. These conditions of tertiary hyperparathyroidism call for subtotal parathyroidectomy. In advanced stages the glands can enlarge to 50 or more times their normal weight. In our hospital we resect all but 50 to 70 mg. of tissue. By transplanting this remnant in forearm muscles, we can (1) check its viability, (2) monitor the amount of PTH produced, and, if necessary, (3) easily gain access to resect more tissue should it continue its hyperplastic growth.

HYPOPARATHYROIDISM

Classification and clinical features. Hypoparathyroidism, characterized by hypocalcemia and hyperphosphatemia, can result from loss of glandular function or from end-organ resistance to PTH action. Hypoparathyroidism most commonly occurs after removal of the glands or damage to their blood supply during thyroid surgery. Within a few hours neuromuscular irritability emerges as muscle spasms or cramps and paresthesias, particularly of the hands, face, and feet. Tapping the facial nerve results in facial muscle contractions (Chvostek's sign), whereas application of a partially inflated blood pressure cuff leads to carpopedospasm (Trousseau's sign). Pronounced hypocalcemia can induce laryngeal spasm and convulsions. This syndrome can be transient or permanent. Hypocalcemia often occurs in the 24 to 48 hours immediately after removal of a parathyroid adenoma. Although usually transient, this relative hypoparathyroidism can require treatment for months, especially when the bones have suffered chronic calcium "starvation" from extensive dissolution.

Treatment. For acute hypocalcemia, intravenous calcium gluconate will bring immediate relief. This is later changed to oral calcium lactate or other calcium salts (5 to 15 gm./day).

Vitamin D remains the keystone of long-term treatment. (Commercial PTH induces antibodies that make it ineffective.) The newest form is 1,25-$(OH)_2$ vitamin D_3, now available commercially. It has distinct advantages: small doses (daily dose about 0.5 to 1 μg./day), rapid action (within hours), and similarly rapid withdrawal. This final active metabolite of vitamin D_3 remains independent of renal conversion and therefore effective regardless of renal function.

Idiopathic hypoparathyroidism. The rare disease idiopathic hypoparathyroidism attacks in childhood or middle age. Cataracts, basal ganglia calcification, mental retardation, and cutaneous involvement such as candidiasis, brittle nails, and patchy hair characterize the childhood disease. Usually the glands are absent or atrophic. Symptoms often are chronic and insidious in onset, particularly in the adult.

Pseudohypoparathyroidism. Pseudohypoparathyroidism is an interesting example of end-organ (kidney) resistance to the effects of a hormone. These patients have all the chemical and clinical features of hypoparathyroidism yet have elevated PTH levels. The kidneys of these patients fail to give the normal phosphaturic response to PTH. This genetic disease also includes peculiar skeletal abnormalities (stunting, short metacarpals) that distinguish it from the idiopathic form.

15
The Adrenal Glands

Richard D. Liechty

Nature has fashioned the mammalian adrenal gland in a curious way. Taking two separate embryological tissues, it has fused them, as adrenal cortex (mesoderm) and medulla (ectoderm), into one gland. Despite this anatomical merger that allows the cortex to bathe the medulla with the body's richest concentration of steroids, man and other mammals do perfectly well without the medulla. Perhaps nature, in our evolutionary past, has devalued the biological ties indicated by the anatomical fusion of adrenal cortex and medulla. Whatever the reason, most scientists today believe that the adrenal medulla (which secretes epinephrine and norepinephrine in a ratio of 4:1) has no more physiological significance than other sympathetic ganglia that secrete catecholamines. In contrast, the cortex maintains critically important functions. Together, man's two adrenal glands weigh only about 14 gm., but without the functioning cortex and its hormones, man dies.

PHYSIOLOGY
Adrenal hormones

The adrenal medulla is the body's chief source of epinephrine. Epinephrine and norepinephrine together increase cardiac rate and stroke volume (B receptors). They increase depth and rate of respiration and constrict cutaneous and renal vessels (A receptors). In addition to these cardiovascular and respiratory effects, catecholamines regulate body fuels. They suppress insulin and stimulate glucagon, thus elevating blood glucose. They also release fatty acids from fat deposits. Consequently, they provide immediate calories (glucose) and

begin the body's anticipated conversion to long-term calories (fats). In the fight-or-flight reaction catecholamines have an initial and crucial role.

Three main types of hormones are secreted by the adrenal cortex: (1) glucocorticoids, (2) mineralocorticoids, and (3) sex steroids. All three originate from the cholesterol molecule. Enzymes within the cells of the adrenal cortex change the chemical structure of cholesterol to produce corticosteroids.

Hypothalamic-pituitary-adrenal triangle

Both the glucocorticoids and the sex steroids are under hypothalamic-pituitary control. ACTH (adrenocorticotropic hormone) released by the pituitary gland, in response to corticotropin-releasing factor (CRF) from the hypothalamus, stimulates the adrenal cortex to produce both glucocorticoids and sex steroids. (Mineralocorticoids are largely independent of pituitary control.) Glucocorticoids (chiefly cortisol), in turn, block ACTH secretion at the pituitary and CRF at the hypothalamic level. This is the reciprocal, negative feedback mechanism (similar to the pituitary-thyroid relationship) that is vital to understanding adrenal physiology.

Corticosteroid hormones
Glucocorticoids

The chief glucocorticoid in the body is cortisol (hydrocortisone). Glucocorticoids increase glycogenolysis (breakdown of glycogen to glucose), convert proteins to glucose, and have an antiinflammatory action. In large amounts they increase fat deposition and cause weakness (from destruction of muscle protein) and water retention. Their most important action is in protecting the body against stress. The exact mechanism of glucocorticoids in response to stress is not known. They probably act on the vascular tree by dilating small vessels, thus increasing blood volume. They make energy available in the form of glucose and free fatty acids. Some believe that protection of lysosomal membranes is a vital cellular function. Another theory relates glucocorticoid action to their inotropic effect on myocardium, which increases cardiac output.

Mineralocorticoids

Aldosterone is secreted chiefly in response to decreased blood volume mediated by renal receptors. It acts to retain sodium and water and to excrete potassium. In concert with ADH (antidiuretic hormone) and renin-angiotensin, it maintains body fluid volume at a constant level.

Aldosterone and water balance. In the normal person the adrenal gland secretes aldosterone, the body's main mineralocorticoid, chiefly in response to decreased blood volume. The kidney's juxtaglomerular apparatus senses the volume deficit and secretes renin, which in turn releases angiotensin I. Enzymes, chiefly in the lungs, rapidly convert angiotensin I to angiotensin II. Angiotensin II, a powerful vasoconstrictor by itself, stimulates the adrenal gland to synthesize and release aldosterone. Acting on the distal convoluted tubule, aldosterone retains Na^+ (and H_2O) and excretes K^+. Thus in normal man the kidney and adrenal gland combine two mechanisms to ensure normal blood volumes through varying states of hydration, electrolyte concentration, and position. Although low Na^+, high K^+, and ACTH also stimulate aldosterone, the most powerful influence is angiotensin II. Acting as a feedback, the aldosterone build-up and increased water volume suppress or turn off renin secretion.

Antidiuretic hormone (ADH). The aldosterone-angiotensin mechanism has a powerful ally in the hypothalamic-posterior pituitary area. Responding chiefly to dehydration (increased osmolality), osmoreceptors in the hypothalamus stimulate release of pituitary-stored ADH. ADH, acting on the renal collecting ducts, causes reabsorption of H_2O. Severe volume deficits (sensed in the heart and large arteries) also elevate ADH, since nature attempts to protect volume at all costs even in the face of hypo-osmolality. Coupled to the osmoreceptor cells, a thirst center signals severe thirst synchronous with water conservation. Thus two main neurohormonal centers, in the brain and paravertebral gutters, protect the body's water balance.

Sex steroids

Androgens, estrogens, and progesterone are produced by the adrenal cortex in small amounts. When they are secreted in excess, they cause virilization (the adrenogenital syndrome) or, rarely, feminization. They do not suppress ACTH, and they are not essential to life.

Adrenocortical hormone similarities and differences

In the confusing welter of steroid hormones occurring in the body (more than 30 have been isolated) and the dozens of commercial steroid preparations, many students feel lost. Certain principles will help clear their understandable confusion:

1. All steroids have three basic actions: (a) "metabolic" or glucocorticoid, (b) mineralocorticoid, and (c) sex steroid.
2. Some overlapping of actions occurs with most corticosteroids; e.g., cortisol, primarily a glucocorticoid and the "mother steroid" in the body, will show mineralocorticoid effects (water retention) and sex steroid effects (acne, hirsutism) if given in large enough amounts.
3. Suppression of ACTH is primarily a function of glucocorticoids; e.g., new, synthetic anti-inflammatory steroids with advertised "decreased side effects" means that they have less water retention and masculinizing effects—but remember, their glucocorticoid properties are very much evident, and they strongly suppress ACTH.

A "triangle of steroid activity" is a helpful device in understanding basic steroid physiology (Fig. 15-1). All steroid preparations may be placed somewhere in this triangle corresponding to their actions.

DISEASES OF THE ADRENAL CORTEX
Addison's disease (adrenocortical failure)

Any process that destroys or suppresses the adrenal cortex (or the hypothalamic-pituitary ACTH centers) will cause Addison's disease. Adrenocortical infections (meningococcosis, tuberculosis), cortical atrophy (probably of autoimmune origin), and surgical adrenalectomy can cause Addison's disease. One of the most common causes is suppression of ACTH from long-term steroid therapy. Other causes are hereditary and congenital, hemorrhage (from sepsis, from anticoagulants, or during pregnancy), or pituitary insufficiency.

Clinically, Addison's disease appears in the adult as *chronic insufficiency, acute adrenal failure,* or an intermediate state between these two.

Chronic addisonian patients have dark pigmentation, weakness, hypotension, apathy, nausea,

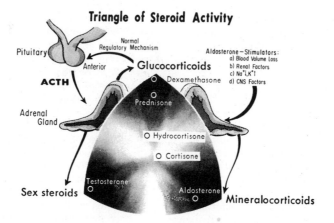

Fig. 15-1. Adrenocortical hormone activity is demonstrated by triangle with three main types of cortical hormones at apices. Overlapping of functions (glucocorticoid, mineralocorticoid, and sex steroid) occurs with most steroid compounds. Approximate overlapping of functions is illustrated by several steroids placed within this triangle.

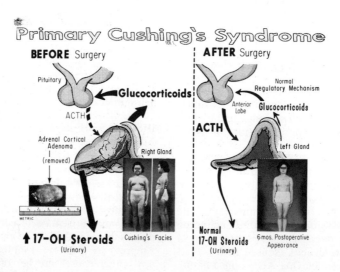

Fig. 15-2. Cushing's syndrome caused by adrenal adenoma. ACTH is suppressed by excess glucocorticoids. After tumor was removed, normal pituitary-adrenal balance resumed. Insets show cushingoid effects in 9-year-old girl and postoperative appearance 6 months after removal of benign adrenal adenoma.

vomiting, weight loss, abdominal pain, hyponatremia, hypoglycemia, and hyperkalemia. They show decreased plasma cortisol levels and urinary 17-OHCS excretion. *Inflexibility* best describes these patients. Any stress, such as an operation or potent drugs, can throw them into shock. Infections will cause critically high fevers with subsequent shock and death unless patients receive vigorous steroid replacement.

Acute adrenal failure comes on suddenly with fever, abdominal symptoms, coma, and shock. Sudden discontinuance of steroids after long-term administration is a common cause of acute adrenal failure. This critical condition demands immediate treatment with intravenous cortisol, 300 mg. (or more) in the first 24 hours, with gradual tapering doses. Maintenance cortisol doses average 25 to 50 mg./day orally.

Patients receiving steroids for long periods of time often pose problems for the surgeon. Some patients can receive large doses of steroids for several months and still maintain an effective adrenal stress response, whereas others receiving smaller doses over shorter intervals may not. In any emergency situation (lacking time to evaluate the pituitary-adrenal integrity) the surgeon should support these patients with full "stress doses" of steroids (300 mg. cortisol/day). Little harm comes from short interval "burst" therapy, but catastrophe may follow if the surgeon overlooks the vital importance of steroid replacement in patients with marginal adrenal reserves.

Cushing's syndrome

Cushing's syndrome is caused by excess quantities of glucocorticoids, mainly cortisol. It may occur from any of the following causes:

1. Adrenal hyperplasia secondary to excess ACTH stimulation from a pituitary tumor (either a basophilic or chromophobic adenoma) or functional pituitary overactivity probably caused by excessive hypothalamic activity. This is called *Cushing's disease.*
2. Ectopic Cushing's syndrome—some extraadrenal cancers (cancer of the lung, pancreas, thyroid gland, parotid gland, liver, and thymus) secrete large amounts of ACTH that cause Cushing's syndrome. These cancers are usually inoperable.
3. A functioning tumor (Fig. 15-2), either an adenoma or a carcinoma, of the adrenal cortex.
4. Administration of large quantities of glucocorticoid drugs (e.g., cortisone).

About 70% of all spontaneous cases of Cushing's syndrome result from hyperplasia, 20% from tumors, and 10% from ectopic ACTH.

The clinical picture is the same: amenorrhea, moon face, truncal obesity, muscular loss and weakness, hirsutism, acne, diabetes mellitus, skin atrophy, hypertension, abdominal striae, ecchymoses, osteoporosis, and mental disturbances (depression to frank psychoses).

Laboratory tests

Diagnosing Cushing's syndrome. The *overnight dexamethasone suppression test* is the most valuable single screening test for Cushing's syndrome. Dexamethasone, 1 mg. taken at midnight, will lower morning plasma cortisol levels below 5 µg./dl. in normal people (normal values, 5 to 20 µg./dl.). Patients with Cushing's syndrome have values usually above 10 µg./dl. after suppression.

Urinary 17-hydroxycorticosteroids (17-OHCS) average 5 to 10 mg./24 hr. in normal people. High levels, especially when they fail to suppress with dexamethasone, indicate Cushing's syndrome. (See Table 15-1.)

Urinary free cortisol (normal: 80 to 400 µg./day) correlates more closely than 17-OHCS with cortisol secretion rates. It is becoming the most dependable test.

Loss of diurnal plasma cortisol variation is a sign of Cushing's syndrome. Normal people show elevated plasma cortisol levels in morning blood samples and depressed afternoon levels. Patients with Cushing's syndrome show little or no diurnal variation.

Differentiating the cause of Cushing's syndrome. After the physician makes the diagnosis of Cushing's syndrome with one or more of the previously mentioned tests, he should attempt to define the cause. Table 15-1 summarizes these tests. ACTH will invariably stimulate the normal and hyperplastic glands but will stimulate tumors variably since their output is largely autonomous. The lower dose (2 mg./24 hr.) dexamethasone suppression test differentiates normal patients from those who have *any form* of Cushing's syndrome. The higher dose (8 mg./24 hr.) test differentiates adrenal hyperplasia from adrenal tumors.

The metyrapone test checks the integrity of the hypothalamic-pituitary-adrenal triangle, thus providing another good differentiation between adrenal hyperplasia and adrenal tumors. Metyrapone blocks the final step in cortisol production in the normal or hyperplastic cortex while allowing the precursors of cortisol to be produced. (These precursors are measured as 17-OHCS in the urine.) But these precursors cannot block ACTH; only cortisol has this ability. Thus metyrapone removes cortisol suppression of ACTH. Normal patients and those with hyperplasia respond by excreting increased amounts of urinary 17-OHCS. Patients with adrenal tumors, given metyrapone, continue to secrete excess cortisol unabated, therefore they show no variation in 17-OHCS excretion. Patients with ectopic ACTH-producing tumors continue to secrete the same excessive amounts of ACTH, despite metyrapone. Large amounts of exogenous ACTH will suppress pituitary ACTH; ectopic ACTH production acts similarly. They have lost the normal hypothalamic-pituitary-adrenal triangle. Therefore patients with ectopic Cushing's syndrome, given metyrapone, will not produce increased amounts of urinary 17-OHCS.

Plasma ACTH measurements (by radioimmunoassay) also reliably separate the causes of Cushing's syndrome. Patients with adrenal tumors have low ACTH plasma levels; those with hyperplasia or ectopic ACTH production have high levels.

X-ray examination. Although skull films with tomograms will show large pituitary lesions, CT scans have greater precision in detecting smaller (<10 mm) tumors. In detecting adrenal lesions scintigraphy with iodocholesterol (NP-59) and CT scans are the most useful diagnostic procedures. Echography, venography, and arteriography are less popular now. The latter two share the disadvantages of being invasive procedures. Nuclear magnetic resonance scans provide images similar to CT scans but with better resolution.

Treatment. The treatment of Cushing's *syndrome* caused by tumors is clear-cut: excision of the tumors, if possible. But treatment of Cushing's *disease* is controversial. Two modalities aim at lowering excess ACTH, two others at ablating cortical tissue.

Irradiation of the pituitary. Conventional irradiation often takes several months to control the disease, and later recurrences are common. High-energy proton beam irradiation, available in only a few centers, is more effective. Irradiation may, of course, destroy other pituitary cells.

Pituitary microsurgery. Some reports indicate a high incidence (80%) of microadenomas and excellent responses from transsphenoidal excision of these minute tumors. Other pituitary functions can often be simultaneously preserved. Pituitary microsurgery has become the first-line therapy. At present only a few institutions have substantial experience with this procedure.

Surgical adrenalectomy. Adrenalectomy controls excess cortisol but not excess ACTH. After adrenalectomy, about 10% to 20% of the patients will develop symptomatic pituitary enlargements (Nelson's syndrome). Thus all postadrenalectomy patients require periodic reassessment of pituitary status. Bilateral adrenalectomy has three main advantages: it can rapidly control florid Cushing's disease, it does not directly threaten other pituitary functions, e.g., fertility, and it is more widely available.

Drugs. o,p'-DDD, a cortical toxin, selectively lyses cortisol-secreting cells and partially sup-

Table 15-1. Laboratory methods used to differentiate the causes of Cushing's syndrome*

	Normal	Hyperplasia	Tumor	Ectopic ACTH
1. Plasma cortisol	10-25 μg./dl. Rhythmic	↑ No rhythm	↑ No rhythm	↑ No rhythm
2. Plasma ACTH	0.1-.04 mU./dl.	↑	↓	↑
3. 17-OHCS In 24-hr. urine collection	5-10 mg./24 hr.	↑	↑	↑↑
4. Urinary free cortisol	80-400 μg./24 hr.	↑	↑	↑
5. Stimulation 25 units ACTH I.V. over 8 hr.	↑	↑↑	↔	↔
6. Suppression a. Dexamethasone by mouth 0.5 mg. q.6h. for 48 hr.	↓ >50%	↔ or ↓	↔	↔
b. Dexamethasone by mouth 2 mg. q.6h. for 48 hr.		↓ >50%	↔	↔, occasionally ↓
7. Metyrapone (SU-4885) 30 mg./kg. I.V. over 4 hr.	↑	↑↑	↔	↔

24-hr. urine collections are completed:
    ACTH: 24 hr. after ACTH begun
    Dexamethasone: in the second 24-hr. period of dexamethasone administration
    Metyrapone: 24 hr. after metyrapone begun

*Key: ↑ increased; ↓ decreased; ↑↑ greatly increased; ↔ unchanged.

presses ACTH. Although it is an excellent treatment for functioning adrenal cancer, its place in treating hyperplasia remains less certain because of many side effects (nausea, diarrhea, vomiting, cerebral dysfunctions, and gynecomastia). (See Chapter 11.)

Aldosteronism

Hyperplasia, or tumors, can arise from any of the three cortical cell types. Although the glomerulosa layer may become hyperplastic, it usually forms single adenomas that secrete excess aldosterone. Hypertension results and, although uncommon, is surgically curable.

Hyperaldosteronism and hypertension coexist in two clinical situations: (1) *primary aldosteronism,* which usually responds to adrenalectomy, and (2) *secondary aldosteronism,* from extra-adrenal causes.

Primary aldosteronism. Accounting for about 1% of all cases of hypertension, primary aldosteronism gives the following clinical picture: hypertension, headaches, polydipsia, polyuria, muscle weakness, partial paralysis, and the ECG changes of hypokalemia. Sodium retention and excessive potassium excretion are the two underlying mechanisms responsible for these symptoms and signs.

Laboratory tests show elevated serum Na^+, alkalosis, depressed K^+, increased serum and urine aldosterone, and low serum renin. Increased blood volume and aldosterone levels suppress serum renin.

The pathological changes of primary aldosteronism occur in the outer, glomerulosa layer of the adrenal cortex as (1) solitary aldosterone-producing adenomas (APA) or (2) idiopathic adrenal hyperplasia (IAH). APA accounts for 75% of primary aldosteronism and IAH for 25% (Fig. 15-3).

Ruling out secondary aldosteronism. Any disease that stimulates renin also elevates aldosterone: renal artery stenosis, intrinsic renal ischemia, juxtaglomerular hyperplasia, etc. Secondary aldosteronism always involves increased renin levels; pure primary aldosteronism, never. Thus renin and aldosterone determinations help select those patients (from the millions of hypertensives) who have potentially curable, aldosterone-induced hypertension (Table 15-2).

Table 15-2. Serum renin and urinary aldosterone relationships in three main types of hypertension*

Cause of hypertension	Serum renin	Urinary aldosterone
Renovascular	↑	↑
"Essential"	↔	↔
Aldosteronism	↓	↑

*Key: ↑ increased; ↓ decreased; ↔ unchanged.

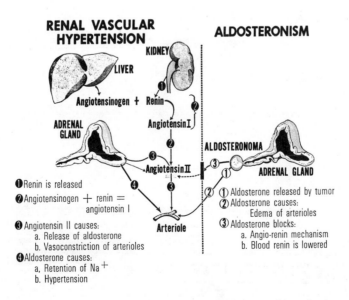

Fig. 15-3. Comparison of mechanisms causing renal vascular hypertension and primary aldosteronism.

Table 15-3. Characteristics of adenomas and hyperplasia

Symptoms	Aldosterone-producing adenomas (APA)	Idiopathic adrenal hyperplasia (IAH)
Blood pressure ↑	Often severe	Moderately high
Aldosterone, Na$^+$, Total CO$_2$	High	Moderately high
Renin, K$^+$	Low	Moderately low
Aldosterone levels after standing	Decreased	Unchanged or increased
CT scan	Single tumor	Bilateral enlargement
Iodocholesterol scan	Uptake in single tumor	Bilateral uptake
Venous sampling (aldosterone)	Unilateral increase	Bilateral increase

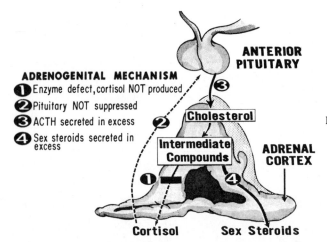

ADRENOGENITAL MECHANISM

❶ Enzyme defect, cortisol NOT produced

❷ Pituitary NOT suppressed

❸ ACTH secreted in excess

❹ Sex steroids secreted in excess

ANTERIOR PITUITARY

Cholesterol

Intermediate Compounds

ADRENAL CORTEX

Cortisol

Sex Steroids

Fig. 15-4. Mechanism of adrenogenital syndrome.

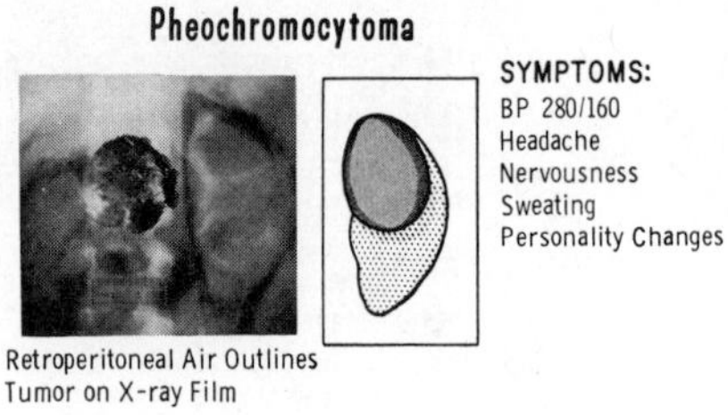

Fig. 15-5. Left adrenal pheochromocytoma outlined by retroperitoneal CO$_2$ insufflation.

Pheochromocytoma

SYMPTOMS:
BP 280/160
Headache
Nervousness
Sweating
Personality Changes

Retroperitoneal Air Outlines Tumor on X-ray Film

Differentiating adenomas from hyperplasia. Because patients with adenomas respond well to excision and those with hyperplasia respond poorly, attempts to separate them become vitally important. The characteristics in Table 15-3 help differentiate these two pathological causes.

Treatment. With more than 95% accuracy, the above clinical and laboratory data will differentiate APA from IAH. After excision of an aldosteroma, 90% of the patients will become normotensive. Patients with hyperplasia respond best to spironolactone. Since bilateral adrenalectomy fails to relieve hypertension in many patients, it should be reserved for only those patients refractory to medical treatment.

Adrenogenital syndrome

In the steps of cortisol synthesis a branching chain is responsible for the formation of the sex steroids (Fig. 15-4). In some children a defective enzyme system allows the sex steroids to be produced while cortisol production is blocked. One can anticipate the chain of events that ensues. In the absence of cortisol, the main inhibitor of ACTH from the anterior pituitary, the anterior pituitary produces excess amounts of ACTH and thus stimulates the secretion of more sex steroids (that cannot suppress ACTH). The overall result is a masculinizing effect. In children the treatment is simply giving cortisol or other glucocorticoids that supply bodily needs while blocking the secretion of excess ACTH. This cuts off all stimulation to the abnormal pathway for sex steroid production. Virilizing symptoms that appear in adult life are strongly suggestive of an adrenal or ovarian tumor.

DISEASES OF ADRENAL MEDULLA
Pheochromocytoma

Pheochromocytoma is a rare tumor arising from the nervelike tissue of the adrenal medulla. Bilaterality, malignancy, and extra-adrenal location each occur in roughly 10% of the cases. Thus it has

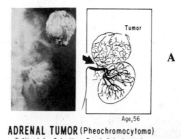

ADRENAL TUMOR (Pheochromocytoma)
Outlined by Selective Renal Arteriography

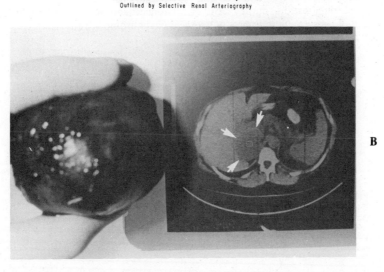

Fig. 15-6. A, Left adrenal pheochromocytoma outlined by dye injected into left renal artery. **B,** Right adrenal tumor *(outlined by arrows)* on CT scan.

been called the "10% tumor." Extra-adrenal pheochromocytomas usually arise from the abdominal sympathetic ganglia, but they may originate within the chest, cranium, or even the bladder wall. Increased production of epinephrine and norepinephrine is responsible for the clinical picture that features the two main types of symptoms—*hypermetabolic* and *neurological*. These symptoms (and signs) are nervousness, sweating, palpitation, headache, weakness, weight loss, syncope, psychic disturbances, and hypertension (Fig. 5-5). The tumors have been reported in all age groups from the newborn to the aged. The patients are usually thin, and about 50% will show abnormal glucose tolerance curves or glycosuria. Neurofibromas coexist in some patients with pheochromocytomas. The symptoms come in "attacks" in about half the cases. Pheochromocytomas tend to be familial. Coappearing with medullary thyroid cancers, parathyroid adenomas, and a Marfan-like body build, they form a multiple endocrine adenopathy with autosomal dominant transmission.

Diagnosis. The most difficult problem is diagnosis. Among the many patients with hypertension, the patient with a pheochromocytoma is sometimes hopelessly obscured. Diagnostic work-ups are costly and time consuming. Thus suspicion and selection are vital diagnostic requisites. Hypertension associated with childhood, glycosuria, pregnancy, orthostatic hypotension, neurofibromas, paroxysmal sweating and headaches, and wide variations in blood pressure recordings should evoke suspicion.

Laboratory tests. Elevated urinary metanephrines, vanillylmandelic acid (VMA), and free catecholamines provide a diagnostic accuracy of over 90%. Quantification of these metabolic products of the epinephrines has largely replaced the more hazardous histamine provocative test and the adrenergic blockade test. Intravenous pyelograms, computerized tomography (CT scans), and selective arteriography will help localize these tumors (Fig. 15-6).

A new specific radionucleotide, [131]I-*meta*-iodobenzylguanidine (MIBG), concentrates in chromaffin cells and has localized pheochromocytomas within the adrenal glands and in ectopic sites. Because it tests adrenal medullary *function*, it can distinguish functioning from nonfunctioning tissue. This provides the surgeon with vital preoperative data. For example, in adrenal medullary hyperplasia, the medulla enlarges at the expense of the adrenal cortex. Even a tenfold medullary enlargement can be missed by ultrasound or CT scans, whereas MIBG will clearly show it.

Treatment. Surgical excision is usually curative. Because 10% of these tumors are bilateral and 10% are extra-adrenal, most surgeons prefer the abdominal approach. Preoperative preparation (for 10 to 14 days) with alpha-blocking agents (phenoxybenzamine [Dibenzyline]), which decrease blood pressure, increase blood volume, and reverse myocardial damage, provides a smoother operative and postoperative course. Beta-blockade with propranolol is added (but only after alpha-blockade) for tachycardias, or arrhythmias, or both.

Some metastatic tumors have responded to MIBG, an exciting new development that simulates the response of thyroid cancer to radioactive iodine.

Bilateral medullary hyperplasia

Bilateral medullary hyperplasia, a rare occurrence, can mimic the clinical characteristics of pheochromocytoma.

The Breast

Richard D. Liechty

Diseases of the breast originate from four basic pathological processes: disturbances of hormonal activity, irritant effects of retained secretions, infections, and tumors. These processes produce a variety of symptoms, including a large measure of anxiety. From a clinical standpoint the most frequent complaint, by far, is that of a mass. The overwhelming significance of any breast mass to the anxious patient and to the concerned physician is the potential threat of cancer. The differential diagnosis and treatment of the three common types of breast masses (mammary dysplasia, fibroadenoma, and cancer) are our major concerns in this chapter.

ANATOMY

The glands of the breast arise from the skin and are similar to sweat or sebaceous glands. About 15 to 25 branching epithelial channels form in early life (Fig. 16-1, *A*). At puberty a resurgence of growth results in the formation of lobes with each main duct emptying into the nipple. Lymphatics within the breast drain into the axillary nodes, internal mammary nodes, supraclavicular nodes, and the nodes in the second and third intercostal spaces (Fig. 16-1, *B*).

Supernumerary breasts or nipples occur along the milk line (Fig. 16-2). Cancer has been known to

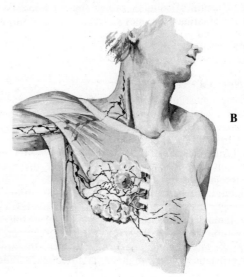

A

B

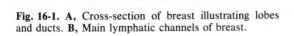

Fig. 16-1. A, Cross-section of breast illustrating lobes and ducts. **B,** Main lymphatic channels of breast.

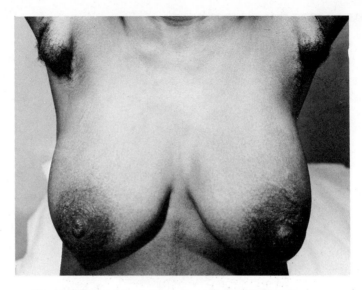

Fig. 16-2. Bilateral breast tissue in axillae of 22-year-old woman.

originate in extra breast tissue occurring in the axilla. Extra breast tissue should be removed for diagnostic or cosmetic reasons.

Physiology

Most women develop some swelling, mild pain, and tenderness of the breasts in a cyclical fashion at the time of menstrual flow. Estrogens stimulate duct cells the first 2 weeks of the cycle. Progesterones stimulate acini (glandular structures) the last 2 weeks. In pregnancy this process is repeated but in terms of months rather than weeks. Estrogens stimulate the duct cells for the first 4 to 5 months, and progesterones continue until delivery. Prolactin (from the pituitary) induces lactation after delivery.

GYNECOMASTIA

Gynecomastia (enlargement of the male breast) is often seen in pubertal boys, probably from sensitized breast tissue overresponding to a changing hormonal environment. It is usually unilateral, transient, and *never* malignant. Gynecomastia in the adult male is characterized by a firm, discrete subareolar disk of breast tissue that is less often unilateral. It usually results from similar functional endocrine disturbances and only rarely from testicular tumors or hyperfunctioning adrenal or pituitary tumors. Severe liver disease (failure to metabolize estrogens), long-term estrogen therapy (for prostatic cancer), digitalis, methyldopa, street

drugs, and starvation may induce gynecomastia. In teen-agers, the surgeon excises gynecomastia for cosmetic (psychological) reasons; in the adult, to rule out cancer (especially when the lesion is unilateral).

HYPERTROPHY

Neonatal hypertrophy commonly occurs in both male and female infants because of maternal estrogenic stimulation. It usually subsides within 6 months.

Virginal hypertrophy occurs as normal bilateral enlargement of the breasts during puberty. Excessive growth occasionally causes painful and disfiguring enlargement; reduction mammoplasty is necessary in the extreme cases. Precocious breast hypertrophy, seen in the first 5 years of life, is almost always caused by estrogen-producing tumors of the endocrine system.

BREAST MASSES

Which masses are significant? Many breasts have granular or nodular tissues that blend into a "background." The significant masses are "three-dimensional" and appear to stand apart from this "background" breast tissue. Such distinct masses should be removed and studied histologically (Fig. 16-3).

Diagnosis. The finding of these masses depends almost entirely on the examiner's palpatory skill. The early breast cancers appear only as a lump.

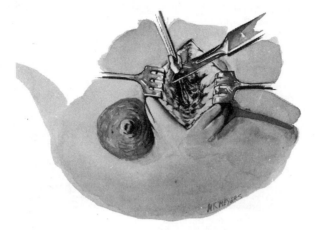

Fig. 16-3. Open excision biopsy of breast mass. Frozen section microscopy done immediately for specific diagnosis.

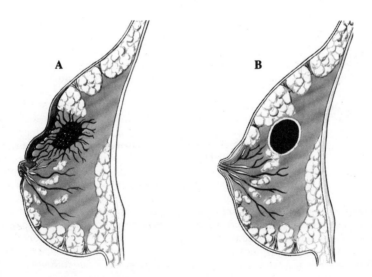

Fig. 16-4. Mammography. **A,** Malignant mass—ragged borders, skin thickening, stippled calcifications, and nipple retraction. **B,** Benign mass—smooth borders, no calcifications, and normal skin.

When obvious skin retraction, fixation, or ulceration appears, the tumor is far advanced. Transillumination is of no help.

Self-examination is often helpful, but difficult because the woman who examines her breast has no basis for comparison or interpretation. Even among nurses, self-examination is fraught with doubts and anxieties that only an experienced physician can resolve.

Mammography. Radiographs of the breast have proved effective in diagnosing breast cancer. Radiographic signs of malignancy are ragged, tentacled borders, finely stippled calcifications, and thickened overlying skin (Fig. 16-4). Unfortunately this procedure is time consuming and costly and demands highly skilled personnel. Many physicians use mammography to screen high-risk patients (those with family history of breast cancer; those with cancer of opposite breast) or exceptionally anxious patients, but mammography's most appealing potential lies in screening all patients *before* they develop palpable masses. Recent studies confirm that these radiographically detectable, early cancers have less nodal metastases and less 5-year mortality. Xeroradiography features a charged plate that forms an electrical image corresponding to the x-ray image. This image, captured on special paper, shows finer details than x-ray film. Experts report over 95% accuracy with xeroradiography. Because of dense breast tissue, young women defy reliable diagnosis (except for calcifications) by either method.

Thermography. Thermography depends on sensitive heat-measuring sensors to detect increased metabolic activity (thus increased heat) over cancers. Thermography currently remains an investigative procedure.

Mammary dysplasia, fibroadenoma, and cancer
Mammary dysplasia (chronic cystic mastitis)

Mammary dysplasia occurs in at least one third of all women (Fig. 16-5). The cause is an abnormal reaction of the breast tissue to cyclical stimulation and withdrawal of hormones. The *symptoms* are bilateral breast pain, tenderness, nodularity, and fullness that is maximal just before menstrual flow. Cysts and fibrous or epithelial tissue hyperplasia form masses that resemble cancer. In years past clinicians debated the malignant potential of mammary dysplasia, but this controversy has largely been resolved. Current evidence indicates that it may be associated with a higher incidence of breast cancer than is normal breast tissue, especially the types with predominant proliferation of ductal epithelium.

Treatment. *Pain and tenderness* occur in women just before their menstrual periods. Firm support

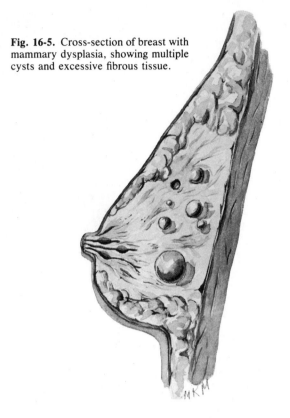

Fig. 16-5. Cross-section of breast with mammary dysplasia, showing multiple cysts and excessive fibrous tissue.

helps most. Androgens may benefit extreme cases, but usually sympathetic counseling is all that is required.

Three-dimensional, solid *masses* should be excised and studied microscopically. Cysts should be aspirated (Fig. 16-6). At least 80% will disappear permanently after aspiration. This simple and safe office procedure avoids the psychological traumatic effects of hospitalization (often repeated) for biopsy diagnosis. If the cysts refill, excision biopsy will rule out cancer. In rare instances, after multiple recurrences and biopsies, simple mastectomy may be indicated to allay permanently the fears of breast cancer in exceptionally anxious patients, or if the biopsies show excessive epithelial ductal hyperplasia. *Subcutaneous mastectomy,* through inframammary incisions, will remove virtually all breast tissue while preserving skin and nipples. Younger women especially benefit from this procedure and subsequent insertion of prosthetic implants.

Nipple discharge is often a frightening symptom to women who have been made cancer-conscious by articles in lay periodicals. If a dominant mass occurs concurrent with the discharge, the mass should be biopsied. If the discharge is not bloody

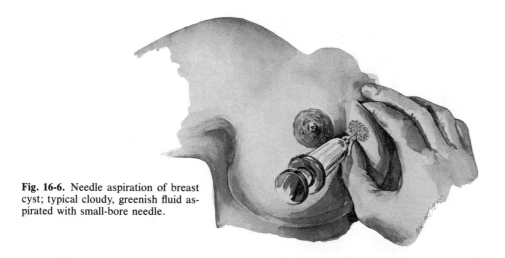

Fig. 16-6. Needle aspiration of breast cyst; typical cloudy, greenish fluid aspirated with small-bore needle.

and no mass is present, the patient should be reassured and have periodic examinations. Cytological studies have been unrewarding in our experience.

If the discharge is bloody, probing of the duct and excision of the lobule of breast tissue draining into the involved duct will allow histological examination to determine the need for more extensive resection (Fig. 16-7). Bleeding is usually caused by an intraductal papilloma, which is *not* a premalignant tumor. If the patient is past the menopause and no intraductal papilloma is found to account for the bleeding, a simple mastectomy will effectively rule out cancer. The likelihood of bloody nipple discharge being caused by cancer increases after the menopause.

Fibroadenoma

Fibroadenoma, a firm, freely movable lesion (Fig. 16-8), occurs in women most frequently in the early twenties. Fibroadenomas are usually smooth walled and solitary, although 10% to 15% are multiple. Bacause they are dominant lumps and also may evolve into *cystosarcoma phylloides,* a bulky tumor that rarely metastasizes, fibroadenomas should be excised.

Cancer

Incidence. One out of eleven American women (9%) will develop breast cancer. About 115,000 new cases of breast cancer in the United States are estimated for 1984. The age-adjusted mortality has remained almost the same for the past 50 years, despite aggressive new treatment methods. This inexorable statistic has stimulated current reappraisals of breast cancer therapy.

Epidemiology and etiology. The epidemiology of breast cancer includes many factors, some of which are endocrine, heredity, geography, economic status, race, preexisting pathosis, and possibly diet.

Endocrine and heredity. Unmarried women, nulliparous women, and parous women who have never nursed run a higher risk of breast cancer. But pregnancy before age 30 or early artificial menopause apparently decreases this risk. Breast cancer shows a definite familial tendency. Daughters whose mothers have had breast cancer have at least a threefold increase in their risk of developing it.

Geography and economic status. Japanese women have the world's lowest incidence of breast cancer, Danish women the highest. Some relate this to decreased subcutaneous fat in the Japanese, others to less fat in the Japanese diet. Some evidence links hypothyroidism to breast cancer, but definite proof of this relationship remains elusive. White women of higher socioeconomic status seem more vulnerable to breast cancer than black women of lower status. This vulnerability may be related to both fertility and nursing.

Infections. Viruslike particles have been traced from the mother's milk of mice to infant mice that subsequently developed breast cancer. Since similar particles have appeared in human milk from patients with breast cancer, a history of breast cancer should interdict women from nursing.

Contraception. About 60 million women have taken contraceptive medications since they were introduced in 1960. Up to now, these women have shown no increased frequency of developing breast cancer.

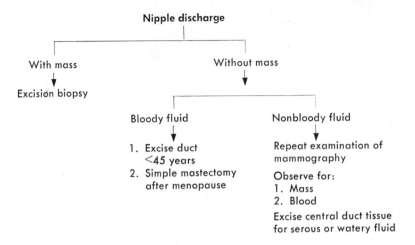

Nipple discharge

With mass → Excision biopsy

Without mass

Bloody fluid
1. Excise duct <45 years
2. Simple mastectomy after menopause

Nonbloody fluid
Repeat examination of mammography
Observe for:
1. Mass
2. Blood
Excise central duct tissue for serous or watery fluid

Fig. 16-7. Management of patient with nipple discharge.

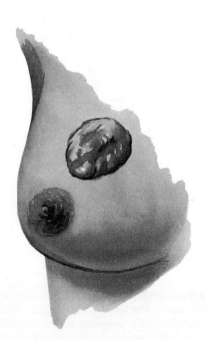

Fig. 16-8. Large fibroadenoma of breast.

Sex and age. The 100:1, female:male sex ratio of breast cancer is well known. This ratio probably relates to high levels of female estrogens. Breast cancer incidence rises with age, though a slight leveling of the rate marks the menopausal years. Although 75% of all breast cancer strikes patients 40 years of age and over, *breast cancer remains the leading killer of the young mother.*

Trauma. Trauma probably plays no causative role in breast cancer.

Besides providing many interesting facts about breast cancer, epidemiological research may prove most useful in pointing to those areas where other types of research can explore most effectively.

Patterns of growth. Some patients with breast cancer die in just a few months; others survive for years with advanced disease. We have followed one patient in whom the disease has smoldered for almost 30 years. This wide range in activity probably represents a varying relationship between tumor and host. Studies based on the time required for breast tumors to double in size reveal that three fourths of the life of an average breast cancer (8 years) is preclinical (before it reaches 1 cm. in diameter). Thus, before it is palpable, the future course of breast cancer is probably established. The type of cancer and the resistance of the host ("host-tumor relationship") are the decisive factors in prognosis. Metastasis to the upper axillary nodes portends decreased host resistance or perhaps increased malignant potential of the tumor.

Pathology. The breast is composed of ducts and glands (acini) along with fibrous tissue and fat; 95% of breast cancer arises in the ducts, and 5% is of acinar origin.

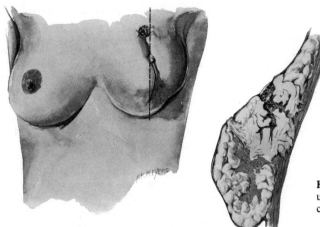

Fig. 16-9. Advanced breast cancer showing skin ulceration, nipple retraction, deformity of breast contour, and fixation to chest wall.

Table 16-1. Types of breast cancer

Pathological types	% of all breast cancers	Patients with positive nodes; % at diagnosis	Prognosis
Infiltrating ductal with fibrosis	78	60	Usually poor to variable
Infiltrating lobular	9	60	Variable
Medullary	4	44	More favorable
Colloid	3	32	
Comedocarcinomas	5	32	
Papillary infiltrating	1	17	
Paget's Inflammatory	Variants of ductal cancers (see text)		

Location. Cancer of the breast originates most often in the upper outer quadrant (40%) and in the subareolar area (25%). Breast cancers probably arise from multicentric areas of neoplastic change. Premalignant changes are not uncommonly seen throughout a breast removed for one locus of malignancy. Lobular cancer is often bilateral.

Types of cancer. Table 16-1 illustrates the types of cancer of the breast. About 80% will have profound sclerosing changes (desmoplasia), which give breast cancer its typically hard and gritty (scirrhous) characteristics (Fig. 16-9).

Although breast cancer can be classified into prognostic patterns, any of these types of cancer may metastasize and kill. *Inflammatory cancer* is singled out only because of its astonishing ability for rapid growth and spread that mimics inflammation—thus its name. *Paget's disease* features a chronic eczematous lesion of the nipple usually with extension to adjacent skin. A duct carcinoma, of relatively low malignancy, underlies the skin

changes. The Paget cells, seen microscopically, are metastatic tumor cells.

Grading. Attempts to predict the course of breast cancer from histological appearance of the cells, except for the favorable types (Table 16-1), are unreliable and unrewarding.

Metastasis. Regionally, breast cancer spreads most commonly to (1) axillary nodes, (2) internal mammary nodes, (3) supraclavicular nodes, and (4) skin. Distant metastases occur in descending order to (1) chest (lungs, pleura, ribs), (2) bones, (3) liver, (4) adrenal glands, (5) brain, and (6) ovaries.

Staging. Staging defines the extent of the disease and thus determines both treatment and prognosis. Clinical staging is important, since this determines what kind of treatment each patient will have.

Clinical staging for cancer of the breast follows:

Stage I	Limited to breast
Stage II	Regional node involvement
Stage III	Distant metastases

Many errors between the palpating hand and the microscope appear after the breast is removed and examined pathologically. Small axillary nodes invaded by tumor may be impossible to palpate, and, conversely, in about 1% of cases, involved axillary nodes may appear before the cancer in the breast is palpable (occult breast cancer). Size alone does not determine operability or prognosis; e.g., medullary cancers may grow to a large diameter while remaining localized to the breast. They often have an excellent prognosis. Similarly, the location of the cancer (whether in the upper-outer quadrant or elsewhere) has little prognostic significance.

Clinical staging is only a crude attempt to determine whether an operation will benefit the patient. Edema of the skin, large axillary metastases, ulceration, fixation, or a very rapid growth rate are all gloomy harbingers of prognosis. Routine preoperative chest roentgenography and mammography of the opposite breast help to rule out lesions in those areas. When findings are suggestive of distant metastases, additional tests should include bone scans (for bone pain), liver scans (for abnormal liver function), and brain scans (for central nervous system dysfunctions). Only the surgeon, weighing all these factors and considering the overall condition of the patient, can make the final decision of whether an operation will benefit the patient (Table 16-2).

Treatment and prognosis. Medical literature bulges with studies of breast cancer treatments. Students often become lost in the massive, sometimes conflicting data. Some of these issues may be clarified when the operative procedures are defined.

Simple mastectomy is excision of (most) breast tissue including skin and nipple. *Total mastectomy* refines the definition to include removal of all breast tissue from midline sternum and the supraclavicular space to the lateral edge of the latissumus dorsi and inferiorly to the costal margin. *Radical mastectomy* is excision of all breast tissue, pectoral muscles, and axillary contents, *en bloc*. *Modified radical mastectomy* is radical mastectomy including axillary dissection but sparing the pectoral muscles. *Extended radical mastectomy* includes radical mastectomy *and* excision of the internal mammary nodes with medial portions of the second through the fifth ribs.

For three decades controversy has raged over whether simpler treatments (simple mastectomy and irradiation) are as effective as more radical ones. Several prospective, randomized studies, including a 34-institution National Surgical Adjuvant Breast Project (NSABP), have largely settled these issues.

Studies from Europe and the United States show that simple mastectomy with irradiation is as effective as (1) radical mastectomy with irradiation or (2) extended radical mastectomy alone.

Using data from Canada and the United States, the NSABP study shows that radical mastectomy offers no special advantages. In patients with clinically negative axillary nodes, three different treatments, radical mastectomy, total mastectomy plus irradiation, and total mastectomy followed by axillary dissection (when nodes became palpable), showed no significant differences either in survival or in treatment failure (tumor in local, regional, or distant site). Similarly, in patients with positive nodes radical mastectomy and total mastectomy followed by irradiation showed no statistical differences.

Because of these studies, surgeons have largely abandoned classical radical mastectomy in favor of modified radical mastectomy. This modified procedure produces less postoperative arm edema, fewer wound problems, and better cosmetic results.

Radiotherapists now have evidence that they can treat *primary* breast cancer effectively. After irradiation these patients show no increased incidence of second malignancies in the treated breast, and survivals at 5, 10, and 20 years approximate those after surgical treatment. Radiotherapy, then, provides an excellent alternative, especially for patients who adamantly refuse operative procedures.

Although it decreases local recurrences, radiotherapy, either pre- or postoperatively, adds nothing to the 5-year survivals after modified radical mastectomy.

Adjuvant therapy. Because some years ago surgical or irradiation treatments or both reached a stable plateau, investigators turned their attention to chemotherapy. In theory this therapy strikes metastatic cells at an early stage. It adds chemotherapy to surgical therapy, when cells might be especially vulnerable. Beginning with mastectomy and continuing for up to 2 years, chemotherapy has clearly increased the disease-free intervals and survivals. The most effective drugs so far include

Table 16-2. Survival rate comparison in treated and untreated patients

	Years of survival	
	5	10
Untreated patients (%)	20	5
Radical mastectomy (%)		
Negative nodes	80	65
Positive nodes	50	30

5-fluorouracil (5-FU), methotrexate, and cyclophosphamide (Cytoxan) in combination.

Remember that, despite the apparent benefits of adjuvant therapy, breast cancer still kills most of its victims. The inexorable host-tumor relationship remains the dominant, controlling force. Fortunately, we have the means now to treat local exacerbations of the disease (Fig. 16-10) and to prolong life, but total cure or total prevention remains the ultimate goal. With adjuvant therapy, perhaps investigators have taken an important early step.

Palliation of advanced breast cancer. About 70% of all breast cancer patients, including operable cases, have or will develop metastases from their cancer. Palliation therefore is a most important concern to both patient and physician.

Radiotherapy. Radiotherapy is most effective in treating *localized* lesions of bone or soft tissue. If the metastatic tumor can be arrested in this manner, systemic therapy with hormones or chemical agents is held in reserve. Some metastases have been controlled for over 10 years with x-ray therapy alone.

Hormone therapy. Hormone therapy (Fig. 16-11) is utilized to treat diffuse metastases. Remission rates average about 30% to 35%. The exact mechanisms of hormonal response are unknown, but two factors seem pertinent and helpful in planning hormonal treatment: (1) the menopausal age of the patient and (2) the addition to, or subtraction from, these patients of estrogens. Premenopausal patients respond best to estrogen withdrawal (oophorectomy) or to estrogen antagonists, either tamoxifen or nafoxidine. Postmenopausal patients respond best to estrogens. Both androgens and estrogens are produced by the adrenal cortex, and they can be suppressed by cortisone administration or ablated by hypophysectomy or adrenalectomy. Medical adrenalectomy with aminoglutethimide has produced excellent responses in some patients. This drug provides a solid alternative to surgical adrenalectomy. Each of these therapies changes the internal hormonal environment of the patient. Theoretically, this change in turn alters the growth pattern of the cancer (Fig. 16-12).

In general, slower growing tumors, tumors that involve bone or soft tissues, tumors that occur just before menopause, or tumors that occur at least 4 years after menopause respond better to hormone manipulation. Tumor tissues that have estrogen or progesterone receptors or both may predict the greatest percentage of responders. If both are present, remission rates will double (60% to 70%). Tumors that grow rapidly or involve brain or liver respond poorly. Therapy should be continued for at least 3 months, because evidence of objective remission is delayed in some patients. Patients who respond will survive about three to four times longer than nonresponders.

Except for rare instances, the physician should advise major gland ablation only for hormonally responsive cancers. In assessing each patient, he must weigh the chance for remission against operative risk and the hormonal consequences after hypophysectomy or adrenalectomy (thyroid, steroid, and vasopressin replacement). Ideally, the candidates for major ablations should have responded to castration, should bind both estrogen and progesterone, and should have a slow growth rate.

Chemotherapy. Cyclophosphamide (Cytoxan),

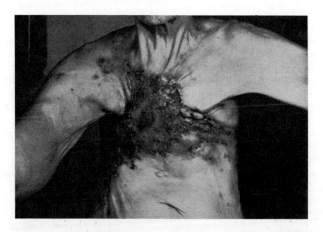

Fig. 16-10. Far-advanced, untreated, ulcerating breast cancer in elderly female.

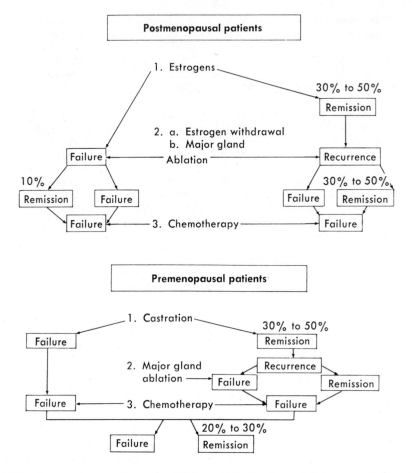

Fig. 16-11. Therapeutic steps in sequential treatment of advanced breast cancer in pre- and postmenopausal women.

prednisone, vincristine, doxorubicin (adriamycin), methotrexate, and 5-fluorouracil in combination have induced responses in about half the patients. Combination treatment, compared to any one drug, increases the percentage of patients responding as well as the average length of response. But remissions are often discouragingly brief, a mean duration of 8 to 10 months.

LESS COMMON BREAST DISEASES
Male breast cancer

Male breast cancer accounts for less than 1% of all breast cancers. It advances somewhat more rapidly in the male, but the 5-year cure rate is about the same as in the female. Mastectomy, hormone therapy, and irradiation are also used in the male. Orchiectomy followed by estrogen ther-

apy (and adrenalectomy) have produced some remissions in advanced stages.

Pregnancy and breast cancer

Breast cancer during pregnancy, a rare occurrence, has a less favorable prognosis than in other women matched for age and stage of the cancer. During the first half of pregnancy, patients should be treated surgically. During the last half, with early lesions, operations can be postponed until after delivery. Advanced lesions often demand abortion, suppression of lactation, and aggressive treatment of the cancer.

Infections

Acute infections usually occur during lactation and are treated like any other infection, with

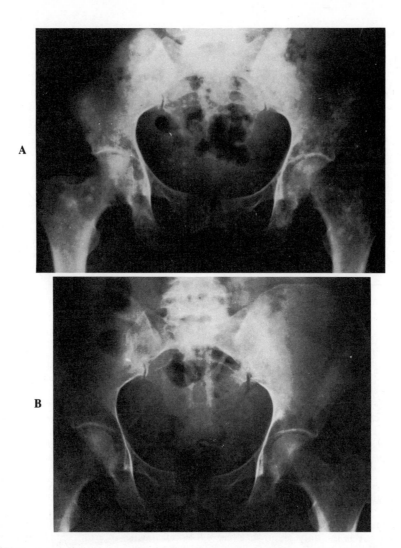

Fig. 16-12. A, Advanced breast cancer (52-year-old female). Notice extensive metastases to pelvis. **B,** Same patient 2½ years later after steroid therapy. Metastases have almost vanished. Patient died 1 year later.

incision, drainage, and antibiotics when indicated. Less commonly, breast infections occur in the newborn, presumably caused by maternal hormone stimulation of breast tissue.

Tuberculosis and other chronic granulomatous lesions are curiosities that must be diagnosed by biopsy or culture.

Traumatic fat necrosis

Traumatic fat necrosis occurs after injury and can usually be diagnosed by history or signs of hemorrhage. Subsequent fibrosis may require biopsy to differentiate these firm areas from cancer.

Plasma cell mastitis

Plasma cell mastitis is a rare disease that mimics inflammatory breast cancer because it produces pain, skin induration, and erythema. It usually occurs in women below 40 years of age and responds to radiation therapy. Biopsy and histological diagnosis are essential for the diagnosis.

Mondor's disease

Mondor's disease is a phlebitis of the superficial veins, usually in the outer quadrants of the breast. This uncommon condition usually begins with pain and terminates in venous thrombosis that slowly resolves.

Liver and Biliary Tract

Robert T. Soper
Nelson J. Gurll

The liver and bilary ducts form a functional unit directing numerous metabolic and excretory processes that are essential to life. The liver has many unique features:

1. It is the largest internal organ in the body, weighing 1.5 kg. in the adult.
2. It is the chemical center regulating at least 40 to 50 metabolic processes ranging from detoxification to synthesis and excretion, and probably many others that are presently unknown.
3. Its unusual blood supply provides inflow of both arterial (hepatic) and venous (portal) blood from two different vascular systems (systemic and portal, respectively).
4. The liver therefore is the only organ that has large inflow arteriovenous shunts, an admixture that occurs in the hepatic sinusoids.
5. It is composed of two lobes, right and left, with a different boundary line separating the anatomical lobes (at the falciform ligament) from the functional lobes (entirely within the right anatomical lobe, at about the position of the gallbladder fossa).
6. It possesses an enormous functional reserve and prodigious regenerative capability. In the experimental animal 80% of the liver can be removed without detectable impairment of function, with regeneration virtually to normal size occurring in 3 to 4 weeks.

These unusual features make the liver and biliary tract one of the organ systems most vital to life and largely dictate the role played by the surgeon in caring for patients with hepatic disease.

ANATOMY
Liver

The liver, one of the best protected organs in the abdominal cavity, is guarded anteriorly and laterally by the lower rib cage and superiorly by the muscular diaphragm. Furthermore, it is anchored superiorly and inferiorly by the ramifying vascular and ductal structures that pass vertically through it. Quite dense peritoneal ligaments attach the superior and posterior surfaces of the liver to the inferior surface of the diaphragm, encompassing a large triangular area of liver devoid of peritoneum and known as the "bare area"; the bare area is attached directly to the diaphragm by areolar tissue and also contains the hepatic veins, which return blood to the inferior vena cava. The falciform ligament, which contains the ligamentum teres and divides the liver into its anatomical right and left lobes, anchors the liver to the anterior abdominal wall down to the umbilical level. The lesser omentum connects the inferior surface of the liver with the duodenum and stomach, and the hepatorenal ligament attaches the inferior and posterior surfaces of the liver to the right kidney, adrenal gland, and inferior vena cava. All these ligaments and tubular structures tend to anchor the liver securely to the surrounding structures and prevent rapid dislocation during trauma.

The blood supply to the liver comes from two sources (Fig. 17-1). Venous blood returns from the entire gastrointestinal tract through the portal vein, which accounts for 75% of the blood flow to the liver, delivered with a relatively low pressure (5 to 15 cm. water) and oxygen content but rich in

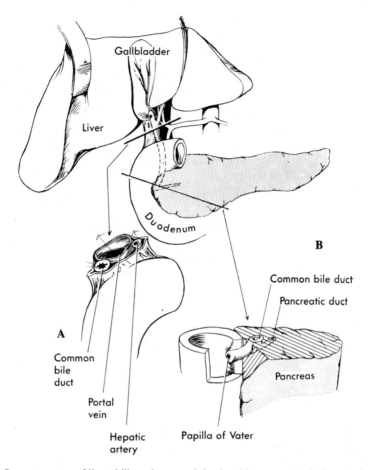

Fig. 17-1. Gross anatomy of liver, biliary ducts, and duodenal loop area. **A,** Intimate relationship of common bile duct, portal vein, and hepatic artery. **B,** Relationships of common bile duct, pancreatic duct, pancreas, and duodenum.

products of digestion. The arterial inflow comes through the hepatic artery under high arterial pressures and rich in oxygen but delivers only 25% of the afferent blood to the liver. Both of these vessels enter the inferior surface of the liver in juxtaposition to the major bile duct (Fig. 17-1, *A*), constituting a triad of structures of extreme importance to the surgeon during operations on the duodenum, stomach, and biliary system. Each of these structures divides into a right and left branch to service the two functional lobes, the dividing line of which lies entirely within the right anatomical lobe in the area of the gallbladder fossa.

The microscopic anatomy of the liver is epitomized by the smallest functional hepatic unit or lobule (Fig. 17-2). It is composed of a central vein that contains venous blood efferent from the liver to the inferior vena cava and thence to the right side of the heart. Surrounding the central vein are radially arranged polygonal hepatic cells that perform most of the chemical and excretory work of the liver. Between the radiating cords of liver cells are the hepatic sinusoids, which are lined by endothelial and specialized Kupffer cells of the reticuloendothelial system; these sinusoids are supplied by tiny lobular end branches from both the portal and hepatic vessels. The bile canaliculi likewise are juxtaposed between the cords of liver cells and coalesce in the perilobular spaces into cholangioles and tiny biliary ductules. These in

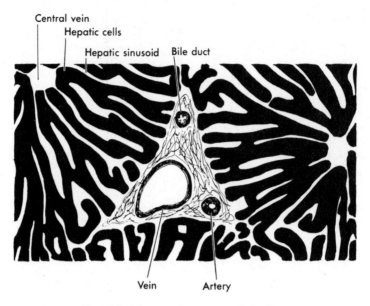

Central vein
Hepatic cells
Hepatic sinusoid   Bile duct

Vein   Artery

Fig. 17-2. Microscopic anatomy of the liver.

turn converge to form the right and left hepatic ducts, which emerge from the inferior surface of the liver with the hepatic and portal vessels.

Biliary ducts

The two main biliary ducts emerging from the inferior surface of the liver join to form the common hepatic duct, which becomes the common bile duct when joined by the cystic duct from the gallbladder (Fig. 17-1). The common bile duct then enters the head of the pancreas and empties into the medial or concave surface of the second portion of the duodenum through a thickening in the muscle of the duodenal wall known as the sphincter of Oddi (Fig. 17-1, *B*). The ampulla of Vater is a dilatation of the terminal portion of the common bile duct just proximal to the sphincter of Oddi, and it is the site of entry of the main pancreatic duct when a so-called common channel (of bile and pancreatic juice) exists. The main pancreatic duct may empty independently into the duodenum.

The common bile duct is 6 to 8 mm. in diameter and occupies the free edge of the lesser omentum, lying anterior to the aperture into the lesser sac known as the foramen of Winslow. The hepatic artery lies medial to the common duct, its right hepatic branches crossing posterior to the common hepatic duct in transit to the right lobe of the liver. The cystic artery is a branch of the right hepatic artery. The portal vein lies posterior and between the common duct and hepatic artery. Abnormalities

of positions and relationships of these ducts and vessels are common.

The gallbladder is a pear-shaped hollow organ with a normal capacity of approximately 50 ml. It lies within the depression on the inferior surface of the right lobe of the liver known as the gallbladder fossa, roughly marking the division between the *functional* right and left hepatic lobes. The rounded fundus of the gallbladder protrudes below the sharp edge of the right liver lobe and is continuous with the slightly larger body, which then narrows into the neck of the gallbladder. Often the neck of the gallbladder is sacculated into a structure known as *Hartmann's pouch,* where stones are commonly sequestered.

The cystic duct connects the gallbladder to the common bile duct and is characterized by a tortuous and narrow channel filled with spiraling mucosal folds known as the valves of Heister. It is understandable why gallstones so frequently become impacted in the cystic duct when one considers its tortuous and relatively small lumen.

The gallbladder wall has serous, fibromuscular, lamina propria, and mucosal layers from without inward. The biliary duct walls are thinner and contain few, if any, muscular elements. The bile duct serves as a simple conduit. Bile flow is the result of pressure produced by elaboration of bile from the hepatocytes and contractions of the gallbladder. The colicky pain of obstruction results from distention of the bile duct. Veins and lymphatics of the gallbladder may enter the liver directly.

PHYSIOLOGY
Liver

The polygonal liver cell is responsible for the majority of the important metabolic, detoxifying, and secretory functions of the liver. The Kupffer cells are mainly concerned with phagocytosis but also produce gamma globulin, which is important in immune defense mechanisms.

Bile formation

Bile is excreted by the liver at an irregular rate, averaging approximately 40 ml./hr. Liver bile is a dilute, slightly alkaline, and only mildly pigmented material composed largely of water (97%), bile salts (2%), bilirubin, cholesterol, phospholipids, and minute amounts of calcium and other electrolytes.

Bilirubin is formed from the catabolism of hemoglobin in mature erythrocytes by the reticuloendothelial system, especially spleen and bone marrow. The bilirubin, bound to albumin, is transported in the circulation to the liver where it is conjugated. After conjugation, the water-soluble bilirubin diglucuronide is excreted into the bile canaliculi and passes into the biliary ducts.

Bile salts are water-soluble substances formed by liver cells from cholesterol and are conjugated to glycine or taurine. Cholesterol is excreted into bile by the liver cells. Cholesterol is totally insoluble in aqueous systems and would immediately precipitate were it not acted on by the bile salts and phospholipids. Lecithin, the chief phospholipid in bile, combines with cholesterol to form liquid crystals. In turn, bile salts exert a detergent-like effect to break these insoluble liquid crystals into small soluble aggregates called mixed micelles. The hepatic secretion of cholesterol, lecithin, and bile salts in ideal ratios prevents cholesterol from precipitating in bile as stones. Bile salts are conserved by their reabsorption from the intestine (mainly distal ileum) into the portal system where they are re-excreted into the bile (enterohepatic circulation).

If the ductal system is obstructed, bile is regurgitated into the general circulation. Conjugated bilirubin is excreted by the renal glomerulus to lend the golden yellow color to the urine so characteristic of obstructive jaundice. Unconjugated bilirubin cannot pass the glomerular endothelium; therefore the jaundice associated with excessive breakdown of red blood cells (hemolytic jaundice) is acholuric (colorless urine). Excessive levels of bile salts in the serum are precipitated in the skin, causing pruritus associated with obstructive jaundice and biliary cirrhosis.

Carbohydrate metabolism

The liver converts monosaccharides absorbed from the intestine into glycogen, the chief form of carbohydrate storage in the body. Glycogen can be broken down into glucose and pentoses, which can be utilized for energy and synthesis of nucleic acids, fats, and proteins.

Fat metabolism

Fatty acids and neutral fats are both synthesized and catabolized by the liver. The liver is the principal site of cholesterol synthesis and esterification. Production and degradation of phospholipids and lipoproteins also occur in the liver.

Protein metabolism

Amino acids are transported from the intestine to the liver where new protein molecules are formed and different amino acids are created; some of the amino acids are deaminized and converted into carbohydrate or fat. Most clotting factors are made in the liver. Serum albumin, prothrombin, and fibrinogen are three important proteins manufactured by the liver cell. The ammonia resulting from deaminization is synthesized to urea for excretion by the kidney.

Steroid synthesis and metabolism

Steroids containing the phenanthrene ring (cholesterol, estrogen, cortisone, bile acids) are synthesized (cholesterol, bile acids) and metabolized (estrogen, cortisone) to inert metabolites by the liver.

Detoxification

Ammonia from protein metabolism is converted to urea. Morphine and barbiturates are metabolized to inactive forms and excreted by the liver.

The bile is the major excretory pathway for iodinated phenolphthalein compounds (iopanoic acid [Telepaque] or iodipamide [Cholografin]), certain dyes (sulfobromophthalein [Bromsulphalein], rose bengal), and some enzymes (alkaline phosphatase) to form the basis for diagnostic tests of hepatic and biliary tract function.

Biliary ducts

Approximately 1 L. of bile is produced each day by the liver at a pressure of 25 to 30 cm. of water (Fig. 17-3). The sphincter of Oddi maintains this head of pressure by tonic contraction. During periods of fasting, much of the bile is diverted into the cystic duct for storage within the gallbladder. Here the bile is concentrated 10 to 15 times by absorption of water and electrolytes such that the solid content of the gallbladder bile approaches 10% to 15% as contrasted to 2% to 3% in the bile as

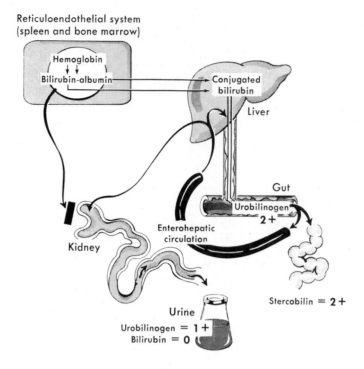

Fig. 17-3. Normal bilirubin metabolism.

it is excreted by the liver. With the entrance of hydrochloric acid and food into the duodenum during a meal, the hormone cholecystokinin is excreted, which causes the sphincter of Oddi to relax and the gallbladder to contract, emptying its bile into the common duct for delivery to the duodenum.

Bile is important to normal digestion principally because it emulsifies and saponifies ingested fats to improve their digestion and absorption from the intestine; fat-soluble vitamins A, E, D, and K require emulsification for normal absorption. Lipolytic and proteolytic enzymes within the succus entericus are activated by bile. Bile increases the absorption of iron and calcium, increases intestinal motility, and is bacteriostatic for many gastrointestinal tract organisms.

After reaching the intestine, colon bacteria reduce bilirubin to urobilinogen and then to stercobilin, to give the brownish pigmentation characteristic of normal stools. Some of the urobilinogen and more than 95% of bile salts are reabsorbed into the portal circulation from the intestine (so-called enterohepatic circulation) where much of it is conserved to produce more bile, and a fraction enters the general circulation; small amounts of urobilinogen are normally excreted in the urine.

Obstruction of the biliary tract (obstructive jaundice) prevents bile from reaching the intestine, producing gray-colored stools that are bulky and fatty because of the poor digestion and absorption of dietary fat; reduced absorption of the fat-soluble vitamin K will cause a hemorrhagic tendency if existent for a long enough period of time. Anorexia, weight loss, osteoporosis, and an iron-deficiency anemia are commonly seen with long-standing absence of bile from the intestine.

Tests of liver and biliary tract function

Literally dozens of different tests on blood, urine, duodenal drainage, and stool measure, directly or indirectly, different aspects of hepatic and biliary tract function (Table 17-1). Because of the enormous functional reserve of the liver, widespread and far-advanced liver disease may occur before distinctive changes are seen in many of these tests. Furthermore, the results of the tests vary from time to time as the disease waxes and wanes, and some functions of the liver may be severely curtailed while others proceed normally, at least according to our limited ability to measure them.

Liver function tests are most commonly performed to differentiate among the three major

Table 17-1. Liver function tests

Liver function tests	Normal	Hemolytic jaundice	Parenchymal jaundice	Obstructive jaundice
Bilirubin				
Serum				
Direct	0.2-0.5 mg./dl.	Normal	Increase	Pronounced increase
Indirect	0.2-0.5 mg./dl.	Increase	Increase	Normal early
Urine				
Urobilinogen	1+	4+	1+	0
Bilirubin	0	0	2+	4+
Stool stercobilin	2+	4+	1+	0
Serum alkaline phosphatase	120 mU./ml.	Normal	Increase	Pronounced increase
Serum albumin	4-5 gm./dl.	Normal	Decrease	Normal early
Prothrombin time	12-14 sec. or 85%-100% of normal control	Normal	Prolonged	Normal early Prolonged late
Bromsulphalein	3%-5% remains in 45 min.	Normal	Increase	Increase
Serum glutamic oxaloacetic transaminase (SGOT)	7-40 mU./ml.	Normal	Increase	Normal to slight increase

types of jaundice: parenchymal hepatic disease, extrahepatic biliary ductal obstruction, and hemolytic jaundice. They help in measuring advanced degrees of hepatic insufficiency and indicate the trend of hepatic disease or the residual liver damage after recovery. Tests of liver function help in evaluating the risk that liver or biliary surgery imposes on the patient. A few of the more commonly employed tests are described in some detail in the paragraphs that follow.

Tests of liver excretory function

Serum bilirubin. Total serum bilirubin normally varies from 0.4 to 1 mg./dl. The direct-acting fraction represents bilirubin that has been conjugated with glucuronic acid in the liver, and the indirect fraction represents bilirubin tied to albumin before conjugation. A normal total value is dependent on normal rates of red blood cell breakdown, conjugation and excretion by the liver, and passage through the biliary ducts to the intestine. Abnormalities of any one of these three steps involved in bilirubin metabolism might alter these levels. *Extrahepatic* obstruction classically produces an elevation of the total and direct bilirubin, whereas *hemolytic* jaundice will elevate the total and indirect fraction. *Parenchymal* liver disease is associated with elevation of total bilirubin and generally both its direct and indirect fractions.

Serum alkaline phosphatase. The normal value of this enzyme is from 3 to 13 King-Armstrong units or 1 to 4 Bodansky units, or less than 120 mU./ml. in most automated methods of analysis. The enzyme is released by rapidly metabolizing cells in many organ systems of the body, especially in bone, pancreas, and liver. It is excreted by the liver into the bile and is ultimately lost from the body in the stool. Elevation of serum alkaline phosphatase occurs with extrahepatic biliary tract obstruction and to lesser degrees with hepatic cellular disease, liver metastases, hyperparathyroidism, bone tumors, and Paget's disease of bone. Differentiation from bony disease may be helped by determination of 5'-nucleotidase or leucine amino peptidase.

Urine and stool bile and urobilinogen. Urobilinogen is partially reabsorbed in the enterohepatic circulation and partially excreted in the stool; small amounts are normally present in both the stool and the urine. Urobilinogen may be measured by simple gross or fairly sophisticated quantitative tests. Extrahepatic obstruction of the biliary ducts is associated with no urobilinogen or bilirubin in the stool (acholic stool) and no urobilinogen but increased amounts of conjugated bilirubin in the urine. With increased hemolysis, the amounts of both urobilinogen and bilirubin are increased in the stool, whereas in the urine the urobilinogen is increased; there is no bilirubin in the urine, since unconjugated bilirubin is not excreted by the kidney.

Metabolic function tests

Serum albumin. Serum albumin is one of the proteins manufactured by the liver cells. The normal serum albumin level is 4.5 to 5 gm./dl. of serum, and the albumin:globulin ratio in the serum is generally above 1. Chronic liver cellular damage is associated with a lowering of the serum albumin and a decrease or reversal of the albumin:globulin ratio.

Prothrombin time. Prothrombin is manufactured by the liver cells when adequate amounts of vitamin K are present. A deficiency of vitamin K occurs with prolonged obstructive jaundice (no bile to emulsify and aid in the absorption of the fat-soluble vitamin K) or chronic hepatocellular disease, resulting in inadequate production of prothrombin and prolongation of the prothrombin time. Normal prothrombin time is about 12 to 14 seconds. An elevated prothrombin time signals the need for parenteral vitamin K administration in the preoperative patient, a return to normal indicating adequate liver cell reserve, and perhaps a less bloody operation.

Bromsulphalein test. Bromsulphalein, a dye, is metabolized by the liver cell and excreted in the bile very rapidly; only 3% to 5% remains in the serum 45 minutes after intravenous administration. Elevation of the amount of Bromsulphalein present 45 minutes after administration is a rather sensitive indicator of hepatocellular damage.

Serum glutamic oxaloacetic transaminase (SGOT). SGOT is present in liver, heart muscle, skeletal muscle, kidney, and pancreas and may be elevated after injury to any of these organs. In reference to the liver, greatest elevations of this enzyme occur with hepatocellular injury (parenchymatous jaundice), and very slight elevations accompany hemolytic or obstructive jaundice.

Jaundice

Jaundice is a yellowish discoloration of the skin, sclera, body surfaces, and secretions. It can be detected on clinical examination when the serum bilirubin rises above 2.5 mg./dl. Three major classifications of jaundice are based on the nature and site of the disturbance of bilirubin metabolism:

1. *Excessive hemolysis* of red blood cells (hemolytic, acholuric, prehepatic jaundice)
2. *Hepatocellular (parenchymatous) disease,* which inhibits bilirubin conjugation (hepatocellular, retention, intrahepatic, or medical jaundice)
3. *Obstruction* of bile flow occurring anywhere from the canaliculi on down the biliary tract into the intestine (obstructive, regurgitation, posthepatic, extrahepatic, or surgical jaundice)

In *hemolytic jaundice* (Fig. 17-4) an excessive lysis of red blood cells causes increased production of bilirubin by the reticuloendothelial cells in the spleen and bone marrow; more bilirubin is produced than can be excreted by the normally functioning hepatic excretory mechanisms. The excess of nonconjugated bilirubin in the serum cannot be excreted in the urine but elevates the *indirect* fraction of bilirubin in the serum, with normal *direct*-acting fraction. The tests for hepatocellular function are normal, but excessive amounts of *urobilinogen* in the urine and stool and bilirubin (stercobilin) in the stool are diagnostic. Hemolytic jaundice is seen in congenital spherocytosis, thalassemia, septicemia, transfusion with mismatched blood, and after certain venomous snake bites. Treatment is directed at the cause of the hemolysis rather than the jaundice per se, and it is nonsurgical except for the definitive treatment of congenital spherocytosis (splenectomy).

Intrahepatic or *parenchymatous jaundice* (Fig. 17-5) is seen with liver infections (hepatitis), exposure to hepatotoxic agents (chloroform, arsenicals, occasionally chlorpromazine), and in the terminal stages of liver failure. Acute viral hepatitis is characterized by elevated SGOT and SGPT in the serum, but with chronic hepatic disorders the liver function tests are seldom diagnostic. There is a moderate elevation of both the direct and indirect serum bilirubin with decreased serum albumin levels, a mild increase in the alkaline phosphatase, and prolongation of the prothrombin time (with a poor response to vitamin K). Treatment is nonsurgical and largely supportive until the disease has run its course.

Obstructive jaundice (Fig. 17-6) results from interference of bile flow somewhere within the biliary ductal system. Most of these obstructions occur within the extrahepatic ducts and are amenable to surgical bypass or removal of the obstruction; therefore differentiation from the other two major types of jaundice becomes very important. In obstructive jaundice the stool is clay colored or very lightly pigmented, the stool and urine urobilinogen are diminished or absent, and the bilirubin (chiefly the direct fraction) is elevated. The hepatocellular tests are normal early, but with increasing duration of jaundice liver cellular damage occurs.

Stones within the common bile duct (choledocholithiasis) are the most common cause of extrahepatic obstructive jaundice, generally associated with pain and fluctuation in the intensity of the jaundice. Strictures of the bile ducts most commonly result from duct injury during cholecystectomy. The resulting jaundice tends to be fluctuating, essentially painless, and often associated with fever and cholangitis. Cancers of the bile ducts,

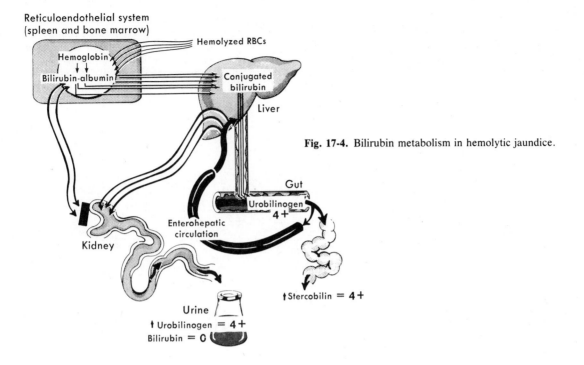

Fig. 17-4. Bilirubin metabolism in hemolytic jaundice.

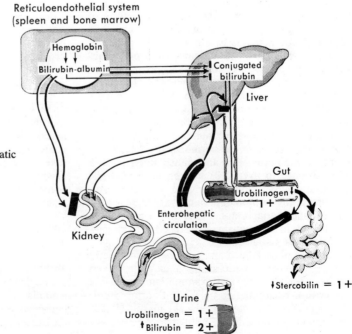

Fig. 17-5. Bilirubin metabolism in intrahepatic jaundice (hepatitis).

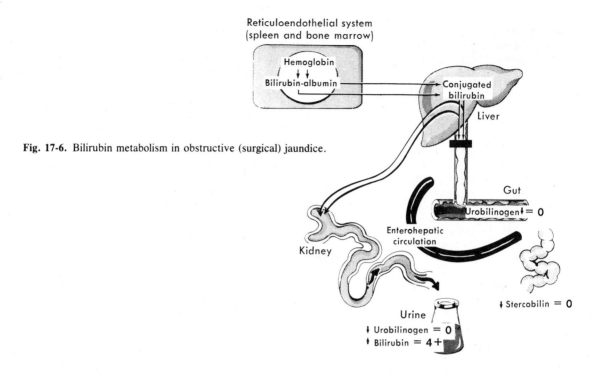

Fig. 17-6. Bilirubin metabolism in obstructive (surgical) jaundice.

ampulla of Vater, and head of the pancreas characteristically produce a progressively deepening and painless jaundice. Jaundice can also result from acute or chronic pancreatitis. Congenital atresia of the bile ducts is one of the two chief causes of *jaundice in the newborn*. It must be distinguished from neonatal hepatitis by early laparotomy.

Occasionally with the administration of certain drugs (chlorpromazine, arsenicals), with sepsis, and during the acute course of hepatitis, the intrahepatic cholangioles becomes obstructed by edema and inflammation to produce a variety of obstructive jaundice indistinguishable biochemically from extrahepatic obstructive jaundice, the so-called *cholestatic* jaundice. Furthermore, the longer obstructive jaundice from any cause persists, the more damage to liver cells will ensue from back pressure, regurgitation of bile, and infection; tests of hepatocellular function become progressively altered, and the laboratory tests therefore become less helpful in distinguishing obstructive from parenchymatous jaundice.

The type of jaundice can be diagnosed correctly in 75% to 80% of patients by a carefully taken history, complete physical examination, and a few simple tests performed on the patient's urine, stool, and blood. In the remaining 20% the more sophisticated liver function tests, cholangiography, liver

biopsy, or even exploratory laparotomy may be necessary to make a correct diagnosis.

Although not an emergency, the work-up of a jaundiced patient should proceed expediently, and a decision regarding the need for surgical exploration should be made as early as possible. The complications of untreated and long-standing jaundice are biliary cirrhosis, cholangitis, bile nephrosis, and ultimately both hepatic and renal failure. All have high morbidity and mortality.

SURGICAL DISEASES OF THE LIVER

Although the liver is often *damaged* by surgical disease (extrahepatic obstructive jaundice) or becomes secondarily involved by surgical disease (liver metastases from a primary intestinal neoplasm), and although liver disease can produce secondary changes that require surgical treatment (splenectomy, esophageal varices ligation, and portasystemic shunts for portal hypertension), few diseases *of* the liver are treated by operations *on* the liver.

Trauma

The liver is commonly injured by penetrating wounds of the abdomen and chest (stabbings, high-velocity missiles), and it ranks third among the intra-abdominal organs injured by nonpenetrating abdominal trauma. Even minor trauma may severely damage a liver enlarged by disease. The right anatomical lobe of the liver is larger and more exposed than the left and is therefore more frequently traumatized. Associated injuries to the right rib cage and other intra-abdominal organs often overshadow the hepatic injury.

Traumatic rupture of the liver results in intra-abdominal spillage of blood and bile with signs of shock and peritoneal irritation proportionate to the volume and speed of extravasation. Pain is initially localized to the right upper abdominal quadrant, then becomes more generalized, and often is referred to the right shoulder tip. Abdominal tenderness and guarding follow the pain, with percussion dullness and occasionally a palpable mass (hematoma). Paralytic ileus with abdominal distension occurs late.

Flat and decubitus plain roentgenograms of the chest and abdomen may reveal fractured ribs, a mass, or elevation of the right hemidiaphragm—all suggestive of liver injury. Peritoneal lavage should be performed if four-quadrant paracentesis fails to reveal blood.

Treatment of minor degrees of hepatic trauma is nonsurgical with bed rest, analgesics, and supportive care. Occasionally delayed subcapsular liver hematomas may rupture; thus observation of the patient for 1 to 2 weeks is advisable. The surgical goals in the treatment of more serious liver injuries are to debride devitalized tissue and to control bleeding. Actively bleeding lacerations are best stopped by direct suture of identifiable vessels. Control may require exploration of the laceration and even hepatic artery ligation. Parenchymal damage resulting from stellate lacerations and blunt injuries is treated by wide débridement. Lobectomy is rarely required and mortality is higher than with débridement. Extensive drainage of the damaged area is of paramount importance. T tube decompression of the biliary tree is associated with complications and is generally not indicated.

Surgical infections of the liver
Pyogenic liver abscess

Better diagnosis and treatment of infections have greatly reduced the incidence, morbidity, and mortality of pyogenic liver abscesses. Most begin as small microabscesses in the portal triads, which then progress to destroy liver cells and coalesce into gross abscesses. Selective antibiotic therapy administered during the microabscess stage probably reverses the infection and is the best explanation for the lowered incidence of frank abscesses.

The origin of 10% to 15% of the pyogenic liver abscesses is unknown; the majority of the re-

mainder originate in some portion of the gastrointestinal tract with spread through the portal vein (septic pylephlebitis) to secondarily involve the liver. Acute suppurative appendicitis is the chief offender; diverticulitis, ulcerative colitis, and enteritis are less common contributors. Ascending infection from a partially obstructed extrahepatic biliary tree (cholangitis) is the next most common source. Coliform organisms understandably are responsible for most pyogenic liver abscesses. Staphylococcal liver abscesses arise from systemic infections (osteomyelitis, carbuncles) and reach the liver through the hepatic artery.

The early clinical features are dominated by signs and symptoms of the causative extrahepatic infection. Right upper quadrant distress heralds hepatic abscess progressing to pain, spiking fever, sweating, shaking chills, and a palpably enlarged and tender liver. Mild jaundice may complicate the picture late in the clinical course and in general is an unfavorable prognostic sign.

The laboratory tests show anemia and leukocytosis with a shift to the left in the differential white blood cell count. Roentgenograms reveal an elevated and relatively immobile right hemidiaphragm with an enlarged hepatic shadow. Blood cultures are positive unless antibiotics have been given. Liver scintiscans may disclose a filling defect provided that the abscess is more than 2 or 3 cm. in size and is located fairly near the surface. Selective hepatic arteriography may reveal defects smaller than the resolution of a scintiscan. The defects are avascular in contrast to most hepatic tumors.

Diffuse bacterial insults to the liver are critical diseases. Antibiotics and supportive care are always indicated. Pyogenic liver abscesses should be treated by surgical drainage, though occasionally simple aspiration of smaller abscesses combined with specific antibiotics is sufficient.

Amebic abscess

Acute amebic colitis is common in tropical and less developed countries; about 10% of cases will be complicated by amebic liver abscesses if not properly treated. There is no history of dysentery in one half of cases of amebic liver abscess. Trophozoites of the parasite *Entamoeba histolytica* gain access to the portal venous tributary through the involved colon wall and migrate to the liver, where liquefactive necrosis of liver tissue occurs with coalescence into larger cavities. These abscesses are composed of necrotic liver tissue of a chocolate-red color often likened to anchovy paste. The offending parasite can usually be found in the wall of the abscess cavity, and with proper treatment it becomes encapsulated and calcified in time. If untreated, the abscesses may enlarge and perforate into the abdominal cavity or burrow through the diaphragm and empty into the thoracic cavity.

The clinical and laboratory findings resemble those of pyogenic liver abscesses except that the white blood cell count is lower, with less of a shift to the left in the differential count. Eosinophilia may be present. The liver complication may occur weeks after the colonic phase, which is often minor and unrecognized. Sigmoidoscopic examination and scrapings from the superficial mucosal ulcerations and warm stool examinations will usually reveal the amebas.

When the diagnosis of amebic hepatitis is made or suspected, the patient should be treated with metronidazole (Flagyl), 750 mg. orally three times a day for 10 days. A dramatic improvement in the patient's condition confirms the diagnosis and is therapeutic as well. Large amebic abscesses can be aspirated percutaneously. If the signs of liver infection worsen, laparotomy is necessary for confirmation of diagnosis; aspiration of the amebic abscess is preferable to open drainage for fear of a more general contamination of the peritoneal cavity by external drainage.

Cysts and tumors of the liver
Simple cysts

Liver cysts may be associated with cysts of the kidneys and may be multiple and small or single and large. They are thin-walled and filled with watery, colorless fluid. The larger cysts are treated by total or partial excision or drainage into the peritoneal cavity or intestine. Their main importance lies in distinguishing them from neoplasms, primary or metastatic to the liver.

Echinococcus cysts

Echinococcus cysts of the liver are common in sheep-growing countries of the world where man serves as the intermediary host in the life cycle of the dog tapeworm *(Echinococcus granulosus)*. The tapeworm within the dog intestine sheds eggs that are excreted and ingested by sheep or man (especially children), with secondary involvement of the liver and lung from intestinal migration. Echinococcus liver cysts, usually slow-growing, may reach a large size with rupture into the free peritoneal cavity, lung, or bile ducts.

Eosinophilia occurs frequently, and complement fixation tests are specifically diagnostic. Plain roentgenograms often reveal calcification in the cyst wall. Surgical treatment consists in excision after careful evacuation of the cyst contents by aspiration and injection of 20% to 30% sodium

chloride or 0.5% sodium hypochlorite to kill the scoleces.

Benign tumors of the liver

Hemangiomas, fibromas, and hamartomas occasionally arise in the liver and must be distinguished from metastatic or primary malignant neoplasms. Large hemangiomas of the liver are removed if they are traumatized (hemorrhage) or sequester large amounts of blood.

Hepatic adenomas are benign tumors whose incidence seems to be increasing because of the use of oral contraceptives. These lesions should be resected (usually by hepatic lobectomy) because they are frequently attended by life-threatening complications such as rupture and bleeding.

Malignant tumors of the liver

The most common malignant tumor of the liver is *metastatic* from primary neoplasms occurring in the stomach, colon, breast, and pancreas. The gastrointestinal tract metastases reach the liver through the portal vein, and others reach the liver through the hepatic artery. Direct spread from primary malignancies of the gallbladder, stomach, and other organs adjacent to the liver also occurs.

The majority of liver metastases are multiple and involve both lobes; only rarely are metastases localized so that resection can be considered. The exceptions to this treatment rule are liver metastases from malignant carcinoids or the Zollinger-Ellison type of pancreatic neoplasms, in which partial resection of the liver metastases is indicated to palliate the functional hormonal effects of the metastases. Radiotherapy of hepatic metastases is rarely indicated because of the severe symptoms (anorexia, nausea, vomiting) that occur when liver tissue is irradiated and because of the relentless (and hopeless) course of liver metastases. Chemotherapeutic agents occasionally produce palliation, especially when delivered directly into the portal vein or hepatic artery by indwelling catheters.

Primary malignant lesions of the liver are rare in the United States but are common among certain ethnic groups such as the Chinese and the African Bantu. Hepatomas arise from the liver cells and are almost invariably preceded by years of cirrhosis, hemochromatosis, or some other such chronic primary inflammatory liver disease. Cholangiocarcinomas arise from the intrahepatic bile duct cells and are not necessarily a sequela of chronic liver disease.

Symptoms of primary malignant liver tumors are insidious and nonspecific at first, including weight loss, anorexia, and low-grade fever. Liver enlargement (nodular or localized) follows with ultimate development of ascites and jaundice. The serum alkaline phosphatase is characteristically high. Treatment is usually futile. Although cholangiocarcinomas localized to one lobe are amenable to hemihepatectomy, the prognosis is poor. Chemotherapeutic agents may offer some palliation.

Portal hypertension

The pressure within the portal vein varies between 5 and 15 cm. of water, depending on position, exertion, and other variables. Portal venous pressure consistently above 20 cm. of water pressure indicates portal hypertension. Portal hypertension occurs whenever the flow of blood within the portal vein is impeded or obstructed; such obstruction can occur at three major sites:

1. *Intrahepatic obstruction*. Intrahepatic obstruction is the most common cause of portal hypertension and is almost always caused by cirrhosis (of varying types) of the liver. Alcoholism generally precedes cirrhosis among adults in this country, though among nondrinkers and children previous severe hepatitis with *postnecrotic cirrhosis* is the most likely precursor. The fibrosis and scarring that occur with any type of cirrhosis inhibit the transport of blood into the central veins of the hepatic lobules, leading to stasis and increased pressure within the portal venous system.

2. *Subhepatic obstruction*. Obstruction of the portal vein is the most common cause of portal hypertension among children and very young adults. Portal vein obstruction may result from the following: (a) an extension of the normal postnatal obliterative mechanisms in the umbilical vein and ductus venosus, (b) neonatal septic pylephlebitis (from omphalitis), (c) sepsis of other origin, or (d) occasionally a congenital malformation (cavernous transformation) of the portal vein. Whatever the cause, the portal vein obstruction inhibits passage of its blood *to* the liver.

3. *Suprahepatic obstruction*. Obstruction within the hepatic veins or the vena cava itself results in stasis of blood within the liver that is transmitted to the portal venous system leading into the liver. The obstruction may result from thrombosis (*Budd-Chiari syndrome*) or from tumors. It is the least common of all causes for portal hypertension, accounting for about 1% of cases.

Regardless of the site of the block in the venous drainage, the increasing volume and pressure of blood within the portal venous system produce a nonspecific group of secondary clincial disorders that are grouped together under the title of *portal hypertension*.

The most serious symptoms are caused by enlargement and collateralization of the vessels that connect the portal and the systemic venous systems. Normally these collateral veins are small and carry minute amounts of blood under low pressure. The naturally occurring portasystemic venous shunts are as follows: *esophageal veins* (which carry portal blood into the azygos system), *hemorrhoidal veins* (which carry portal blood into the pudendal and iliac veins), and *umbilical veins* (which carry portal blood to the anterior abdominal wall veins). There are innumerable other unnamed collaterals in the retroperitoneal spaces adjacent to the kidneys and spleen. The dilatation and increase in venous pressure within all of these systems may then result in:

1. *Esophageal varices*. Esophageal varices protrude into the lumen of the esophagus, where ulceration results from irritation of food, tubes, or acid-peptic factors. Massive and potentially lethal upper gastrointestinal bleeding is a dreaded result. Diagnosis is confirmed by esophagram (Fig. 22-2) and esophagoscopy.

2. *Hemorrhoids*. Hemorrhoids may prolapse and bleed.

3. *Caput medusae*. In this condition the abdominal wall collaterals may increase in size, radiating outward from the umbilicus.

A second major effect of portal hypertension is on the spleen (discussed in Chapter 19). It is characterized by splenomegaly and hypersplenism with anemia, leukopenia, and thrombocytopenia.

The final effect of portal hypertension is increased production of ascitic fluid, associated with the suprahepatic or intrahepatic blockage. Poor drainage of the lymphatics of the liver capsule with "bleeding" of this lymph fluid into the free peritoneal cavity is the probable cause. There is also increased formation of hepatic and splanchnic lymph. Additional causes for ascites often accompany portal hypertension associated with primary liver disease and include hypoalbuminemia and sodium and water retention because of endocrine and renal factors.

Portal hypertension attributed to primary liver disease may be complicated by hepatic coma from liver decompensation. This is especially likely to occur when large amine loads are thrust on a poorly functioning liver (by massive gastrointestinal tract hemorrhage from gastritis, ulcer, or esophageal varices). The liver cells are incapable of handling the amine load resulting from the bacterial digestion of blood proteins in the gastrointestinal tract, or these amines are shunted through portasystemic collaterals into the systemic circulation without passage through the liver. Resulting hyperammonemia may be responsible for many central nervous system manifestations of hepatic failure (coma, liver flap). Other possible mechanisms for hepatic coma involve the production of certain amines and amino acids that can act as false neurotransmitters.

Clinical features. Massive upper gastrointestinal tract bleeding is the most frightening manifestation of portal hypertension especially as the vomiting of blood (hematemesis). Consequent hypovolemia and hyperammonemia superimposed on severe liver disease may be lethal. Bleeding from esophageal varices in patients with subhepatic obstruction (normal liver function) is tolerated much better. Caput medusae is an interesting diagnostic adjunct to the diagnosis of portal hypertension but is not clinically significant. The enlarged and bleeding hemorrhoids, often a nuisance, are not a serious threat to the patient's life and are seldom treated surgically.

Signs of impending liver failure often occur after gastrointestinal tract bleeding in patients with liver disease; concurrent jaundice is a grave prognostic sign. Ascites may be the outstanding clinical feature of patients with suprahepatic obstruction.

Diagnosis and differential diagnosis. Massive upper gastrointestinal tract bleeding from esophageal varices must be distinguished from blood originating within the stomach and duodenum (Chapter 22). Peptic ulcer of the stomach or duodenum and gastritis are the most common lesions to be differentiated, though carcinoma of the stomach in the older patient must also be ruled out. Distinguishing a bleeding peptic ulcer from esophageal varices is difficult, especially if the patient has cirrhosis, since cirrhotic patients have a 7 to 10 times greater incidence of peptic ulcer than the general population does. To complicate the picture further, peptic ulcer or gastritis and esophageal varices may coexist.

If most of the blood is effortlessly vomited and little appears rectally, esophageal varices are likely to be the site of bleeding; on the other hand, bleeding that occurs mainly as tarry stools (melena) with little blood in the stomach is most likely to be duodenal (and peptic) in origin. Hemorrhage originating in the stomach may present with significant hematemesis and tarry stools concomitantly. Differentiation among these three sites of bleeding is important because of the different approaches in management.

Careful attention to the history of previous acid-peptic diathesis plus a history of current or previous alcoholism or hepatitis is important. Chil-

dren and nondrinkers who have never had hepatitis most likely have subhepatic blockage. Physical examination should be directed toward finding stigmas of liver disease such as jaundice, reddened palms, spider hemangiomas, caput medusae, ascites, hepatosplenomegaly, and hemorrhoidal varices.

Prothrombin time, Bromsulphalein retention, and serum ammonia tests may be helpful. If they are abnormal, the diagnosis of cirrhosis can be presumed, and treatment with vitamin K is begun. Gastric intubation and lavage are helpful in assessment of the volume of blood loss. Emergency esophagogastroscopy is indicated, since patients with varices are often found to be bleeding from other sources. Emergency upper gastrointestinal barium studies are performed if the patient's condition stabilizes. Central venous pressure and urinary output should be monitored.

Emergency treatment. The initial treatment of bleeding esophageal varices is aimed at stabilization of the circulating blood volume with fluid and blood. Fresh blood is preferable to bank blood because of its higher platelet content and other support of the blood coagulation mechanism. Control of bleeding can be attempted by balloon tamponade, vasopressin infusion, injection sclerotherapy or operation.

A triple-lumen rubber tube, *Sengstaken-Blakemore tube* (Fig. 22-3). is helpful in both differential diagnosis and treatment of bleeding esophageal varices. The tube is passed into the stomach, and the gastric balloon, inflated with 250 cc. of air, is pulled up snugly against the esophagogastric junction. Compression of the gastroesophageal collaterals by this maneuver commonly arrests bleeding from esophageal varices. The inner lumen of the tube allows continued gastric aspiration and lavage. If bleeding ceases, its origin from esophageal varices is confirmed. Also, if blood continues to well up into the hypopharynx with the gastric balloon in place, esophageal varices are probably responsible. These can be tamponed temporarily by inflation of the esophageal balloon with air to a pressure of 30 to 40 mm. Hg. The Sengstaken-Blakemore tube is left inflated for 24 to 36 hours. This respite allows time for diagnostic work-up and stabilization of the patient. The esophageal and gastric balloons must be deflated gradually. The tube is removed if bleeding does not recur in the next 24 hours. Pressure necrosis of gastric or esophageal surfaces may result if the Sengstaken-Blakemore tube remains in place for longer than 48 to 72 hours.

Treatment of the patient during the period of tube inflation should include blood transfusions, vitamin K, neomycin to reduce the bacterial flora

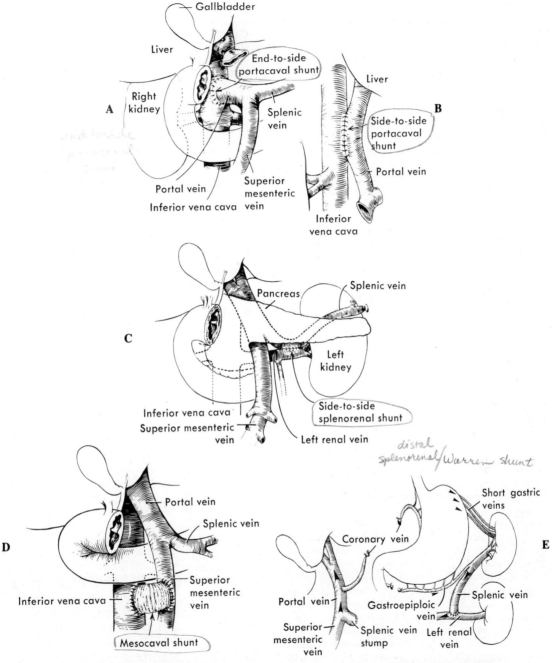

Fig. 17-7. Major types of shunting operations performed for portal hypertension and esophageal varices bleeding. **A,** End-to-side portacaval shunt (end of divided portal vein anastomosed to side of inferior vena cava). **B,** Side-to-side portacaval shunt (portal vein not divided, some blood flows retrogradely from liver into inferior vena cava). **C,** Side-to-side splenorenal shunt (splenic vein anastomosed to left renal vein). **D,** Mesocaval shunt (superior mesenteric vein connected to inferior vena cava by knitted Dacron graft 18 to 20 mm. in diameter, 5 to 8 cm. in length). **E,** Distal splenorenal or Warren shunt (with portoazygous disconnection to ensure drainage of esophagogastric variceal blood through spleen and splenic vein into left renal vein).

(responsible for liberating the amines from the blood proteins), lactulose, and vigorous laxation and enemas to remove the residual blood from the gastrointestinal tract. Intravenous glucose and vitamin B support the diseased liver. Peritoneal dialysis or exchange blood transfusions may be helpful if liver failure seems imminent.

If bleeding from the esophageal varices resumes after deflation of the tube, the gastric and esophageal balloons are quickly reinflated and preparations made for emergency sclerotherapy or portasystemic shunting. The constant intravenous infusion of vasopressin is extremely effective in controlling variceal bleeding during preparation for definitive operation and sometimes is followed by long-term cessation of bleeding. It should not be used concurrently with balloon tamponade because of the cumulative morbidity and mortality.

Emergency portasystemic venous shunting procedures carry a high mortality, and every effort is made to control acute bleeding, followed by intensive medical treatment, in preparation for elective portasystemic shunting. Injecting the esophageal varices through an endoscope with an agent that rapidly induces clotting (sclerotherapy) has been resurrected, is effective in controlling bleeding, and has achieved widespread use as an alternative to emergency operation.

Definitive treatment. Surgical procedures are available for prophylactic and more definitive treatment of good-risk patients with hypersplenism and portal hypertension. Patients with serious liver disease who have already had one episode of major hemorrhage from esophageal varices run a 50% risk of being dead within a year from a second massive hemorrhage. On the other hand, patients with subhepatic portal obstruction almost never die from major esophageal hemorrhage provided that adequate blood replacement and supportive care are available.

The mortality for the major portasystemic venous shunt operations (Fig. 17-7) is about 10%; the highest mortality is seen in patients with intrahepatic block with a serious degree of liver impairment. Good-risk patients have a serum bilirubin less than 3 mg./dl., serum albumin greater than 3 gm./dl., Bromsulphalein (BSP) retention less than 30%, and prothrombin time more than 50% of normal after the administration of vitamin K; they will not have ascites and should be less than 60 years of age. These are useful guidelines in the selection of candidates for portasystemic shunt procedures.

Work-up of a patient who is a candidate for operation includes careful esophagogastroscopy to verify the presence of varices and the absence of concomitant peptic ulcer, selective arteriography

with careful attention to the venous phase to visualize vascular anomalies and the patency of the portal system, and percutaneous splenoportography in selected patients in whom the question of portal pressure or the state of the portal venous system is unclear. This information is vital in both the timing and the selection of the proper shunting operation.

Definitive operations. The only portasystemic shunts possible for patients with subhepatic obstruction are the splenorenal or mesocaval shunts (Fig. 17-7). Splenectomy is often done at the time of side-to-side splenorenal shunt (Fig. 17-7, *C*) but is seldom indicated as the sole treatment of portal hypertension because the thrombosis of the splenic vein that inevitably occurs obviates later splenorenal shunt should that become necessary. After successful portasystemic shunting, the spleen decreases in size and returns to normal function.

Five types of portasystemic venous shunts are commonly used in patients with intrahepatic portal block. The end-to-side (Fig. 17-7, *A*), or side-to-side (Fig. 17-7, *B*) anastomosis of the portal vein just below the liver to the inferior vena cava is a commonly used shunt. When the portal vein is thrombosed, the splenorenal shunt may be performed (Fig. 17-7, *C*). The mesocaval shunt (Fig. 17-7, *D*) has the advantage of relative technical simplicity (as compared to side-to-side splenorenal and portacaval shunts). The distal splenorenal shunt (Fig. 17-7, *E*) has a lower incidence of death from encephalopathy than other portasystemic shunts but is less effective in preventing further bleeding.

Prognosis. The benefit of any of the shunting procedures depends on maintained patency of the anastomosis, since thrombosis is followed by a recrudescence in the portal hypertension and its serious sequelae. After a successful portasystemic shunt, the prognosis in patients with subhepatic block is excellent, whereas that in patients with intrahepatic obstruction and cirrhosis is dependent on the liver disease itself. Survival is better in alcoholic cirrhotics who manage to abstain from alcohol.

SURGICAL DISEASES OF THE BILIARY DUCTS AND GALLBLADDER

Operations on the gallbladder and biliary tree rank next to hernia repair and appendectomy in frequency of abdominal operations performed in the United States. Most of the biliary tract disorders arise from the complications of gallstones. Many Americans harbor gallstones at autopsy, with the frequency reaching 30% in females and 10% in males about 65 years of age.

Meticulous dissection in a bloodless operative

field and absolute identification of anatomical structures are laudable principles in any surgical procedure, but never are they so vital as in gallbladder and biliary tract operations (Fig. 17-1). The closeness to the portal vein, hepatic arteries, and other structures vital to life, the propensity for congenital anatomical variations, and the obliteration of landmarks imposed by inflammation combine to emphasize the need for strict adherence to these general principles. Biliary tract surgery in the infant and young child is further complicated by a spectrum of diseases different from that in the adult, plus the additional technical problems imposed by size.

Congenital anomalies

The liver and biliary tree arise embryologically as a diverticulum from the ventral aspect of the foregut at the 3 mm. embryo stage; the lumen early becomes solidified by cellular accumulations but later recanalizes. Liver cells and supporting mesenchymal tissue proliferate beneath the developing diaphragm. Abnormalities in development are common, thus explaining the anatomical variations of the biliary ducts and their relationship to the hepatic artery, portal vein, and pancreatic ducts that are encountered at operation.

Neonatal jaundice is clinically apparent in about 50% of term babies and 80% of premature babies. In almost all of them, fortunately, it is transient and insignificant. The age of onset of jaundice has some bearing on cause and prognosis:

1. Jaundice beginning on the first day of life generally results from intrauterine hemolysis, most often with Rh incompatibility (erythroblastosis fetalis) and less frequently with major ABO blood group incompatibility between the fetus and the mother.
2. Jaundice that is first apparent on the second or third day of life is almost always "physiological," with rapid and spontaneous resolution.
3. Jaundice arising on days 3 to 7 of life is most commonly caused by infections (sepsis, syphilis, toxoplasmosis, cytomegalic disease) and drugs (vitamin K, sulfonamide drugs), but occasionally it may result from hematoma absorption and thrombocytopenic purpura.
4. Jaundice becoming apparent at or beyond 2 weeks of life may be caused by neonatal hepatitis, infections (sepsis, syphilis, herpes, toxoplasmosis), metabolic storage disorders (Gaucher's disease, Niemann-Pick disease), or galactosemia. Extrahepatic obstructive jaundice occurs less often and results from bile inspissated within the ducts, atresia of the ductal system, or choledochal cyst.

Differential diagnosis of jaundice arising at 2 to 3 weeks of age rests between hepatitis and obstructive jaundice. The other medical causes for jaundice can generally be diagnosed or ruled out. Differentiation between hepatitis and extrahepatic obstructive jaundice is difficult (if not impossible) by physical examination or laboratory tests; therefore, if the jaundice persists for 4 to 6 weeks, exploratory laparotomy is required. Open-liver biopsy with frozen section evaluation will quickly establish the diagnosis of hepatitis on the basis of giant cells and lack of bile duct proliferation, and no further exploration is necessary. If the liver biopsy is not diagnostic, the surgeon must determine ductal patency by cholangiograms and surgical dissection.

The *inspissated bile syndrome* results from a plug of tenacious and thick bile somewhere within the ductal system. Some cases are associated with previous hemolytic disorders, and others complicate neonatal hepatitis. Cholangiograms obtained after the ductal system is flushed with saline introduced through a needle or catheter in the fundus of the gallbladder are both diagnostic and therapeutic.

Congenital atresia of the bile ducts is characterized by partial or complete obliteration of some portion of the biliary tree. In only about 10% will the obstruction be correctable: a block in common bile duct or gallbladder with dilated proximal ducts draining bile. Surgical bypass is carried out by means of choledochojejunostomy. Until recently, the other 90% of babies with biliary atresia died of liver failure within 2 years. However, Japanese surgeons have developed the Kasai operation (hepatic portoenterostomy), which cures 20% to 40% of these patients. A button of tissue is removed from the liver hilum where the intrahepatic bile ducts converge, to which the jejunum is anastomosed. The operation succeeds if there are bile-containing ducts within the liver hilum but not if the intrahepatic ducts are sclerosed or nonexistent.

Choledochal cyst is a cystic dilatation of the supraduodenal portion of the common bile duct containing stagnated bile (and often stones). A tiny and poorly functioning connection to the duodenum at the ampulla of Vater is usually seen. Whether the cyst is truly congenital (because of developmental difficulties) or it arises secondary to abnormal ductal anatomy, which allows pancreatic juice to enter the common bile duct, is unknown. In any event, the complications of gallstone formation, cholangitis with biliary cirrhosis, and perforation have all been reported.

Choledochal cyst commonly presents as a right upper quadrant abdominal mass in a child or young adult with recurrent bouts of mild jaundice and attacks of right upper abdominal pain. Oral chole-cystography reveals displacement of the gallbladder; upper gastrointestinal tract barium studies reveal a downward and medial displacement of the duodenum. Use of ultrasound is diagnostic. These cysts are best treated by excision and biliary-enteric drainage since their malignant degeneration has been described.

Gallstones

Gallstones produce the majority of surgical diseases of the gallbladder and biliary ducts (Fig. 17-8). The incidence of gallstones varies with different races, geographical locations, and dietary habits. All autopsy studies have shown a distinct relationship to age with frequency increasing with advancing age. A striking sex relationship is also noted; women harbor stones three times more often than men and at a younger age. Gallstones almost invariably arise within the gallbladder and only secondarily involve the common bile duct. A higher than normal incidence of gallstones occurs with pregnancy, diabetes, pancreatitis, cirrhosis, obesity, and hypothyroidism. About 10% to 15% of gallstones are radiopaque.

Two main types of gallstones are recognized:

1. *Cholesterol stones.* Stones containing 60% to 95% cholesterol by dry weight are the most common type of gallstones (75% of all). The noncholesterol component of such gallstones is predominately inert material with small amounts of bile pigment and calcium. They are generally multiple, faceted by indentations created by their neighbors, and firm and contain concentric laminations suggestive of periodic deposition. Occasionally cholesterol stones present as a single, large, smooth, soft, yellow-white stone containing almost pure cholesterol arranged in a radiating manner. *Cholesterosis of the gallbladder* is a specific pathological entity in which many tiny plaques of cholesterol are present within heaped-up mucosal folds in the gallbladder dotting the interior lining of the gallbladder; since they resemble the seeds of a ripe strawberry, the term *strawberry gallbladder* is often used.

2. *Pigment stones.* Pigment stones are multiple, soft, and black and resemble fine particles of sand. They are composed of bilirubin or biliverdin and may develop from antecedent cirrhosis, chronic hemolysis, or bile stasis with or without infection. Whereas cholesterol stones are most common in Western civilizations, pigment stones are more frequent in countries where thalassemia, con-

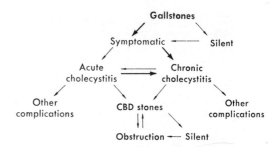

Fig. 17-8. Natural history of gallstones. *CBD*, Common bile duct.

genital spherocytosis, sickle cell anemia, and certain parasitemias are common.

Although the precise cause of gallstones is poorly understood, four etiological factors are present, to varying degrees, in most patients with cholelithiasis.

1. *Metabolic.* Cholesterol stones are commonly associated with diabetes mellitus, obesity, pregnancy, and hypothyroidism. Although these same conditions are associated with increased levels of cholesterol in blood, hypercholesterolemia itself has not been clearly established as the cause of cholesterol stones in these patients. Pigment stones are associated with hemolytic disorders such as thalassemia, congenital spherocytosis, and sickle cell anemia.

2. *Chemical.* Cholesterol is insoluble in water and is held in emulsion by combining with lecithin and bile salts to form tiny soluble micelles. Thus the concentration of bile cholesterol, lecithin, and bile salts control cholesterol solubility. Chronic elevation of bile cholesterol (as seen in the American Indian or the morbidly obese) or reduction of bile salts (as seen in ileal resection and inflammatory bowel disease) frequently result in cholesterol gallstone formation. Once a nidus of cholesterol is present, additional cholesterol will be precipitated during those periods of each day when bile is super-saturated with cholesterol even in normal persons.

3. *Stasis.* Stagnation of bile flow favors precipitation of the emulsified solids. Stasis of bile occurs during pregnancy and is proximal to tortuous or narrowed portions of the ductal system.

4. *Inflammation.* Inflammation is almost always associated with cholelithiasis. The inflam-

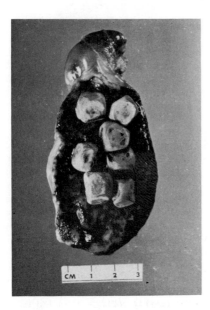

Fig. 17-9. Large gallstones causing acute cholecystitis.

matory exudate of mucus, cellular debris, and fibrin is believed to be incorporated within the substance of developing stones; inflammatory edema also can narrow the ducts, thereby encouraging stasis and obstruction to perpetuate the cycle. β-Glucuronidase released by certain gram-negative organisms leads to deconjugation of the soluble bilirubin diglucuronide to insoluble bilirubin, which can precipitate and form the nidus for precipitation of cholesterol or more bilirubin with resultant stone formation.

Acute cholecystitis

Acute cholecystitis is triggered by *obstruction* to the outflow of bile from the gallbladder (Fig. 17-9). The point of obstruction is commonly within the tortuous cystic duct, most often because of stone impaction. Less common causes of cystic duct obstruction are inflammatory edema, neoplasm, and rarely volvulus of an abnormally formed gallbladder suspended from a mesentery. Acute cholecystitis is basically a *chemical* inflammation. Bacterial inflammation may occur secondarily from organisms within the bile (coliform in type) or organisms that reach the gallbladder through lymphatics and vessels.

Early in the course of acute cholecystitis the gallbladder becomes distended with bile and later develops mucosal ischemia from pressure. Its wall becomes thicked, edematous, and injected, and an acute cellular inflammatory reaction develops rapidly. The cycle is self-perpetuating until and unless the obstruction to outflow is relieved. Migration of the omentum and adjacent organs to the inflamed gallbladder occurs, with fixation of the serosal surfaces to each other by vascular adhesions. These serve as tampons to prevent the inflammation from reaching the general peritoneal cavity. *Empyema of the gallbladder* is a descriptive term applied to the acutely inflamed, totally obstructed gallbladder to which bacterial contamination (with a purulent exudate) has been added. Complications will occur rapidly unless the obstruction is relieved.

Complications of acute cholecystitis occur in 10% to 15% of cases if treatment is inadequate or delayed. Increasing intraluminal pressure of the inflamed gallbladder produces ischemia, ulceration, necrosis, and perforation of its wall. Pericholecystic collections of bile or pus will result if the walling-off processes are adequate, or contamination of the general peritoneal cavity will result if progression is unduly rapid or if the defense mechanisms are lacking.

In the other 85% to 90% of patients with acute cholecystitis, the cystic duct obstruction is relieved spontaneously (by a "ball valve" disimpaction of the stone) to abort the current attack. However, the stage is set for recurrences.

Clinical features. Acute cholecystitis is often preceded by a rather nondescript history of postprandial bloating, indigestion, food intolerance, and varying degrees of right upper abdominal quadrant pain.

The acute attack begins suddenly, often a few hours after ingestion of a large or fatty meal. The chief symptom is pain, initially colicky but later sustained. It is located in the right subcostal or epigastric region but is frequently referred to the tip of the right scapula. The pain is aggravated by pressure, but contrary to many other inflammatory intra-abdominal conditions the patient is often more comfortable when up and about. Nausea, bilious vomiting, abdominal distension, and belching or flatulence are commonly associated. Later in the attach, fever and mild jaundice are often noticed.

Physical examination reveals an acutely ill patient with upper abdominal tenderness and guarding, most pronounced in the right subcostal area. Gentle palpation of this area may suddenly stop the patient's inspiratory effort (positive *Murphy's sign*). The tender, globular gallbladder with adherent colon and omentum can be palpated in almost one third of the patients with adequate relaxation and analgesia.

Urinalysis is normal unless dehydration with

ketosis is present. The white blood count is elevated to 15,000/cu. mm. or above, with a pronounced shift to the left in the differential count. The serum bilirubin level may be elevated to 2 to 3 mg./dl., the borderline of scleral icterus, and occasionally as high as 6 mg./dl. Plain roentgenograms of the abdomen often show a localized paralytic ileus and calcified stones in 10% to 15% of patients.

Differential diagnosis. The differential diagnosis of acute cholecystitis may be difficult. Acute appendicitis must be considered, but in this disease the evolution of the acute episode is slower, and the maximal signs of inflammation are anatomically lower than in acute cholecystitis. Right lower lobe pneumonia and pleurisy are extremely difficult to differentiate. Rales, a pleural friction rub, or radiographic evidence of pneumonia are suggestive of pulmonary disease. Acute pancreatitis can be especially confusing and occasionally is associated with acute cholecystitis. Radiation of pain to the back, elevated serum amylase level, maximal tenderness in the epigastrium or left upper abdominal quadrant, pronounced tachycardia, and shock favor the diagnosis of pancreatitis. Confusion about the diagnosis can be resolved in favor of acute cholecystitis with a biliary scintiscan (technetium-labeled derivatives of iminodiacetic acid, IDA) showing tech-

netium in the biliary ducts and not in the gallbladder, since acute cholecystitis is attributable to obstruction of the cystic duct, usually by stone, in 95% of cases; the obstruction prevents the flow of radioisotope medium into the gallbladder. Duodenal ulcer, pyelonephritis, and myocardial infarction are sometimes confused with acute cholecystitis.

Treatment. The treatment of acute cholecystitis in most is initially nonoperative: nasogastric suction, intravenous fluid and electrolyte replacement, analgesia (with drugs that do not produce smooth muscle sphincter spasm, as morphine does), bed rest, and antispasmodics. Antibiotics are not given early, since this is primarily a chemical infection. When improvement is prompt (6 to 8 hours), nonoperative treatment is continued. In most cases the acute episode subsides. Cholecystectomy is planned in 6 weeks when inflammation has resolved and a more complete work-up (including oral cholecystography) has been done.

Exploratory laparotomy is indicated in patients with toxemia, advanced disease, a palpable tender gallbladder, or persistence or worsening of symptoms with nonoperative management. In the very elderly, obese, or poor operative risk patient, simple evacuation of the distended gallbladder contents by trochar suction is performed, with

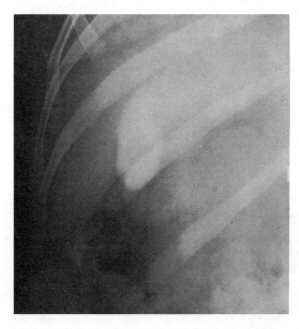

Fig. 17-10. Large, solitary gallstone producing filling defect in functioning gallbladder on oral cholecystography.

removal of the obstructing stones and tube drainage of the gallbladder *(cholecystostomy)*. Cholecystectomy is carried out on a nonemergency basis some weeks later after complete recovery.

In the good-risk patient immediate cholecystectomy can be done provided that the inflammatory reaction is limited enough to allow meticulous and orderly anatomical dissection of the ductal structures. Some have advocated acute cholecystectomy for all patients with acute cholecystitis. Common bile duct exploration is undertaken if a common duct stone is suspected. Intraoperative cholangiography should be performed to rule out common duct stones, which may be asymptomatic. Should the acuteness of the inflammatory reaction make dissection difficult, simple cholecystostomy is preferable to cholecystectomy even in the good-risk surgical candidate.

Chronic cholecystitis

Over 90% of patients with chronic cholecystitis have stones in the gallbladder. The gallbladder is generally rather small and invariably has fibrosis and other evidence of chronic inflammation in its wall. Many previous episodes of indigestion, food intolerance, and acute or subacute attacks of right upper abdominal pain characterize chronic cholecystitis.

Occasionally the cystic duct becomes totally obliterated by fibrous scar tissue. In the absence of infection the bile pigment is absorbed during the ensuing weeks, and the gallbladder becomes slowly and progressively more distended with secreted mucus *(white bile)*. This phenomenon is called *hydrops of the gallbladder* and may be thought of as the "sterile" and slowly evolving counterpart of empyema of the gallbladder. It is the only variety of chronic cholecystitis in which the gallbladder is palpable on physical examination. *White bile,* devoid of pigment, is characteristic of any long-standing and complete obstruction of the biliary tree.

Physical examination of the patient with chronic cholecystitis is seldom diagnostic. Blood and urine studies are of little help. Oral cholecystography commonly fails to visualize the gallbladder. If the gallbladder is still functioning, the nonradiopaque stones will stand out as filling defects (Figs. 17-10 and 17-11). Sonography may reveal gallstones or evidence of chronic gallbladder disease (thick wall or shrunken gallbladder). In some patients laboratory support for the clinical diagnosis comes only from duodenal drainage and cholecystokinin cholangiography. Because the majority of the patients are middle-aged or elderly, barium studies of the upper and lower gastrointestinal tracts are

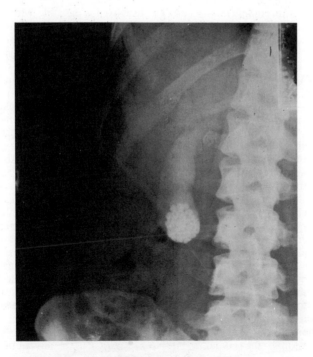

Fig. 17-11. Multiple, calcified gallstones.

often performed to rule out peptic ulcers, gastric and colonic neoplasm, hiatus hernia, and other conditions that may mimic the nondescript clinical features of chronic cholecystitis. Electrocardiographic examination should be performed in patients with a history of heart disease.

Treatment of symptomatic chronic cholecystitis is clearly surgical. Cholecystectomy is curative and gives the surgeon the opportunity to palpate the common bile duct carefully or evaluate it by means of dye injected through the cystic duct at the time of the operation (*operative cholangiography*) to rule out common bile duct stones.

Silent gallstones

People who are incidentally found to harbor gallstones without symptoms are said to have "silent gallstones." The incidence of silent gallstones is increasing as our population ages and as screening examinations become routine. They pose a treatment dilemma, inasmuch as they are potentially dangerous and yet not immediately or invariably so. Each patient with silent gallstones must be evaluated individually, the low risk of elective operation in patients younger than 65 years being balanced against such factors as the patient's general health, longevity, wishes, and the potential hazard of the gallstones themselves as determined by their size, number, and location. Operation is recommended in patients with diabetes mellitus, where the complications associated with acute cholecystitis are more serious than the slightly increased risks of elective cholecystectomy.

Common bile duct stones (choledocholithiasis)

Overall, about 15% of patients with gallbladder calculi also have stones within the common bile duct, though this association will be found in nearly 50% of those over 80 years of age. They are believed to originate within the gallbladder, with subsequent passage into the common duct. Therefore common duct stones found months or even years after cholecystectomy were probably overlooked at the time of the initial operation. Since repeat operation on a jaundiced patient has high mortality and morbidity, exploration of the common bile duct at the time of cholecystectomy is preferred should any doubt exist about the presence of choledocholithiasis. In other words, it is better to explore the common bile duct unnecessarily at the time of elective cholecystectomy than to overlook retained stones. Even the most experienced surgeons will overlook an occasional common bile duct stone, and despite the strictest criteria for choledochostomy, the common bile

duct will contain no stones when explored in approximately 25% of cases.

The classical indications for common bile duct exploration (choledochotomy) are (1) existing or recent jaundice, (2) a dilated (> 1 cm.) common bile duct, (3) palpable stones within a duct, (4) small stones in the gallbladder with a large cystic duct, (5) filling defects or other abnormalities in the preoperative or operative cholangiograms, and (6) pancreatitis in association with biliary tract disease.

Common bile duct stones cause symptoms from impaction within the distal duct at the ampulla of Vater. A "ball valve" effect produces intermittent obstruction with stagnation and increase in pressure of the bile, colicky pain (from hyperperistalsis), and obstructive jaundice. As the obstruction abates, so do the symptoms and signs. During total obstruction, the stool is acholic or only lightly pigmented and the urine is dark. Secondary infection may produce cholangitis with shaking chills and fever (Charcot fever) and intrahepatic abscesses. Biliary cirrhosis results if the obstruction is chronic.

The clinical features of choledocholithiasis wax and wane with the obstruction. Up to 50% of patients harboring common duct stones have no obvious symptoms. If the gallbladder is present, cholecystitis may dominate the physical findings. *Courvoisier's sign* is negative; the gallbladder is usually not palpable with extrahepatic obstructive jaundice caused by gallstones since a chronically inflamed gallbladder is contracted.

The work-up of the jaundiced patient should include evaluation of the stool for bilirubin and the urine for urobilinogen and bilirubin. The serum bilirubin is elevated, mainly the direct fraction, as well as the serum alkaline phosphatase. Plain abdominal radiography may reveal a radiopaque stone. If the serum bilirubin is above 2 mg./dl., oral cholecystography is futile because the biliary tract will not be visualized. Abdominal sonography or computerized tomography are used to show dilated ducts; then cholestatic jaundice can be ruled out.

Percutaneous transhepatic cholangiography (Fig. 17-12), with injection of radiopaque dye through a long needle inserted into the liver after aspiration of bile, will clearly show the biliary duct anatomy and point of obstruction. The use of the "skinny" (Chiba) needle has obviated the previous problems of blood and bile leak into the peritoneal cavity with resultant peritonitis, and the procedure can be done without the obligation of immediate laparotomy.

Endoscopic retrograde cholangiopancreatography (ERCP). The advent of the fiberoptic duodeno-

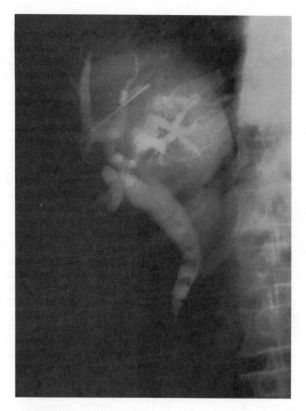

Fig. 17-12. Percutaneous cholangiogram showing multiple stones (filling defects) in dilated common bile duct.

scope has made it possible to cannulate the ampulla of Vater in the awake patient. Contrast material injected through the cannula will identify the cause and site of obstruction.

Choledocholithiasis must be differentiated from the other causes of obstructive jaundice: ductal strictures and carcinomas of the extrahepatic biliary duct, ampulla of Vater, and head of the pancreas. Progressive and unrelenting jaundice associated with fatty stools, hyperglycemia, and an enlarged gallbladder (Courvoisier's sign) is suggestive of carcinoma of the pancreas. Intermittent jaundice associated with occult blood in the stool and a filling defect in the duodenal concavity on upper gastrointestinal tract barium studies favor carcinoma of the ampulla of Vater. Unrelenting jaundice with an enlarged gallbladder but with no evidence of pancreatic exocrine or endocrine dysfunction is suggestive of carcinoma of the extrahepatic biliary tree. Intermittently painful and repeated episodes of jaundice with no palpable gallbladder indicate choledocholithiasis. Strictures

of the common bile duct occur after accidental injury to the duct structures at the time of cholecystectomy; the jaundice is obstructive in type, generally painless, and associated with cholangitis. This history of preceding biliary surgery sets this apart clearly from other causes of obstructive jaundice. Since laparotomy is necessary for diagnosis and treatment of all these conditions, it should not be delayed.

The treatment of choledocholithiasis is surgical removal of stones and temporary drainage of the common bile duct. If the patient is seriously ill, preoperative treatment with vitamins K and B complex, intravenous fluids, electrolytes, and glucose and other supportive measures for a short period of time may be needed. If the gallbladder is present, cholecystectomy should be performed in addition to choledochotomy and removal of all the common bile duct stones. The common bile duct is explored both proximally and distally and is irrigated with saline until the bile is free of debris. A probe is passed through the ampulla and into the

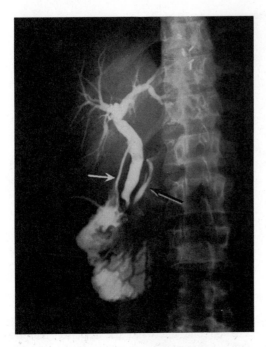

Fig. 17-13. Operative cholangiogram. Dye injected by T tube *(white arrow)* fills entire biliary system and pancreatic duct *(black arrow)* and enters duodenum inferiorly. Faint shadow in center of common bile duct is a retained stone.

duodenum, and the duct is carefully palpated around this probe to be certain that no stones remain. The duct should be closed snugly around a T tube, the short limbs of which are placed into the common bile duct and the long limb exteriorized through a separate stab wound. Operative cholangiograms should then be done through the T tube (Fig. 17-13) to be certain that the common bile duct contains no additional filling defects and that it empties freely into the duodenum. The T tube serves as an external vent for drainage of bile during the first few postoperative days. Cholangiograms are repeated through the T tube before its removal after the tenth postoperative day to assure once again that the biliary ducts are free of stones. A biliary-enteric anastamosis is done if the patient has had a previous common duct exploration.

Postcholecystectomy syndrome

In about 5% to 10% of patients who have had cholecystectomy, some or all of the symptoms that the patient had before the operation (originally ascribed to cholelithiasis) persist or recur. This is referred to as the *postcholecystectomy syndrome*. This syndrome has a number of causes, including an erroneous original diagnosis, an unduly long and dilated cystic duct stump, residual common bile duct stones, biliary dyskinesia, or conditions outside of the biliary tract with similar symptoms (hiatus hernia, duodenal ulcer, pancreatitis). Intravenous or percutaneous cholangiography is helpful in sorting out this problem, often accompanied by barium studies of the upper gastrointestinal tract. Repeat operation is necessary should a dilated cystic duct remnant or residual common duct stone be found.

Carcinoma of the gallbladder and biliary ducts

Carcinomas of the gallbladder and extrahepatic bile ducts are generally associated with cholelithiasis and chronic inflammatory disease of the gallbladder and ducts, but it is not known if the carcinomas are the cause or the result of the stones and inflammation. The cancers arise from the mucosal surfaces as adenocarcinomas.

Carcinomas of the gallbladder spread early to the liver by direct invasion and to the periportal lymph nodes. Because these carcinomas are silent and spread before discovery, surgical cure is possible only when the carcinoma is an incidental finding at the time of operation.

Neoplasms of the bile ducts are even more rare than those of the gallbladder, but because they cause symptoms earlier, the prognosis is better. The duct lumen is abruptly narrowed at the point of the neoplasm with proximal dilatation, stagnation, and ultimately obstructive jaundice. Spread occurs locally to the contiguous viscera and to the liver through the periportal lymphatics and portal vein.

Neoplasms of the extrahepatic bile ducts comprise a small fraction of the patients with total obstructive jaundice. When localized to the distal ductal system and if spread has not occurred, they are amenable to treatment by pancreaticoduodenectomy (Whipple procedure, Chapter 18). The 5-year cure rate with this operation in treatment of carcinomas of the distal biliary ducts (15%) is better than that for carcinoma of the head of the pancreas (5%) but not nearly so good as that for carcinoma of the ampulla of Vater (40%). If incurable surgically, bypass of the obstructed bile duct is carried out by anastomosis of the duct to the jejunum when possible. For tumors located more proximally, effective palliation can be obtained by dilatation and transhepatic intubation of the tumor.

18
Pancreas

Jack R. Pickleman
Jeffrey R. Clark

Diseases of the pancreas are among the most serious and challenging that the surgeon is called upon to treat. Because of its retroperitoneal location, the pancreas has remained relatively secure from radiological investigation until recent years when a wide variety of complex studies have completely revolutionized our management of patients with pancreatic disorders. These tests include ultrasound and abdominal CT scanning, endoscopic retrograde cholangiopancreatography (ERCP), percutaneous transhepatic cholangiography (PTC), and arteriography. To these will soon be added nuclear magnetic resonance (NMR). Today, diagnosis of most pancreatic conditions can be readily made by a combination of these studies. Treatment, however, has lagged behind diagnosis. The retroperitoneal location of the pancreas and its proximity to so many vital structures have thwarted many attempts to ameliorate both benign and malignant diseases, and morbidity and mortality of pancreatic procedures remain high, especially in the hands of the occasional pancreatic surgeon. This chapter focuses on the current state of our knowledge of the diagnosis and treatment of the more common pancreatic disorders.

ANATOMY

Many signs and symptoms of pancreatic disease can be explained by its retroperitoneal location and intimate association with surrounding vital organs and blood vessels (Fig. 18-1). The pancreas weighs 80 grams and lies obliquely across the upper abdomen from the duodenum at L2 to the hilum of the spleen at T10. The head of the pancreas is nestled in the C loop of the duodenum. The distal common bile duct and the superior mesenteric artery and vein are surrounded by pancreatic tissue. Any mass or scarring in the head of the pancreas may cause obstruction of the common bile duct or duodenum. Similarly, duodenal and pyloric ulcers may penetrate the pancreas and cause pancreatitis. The neck of the pancreas lies directly on the portal vein, which is the confluence of the splenic, superior, and inferior mesenteric veins. Pancreatic cancer may directly involve any of these contiguous vessels, rendering the cancer unresectable in the opinion of most surgeons. The body of the pancreas crosses over the unyielding and rigid vertebral column. Blunt upper abdominal trauma (as in a steering-wheel injury) may therefore crush the gland against the vertebrae. Diagnosis of this injury is difficult because the symptoms are vague and the process is confined to the lesser sac. The tail of the gland, intimately associated with the hilum of the spleen, may be easily injured during splenectomy.

Upon opening the abdomen the pancreas cannot be seen because it is covered by the stomach and transverse colon. The surgeon uses several different maneuvers to expose this hidden area. The omentum must be detached from the greater curvature of the stomach to enter the lesser sac and expose the body of the pancreas. During a "Kocher manuever" the surgeon will incise the retroperitoneum just lateral to the duodenum and insert his hand behind the duodenum and head of the pancreas but anterior to the hilum of the right kidney and to the inferior vena cava. This impor-

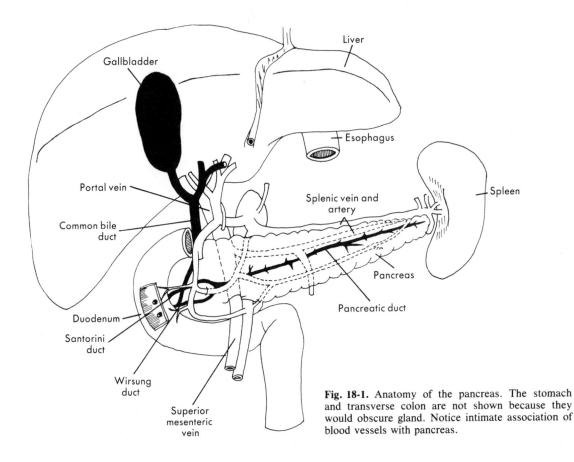

Fig. 18-1. Anatomy of the pancreas. The stomach and transverse colon are not shown because they would obscure gland. Notice intimate association of blood vessels with pancreas.

tant maneuver allows bimanual palpation of the head of the pancreas and manipulation of the distal common bile duct. The tail of the gland can be more adequately examined if the splenic attachments to the diaphram, colon, and kidney are divided and a hand inserted behind the spleen and distal pancreas but anterior to the left kidney. This extensive dissection is necessary for adequate examination of the pancreas.

Any injury to the pancreas, indeed even a biopsy, can release a most potent combination of digestive enzymes into the abdominal cavity. Most surgeons prefer a needle biopsy to a wedge biopsy, and many prefer to insert the needle through the duodenum (transduodenal route). Most operations on the pancreas must be followed by external drainage of these secretions.

The blood supply of the pancreas is shared with the duodenum through the superior and inferior pancreaticoduodenal vessels. These vessels provide an important communication between the coeliac axis and the superior mesenteric artery.

The head of the pancreas cannot be excised without removal of the duodenum, distal part of the common bile duct, and usually the distal part of the stomach. This formidable undertaking is a "Whipple procedure" (Fig. 18-10). The splenic artery and vein, lying directly behind the pancreas, are intimately associated with the body and tail, and through multiple small vessels they nourish this area of the gland. The uncinate process wraps around the superior mesenteric artery and vein and receives fragile branches from these vessels.

Armed with a clear picture of the anatomical relationships of the pancreas, one can now easily understand why

- The most frequent symptom of pancreatic disease is boring back pain.
- A mass in the pancreas (i.e., pseudocyst) may displace the stomach anteriorly and cause satiety.
- Hemorrhage into the pancreas (hemorrhagic pancreatitis) dissects retroperitoneally to the flanks causing bluish discoloration of the skin (Turner's sign).

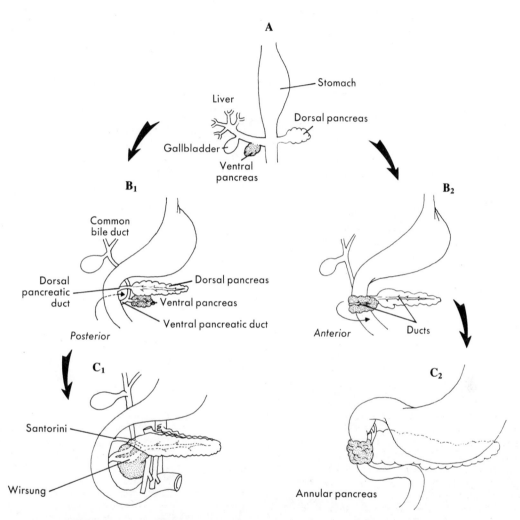

Fig. 18-2. Embryology of pancreas. **A**, Normal development at 4 weeks of gestation. **B₁**, Normal posterior rotation of ventral pancreas. **C₁**, Shaded area represents contribution of ventral pancreas. **B₂**, Abnormal anterior rotation of ventral bud. **C₂**, Final product of abnormal rotation and fusion is annular pancreas.

- Pancreatitis may cause a pseudo-obstruction of the transverse colon because of its proximity (colon cut-off sign).
- Cancer of the pancreas causes obstruction of the common bile duct and a palpably enlarged gallbladder (Courvoisier's sign).

The splanchnic (sympathetic) and vagus (parasympathetic) nerves supply both motor and sensory (visceral pain) fibers to the ducts, acini, and vessels of the pancreas. Surgical or chemical ablation of the plexus of these nerves for control of pancreatic pain has met with limited long-term success.

Lymph drains in all directions radially from the pancreas to the superior mesenteric, hepatic, coeliac, and splenic nodes. Pancreatic cancer disseminates early and extensively along these radial pathways.

In summary, operations on the pancreas may be frustrating because of the following:

1. Retroperitoneal location makes exposure difficult.
2. Soft consistency of the gland and lack of distinct capsule make suturing difficult.
3. The pancreas releases damaging digestive enzymes with even slight injury.
4. Cancer of the pancreas is biologically aggressive and involves vital peripancreatic structures early.

EMBRYOLOGY

The pancreas develops from the ventral and dorsal pancreatic buds, which protrude from the primitive gut in the third and fourth weeks of gestation. The ventral bud rotates posteriorly around the duodenum taking with it the distal common bile duct to join with the dorsal bud. The ventral bud becomes most of the head and duct of Wirsung. The dorsal bud contributes to the head and forms the remainder of the gland and ductal system. If the ventral and dorsal buds incompletely fuse, the ducts will not cross-communicate (pancreas divisum) (Fig. 18-2). Because of this variable embryological development, several different patterns of duct anatomy result (Fig. 18-3).

Ectopic pancreatic tissue can occur anywhere in the gastrointestinal tract but is usually found in the stomach or duodenum or in a Meckel's divertic-

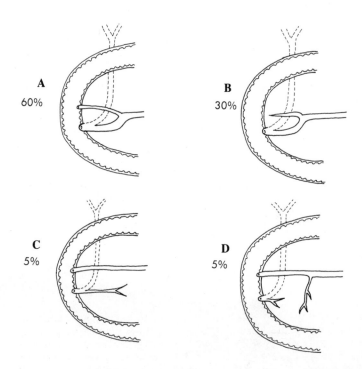

Fig. 18-3. Variations of pancreatic ducts. **A** and **B**, Most common patterns of duct anatomy. **C** and **D**, Two forms of pancreas divisum resulting from incomplete fusion of the ventral and dorsal pancreatic anlage.

ulum. Complications of this abnormally located tissue include obstruction, bleeding, and intussusception.

ANNULAR PANCREAS

Pancreatic tissue surrounding the duodenum, annular pancreas, is a rare cause of duodenal obstruction in both the infant and adult. The probable embryological explanation is anterior, rather than posterior, rotation of the ventral pancreatic anlage, which constricts the duodenum (Fig. 18-2, C_2). This condition is one of the causes of bilious vomiting in newborns. Air in the stomach and first portion of the duodenum, the double-bubble sign, is pathognomonic of duodenal obstruction on roentgenograms. This ring of pancreatic tissue is intimately associated with the duodenal musculature and contains ductal structures. Therefore, division of this ring of tissue, to open the stenotic duodenum, causes a prohibitive incidence of subsequent pancreatitis, pancreatic fistula, and injury to the duodenal wall. Bypass operations, side-to-side duodenoduodenostomy or duodenojejunostomy, are technically easy and give excellent long-term results. Gastrojejunostomy should be avoided because of incomplete duodenal drainage and a potential for ulcer formation at the anastomotic site.

PANCREAS DIVISUM

Pancreas divisum results when the ductal system of the ventral and dorsal pancreatic anlagen fail to fuse, causing independent drainage of the main and accessory pancreatic ducts into the duodenum (Fig. 18-3). Recurrent acute pancreatitis may occur in this condition when the ampulla of the ducts become stenotic. Sphincteroplasty of the abnormal ampullae cures most cases.

PANCREAS PHYSIOLOGY—EXOCRINE FUNCTION

Ninety-eight percent of the pancreas by weight is devoted to exocrine function (acinar cells) and 2% to endocrine function (islet cells). Just as in the regulation of acid secretion by the stomach, so too is pancreatic secretion stimulated by three phases: cephalic, gastric, and intestinal. The cephalic phase, mediated by the vagus nerves and acetylcholine, produces an enzyme-rich secretion. The gastric phase, mediated by gastrin in response to protein in the stomach also results in an enzyme-rich secretion. The intestinal phase is mediated by cholecystokinin-pancreozymin (CCK-PZ) and secretin, both elaborated by the duodenum. Secretin, released in response to acid in the duodenum, results in an alkaline pancreatic secretion of water and bicarbonate (HCO_3^-). The bicarbonate concen-

tration increases as the flow rate increases, maintaining a more constant pH in the duodenum. CCK-PZ is released in response to proteins, fats, and their metabolites in the duodenum and results in an enzyme-rich pancreatic secretion (amylolytic, lipolytic, and proteolytic enzymes) and also causes contraction of the gallbladder. Amylase splits starches into simple sugars; lipase, phospholipase, and esterases attack fats; and trypsin and chymotrysin break down proteins into peptides and amino acids. These enzymes are secreted with inhibitors that are inactivated in the duodenum. This mechanism prevents pancreatic autodigestion. In acute pancreatitis, this mechanism fails, resulting in the autodigestion of the retroperitoneum and pancreas.

DISEASES OF THE PANCREAS
Acute pancreatitis

In the United States, the clear majority of cases of acute pancreatitis are associated with *gallstones* or *alcoholism*. However, other causes exist and must be considered. The causes are as follows:

Alcohol
Gallstones
Trauma
Peptic ulcer
Hyperparathyroidism
Hyperlipidemias—types I & V
Ischemia
Carcinoma
Embryological malformations—pancreas divisum
Viruses
Drugs
   Corticosteroids
   Thiazides
   Azathioprine
   Furosemide

Although the exact pathophysiology of acute pancreatitis is not understood, the resultant local tissue injury is mediated by numerous enzymes. Trypsin not only destroys tissue but also activates other destructive enzymes such as elastase and lecithinase. Vasoactive substances including kinins, kallikrein, and histamine lead to cardiovascular dysfunction and collapse. In the full-blown picture, blood pressure falls and respiratory, renal, and myocardial failure supervene, accounting for the approximate 10% mortality noted in many series.

The presenting *clinical features of acute pancreatitis* are epigastric pain, often radiating to the back, associated with nausea, vomiting, and fever. Local tenderness is common, but frank peritoneal signs are less usual. Ileus is prominent. Unfortunately, several other acute abdominal conditions may give similar signs and symptoms, including perforated duodenal ulcer, acute cholecystitis, and small bowel obstruction; therefore the diagnosis may be difficult. The hallmark of acute pancreatitis is an elevated serum amylase. This is not specific for acute pancreatitis however, and many other acute abdominal conditions may be associated with elevated levels. Further refinements in diagnosis have been sought, such as the amylase/creatinine clearance ratio, but this has yielded mixed results. Urinary amylase levels may likewise be elevated, but this merely reflects increased serum levels. Serum lipase is also elevated, but as this test takes considerably longer to perform than the serum amylase, it is less useful clinically. To further complicate the issue, the recent analysis of amylase isoenzymes has disclosed that many patients admitted with abdominal pain and hyperamylasemia with the presumptive diagnosis of acute pancreatitis have only elevation of the nonpancreatic fraction and in reality do not have pancreatitis.

In the usual situation, the presumptive *diagnosis of acute pancreatitis* is made in a patient with the above clinical signs in whom the serum amylase is elevated and in whom there is no evidence of free air or small bowel obstruction on abdominal roentgenograms. Hypocalcemia, hyperglycemia, and hypertriglyceridemia may accompany the amylasemia. Abdominal roentgenograms usually show only a localized ileus (sentinal loop) or less often a left-sided pleural effusion.

The *treatment of acute pancreatitis* is medical; the cornerstone is adequate fluid replacement to replenish extracellular volume. Large quantities of third-space fluids may be lost initially and must be aggressively replaced to prevent complications. A Foley catheter, central venous pressure catheter, and sometimes a pulmonary artery catheter will be required. The resuscitative end points are normalization of vital signs and urine output. Although the need for nasogastric suction has been questioned as a routine measure, it is probably indicated for all patients with acute pancreatitis to decrease hydrochloric acid stimulation of secretin secretion. On the other hand, the empiric administration of calcium, anticholinergic drugs, and antibiotics has no apparent effect on morbidity. In severe cases, the early institution of total parenteral nutrition may prove beneficial.

Prognosis in patients with acute pancreatitis depends on whether the inflammation is of the edematous variety or the condition has progressed to the hemorrhagic stage in which mortality of up to 90% may be noted. Death may come early from multiple organ system failure or later after the development of pancreatic abscess and resultant systemic sepsis. A number of prognostic signs tend to predict those patients whose courses will be complicated or fatal. These signs are as follows:

Excessive fluid requirements
Falling hematocrit
Elevated white blood count
Elevated blood glucose
Elevated lactate dehydrogenase and SGOT
Elevated blood urea nitrogen
Hypocalcemia
Hypoxemia
Acidosis

Following are indications *for operation* in patients with acute pancreatitis:

Obscure diagnosis
Worsening clinical picture
Trauma
Pancreatic cyst
Pancreatic abscess
Pancreatic ascites

Although most authorities would agree that operation is needed in these circumstances, disagreement surrounds what procedure to use. Peritoneal lavage, either percutaneous or by catheters inserted at celiotomy, appears to dramatically improve some patients, resulting in decreased fluid requirements, improvement in vital signs, and elimination of the need for vasopressor support. Necrotic pancreatic tissue, noticed at celiotomy, requires débridement and extensive sump drainage. Others, especially in France, have championed emergency pancreatectomy in these circumstances, but most would believe that this is unduly hazardous. Some form of intervention seems to benefit the acutely ill patient with multiple system failure, but late deaths from pancreatitis continue to occur.

The commonest complications of acute pancreatitis are *pancreatic abscess, pseudocyst*, and less commonly *pancreatic ascites*. Pancreatic abscess is heralded by sepsis in a patient recovering from an attack of acute pancreatitis and is easily diagnosed by either ultrasound or CT scanning. Treatment includes celiotomy with extensive débridement and sump drainage of the pancreas. Despite optimal treatment, complications are common, redrainage is frequently required, and death occurs in at least 20% of patients. Recent attempts at percutaneous catheter drainage of these abscesses has been disappointing, probably because the cavities contain large pieces of necrotic material, which require operative evacuation.

Pancreatic pseudocysts are lesser sac collections of pancreatic fluid arising during the course of an attack of acute pancreatitis. They are heralded by abdominal pain and a persistent or rising serum amylase level. Diagnosis is readily made by ultrasound. Unless complicated by sepsis, a rising bilirubin, or progressive increase in cyst size, acute pseudocysts may be observed, since 20% to 30% will resolve without treatment. Persistence beyond 4 to 6 weeks makes spontaneous resolution unlikely and calls for operative therapy. Internal drainage through a cyst gastrostomy or Roux-en-Y cyst jejunostomy (Figs. 18-4 and 18-5) is the treatment of choice depending on the location of the cyst. Should operation be required before 4 to 6 weeks for the above indications, external sump drainage alone will be required because the immature cyst wall is too friable for internal anastomosis.

Pancreatic ascites afflicts patients who are recovering from an attack of acute pancreatitis. Because many of these patients are alcoholics, the development of ascites in the past has often been attributed to cirrhosis. However, analysis of the ascitic fluid demonstrating an elevated amylase and a total protein greater than 3 gm./dl. will point to the true cause. Many cases will spontaneously resolve; others will require internal drainage of the associated leaking pseudocyst or pancreatic duct through a Roux-en-Y loop.

Gallstone pancreatitis

One of the most serious complications of gallstones occurs when stones pass into the common duct with resultant impaction at the sphincter of Oddi, pancreatic ductal obstruction, and acute pancreatitis. Clinically these patients have acute pancreatitis, serum amylase levels tend to be in the the very high range (>1,500 IU), and this finding along with gallstones noticed with ultrasound is diagnostic.

Conservative management brings about rapid improvement in about 90% of patients with a cessation of pain and normalization of serum amylase levels within 3 or 4 days. After this, cholecystectomy is performed along with operative cholangiography and common bile duct exploration, as needed. About 85% of patients undergoing such treatment have no common bile duct stones at the time of cholecystectomy, indicating successful passage of the stones through the ampulla into the duodenum. Studies showing recovery of the stones in carefully strained stool specimens have documented this event. Advocates of early operation for gallstone pancreatitis (during the attack of acute pancreatitis) base their approach on evidence that some patients have impacted common duct

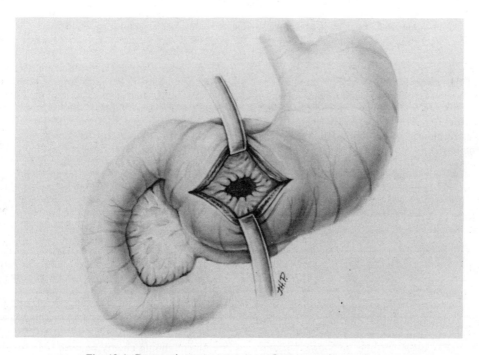

Fig. 18-4. Pancreatic cystogastrostomy for pancreatic pseudocyst.

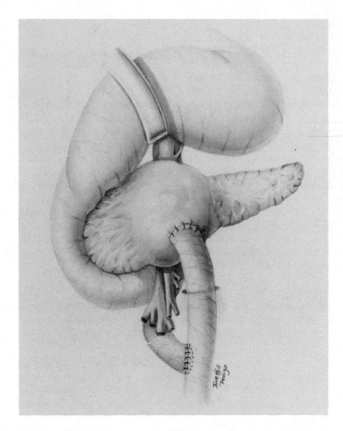

Fig. 18-5. Roux-en-Y pancreatic cystojejunostomy for pancreatic pseudocyst.

stones and will not recover without manual removal of the stones. However, some studies have shown that early operation may lead to an increased mortality and is therefore to be avoided.

If a patient does not promptly recover with conservative means, endoscopic papillotomy may be attempted; this will cause passage of the impacted stones and cholecystectomy can be carried out electively a few days later. Patients who have spontaneously recovered from an attack of gallstone pancreatitis should clearly be advised to undergo cholecystectomy before discharge from the hospital because 30% to 50% of patients will develop recurrent gallstone pancreatitis during the next 6 months if cholecystectomy is deferred.

Chronic pancreatitis

In this country, chronic pancreatitis generally accompanies alcohol abuse, the percentage being from 60% to 100% in several reported series. Other less common causes include gallstones, trauma, and congenital problems. The overriding symptom

is pain, often constant and requiring narcotic analgesics for control. Perhaps 20% of these patients manifest some degree of exocrine insufficiency and over a third are diabetic. Multiple calcifications throughout the pancreas (pancreatic lithiasis) are typical on abdominal roentgenograms. Medical treatment is frequently unsuccessful in this alcoholic population, and operation may be necessary.

The operative procedure depends on the ductal anatomy noted on ERCP. For those patients with a dilated ductal system (Fig. 18-6), a longitudinal pancreaticojejunostomy (Puestow procedure) is utilized (Fig. 18-7). The absence of ductal dilatation indicates subtotal pancreatic resection. Resection entails removal of 80% to 95% of the gland, with sparing of a small remnant in the duodenal sweep to preserve duodenal blood supply. After either operation three fourths of these patients benefit with decreased or no pain. Permanent diabetes mellitus and exocrine insufficiency may accompany surgical treatment however, and such treatment should clearly be used only for incapacitating pain.

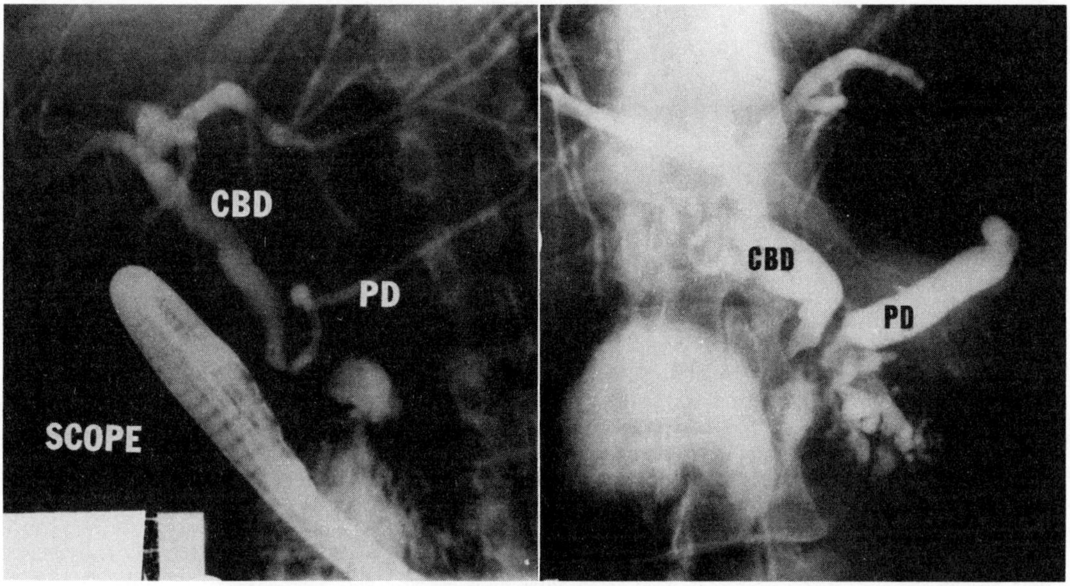

Fig. 18-6. A, Normal common bile duct (CBD) and pancreatic duct (PD) by ERCP (endoscopic retrograde cholangiopancreatography). **B,** Chronic pancreatitis with fibrosis and scarring. The common bile duct (CBD) is obstructed, the main pancreatic duct (PD) is greatly dilated, and there is pronounced ectasia of Wirsung's duct.

Pancreatic trauma

Because of its retroperitoneal location, injuries to the pancreas are less frequent than injuries to other intra-abdominal viscera. Both penetrating and blunt injuries, however, can prove fatal unless treatment is prompt and appropriate. Injuries to the pancreas are equally divided among head, body, and tail, and association with other visceral injuries is common. In patients with penetrating injuries, the pancreatic component is readily detected at celiotomy. The patient sustaining blunt trauma, however, poses a distinct diagnostic problem. Elevation of serum amylase is inconstant in pancreatic trauma. In one review of 74 patients with blunt pancreatic injury, only 71% had an elevated amylase. Likewise, an elevated amylase level in a trauma patient indicates pancreatic injury in only 15% of patients. With wider usage of abdominal CT scanning in trauma cases, this should improve diagnostic accuracy and lead to earlier operation. Similarly, peritoneal lavage may be falsely negative in pancreatic injury, and so information obtained from lavage must be carefully evaluated.

Treatment depends on the location and severity of the injury. Simple contusions and lacerations are readily managed by sump drainage. Distal resection is reserved for those patients who have transection of the gland or severe distal injury. Patients with injuries to the head of the gland associated with major pancreatic ductal injury may be managed by some form of duodenal exclusion, one example of which is shown in Fig. 18-8. In this procedure, the pylorus is ligated with absorbable suture material through a gastrotomy incision and a gastroenterostomy is fashioned. Extensive sump drainage completes the procedure, and within a few weeks the pylorus recanalizes. For extensive injuries of the head of the gland involving the duct and also sometimes the duodenum, a pancreaticoduodenectomy (Whipple procedure) may be necessary. Complications of pancreatic injury are common and include fistula, abscess, and hemorrhage. Death from these complications occurs in 5% to 20% of patients.

Cancer of the pancreas

Cancer of the pancreas is steadily increasing in incidence, and it truly deserves its notoriety as a major unsolved, lethal disease (Fig. 18-9).

With a 5-year survival rate of only 1% to 2%, pancreatic cancer is the fourth leading cause of

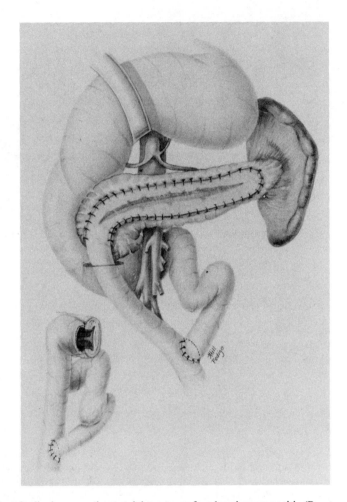

Fig. 18-7. Longitudinal pancreatic cystojejunostomy for chronic pancreatitis (Puestow procedure).

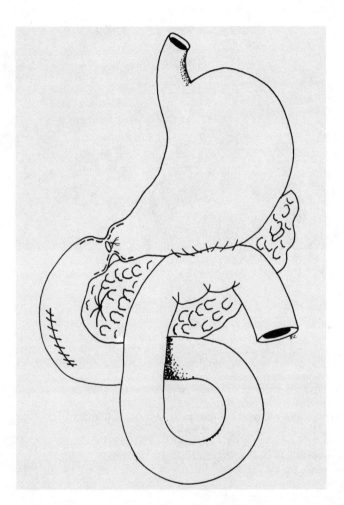

Fig. 18-8. Duodenal exclusion procedure for patients with significant trauma to head of pancreas.

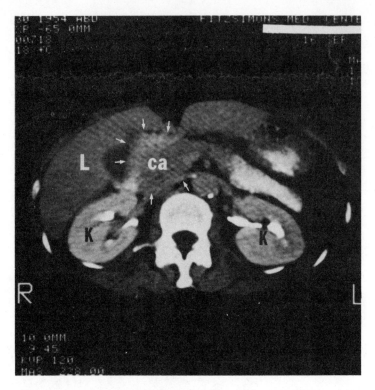

Fig. 18-9. CT scan of cancer in head of pancreas. *L*, Liver; *K*, kidney; *ca*, cancer.

cancer death (behind lung, colon, and breast). Risk factors include advanced age, males, blacks, diabetes, alcoholism, and cigarette smoke. Symptoms of epigastric and back pain, weight loss, anorexia, and jaundice appear late, rendering early diagnosis difficult. Thus, only 15% to 20% of patients have resectable disease at celiotomy. This tumor should be clearly differentiated from the less common periampullary tumors such as carcinoma of the duodenum, ampulla, or common bile duct, in which the prognosis is distinctly better and radical pancreaticoduodenectomy can be curative.

The advent of modern techniques for diagnosing pancreatic disease has brought little improvement in outcome. Treatment in the resectable patient consists in a radical pancreaticoduodenectomy (Whipple procedure) (Fig. 18-10). Because of frequent local recurrences after this procedure, total pancreatectomy has been advocated to eradicate all foci of a possibly multicentric neoplasm and also to eliminate the tenuous pancreaticojejunal anastomosis. However, no evidence, as yet, indicates that patients receiving this operation have an improved outcome. In patients who are not resectable, a biliary bypass (cholecystojejunostomy,

choledochoduodenostomy) or a gastric bypass (gastrojejunostomy) can lead to temporary palliation in the patient's obstructive jaundice and inability to eat (Fig. 18-11). Operative mortality after pancreatic resection is from 10% to 20%, but length of survival (average 12 to 20 months) and quality of life are superior to those seen after bypass procedures (average 3 to 6 months survival).

THE ENDOCRINE PANCREAS
Physiology

Constituting 1% to 2% of the pancreatic mass, about one million pancreatic islets are scattered throughout the pancreas. The islet cells secrete five native (entopic) humoral substances, as shown below:

Entopic cells	Secretion
A-cells	Glucagon
B-cells	Insulin
D-cells	Somatostatin
PP-cells	Pancreatic polypeptide
Enterochromaffin cells	Serotonin

Responding to autonomic nervous system stimuli and to blood levels of glucose, amino acids,

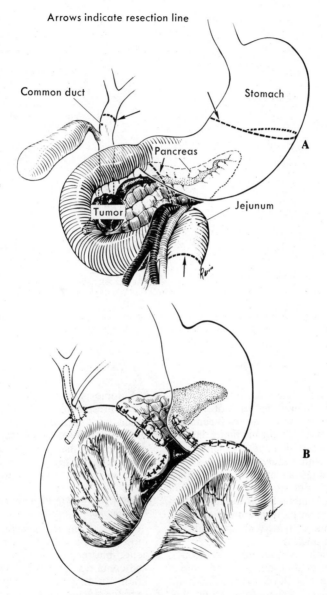

Arrows indicate resection line

Common duct

Stomach

Pancreas

A

Tumor

Jejunum

B

Whipple

Fig. 18-10. Pancreaticoduodenectomy. **A,** Anatomical resection lines. **B,** Completed operation. Three anastomoses: pancreatojejunostomy, choledochojejunostomy, gastrojejunostomy.

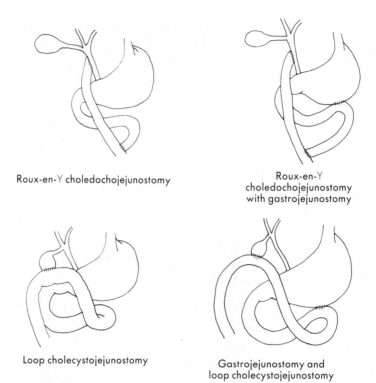

Roux-en-Y choledochojejunostomy

Roux-en-Y
choledochojejunostomy
with gastrojejunostomy

Loop cholecystojejunostomy

Gastrojejunostomy and
loop cholecystojejunostomy

Fig. 18-11. Methods used to bypass unresectable pancreatic cancer. A gastrojejunostomy is added if duodenal obstruction by the cancer is imminent.

fatty acids, and gastrointestinal hormones, the islet cells secrete finely modulated mixtures of insulin, glucagon, and somatostatin. These polypeptides keep the glucose levels within normal limits despite excessive intake or bodily demands (violent exercise). For example, with sudden influxes of glucose, insulin rises and glucagon falls. With sudden demands for glucose, glucagon rises and insulin falls. Somatostatin probably helps modulate the entry of glucose and other nutrients into the bloodstream. The functions of pancreatic polypeptide and serotonin remain unclear.

Extensive intracellular connections (gap junctions) permit the islet cells to communicate internally, thus assuring a high level of coordination. Sensing signals from the brain, from blood nutrients, from gastrointestinal hormones, and from their sister islet cells, the islets deliver a precise mixture of hormones that regulate body fuels, maintaining blood glucose levels at remarkably constant levels between 60 and 170 mg./dl. Teleologically, these monitored levels assure optimum brain function.

Ectopic islet cells sometimes arise within the islets presumably from native cells reverting to other more primitive forms. From these cells, tumors or diffuse hyperplasia may produce ectopic polypeptides that are *not* native to the adult pancreas, e.g., gastrinomas (gastrin) and vipomas (vasoactive intestinal polypeptide).

Endocrine tumors of pancreas
Insulinoma

Arising from the B-cells, insulinomas are the most common entopic tumor. Symptoms of headache, blurred vision, incoherence, convulsions, and coma result from hypoglycemic effects on the brain. In response to hypoglycemia, the body secretes excess catecholamines, which, in turn, cause sweating, weakness, hunger, palpitation, and trembling.

Most patients demonstrate Whipple's triad: (1) signs and symptoms of insulin shock with fasting, (2) fasting blood glucose levels below 50 mg./dl., and (3) relief of symptoms by glucose administration. Newer tests emphasize the insulin-to-glucose

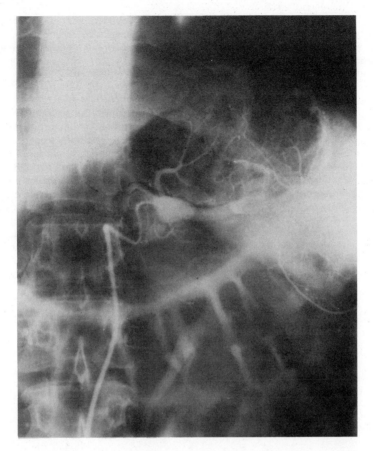

Fig. 18-12. Arteriogram showing staining of insulinoma in pancreatic tail.

ratio. An insulin (normal 5 to 25 microunits/ml.)–to–glucose (normal 60 to 170 mg./dl.) ratio of more than 0.3 during prolonged fasting indicates insulinoma. The reason is that, in normal people, fasting decreases blood glucose levels; consequently, the beta cells, sensing hypoglycemia, should reduce insulin output to undetectable levels. Even slightly elevated insulin levels are inappropriate with fasting glucose levels below 60 mg./dl.

Another test features the suppression of insulin secretion by diazoxide. Diazoxide suppression of insulin with concurrent elevated glucose levels has two functions: (1) it helps make the diagnosis of hyperinsulinism, and (2) it also indicates that diazoxide can control hypoglycemia in specific patients, allowing time for additional localizing studies, if an insulinoma escapes detection at operation.

Localization. Arteriography and newer compu-terized scanning techniques will often localize these tumors (Fig. 18-12). Venous sampling for insulin levels has special usefulness before *reoperations* for insulinomas.

Pathology and treatment of insulinoma

Most insulinomas in adults are single, benign tumors, averaging about 2 cm. in diameter. Ten percent are multiple, and 10% malignant. Diffuse islet cell hyperplasia occurs rarely in adults but is the chief cause of hyperinsulinism in children, especially under 2 years of age.

If these tumors occur in the tail of the pancreas, distal pancreatectomy will remove them. For tumors in the head of the pancreas most surgeons prefer enucleation because it preserves vital endocrine and exocrine functions of the pancreas. Islet cell hyperplasia responds best to subtotal pancreatectomy. When the surgeon cannot palpate a tumor (10% of cases), he should biopsy the pancreatic tail to rule out islet cell hyperplasia. If the patient has previously responded to diazoxide, most authorities would defer blind distal pancreatectomy or more radical procedures, place the patient on diazoxide, and order further localizing studies.

Glucagonoma

Mild diabetes, anemia, venous thrombosis, blackout spells, and necrotizing migratory erythema (the most dramatic feature) characterize this rare syndrome. Elevated plasma glucagon levels make the diagnosis. Most tumors have been malignant. Resection, if possible, or chemotherapy highlight the treatment.

Somatostatinoma

Even more rare than glucagonomas, somatostatinomas have a nonspecific clinical picture that includes diabetes, gallstones, steatorrhea, indigestion, and anemia. Elevated levels of blood somatostatin (with depressed insulin and glucagon levels) make the diagnosis. Up to now, most of these tumors have been malignant.

Gastrinoma (see Chapter 22)

Vipoma (VIPoma, watery diarrhea syndrome)

The ectopic islet cell tumor called vipoma produces profuse, tea-colored, watery diarrhea, dehydration, profound weakness, and sometimes tetany. The basic humoral cause is probably vasoactive intestinal polypeptide (VIP), which mimics the actions of enterotoxic cholera. The massive secretions from small intestine and pancreas overwhelm the absorptive capacity of the colon. Adenoma, carcinoma, and hyperplasia, in decreasing order, account for the pathological causes. Elevated levels of VIP confirm the diagnosis. Excision of localized tumors and subtotal pancreatectomy for hyperplasia keynote the treatment.

19
Spleen

Robert T. Soper
Kevin C. Pringle

The spleen is part of the reticuloendothelial system, filtering blood rather than lymph. At least in the adult it is not vital to life though it does have important immune functions. Traditionally the only operation ordinarily performed on this organ has been its removal, splenectomy.

ANATOMY

The anatomical peculiarities of the spleen dictate much of its importance to the surgeon (Fig. 19-1). Thus it is held loosely in the depths of the left hypochondrium by dense ligaments to surrounding organs (greater curvature of stomach, splenic flexure of colon, inferior surface of left diaphragm). When these ligaments are retracted during operations (on adjacent organs) or stretched suddenly when the spleen is rapidly displaced by external trauma, the fragile splenic capsule may tear. The splenic vein receives many short branches from the adjacent pancreas, anatomical features that generally require splenectomy when the distal part of the pancreas is removed. A portion of the lymphatic drainage of the stomach is through nodes in the splenic hilum, and splenectomy is necessary when curative gastrectomy is performed for carcinoma of the body of the stomach. The splenic vein contributes about one fourth of the portal blood; since this is a two-way street, any increase in portal pressure is transmitted to the splenic pulp. This results in splenomegaly and hypersplenism, which, at times, are the earliest manifestations of portal hypertension.

FUNCTION

The splenic capsule contains elastic fibers that allow considerable fluctuation in size of the organ. The spleen therefore acts as a blood reservoir in lower animals; it stores up to one third of the blood volume for release back into circulation when additional blood is required, as in response to stress or epinephrine release. This is not an important function of the human spleen.

Red blood cells are destroyed in the spleen as they approach the end of their 120-day life-span, with degradation of hemoglobin and salvage of iron. This destruction probably occurs because of increased osmotic and mechanical fragility of the cells with aging. Red blood cells that are excessively fragile for other reasons (spherocytosis) also are trapped and destroyed in the spleen. It is a curious paradox that red blood cells can also be manufactured (extramedullary hematopoiesis) in the spleen, normally during fetal life and abnormally in the adult with chronic bone marrow failure (fibrosis). Extramedullary hematopoiesis produces splenomegaly; bone marrow smears are done before elective removal of a large spleen so that marrow failure as the cause for splenomegaly can be ruled out. In addition to entrapping particles (particularly bacteria) and as part of its reticuloendothelial function, the spleen produces antibodies, lymphocytes, plasma cells, opsonins, tuftsin, and immunoglobulins (IgM, IgG). Splenic IgM is the first antibody produced in response to a new particulate antigen, such as a bacterium. Persons

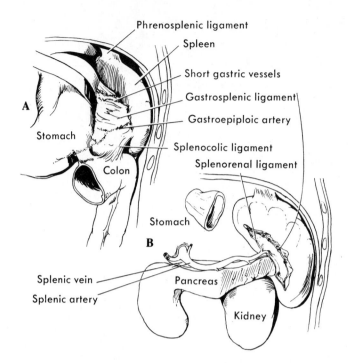

Fig. 19-1. Gross anatomy of spleen and its relationships to surrounding organs. **A,** Note intimate attachments of spleen to diaphragm, stomach, and colon. **B,** Cutaway section showing relationship of spleen to pancreas.

who are asplenic for whatever reason (congenital, sickle cell anemia, or after splenectomy) are subject to bouts of overwhelming sepsis, generally caused by mucopolysaccharide-encapsulated organisms (pneumococci, meningococci, and less commonly *Haemophilus influenzae*), which multiply rapidly and are normally filtered out of circulation by the spleen. This overwhelming sepsis has a 50% to 80% mortality within 24 to 36 hours of onset. Although its incidence is inversely related to age (the younger the asplenic patient, the more susceptible he seems to be) and is more likely to occur within 2 to 3 years after splenectomy, it has been reported in adults up to 15 years after removal of the spleen. Statisticians have calculated that persons without a spleen have a chance of developing overwhelming sepsis 50 times greater than that of the normal population.

Appreciation of these facts has prompted considerable change of attitude toward splenectomy in the past decade. Splenectomy should be avoided when possible during childhood and is undertaken in adults with care. If splenectomy is necessary, prophylactic penicillin or pneumococcal vaccines should be considered postoperatively. All splenectomized patients need to be made aware of the

overwhelming postsplenectomy infection (OPSI) syndrome.

SURGICAL DISORDERS OF THE SPLEEN
Splenic rupture and its causes

The most common indication for splenectomy is hemorrhage after rupture (Fig. 19-2). In descending order of importance splenic rupture is caused by (1) trauma, (2) surgical traction, and (3) softening and enlargement of the spleen because of disease, with subsequent spontaneous rupture.

Trauma

Despite the relatively small size of the spleen, its mobility, and the protection afforded by the left lower rib cage, the spleen is the intra-abdominal organ most susceptible to rupture by trauma. The spleen is more susceptible to injury in the child because of the greater flexibility of the overlying ribs and the relatively larger spleen than that in the adult.

The trauma may be direct or indirect, by a penetrating or a nonpenetrating force. Associated injury to surrounding organs (stomach, colon, pancreas, left kidney) is common, and often splenic rupture is seen with multiple injuries to other parts

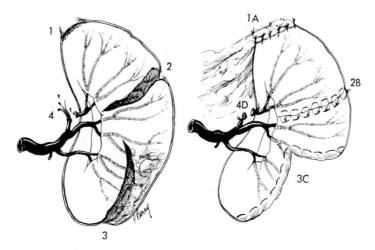

Fig. 19-2. Four types of splenic trauma are shown in left diagram: *1*, avulsion of splenic capsule, as with surgical traction; *2*, transverse laceration of splenic pulp parallels course of intrasplenic vessels; bleeding is minor and no splenic pulp is devascularized; *3*, vertical laceration cuts across vessels; bleeding is brisk and peripheral pulp *(shaded)* is devascularized; *4*, brisk bleeding from major hilar vessels. Repair of four types of trauma is depicted in right diagram: *1A*, suture and omental tamponade; *2B*, mattress suture repair; *3C*, excision and mattress suture closure; *4D*, ligature control of bleeding. Splenectomy is not mandatory.

of the body. The signs and symptoms of splenic injury may be masked by these other injuries. Splenic penetration by missiles is often seen in combat military practice. Nonpenetrating multiple system injury is more common in civilian automobile accidents or falls.

Surgical traction

Iatrogenic tears in the splenic capsule by excessive traction on the tough capsular ligaments are occasionally produced during operations on adjacent organs. Downward traction on the stomach (transabdominal vagotomy or hiatus hernia repair) injures the spleen in about 5% of cases. Better exposure and more gentle traction reduce the frequency of this misadventure.

Spontaneous rupture of a diseased spleen

An enlarged spleen from any cause will be more exposed and therefore subject to rupture by lesser degrees of trauma. A spleen softened by disease, such as malaria or lymphomatous involvement, on occasion ruptures spontaneously. Awareness of this possibility, especially in children subjected frequently to minor trauma, justifies early treatment of the primary disease.

Clinical manifestations. Multiple injuries to other body systems commonly complicate and mask splenic injury. The signs and symptoms of splenic rupture in turn will depend on the amount and rate of blood loss (Fig. 19-2). Thus a complete rupture of the major artery or vein in the splenic hilum produces massive blood loss signaled by profound shock. Lesser degrees of blood loss, as with a transverse laceration of the splenic pulp, are associated with gradually appearing signs of shock, often accompanied by abdominal pain, tenderness, percussion dullness, and an expanding hematoma mass in the left upper abdominal quadrant. The pain is more severe with breathing and may be referred via the phrenic nerve to the left shoulder tip (Kehr's sign, noted in 15% of cases). The left hemidiaphragm is elevated and restricted in its movement. Free blood in the peritoneal cavity may cause loin bulging and shifting dullness and is suggested on rectal examination by a fullness in the rectovesical space. Deepening pallor, rising pulse rate, narrowing pulse pressure, and serial diminution in the hemoglobin and hematocrit reflect the resultant hypovolemia.

In about 15% of patients with traumatic rupture of the spleen, the bleeding is controlled by intrinsic tamponade by the omentum or diaphragm to produce a perisplenic hematoma, or else the hemorrhage is confined beneath the splenic capsule. In this situation the signs of hypovolemia may be minimal or lacking and the abdominal signs may be more localized to the left upper abdominal quadrant. In time this hematoma may resolve entirely, may remain as a splenic cyst, or rarely may rupture secondarily into the free peritoneal cavity with a return of the progressive signs of hypovolemia and spreading hemoperitoneum. Delayed rupture has been reported up to 50 days after injury.

Exploratory laparatomy is the safest and most decisive way to confirm the diagnosis of splenic rupture. Abdominal paracentesis may help confirm the diagnosis of intraperitoneal hemorrhage before laparotomy. Supportive therapy should begin immediately, followed by laparotomy if the patient's condition is unstable.

When bleeding is slower, additional diagnostic study of the patient is possible. A leukocytosis of 15,000 to 20,000/cu. mm. is an early but nonspecific sign of splenic rupture. Serial hemoglobin and hematocrits, which reflect dilution of circulating blood with extracellular tissue fluid to compensate for lost blood, are sometimes helpful. Plain roentgenograms show elevation of the left hemidiaphragm, medial displacement of the gastric air bubble with serration of its greater curvature, and inferior displacement of the air within the splenic flexure of the colon associated with a "ground-glass" tissue density in the left upper abdominal quadrant. When diagnosis is doubtful, splenic scan or angiography may confirm splenic laceration or hematoma.

Treatment. Splenic trauma requires splenectomy when the splenic pulp is smashed beyond repair, when the spleen is devascularized by avulsion of its hilar vessels, or if the patient's general condition is poor from other concurrent injuries. However, because of recent studies that have documented the immunological importance of the spleen at all ages (but especially in children), judicious attempts should be made to salvage traumatized spleens when possible. Avulsion injuries can be safely tamponaded by Gelfoam, Avitene, or omentum. Transverse lacerations are closed by simple mattress sutures. Devascularized segments are excised, and the raw splenic surface is sutured and covered by omentum (Fig. 19-2). Splenic bleeding can cease spontaneously or be arrested surgically; not every traumatized spleen need be removed.

Hypersplenism

The term *hypersplenism* is nonspecific and implies abnormal splenic sequestration of one or more of the formed elements of the blood (RBCs, WBCs, or platelets) (Table 19-1). It is almost always associated with splenomegaly, a depression of the sequestered blood elements, and increased bone marrow production of those elements that are diminished in the peripheral blood.

Hypersplenism may be primary or secondary. In *primary hypersplenism* no other known disease process induces the exaggerated splenic function. Examples include idiopathic (primary or essential) thrombocytopenic purpura, idiopathic (primary) splenic neutropenia or pancytopenia, and congenital spherocytosis. Splenectomy is generally quite effective in the treatment of primary hypersplenism.

In *secondary hypersplenism* the overactivity is caused by another disease process involving the spleen and other portions of the reticuloendothelial system (leukemia, lymphomas, Hodgkin's disease, sarcoidosis, tuberculosis, β-thalassemia major, and the metabolic storage diseases). Splenectomy may temporarily improve the hematological picture in secondary hypersplenism, but it does not affect the course of the primary disease per se. Hypersplenism associated with portal hypertension is the most common form of secondary hypersplenism.

Idiopathic thrombocytopenic purpura

Idiopathic thrombocytopenic purpura is characterized by pronounced diminution in circulating platelets with a resultant bleeding diathesis. It must be distinguished diagnostically from thrombopenia and purpura associated with toxic bone marrow depression (and diminished platelets) caused by a wide variety of agents such as tuberculosis, excessive radiation, leukemia, widespread bony metastases, and bone marrow sensitivity to drugs such as sulfonamides, chloramphenicol, arsenicals, and benzol. Secondary thrombocytopenic purpura is not helped by splenectomy.

Idiopathic thrombocytopenic purpura is more

Table 19-1. Primary hypersplenism*

Disease	Blood	Marrow	Benefit by splenectomy (%)
Idiopathic thrombocytopenic purpura	↓ Platelets	↑ Megakaryocytes	80
Congenital spherocytosis	↓ RBCs	↑ Erythroid elements	100
Primary neutropenia	↓ Neutrophils	↑ Myeloid elements	80
Primary pancytopenia	↓ Formed elements	↑ All precursor elements	80

*↓, Lowered; ↑, elevated.

common in females, children, and young adults. As the name suggests, the basic cause is unknown. Some theories incriminate a hormone from the spleen that prevents platelet release from the bone marrow; others suggest a globulin that agglutinates platelets to increase their splenic sequestration and destruction.

Clinically the disease is characterized by periodic exacerbations of abnormal bleeding manifested by the appearance of petechiae, ecchymoses, and hematomas, which appear either spontaneously or after minor trauma. Surface bleeding can occur into the intestinal or urinary tracts, and menorrhagia is seen in the menstruating female. Hematomas in the intestinal wall can produce obstruction or can serve as the lead point in intussusceptions. The most crippling and lethal bleeding occurs intracranially, and its prevention compels early treatment of this disorder. Large hematomas or hemarthroses are uncommon. This is the only form of hypersplenism that is not commonly (in only about 20% of cases) associated with splenomegaly; furthermore, if thrombocytopenia and splenomegaly are associated, it is likely that one is dealing with a secondary type of thrombocytopenic purpura.

The diagnosis of idiopathic thrombocytopenic purpura is suggested by a positive Rumpel-Leede test: petechiae are produced distal to a sphygmomanometer cuff inflated above venous pressure. The bleeding time is prolonged and the clot retraction is poor, though the coagulation time is normal. Platelet count in the peripheral blood is below 40,000/cu. mm., and the bone marrow smear contains increased numbers of platelet precursors (megakaryocytes).

Initial treatment often consists of steroids and transfusion of platelets or fresh blood collected in a siliconized container; this temporarily prevents additional bleeding. Remissions occur spontaneously and are often induced by steroid therapy, especially in children. The remissions may be permanent.

Splenectomy is indicated if a remission is not achieved or if the disease exacerbates while under steroid maintenance therapy. Splenectomy generally produces a thrombocytosis that reaches its peak between 2 and 12 days postoperatively, followed by a return of the platelet count to near normal ranges. Improvement in clot retraction and bleeding time will likewise occur promptly. Some patients are relieved of their bleeding tendencies even though the platelet count is unchanged.

Splenectomy is curative in about three fourths of patients with idiopathic thrombocytopenic purpura. It will prevent further serious bleeding episodes or will make steroid management easier in the majority of the other patients, even though the platelet counts remain low.

Idiopathic splenic neutropenia and pancytopenia

In the rare *primary* disorders, idiopathic splenic neutropenia and pancytopenia, there is a deficiency in one or all of the formed blood elements within the peripheral blood, associated with an increase in marrow activity in the element or elements deficient peripherally. Further, no other diseases contribute to these changes. Splenectomy is curative.

Much more commonly, these varieties of hypersplenism occur *after* other primary disorders including infections (malaria, sarcoidosis), neoplasms (leukemia, lymphosarcoma, Hodgkin's disease), metabolic storage diseases (Gaucher's disease, Niemann-Pick disease, Hand-Schüller-Christian disease, Letterer-Siwe disease), β-thalassemia major, and portal hypertension. Progressive splenomegaly is characteristic of secondary splenic pancytopenia, and treatment should be directed at the primary disease rather than the spleen. Occasionally splenectomy is indicated when the massive size of the spleen itself produces symptoms or poses a threat to life because of ease of injury. Splenectomy is also done to improve the hematological picture when the latter changes are extreme. Portal hypertension is the most common cause of secondary splenic pancytopenia; the hypersplenism improves with lowering of the portal pressure by portasystemic venous shunts (Chapter 17).

Hemolytic anemias

Hemolysis of red blood cells associated with anemia can be produced in many ways, including transfusion of mismatched blood, septicemia, and exposure to various hemolysins, such as certain snake venoms. Apart from these is a group of disorders in which the spleen is instrumental in destroying red blood cells to cause anemia and splenomegaly. Sickle cell anemia and β-thalassemia major are not often benefited by operation and will not be considered further here.

Congenital spherocytosis

Congenital spherocytosis is the best understood of these so-called hemolytic anemias. In this disorder the red blood cells are morphologically altered to a spheroid rather than a biconcave disk shape. This is genetically determined as a mendelian dominant trait transmitted by either parent. About 20% of cases seem to arise spontaneously, presumably by mutations, but the remainder show a strong family history of anemia and jaundice. However, the gene responsible for the hemolysis exhibits varying degrees of penetrance. Some members of the family have spherocytosis with little evidence of anemia or splenomegaly, whereas others have the full-blown clinical picture with the same degree of spherocytosis. The mechanical and osmotic fragility of the spherocytes is increased; thus they are made more susceptible to entrapment and hemolysis by the spleen.

Characteristically, mild anemia and jaundice with a slightly enlarged spleen are apparent in the first decade of life. Patients with mild forms of the disease may live a normal life-span, though a significant proportion (25%) ultimately develop gallstones because of the chronic hyperbilirubinemia.

Aplastic crises. Patients with more severe forms of spherocytosis will develop intermittent crises, sometimes precipitated by infections. Such crises are characterized by abdominal pain, fever, nausea and vomiting, progressive anemia, acholuric jaundice, and splenomegaly. The peripheral blood reveals spherical erythrocytes on smear with an anemia that reflects the severity of the disorder. Reticulocytosis is expected during the recovery period after a crisis, but the reticulocyte count may fall to zero during a crisis. Recent theory ascribes the crisis to cessation of red blood cell formation in the bone marrow rather than to an increase in hemolysis within the spleen. A splenic hormone may be involved in this mechanism.

The red blood cell fragility test (preferably interpreted after 24 hours of incubation) is the most effective diagnostic study. Hemolysis of the spherocyte begins in 0.75% saline rather than in the 0.45% saline concentration necessary to lyse normal red blood cells. Hemolysis is completed at 0.4% rather than 0.3% saline in the normal person. The indirect serum bilirubin level is elevated and stools are more darkly pigmented than normal, though no bile is present in urine in keeping with the unconjugated nature of the bilirubin. The results of Coombs' test are negative, and a bone marrow smear reveals erythroid hyperplasia.

Initially treatment is directed at tiding the patient over the acute crisis by cautious blood transfusions. Splenectomy cures the serious hemolysis and prevents future crises but does not alter the red blood cell shape or fragility. All patients who are symptomatic should have splenectomy as an elective procedure, since there is no known medical treatment, and spontaneous remissions do not occur when symptoms are pronounced. Cholecystectomy should be carried out at the same time if the patient's condition allows and if cholelithiasis is present.

Acquired anemias

The *other hemolytic anemias* are acquired (or secondary) and are not of particular surgical interest. Idiopathic acquired hemolytic anemia is a condition that belongs among the autoimmune family of disorders with spontaneously arising agglutinins and hemolysins that damage otherwise normal red blood cells. Splenomegaly, hemolysis, and anemia result. The results of Coombs' test are usually positive, the morphological appearance of the red blood cell is generally normal (though cases are reported that do have some spherocytosis), and there is no family history of hemolytic anemia. Steroids are the preferred treatment. Splenectomy is indicated only for those who fail nonoperative treatment.

Miscellaneous

Primary neoplasms of the spleen are extremely rare and generally of mesenchymal tissue origin. Secondary splenic involvement is common in the leukemias and lymphomas, but metastases from carcinomas are almost unheard of.

Cysts of the spleen are rare and may be congenital, associated with liquefaction of old hematomas or parasitic infestations such as hydatid cyst, or caused by a solitary dermoid cyst.

Accessory spleens are miniature duplications of splenic tissue found on routine postmortem examination in about 10% of the population. They are usually located near the splenic hilum or the gastrocolic ligament and are darker than lymph nodes. Interestingly enough, accessory spleens are found in 20% of people with hypersplenism. Hypertrophy probably allows easier detection in hypersplenism. Accessory spleens must be removed at the time of splenectomy for hypersplenism—if left behind, they may undergo hyperplasia and assume the function of the parent spleen. Missed accessory spleens are occasionally a reason for failure of splenectomy in the treatment of hypersplenic conditions.

20
Peritoneum and Acute Abdominal Conditions

Neil R. Thomford

The term *acute abdomen* endures as a valuable method for signaling an apparent intra-abdominal crisis and indicating the diagnostic protocol to be followed. Neither the patient nor untrained observers may perceive the problem as being acute or of serious potential, but for the responsible physician the acute abdomen demands prompt if not immediate evaluation of the patient, a working diagnosis, and early, clear decisions regarding subsequent study and management.

A great number of illnesses have the capacity to produce an acute abdomen. In most instances the syndrome is the result of a local disease process within the abdomen or pelvis. The following are possible causes:

Gastrointestinal
  Appendicitis
  Cholecystitis
  Perforated peptic ulcer
  Pancreatitis
  Diverticulitis of the colon
  Meckel's diverticulitis
  Mechanical obstruction of the intestine
  Granulomatous enterocolitis
  Ulcerative colitis
  Acute gastritis
  Acute hepatitis
  Gastrointestinal hemorrhage
  Gastroenteritis
Gynecological
  Ectopic pregnancy
  Torsion or rupture of ovarian cyst
  Pelvic inflammatory disease
  Gonococcal perihepatitis
  Painful ovulation (mittelschmerz)
  Regurgitation of menstrual blood into peritoneal cavity

Vascular
  Dissecting aneurysm of the abdominal aorta and its branches
  Embolic occlusion of visceral branches of the abdominal aorta
  Nonocclusive mesenteric infarction
  Ruptured aneurysm of the abdominal aorta or one of its intra-abdominal branches
Genitourinary
  Urinary tract infection
  Urinary tract calculus
Systemic disease
  Diabetic acidosis
  Tabetic crisis
  Porphyria
  Sickle cell anemia
  Henoch-Schönlein purpura
Other
  Primary peritonitis
  Mesenteric lymphadenitis
  Intra-abdominal hemorrhage associated with trauma
  Intra-abdominal hemorrhage associated with anticoagulants
  Acute lead poisoning
  Acute adrenal insufficiency
  Herpes zoster
  Rectus sheath hematoma
  Black widow spider bite

In other cases the primary disease is systemic, with abdominal or pelvic manifestations of the illness causing the symptoms and signs. Finally, thoracic diseases, listed as follows, may cause symptoms and signs suggesting an intra-abdominal catastrophe.

Thoracic diseases
  Myocardial infarction
  Acute pericarditis

Pneumonia
Diaphragmatic pleurisy
Pulmonary infarction
Spontaneous pneumothorax
Acute mediastinitis

To arrive at the correct diagnosis the examiner must know the anatomy and innervation of the abdominal tissues and organs, have a thorough understanding of the pathology and pathophysiology of the many causes of the acute abdomen, and be aware of both the potential and the limitations of available diagnostic studies. The rapidity with which the evaluation and decision-making process is accomplished must match the urgency of the situation. The course of action when encountering a patient who is in profound shock from rupture of an abdominal aortic aneurysm will differ from that with a 20-year-old whose symptoms and signs are suggestive of early appendicitis. If the evaluation does not provide the diagnosis, clinical judgment must choose between observation, repeated or added diagnostic studies, or an exploratory operation.

EVALUATION OF THE PATIENT
The history

Acute disease or injury of organs and tissues in the abdomen and pelvis results in either inflammation, obstruction of a hollow viscus, hemorrhage, or any combination of the three. These changes produce one or more symptoms that lead to the patient-physician encounter and the beginning of the evaluation and management of the patient with an acute abdomen.

Pain

Pain is the most common symptom of patients with a clinical picture of the acute abdomen. Sensory nerve pathways from the abdomen include both spinal nerves and the autonomic nervous system. The intercostal branches of spinal nerves 5 through 11 innervate the parietal peritoneum. In addition the phrenic nerve provides sensory innervation to the peritoneal surface of the diaphragm. The innervation of the visceral peritoneum and the abdominal and pelvic organs is provided by the autonomic nervous system.

Because the gastrointestinal tract develops from the midline in the embryo, pain from lesions of the stomach and duodenum is epigastric in location, pain from the midgut is felt in the periumbilical area, and pain from the left colon and rectum is often localized to the hypogastric area. Since the gallbladder and appendix are also of midline derivation, the initial pain from disease of these structures is epigastric and periumbilical, respectively.

Pain may shift position, radiate, or occur as referred pain. When the periumbilical pain of appendicitis "localizes" in the right lower quadrant of the abdomen, this is an example of pain shifting. In this instance the shift results from extension of the inflammatory process through the wall of the appendix to involve the parietal peritoneum, with pain mediated through spinal nerves. Other mechanisms may cause pain to shift in location. Severe epigastric pain from perforation of a peptic ulcer may shift to the right lower quadrant as gastric and duodenal contents spill into the peritoneal cavity and drain into the lower abdomen along the ascending colon. An example of radiating pain is the pain of a ureteral calculus, which often extends from the lumbar region and flank to the inguinal region and the scrotum. Finally, referred pain is the result of two separate anatomical areas being innervated by the same nerve trunk. The brain may then erroneously interpret the site of origin of the pain impulses. Because the phrenic nerve provides sensation for the peritoneal surface of the diaphragm and the skin of the top of the shoulder, subdiaphragmatic irritation may cause shoulder pain.

The character of the pain provides valuable diagnostic clues. Persistent uninterrupted pain characterizes strangulated intestine, whereas "waves" of pain often indicate acute pancreatitis. Intermittent cramps point to mechanical obstruction of the intestine. The severity of the pain may also assist in identifying the disease. Patients with dissecting aneurysms of the abdominal aorta are in great agony and in many instances unable to control themselves and communicate with the physician. Renal colic also causes severe pain, whereas the pain of cholecystitis, pancreatitis, appendicitis, and diverticulitis is less incapacitating. Some significance may also be attached to the patients' response to their pain. Patients with cholecystitis usually "walk the floor," while persons with localized or generalized peritonitis from appendicitis, diverticulitis of the colon, or pelvic inflammatory disease prefer to lie still. When queried, patients with peritonitis will often remark that their pain increases with any sudden movement or jarring of the body.

Vomiting

The presence or absence of vomiting and the character of the vomitus may help determine the diagnosis. Vomiting is relatively common with biliary colic and mechanical obstruction of the gastrointestinal tract. When obstruction occurs in the proximal gastrointestinal tract, vomiting begins early; with obstruction of the distal small intestine or colon, vomiting begins late, if at all, and the vomitus often has fecal qualities. Vomiting is uncommon with perforated ulcer, appendicitis, and pelvic inflammatory disease. The presence or absence of red blood in the vomitus is of critical importance. The significance of finding occult blood in the emesis or gastric aspirate is often more difficult to assess.

Bowel function

Diarrhea is suggestive of gastroenteritis or one of the inflammatory diseases of the colon. Yet some children with appendicitis and patients with hyperperistalsis caused by mechanical obstruction of the small or large intestine have frequent small liquid bowel movements. Cessation of flatus signifies intestinal obstruction. A history of the passage of bright or dark red blood or black, tarry stools must be considered together with the patient's other symptoms. In general, black, tarry stools are suggestive of hemorrhage proximal to or near the ileocecal valve. The passage of significant quantities of red blood through the rectum usually indicates hemorrhage from the colon but may occur with *massive* bleeding from the proximal gastrointestinal tract.

Syncope

Syncope occurs most often with acute abdominal disease when hemorrhage is the major complication of the illness. Syncope *without* pain often accompanies occult hemorrhage into the gastrointestinal tract. Syncope *with* abdominal pain should alert the examiner to probable intraperitoneal or retroperitoneal bleeding.

Menstrual history

No history of an abdominal or pelvic illness in the female is complete without a menstrual history: When did the last menstrual period occur? Was it normal? Is the patient pregnant? Acute pelvic inflammatory disease often occurs at the termination of the menstrual flow; mittelschmerz may be expected at the midpoint of the menstrual cycle, whereas the pain of endometriosis classically occurs during the last 2 to 3 days of the menstrual cycle. Small amounts of blood leaking from endometrial and functional cysts of the ovaries may be accompanied by pain in the pelvic region. When 500 to 1,000 ml. of blood is lost into the peritoneal cavity from rupture of an ectopic pregnancy, blood in the pelvis often results in the urge to urinate. Blood irritating the undersurface of the left hemidiaphragm may cause referred pain to the left shoulder.

Past medical history and system review

The more acutely ill the patient, the more rapidly the physician must act. Under emergency conditions the physician should inquire early about the past medical history. If the patient has had attacks of renal colic, has a history of peptic ulcer, or has known gallstones, this information is vital for quick arrival at a working diagnosis. If the patient presents symptoms suggestive of intestinal obstruction, the diagnosis becomes more likely if he has had a previous abdominal operation. Similarly, if the patient has had an abdominal aortic prosthesis inserted and now has hemorrhage from the gastrointestinal tract, he is presumed to have an aorta-enteric fistula until proved otherwise.

A general review of systems should cover all areas not reviewed when the history of the illness is obtained. Special attention should be given to the cardiovascular and genitourinary systems.

The physical examination

The physical examination must be complete. To exclude any area of the body or any particular part of the physical examination invites diagnostic error. Even in the emergency situation the accomplished clinician who is a keen observer may complete an adequate examination of the patient in the matter of a few minutes.

General observations

The patient's posture, mental status, vital signs, and skin color and temperature, together with inspection of any emesis or rectal discharge, will allow a preliminary opinion as to whether or not the patient's acute abdomen is the result of inflammation, distension of a hollow viscus, or hemorrhage.

Examination of the abdomen

Inspection of the abdomen will identify abdominal distension, asymmetry of the abdomen, an obvious mass, scars from previous operations, bruises or other abnormalities suggestive of trauma, or evidence of a hernia. In rare instances visible peristalsis will be strongly suggestive of a diagnosis of mechanical intestinal obstruction. A bluish discoloration of the navel (Cullen's sign) may indicate blood within the peritoneal cavity, whereas a dusty bluish hue in one or both flanks (Grey Turner's sign) may indicate retroperitoneal hemorrhage.

When time permits, the physician should auscultate the abdomen for a minimum of 1 minute and preferably for 5 minutes to assess accurately the degree and character of peristaltic activity. Hyperactive, high-pitched peristaltic sounds, rushes, and tinkles indicate mechanical obstruction of the intestine, whereas silence as a result of cessation of peristaltic activity points to intra-abdominal inflammatory diseases. Auscultation should include a search for bruits. Percussion may identify tender areas and differentiate between air and fluid as a cause of any abdominal distension. Percussion can identify the large liver of acute fatty infiltration or alcoholic hepatitis, the enlarged spleen, and the distended urinary bladder.

Palpation of the abdomen ordinarily is the most informative method of evaluating the area. Gentleness is essential to distinguish between voluntary guarding and an area of involuntary muscle spasm caused by local irritation of the inner aspect of the abdominal wall. Rebound tenderness, a sign of inflammation of the parietal peritoneum, is elicited when the hand depressing the abdominal wall is quickly removed and pain occurs with the sudden return of the abdominal wall to its normal contour. Palpation should identify organ enlargement or a mass, rule out hernias of the abdominal wall and groins, and assess the aorta and the iliac and femoral arteries.

Examination of the rectum should include both digital examination of the rectum and bimanual palpation of the pelvis and lower abdomen. The pelvic examination of the female patient should include a speculum examination of the vagina and cervix to determine the patency of the cervical os, the nature of the cervical discharge, and the position of the uterus. The bimanual examination should determine the size, contour, and position of the uterus and ovaries. The finding of a purulent discharge from the cervix together with thickening, tenderness, or enlargement of the adnexa signifies pelvic inflammatory disease, whereas a tender mass of one adnexa may represent an endometrioma or an ectopic pregnancy. A number of special physical tests and signs are used by physicians evaluating patients with suspected abdominal or pelvic disease. These tests and signs are described in standard textbooks of physical diagnosis.

Examination of the head, neck, chest, back, and extremities will assist in ruling out causes of the acute abdomen outside the abdomen and pelvis.

Diagnostic procedures

The nature and urgency of the situation as assessed by the examiner will determine which diagnostic studies are done and in what order. The following sequence is appropriate when the patient's condition is stable and adequate time is available.

Bedside procedures

If gastrointestinal disease is suspected, a nasogastric tube may be inserted to determine the nature of the gastric aspirate and the presence or absence of gross or occult blood. Samples of the stool obtained at the time of rectal examination should be examined for gross or occult blood. If the examination indicates the need, a central venous catheter should be inserted to allow monitoring of central venous pressure. (See Chapter 29.)

Abdominal paracentesis in one or more sites may reveal hemoperitoneum. If simple paracentesis is not diagnostic, lavage of the peritoneal cavity with saline and microscopic examination of the aspirate for red blood cells will provide a more definitive answer. Paracentesis may also identify bile, feces, or other contaminants of the peritoneal cavity associated with intra-abdominal accidents.

Laboratory procedures

Minimum laboratory procedures should include hemoglobin concentration, hematocrit, white blood count, differential count, and urinalysis. Added selected laboratory tests may include serum sodium, potassium, and chloride concentrations, serum amylase determination, arterial blood gas analysis, stools for ova and parasites, smears and cultures of the cervical discharge, an electrocardiogram, and studies of blood coagulation, hepatic function, and renal function.

Roentgenograms

Plain roentgenograms of the chest and roentgenograms of the abdomen with the patient in both the supine and the erect position are essential. The chest x-ray examination assists in identifying thoracic causes of the acute abdomen as well as sometimes showing specific x-ray findings of intra-abdominal catastrophes, i.e., free air under the diaphragm associated with perforation of the gastrointestinal tract. In addition, the chest roentgenogram often shows abnormalities that reflect subdiaphragmatic disease, e.g., a left pleural effusion from pancreatitis.

Roentgenograms of the abdomen are perhaps most essential in patients suspected of having mechanical obstruction of the intestine. The history and physical examination may be equivocal and the results of laboratory studies are often within normal limits. In contrast, roentgenograms will show dilated segments of intestine with air fluid levels. When the mechanical obstruction involves the small intestine, the absence of gas in the colon is often as important a diagnostic sign as the dilated loops of small bowel.

Roentgenograms of the abdomen with the patient in the upright position will show free air within the peritoneal cavity in 60% to 75% of patients who have a perforation of the gastrointestinal tract. Other potential findings with plain films of the abdomen include a fecalith of the appendix, a renal calculus (90% are radiopaque), calcifications in the pancreas suggestive of chronic recurrent pancreatitis, and curvilinear calcification of the left wall of the infrarenal aorta suggestive of an abdominal aortic aneurysm. Biliary tract disease may be identified in a small number of patients by identifying calcified gallstones (10% to 15% have sufficient calcium to be seen on plain films).

Other diagnostic studies

Examination of the esophagus and gastrointestinal tract using barium sulfate as a contrast medium is safe unless one suspects perforation of the gastrointestinal tract with the potential for barium to enter the peritoneal cavity. The upper gastrointestinal and barium enema examinations may provide a definitive diagnosis of intestinal obstruction or identify the site and nature of hemorrhage. An intravenous urogram may locate a renal calculus or an obstruction or injury of the urinary tract.

Angiography can disclose embolic occlusion of the superior mesenteric artery or other branches of the abdominal aorta or the site of hemorrhagic lesions of the gastrointestinal tract. Proctosigmoidoscopy may reveal inflammatory disease or neoplasms of the rectum or volvulus of the sigmoid colon.

The development of ultrasound instruments and computerized tomography has provided physicians with noninvasive tests capable of identifying gallstones, cysts of the pancreas and ovary, aneurysms of the abdominal aorta, and other intra-abdominal abnormalities. When clinical findings indicate a possible acute pelvic condition, one of the first diagnostic studies should be an ultrasound examination of the pelvis. Ultrasound is also of special value in identifying gallstones in patients suspected of having acute cholecystitis. Ultrasound and the more recently introduced biliary radionuclide scans can confirm the diagnosis of acute cholecystitis and thereby allow more specific medical therapy and earlier surgical intervention.

Laparoscopy and mini-laparotomy are formal surgical procedures. Although local anesthesia may be used, one must be prepared to proceed with general anethesia. Finally, for those patients who have an acute intra-abdominal problem of unknown nature and whose symptoms, signs, and laboratory findings are suggestive of a threat to life, laparotomy remains the most prudent diagnostic procedure.

THE PERITONEUM AND PERITONITIS

The peritoneum is a single layer of mesothelial cells overlying a loose layer of connective tissue. The parietal peritoneum lines the abdominal cavity and is reflected onto the abdominal viscera as the visceral peritoneum or serosa. Organs and tissues of the abdomen and pelvis lie either within the peritoneal cavity or in the retroperitoneum.

Peritonitis is a response of the visceral or parietal peritoneum or both to any irritation or injury. The local defense reaction includes hyperemia with increased capillary permeability and an influx of leukocytes and fibroblasts. In addition there is a more generalized response of the abdominal tissues to the injury including a "walling off" of the inflamed area by omentum, loops of intestine, and other tissues and organs. To help isolate inflammation, peristalsis decreases.

Primary peritonitis, an uncommon diffuse inflammation of the peritoneum, has no intra-abdominal cause. An illness principally of infants and children, it is almost always caused by a single pathogenic organism, usually pneumococcus, streptococcus, or *Escherichia coli.* Bacteria presumably enter the peritoneal cavity by the genital tract or the bloodstream, or by transmural migration through the wall of the intestine.

The diagnosis of primary peritonitis depends on the analysis of fluid from the peritoneal cavity. An acidic fluid leukocyte count greater than 300/cu. mm. with more than 30% neutrophils is diagnostic of intraperitoneal infection. Isolation of a *single* organism is strongly suggestive of primary peritonitis.

Secondary peritonitis of varying degree is common, accompanying most acute intra-abdominal disease. Bacterial contamination leads all causes. Others include bile, pancreatic juice, blood, or acid released into the peritoneal cavity as a result of intra-abdominal disease or injury.

There is great variation in both the symptoms and the physical findings of secondary peritonitis. With perforation of a duodenal ulcer, the pain is sudden in onset, and rigidity of the muscles of the abdominal wall is soon apparent. In contrast, the pain and tenderness of the common inflammatory conditions of the lower abdomen and pelvis are often insidious in their onset. Fever and an increase in the pulse rate are present in most patients. Pain is the premier symptom. When there is generalized peritonitis, the pain is diffuse. With localized inflammation of the peritoneum, the pain will often allow identification of the site of the peritonitis. With the more localized variety, the point of maximum tenderness and the palpation of a mass are other findings that may allow identification of the origin of the peritonitis. These classical findings of peritonitis may be difficult to interpret in patients who have recently had an abdominal operation and may be absent in immunodepressed patients. Laboratory studies will often include leukocytosis and evidence of dehydration. Radiological examinations may show free air below the diaphragm from a ruptured viscus and adynamic ileus of both the small and large intestine secondary to the peritonitis. When the need for an exploratory operation is in question, needle aspiration or lavage of the peritoneal cavity may confirm the presence of peritonitis but cannot identify localized areas of inflammation.

21
Intestinal Obstruction

Richard D. Liechty
Greg Van Stiegmann

Intestinal obstruction is defined as an interference in the normal movement of the bowel contents through the intestinal tract. Two main types of obstruction occur: (1) *mechanical obstruction,* which arises from structural lesions (adhesive bands, stones, tumors, etc.) that block the bowel lumen, and (2) *paralytic ileus,* which arises from a failure of the neuromuscular propulsive action of the bowel wall. The distinction between these types is vitally important because mechanical obstruction, if unrelieved, may progress to *strangulation* (shutting off of the blood supply to the obstructed segment) or *perforation.* Both of these complications pose a serious threat to life. Paralytic ileus, on the other hand, rarely threatens life and is treated conservatively with gastrointestinal decompression and correction of the factors causing the bowel wall paralysis.

Simple obstruction, in contrast to *strangulation obstruction,* occurs when the blood supply to the obstructed bowel is adequate. *Vascular obstruction* occurs when an impedance to the arterial flow or venous return sets the stage for bowel infarction. In *partial obstruction* the signs and symptoms of bowel obstruction occur, but some passage of bowel contents continues.

MECHANICAL OBSTRUCTION
Site of mechanical obstruction

The small bowel is about 20 feet in length, and the large bowel is 5 feet in length. This 4:1 ratio parallels the ratio of mechanical obstructions that occur in the small and large bowel; 80% occur in the small bowel, and only 20% involve the large

bowel. The student can recall the relative incidence favoring small bowel obstruction by this helpful question: Given a certain amount of traffic, will more accidents occur along a 20-mile two-lane curving highway or along a 5-mile four-lane straighter highway?

Etiology

The "big three" in causation of adult mechanical intestinal obstruction are hernias (incarcerated or strangulated), adhesions, and tumors (Fig. 21-1). Hernias and adhesions together account for about 70% of *all* bowel obstruction. Tumors cause about 15% of all intestinal obstruction, but they are, by far, the most common cause of *large bowel obstruction.* Intussusception, volvulus, obturation (fecal impactions, gallstone ileus), inflammatory lesions, and vascular obstruction make up the remaining causes of adult intestinal obstruction. Intestinal obstruction in the child, limited primarily to congenital defects and intussusception, is discussed in Chapter 28.

Hernias

The various sites of hernias (including incisions) should be inspected and palpated carefully (Fig. 21-1, *C*). Hernias in obese people are often difficult to detect through thick paddings of fatty tissue. Richter's hernias (a knuckle of bowel in the defect) may be deceptively small. If a hernia becomes tense, tender, and nonreducible, the surgeon must assume that it is strangulated. He should operate immediately, reducing it surgically and resecting any necrotic bowel.

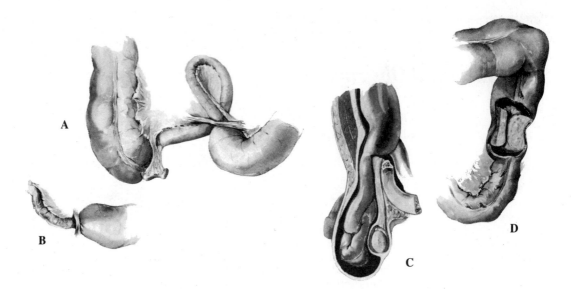

Fig. 21-1. The three leading causes of intestinal obstruction—adhesions, hernias, and tumors. Adhesions causing bowel obstruction. **A,** Fibrous band causing obstruction and volvulus about band. **B,** Fibrous band obstructing segment of small bowel. Notice proximal dilatation. **C,** Inguinal hernia with loop of obstructed small bowel. Notice that obstruction occurs at internal inguinal ring. **D,** Cancer of colon causing bowel obstruction.

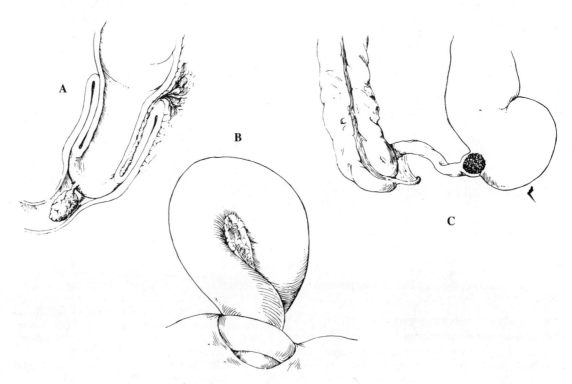

Fig. 21-2. A, Polyp of bowel "leading" an intussusception. **B,** Volvulus of bowel. **C,** Gallstone ileus. Large gallstone obstructing distal ileum.

Adhesions

The incidence of intestinal obstruction caused by adhesions appears to be increasing (Fig. 21-1, *A* and *B*). *Lower abdominal incisions* are more likely to produce adhesive obstructions than *upper abdominal incisions* because the omentum shields the small intestine from the incision in the upper abdomen. About 15% of obstructions caused by adhesions are strangulating. *Closed loop* obstructions, in which a portion of bowel is closed at both ends, threaten perforation from increasing gas pressure (from putrefaction) within the bowel lumen. Early operative release of the obstructing bands can prevent these complications.

Tumors

Neoplasms of the *small bowel* (carcinoma, carcinoid, lymphoma, and benign tumors) are rare causes of obstruction. In contrast, neoplasms cause most obstructions of the colon (Fig. 21-1, *D*) (diverticulitis is next in incidence). Left colon lesions may cause tremendous dilatation of the proximal colon when the ileocecal valve is competent. Because the proximal colon wall is thinned from dilatation and the bowel cannot be prepared preoperatively, decompressive colostomy or cecostomy usually must precede resection of the tumor. In certain cases the obstructing tumor, with bowel and mesentery, can be exteriorized and removed (obstruction resection). (See Chapter 25.)

Intussusception

Intussusception, common in children (Chapter 28), is rare in adults. Polypoid tumors often "lead" the adult intussusception (Fig. 21-2, *A*). Because of these mechanical lesions underlying adult intussusception, we never attempt hydrostatic reduction as in children, but immediately explore and resect the involved bowel.

Volvulus

Volvulus is a twisting of a portion of the gastrointestinal tract on its mesentery. The blood supply is always threatened, if not completely occluded, in this situation (Fig. 21-2, *B*).

Sigmoid volvulus (Fig. 21-3) is the most common type of volvulus because the sigmoid mesentery is long and redundant. In eastern European and some Asian countries sigmoid volvulus is one of the most common causes of bowel obstruction. The high cellulose diet in these areas may be an etiological factor. In western areas sigmoid volvulus usually occurs in older, debilitated patients. Barium enema will often outline the twist. Sigmoidoscopy with insertion of a soft rubber rectal tube usually effects decompression amidst a rush of gas and liquid feces. Operative treatment (detorsion or sigmoid resection) is utilized for recurrence, strangulation, or failure of decompression by a rectal tube.

Cecal volvulus (Fig. 21-4) occurs when the cecal mesentery is long, allowing the cecum free movement within the peritoneal cavity. The twisted cecum containing gas usually (and paradoxically) appears in the left upper abdomen on x-ray examination. Barium enema confirms cecal volvulus and differentiates the contained gas from air within the stomach.

Volvulus of the stomach is rare. It is usually

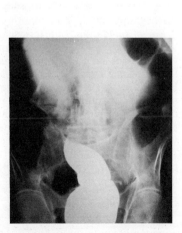
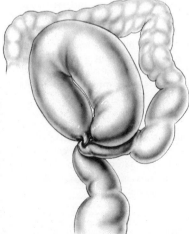

Fig. 21-3. Sigmoid volvulus. Roentgenogram shows large fluid-filled mass and typical bird-beak deformity outlined by barium in distal sigmoid colon. Diagram shows twist.

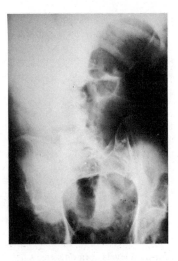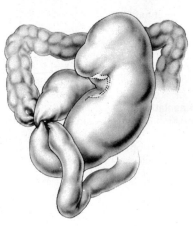

Fig. 21-4. Cecal volvulus. Notice dilated, gas-filled cecum in left upper quadrant on roentgenogram. Diagram shows twist.

associated with paraesophageal hernias. *Small intestinal volvulus* almost invariably results from adhesions. Adhesions pathologically join two portions of the small bowel that form the base of the loop. Volvulus results from a twisting of this loop about the base. *Midgut volvulus,* which occurs almost exclusively in children, involves an abnormality in the embryological rotation and return of the developing intestine (Chapter 28).

Obturation

Obturation results when materials *within* the gut occlude the lumen. *Fecal impaction* and *gallstone ileus* (Fig. 21-2, *C*) are the most common causes of intraluminal obstruction in more advanced countries. Parasitic infections (chiefly *Ascaris lumbricoides,* which may produce a ball of worms) cause intestinal obstruction in less advanced areas. Bezoars of various types are common in patients who are mentally defective.

Inflammatory causes

Tuberculosis, regional enteritis, ulcerative colitis, and amebiasis are the more common causes of intestinal obstruction associated with inflammation. The diagnosis, usually obscure, depends on biopsy and culture specimens.

Vascular obstruction

Vascular obstruction is the reverse, pathologically, of *strangulation obstruction; primary* blood vessel blockage precedes and causes bowel obstruction. (See Chapter 24.)

The final clinical picture is identical to strangulation obstruction. The early stages of vascular obstruction feature extreme abdominal pain, which comes on abruptly (with crescendos) before becoming steady, and vomiting and diarrhea. Many patients, perhaps one third, give a prior history of crampy pains after meals.

The diagnosis of vascular obstruction is difficult especially in older patients, in whom it occurs frequently. The onset may be deceptively subtle with minimal symptoms. In younger patients the onset is frequently sudden and confusing. A thorough knowledge of the patient and of the possible antecedent causative factors gives the physician the best opportunity to make this diagnosis.

Embolism (cardiac or arteriosclerotic), *increased venous pressure* (abdominal tumor, cirrhosis, congestive heart failure), *hypercoagulability* (polycythemia, some cancers), or *vascular diseases* (collagen diseases, vasospastic diseases, prolonged infections, or trauma) should be considered in the differential diagnosis. Arteriograms will often pinpoint the obstructed artery. Immediate operation, with embolectomy when possible, and bowel resection (often massive) are the only therapeutic options. In older patients the mortality is extremely high.

Clinical features

Symptoms. Pain, obstipation, distension, and vomiting keynote the patient's symptoms in intestinal obstruction.

Pain is typically crampy and intermittent, result-

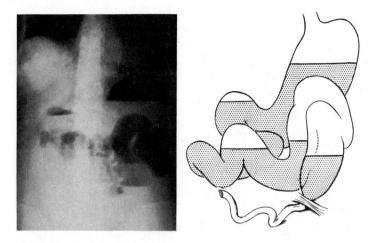

Fig. 21-5. Mechanical bowel obstruction. Localized air-fluid levels seen on upright film of abdomen. Diagram shows dilated proximal bowel and stomach, air-fluid levels, and adhesive band causing obstruction.

ing from forceful contraction of the bowel wall musculature attempting to push fluid and gas past the obstruction. Continuous pain usually signifies strangulation or perforation. Vomiting temporarily relieves the pain from upper gastrointestinal obstructions as bowel distension is ameliorated. In colon obstruction the crampy pains occur at longer intervals than with small bowel obstruction.

Because intestinal obstruction may be only partial or intermittent, *obstipation* is not absolutely necessary to make the diagnosis of intestinal obstruction. Gas or feces in the bowel segment distal to the obstruction may pass in small amounts, especially in response to enemas. However, complete obstruction usually produces eventual failure to pass either gas or feces.

Distension, to some degree, always accompanies obstruction. In high (proximal small bowel) obstruction, distension is minimal. In lower obstructions, distension is massive because of the greater amount of bowel that is filled with gas and liquid.

In high obstruction *vomiting* occurs as an early symptom because the upper small bowel receives bile and pancreatic and gastric juice (in addition to its own secretions) and is poorly absorptive. In obstructing lesions of the low ileum or colon *feculent vomiting* results from stagnation and bacterial putrefaction and strongly suggests the low site of obstruction. In obstruction of the colon with a competent ileocecal valve, vomiting seldom occurs as a "backup" phenomenon, but it does result on a reflex basis.

Laboratory diagnosis

X-ray examination. Plain films of the abdomen taken with the patient in the upright (or decubitus) and supine positions are the most important aids in the diagnosis of intestinal obstruction. Small intestinal gas and fluid levels in the adult patient invariably indicate mechanical intestinal obstruction (Fig. 21-5). This pattern usually appears within 12 hours of the onset of symptoms. Air and fluid levels throughout both large and small bowel indicate adynamic (paralytic) ileus.

Plain films of the abdomen may also show free air in the peritoneal cavity (from perforation of a hollow viscus), calculi in the biliary or renal areas, fecaliths, tumors, or radiopaque foreign bodies. Barium enemas help to localize the area of colon obstruction. In suspected cases of obstruction, radiologists use oral barium cautiously because of the threat of inspissation of the barium above the obstruction.

Blood studies. Elevations in the hemoglobin and hematocrit commonly indicate dehydration and hemoconcentration. The white blood count is usually elevated, with a shift to the left, especially with strangulation obstruction.

Urinalysis. A high specific gravity and ketonuria indicate a common complication of intestinal obstruction: dehydration and fluid sequestration. Adynamic ileus may be caused by *diabetic acidosis* or *primary renal disease.* Glycosuria or proteinuria (with abnormal cellular elements in the urine) should always indicate the possibility of these diseases.

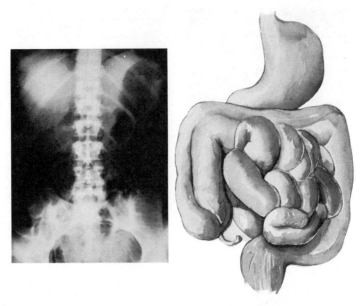

Fig. 21-6. Paralytic ileus. Upright film of abdomen shows dilated small and large intestine. Gas is scattered diffusely throughout intestinal tract. Diagram shows diffuse intestinal dilatation.

Blood chemistry. Amylase may be slightly elevated in intestinal obstruction. Usually, electrolyte determinations guide preoperative fluid replacement. (See Chapter 3.)

PARALYTIC ILEUS (ADYNAMIC ILEUS, NEUROGENIC ILEUS)

In evolutionary terms *paralytic ileus* is a protective mechanism that "splints" the gastrointestinal tract after abdominal injury. It prevents the muscular contractions of the gastrointestinal tract from continuously pouring out noxious bowel contents into the peritoneal cavity after a hollow viscus is perforated, thus allowing the perforation to seal.

Etiology

Four general causative mechanisms for paralytic ileus are as follows:

1. *Direct peritoneal irritation* from any source: acute cholecystitis, pancreatitis, appendicitis, perforation of a hollow viscus, or any abdominal operation (this is the commonest cause)
2. *Extraperitoneal irritation:* pneumonitis, hemorrhage, fractured ribs or spine, trauma to retroperitoneal nerves, renal lesions, etc.
3. *Systemic imbalances:* infections, electrolyte imbalance, shock, myxedema, Addison's disease, uremia, diabetes, or porphyria

4. *Neurogenic disorders:* spinal cord lesions, severe strokes, or central nervous system trauma

Bowel sounds are absent, and gas appears scattered throughout the gastrointestinal tract (Fig. 21-6). Nasogastric suction, correction of the mechanisms causing the paralytic ileus, and parenteral fluid replacement keynote the treatment.

DIFFERENTIAL DIAGNOSIS
Simple versus strangulation obstruction

Since strangulation obstruction requires immediate operative treatment, the physican must constantly look for these five diagnostic points: (1) when intermittent, colicky pain become steady and unrelenting, (2) when abdominal tenderness (and rebound) become evident, (3) when a mass becomes palpable, (4) when the temperature and pulse increase, and (5) when laboratory studies suggest acute inflammation. In brief, the "warm" abdomen changes dramatically to the hot abdomen when strangulation of the bowel occurs. Diagnostic laparotomy is a certain method for determining strangulation obstruction in the difficult diagnostic case.

Mechanical obstruction versus paralytic ileus

In *paralytic ileus* an obvious cause of the ileus is usually evident, such as acute peritonitis from

Table 21-1. Comparison of paralytic ileus and mechanical obstruction

	Paralytic ileus	*Mechanical obstruction*
Cause	Peritoneal irritation Extraperitoneal irritation Neurogenic disorders Metabolic disorders	Hernia Adhesions Tumors Volvulus Intussusception Obturation Inflammation
Site	Entire bowel is dilated	Dilatation proximal to obstruction
Clinical findings	Distension, vomiting, obstipation; silent abdomen; abdomen may or may not be tender	Crampy pain, distension, vomiting, obstipation, hyperactive bowel sounds at first; later bowel may be silent
X-ray findings	Gas throughout (Fig. 21-6)	Gas and fluid proximal to obstruction No gas distal to obstruction (Fig. 21-5)
Treatment	Conservative with treatment of the cause of the ileus	Operative release or bypass of the obstruction
Prognosis	Usually good after correction of cause; strangulation and perforation are *not* a threat	Strangulation or perforation constant threat until obstruction relieved

appendicitis, pancreatitis, cholecystitis, gastroenteritis, abdominal surgery, pneumonitis, or trauma (Figs. 21-5 and 21-6). The abdomen is silent. When the cause of the ileus is not associated with peritonitis, the abdomen is painless and nontender. The roentgenogram of a paralytic ileus shows gas distributed evenly throughout the large and small bowel (Fig. 21-6). Roentgenograms of the abdomen are not infallible, however. Because any condition that causes peritonitis also causes some degree of paralytic ileus, these abdominal disorders mimic strangulation obstruction. The abdominal roentgenograms are usually the only objective method, other than a diagnostic laparotomy, for differentiating paralytic ileus (associated with peritonitis) from strangulation obstruction (Table 21-1).

Small versus large bowel obstruction

Differentiating colon from small bowel obstruction depends on radiographic evidence, either plain abdominal roentgenograms or barium enema demonstration of an obstructing lesion of the colon. Differentiation is important so that the patient (and his family) can be prepared for a colostomy, if it is necessary. Clinical localization, though less accurate, is also possible. Obstruction in an older patient, with no hernia or history of previous abdominal operations, and with distension and no vomiting, usually indicates carcinoma of the large bowel. Sharp frequent abdominal cramps, severe vomiting, and early fluid and electrolyte imbalance are suggestive of small bowel obstruction.

PATHOPHYSIOLOGY

Simple intestinal obstruction causes death, if untreated, because of two factors: (1) *distension* of the bowel proximal to the obstruction and (2) *dehydration*.

Distension

Distension of the proximal bowel constantly threatens ischemia of the involved bowel wall. Violent contractions of the proximal bowel wall attempting to force bowel contents past the obstruction ultimately cause edema of the bowel wall. An edematous bowel wall loses some of its absorptive capacity while secretions (and edema fluid) increase. Anxiety, pain, and nausea cause increased aerophagia (air is mostly nitrogen, which is poorly absorbed). Thus intraluminal pressure (both gas and fluid) builds up to the point where it compresses the small vessels in the bowel wall, and eventually it exceeds the capillary perfusion pressure. Consequent ischemia causes further edema and results in bowel wall necrosis, perforation, and peritonitis. As this final phase approaches, the edematous, stretched, and thinned bowel wall loses its power to contract. The patient no longer complains of cramping pains, and the abdomen is forebodingly silent. Thus every case of "simple" obstruction will ultimately become "self-strangulating" obstruction if proximal bowel distension is not relieved.

Dehydration

Dehydration occurs rapidly because oral intake is impossible and water and electrolytes are lost by (1) vomiting, (2) increased net secretions from the gastrointestinal tract (because the reabsorptive power of the mucosa is impaired), and (3) edema of the bowel wall with transudation into the peritoneal cavity.

As strangulation approaches, bacteria and their toxins escape into the peritoneal cavity, causing edema of the parietal peritoneum, venous thrombosis with more anoxia, and eventually endotoxic shock. When strangulation precipitates the bacterial phase of intestinal obstruction, all the lethal effects of diffuse peritonitis are suddenly superimposed on an already critically ill patient. The mortality is understandably high.

TREATMENT OF MECHANICAL BOWEL OBSTRUCTION

The treatment of bowel obstruction is keyed to the pathophysiological developments, but *in reverse order. Dehydration* and *proximal bowel distension* initiated by the obstruction must be treated first, and the *obstruction* is relieved subsequently.

Dehydration

Severe dehydration poses the serious threat of hypovolemia and shock; this threat is heightened by the vasodilator effect of anesthetics, which causes further decrease in circulating blood volume. Thus replacement of these abnormal fluid losses is a vital first step in the treatment of bowel obstruction. In estimating the amount of replacement fluids, the physician must realize that obstructed patients lose fluids from (1) increased net secretions into the bowel lumen, (2) transudation, (3) edema (bowel wall, mesentery), and (4) vomiting. When signs of shock appear in advanced stages of bowel obstruction in the adult, the patient has lost at least 5 or 6 L. of fluid.

Proximal bowel distension

Intestinal intubation with suction to remove gas and fluid accumulation keynotes the treatment of bowel distension. Surgeons use nasogastric tubes, long intestinal tubes, or tubes inserted directly (at laparotomy) to decompress the distended gastrointestinal tract.

Nasogastric versus long-tube decompression

In proximal small bowel obstruction nasogastric suction is adequate to relieve intestinal distension. In lower obstructions many surgeons cite the advantage of the long intestinal tube in more completely decompressing the dilated loops of bowel, thus decreasing pressure on the stretched and edematous bowel wall. Subsequent operative correction of the obstruction is aided by the flattened, decompressed small bowel. Several long and trying hours may be required to pass a long tube into the lower small bowel; thus other surgeons favor nasogastric intubation with immediate operative decompression and removal of the obstruction.

Intestinal intubation as definitive treatment

In a minority of instances long-tube decompression may relieve intestinal obstructions completely (usually those caused by adhesions). This treatment requires several days of suction and intravenous feedings (and immobility) to be certain that the obstruction is relieved. During this treatment, the threat of recurrent obstruction constantly plagues both surgeon and patient alike. Because of the hardship and uncertainty of this treatment, most surgeons lack enthusiasm for the conservative treatment of mechanical bowel obstruction.

Removal of the obstruction—operative treatment

The final goal in treating mechanical bowel obstruction is removal of the obstruction. Strangulating or potentially strangulating lesions (hernia, volvulus, intussusception in older patients, and complete obstruction because of adhesions or closed-loop obstructions) demand emergent operative treatment. With partial or early obstructions, the surgeon has valuable time for diagnostic studies.

SMALL BOWEL OBSTRUCTIONS

Since most small bowel obstructions are extrinsic, the surgeon can easily lyse adhesions or reduce hernias. If the small bowel is necrotic, he can safely resect it, since the small bowel is relatively sterile. Bypass operations (enteroenterostomies or enterocolostomies) are useful in complicated situations such as multiple dense adhesions in critically ill patients. To prevent recurrent obstructions, some surgeons pass a long tube with an inflatable balloon (Baker tube) into the proximal jejunum and manipulate it to the cecum. It serves as an internal stent to allow adhesion to form without sharp kinking of the small bowel.

LARGE BOWEL OBSTRUCTIONS

The majority of large bowel obstructions (in contrast to those of the small bowel) are caused by intrinsic lesions (cancer or diverticulitis). Most obstructions of the colon occur in the sigmoid area because (1) this is the most common site for both cancers and diverticulitis and (2) the sigmoid lumen is smaller and the feces are more solid than in the more proximal colon.

Closed loop obstructions

Because the ileocecal valve is competent in about 50% to 60% of all people, *closed loop* bowel obstructions occur in a similar percentage of all large bowel obstructions. Roentgenograms of the abdomen show gross dilatation of the colon between the one-way cecal valve and the obstructing lesion. Immediate operative decompression key-notes the treatment. Foolish reliance on long-tube decompression of the small bowel may cause a deadly delay. Mounting gas pressure from putrefaction within the closed loop will eventually burst through the thinned bowel wall (usually the cecum) contaminaing the peritoneal cavity with toxic bowel contents.

Incompetent ileocecal valve obstruction

When the ileocecal valve permits regurgitation, the distal obstruction differs very little clinically from a low small bowel obstruction. Barium study of the distal colon will usually detect the colonic site of obstruction.

Large bowel decompression

Because the large bowel teems with bacteria and the weakened colonic wall holds sutures poorly, primary anastomosis is always hazardous (Chapter 25). (Infection jeopardizes any anastomosis.) Proximal colostomy is a safe and simple procedure, decompressing the bowel and totally bypassing gas and feces through the abdominal wall. Cecostomy differs from colostomy in providing only a vent through the abdominal wall; it does not provide a bypass for *all* the cecal contents.

In certain cases when sufficient mesentery provides adequate mobility, the colon lesions may be *exteriorized* and removed (obstructive resection). The proximal and distal portions of the colon remain above the skin and may be subsequently reunited.

22
Gastrointestinal Hemorrhage

James A. Schulak
Robert J. Corry
Robert T. Soper

Massive hemorrhage from the gastrointestinal tract continues to represent a major diagnostic and therapeutic challenge, enlisting the cooperative efforts of surgeon, endoscopist, and radiologist. Bleeding that is either small in volume or occurs abruptly and then ceases, though not life-threatening in itself, may be the harbinger of more serious gastrointestinal tract disease such as cancer. Although massive bleeding is more common from the upper gastrointestinal tract, its management is sometimes even more challenging when it occurs from a colonic source.

Regardless of the cause, location, or rate of gastrointestinal hemorrhage, the patient must be approached in a logical, stepwise manner, the immediate goal being to stop the bleeding and the ultimate goal to eliminate its cause. For the patient with a massive hemorrhage, the first priority is to prevent exsanguination. Precise diagnosis and definitive management remain important but are less urgent considerations.

Three fundamental evaluations are required for each patient with gastrointestinal hemorrhage: (1) the volume and rate of blood loss, (2) the location and specific lesion producing the bleeding, and (3) the general condition of the patient.

The *volume and rate of blood loss* must be determined with a fair amount of accuracy since therapy will have to be instituted immediately in the patient with massive bleeding. The triad of hematemesis, hematochezia, and hypovolemia indicates massive gastrointestinal bleeding and requires urgent treatment, as discussed later in this chapter. Signs and symptoms of hypovolemia including weakness, pallor, sweating, dizziness, tachycardia, and extreme thirst signify massive bleeding. A nasogastric tube should be passed immediately to evacuate the stomach and measure the rate of blood loss. If the rate of bleeding slows as measured by vital signs, hematocrit determinations, the number and character of stools, and the volume of nasogastric aspirate, a more elaborate diagnostic work-up can be instituted. In patients with slow gastrointestinal bleeding, serial hematocrit determinations are probably the most reliable measurement of the rate of blood loss.

The *location* and the *specific lesion* producing the bleeding should be ascertained as soon as possible in the patient with massive hemorrhage. Most patients with brisk upper gastrointestinal bleeding have hematemesis and thus the differential diagnosis between lower and upper gastrointestinal bleeding is made by history. When hematemesis has not occurred in the presence of massive hematochezia, aspiration of bile from the stomach usually indicates a source of bleeding below the ligament of Treitz. As discussed in detail later, endoscopy or angiography is usually necessary to determine the precise source of hemorrhage preoperatively.

The *general condition of the patient* should be assessed as quickly as possible because the so-called poor-risk patient will require a more precise diagnostic and therapeutic approach than the good-risk patient without cardiovascular disease or diseases of other systems.

For the purpose of clarity this chapter will deal first with upper gastrointestinal bleeding and second with lower gastrointestinal bleeding and will emphasize general principles, rather than being an attempt to either deal thoroughly with the basic disease processes or outline a complex formula to manage gastrointestinal hemorrhage.

UPPER GASTROINTESTINAL HEMORRHAGE

Massive upper gastrointestinal hemorrhage produces signs of acute hypovolemia following closely on the heels of both hematemesis and hematochezia. For all practical purposes, this type of bleeding is equally distributed among peptic ulceration, gastritis, and ruptured esophageal varices, with the bleeding ulcer being slightly more common than the other two.

Unusual causes of massive upper gastrointestinal hemorrhage are worthy of brief mention so that they will not be forgotten in the haste of the moment. *Oronasopharyngeal bleeding* may be suspected if the patient appears to be swallowing blood; bleeding can be quite massive but usually stops with direct tamponade. *Hematobilia* can be diagnosed only by angiography or choledochotomy but should be suspected when there are symptoms and signs of hepatobiliary disease or history of previous blunt hepatic trauma. Bleeding as a complication of a *cholecystoduodenal fistula* is an uncommon entity usually diagnosed at laparotomy. Likewise, the possiblity of an aortoduodenal fistula should be considered in any patient with an aortic prosthesis. The *Mallory-Weiss syndrome* is most commonly diagnosed at gastroesophagoscopy. *Bleeding disorders* should be considered in all cases and an accurate history, inspection for cutaneous bleeding, and laboratory bleeding studies should be carried out. (See Chapter 4.)

General considerations of diagnosis and management

Massive blood loss from peptic ulcer eroding into the left gastric or gastroduodenal artery, hemorrhage from gastritis, or a ruptured esophageal varix can all result in hypovolemic shock. Usually a history of ulcer pain or previous bleeding from an ulcer can be elicited from the patient or his family, which enables the physician to place high priority on peptic ulcer as a source of hemorrhage. However, a patient may bleed from an acute duodenal ulcer without a previous history.

Similarly, a history of cirrhosis, chronic alcoholism, or remote hepatitis alerts the physician to consider bleeding esophageal varices, particularly if physical signs point to evidence of hepatic dysfunction such as caput medusae, jaundice, spider angiomas or ascites. It must be emphasized, however, that the patient with the liver disease is also prone to develop gastritis.

The patient who has been generally well but who has had a recent history of ingesting alcohol, aspirin, or indomethacin may have hemorrhagic gastritis. Physical examination usually does not help differentiate duodenal ulcer from gastritis.

The first priority in the patient with massive upper gastrointestinal hemorrhage is intravenous insertion of two 15-gauge needles or plastic cannulas for rapid transfusion of volume expanders followed by blood. A No. 36F Ewald tube is then passed into the stomach for gastric lavage with iced saline. Occasionally, the bleeding will stop with vigorous lavage and evacuation of stomach blood clots.

The most important diagnostic maneuver in the patient with massive upper gastrointestinal bleeding is endoscopy, preferably with a flexible fiberoptic esophagogastroscope. If bleeding is present during the examination, its source and magnitude can be determined simultaneously, and in some cases control can also be attempted. For example, if bleeding esophageal varices are encountered, not only is the diagnosis made with certainty but also definitive therapy can be administered by injection of sclerosing agents. In the presence of somewhat localized gastritis or bleeding peptic ulcer, the endoscopist can attempt control of hemorrhage by applying electrocautery through the endoscope. It should be emphasized, however, that this procedure has the potential hazard of perforation if applied inappropriately.

Once diagnosis is established, subsequent management is instituted, as shown schematically in Fig. 22-1. It is unusual for pulsatile hemorrhage from the gastroduodenal or left gastric artery to stop with iced lavage; in that situation the patient will require urgent surgical intervention. On the contrary, bleeding from minor or small vessels often justifies a period of further medical management. Initially iced saline lavage is continued, but intensive antacid therapy may be more important. Gastric pH should be measured hourly by aspiration through a No. 18 sump nasogastric tube. The antacid regimen is adjusted to achieve a neutral pH. Systemic administration of histamine receptor–blocking agents such as cimetidine may be helpful to achieve this goal.

Angiography

Although the flexible fiberoptic esophagogastroscope has substantially increased the diagnostic accuracy of bleeding lesions of the esophagus, stomach, and duodenum, angiography provides added dimensions to both diagnosis and therapy. Therefore, if bleeding persists and the definitive diagnosis is not made endoscopically, or if the diagnosis is made and the patient is a poor opera-

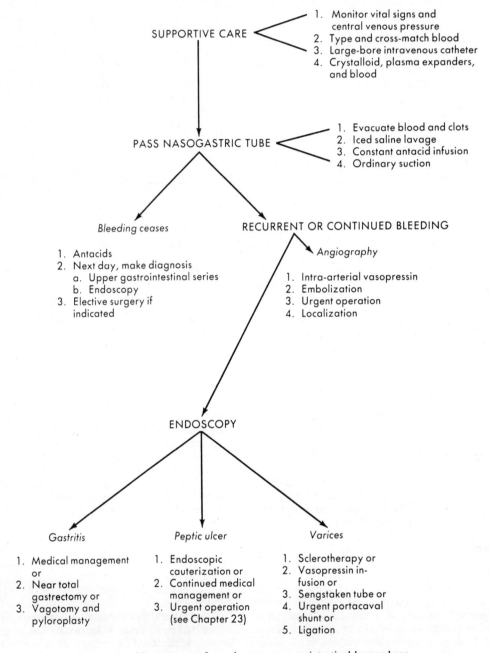

Fig. 22-1. Management of massive upper gastrointestinal hemorrhage.

tive risk, emergency angiography should be carried out. The skilled angiographer can selectively cannulate the left gastric artery, infuse vasopressin (Pitressin), and frequently stop the bleeding of hemorrhagic gastritis; he can cannulate the gastroduodenal artery and infuse either preformed blood clot or vasopressin to stop duodenal ulcer bleeding; and he can cannulate the superior mesenteric artery and infuse vasopressin to lower portal pressure and stop variceal bleeding. When the bleeding is at a rate of 30 ml./hr., angiography will frequently show bleeding from shallow lesions not easily seen endoscopically.

Peptic ulceration

When hemorrhage occurs from a peptic ulcer, whether the source is in the stomach or the duodenum, the immediate aim is to control the bleeding. The diagnosis can usually be made by history unless bleeding is occurring for the first time as the symptom of an acute stress ulcer. Physical examination and laboratory studies are usually of little help.

If the bleeding stops as a result of gastric lavage or if bleeding has stopped before admission to the hospital such that a nasogastric tube aspirate yields only old or changed blood, gastroscopy may be deferred and angiography will not be helpful. The patient should be managed with gastric suction to decompress the stomach, and gastric pH neutralization as outlined previously. An upper gastrointestinal contrast radiographic study may be safely performed if bleeding has not recurred for 12 hours. If bleeding recurs, endoscopy or angiography should be carried out to identify the precise source of bleeding.

Once the diagnosis of peptic ulcer is made by any of these measures, it is treated either medically or operatively depending on the previous history of bleeding, pain, and chronicity. A second episode of bleeding while the patient is hospitalized on intensive medical therapy usually justifies an operation. The choice of operation, discussed in Chapter 23, is designed to reduce gastric acidity and prevent recurrence of peptic ulcer disease.

Esophageal varices

The diagnosis of bleeding from a ruptured varix is suggested in the patient with upper gastrointestinal hemorrhage who has a history of chronic alcoholism or chronic liver disease. Frequently the patient is in a precomatose state and physical examination reveals mild jaundice, ascites, and muscle wasting. Definitive diagnosis of variceal hemorrhage is made by esophagoscopy. A barium swallow that will outline the extent of the varices is more useful when the patient is not bleeding (Fig.

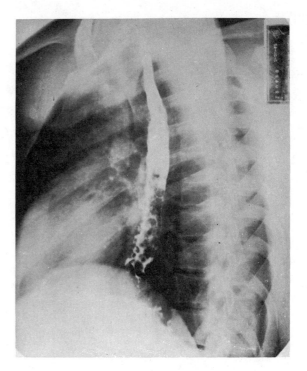

Fig. 22-2. Barium in esophagus outlining large esophageal varices.

22-2). Occasionally patients with portal hypertension bleed from hemorrhagic gastritis rather than from varices, though its frequency is probably exaggerated; endoscopy and angiography may help make this decision.

Emergency management of the patient with bleeding varices is directed toward stopping the hemorrhage as soon as possible. In addition to the deleterious effects of blood loss and shock common to all patients with upper gastrointestinal bleeding, hepatic encephalopathy may also ensue because of the large amount of ammonia released by the bacterial action on intraluminal blood. Therefore, coincident with attempts to control the hemorrhage, efforts should be made not only to rid the gastrointestinal tract of blood by vigorous catharsis but also to impede its breakdown. This latter goal can be achieved by administration of either poorly absorbed antibiotics, such as neomycin, that reduce the bacterial flora of the colon, or unabsorbed sugar, such as lactulose, that decrease ammonia production by interfering with bacterial metabolism.

Massive variceal bleeding usually will not stop with gastric lavage alone necessitating additional

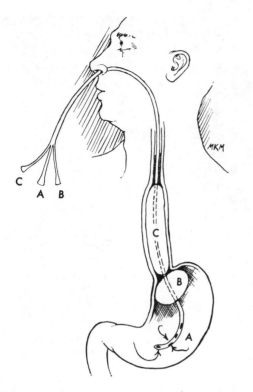

Fig. 22-3. Sengstaken-Blakemore tube. Triple-lumen tube: *A*, gastric suction; *B*, balloon in gastric fundus; *C*, balloon in lower esophagus. Tube is passed into stomach, inflated gastric balloon is snugged up to esophageal junction, and esophageal balloon is then inflated to compress varices.

nonoperative measures. Triple-lumen tubes (Fig. 22-3) can be used to effectively tamponade the bleeding site by inflating either or both the gastric and esophageal balloons. The potential for significant complications such as ischemia of the gastroesophageal junction or perforation of the esophagus has led to replacement of this technique with either pharmacological intervention or endoscopic sclerotherapy. Nevertheless, balloon tamponade may be a lifesaving maneuver in some cases, especially in the face of failure of these latter modalities.

Pharmacological control of bleeding varices has been widely reported using infusion of vasopressin (pitressin), which lowers portal pressure by reducing splanchnic blood flow. Although early experience dictated intra-arterial infusion through the superior mesenteric artery, it has been clearly demonstrated that simple intravenous administration is as effective and eliminates the need for a skilled angiographer. Pitressin is administered as a 20-unit bolus followed by hourly infusion of 0.2 to 0.4 units/ml/hr. This approach has been successful in at least temporarily halting variceal hemorrhage in approximately 70% of patients.

Endoscopic sclerosis of bleeding varices is an alternative method of managing the acute bleeder. Although sclerotherapy is easier to accomplish in nonbleeding patients, with practice it can be performed in the active bleeder by most endoscopists with a success rate of approximately 75%. Several courses of therapy may be needed to obliterate the entire variceal network, during which time rebleeding can occur. Nevertheless, repeat procedures are usually well tolerated by the patient, and so this form of therapy is made the procedure of choice in many medical centers.

Surgical approaches to acute variceal hemorrhage include portasystemic shunting, esophagogastric devascularization procedures as described by Sugiura in Japan, simple esophageal transection with the EEA stapler and transesophageal variceal ligation. Both emergency portacaval shunting and variceal ligation have high mortality, approaching 50% in patients with poor liver function, thus reducing their usefulness. Because only limited experience has been reported for use of the various devascularization procedures in the typical poor-risk cirrhotic patient, these techniques cannot yet be recommended as procedures of choice.

Long-term management of patients with bleeding varices after control has been achieved through nonoperative measures remains controversial. Elective portasystemic shunts in good-risk patients carry a low mortality, have a negligible rebleeding rate, but are complicated in many by the late development of encephalopathy. Distal splenorenal shunts somewhat obviate this problem but may have a higher recurrence of bleeding because of their somewhat poorer decompression of the splanchnic venous system. Esophagogastric devascularization is a difficult and potentially dangerous operation that should only be attempted by those with experience. On the other hand, sclerotherapy may be repeated as needed, does not further compromise function of the diseased liver, and is safe, making it a highly attractive alternative to the various surgical alternatives.

Gastritis

Massive hemorrhage from erosive gastritis is a common cause of upper gastrointestinal bleeding that is frequently encountered in patients experiencing stress as with extensive burns, sepsis, trauma, and previous major operations. In others, the history will often reveal recent or chronic ingestion of substances that are toxic to gastric mucosa such as aspirin, indomethacin, steroids, or alcohol. Diagnosis is made exclusively with gastroscopy and more often than not reveals diffuse disease, precluding both endoscopic coagulation and limited resection.

Management of hemorrhagic gastritis should be nonoperative because the majority of cases will stop bleeding spontaneously. Medical management is similar to that for peptic ulceration and includes evacuation of gastric blood clots, iced saline lavage, sedation, and blood replacement. Early neutralization of gastric acidity with intensive antacid therapy adjusted according to hourly gastric pH values is of utmost importance. The histamine-receptor antagonists cimetidine and ranitidine have been helpful in this respect, though their use alone may not be adequate in the face of severe bleeding and therefore should be used in concert with topical antacids. As with variceal hemorrhage, administration of vasopressin may also be helpful in controlling difficult cases. This drug may be administered intravenously or through selective cannulation of the left gastric artery at the time of angiography.

Fortunately, surgical intervention is not often necessary because the appropriate operation for hemorrhagic gastritis is controversial. Near total gastrectomy enjoys the lowest rebleeding rate but is a major undertaking that is not without complication. Vagotomy and pyloroplasty with oversewing of individual bleeding points through a large gastrotomy is better tolerated by the extremely sick patient but is accompanied by a greater probability of recurrent hemorrhage. Thus individualization is the best policy. For example, one might select the latter procedure for patients who can best tolerate a rebleed should it occur and paradoxically reserve gastric resection for those least likely to endure a second operation.

Other causes of upper gastrointestinal hemorrhage

Aberrant blood vessels, tumors undergoing necrosis, aorticoduodenal fistulas, and lesions of the small intestine including vascular malformations and Meckel's diverticulum are managed with ad hoc operations applicable to the particular lesion. Recurrent slow bleeding from chronic peptic ulcer disease is usually diagnosed by contrast studies of the upper gastrointestinal tract and is managed by the operation appropriate to the disease entity.

LOWER GASTROINTESTINAL BLEEDING

Rarely is colonic bleeding massive and life threatening; more commonly it is slow and intermixed with stool. Persistence of chronic rectal bleeding warrants an immediate and thorough investigative work-up to establish its cause. In this situation the bleeding is not the problem, but its cause can be serious and life threatening.

Massive colonic bleeding

It must be emphasized at the outset that an upper gastrointestinal source of bleeding should be eliminated as a possibility in the patient with massive rectal bleeding. Aspiration of clear bile from the stomach for all practical purposes establishes the source of bleeding as being located at least below the ligament of Treitz.

History is not usually as helpful as it is in upper gastrointestinal bleeding, and the physical examination may be equally unrevealing. The most common causes of massive lower gastrointestinal bleeding are angiodysplasia of the right side of the colon and diverticula, and these should be highly suspect, especially in the elder patient. Numerous other conditions, however, can often produce brisk rectal bleeding such as *internal hemorrhoids,* an ulcerating *colonic neoplasm, colonic ischemia, ulcerative colitis,* and in rare instances *superficial erosions* of the colon, or *Crohn's colitis.* Although it is said that diverticulitis does not bleed, we have observed several patients with massive hemorrhage coincident with acute diverticulitis.

As with upper gastrointestinal bleeding, plasma expanders followed by blood transfusions should be instituted immediately while diagnostic measures are undertaken. Anoscopy and sigmoidoscopy with adequate facilities to aspirate blood should be undertaken as soon as possible. If the bleeding arises above the end of the sigmoidoscope and is persistent and massive, selective arteriography should be immediately carried out. Inferior mesenteric artery followed by superior mesenteric artery injection of contrast material frequently identifies the source of bleeding. When the bleeding point is identified and is localized to either the left or the right colon, continuous intra-arterial infusion of vasopressin is begun. Success with this technique has eliminated the need for urgent laparotomy and colon resection in many patients. If bleeding is not controlled or if it recurs, limited resection of the appropriate segment of bowel can be carried out.

In the event that angiography is not available or has been unsuccessful in either localizing the bleeding site or controlling the hemorrhage with vasopressin infusion, surgical management is necessary. Before operation, however, an attempt to localize the bleeding site with radionuclide scintigraphy may be useful. Both technetium 99m–labeled sulfur colloid and technetium 99m–labeled red blood cells have been demonstrated to detect and localize acute lower gastrointestinal bleeding. Alternatively, some have advocated the use of emergency barium enema because this may not only reveal an obvious lesion thus allowing for a more limited resection, but also may actually effect control by tamponading the bleeding site.

Laparotomy attempts to localize the hemorrhage by segmental clamping of the colon are theoretically attractive but have generally been disappointing. Similarly, endoscopic examination of the colon at operation through a colotomy is also frequently unsuccessful and has the disadvantage of spilling feculent material into the peritoneal cavity. Usually therefore it is necessary to carry out a total abdominal colectomy with either ileorectal anastomosis or end ileostomy in order to ensure resection of the offending segment of colon. More limited resection may be indicated if angiodysplasia is suspected because this entity occurs most commonly in the right side of the colon and certainly if preoperative attempts at localization were successful.

Chronic lower gastrointestinal bleeding

Slow and recurrent or persistent colonic bleeding is suggested by history of blood passed rectally in a patient with chronic anemia. Bright red rectal blood indicates a point of origin within the anus or rectum, especially when it coats the outside of stool. Anal fissures, hemorrhoids, and low-lying carcinomas are the most likely sources of this type of slow rectal bleeding. Tarry-appearing material or dark blood intermixed with stool suggests a right colonic or small bowel origin. Bloody diarrhea mixed with mucus suggests *ulcerative colitis, granulomatous enterocolitis,* or *amebic colitis.* The diagnostic work-up is performed with dispatch but not as an emergency. Careful rectal examination, anoscopy, and sigmoidoscopy should be carried out when the patient is first seen. These procedures will confirm the diagnosis of numerous conditions including hemorrhoids, fissures, ulcerative colitis, and about three fifths of the colonic neoplasms. The next diagnostic maneuver should be a barium enema, usually with air contrast. This procedure will confirm the diagnosis of colonic diverticulosis, neoplasms above the reach of the sigmoidoscope, chronic ulcerative colitis, and colonic polyps.

If these procedures fail to reveal the diagnosis of the bleeding, colonoscopy should be carried out. When performed by an experienced operator, diagnostic colonoscopy carries little morbidity. Furthermore, transcolonoscopic removal of polyps may make obsolete the endless debate about the neoplastic state of polyps.

23
Stomach and Duodenum

Israel Penn

Three disorders of the stomach and duodenum—peptic ulcer, gastric cancer, and hypertrophic pyloric stenosis—completely overshadow all other diseases that involve these important digestive organs. The main concerns of this chapter are peptic ulcer and gastric cancer. Hypertrophic pyloric stenosis is discussed in Chapter 28. The less common diseases of the stomach and duodenum are mentioned at the end of this chapter, as also is gastric surgery for the treatment of morbid obesity.

PEPTIC ULCER

A peptic ulcer is any gastrointestinal ulcer caused by contact with acid-pepsin secretions. Patients with pernicious anemia (total anacidity) very rarely get peptic ulcers. Although acid-pepsin secretions link the three main types of peptic ulcers, important differences separate them. The student should envision these three main classifications as follows:

1. Duodenal ulcer diathesis (duodenal, pyloric channel, and synchronous gastric and duodenal ulcers)
2. Chronic gastric ulcer
3. Acute gastric mucosal ulcerations

Peptic ulceration may also occur in the lower esophagus in patients with reflux esophagitis; in the jejunum in severe cases of the Zollinger-Ellison syndrome (see below) or after anastomosis of the stomach to the jejunum; or in the ileum in patients who have a Meckel's diverticulum containing ectopic gastric mucosa.

Gastric physiology
Stimulation of gastric secretion

A combined vagal-antral phase increases gastric secretion as follows. Stimuli from the brain (hunger—thought, sight, smell, and taste of food) travel along the vagus nerves to (1) incite the gastric parietal and chief cells to secrete acid and pepsin, and (2) stimulate the antral G-cells to release gastrin, a secretory hormone that also stimulates the parietal and chief cells. Thus nervous stimuli trigger a dual mechanism that heightens gastric secretion. Distension of the antrum by food also stimulates gastrin release, as do various secretagogues (peptones and amino acids from food). These overlapping mechanisms of gastric secretion potentiate one another.

Inhibition of gastric secretion

As digestion in the stomach ceases, several factors inhibit gastric secretion. Vagal activity decreases, and as the stomach empties, antral distension, an important stimulus to gastrin release, subsides. The low pH reached in the antrum also inhibits gastrin release. The acid contents of the stomach, as they flow into the duodenum, trigger release of a hormone (secretin) that inhibits both gastric secretion and motility. Acid, fat, and hypertonic solutions, as they enter the duodenum, all suppress gastric secretion (possibly by release of enterogastrone or gastric inhibitory peptide). Thus in normal people a remarkable mechanism stimulates gastric secretion during hunger and food intake and shuts it off as the food leaves the stomach.

The mucosal barrier

The answer to the question, Why doesn't the corrosive gastric content digest the stomach wall? rests on the concept of a gastric mucosal barrier, a secreting, dynamic "containing wall" capable of maintaining an H^+ hydrogen-ion gradient (stomach to blood) of about 2,000,000:1.

This wall features a layer of mucus acting chiefly as a lubricant and weak buffer and, most important, a layer of highly specialized, tightly joined, columnar cells that prevent back-diffusion of acid. A rich blood supply supports both of these layers and allows the mucosal cells to replace themselves within 48 hours, if injured. Much current research has centered on this mucosal layer and its blood supply. From these studies new theories have emerged to explain how gastric ulcers arise in tandem with low gastric acidity and why acute gastric mucosal ulcers accompany shock and stress.

Duodenal ulcer

Incidence. The incidence in different parts of the world varies from 1% to 20% of the population. Duodenal ulcers occur in all age groups. Men are more frequently affected than women, especially in the younger age groups (Fig. 23-1).

Cause. Excess secretion of acid and pepsin keynotes the pathogenesis of duodenal ulcer. This is attributable in part to an increased number of functioning parietal cells, which may be hereditary, or to hyperplasia as a result of chronic stimulation. Hypersecretion may also result from a high secretory drive or from an increased sensitivity of the parietal cells to a normal drive. Reduction of duodenal buffers may contribute to ulceration.

Most experienced clinicians accept psychological factors as the most common link in the genesis of duodenal ulcers. Chronic psychic stress (e.g., the hard-driving, ambitious person) undoubtedly augments gastric secretion through brain centers and the vagus nerves. Duodenal ulcer traits run through families, especially those members sharing blood group O. The role of diet (e.g., coffee drinking) remains debatable. Excess alcohol intake may increase gastric secretion and the incidence of duodenal ulcer. For unknown reasons patients with pulmonary emphysema suffer a three fold increase in duodenal ulcers.

Clinical features. The classical symptom is a gnawing pain in the upper abdomen an hour or two after meals, sometimes radiating to the back and relieved by food. Some patients complain only of vague discomfort—a feeling of hunger or cramps. The pain frequently awakens patients from sleep and is relieved by milk or antacids. An important feature is periodicity of the pain. Attacks lasting for several weeks are interspersed with months of complete freedom from symptoms. An occasional patient will bleed severely yet deny any prior pain. The only common physical finding is mild tenderness in the right upper abdomen.

Laboratory examination. Overnight collections of gastric secretions show a two- to fivefold increase in volume and concentration of acids (Table 23-1). Barium x-ray studies of the stomach and

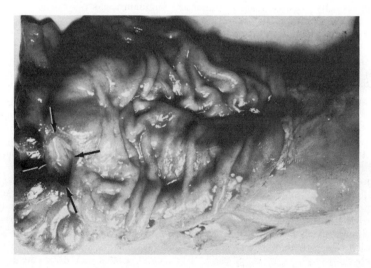

Fig. 23-1. Duodenal ulcer. Opened stomach on right; duodenal ulcer with sharply demarcated edges on left.

duodenum will usually show an ulcer crater or scarring in the proximal portion of the duodenum (duodenal bulb). Endoscopic examination of the duodenum will confirm the diagnosis in problem cases.

Treatment. Effective medical treatment involves drastic reduction of acid secretion by the use of intensive antacid therapy (as frequently as every hour) or the use of histamine (H_2) receptor blockers, such as cimetidine or ranitidine, given for a period of 6 to 8 weeks. The majority of duodenal ulcers heal with these measures. It is debatable whether reduction of smoking and ingestion of alcohol, coffee, and tea play a significant role in the reduction of acid secretion.

An alternative therapy to acid reduction is sucralfate (a complex of sulfated sucrose and aluminum hydroxide). This adheres to proteinaceous exudate at the ulcer site and forms a protective coating that shields the ulcer from acid, pepsin, and bile salts. High healing rates have been obtained in controlled trials.

Surgical therapy is indicated for the small percentage of patients who develop complications, listed in order of frequency:

1. *Bleeding*. Surgical treatment is indicated for severe, persistent, or recurrent bleeding. The decision for surgical therapy depends on such factors as the patient's age, general health, length of ulcer symptoms, and presence or history of other ulcer complications (see Chapter 22).
2. *Perforation*. An ulcer may perforate the duodenal wall, releasing caustic duodenal contents into the peritoneal cavity. Severe peritonitis with a boardlike abdomen and shock results, requiring emergency closure of the perforation or a definitive ulcer operation in selected patients who are in good condition and have slight peritoneal contamination.
3. *Obstruction*. Chronic duodenal ulcers may cause gastric outlet obstruction from edema and severe scarring, with symptoms of nausea, vomiting, weight loss, and metabolic alkalosis. Obstruction causes stasis and excites the antral phase to increase gastric secretion. A vicious cycle results, which often must be interrupted by surgical correction.
4. *Intractability*. Intractability used to be the major indication for surgery. Currently with effective medical therapy few patients need surgery for this indication. Operation is reserved for those who cannot comply with the medical regimen or have severe side effects from the medications.

In general, duodenal ulcers need not be removed. If the conditions causing duodenal ulcers are corrected by the surgical procedure, the ulcers will heal.

Theoretically the ideal surgical treatment for duodenal ulcer is (1) division of the vagus nerves (vagotomy) to control the vagal-antral phase and (2) antrectomy (distal gastric resection) to control the antral phase. Since vagotomy along interferes with gastric emptying and leads to stasis, with nausea, vomiting, weight loss, and recurrent ulceration, antrectomy or some drainage procedure must complement it.

Three operations will improve gastric emptying:

1. Pyloroplasty (longitudinal division of the pyloric muscle with transverse closure) widens the gastroduodenal junction (Fig. 23-2, *A*).
2. Gastrojejunostomy (anastomosis of the stomach to the jejunum) provides an alternative opening from stomach into small bowel (Fig. 23-2, *B*).
3. Gastroduodenostomy (anastomosis of stomach to duodenum, the Jaboulay procedure) bypasses the pylorus.

None of these emptying procedures sacrifices any of the stomach; its reservoir capacity remains unaltered.

Vagotomy plus antrectomy, or one of the emptying procedures, has largely replaced the older surgical operations for duodenal ulcers, which involved removal of large portions (up to 80%) of the stomach (Fig. 23-2, *C* and *D*). The newer procedures are as effective as yet safer and technically easier to perform than extensive gastric removal. Extensive gastric resections may produce undersirable side effects in 25% of patients (dumping syndrome, chronic weight loss, diarrhea, malabsorption, anemia, metabolic bone disease, bilious vomiting, alkaline reflux gastritis, and an increased incidence of gastric cancer). These complications are less frequent after vagotomy with antrectomy or drainage.

Table 23-1. Approximate average values of volume and acidity in 12-hour collection of gastric juice for conditions listed

	12-hour nocturnal aspiration of stomach	
	mEq. of HCl	*Volume of secretion (ml.)*
Normal	20	200
Duodenal ulcer	60	500
Gastric ulcer	12	150
Zollinger-Ellison syndrome	100 or more	1,000 or more
Gastric cancer	8	100

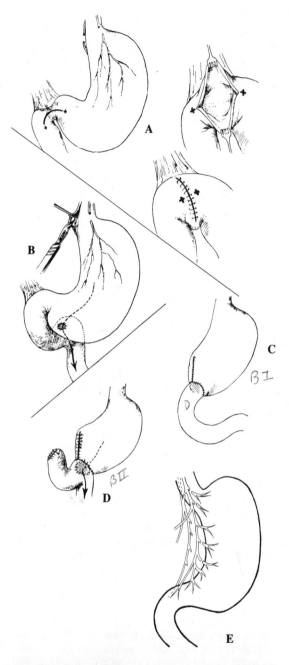

Fig. 23-2. Surgical treatment of peptic ulcer. **A,** Vagal nerve division and pyloroplasty. **B,** Vagal nerve division and gastrojejunostomy—arrow shows new exit for gastric contents. **C,** Billroth I partial gastric resection—stomach is anastomosed to duodenum. **D,** Billroth II partial gastric resection—duodenal stump is closed and stomach is anastomosed to jejunum. **E,** Highly selective vagotomy. Notice preservation of fibers supplying antrum and pylorus.

In the standard type of vagotomy or truncal vagotomy (Fig. 23-2, *A* and *B*) the nerve trunks are divided as they lie on the lower esophagus. Not only is the acid-secreting area denervated, but also the antrum, pylorus, liver, gallbladder, pancreas, and other organs. Side effects of the vagotomy (diarrhea, increased incidence of gallstones) and of antrectomy or drainage (mostly dumping and alkaline reflux gastritis) have led to the introduction of highly selective vagotomy (HSV) or parietal cell vagotomy (Fig. 23-2, *E*) in which branches to the lower esophagus and upper stomach are divided, denervating the parietal cells only. Because the antrum and pylorus remain innervated, the stomach empties normally and drainage is unnecessary. Although HSV reduces the usual side effects of vagotomy, it is complicated by a higher incidence of recurrent ulcers than that seen with the other types of vagotomy.

Recurrence. Depending on the type of operation, recurrent or stomal ulcerations may occur in 1% to 15% of patients. Recurrences usually indicate incomplete vagotomy or inadequate drainage. Other causes include insufficient resection of the acid-bearing portion of the stomach, retention of antral mucosa, hyperparathyroidism, or the Zollinger-Ellison syndrome. Diagnosis of stomal ulceration is based on the history, barium studies, and endoscopy. Complications of stomal ulcers include obstruction, hemorrhage, perforation, and gastrojejunocolic fistula. Some recurrent ulcers will heal after treatment with cimetidine or ranitidine. Those occurring after incomplete vagotomy respond well to transthoracic vagotomy. Sluggish gastric drainage, detected by barium studies, often necessitates refashioning of the gastric outlet.

Chronic gastric ulcer

Incidence. Clinically, gastric ulcer is three to four times less common than duodenal ulcer. It occurs more frequently in the middle aged and elderly and about equally in men and women.

Cause. About 80% of gastric ulcers appear in stomachs that secrete normal or decreased acid. Evidence points to a defective mucosal barrier and back-diffusion of acid (from stomach lumen into the mucosa) as the immediate cause. A defective pyloric sphincter allows bile to reflux into the stomach and disrupt the vital mucosal barrier; the resulting chronic gastritis precedes most gastric ulcers.

The other 20% of gastric ulcers usually occur just inside the pylorus or are associated with duodenal ulcers near the pylorus, causing pylorospasm or obstruction. These ulcers, arising in a hyperacidic environment, belong in the duodenal ulcer group.

Table 23-2. Comparison of duodenal and gastric ulcers

	Duodenal ulcer	*Gastric ulcer*
Cause	Increased acid secretion, increased gastrin, defect in acid disposal	Abnormal pyloric sphincter–bile reflux gastritis, increased back diffusion of hydrogen ion
Location	Duodenum	Stomach
Age	Younger (30 to 50 years)	Somewhat older
Sex	Male:female, 7:1	Male:female, 1:1
Incidence	1% to 20%	1% to 5%
Symptoms	Much the same	
Malignancy	Rare	5%
Free HCl (12-hr. night secretion)	60 mEq. (average)	12 mEq. (average)
Medical treatment	Excellent (successful in over 90%)	Poor (successful in 50%)
Surgical treatment	Vagotomy and antrectomy or emptying procedure, parietal cell vagotomy	Removal of the ulcer with limited partial gastrectomy

Several drugs may disrupt the mucosal cell barrier or the protective mucus. Aspirin, phenylbutazone, indomethacin, reserpine, and steroids are the chief offenders, in addition to the antiarthritic drugs ibuprofen, tolmetin, and naproxen.

Clinical features. The clinical picture of gastric ulcer simulates that of duodenal ulcer. Gastric ulcers tend to occur in patients who are older and of lower social status than those with duodenal ulcers. The pain localizes more often to the left upper quadrant and sometimes is provoked by food or hot or cold liquids. Gastric ulcers are more worrisome than duodenal ulcers because about 5% of gastric ulcers are malignant; duodenal ulcers are virtually never malignant (Table 23-2).

Laboratory examination. Overnight collections of gastric secretions show a decrease in both volume and concentration of acid in gastric ulcer as compared to duodenal ulcer (Table 23-1). Barium x-ray studies often show an ulcer crater in the stomach (Figs. 23-3 and 23-4). Gastroscopy with multiple biopsies or gastric washings with careful cytological studies help to exclude cancer.

Treatment. The same conservative treatment is tried for gastric ulcer as for duodenal ulcer. During the period of therapy, aspirin and other barrier-breaking drugs must be stopped. Because gastric ulcers may be malignant, the physician must recommend operation if the ulcer fails to heal after 6 weeks of treatment. About 50% of benign gastric ulcers fail to respond satisfactorily to medical treatment and must ultimately be treated surgically. Indications for surgery are failure to heal, suspicion of malignancy, recurrence, persistent bleeding, perforation, and obstruction. This last complication rarely occurs except with pyloric channel ulcers.

Removal of the distal half of the stomach gives excellent results for gastric ulcer. (The antrum is of course removed in this procedure.) A Billroth I reconstruction is preferred, since it reduces the risk of bile gastritis, iron deficiency, and afferent loop syndrome. The recurrence rate is negligible.

In patients with pyloric channel ulcers or combined gastric and duodenal ulcers surgical treatment is the same as for duodenal ulcers.

Acute gastric mucosal ulcers (AGM ulcers or stress ulcers)

Cause. AGM ulcers arise in critically ill patients after varied insults including shock, burns, sepsis, operations, and drugs. *Ischemia* and a *damaged mucosal barrier* are the common denominators underlying these superficial erosions. Almost all patients in severe shock will show AGM ulcers. Ischemia disrupts the vital mucosal barrier; ileus, with reflux of bile, adds to the mucosal damage. Gastric acid diffuses through the impaired mucosa, and ulcers–often multiple–result.

Clinical features. Upper gastrointestinal bleeding that develops in a critically ill patient with no prior history of peptic ulceration should indicate AGM ulcerations. Because of clots within the stomach and the superficial nature of AGM erosions, diagnostic barium studies often fail to detect them. Gastroscopy and celiac arteriography help to localize the bleeding site or sites.

Treatment. Prevention is probably the most important measure. The physician should anticipate these ulcers in any critically ill patient. Continuous nasogastric suction with instillation of antacids helps in neutralizing gastric acidity. Cimetidine is a useful adjunct because it reduces the need to give large amounts of antacids, which can cause undesirable side effects. However, cimetidine alone does not give adequate protection. Concurrent

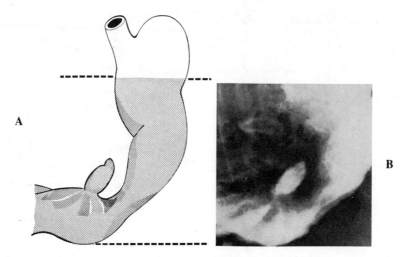

Fig. 23-3. Benign gastric ulcer. **A,** Diagram of x-ray findings. **B,** Upper G.I. series showing gastric folds radiating away from ulcer and sharp margins that are not elevated.

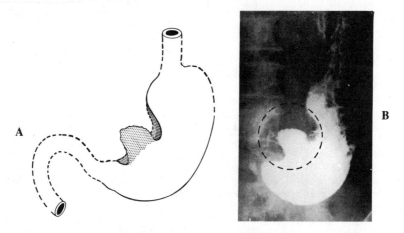

Fig. 23-4. Malignant gastric ulcer. **A,** Diagram of x-ray findings. **B,** Upper G.I. series showing no radiating folds and heaped-up ulcer margins.

treatment of shock, sepsis, etc. will relieve gastric ischemia.

If a patient presents with bleeding AGM ulcers, treatment consists of blood volume replacement, gastric lavage, and neutralization of gastric acid. If hemorrhage persists or recurs, bleeding points may be controlled by transendoscopic laser photocoagulation using the neodymium-YAG laser. Alternatively, arteriography may be used to localize the bleeding site, and in suitable cases, selective infusion of Pitressin into the left gastric artery may induce spasm and thrombosis of the bleeding vessel. The associated decrease in mucosal perfusion

does not cause further ulceration if the gastric contents are kept alkalinized during this treatment. If these conservative means fail, most surgeons rely on vagotomy with gastric resection and pyloroplasty (and oversewing the bleeding sites) to stop the bleeding. Severe hemorrhage sometimes demands total or near-total gastrectomy.

Peptic ulcers from other causes
Zollinger-Ellison syndrome

A rare syndrome of recurrent, severe ulcer disease, the Zollinger-Ellison syndrome emphasizes the importance of gastrin in gastric secretion;

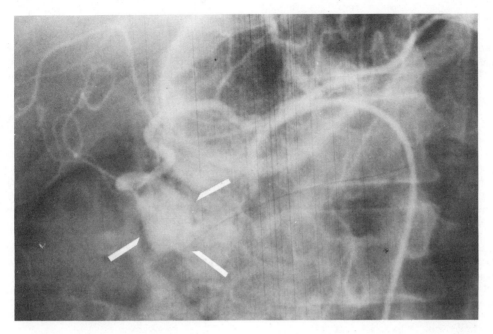

Fig. 23-5. Angiogram demonstrating 2.5 cm. solitary tumor in head of pancreas. Fasting serum gastrin was 4,300 pg./ml.

it explains the frustrating phenomenon of recurrent ulceration in some patients who have had adequate previous treatment.

The cause is a gastrin-secreting nonbeta islet cell tumor of the pancreas (Fig. 23-5). Gastric secretion is enormous (the 12-hr. volume is over 1,000 ml., and free HCl is over 100 mEq.). Serum gastrin levels in these patients average over 600 pg./ml. (normal: 200 pg./ml.). Also the basal acid secretion is high, usually 60% or more of maximal acid output (after stimulation with betazole [Histalog]). As the tumors are frequently multiple and microscopic in size or are malignant and have already metastasized, excision is seldome curative except in the occasional patient with a solitary lesion usually in the duodenum. Until recently the only effective treatment was a total gastrectomy that removed the target organ.

Cimetidine or ranitidine effectively controls the hyperacidity and symptoms and must be given indefinitely. Because of the prodigious doses needed to control symptoms, some surgeons add highly selective vagotomy to the treatment with the aim of reducing drug dosage and side effects. Because the tumors are of low-grade malignancy, patients may survive for many years after effective control of gastric hypersecretion.

Hyperparathyroidism

Because hypercalcemia increases gastric secretion, patients with hyperparathyroidism develop a higher than normal incidence of duodenal ulcers. These usually fail to respond to medical therapy but subside with treatment of the hyperparathyroidism.

Multiple endocrine adenopathy

Two main syndromes involving adenomas of endocrine glands have been described: MEA I (parathyroid, pituitary, and pancreas) and MEA II (parathyroid, adrenal medulla, and thyroid C-cells). The boundaries of these syndromes are currently not nearly so distinct as previously described. Both entities are associated with peptic ulcerations, probably because of hyperfunctioning parathyroid (parathormone) and pancreatic (gastrin) tissues.

GASTRIC CANCER

Stomach cancer currently makes up 3% of malignancies in the population of the United States. Although the incidence is decreasing for unknown reasons, about 25,000 new cases of gastric cancer occur each year.

Carcinoma of the stomach

Pathology. The varieties of gastric carcinoma are carcinoma in situ (rare), superficial spreading carcinoma (rare), ulcerative (28%), fungating or polypoid (23%), infiltrative (13%), and advanced (33%). Linitis plastica (leather bottle stomach), a diffuse form of the infiltrative variety, has a poor prognosis. The gross appearance of these tumors correlates poorly with their histology.

In decreasing order of frequency the sites most often involved are the pylorus and prepyloric region (about half of all cases), the body of the stomach, and the area of the cardia.

There are two basic histological types—intestinal and diffuse. The former, usually well differentiated and often accompanied by intestinal metaplasia, has a better prognosis. The latter, less well differentiated and infrequently accompanied by intestinal metaplasia, has a poorer prognosis.

Spread. Regional lymph node metastases are present in 90% of cases at autopsy and 70% of surgical specimens. Metastases commonly involve nodes along the greater and lesser curvatures and around the pylorus, celiac axis, and porta hepatis. Cancers in the upper stomach also spread to splenic hilar and peripancreatic nodes. Rarely, cancer cells invade the left supraclavicular nodes (Virchow's nodes), presumably through the thoracic duct.

Microscopic metastases may extend submucosally and subserosally for surprising distances. Gastric cancer often invades the pancreas, liver, and transverse colon. Hematogenous spread occurs most frequently to the liver and lungs. Tumor cells may shed and grow on peritoneal surfaces as multiple implants and may cause massive ascites. Deposits on the pelvic floor are known as Blumer's shelf and on the ovary as Krukenberg's tumor.

Staging. The following system of clinical staging helps in treatment and prognosis:

Stage I. Cancer confined to stomach
  A. Cancer confined to mucosa
  B. Cancer extending to but not through serosa
  C. Cancer extending through serosa with or without invasion of adjacent structures
Stage II. Diffuse involvement of gastric wall (linitis plastica) or involvement of regional lymph nodes
Stage III. Involvement of regional nodes remote from the tumor or on both gastric curvatures
Stage IV. Distant metastases

This system gives a reasonably accurate idea of prognosis, e.g., stage IA has an excellent prognosis, stage IV a dismal one.

Clinical characteristics. Specific or early symptoms are notoriously lacking in cancer of the stomach. Epigastric pain, weight loss, anorexia, vomiting, fatigue, and anemia occur insidiously and are often ignored. Dysplasia occurs with lesions in the cardia. A mass is palpable in one third of the patients. Hepatomegaly raises suspicion of liver metastases. Males outnumber females about 3:1. Diseases that may precede and predispose to cancer of the stomach include pernicious anemia (achlorhydria), gastric polyps, and chronic atrophic gastritis.

Diagnosis. Cancer of the stomach is suspected from x-ray evidence, gastroscopy findings including biopsy, and cytological evidence of malignant cells in the gastric aspirate.

Treatment. Surgical excision of the lesion and involved nodes is the only treatment of definite value. Radiation therapy offers little help.

Prognosis. If all the tumor can be removed, with no spread beyond the stomach, up to 50% of these patients will live 5 years. However, because of the lack of early symptoms, the rich lymphatic supply, and the aggressiveness of these tumors, less than 10% of all patients with gastric carcinoma survive 5 years.

Sarcoma of the stomach

Sarcomas account for about 3% of all malignancies of the stomach. Lymphomas, the most common type, occur primarily in the stomach or as manifestations of a generalized process. Grossly they appear as mucosal thickenings, multiple nodules, or a single polypoid growth. Since lymphomas are radiosensitive and gastric carcinoma is not, biopsy of gastric tumors for specific diagnosis is often indicated even when the lesions appear far advanced. Treatment consists of radical resection followed by postoperative radiotherapy. Chemotherapy may be needed in patients with extensive lesions. Leiomyosarcoma, a rare cancer, responds best to excision.

MISCELLANEOUS CONDITIONS OF STOMACH AND DUODENUM
Gastric polyps

Polyps in the stomach are rare, except in patients with pernicious anemia. Usually single, they may number in the hundreds. Malignant potential increases with the size of the polyps. Those over 2 cm. are likely to be malignant and should be removed.

Multiple benign polyposis (Peutz-Jeghers syndrome), an inherited syndrome, may involve the stomach as well as other parts of the gastrointestinal tract. It is associated with melanin spots of the lips and buccal mucosa. Conservative treatment is usually indicated.

Duodenal diverticula

Duodenal diverticula are outpouchings in the duodenum. Although common, they usually cause no symptoms and should be left alone unless they are a suspected cause of bleeding or inflammation, both of which are rare complications.

Gastritis

Inflammation of the stomach wall may occur after dietary indiscretions, especially after an increased intake of alcohol. *Atrophic gastritis*, associated with hypochlorhydria or achlorhydria, may cause malabsorption of vitamin B_{12}. The thinned atrophic mucosa is clearly visible during gastroscopy. Enlarged rugal folds, often present in the Zollinger-Ellison syndrome, indicate *hypertrophic gastritis*. After operations that destroy or bypass the pylorus, duodenal contents sometimes reflux into the stomach causing *reflux gastritis*, with epigastric pain, anemia, and weight loss. Although usually responsive to medical therapy, this condition, if it becomes intractable, may necessitate surgery to divert duodenal contents away from the stomach.

Mallory-Weiss syndrome

Mallory-Weiss syndrome is an uncommon complication of severe vomiting that results in a laceration through the mucosa of the esophagogastric junction. Surgical suture of the laceration is sometimes necessary to stop bleeding.

Dumping syndrome

Dumping occurs to some extent in about 10% to 20% of patients who have gastric operations involving pyloric bypass or destruction. This syndrome features two types of symptoms, gastrointestinal and hemodynamic. Gastrointestinal symptoms include nausea, vomiting, abdominal pain (fullness, cramps), and diarrhea. Hemodynamic symptoms are weakness, fatigue, palpitations, sweating, pallor, and sensation of warmth. These symptoms begin within 30 minutes after a meal; they usually last less than 60 minutes. The intensity of dumping symptoms varies widely.

Although the precise cause remains unknown, the basic trigger seems to be rapid distension of the jejunum from hyperosmolar fluid rushing (or dumping) into it. Investigators are less certain about the hemodynamic aspects of dumping. Older theories cite the importance of hypovolemia from plasma elements pouring into the jejunum in response to the sudden hyperosmolar load. Newer theories, focused on chemical mediators released from the distended mucosa, have implicated both serotonin and bradykinin.

Treatment consists of a high protein-low carbohydrate diet, recumbency after meals, and withholding fluids during meals. Symptoms improve with time as patients adjust to their postgastrectomy state; less than 5% of patients have protracted dumping. Thus operative treatment should be reserved for patients with severe and chronic

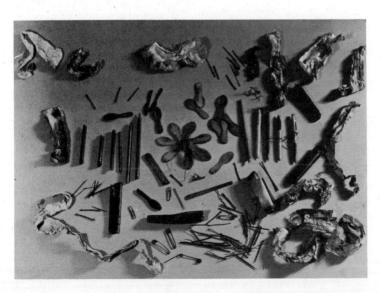

Fig. 23-6. Foreign bodies removed from stomach of mentally defective patient.

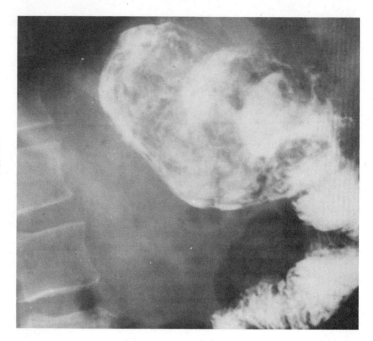

Fig. 23-7. Large filling defect in stomach on barium meal study caused by phytobezoar that developed following vagotomy and Billroth I partial gastrectomy.

symptoms. Interposition of a short reversed segment of jejunum between the gastric remnant and the small bowel helps to slow the rush of fluid into the jejunum.

Foreign bodies

Children or mental incompetents may swallow an astonishing variety of foreign bodies (Fig. 23-6). Most pass through the gastrointestinal tract in 3 to 4 days without symptoms or complications. *Trichobezoars* are hair balls that accumulate in the stomach from chronic hair ingestion. *Phytobezoars* are accretions of indigestible food fibers. Gastrectomy, particularly when accompanied by vagotomy (poor gastric drainage) (Fig. 23-7), improper mastication, and diets high in cellulose, favors their formation. Cellulase or other enzymes may break up the mass.

Gastric operations for morbid obesity

Morbid obesity is a condition in which a person is at least 100 pounds overweight or whose weight exceeds twice the ideal weight. It affects 7% of females and 5% of males in the United States. Most likely causes are a genetic predisposition and excessive intake of food arising from overactive appetite centers in the midbrain. It is refractory to medical treatment. Complications include adult onset diabetes, hypertension, ischemic heart disease, cerebrovascular accidents, varicose veins, restrictive lung disease, hernia, osteoarthritis, accidents, sleep apnea, and gallstones. Death rates are 11 times greater than in the nonobese.

The aim of surgery is to reduce daily intake of food to less than 800 calories until weight reduction is achieved and to prevent the complications of morbid obesity. All gastric operations are designed to create a small proximal gastric pouch (capacity 50 ml.) that empties slowly through a small opening, not greater than 1 cm. Eating brings on a feeling of early satiety. Gastric bypass consists in constructing a small gastric pouch that drains into a loop of jejunum. Disadvantages are high operative morbidity, stomal ulcers in 5% of patients, and uncertainty as to future problems associated with bypass of most of the stomach and duodenum. The more popular operation is gastroplasty in which two rows of staples form a small (50 cc.) pouch, with a 1 cm. outlet, in the upper stomach. Various measures are used to reinforce the outlet, since a cause of failure in the past has been gradual dilatation of the pouch and the outlet permitting egress of excessive quantities of food. These operations achieve 50% loss of excessive weight in 75% of patients treated. Postoperative complications include gastric leaks, outlet stenosis, wound infections, and rarely vitamin deficiencies.

24
Small Intestine

Robert T. Soper
Siroos S. Shirazi

The small intestine is the longest segment of the gastrointestinal tract, extending from the pyloric sphincter to the ileocecal sphincter or valve. Curiously enough, although the small bowel is frequently operated on (resection, bypass, decompression, lysis of adhesions, placement of indwelling catheters for suction or feeding purposes), few of these operations are done *on* the small bowel for diseases that originate *within* the small bowel. Thus duodenal ulcer is caused by acid-peptic factors originating within the stomach with the major effect on the duodenum; mesenteric vascular occlusion infarcts and perforates the small bowel but originates primarily as a vascular lesion; small bowel obstruction is most commonly caused by extrinsic factors (hernias, adhesions) not of primary origin from the small bowel itself. Numerically, few surgical diseases primarily arise *within* the small intestine itself.

ANATOMY

The small intestine measures 7 to 8 m. in the adult and a surprisingly long 200 cm. in the newborn infant. Its subdivisions (duodenum, jejunum, and ileum) are continuous, and only the duodenojejunal junction is marked clearly (by the ligament of Treitz).

The duodenum begins at the pylorus, measures roughly 25 cm. in length, and is largely retroperitoneal. It receives the contents of the stomach proximally, and the bile and pancreatic enzymes in the concave mesenteric surface of its second portion, which is occasioned by embryological rotation. It can be mobilized partially by the *Kocher maneuver*, which divides the peritoneal attachments to its convex surface. The juxtaposition of large vessels, pancreas, and vital duct structures makes surgical manipulations of the duodenum hazardous and necessitates removal of the distal stomach, common bile duct, and pancreatic head if the duodenum must be resected. (See discussion of the Whipple procedure, Chapter 18.)

In contrast, the jejunum and ileum are suspended freely in the peritoneal cavity by the dorsal mesentery and are therefore easy to inspect, manipulate, and resect at laparotomy. The jejunum encompasses the proximal 40% of the bowel from the ligament of Treitz to the ileocolic valve, and the ileum makes up the remainder. The junction between the two is not clearly defined. In general, the jejunum has (1) a larger lumen, (2) thicker walls, (3) larger and more numerous transverse mucosal folds (*valvulae conniventes*), and (4) a better blood supply delivered through fewer vascular arcades than the ileum.

Arterial blood to the small intestine is supplied entirely from the superior mesenteric artery and largely through end arteries. There is little collateral blood flow to the small bowel, in striking contrast to the stomach and colon, and therefore vascular occlusion is more likely to produce bowel infarction.

Venous blood from the small bowel carries fluid end products of digestion to the liver through the portal vein. The small bowel lymphatics, or *lacteals*, travel in the mesentery and collect retroperitoneally into the *cisterna chyli*; they transport products of fat digestion (chyle) into the systemic venous system through the thoracic duct.

The nerve supply to the small bowel is entirely

from the autonomic nervous system. The efferent nerves ensure coordinated aboral peristaltic waves to carry intestinal contents downstream during digestion. The sensory afferents localize and discriminate pain of small bowel origin very poorly as a dull, vague aching in the epigastrium or periumbilical area of the abdomen.

The wall of the small intestine is composed of four layers:

1. The inner mucosa is composed of simple columnar epithelium with innumerable intestinal glands, the absorptive surface being increased enormously by the presence of villi, plus the mucosal folds known as the *valvulae conniventes.*
2. The submucosa consists of fibrous and supporting tissue and is richly supplied by the intrinsic vascular and nervous elements of the intestine.
3. The outer longitudinal and inner circular muscle layers contribute the peristalsis necessary to propel intestinal material downstream.
4. The outer serosa is visceral peritoneum that, in its pristine state, allows free motion of the intestine, provides an impermeable barrier to the passage of bacteria to the peritoneal cavity, and adds considerably to the suture-holding qualities of the bowel wall.

PHYSIOLOGY

During intrauterine life, the intestine functions as an integral part of normal amniotic fluid circulation. Amniotic fluid is swallowed by the fetus, and a portion is absorbed, utilized, and then excreted as urine back into the amniotic fluid. Interruption of this cycle at any stage results in retention of abnormal amounts of amniotic fluid, a condition known as *polyhydramnios:* 50% of babies born of mothers with polyhydramnios will have major congenital anomalies that interfere with this circulatory system, including hydrocephalus, anencephaly, myelomeningocele, upper gastrointestinal tract obstruction, and congenital hydronephrosis.

In postnatal life the small intestine has digestive and absorptive functions. In the adult, 8 to 10 L. of digestive secretion are produced daily in the oral cavity, stomach, small bowel, pancreas, and liver to aid enzymatic breakdown of ingested food to molecules small enough to be absorbed. The small bowel adds somewhat to the digestive secretions and propels the succus entericus downstream in an orderly and relatively slow manner. After digestion has been completed, the mucosal surface of the small intestine absorbs water, electrolytes, and the basic breakdown products of the food. Fat travels through the lacteals and lymphatic ducts to the superior vena cava, and the bulk of the remaining products is conveyed to the liver through the portal venous system for further metabolic alteration. Normally up to 98% of the liquid volume of the succus entericus is absorbed, largely from the lower portion of the small intestine.

Resection or bypass of up to 50% of the small intestine is generally followed by an initial period of diarrhea and weight loss but is compatible with perfectly normal subsequent growth and development, regardless of age at the time of operation. Chronic diarrhea, anemia, osteomalacia, and varying degrees of malnutrition, at least temporarily, occur after loss of more than half of the small intestine.

SURGICAL DISEASES OF THE SMALL INTESTINE

The majority of operations performed on the small bowel are done because of peptic ulcers, or intestinal obstruction (including those of congenital origin), or as a necessary part of operations primarily on the colon; these entities are properly discussed in their own specific chapters and are not considered further here. The remainder of this chapter is therefore devoted to that small fraction of surgical diseases arising primarily within the small intestine.

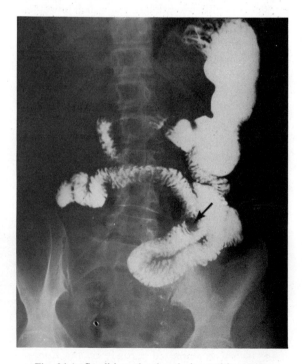

Fig. 24-1. Small bowel polyp designated by arrow.

Neoplasms

The small intestine is singularly free of neoplasms, both benign and malignant, as compared with the esophagus, stomach, and colon. The reasons for this discrepancy are unknown. They comprise well under 5% of all primary neoplasms of the gastrointestinal tract. Benign tumors include polyps, villous adenomas, myomas, leiomyomas, fibromas, lipomas, and aberrant gastric or pancreatic tissue. They commonly are asymptomatic and are found incidentally at autopsy or laparotomy. They become symptomatic by ulcerating the overlying mucosa with bleeding or by acting as the leading point for small bowel intussusception; the larger tumors may obstruct the lumen. Diagnosis is made at laparotomy, but occasionally the tumors show as filling defects in the barium column during small bowel x-ray examination (Fig. 24-1). Duodenal lesions can now be viewed by the flexible fiberoptic endoscope, allowing precise preoperative biopsy diagnosis (Fig. 24-2). Lesions of the jejunum and ileum require laparotomy for diagnostic confirmation and surgical excision.

The *Peutz-Jeghers syndrome* is the association of intestinal polyps with melanin spots on the mucosa of the lips, mouth, and anus. The disorder is inherited on a genetic basis. The polyps are generally localized to the small intestine and are from one to five in number; occasionally they are more numerous and are located within the stomach or colon. Malignant degeneration is extremely unusual with the Peutz-Jeghers type of polyp, and surgical treatment is undertaken only when the polyps produce symptoms.

The most common malignant neoplasm of the small intestine is the *adenocarcinoma,* about one half of which are primary within the duodenum. Bleeding and obstruction are the most common signs and often occur late in the evolution after metastasis has already occurred. *Lymphosarcomas* are the next most common variety, generally occurring in children and young adults and often in association with widespread disease.

The signs of small bowel malignancy in roughly descending order of frequency are intestinal obstruction, gastrointestinal tract bleeding, an abdominal mass, and perforation. Diagnosis is made at laparotomy, but plain and barium contrast studies of the intestine may be helpful. Treatment is wide surgical resection of the involved bowel and its draining lymphatic pathways when possible and if distant metastasis has not already occurred. X-ray therapy is useful in additional treatment of lymphomas. Local resection or bypass occasionally palliates incurable neoplasms. The overall 5-year survival rate is from 10% to 15%, the

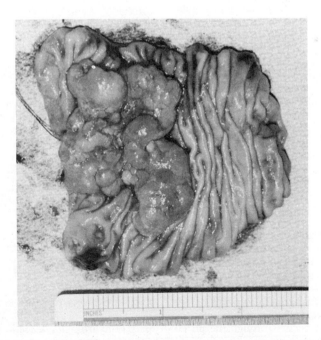

Fig. 24-2. Benign villous adenoma resected from third portion of duodenum; seen preoperatively by fiberoptic endoscopy.

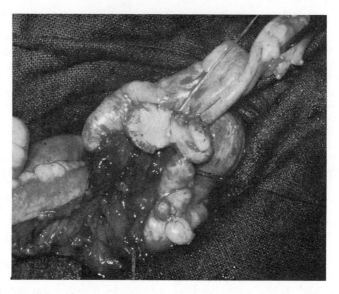

Fig. 24-3. Carcinoid tumor at base of appendix. Probe *(upper white line)* points to yellow-white tumor, which has been sectioned. Appendix is retracted toward upper right of field.

prognosis for lymphosarcoma being materially better than that for primary small bowel adeno-carcinoma.

Carcinoid tumors (Fig. 24-3) arise from argen-taffin cells near the base of the intestinal glands. They are most commonly found in the appendix, with the small intestine next in frequency. However, they can arise anywhere within the gastrointestinal tract, and pulmonary carcinoids have occasionally been reported. Carcinoid tumors are yellow or gray; the cells have a columnar arrangement and stain with chromic acid to allow a specific histological diagnosis.

Carcinoid tumors may be either benign or malignant, probably related more to the time at which they are discovered than to any inherent difference in malignant potential. This supposition is supported by the observation that although 60% of carcinoid tumors arise within the appendix, they are never malignant in this location; they probably produce early obstruction of the very small appendiceal lumen that initiates signs of appendicitis leading to prompt surgical excision and cure. On the other extreme, carcinoid tumors arising in the small intestine are almost always malignant by the time of discovery. The larger lumen of the intestine allows years of undetected growth to occur before symptoms are produced and surgical treatment is carried out. Metastasis occurs through the portal venous system to the liver.

The *carcinoid syndrome* is seen only when malignant carcinoids have *metastasized* widely to the liver or other extraportal sites such as the lungs; it is present in about 25% of reported malignant carcinoids. The clinical features of the *carcinoid syndrome* are periodic attacks of (1) colicky abdominal pain with diarrhea and weight loss, (2) flushing of the face, neck, and torso, and (3) asthmatic wheezing. Late in the course of the carcinoid syndrome, pulmonic or tricuspid valvular stenosis develops gradually, leading to cardiac failure and death.

Argentaffin cells normally produce minute amounts of hydroxytryptophan (as an intermediate in the biosynthesis of serotonin), which is believed to play a role in hemostasis and maintenance of smooth muscle tone in blood vessels and intestine. Carcinoid tumors synthesize enormous amounts of serotonin that, however, are altered and "detoxified" by the liver so long as the venous drainage goes into the portal system. However, large hepatic or extraportal metastases secrete serotonin directly into systemic blood to induce the smooth muscle contractions responsible for the characteristic signs and symptoms previously related. The reason for the periodicity of attacks is unknown. Diagnostic confirmation is provided by demonstration of excessive levels of serotonin in the serum (5-hydroxytryptamine, or 5-HT) or its degradation products (5-hydroxyindoleacetic acid, or 5-HIAA) in the urine. Serotonin is also excreted by the lungs into expired air, explaining why valvular disease is limited selectively to the valves on the right side of the heart.

Malignant carcinoids are the exception to the rule that the metastases of incurable primary intestinal neoplasms should not be resected. Malignant carcinoids grow slowly, and removal of portions of the metastases may provide gratifyingly long relief from the distressing and ultimately serious (or fatal) effects of hyperserotoninemia.

Trauma

The small intestine is damaged by both *penetrating* and *nonpenetrating* abdominal trauma, often in association with other visceral injuries. The penetrating missile may perforate intestine or produce mesenteric vascular injury, ranging from a minor hematoma confined to the mesentery to massive hemorrhage into the free peritoneal cavity with shock and serious compromise to the blood supply of the involved segment of intestine. Plain supine and decubitus abdominal roentgenograms will often show free air and will locate the missile if it has been retained in the body to help map out the pathway traversed. Laparotomy is almost always indicated with a painstaking and orderly inspection of the entire peritoneal cavity for injury. The missile need not be removed, but damage to the viscera must be repaired. Minute or sharply demarcated puncture wounds of small intestine may be turned in, but large or ragged lacerations and severely contused or devascularized bowel require resection and anastomosis. Mesenteric bleeding must be controlled by pressure or ligature. Because of the chemically irritating and septic content of the small intestine, the peritoneal cavity should be lavaged, suctioned, and drained and appropriate antibiotics administered postoperatively if spillage has occurred.

The mortality for nonpenetrating abdominal trauma is approximately three times that for penetrating injuries, probably because there are less compelling indications for exploratory laparotomy in the former. The intestine ranks fourth behind the spleen, kidneys, and liver in frequency of damage by nonpenetrating abdominal trauma. The jejunum and ileum are relatively mobile and tend to slide away and escape injury from a nonpenetrating blow, though sudden dislocation may indeed lacerate the small bowel mesentery. The duodenum and duodenojejunal junction are anchored retroperitoneally and cannot escape, resulting in a much higher incidence of injury. This is especially true for the fourth part of the duodenum, trapped between the wounding blow anteriorly and the rigid second lumbar vertebra posteriorly. Intramural hematoma and laceration are the common duodenal injuries incurred in this manner. If the duodenum is lacerated beneath its peritoneal cover, extravasation of duodenal contents occurs retroperitoneally.

Intramural *duodenal hematomas* produce symptoms by obstructing the lumen, which may take several hours or even days to complete. Diagnosis is suggested by narrowing of the lumen and a "coil spring" appearance of the duodenal mucosa on upper gastrointestinal barium roentgenograms. Surgical treatment consists in evacuating the hematoma through a serosal incision, careful inspection for a break in the mucosa, and drainage. Operative therapy is indicated only if 5 to 7 days of intravenous fluids and nasogastric suction fail to relieve the obstruction.

The diagnosis of retroperitoneal laceration of the duodenum may be extremely difficult to estabish, though the plain abdominal roentgenogram often shows obliteration of the right kidney profile and small bubbles of gas above the kidney. In view of the subtle clinical signs and the disastrous results of untreated duodenal laceration, any patient with a nonpenetrating abdominal injury must be hospitalized and observed very closely. Diagnostic laparotomy should be carried out if his condition does not promptly improve. The laparotomy is not complete without a Kocher maneuver being performed to allow inspection of the retroperitoneal duodenum and exploration of the lesser sac to look for associated pancreatic injury. Duodenal lacerations are closed, and the area is generously drained.

People involved in automobile accidents while wearing abdominal seat belts suffer a peculiar type of subtle injury to the abdomen that deserves special mention. Rapid deceleration whips the upper part of the torso forward, and if the seat belt is above the pelvic bony girdle (where it generally is), it momentarily traps the viscera against the vertebral column and imposes many different shearing and compression injuries to gut and mesentery. The abdominal injuries most commonly seen are mesenteric hematoma, devascularization of bowel, severe damage leading to rupture of the bowel wall, and delayed ecchymosis and hemorrhage of the abdominal wall in a beltlike area. Symptoms are likely to be slow in onset and often are overshadowed by other injuries. Any automobile accident victim who bears the ecchymotic imprint of a seat belt injury on his abdomen and who develops late abdominal pain, distension, paralytic ileus, or slow return of gastrointestinal function is a prime candidate for serious visceral injury. Repeated abdominal examinations, x-ray examinations, and paracenteses are often helpful in confirming this diagnosis, but laparotomy often must be the final arbiter.

Infections

None of the primary infections of the small intestine or its mesentery is treated primarily by surgical means, but often the symptoms produced by them mimic surgically treated diseases (appendicitis) or are complications of hospitalized patients (pseudomembranous enterocolitis).

Acute gastroenteritis

Acute gastroenteritis is generally caused by food poisoning or virus infections, and in North America it is less commonly caused by dysentery (*Shigella, Salmonella*) or paratyphoid infection, and very rarely by typhoid fever. Profuse vomiting and diarrhea are associated with colicky abdominal pain, diffuse abdominal tenderness, and hyperactive bowel sounds. Attention to these features on physical examination will in most cases adequately distinguish gastroenteritis from appendicitis. The temperature is often elevated, but tachycardia is not seen until the late stages of the disorder when the patient becomes dehydrated. Stool culture and serum agglutination tests are helpful in the diagnosis, and leukopenia is a characteristic finding with both typhoid and viral infections.

Primary intestinal tuberculosis

Primary intestinal tuberculosis is extremely rare in countries that have eliminated bovine tuberculosis and controlled human pulmonary tuberculous infection. Intestinal tuberculosis involves the distal small bowel and cecum with a granulomatous mass and is best treated by chemotherapy in a tuberculosis sanatorium; obstructive complications of the tuberculous mass may require surgical bypass.

Tuberculous peritonitis

Tuberculous peritonitis is a bland form of peritonitis that is self-limiting in its course; it is characterized by yellowish deposits on the mesenteric surface that are composed of typical tubercles. The diagnosis is confirmed by biopsy of one of the tubercles. Intestinal tuberculosis is often the source of peritoneal involvement, though hematogenous spread may be responsible.

Mesenteric lymphadenitis

Mesenteric lymphadenitis is a hyperplastic enlargement of mesenteric lymph nodes, generally seen only in children and young adults, which produces pain difficult to distinguish from that of appendicitis. It is probably caused by a viral enteritis (adenovirus) with secondary mesenteric lymph node involvement. The clinical picture is characterized by central and right lower quadrant abdominal pain in a mildly febrile child who commonly has evidence of pharyngitis or tonsillitis.

Abdominal tenderness is maximal in the right lower abdominal quadrant or right paraumbilical area without sharp localization or signs of peritoneal irritation. The enlarged nodes can be palpated as irregular, tender nodules if the patient is adequately relaxed. Treatment is supportive, and the patient is observed to be certain that signs of appendicitis do not supervene. Exploratory laparotomy is indicated when appendicitis cannot be ruled out, at which time prophylactic appendectomy is recommended to avoid subsequent confusion should the disease recur.

Acute necrotizing enterocolitis

Acute necrotizing enterocolitis (pseudomembranous enterocolitis) (Fig. 24-4) is a fulminating infection of the small bowel or colon that is sometimes caused by an overgrowth of staphylococci but may also occur in the absence of any cultured pathogen. The clinical settings favoring the development of acute enterocolitis are chronic low-grade intestinal obstruction (children with Hirschsprung's disease) or cases in which treatment with broad-specturm antibiotics has upset the balance of the intestinal flora to allow overgrowth of bacteria in the gastrointestinal tract. There is widespread denudation of the intestinal mucosa, especially in the small bowel, with edema and inflammation of the wall and pooling of large amounts of fluid within the bowel lumen.

Acute enterocolitis is characterized by the sudden onset of profuse diarrhea containing desquamated mucosa and blood that is associated with a high fever, tachycardia, nausea and vomiting, abdominal pain, and tenderness. Dehydration, electrolyte imbalance, and hypovolemic shock quickly occur from the massive amounts of fluid entrapped in the bowel lumen, which may not become evident as diarrhea for several hours because of an adynamic ileus. Hypovolemic and septic shock is the most common cause of death.

Treatment must be heroic, with rapid replacement of fluids, electrolytes, and blood. Nasogastric suction is begun, and cleansing enemas are given to expel the fluid retained within the bowel lumen. Antibiotics to which staphylococci are sensitive (penicillinase-resistant penicillin, vancomycin) should be given if stool smear and culture suggest an overgrowth of staphylococci. Steroids and fecal enemas are sometimes helpful. In patients harboring chronic intestinal obstruction, the obstruction should be relieved as soon as possible.

Granulomatous (transmural) enterocolitis

The term *granulomatous (transmural) enterocolitis* includes regional enteritis, regional ileitis, regional ileocolitis, and Crohn's disease. It is pref-

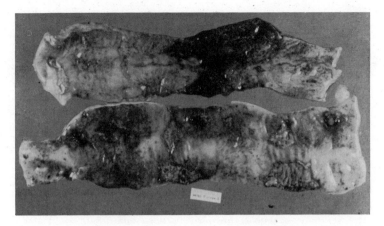

Fig. 24-4. Acute necrotizing enterocolitis. Notice hemorrhage, edema, superficial ulceration, and exudation of mucosa.

erable to the older terms of Crohn's disease or regional enteritis because a granulomatous reaction is the most characteristic microscopic feature of the disorder, and it can indeed involve all layers of any or all portions of the intestine. It was first described in 1932 by Crohn and his associates as a specific entity distinct from tuberculous enteritis and other less specific infectious disorders of the intestine.

Granulomatous enterocolitis is an uncommon disease that affects principally young adults. It is rare among blacks and has an equal sex incidence. The cause of the disease is unknown, though allergic, infectious, and autoimmune factors have been suggested as contributing factors.

Granulomatous (transmural) enterocolitis either originates in, or is totally confined to, the distal ileum in the majority of cases. Spread commonly occurs proximally and occasionally distally to the colon. During the latter stages it often has multiple sites of involvement with uninvolved "skip areas" intervening. In early phases the bowel mucosa ulcerates and the wall becomes grossly thickened, erythematous, and edematous, with thickening of the adjacent mesentery and rubbery enlargement of the mesenteric lymph nodes. At this stage the outstanding histological features are mucosal ulceration, submucosal lymphoid hyperplasia, and transmural lymphangiectasis, infiltrates of inflammatory cells and eosinophils, sclerosing lymphangitis, and granulomas without caseation. Involvement of all layers of the bowel wall justifies the descriptive term *transmural* and, when this peculiar disease attacks primarily the colon, serves to distinguish it from the primarily mucosal inflammation of chronic ulcerative colitis.

If limited to the ileum, the early stages of acute granulomatous enterocolitis often mimic appendicitis and are distinguished only at laparotomy. If the cecal base is not involved, prophylactic appendectomy may be safely performed at this time, along with confirmatory biopsy of a mesenteric lymph node. Approximately 50% of such cases will have spontaneous subsidence of the small bowel inflammation, with lengthy periods of remission.

In later stages of the disease, the edema and erythema of the involved bowel wall are replaced by fibrous tissue with rigidity, contracture, and narrowing of the lumen (Fig. 24-5). A moderately tender mass can usually be palpated at this stage, which is clinically manifested by periodic bouts of crampy abdominal discomfort and diarrhea associated with weight loss and anemia caused by occult blood loss in the stool. Fever and leukocytosis parallel the activity of the disease, and for unknown reasons perianal abscesses and fistulas are common.

The later stages of transmural enterocolitis are characterized by abscess formation and inflammatory involvement of adjacent viscera leading to both external and internal fistulas. The viscera more commonly involved in these fistulas are small bowel, bladder, and sigmoid colon, with varying symptoms related to the fistulas. The signs and symptoms of chronic low-grade intestinal obstruction (caused by the extreme narrowing of the lumen) are often superimposed.

The course of granulomatous enterocolitis is characterized by chronicity and periods of remissions and exacerbations. Generally speaking, the younger the patient and the more acute the onset,

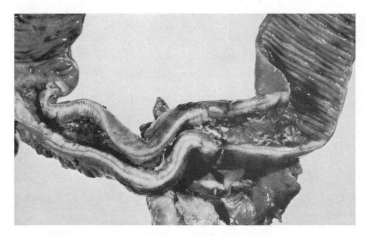

Fig. 24-5. Chronic granulomatous enterocolitis (regional ileitis) with scarring, rigidity, and thickening of bowel wall and narrowing of lumen. (From Anderson, W.A.D., and Scotti, T.M.: Synopsis of pathology, ed. 10, St. Louis, 1980, The C.V. Mosby Co.)

the more guarded the prognosis must be in terms of later recurrences and complications.

The diagnosis of transmural enterocolitis is generally confirmed by contrast (barium) x-ray examination. The early radiographic signs include a modest degree of narrowing of the lumen associated with flattening and a raggedness of the mucosal pattern with puddling of barium. Later stages are extreme narrowing of the lumen, referred to as the *string sign* (Fig. 24-6), with dilatation of the proximal loops according to the degree of intestinal obstruction present. Occasionally fistulas or extravasation of barium into abscess cavities is seen. Barium enema with retrograde filling of the distal ileum occasionally is helpful in the diagnosis of transmural ileitis.

Treatment of granulomatous enterocolitis is nonoperative until and unless complications occur. Indications for operative treatment are the development of intestinal obstruction, fistulas, intraabdominal abscesses, and hemorrhage, or if the patient's general well-being is severely compromised by chronic malnutrition, anemia, pain, and debility. Malignant degeneration rarely occurs. In large series of cases, over one half will ultimately require surgical intervention.

Specific treatment for granulomatous enterocolitis is nonexistent. Evaluation of different forms of therapy is difficult because of the unpredictable and remitting course of the disease. Corticosteroids or ACTH, a nutritious and low-residue diet, supplements of vitamins and iron, ingestion of nonabsorbed sulfonamides (Azulfidine), rest, and symptomatic treatment for diarrhea are all employed in the nonoperative treatment of granulomatous enterocolitis. Operative treatment is directed to the specific complication or indication for surgery, including resection of the involved intestine. Recurrence of the disease in previously uninvolved bowel can be expected in fully one fourth to one third of patients who are followed for many years after surgical treatment. Repeated resections and bypassing procedures are fraught with nutritional and metabolic disturbances in themselves, thus warranting intensification of nonoperative treatment and avoidance of operative therapy when possible.

Vascular diseases
Superior mesenteric vascular occlusion

Occlusion of the superior mesenteric artery and vein may occur singly or together, because of a host of disparate influences. Trauma, stagnation of flow, compression, a state of hypercoagulability, and atheromatous plaques favor thrombosis. Occlusion also may occur from emboli originating within the left side of the heart, generally associated with auricular fibrillation. Rarely is the superior mesenteric vein alone thrombosed, but venous thrombosis predictably occurs after occlusion of the arterial inflow. The inferior mesenteric vessels are rarely involved.

Occlusion of the superior mesenteric vessels produces vascular compromise of that segment of small intestine distal to the point of occlusion; the more proximal the occlusion, the longer the seg-

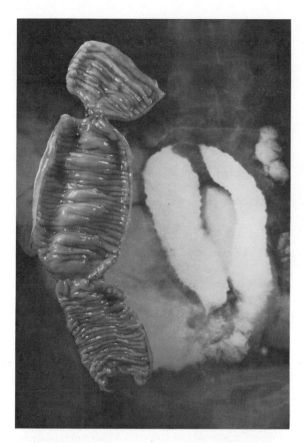

Fig. 24-6. Granulomatous enterocolitis (regional ileitis). "String sign" and uninvolved "skip areas" illustrated in distal ileum superimposed on barium study.

with vomiting, shock, and later the passage of blood-tinged stool. Signs of peritoneal irritation ensue as transudation of fluid and bacteria into the peritoneal cavity occurs.

Prime candidates are the very elderly with advanced generalized arteriosclerosis, patients with thrombocytosis (postsplenectomy) or who are recuperating from operations on the aorta or portal vein, and patients with recent fibrillation (often associated with mitral stenosis).

Physical examination reveals a distended abdomen with dullness to percussion and generalized tenderness, often with guarding and rebound. Bowel sounds are absent and rectal digital examination may reveal bloody stool. Often a vague central abdominal mass is palpable. Plain flat and decubitus x-ray studies of the abdomen are not very helpful in the diagnosis.

Diagnosis and treatment are made at early laparotomy after nasogastric suction and rapidly administered supportive treatment in the form of intravenous fluids, electrolytes, blood, and antibiotics. Thrombectomy, embolectomy, endarterectomy, and arterial bypass are indicated if frank necrosis has not occurred, but generally the surgeon's efforts are limited to resection of frankly necrotic intestine. Prognosis is poor unless the infarcted intestine is short, or unless the occlusion can be corrected before bowel necrosis occurs.

Abdominal angina and *postprandial intestinal angina* are terms used to describe a clinical syndrome associated with gradually developing superior mesenteric artery insufficiency generally caused by atheromatous plaques. Intestinal ischemia follows the stimulus to intestinal secretion and activity provoked by ingestion of a large meal. Retrograde aortic angiography demonstrates narrowing at the takeoff of the superior mesenteric artery from the abdominal aorta. Direct arterial reconstructive surgery relieves symptoms and may avert the later development of total occlusion.

Superior mesenteric artery syndrome

The superior mesenteric artery syndrome is characterized by obstruction of the distal duodenum where it is compressed by the superior mesenteric artery against the unyielding second lumbar vertebral body posteriorly. The obstruction may be acute, or chronic and intermittent. Epigastric distension and bilious vomiting parallel the degree and acuteness of the duodenal compression. Diagnosis is suggested by a very carefully performed barium upper gastrointestinal tract x-ray series demonstrating a dilated stomach and duodenum with abrupt narrowing at the point where the duodenum crosses under the vessel. Normal small bowel is seen distal to this point. Differentiation from other

ment of bowel that will be involved. Primary venous occlusion is associated with a "wet gangrene" type of reaction with noticeable hemorrhage and edema of the involved bowel and an effusion of sanguineous fluid from its surface. Arterial occlusion produces initial blanching of the intestine with venous stagnation subsequently inducing a blue-red discoloration. The intestine becomes slightly distended and hypotonic because of paralytic ileus that, with continued ischemia, progresses to perforation and peritonitis. Bowel infarction is generally limited to the jejunum, ileum, and right colon, even when the superior mesenteric artery is occluded at its takeoff from the aorta, because of collateral arterial blood flow to duodenum and colon.

Clinically, acute occlusion of the superior mesenteric vessels is characterized by rapid onset of abdominal tenderness and distension associated

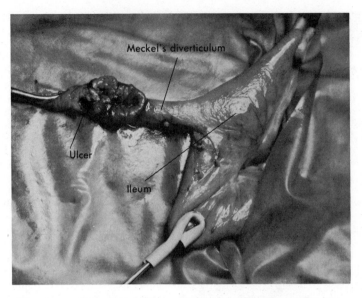

Fig. 24-7. Meckel's diverticulum opened to show bleeding peptic ulcer.

types of duodenal obstructions (intrinsic stenotic membrane) is made at the time of laparotomy, and the obstruction is bypassed by a side-to-side duodenojejunal anastomosis.

Diverticula
Meckel's diverticulum

Meckel's diverticulum (Fig. 24-7) is the most common type of small bowel diverticulum, occurring in 2% of the general population. It represents a persistence of the atavistic structure known as the vitellointestinal tract (omphalomesenteric duct), which connects the distal ileum to the yolk sac early in embryonic life. The vitellointestinal tract normally obliterates and disappears entirely by the seventh week of gestation. Persistence of the entire tract is rare but is manifested early in life by drainage of ileal content at the umbilicus. Diagnosis is confirmed by injection of the fistula with radiopaque material to show a connection with the distal ileum. If the lumen of the retained tract is obliterated, the anomaly appears as a fibrous cord between the ileum and the umbilicus; the diagnosis is made incidentally at laparotomy or when small bowel obstruction occurs because of external compression by the fibrous cord.

The most common remnant of the vitellointestinal tract is persistence of its proximal end, known as Meckel's diverticulum. It is represented by a blind diverticulum situated on the antimesenteric border of ileum, which in the adult is located about

2 feet proximal to the ileocecal valve. The majority of these common types are asymptomatic and are discovered incidentally at autopsy or laparotomy.

The symptoms of Meckel's diverticulum are produced by peptic ulceration, intussusception, or diverticulitis. About 50% of the symptomatic diverticula (and about 15% of all Meckel's diverticula) contain ectopic gastric mucosa that secretes hydrochloric acid directly on unprotected adjacent ileal mucosa. Peptic ulceration occurs with pain, bleeding, inflammation, or sometimes perforation. Dark red to tarry blood passed rectally is the most common complaint prompting surgical consultation. The diverticulum may become inverted into the lumen of the ileum to provide the leading point of an ileoileal intussusception, with ultimate symptoms of intestinal obstruction and currant jelly type of bloody stools. Most Meckel's diverticula are wide necked and drain readily, but occasionally the neck is narrow with poor drainage of intestinal material producing primary diverticulitis.

The diagnosis of Meckel's diverticulum is virtually impossible by barium contrast x-ray examination. Abdominal scan after infusion of ^{99m}Tc may show a "hot spot" of uptake in Meckel's diverticulum, provided that it contains functioning ectopic gastric mucosa. Asymptomatic Meckel's diverticula are discovered incidentally at exploratory laparotomy carried out for other purposes, and the symptomatic ones are found at laparotomy undertaken for symptoms produced by the various complications. Appendicitis is the most common presumptive diagnosis when pain, inflammation, and perforation are the symptoms. Treatment is complete surgical excision.

Other small bowel diverticula

Diverticula of the small bowel unrelated to the vitellointestinal tract remnant usually arise from the mesenteric surface and are much more common in the duodenum than in the jejunum or ileum. Duodenal diverticula are said to be present in 6% of patients who have upper gastrointestinal tract barium studies performed, but they are present in about 20% of cadavers at autopsy. Duodenal diverticula commonly arise at or near the ampulla of Vater, are generally single, and are rarely symptomatic. They must be distinguished clinically from other, much more common, symptom-producing lesions of the pancreas, stomach, and biliary tract.

Jejunal and ileal diverticula are likely to be multiple. Large diverticula may cause diarrhea, weight loss, and malabsorption-like states attributed to stagnation of contents producing inflammation, infection, and ulceration. Small bowel diverticula are diagnosed from barium x-ray series as sacculations that readily fill with barium.

Symptomatic diverticula of the jejunum and ileum are uncommon, but they are treated surgically with ease by resection of the involved segment of the bowel. Duodenal diverticula are more frequent, less commonly symptomatic, and dangerous to approach surgically because of the relative inaccessibility of the duodenum. Resection or inversion of duodenal diverticula must be done with infinite care and meticulous dissection, with the common bile duct protected by cannulation when necessary. For these reasons, conservatism is the rule in the treatment of duodenal diverticula.

25
Large Intestine

George E. Block
Richard D. Liechty

Diseases of the colon range from congenital malformations to degenerative processes. They include developmental defects (aganglionosis, Hirschsprung's disease), trauma, inflammation (specific or nonspecific), neoplasia, and degeneration of colonic musculature or vasculature.

Of all the organs in the body, none harbors a more septic internal environment. Proper surgical management of colonic disease demands an understanding of this milieu and the diseases that arise within it.

GENERAL PRINCIPLES

Sigmoidoscopy. No physical examination of an adult patient is complete without a sigmoidoscopic examination. This examination may allow inspection of the lumen of the distal 25 to 30 cm. of the gut and is theoretically capable of disclosing up to 70% of the neoplasms of the large bowel, sites of hemorrhage, or local inflammation. Examination of at least the distal 10 to 15 cm. is easily accomplished and allows detailed inspection of that portion of the colon where roentgenograms are notoriously inaccurate or inadequate. This examination may also be performed in severely ill patients before emergency operation in order to disclose or rule out sites of hemorrhage, perforations, or neoplasm, and it may aid in decompressing or evacuating the lower gut.

This procedure is performed as follows:

1. Sigmoidoscopy may be performed with the patient in the Sims or jackknife position or with the hips flexed on a table.
2. A prepackaged enema 30 minutes before the examination provides a clean field. (If a patient has had a bowel movement within 2 to 3 hours, an enema is not always necessary.)
3. Constant reassurance by the examiner immensely aids relaxation and the ease of the examination.
4. Rectal examination followed by pressure from within the rectum toward the perineal body for several seconds relaxes the anal sphincters.
5. The scope is introduced and, under *direct vision,* advanced. After advancing as far as possible it is withdrawn slowly, and the entire bowel wall circumference is methodically scanned.
6. This procedure may be uncomfortable, but it should *never be painful!* One painful experience may, unfortunately, destroy a patient's enthusiasm for subsequent examinations. The lower 10 to 15 cm. (where x-ray examination is the least accurate) is the most important area to be visualized. Painful (and dangerous) forcing of the sigmoidoscope beyond 10 to 15 cm. (where a natural curve often impedes progress) is indefensible.

Diagnostic value. About 60% of both polyps and carcinomas of the large intestine arise within reach of the sigmoidoscope (25 cm.). Sigmoidoscopy allows inspection of the mucosa, biopsy of suspicious growths, smear and culture of ulcers, and introduction of tubes to decompress the bowel. It is helpful in the diagnosis of benign and malignant neoplasms and inflammatory disorders that involves the distal large bowel. Endoscopy for dis-

Table 25-1. Comparison of types of colostomies

Type	Advantages	Disadvantages
Loop (proximal to lesion)	Sterile procedure; rapid and simple; easy closure	Fecal "spillover"; large cumbersome stoma; in perforations, feces in distal limb may continue peritoneal soilage; more stages to surgical treatment
Divided limb (proximal to lesion)	No fecal "spillover"; small stoma, easily cared for	Contaminated field; later colostomy closure is more difficult; technically more difficult; in perforations, feces in distal limb may continue peritoneal soilage; more stages to surgical treatment
Exteriorization of lesion itself	Well adapted to perforations (no fear of continued fecal contamination); double-barreled colostomies simplify closure; removed lesions allow histological diagnosis; fewer operations required	Technically often difficult; limited to mobile areas of colon; cancer operations are often compromised; double-barreled stoma is clumsy

eases of the anal canal is discussed in the next chapter.

Colonoscopy. Colonoscopy requires meticulous preparation of the gut, is used to inspect only the mucosa of the lumen, and is generally not suitable for the diagnosis of massive hemorrhage or complete obstruction. Present or threatened perforation of the bowel is, in general, a contraindication to colonoscopy. The fiberoptic colonoscope permits visualization of the entire colon and allows biopsy of large lesions and removal of small ones.

Colonic bypass procedures. Colostomies divert the fecal stream through the abdominal wall and away from areas of the distal colon that are *obstructed, perforated, severely traumatized, infected* (diverticulitis), or the site of *difficult, tenuous anastomoses*. Notice that in all these conditions *perforation* or *erosion* exists or threatens.

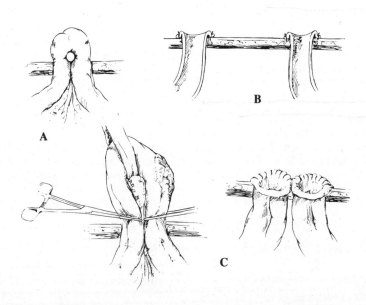

Fig. 25-1. Types of colostomies. **A,** Loop colostomy unopened. **B,** Divided limb colostomy. **C,** Exteriorization of diseased portion of colon; *on left,* segment of colon with tumor is brought out through abdominal wall incision—specimen is removed above clamps; *on right,* clamps are later removed—colon ends sutured to skin.

Perforation of the colon engenders *continued contamination,* which may result in generalized peritonitis and death. Colostomies are not done if resection and primary anastomosis of the lesion can be performed safely.

Three main options in designing colostomies are available (Fig. 25-1 and Table 25-1): (1) the *loop colostomy,* (2) the *divided limb colostomy,* and (3) *exteriorization* of the diseased poriton of the colon.

Loop colostomy. Loop colostomies are technically simple procedures in which a segment of colon (usually transverse colon) is brought out through a small incision in the abdominal wall (Fig. 25-1, *A*). A small rod or tube under the loop supports it until healing takes place. If the proximal portion is distended with gas, aspiration with a needle or a small rubber catheter will immediately decompress it. This is essentially a sterile procedure since the bowel lumen is not entered until the wound is closed. The exteriorized loop may be opened and "matured" by suturing of the mucosa of the bowel to the skin at the termination of the operative procedure. Although subsequent "spillover" may result, excessive gas pressure in the distal limb is immediately and permanently relieved. Loop colostomies should be considered temporary, with anticipated closure at a later date. Loop colostomy closure is technically simple.

Divided limb colostomy. Divided limb colostomies (Fig. 25-1, *B*) prevent "spillover" of fecal material, but since the colon must be divided, some operative contamination invariably results. With careful technique, however, contamination is minimized. The divided bowel ends are exteriorized through separate incisions. Divided limb colostomies require more dissection than loop colostomies, but the resultant proximal stoma is smaller, more esthetic, and easier to fit with a colostomy appliance. Divided limb colostomies are preferred when permanent fecal diversion is desired.

Exteriorization. Exteriorization is often the safest and most rapid method of fecal diversion. However, it requires an adequate length of mesentery (natural or tailored) and implies a second operation to close the resultant stomas. Exteriorization is best used for perforation but may be adapted to obstructing or perforated colon cancers if the surgeon meticulously dissects the entire lymph node–bearing colonic mesentery (Fig. 25-1, *C*).

INFLAMMATORY DISEASES
Appendicitis

For a full description of appendicitis, see Chapter 28. Some of the features associated with adult appendicitis are mentioned briefly here.

Although appendicitis chiefly afflicts the young, no age is immune. The basic initiating factor in

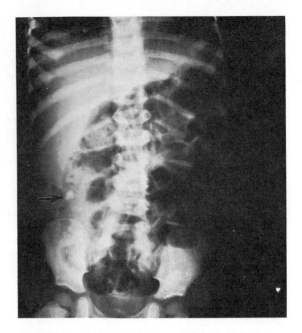

Fig. 25-2. Arrow marks fecalith in appendix.

most adult appendicitis is *obstruction* secondary to a fecalith (Fig. 25-2), impacted within the appendiceal lumen. Obstruction of the left colon from carcinoma has been cited as a precipitating factor in adult appendicitis, presumably because of increased intraluminal pressure in the colon. Perforation of the appendix is less common in adults than in children. (It is most common below 2 years of age.) In the aged patient the response to appendicitis may be deceptively mild. In some older patients, for example, the white blood cell count and temperature remain normal with acute suppurative appendicitis. However, pain and tenderness are remarkably constant factors in appendicitis, regardless of the age. In the adult patient a fistula occurring after appendectomy should always be suggestive of distal colonic obstruction usually from a neoplasm or an inflammation. The obstruction must be relieved before the fistula will close.

A perforated carcinoma of the cecum or terminal ileitis (Crohn's disease) often mimics acute appendicitis.

Diverticulosis and diverticulitis

Incidence. Diverticulosis occurs in about one third of all adults. (This incidence increases with age.) About one sixth of all persons with diverticulosis will develop symptoms of diverticulitis. Operation is required for the *complications* of the

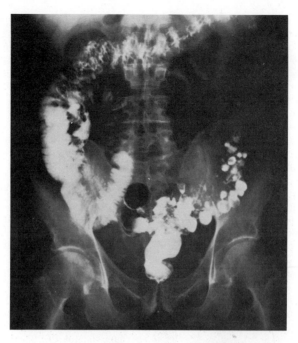

Fig. 25-3. Sigmoid diverticulitis. Globular collections of barium within diverticula.

disease (perforation, obstruction, hemorrhage, fistula, and abscess).

Site. Diverticulosis has a predilection for the sigmoid and distal descending colon (about 80% of patients) (Fig. 25-3). The reason for this relationship is not clear (firmer feces and increased pressure in the sigmoid loop may be important). Diverticula are usually (1) acquired and (2) appear where blood vessels penetrate the colonic wall. Since vessels normally course through the bowel wall in the mesenteric border and beneath appendices epiploicae, diverticula most commonly appear in these areas, though no part of the bowel wall is immune. Diverticula rarely occur in the rectum.

Epidemiology. Diverticulosis chiefly afflicts developed societies. Lack of dietary roughage may play a leading role in causation. Other probable factors include aging, obesity, genetic trait, and chronic constipation.

Pathology. Although the area of diverticulitis is usually less than 10 inches in length, it may extend to include the entire colon. Obstruction of the neck of the diverticulum (by feces or barium) initiates diverticulitis. Inflammation and consequent edema in the bowel wall may constrict adjacent diverticula, inducing "secondary diverticulitis." This process may continue as a chain reaction limited only by the extent of diverticulosis. Massive *lower*

gastrointestinal bleeding (the most common cause is diverticulosis) results from anatomical proximity of the diverticulum and the blood vessel that accompanies it through the bowel wall.

The inflammatory process causes some degree of bowel narrowing and may progress to complete bowel obstruction that mimics carcinoma. Abscesses, fistulization to adjacent structures, or perforation often complicates the course of diverticulitis. Pericolitis and edema of the mesentery invariably accompany the inflammation. Muscular hypertrophy of the bowel wall usually coexists with these findings. Most evidence points to this hypertrophy as associated with the inflammation and not a primary cause of the diverticula.

Clinical course. Clinical signs and symptoms vary with the pathological stages and complications that have been described. Left lower quadrant pain, fever, and altered bowel habits (small-caliber stools or diarrhea) are common. Symptoms of pyuria (frequency, dysuria, urgency) are caused by the inflammatory mass impinging on the urinary bladder or forming a fistula into the bladder. A mass is sometimes palpable in the left lower quadrant or on pelvic or rectal examination.

Barium enema examination may show normal mucosa in the typically funnel-shaped constricted area, but this seldom, if ever, absolutely rules out carcinoma. (Some sigmoid cancers may also cause pain, fever, and a mass.) Sigmoidoscopy is of little help in the diagnosis of diverticulitis and the differential between an obstructing cancer and obstructing diverticulitis may be made by elective colonoscopy. Diverticulitis usually runs an intermittent course of remissions and exacerbations over periods of months or years, but we have seen acute perforation with *no* previous warning signs or symptoms.

Treatment. Medical treatment includes bed rest, broad-spectrum antibiotics appropriate to aerobic or anaerobic organisms, nasogastric suction, and sedation. This regimen may result in the subsidence of the acute attack, and bulk-forming laxatives and bulky diets may prevent further attacks of the disease. Should recurrent attacks or complications arise (perforation, hemorrhage, fistula, obstruction, abscess), operation is indicated. Resection and primary anastomosis are the treatment of choice for those patients undergoing elective operation after meticulous preparation of the bowel. With obstruction or perforation, *exteriorization-resection* is the treatment of choice. In some cases with severe inflammation, exteriorization or primary resection is not possible, and in these cases a three-stage operative treatment is elected:

1. The obstruction is relieved by a *proximal colostomy.*
2. After the inflammation subsides (3 to 6 months), the *diseased segment is resected* and the colon ends are anastomosed.
3. After subsequent healing of the anastomosis (in 4 weeks), the *colostomy is closed* as the final stage.

When operation is indicated for massive hemorrhage, the offending segment is resected or exteriorized. In some persons requiring emergency operation for massive hemorrhage, the site of hemorrhage is not identified. In these patients the site of hemorrhage may occasionally be disclosed by selective angiography of the inferior mesenteric artery. In this rare situation the affected site alone may be resected. If the site of massive hemorrhage is not disclosed, an abdominal colectomy

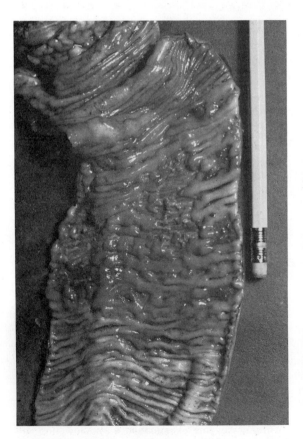

Fig. 25-4. Ulcerative colitis. Notice shallow ulcers oriented longitudinally and areas of edematous mucosa.

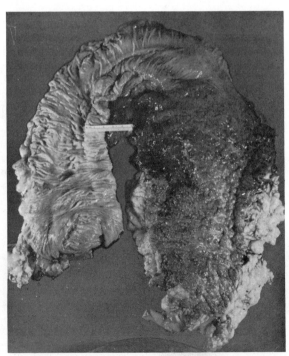

Fig. 25-5. Ulcerative colitis. There is diffuse involvement of half of specimen and pronounced pseudopolyposis.

with ileoproctostomy is recommended for these patients.

Mucosal (ulcerative) colitis

Idiopathic ulcerative colitis, or mucosal colitis, is an inflammatory disease of unknown cause that is confined to the colon and rectum and usually affects the entire large bowel, with the most pronounced disease in the distal portion. The idiopathic inflammation may be a consequence of abnormal responsiveness of the patient to his internal or external environent, exposure to a foreign agent, or both. Exogenous agents such as polysaccharides, specific bacteria, and bacterial products have been suggested, but not identified, as the cause of the disease. Similarly, vascular, neurogenic, lymphatic, and degenerative abnormalities have also been suggested as a cause of colitis. Up to now, no specific entity has been universally accepted as the cause of ulcerative colitis.

Pathology (Figs. 25-4 and 25-5). The pathological findings, most noticeable in the mucosa, feature inflammatory cells, ulcerated areas, and many small microscopic crypt abscesses. The submucosa is edematous with evidence of fibrosis. The seromuscular layer shows significantly little abnormal

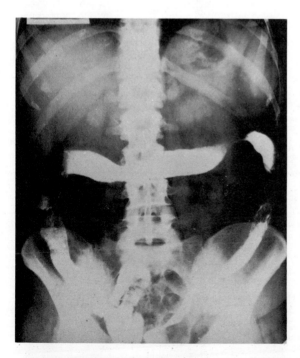

Fig. 25-6. Ulcerative colitis. Barium enema shows contraction, foreshortening, ragged mucosa, and loss of haustral markings.

reaction except in areas of perforation or abscess formation. The pathological findings vary with the clinical course. In the fulminant variety little mucosa remains and the outer colonic layers are edematous and infiltrated by inflammatory cells. In the chronic form the colon is contracted and the mesentery is fibrotic (Fig. 25-6), shortened, and edematous. Ulcerations may coalesce leaving islands of intact or proliferated mucosa known as pseudopolyps.

In the majority of patients the rectum is involved with or without retrograde involvement of the remainder of the colon. The so-called "backwash" ileitis is a nonspecific inflammation undoubtedly attributable to the propinquity of the terminal ileum to the inflamed colon. In this entity no specific mucosal lesion is found, and it is a reversible phenomenon.

Cancer of the colon develops in 4% to 6% of patients with chronic ulcerative colitis. Certain subsets of the colitic patients are identified as being particularly cancer prone: patients with pancolitis, patients whose colitis occurred during adolescence or younger, and patients whose disease has been present 10 years or longer. If all three of these factors are operative, the lifetime cancer risk exceeds 40%. Those patients likely to develop a colon cancer associated with colitis may be identified by certain cytological changes or by random biopsies of the colonic mucosa. The appearance of dysplasia or carcinoma in situ is indicative of the tendency to colitic cancer. Patients with cancer of the colon arising in ulcerative colitis have the same prognosis as their noncolitic counterparts.

Clinical course. Ulcerative colitis can occur from early childhood to late life but it is characteristically a disease of the second and third decades. It may be fulminant or chronic with exacerbations and remissions occurring over a period of years. In the fulminant presentation a bloody diarrhea with concomitant protein and blood loss characterize the disease, as well as fever, abdominal cramps, distension, and electrolyte loss. A particularly virulent form of ulcerative colitis occurs as *toxic megacolon*. In this entity there is transmural progression of the disease with destruction of the myenteric plexus; the colon passively dilates from swallowed and fermented gas. Roentgenograms of the abdomen will reveal an immensely dilated colon with asymmetrical ulcers shown in relief. Toxic megacolon is usually associated with severe constitutional manifestations of the disease subsequent to blood, protein, and electrolyte deficiencies and local septic complications.

Abnormalities of other organs such as uveitis, arthritis, stomatitis, cirrhosis, and biliary duct fibrosis accompany many chronic cases of mucosal colitis. The precise cause and relationship of these associated ailments remain obscure, but metastatic sepsis has been implicated in a number of these entities. The diagnosis of mucosal colitis is confirmed by the clinical course, the appearance of the mucosa on sigmoidoscopy, biopsy of the rectal mucosa, and the absence of specific pathogens on culture and biopsy.

Treatment. Medical treatment is successful in the majority of cases with ulcerative colitis, but 30% of the patients with ulcerative colitis will eventually require operation. The medical treatment includes sedation, repletion of specific deficiencies, bowel rest, and anti-inflammatory agents such as sulfasalazine (Azulfidine) and corticosteroids. Operation is indicated for toxic megacolon, severe hemorrhage, perforation, fistula or abscess formation, failure of medical treatment, relapsing chronic colitis, or when cancer is suspected or present. The treatment of ulcerative colitis is total proctocolectomy in one or two stages with the establishment of a permanent ileostomy. Various attempts at preservation of the rectum for eventual anastomosis have failed.

In selected persons, however, preservation of the rectal musculature with total excision of the rectal mucosa allowing an anastomosis of the terminal ileum to the anus through a muscular cuff of the rectum has achieved a varying degree of success for voluntary defecation. These patients have from five to 20 stools per day. An ileal pouch is usually constructed proximal to the ileoanal anastomosis. This procedure, the endorectal pull-through procedure, is not indicated when operation is done on an emergency basis for such entities as hemorrhage, fulminant colitis, or toxic megacolon.

Another attempt to avoid a noncontrolled stoma is the so-called continent ileostomy, or Kock ileostomy. In this procedure a prestomal pouch is constructed intra-abdominally and the patient defecates by irrigating the pouch through the stoma and its nipple valve several times per day. This procedure found wide initial acceptance, but its failure rate (reoperation in over 30% of the cases) has dimmed enthusiasm.

Transmural colitis (granulomatous colitis, Crohn's disease) (see Chapter 24)

We know now that transmural colitis involves the colon in up to 50% of all cases previously believed to be exclusively mucosal colitis. Patients with transmural colitis have much the same symptoms as those with mucosal colitis, i.e., diarrhea, abdominal cramps, and fever. We cannot differentiate between the two diseases from symptoms, but we can get help from clinical findings as outlined in Table 25-2.

The symptoms of mucosal and transmural colitis are identical; the medical treatment is also the same. Why should we bother to distinguish them? Because a precise diagnosis helps the clinician to anticipate complications, including cancer, plan the operation, and justify radical procedures (total colectomy and ileostomy) when necessary.

Diagnosis (Table 25-2). Ulcerative colitis is associated with bloody stools, rectal involvement, episodes of toxic megacolon, and the occasional development of cancer. Perianal and internal fistulas are commonly associated with Crohn's colitis, whereas carcinoma is rare. When performing an emergency operation, the surgeon often lacks preoperative information to make an accurate diag-

Table 25-2. Comparison of ulcerative colitis and Crohn's colitis

Diagnostic features	Ulcerative colitis	Crohn's colitis
Distribution	Continuous with rectum	Often discontinuous (segmental)
Rectum	Almost always involved	Often normal
Internal fistulas	Rare	Frequent
Strictures	Uncommon: suggests carcinoma	Frequent
Mucosa	Shallow ulceration may have pseudopolyps	Longitudinal fissures, cobblestone appearance
Symmetry	Symmetrical	Asymmetrical (one wall involvement)
Terminal ileum	Normal	Usually involved
Megacolon	Frequent	Less common
Colon perforation	Common	Infrequent
Operative findings		
Serositis	Absent	Common
Inflammatory masses	Rare	Frequent
Enlarged mesenteric lymph nodes	Infrequent	Usual
Anal lesions	Nonspecific	Common with granulomas present

nosis. Even postoperatively definite diagnosis will not be established in approximately 5% of patients. The appearance of the colon at the time of operation is helpful. If the diagnosis is not apparent, the surgeon must make every effort to preserve the rectum at the initial operation unless there is overwhelming rectal involvement.

Treatment. Ulcerative colitis responds to medical treatment in two thirds to three fourths of the patients. Crohn's colitis is less likely to respond to medical treatment. Crohn's colitis infrequently develops into toxic megacolon. Although cancer has been reported in Crohn's colitis, it is extremely rare and strictures may be considered benign. Similar strictures in ulcerative colitis must be considered as a carcinoma until proved otherwise.

Total colectomy and permanent ileostomy cure the patient with ulcerative colitis. A similar operation for Crohn's colitis will eventually result in recurrences in the neoileum in 10% to 16% of the patients, usually depending on the extent of initial small bowel disease.

Specific infections
Pseudomembranous colitis

Pseudomembranous colitis is discussed in Chapter 24.

Amebiasis

Amebiasis of the colon is uncommonly seen in our country, with the exception of inmates in mental institutions. Amebic infiltrates have a predi-

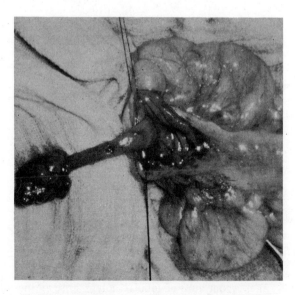

Fig. 25-7. Adenomatous polyp of colon on long stalk.

lection for the rectum and cecum. They may mimic carcinoma, or a diffuse amebic colitis may be confused with ulcerative colitis. Sigmoidoscopic examination with biopsy specimens and stool cultures usually confirms the diagnosis. Emetine and other antiamebic drugs control most cases. Complications such as the development of toxic megacolon or perforation with peritonitis or abscess formation necessitate operation.

Tuberculosis

Tuberculosis of the colon is almost always associated with pulmonary tuberculosis. A primary form, probably of bovine origin, seldom arises in our country. The typical granulomatous nature of tuberculosis involves, in the large bowel, chiefly the cecum and right colon. Although the diagnosis can be suspected preoperatively, it is seldom confirmed except at operation. When obstruction occurs, resection of the involved portion of the large bowel may be necessary. Antituberculous drugs must be used to control the systemic infection.

Bacillary infections

Bacillary infections may be confused clinically with chronic ulcerative colitis. The sigmoidoscopic findings are also similar, but bacterial culture establishes the diagnosis of bacillary dysentery.

An overgrowth of *Clostridium difficile* after administration of many of the common antibiotics may result in pseudomembranous enterocolitis or colitis. This diagnosis may be established by serological detection of the offending organism, which is best treated by cessation of the inducing antibiotic and the substitution of oral vancomycin.

Actinomycosis

Actinomyces bovis is a rare cause of human intestinal disease, though it is a relatively common inhabitant of the gastrointestinal tract. Biopsy, cultures, or hanging-drop preparations usually reveal the diagnosis. Persistent (and confusing) abdominal wall fistulas may occur, sometimes months after an operation. Treatment with new penicillin preparations has been gratifying.

NEOPLASMS

Adenomatous polyps and adenocarcinoma are the most common tumors of the colorectum. Although polyps may bleed and occasionally cause bowel obstruction, their overwhelming significance resides in the possibility of associated malignancy.

Polyps

Polyps are sessile or pedunculated (Fig. 25-7). About 70% arise within range of the sigmoido-

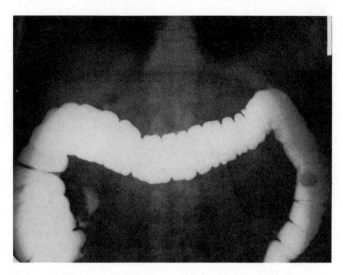

Fig. 25-8. Polyp of colon shows as filling defect on barium enema.

Table 25-3. Comparison of polyps of the large bowel

Type	Frequency	Site	Malignancy	Treatment
Tubular	Most common polyp; 10% of all adults; increases with age	Rectosigmoid 70%	Premalignant	Endoscopy and biopsy excision; excise larger upper colonic polyps
Villous	Relatively common in the aged	Rectosigmoid 80%	About 25% malignant Increases with size	Total biopsy; radical operation if malignant
Juvenile	Common in first decade; rare in adults	Chiefly rectum	Never	Excise only for bleeding, intussusception, diagnosis
Hereditary familial	Very rare	Scattered	100%	Total or near-total colectomy
Peutz-Jeghers	Very rare	Chiefly small bowel	Never (?)	Excise for bleeding or obstruction

scope and most of the others are visible through the colonoscope. Barium studies, especially air-contrast studies, outline most polyps in the upper colon (Fig. 25-8 and Table 25-3). Five chief types of polyps are seen: tubular, villous, juvenile, hereditary familial, and those associated with the Peutz-Jeghers syndrome.

Pseudopolyps

Pseudopolyps are discussed in the section on mucosal, or ulcerative, colitis, p. 241.

Adenomatous polyps

Tubular adenomatous polyps (polypoid adenomas, pedunculated polyps) are without question the most common polyps.

Age. Tubular polyps reach a peak incidence during the eighth decade. Below 20 years of age they are nonexistent (except for genetically induced multiple polyposis). Tubular polyps are more common in males than in females.

Site. About 70% of tubular polyps arise in the rectosigmoid area. A similar occurrence for carcinomas is suggestive of a casual relationship between adenomatous polyps and colorectal carcinoma.

Incidence. The incidence of tubular polyps varies with age. Clinical studies indicate that above 40 years about 10% of patients have rectosigmoid polyps. Autopsy studies indicate a much higher incidence (20% to 50%). Multiple polyps (2 to 10 polyps) occur in about 30% of all patients with polyps.

Malignant potential. The potential for malignancy is the most important factor concerning polyps. Advocates for the malignant potential of polyps cite as corroborative evidence the striking parallelism between polyps and cancer in (1) location, (2) age and sex incidence, (3) frequent association of polyps and cancer, (4) the absolute 100% incidence of cancer with familial polyposis, and (5) the occasional finding of an invasive cancer arising in an adenomatous polyp.

At the present time the evidence is overwhelming that tubular adenomatous polyps and villous adenomatous polyps are premalignant. There is general agreement that wide-based polyps and large polyps (greater than 2 cm. in diameter) are often sites of occult malignancy and should be totally excised for whole-mount examination.

Treatment. *Sigmoidoscopic removal* of polyps is usually safe and simply accomplished. Wide-based rectal polyps are removed by transanal excision (after sphincter dilatation) and direct suture closure.

Colonoscopy has added a dramatic new dimension to upper colonic polypectomy (or biopsy). Experienced colonoscopists can reach the cecum in about 90% of all patients, and they can successfully visualize (and biopsy or excise) an even larger percentage of polyps within the distal colon. By preempting laparotomy, colonoscopy has made polypectomy safer for many patients and allowed biopsies of wide-based polyps that help select those lesions that require laparotomy and excision.

Celiotomy and polypectomy. Polyps that defy visualization and excision by sigmoidoscopy or colonoscopy necessitate celiotomy and polypectomy. Multiple polyps throughout the colon require abdominal colectomy with ileosigmoid or ileorectal anastomosis as indicated. The premalignant potential of adenomatous polyps demands an aggressive course of removal.

Laparotomy and polypectomy. The student should realize that repated diagnostic barium enema studies and endoscopy are time consuming, costly, and uncomfortable. For those patients who accept repeated examinations reluctantly or diffidently, laparotomy may prove to be the most prudent plan.

Villous adenomas

Villous adenomas (villous papilloma, villous tumor, papillary adenoma, and true papilloma) are velvety, broad-based tumors that may grow to encircle the bowel. About 80% reside in the rectum. In contrast to cancer, which they resemble, they are usually soft and pliable, so soft, in fact, that they can be missed by digital examination of the rectum.

Malignant potential. Although some surgeons look upon villous adenomas as malignant tumors per se, only about one fifth of the tumors are actually malignant. The percentage increases with the size of the tumor so that tumors of 5 cm. or more may be considered to always harbor an occult carcinoma.

Treatment. Most villous adenomas (1) occur in older persons, (2) occur in the rectum, and (3) have broad bases (therefore small biopsy specimens are inconclusive). Combined abdominoperineal resection, which would be required for most of these rectal lesions if malignant, carries an imposing mortality in aged patients. Therefore *total biopsy* of the tumor with frozen-section diagnosis of several cross sections of the tumor helps greatly in the determination of whether radical resection is necessary. If the lesion is benign, nothing more need be done: if it is malignant, a cancer operation is performed. In some critical-risk patients focal cancer has been treated by such local resections alone—or cauterization—in deference to the forbidding mortality of radical operations.

In no instance has malignant recurrence occurred after total biopsy of benign tumors in our experience. In rare instances severe fluid and electrolyte problems have been caused by the copious diarrhea (mucorrhea) that these patients so frequently exhibit. Potassium loss is especially high. Large tumors can be removed by spreading the sphincters and direct excision. Coccygectomy and posterior proctotomy help to expose lesions high in the rectum.

Juvenile polyps

Juvenile polyps are hamartomas, not true neoplasms. Grossly they are smooth, round, and cherry red and exude mucus when cut across; microscopically they are characterized by mucoid cystic spaces with a large amount of interstitial fibrous tissue. Generally single, they occur most frequently in the first decade of life and tend to disappear spontaneously. Because of bleeding they may be a persistent nuisance. They rarely induce intussusception, and *malignancy never occurs* in juvenile polyps. Biopsy excision to control bleeding or to differentiate familial polyposis should be the extent of treatment. Indiscriminant radical

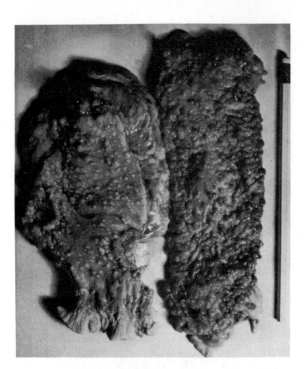

Fig. 25-9. Multiple polyposis of colon.

colectomy for juvenile polyposis is a surgical tragedy. The polyps in a patient with multiple or scattered polyps will almost invariably share the same histological pattern; thus, if the physician can prove microscopically that one accessible polyp is of the juvenile variety, he need not remove any others unless they are symptomatic.

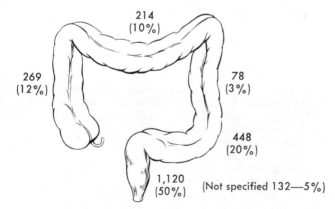

Fig. 25-10. Sites of 2,261 colorectal cancers at University of Iowa Hospitals, 1940 to 1960.

Familial polyposis

Familial polyps will become malignant in 100% of the instances. This rare inheritable trait is autosomal dominant and may be transmitted by either parent (Fig. 25-9). The polyps rarely appear before adolescence, and in some instances they appear sporadically because of a mutant gene.

Treatment. Either total removal of the rectum and colon with ileostomy or total colectomy with preservation of the rectum (an ileoproctostomy) must be performed. It is generally accepted that if there are fewer than 20 polyps in the rectum as encountered by proctoscopy an ileorectal anastomosis is "safe." The experience of several centers does not bear this out, however, and it is advisable to remove all rectal mucosa. The advent of the endorectal pullthrough operation is ideal for patients with familial polyposis so that the voluntary sphincter may be preserved with all the premalignant mucosa excised.

After he diagnoses familial polyposis, the physician's responsibility includes surveillance of all other members of the family who might carry the inheritable trait.

Peutz-Jeghers syndrome

Peutz-Jeghers syndrome is discussed in Chapter 24.

Adenocarcinoma

Adenocarcinoma of the colon and rectum rivals lung cancer as the most common killing cancer in humans. About 60% of these tumors lie within range of the sigmoidoscope; now that the colonoscope can reach the remaining 40%, diagnostic efficiency should improve (Fig. 25-10).

Epidemiology. Mortality for colorectal cancer is high in North America, western Europe, Australia, and Israel and in patients with ulcerative colitis or familial polyposis. Colorectal cancer is uncommon in Asia and Africa. Burkitt hypothesizes that low-fiber, high-sugar diets induce colon and rectal cancers.

Age. The relative incidence of colorectal cancer increases with age; 90% appear in patients past 40 years of age. Under 30 years of age, familial polyposis and ulcerative colitis often coexist. The prognosis in youthful cases (mostly mucoid carcinoma) is poor.

Symptoms. Alteration in bowel habits, blood in or with the stools, obstruction, and anemia keynote the symptoms. *Anemia* is most common with right-sided colon lesions because the tumors are characteristically polypoid, and the ileal contents that bathe these tumors are caustic (Fig. 25-11, *A*). An unexplained iron-deficiency anemia in an adult over the age of 40 must be considered to be a gastrointestinal neoplasm until proved otherwise.

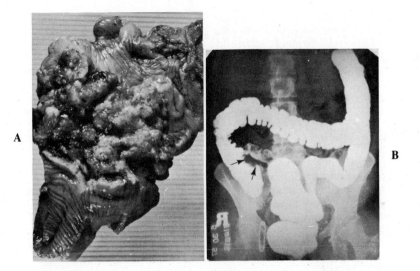

Fig. 25-11. A, Polypoid, ulcerating carcinoma of cecum. Distal ileum at left. **B,** Barium enema with arrows marking filling defect of cecal carcinoma.

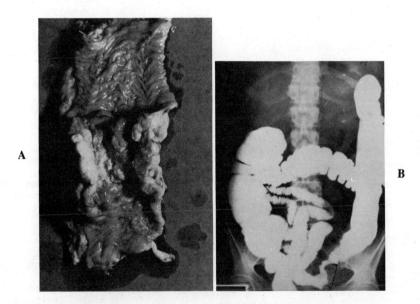

Fig. 25-12. A, Annular, constricting carcinoma of sigmoid colon. **B,** Barium enema outlining "apple core" defect of sigmoid carcinoma shown in **A.**

Obstruction predominates in left-sided colon lesions because of a narrower lumen, firmer feces, and a characteristic annular lesion at this location (Fig. 25-12, *A*).

Diagnosis. *Physical signs* are often scant. Masses are sometimes palpable, most often by rectal examination, and stools usually show blood, sometimes grossly but most often in the occult form. Endoscopy greatly aids early diagnosis.

The adoption of the "Hemocult" examination for occult blood in the stool has added greatly to the early diagnosis of carcinoma of the colon. For this the patient merely abstains from meat for 3 days and sends to his physician paper folders containing minute specimens of stool. A "positive" report for occult blood is then followed up by appropriate examination. It has been gratifying to see the patient and physician response to this easy and inexpensive examination, and it has resulted in the detection of many early carcinomas and polyps.

Barium enema examination and colonoscopy help detect colonic cancers above the reach of the sigmoidoscope (Figs. 25-11, *B*, and 25-12, *B*).

Differential diagnosis. Since large polyps that resemble carcinomas should be removed (Fig. 25-13), they present few diagnostic problems. Distinguishing diverticulitis from cancer, usually in the sigmoid colon, is the major diagnostic problem. Even at laparotomy some cases defy diagnosis until the specimen is opened. (Cancers always involve mucosa; diverticulitis causes mucosal edema.) Since diverticulosis and cancer of the colon may coexist, barium studies seldom exclude carcinoma absolutely. Colonoscopy often will. If, however, the diagnosis remains in question, the surgeon must assume the "worst" and perform an appropri-

ate cancer operation. This will obviously cure the complication of the diverticulitis and give the greatest chance for cure in any cancer.

Tuberculosis and other infections and benign tumors (lipoma, fibroma, mucocele of the appendix, endometriosis) are on rare occasions mistaken for carcinoma of the colorectum. In all such cases, biopsy diagnosis must exclude colorectal cancer.

Metastases. Metastases from large bowel cancers spread in a number of ways: (1) intramurally, (2) lymphatic spread, (3) venous spread, (4) implantation within the bowel lumen—often by the surgeon at the time of resection, (5) direct extension, and (6) transperitoneal spread. Two factors that influence the prognosis of a colorectal lesion are the depth of penetration of the bowel wall by the tumor and the presence or absence of regional lymph node metastases. Several classifications are used to describe colorectal cancers. These are as follows:

Dukes' classification	*Extent of disease*	*5-year survival (%)*
A	Confined to bowel wall	80-90
B	Extension into pericolic tissues; nodes—negative	50
C	Involving adjacent structures; nodes—positive	20

Astler-Coller classification	*Extent of disease*
A	Confined to mucosa
B1	Extension into the muscularis propria; nodes negative
B2	Penetration of the muscularis propria; nodes negative
C1	Extension to the muscularis propria; nodes positive
C2	Penetration of the muscularis propria; nodes positive

TNM classification	*Extent of disease*
T1	Mucosal or submucosal involvement
T2	Involvement of the muscular wall
T3	Involvement of all layers of the colon with extension to immediately adjacent structures
T4	Fistula present
T5	Tumor is spread by direct extension beyond the immediately adjacent organs or tissues
N0	Regional nodes not involved
N1	Regional nodes involved
M0	No known distant metastases
M1	Distant metastases present

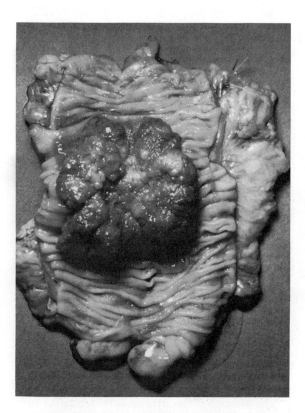

Fig. 25-13. Large polypoid carcinoma of colon.

T designates primary tumor, *N* designates lymph nodes, and *M* designates distal metastases. Example: A modified Duke's B2 would be under the TMN classification T2 N0 M0. Survival is inversely proportional to extent of disease by any staging method.

Treatment. The aim of treatment of colorectal cancer is to remove the cancer with its areas of local extension and areas of lymphatic spread (Table 25-4). During these procedures, early ligation of the venous return and ligation of the bowel above and below the tumor have been advocated to help prevent operative dissemination of cancer cells. Up to now neither laboratory nor clinical proof indicates that either of these two maneuvers substantially decrease local or systemic recurrences.

Operations are designed to remove the lymph node–bearing tissue, contiguous bowel, and any adjacent organs involved by the tumor such as small bowel, bladder, uterus, etc.

Major colonic resections are preceded by a thorough cleansing of the bowel by (1) a clear liquid diet, (2) a laxative, and (3) enemas. An attractive alternative to this is the oral administration of large amounts (5 to 7 liters) of a balanced saline solution containing potassium before operation for patients whose tumor is not obstructing the gut. Obviously, patients with congestive heart disease or kidney failure are not candidates for such massive fluid administration. For healthier patients this has proved to be an excellent and rapid method for mechanical cleansing. Most surgeons use some type of preoperative antibiotics to reduce the concentration and total number of gut organisms. The prophylactic antibiotics may be utilized either orally or systemically. If systemic antibiotics are adopted, no more than two postoperative doses are necessary, but the preoperative dose must be given early enough so that an adequate blood-and-tissue level are present at the time of incision. Whether or not systemic or oral antibiotics are utilized, all surgeons agree that a thorough mechanical cleansing is the most important factor in the preoperative preparation of the colon.

Prognosis. Results vary with age, extent of tumor, pathological type of tumor, location of tumor, the presence or absence of involved nodes, associated diseases (ulcerative colitis or familial polyposis), and the operation performed. A summation of the prognostic importance of these factors follows, highlighted (as in many other cancers) by the presence or absence of involved lymph nodes:

1. Without positive lymph nodes, the 5-year survival is about 80%; with positive lymph nodes, the 5-year survival is about 60%. In *all* cases the 5-year survival is more than 50%.
2. Transverse colon cancers have a poor prognosis.
3. Men and blacks show a poorer prognosis in all age groups.
4. Large bowel cancers in young people (below 40 years) have a poor prognosis.
5. Rectal cancers that originate *above* the peritoneal reflection have a better prognosis than those that originate *below* the peritoneal reflection.
6. Obstructing and perforating cancers of the colon have a poor prognosis.
7. If the colon is not removed in *familial polyposis*, almost all patients will develop cancer by 50 years of age.
8. Cancer associated with chronic mucosal colitis is especially vicious.
9. Radiation therapy decreases pain in many advanced cases, but neither radiation nor chemotherapy increases survival.

Table 25-4. Operations for colorectal carcinoma

Tumor site	Operation	Anastomosis or colostomy
Cecum, ascending colon	Right colectomy	Ileum to midtransverse colon
Hepatic flexure	Right and transverse colectomy	Ileum to midtransverse or left transverse colon
Transverse colon	Right, transverse, and upper left colectomy	Ileum to upper descending colon
Splenic flexure	Right, transverse, and upper left colectomy	Terminal ileum to descending colon
Descending colon, sigmoid colon	Left colectomy	Left transverse colon to rectosigmoid
Rectum	Left lower colectomy with low anastomosis or anal anastomosis; abdominoperineal resection	Descending colon to rectal stump; terminal sigmoid colostomy

TRAUMA

Trauma to the large bowel may be *penetrating* or *blunt*. *Penetrating* wounds may occur from *outside* (knife wounds, missile wounds) or *inside* from objects inserted into the rectum (thermometers, sigmoidoscopes, enemas) or swallowed (safety pins, toothpicks, fishbones). *Blunt trauma* is most common from automobile accidents in civilian life and from blast injuries in combat military personnel. Improperly worn seat belts (which ride too high) can themselves induce intra-abdominal injury.

Diagnosis. The extent of *penetrating* wounds from the outside is usually indeterminant from examination of the wound. Probing small abdominal wall wounds is misleading, since contraction of the musculofascial layers overrides and obscures the original tract. Most penetrating abdominal injuries demand immediate laparotomy.

In all instances of abdominal trauma two serious threats arise; (1) *bleeding* and (2) *perforation*. If sufficient blood is lost (1,000 to 1,500 ml.), shock occurs. The bleeding vessel must be ligated. With losses of lesser amounts of blood, the findings are more subtle. In these instances, paracentesis or peritoneal lavage (500 to 1,000 ml. of balanced salt solution through a peritoneal dialysis catheter, then evacuated by placement of the bottle on the floor) gives the most accurate information. Blood (above 100,000 RBC/cu. mm.), bile, bacteria, or amylase indicates intraperitoneal disease.

Perforation is suggested by abdominal pain and tenderness (the "acute abdomen," discussed in Chapter 20). The diagnosis of perforation of a hollow viscus is not always easy, since trauma to the abdominal wall may induce both pain and tenderness within the wall itself.

Plain and upright films of the abdomen are helpful, since free peritoneal air is diagnostic of perforation of a hollow viscus. Negative films for free air, however, do *not* rule out perforation since small amounts of free air may be overlooked. Thus frequent, repetitive examinations, abdominal films, and peritoneal lavage form the core of successful management of the patient with possible colon damage.

Treatment. When intraperitoneal hemorrhage or perforation is diagnosed, operative treatment must be immediate. In perforation the elapsed time since the injury determines treatment. When the patient arrives soon (within 4 to 6 hours) after the wound and peritoneal soilage is limited, simple closure of the wound may suffice. When the patient arrives late and peritoneal soilage is extensive, exteriorization of the damaged bowel segment (when possible) or a diverting colostomy when exteriorization is technically difficult are the treatments of choice. In penetrating wounds of the abdominal wall, when uncertainty exists concerning intraperitoneal damage, watchful waiting and diagnostic laparotomy are the two main therapeutic options. Laparotomy is, of course, the most certain plan, but under battlefield conditions or with multiple-person injuries in civilian practice, the physician must sort out the patients who require operation from those he can keep under observation. In battle wounds, high-velocity missiles may damage a wide area around the wound because of shock waves. Wide débridement of the bowel wall before closure helps prevent necrosis.

26
Anorectum

Samuel D. Porter
Richard D. Liechty

In terms of physical agony (from painful anorectal disorders) or mental anguish (from concern with bowel function or cancer) the anorectum assumes an importance that belies its insignificant anatomical status; e.g., hemorrhoids are one of the commonest of all human ailments. The pain from one small, thrombosed, external hemorrhoid can completely overwhelm an otherwise healthy person.

In our cancer-conscious generation, fresh blood on the toilet paper or a lump appearing at the anus sends patients trembling to their physicians, even though both signs often result from simple hemorrhoids.

The anorectum, the site of a variety of disorders (both simple and complex), is an area of understandable patient concern.

ANATOMY

Pertinent anatomical points are shown in Figs. 26-1 and 26-2:

1. The anatomical *key* to the anorectum is the *pectinate line*.
2. *Above it* pain sensation is absent, blood drains to the portal system and vena cava, and lymph drains along the superior rectal vessels or lateral to the obturator or iliac nodes.
3. *Below* the pectinate line pain is notably present, blood drains to the inferior vena cava, and lymph drains to the inguinal nodes.
4. *Anal glands* empty into anal crypts at the pectinate line. When obstructed or infected, these glands become the source of abscesses and fistulas.

PHYSIOLOGY

When the rectosigmoid colon distends with feces, autonomic nerve impulses stimulate the colon to contract involuntarily, forcing the feces toward the anus. Voluntary relaxation of the tonically contracted puborectalis and external sphincter muscles permits this passage.

Chronic or injudicious use of laxatives thwarts this remarkably efficient mechanism by stimulating the colon when the rectum is *not* distended with feces. This process, repeated many times, results in temporary loss of the natural response. Thus habitual laxative (or enema) use becomes physiologically disrupting in the vain effort to "regulate" (or coerce) bowel movements.

When laxatives liquefy the stool, another disruption occurs. Normal stools (the consistency and shape of bananas) gently compress the anal canal, "milking" the anal glands and crypts. Chronically liquid stools lack this milking effect. Thus liquid stools bathe the crypts and glands with bacteria; chronic cryptitis and anal gland infection result. The increased frequency of anal disease in patients who practice chronic self-purgation is, we are convinced, more than coincidental.

Regular bowel movements are obtained by a balanced diet, exercise, adequate fluid intake, and heed to nature's demands. Laxatives and enemas for constipation in an otherwise healthy person should be condemned for what they are—nostrums.

EXAMINATION

In no other area of the body is physical examination more important than in the anus and rectum.

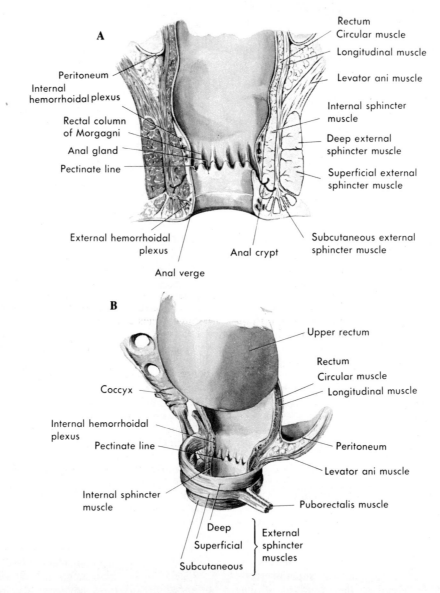

A

Peritoneum
Internal hemorrhoidal plexus
Rectal column of Morgagni
Anal gland
Pectinate line

External hemorrhoidal plexus
Anal verge
Anal crypt

Rectum
Circular muscle
Longitudinal muscle
Levator ani muscle
Internal sphincter muscle
Deep external sphincter muscle
Superficial external sphincter muscle
Subcutaneous external sphincter muscle

B

Coccyx
Internal hemorrhoidal plexus
Pectinate line
Internal sphincter muscle
Deep
Superficial
Subcutaneous
External sphincter muscles

Upper rectum
Rectum
Circular muscle
Longitudinal muscle
Peritoneum
Levator ani muscle
Puborectalis muscle

Fig. 26-1. A, Vertical section of anorectum. **B,** Anorectum. Three-dimensional diagram showing relationship of external sphincter to internal sphincter; notice that superficial portion of external sphincter inserts into both coccyx and pubis.

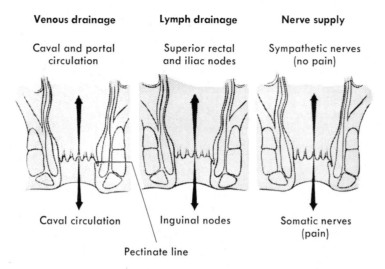

Venous drainage   **Lymph drainage**   **Nerve supply**

Caval and portal circulation   Superior rectal and iliac nodes   Sympathetic nerves (no pain)

Caval circulation   Inguinal nodes   Somatic nerves (pain)

Pectinate line

Fig. 26-2. Pectinate line marks important differences in nerve supply, venous drainage, and lymph drainage.

For complete examination, three important elements are good illumination, proper positioning, and patient cooperation.

Inspection of the perianal area can yield much information. Excoriations from scratching (in pruritus), fissures, external fistulas, external hemorrhoids, abscesses, and occasionally tumors can be seen.

Digital examination of the rectum should be an integral part of *all* physical examinations except when preempted by pain (anal fissure). In this situation the digital examination is performed with anesthesia or is deferred until acute inflammation subsides. Sphincter tone, prostatic size, point tenderness, extrinsic or intrinsic rectal masses, pelvic hernias, or a "rectal shelf" (tumor deposits in the cul-de-sac) is noted. Remember that *many large bowel malignant tumors can be palpated by rectal examination*. A specimen of stool from the examining finger is immediately available for testing for occult blood.

Anoscopy is carried out simply and without prior enemas. The diseases of the anorectum that can be observed or palpated are discussed in the next section. (Sigmoidoscopy is discussed in Chapter 25.)

DISEASES OF THE ANORECTUM
Hemorrhoids

Internal hemorrhoids are dilated veins of the superior and middle rectal plexuses that occur above the dentate line and underlie mucosa. *External hemorrhoids* are dilated inferior rectal veins

that lie below the dentate line and are covered by squamous epithelium. Factors that increase pressure in these venous systems are theoretically responsible for development of hemorrhoids. The common ones are constipation, straining at stool, hereditary varicose tendencies, pregnancy, prolonged upright position, abdominal or pelvic tumors, and portal hypertension. Chronic anal infection from colitis and ileitis, or chronic laxative usage may also dilate the vein walls by causing chronic cryptitis and anal vein phlebitis with consequent dilatation.

Bleeding, protrusion, dull *pain,* and *pruritus* (in any combination) characterize uncomplicated hemorrhoids. Thrombosis or acute prolapse (with edema or ulceration) is exquisitely painful. Toxic symptoms may accompany acute episodes.

The diagnosis is usually obvious from inspection, but diagnostic efforts must *always* include barium studies and sigmoidoscopy to rule out other large bowel disease. Many patients with colon cancer have had hemorrhoidectomies *shortly before* the cancer was diagnosed.

Treatment. The three common indications for hemorrhoidectomy are *pain, prolapse,* and *bleeding.* Since most adults eventually develop hemorrhoids, excision is advised only when symptoms warrant the risk and inconvenience.

Treatment of an acutely thrombosed external hemorrhoid is incision and evacuation of the painful clot, followed by warm sitz baths. Small internal hemorrhoids may be injected with a sclerosing solution with good success. This promotes microthrombi formation and ultimate fibrosis of the hemorrhoid. Sodium morrhuate and 5% phenol in oil are commonly used solutions for injection. Rubber band ligation of internal hemorrhoids is now the preferred treatment.

Larger external hemorrhoids and internal hemorrhoids, which are symptomatic, are surgically excised. All methods of hemorrhoid removal have the same goal: the complete removal of the hemorrhoids with preservation of an intact, functional anus.

After hemorrhoidectomy an important problem is control of pain. Pain followed by perianal muscle spasm induces many postoperative complications, such as urinary retention, constipation, fecal impaction, and pulmonary difficulties caused by immobilization. Pain is alleviated by warm, moist packs, adequate analgesia, and maintenance of a soft stool. Gentle daily digital dilatation for several days promotes normal healing and discourages stenosis.

Anal fissure

Anal fissures are slitlike ulcers in the anal mucosa. They are, of course, always infected. The commonest causes are (1) trauma, usually from passage of hard stool, (2) cryptitis, in which the anal crypts become inflamed and subsequently develop a mucosal break that extends distally, and (3) ulceration of mucosa over a thrombosed hemorrhoid. Spasms of the anal sphincters (by decreasing blood flow) help sustain anal fissures.

These fissures occur most frequently in the posterior midline. A "sentinel tag," a small projection of skin, usually lies just below and marks the fissure.

Severe pain with defecation and blood-streaked stools characterize anal fissures. The anus is, of course, greatly sensitive to digital examination.

Anal fissures are treated conservatively by scrupulous anal hygiene, hot sitz baths, and stool softeners. If the fissure does not heal within 3 weeks, *sphincter dilatation* (under anesthesia), *fissurectomy*, and *partial sectioning* of the *internal sphincter* or the *external sphincter* (subcutaneous portion) are the operative options. These procedures used alone or in combination are advocated with varying degrees of enthusiasm. They have in common relaxation of the sphincter mechanism. We prefer internal division of the partial sphincter. With sphincter muscle spasm relieved, stool passage is easier, which aids healing. Complicated fissures occasionally progress to abscesses, fistulas, or anal stenosis.

Anorectal abscesses and fistulas

Since fistulas are the result of perianal abscesses, these diseases are discussed together. *Perianal abscesses* almost invariably result from infected anal glands that erode into underlying tissues. Chronic use of purgatives, regional enteritis, and ulcerative colitis have liquid stools in common, as a probable causative factor. Uncommon infections (actinomycosis, tuberculosis, other fungal diseases), pelvic inflammatory disease, prostatitis, and cancer may rarely be associated.

Fig. 26-3 shows the common locations of these abscesses. Opinions vary as to frequency of occurrence in various anatomical sites. The ischiorectal abscess is probably the most common.

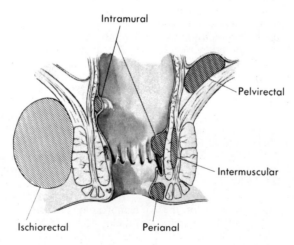

Fig. 26-3. Location of pelvirectal and perirectal abscesses. Infections in anal crypts are usual source.

Early symptoms of dull rectal aching and mild systemic complaints progress to severe, throbbing perianal pain with fever, chills, and malaise. A fluctuant, "pointing" area is not always apparent because of the thick perianal skin. Redness, tenderness, and a generalized bulging are the usual findings. Prompt incision and drainage *without* waiting for fluctuation (as in other subcutaneous infections) can prevent serious extensions. We have seen mutilating extensions that involved thighs, scrotum, and even the abdominal wall. Because of severe pain, general or regional anesthesia is preferable, but some surgeons drain perirectal abscesses under local anesthesia.

Supralevator abscesses. Supralevator abscesses are uncommon. Anal gland infections and pelvic or intraperitoneal infections engender these abscesses.

Intramural abscesses. Intramural abscesses cause little discomfort since the bowel wall has no pain sensation. They are drained through a sigmoidoscope. Pelvirectal abscesses are drained through the skin. Drains are always brought out through *external* incisions.

Perirectal fistulas. Most perirectal abscesses, after drainage, eventually heal with no sequelae. But those that fail to heal primarily evolve into fistulas. The external opening may close temporarily only to recur when pus accumulates in the tract and eventually the tract becomes lined with epithelium. Multiple openings ("pepper pot anus")

complicate some cases. Extensions to the urinary tract, perineal area, thighs, or bone may occasionally occur.

Usually the fistulous tract follows a variable course, but a few general rules are available for simplification:

1. The primary or internal opening is usually found in one of the anal crypts.
2. Most lie at one side or the other of the posterior midline.
3. If the cutaneous opening is anterior to a *transverse* line drawn through the anus, the internal opening is on a radial line directly into the anorectum. If the cutaneous opening is posterior to the line, the internal opening will probably be in the posterior midline (Fig. 26-4, *A*).

Symptoms are usually confined to intermittent swelling, drainage, pruritus, and varying discomfort. The history of an abscess is of obvious help in the diagnosis.

The cutaneous opening is characteristically a slightly raised, gray-pink papule of granulation tissue. In time scarring along the tract becomes palpable. A probe can sometimes be passed through the fistula to the pectinate line. This is ordinarily not painful. Common courses of anal fistulas are shown in Fig. 26-4, *B*.

Simple, early fistulas are incised with saucerization (excision of the overhanging margins) of the tract. In severely scarred fistulas, excision of the

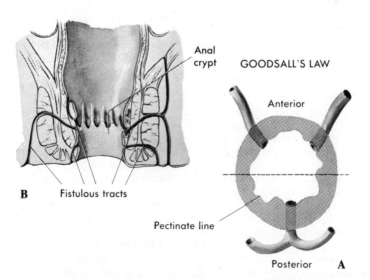

Fig. 26-4. A, Anorectal fistulas. Location of external fistulous opening is key to position of internal opening. **B,** Common courses of anorectal fistulous tracts. Internal (primary) opening is almost always in crypt; fistulas are usually single and involve only portions of sphincter muscles; multiple fistulas or fistulas that involve all external sphincter muscles are less common.

tract, leaving the skin open, is the best method of removal. In either case the internal opening must be obliterated or the fistula will recur. If the fistula follows a course that necessitates cutting of the sphincter, the incision must traverse the muscle fibers perpendicularly and *at only one level;* none of the muscle should be removed.

If the fistula is the result of carcinoma, tuberculosis, Crohn's disease, or mucosal colitis, the primary disease must of course receive treatment priority. Most surgeons are extremely reluctant to perform anorectal operations on patients with mucosal colitis or Crohn's disease because of local recurrence with failure of wound healing.

Pruritus ani

Pruritus ani, intense itching of the perianal area, is a symptom, not a disease. Common and frequently dibilitating, it offers a constant therapeutic challenge. A busy general practitioner will see numerous patients every month with this complaint.

A classification of etiological factors is listed below:

Surgical: Hemorrhoids, fissures, fistulas, prolapse, cryptitis, neoplasm
Nonsurgical:
   Local: Dermatitis, bacterial, fungal, contact; pinworms, antibiotic irritation
   Systemic: Jaundice, diabetes, psoriasis, syphilis, seborrheic dermatitis, leukemia
   Idiopathic: Including psychophysiological

With such a broad spectrum of causes, the necessity for cultures and other pertinent laboratory tests is obvious.

Treatment. Underlying anatomical factors are treated surgically (fissures, fistulas, hemorrhoids, or neoplasm). Similarly, in systemic conditions, such as diabetes or jaundice, or with local irritants and infestations, such as antibiotics or pinworms, the offending cause is specifically treated. "Smothering" symptoms with local treatments (for specific disorders) is unacceptable.

Even after extensive search a cause of pruritus ani often remains elusive. *Idiopathic pruritus* accounts for approximately half of the patients seen. The single common denominator in all patients with this complaint is feces being excreted through the anus and thus perianal fecal irritation. Immaculate perianal hygiene alone will often relieve the itching. The perianal area should be washed with water and dried with cotton or a soft cotton cloth. Cornstarch applications help to keep the area dry. Hydrocortisone ointment, 1%, is nonspecific, but

usually helpful. Many patients suffer from anxiety states.

Subcutaneous alcohol injections, radiation therapy, and presacral neurectomy are heroic treatments reserved for a very few, truly intractable patients with pruritus ani.

Prolapse of the rectum

The three types of rectal prolapse (Fig. 26-5) are: (1) mucosal prolapse, (2) rectal intussusception, and (3) true prolapse.

Mucosal prolapse (Fig. 26-5, *B*) occurs with an intact sphincter and involves extrusion through the anus of *rectal mucosa* only. The remainder of the wall is not involved. It becomes symptomatic because of irritation and occasionally ulceration of the prolapsed tissue. Soiling results from mucosal secretions. This condition is common in infancy (theoretically because of the lack of sacral curvature) and in the aged. Infant prolapse almost invariably disappears by 5 years of age. In the adult radial incisions, similar to hemorrhoidectomy incisions, result in scarring, which holds redundant mucosa in place.

Rectal intussusception (Fig. 26-5, *C*) involves protrusion of the entire rectal wall, without a peritoneal sac. It starts above the pectinate line. The palpable full-thickness wall in the prolapsed portion and *concentric* folds distinguish it from mucosal prolapse. A sulcus can be palpated along the periphery of the prolapsed part of the anal ring that is *not* present in true prolapse.

True prolapse (Fig. 26-5, *D*) occurs by herniation of the pelvic peritoneum through the pelvic diaphragm, the anterior rectal wall, and the anus. The anal sphincter tone is poor. True prolapse occurs mainly in infants, men in their twenties or thirties, and woman at any age. In men it probably represents a congenital weakness because the prostate and seminal vesicles lend adequate support anteriorly to prevent herniation.

Several operations have been devised for correction of intussusception and true prolapse, and, as is usually the case when several operations are used for a particular condition, all leave something to be desired. The operations that give the best results utilize obliteration of the peritoneal sac, shortening and fixation of the rectosigmoid colon, and approximation of the levator ani muscles.

Specific infections

Specific infections of the anorectum are uncommon yet must be remembered when sinus tracts, ulcers, or tumors appear that defy the usual categorization or treatment. The venereal diseases listed in Table 26-1 may be the offenders in such instances.

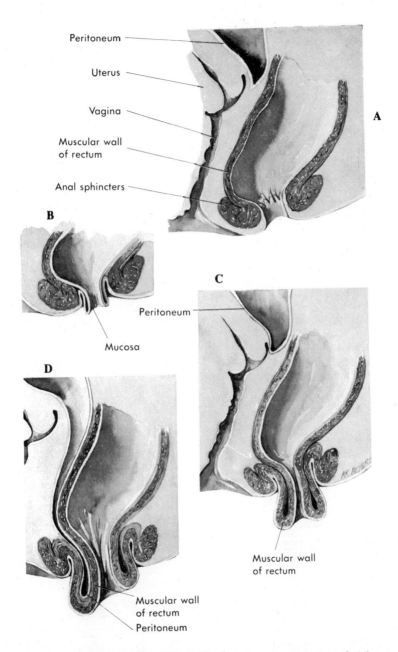

Fig. 26-5. Rectal prolapse. **A,** Normal. **B,** Mucosal prolapse most common type of prolapse; mucosa shows radial folds. **C,** Rectal intussusception; all layers of rectal wall prolapse—peritoneum does not. **D,** True prolapse; all layers of rectal wall prolapse; peritoneum descends as hernial sac anteriorly. Both **C** and **D** show concentric folds from accordion-like effect of mucosa that has not been depicted.

Table 26-1. Venereal diseases

Type	Cause	Diagnosis	Treatment
Lymphogranuloma venereum	Virus	Frei test; biopsy	Noneffective
Condyloma acuminatum	Virus	Biopsy; multiple warts	Podophyllin (25%); electrocautery
Syphilis	Spirochetes	Biopsy; dark-field examination	Penicillin ⎱ Other antibiotics
Gonorrhea	Bacteria	Smear; intracellular diplococci	Penicillin ⎰

Anorectal tumors

Basal cell carcinomas and *melanoma* of the anus are curiosities treated by wide excision (as in other parts of the body) with or without preoperative irradiation.

Epidermoid carcinoma of the anus occurs in the elderly, is associated with chronic infection (an excellent reason for biopsy of chronic lesions), and metastasizes to pelvic and inguinal nodes. (Inguinal nodes are also involved with anal infections.) Radical abdominoperineal resection with resection of involved inguinal lymph nodes (or, in low, early lesions, conservative resection) appears to offer about the same 5-year survivals as rectal adenocarcinoma.

Pilonidal sinus

Although not arising from the anorectum, pilonidal disease often enters the differential diagnosis of anorectal diseases; it can mimic anorectal abscesses or fistulas.

As the name suggests, a nidus of hair is almost invariably found within these sinus tracts. Almost all the hairs enter the sinus *root end first.* Hair scales pointing away from the root end (like feathers on an arrow) apparently are driven inward by a rolling action between the buttocks. Hair *follicles* or other skin appendages are *never* found within the sinus walls. These lesions occur in the intergluteal region of young hirsute males and less commonly in females. Pilonidal disease is common in young military personnel. It almost never occurs in person 45 years of age or older. An analogous pilonidal sinus occasionally afflicts the hands of barbers by indriven hairs.

Infection with rupture through the skin (which forms sinuses), chronicity, and recurrence keynote the problem. Simple incision and drainage of infected cysts and excision with open healing of chronic sinuses have evolved, since World War II, as the most prudent treatment. Excision with primary closure is preferred by some surgeons.

27
Abdominal Hernias

Robert T. Soper
Kevin C. Pringle

A *hernia* is an abnormal protrusion of an organ or tissue through an aperture, or opening. Thus the brain may herniate through the foramen magnum or the lung through a thoracotomy incision. Usually, however, the word is restricted to describe an abdominal hernia, i.e., an abnormal opening in the abdominal wall through which protrusion of intra-abdominal viscera occurs.

Hernial apertures, or openings, generally represent defects in the musculofascial tissues surrounding and supporting the abdominal cavity. These defects may be congenital or acquired. A pouch of peritoneum (the hernial sac) pushes through the fascial defect (the hernial ring) and then abdominal contents enter this sac because of continuity with the intra-abdominal cavity. The neck of the hernia sac is that portion protruding through the musculofascial defect and defining its narrowest dimension. The omentum, small bowel, large bowel, stomach, and urinary bladder are the most common organs that herniate into hernia sacs in roughly descending frequency.

The status of the contents of the hernial sac is of extreme clinical importance and is defined by the following descriptive adjectives:

1. A *reducible* hernia is one in which the organs contained within the hernia sac can be returned to the abdominal cavity.
2. An *irreducible* hernia is one in which the hernia sac contents cannot be returned to the abdominal cavity without operative reduction.
3. An *incarcerated* hernia (Fig. 27-1, *B*) is synonymous with an irreducible hernia. Neither

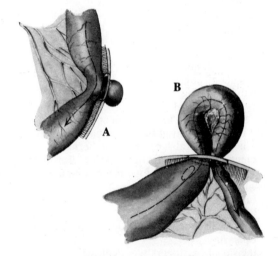

Fig. 27-1. A, Richter's hernia. Only a portion of bowel passes through hernial ring; arrow indicates that bowel need not be obstructed mechanically even with strangulation. **B,** Incarcerated hernia. Distended bowel in hernia cannot return to abdomen through narrow fascial defect.

of these terms implies intestinal obstruction or vascular interference.

4. A *strangulated* hernia is one in which the blood supply to the herniated viscus is compromised. Infarction of the viscus occurs if surgical reduction is not promptly carried out. If intestine is involved, obstruction is gener-

ally present. A strangulated hernia is generally irreducible or incarcerated, but an irreducible hernia is generally *not* strangulated.

Further definitions might clarify certain points about hernias for the student:

A *ventral* hernia is one that occurs through the ventral abdominal wall and generally includes umbilical, epigastric, and incisional hernias.

An *incisional* hernia is one that occurs through an incisional wound that fails to heal completely. Thus an incisional hernia is also a ventral hernia, provided that the incision is made through the ventral abdominal wall.

Richter's hernia (Fig. 27-1, *A*) is herniation of only a part of the circumference of bowel through a fascial defect; it is especially dangerous because strangulation can occur *without* complete mechanical intestinal obstruction. It is most commonly found in femoral hernias because of the small size and sharp and relatively inflexible nature of the fascial ring in this area.

Littre's hernia appears to be similar to Richter's hernia, but it should be restricted to the herniation of Meckel's diverticulum through a fascial ring.

A *sliding* hernia (Fig. 27-2) is one in which a portion of the sac of a hernia is made up of the herniating viscus itself. Its importance lies in the fact that attempts at surgical removal of the entire sac will, of course, remove or injure the viscus which is "sliding." The most common sliding hernias involve the bladder in direct inguinal hernias, the sigmoid colon in left indirect inguinal hernias, and the cecum in right indirect inguinal hernias.

The anatomical location of a hernia is a convenient method of identification or classification. The following is a list of the more common hernias according to *location:*

Inguinal (indirect or direct)
Femoral
Umbilical (infantile, adult, or omphalocele)
Epigastric
Incisional (postoperative, ventral)
Pelvic
Lumbar
Diaphragmatic (congenital or hiatal)

INGUINAL

The surgical treatment of inguinal hernia is the most common major operation performed in the United States. Inguinal hernias are 20 times more common in males than in females because of the defect in the abdominal wall occasioned by descent of the testis into the scrotum in the male and also perhaps because of the protection to the inside of the lower ventral abdominal wall afforded by the uterus in females.

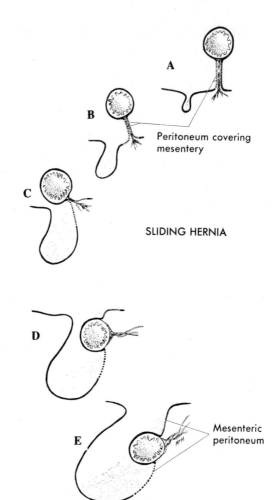

Fig. 27-2. Sliding hernia. Simple hernia evolves in **A** and **B**. It begins to "slide" with one mesenteric leaf in **C** and the bowel itself in **D**. In its final evolution in step **E**, bowel and both mesenteric leaves are part of hernial sac.

Inguinal hernias are of two types: indirect and direct. The fascial defect in an indirect inguinal hernia (Fig. 27-3) lies *lateral* to the inferior deep epigastric artery, and the defect in the direct hernia (Fig. 27-4) lies *medial* to this structure. Usually the indirect type has a preformed or congenital sac, occurs in the infant to young adult male, and is more symptomatic and more prone to develop complications; in contrast, the direct inguinal hernia is much less common, is seen in the elderly male as part of the "wear and tear" process of aging, almost never becomes complicated by strangulation, is generally less symptomatic, and is

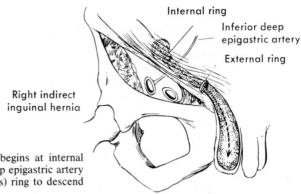

Fig. 27-3. Right indirect inguinal hernia. Hernial sac begins at internal (deep, or abdominal) inguinal ring lateral to inferior deep epigastric artery and exits from inguinal canal at external (subcutaneous) ring to descend into scrotum. Sac lies anteromedial to cord structures.

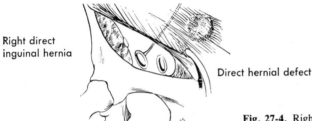

Fig. 27-4. Right direct inguinal hernia. Hernial sac arises in Hesselbach's triangle medial to inferior deep epigastric artery and just above pubic tubercle. It does not descend into scrotum.

almost unheard of in the female. The distinction between the two is perhaps academic in the good-risk patient, since both should be corrected surgically at an elective time. However, in the poor-risk elderly patient the distinction between the two becomes important in the selection of the appropriate treatment; a low-risk direct hernia in a high-risk patient might better be treated by a well-fitted truss or other conservative methods.

Indirect

Etiology. Most indirect inguinal hernias arise because of retention or imperfect obliteration of the *processus vaginalis,* the embryological outpocketing of peritoneum that precedes testicular descent into the scrotum. The testis originates along the urogenital ridge in the retroperitoneum and migrates caudad during the second trimester of pregnancy to arrive at the internal inguinal (abdominal) ring at about the sixth month of intrauter-

ine life. During the last trimester, it proceeds through the abdominal wall via the inguinal canal and descends into the scrotum, the right slightly later than the left. The processus vaginalis then normally obliterates postnatally except for that portion surrounding and serving as a covering for the testicle (tunica vaginalis). Failure of this obliterative process results in an indirect inguinal hernia at birth or during the first few months or years of life (coincident with the highest age peak of incidence of this hernia). The incidence then diminishes to rise again in young adult males. Herniation at this latter age probably results from the stress of muscular activity and the increase in intra-abdominal pressure forcing open a previously imperfectly obliterated processus vaginalis. Indirect inguinal hernias seldom arise after 40 years of age, underscoring the importance of this congenital, or preformed, sac in its genesis.

A hydrocele is an unobliterated processus

vaginalis in which the communication with the peritoneal cavity is large enough to allow peritoneal fluid to enter but not large enough to admit bowel. About 15% of inguinal hernias in infants and children are preceded by a hydrocele, but most hydroceles in the very young disappear spontaneously as the continuing obliterative process closes off the peritoneal connection. Hydroceles do not require treatment unless they persist into childhood; surgical treatment involves simply dividing and ligating the communicating tract.

Diagnosis. Early complaints of indirect inguinal hernia include a bulge or swelling in the groin that appears only when the patient strains, cries, or assumes an upright position and that disappears when reclining. Commonly the bulge is associated with a nagging, dull discomfort locally. Occasionally forceful straining or lifting precipitates an acute hernia, heralded by sudden groin discomfort and a bulge in the area. With time, the groin bulge increases in size and pursues an oblique course from the internal inguinal ring downward and medially along the course of the inguinal canal, and when it descends to the bottom of the scrotum it becomes a *complete* or *scrotal* hernia.

Physical examination is the key to diagnosis. An oblong swelling in the groin that appears with standing and straining and extends downward and medially into the scrotum, disappearing in a reverse direction on assumption of the supine position, is the classical finding. Inversion of scrotal skin by the examining index finger confirms that the external (subcutaneous) inguinal ring has been dilated by the hernia. Asking the patient to cough or strain (cough impulse) will bring down the bowel or the end of the sac against the end of the examining finger. After an indirect inguinal hernia has been completely reduced, finger pressure over the internal (abdominal) inguinal ring (located 1 cm. superior to the midpoint of a line drawn from

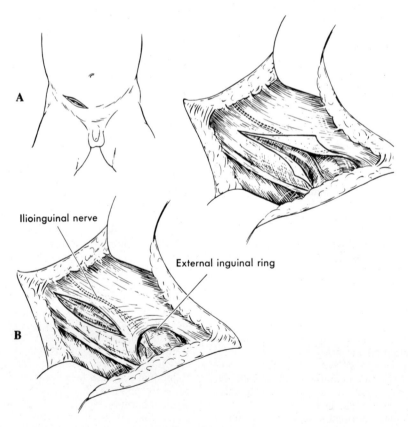

Fig. 27-5. Repair of right indirect inguinal hernia in infant. **A,** Groin-crease skin incision. **B,** Incision in external oblique aponeurosis exposes hernia and cord structures; ilioinguinal nerve should be protected.

the anterosuperior iliac spine to the pubic tubercle) prevents recurrence unless a direct hernia coexists (so-called *pantaloon* hernia).

Treatment. Indirect inguinal hernias should be repaired surgically unless specific contraindications exist because of the discomfort that they evoke, the certainty that once established they will persist and even become larger with time, and the constant threat of complications of the hernia. In the infant and young child adequate surgical treatment (Fig. 27-5) consists of simple division of the sac with high ligation of the sac neck. There is usually no need for fascial reconstruction, since the basic defect is the sac itself rather than a deficiency of the supporting musculoaponeurotic structures. The distal sac can be left in situ as normal cord and testicular coverings.

In the older child or young adult division and closure of the neck of the sac are carried out after reduction of the herniated viscera. In addition, the abdominal ring (aperture in the transversalis fascia) is snugged up closely around the carefully identified (and undamaged) cord structures over the top of the ligated sac. In those hernias that through neglect have grown to enormous proportions, destroying a good part of the supporting transversalis fascia and displacing the inferior deep epigastric vessels medially, a more extensive fascial repair is necessitated after the sac has been ligated. Reattachment of the fresh superior edge of transversalis fascia to Cooper's ligament and the prefemoral fascia (McVay operation) is one of the more popular operations designed to restore the integrity of the musculoaponeurotic support. Recurrence of the hernia is seen in only 1% to 2% of the smaller hernias of infancy and childhood and in up to 5% of the very large hernias of adulthood.

Complications

Incarceration. Acute incarceration of a previously reducible hernia is associated with local pain and, if not reduced promptly, may produce edema and increased pressure at the narrowed sac neck with strangulation of the herniated viscera. Acute incarceration sometimes heralds the onset of the inguinal hernia, especially in the infant and young child. Nonoperative reduction may be attempted, provided that the irreducibility is only a few hours in duration and there is no localized tenderness, redness, or signs of intestinal obstruction to suggest early strangulation. To accomplish mechanical reduction, the patient should be placed in the supine position with the hips flexed and the foot of the bed elevated; a sedative or analgesic agent will help produce relaxation, after which gentle pressure over the hernia is applied.

If gentle attempts at manual reduction are unsuccessful or there is any suggestion of early strangulation, surgical correction of the hernia must be carried out as an emergency. The techniques of repair are the same, namely, opening the sac, careful inspection of the herniated viscera to assure their viability, after which they are reduced

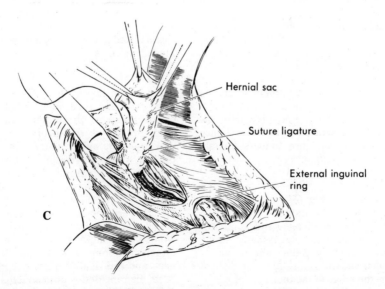

Fig. 27-5, cont'd. C, Hernial sac has been separated from cord structures and divided, and contents have been reduced; suture-ligature is closing neck of sac.

into the intraperitoneal cavity, high ligation and division of the sac neck, and fascial repair if indicated.

A long-standing hernia often becomes less completely reducible and ultimately may be completely irreducible or incarcerated. A chronically incarcerated hernia is not likely to be symptomatic, nor does it carry the threat of immediate strangulation. It often indicates that the hernia is really a sliding hernia (Fig. 27-2) rather than the more common nonsliding type. Surgical repair of a sliding hernia is more complicated in that complete sac dissection and division and closure of the sac neck are impossible because a portion of the sac wall itself is composed of the sliding viscus. Only that portion of the sac not made up of viscus can be excised, and the entire remaining sac and its sliding viscus must then be reduced en masse; repair of the musculoaponeurotic supporting tissue can then be made superficial to the sac to prevent its recurrence. The morbidity, mortality, and recurrence after surgical repair of a sliding hernia are all higher than with a nonsliding hernia and justify early hernia repair before the sliding hernia has time to develop.

Strangulation. A hernia is more likely to strangulate if it has a capacious sac with a rather narrow sac neck surrounded by a rigid and unyielding fascial ring. Pressure at the ring first slows venous return, producing stasis and edema, thereby ensuring irreducibility. An inflammatory response adds to the vicious cycle and culminates with impedance of arterial inflow to the strangulated viscus with necrosis and gangrene. Small intestine is the most commonly strangulated viscus and is, of course, associated with mechanical intestinal obstruction at this point. Delaying surgical repair by attempts at forceful reduction will further traumatize the friable viscus, often resulting in perforation and spreading peritonitis. Surgical treatment should be undertaken promptly by resection of the strangulated organ, followed by anatomical repair of the hernia. The morbidity, mortality, and recurrence after strangulated hernias are understandably higher than for nonstrangulated types.

Direct

Direct inguinal hernia (Fig. 27-4) is only about one fifth as common as the indirect counterpart, originates after 40 yeares of age, and is almost never seen in the female. The bulge is medial to the inguinal canal just above the pubic tubercle and is likely to be circular and diffuse, rather than distinct and elongated as the bulge in the indirect variety is. The fascial edges are indistinct in keeping with its origin as a gradual and diffuse weakening of the fascia transversalis in Hesselbach's triangle, associated with aging and increasing intraabdominal pressure from coughing (asthma), straining to micturate (prostatism), obesity, constipation, and nutritional defects. This very fact, however, is the reason direct inguinal hernias, though uncomfortable, rarely become complicated by incarceration. As they get larger, the bladder commonly "slides" into the medial edge of the direct hernia sac, a factor that must be remembered at the time of surgical repair.

On physical examination the distinction between the indirect and direct hernias is not difficult. When the examining finger is placed through the external (subcutaneous) ring and then directed posteriorly, the weakness in the fascia transversalis forming the floor of the inguinal canal is the most distinctive finding. After reduction, finger pressure over the internal (abdominal) ring does not prevent a direct hernia from appearing immediately when the patient strains or stands. Direct hernia sacs have no direct relationship to the testicular cord structures, nor do they commonly descend into the scrotum. In view of the low complication rate, a direct inguinal hernia may be conservatively treated in the high-risk, debilitated patient. A well-fitted truss, though cumbersome, can relieve the symptoms.

The more expedient treatment consists of surgical repair. Direct inguinal hernia sacs are simply reduced and the defect in the floor of the inguinal canal is repaired when one brings down the strong superior margin of fascia transversalis and reattaches it by suture to Cooper's ligament medially and to the prefemoral fascia laterally (McVay repair). Recurrence rates are twice as high as with indirect hernias.

FEMORAL

A femoral hernia (Fig. 27-6) is one that occurs through an enlarged femoral ring, the medialmost compartment of the femoral canal. The femoral canal lies below the inguinal (Poupart's) ligament and above the pubic bone and is bounded medially by the rather unyielding lacunar ligament. The contents of the femoral canal from lateral to medial spell out the word *nave* (standing for femoral *n*erve, *a*rtery, *v*ein, *e*mpty space). It is through this empty space that a femoral hernia occurs.

Femoral hernias occur more commonly in women than in men and are probably acquired rather than congenital. The narrowness of the sac neck and the rigidity of its boundaries predispose to its high incidence of irreducibility, strangulation (up to 20%), and Richter's type of strangulated hernia (Fig. 27-1, *A*). It is understandable why

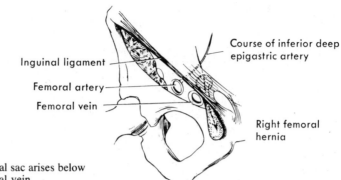

Fig. 27-6. Right femoral hernia. Hernial sac arises below inguinal ligament and medial to femoral vein.

Table 27-1. Inguinofemoral hernias

	Femoral	*Indirect inguinal*	*Direct inguinal*
Age at onset	Young to middle-aged adult	Infant, child, young adult	Middle to old age
Sex	Female > male	Male 20:1	Almost always male
Cause	Congenital (?)	Congenital	Wear and tear
Incidence	Uncommon	Most common	Second most common
Origin	Femoral canal	Internal inguinal ring	Hesselbach's triangle
Neck size	Small, rigid	Small to medium	Large
Course of sac	Variable	Oblique to scrotum	Local protrusion
Incarceration	Common	15%-20%	Rare
Strangulation	Common	5%-10%	Hardly ever
Sliding	Rare	Common if longstanding; right—cecum, left sigmoid	Common (bladder)
Treatment	Always surgical	Always surgical	Surgical if symptomatic

symptoms occur earlier and why prompt surgical treatment should be carried out more urgently than with inguinal hernia.

Initially the bulge of a femoral hernia lies below the inguinal (Poupart's) ligament medial to the femoral arterial pulse. However, as the sac enlarges with time, it is likely to turn upward anterior to the inguinal (Poupart's) ligament and then present as an inguinal swelling difficult to distinguish from an indirect inguinal hernia. Careful inspection will often reveal that its neck is located low and that reduction occurs in a different direction from the indirect inguinal hernia.

Surgical repair is the only recommended treatment for femoral hernia, preferably undertaken before complications occur. The surgical approach is through the same skin incision (inguinal crease) as that used for the two more common types of inguinal hernias, and the essentials of repair are the same, namely, opening of the sac, reduction of the herniated contents, ligation and high closure of the sac neck, and reattachment of the fascia transver-

salis to Cooper's ligament to close off completely the empty space in the femoral canal without compromise to the femoral vein.

Table 27-1 compares and contrasts the three varieties of inguinofemoral hernias.

Differential diagnosis of inguinofemoral masses

The three types of inguinofemoral hernias (direct inguinal, indirect inguinal, and femoral) can often be distinguished from one another on careful physical examination, and they *must* be distinguished carefully from other disorders that produce swelling in the same general area. A few of the more common considerations in differential diagnosis of inguinofemoral masses are discussed briefly:

1. *Hydrocele* of the cord or testis or both (pp. 261 and 300) is distinguished from indirect inguinal hernia by the fact that it cannot be quickly reduced, is not attended by discomfort, transilluminates brilliantly, and often is associated with a thickening of the cord structures above the hydrocele.

2. *Undescended testis:* Careful palpation of the scrotal sac should make the diagnosis of cryptorchidism clear. When the testis is within the inguinal canal, it is palpated as a firm mass that cannot be brought down by traction to within the scrotum; this distinguishes it from simply a high-riding or retractile testis that, with gentleness, persistence, and often exposure to warm water, can be brought down into the scrotum and is not truly undescended. Cryptorchidism is almost invariably associated with an indirect inguinal hernia that in itself commonly justifies early surgical treatment of the hernia and concomitant replacement of the testis within the scrotum.

3. *Inguinal lymphadenitis:* Enlarged inguinofemoral lymph nodes generally are multiple rather than solitary and are sometimes tender. The site of infection within the extremity or perineum resulting in the inguinal node enlargement should be apparent on examination. The nodes do not become reduced or transmit a cough impulse.

4. *Varix of upper greater saphenous vein:* A localized varix or thin-walled enlargement of the proximal portion of the greater saphenous vein presents as a soft swelling below the inguinal ligament that is commonly confused with femoral hernia. It is generally associated with varicosities of the rest of the saphenous system. It transmits a cough impulse that is felt in the remainder of the dilated vein, and percussion of the veins transmits a percussion thrill to the varix to distinguish this clearly from femoral hernia. The varix swelling promptly disappears when the patient is recumbent.

5. *Lipoma of the cord:* A lipoma surrounding the cord structures is difficult to distinguish from indirect inguinal hernia. It occasionally is associated with a hernia and constitutes part of the inguinal canal swelling. Lipoma of the cord is not reducible, is not painful, and does not transmit a cough impulse.

UMBILICAL

There are three general types of umbilical hernia that differ greatly in causation, prognosis, and tratment: omphalocele, infantile hernia, and adult hernia (Table 27-2).

Omphalocele

An *omphalocele* is not a true hernia because its covering is made up of amniotic sac, it has no true inner peritoneal lining or skin covering its outer surface; it really represents a failure of the extracoelomic midgut to return to the peritoneal cavity after the tenth to twelfth week of intrauterine existence (p. 284). The prognosis of an omphalocele is grave because of its propensity to rupture, a high incidence of associated congenital anomalies elsewhere, and extreme difficulty in reducing the herniated viscera even at operation. Surgical treatment is aimed at excision of the sac and closure of the abdominal wall in layers, when the contents can be reduced without tension and the defect in the abdominal wall is not large.

If the viscera cannot be safely reduced, even after the abdominal cavity has been enlarged by manual stretching of the abdominal wall, it is best to suture a Dacron-reinforced sheet around the defect and over the herniated viscera. This so-called silo affords a physiological covering to the viscera, allowing their staged reduction into a gradually expanding abdominal cavity. Complete reduction is achieved by 7 to 10 days of age, allowing safe skin and fascial closure after removal of the silo.

Table 27-2. Umbilical hernias

	Omphalocele	Infantile	Adult
Age at onset	Newborn (premature)	Newborn (premature)	Middle to elderly
Sex	Equal	Equal	Female > male
Race	Equal	Black > white	Equal
Incidence	Rare	Very common	Common
Cause	Congenital	Congenital	Wear and tear
Skin cover	None	Intact	Intact
Other anomalies	Frequent	Average	Average
Neck size	Large	Small to large	Often small
Incarceration	Rare	Rare	Frequent
Strangulation	Rare	Rare	Frequent
Treatment	Surgical	Observation	Surgical

Infantile

Infantile umbilical hernia is very common, occurring in upwards of 5% of white infants and 20% of black infants. The incidence is higher among premature than among term infants. It represents protrusion of a hernia sac through an aperture created when the umbilical vessels thrombose and rapidly involute at the time of delivery. Because the infantile type of umbilical hernia almost never becomes complicated by incarceration or strangulation and almost always disappears spontaneously by the seventh year of life, the indications for surgical repair are few. Trusses do not speed resolution of an umbilical hernia and may even entrap and irritate herniated intestine; their use is therefore discouraged. In the occasional case that is symptomatic, becomes incarcerated or strangulated, or is so large as to predispose to external trauma, surgical repair is indicated.

Adult

The adult type of umbilical hernia occurs more commonly in the obese and multiparous female. It originates through a dilated and weakened umbilical ring or through a weak spot in the linea alba just above the umbilicus. Adult hernias in this region are dangerous because, like the femoral hernias, the neck remains small and unyielding despite often a very capacious hernia sac. This results in a high incidence of incarceration and strangulation, a feature that demands early surgical repair.

The surgical treatment of umbilical hernias is carried out through a curving infraumbilical incision; the sac is opened, the contents are reduced, and the neck of the sac is closed flush with its entrance into the abdominal cavity. The fascia surrounding the resultant defect is then brought together and often overlapped (imbricated) for a two-layer repair.

EPIGASTRIC HERNIA

Epigastric hernias occur in the linea alba between the xiphoid process and the umbilicus. These hernias are probably initiated by properitoneal fat protruding through apertures created by perforating vessels, which then gradually enlarge with continuing stress (a rise in intra-abdominal pressure) to allow a peritoneal sac to protrude. They cause local pain and tenderness, even though small in size, and are generally seen in middle-aged men doing manual labor. The pain can mimic other types of intra-abdominal surgical disease that must be ruled out before elective hernia repair is undertaken. The repair consists in excision and closure of the sac and repair of the defect in the fascia.

INCISIONAL HERNIA

An incisional hernia is one that occurs through an old operative incision in the abdominal wall that has become partially dehisced. Incisional hernias develop more commonly in vertical than in transverse incisions and in patients with poor wound healing, *postoperative wound infections,* or conditions causing increased intra-abdominal pressure. Poor wound healing may occur because of faulty surgical technique (placement of sutures too close to the edges being apposed, use of too small or too large suture material, knots tied so tightly as to necrose abdominal wall layers, knots becoming untied, or interruption of a running suture that then unravels for the length of the incision). Hematomas and infections of the wound produce delayed and imperfect healing; foreign bodies brought through the wound (drains, catheters) prevent sound approximation of wound edges and are associated with a high incidence of herniation. Postoperative cough, distension, and hiccups all greatly elevate intra-abdominal pressure and place undue strain on the sutures, which may then give way to initiate an incisional hernia.

The symptoms are those of a variable-sized swelling in an old incision line, generally attended by only mild symptoms of local discomfort. Incarceration is fairly common, but strangulation is rare because of the large size of the sac neck.

Treatment is generally surgical, though satisfactory control of moderate-sized hernias can be afforded by girdles or trusses for the poor-risk patient. Small and symptomatic hernias should be repaired surgically because of danger of strangulation, and the large and diffuse ones should be repaired because of failure of control by binders or girdles. In the large hernias with attenuated fascia, fascial grafts and prosthetic replacement to bridge gaps in the fascia are commonly necessary.

LUMBAR HERNIA

Most lumbar hernias are really incisional hernias occurring in old nephrectomy incisions. However, occasionally they occur spontaneously either just above the iliac crest posteriorly or just below the twelfth rib. The hernias generally remain reducible, do not tend to strangulate, and can usually be controlled by a corset or belt.

RESPIRATORY DIAPHRAGMATIC HERNIAS

The respiratory diaphragm separates the thoracic from the abdominal cavity and is breached by the esophagus, the aorta, and the inferior vena cava. It is an extremely important muscular organ that assists in respiratory efforts and can remarkably affect pressures within the thoracic and ab-

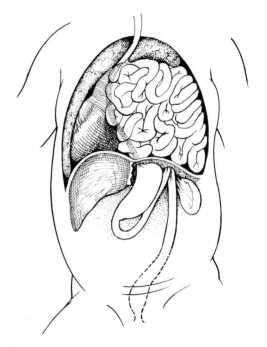

Fig. 27-7. Typical left-sided Bochdalek hernia with air-filled midgut in left pleural cavity. Midline structures (esophagus, heart) are displaced to right side and both lungs are compressed. Liver underlies right hemidiaphragm, accounting for lower incidence of right-sided Bochdalek hernia.

dominal cavities and vessels. It is formed embryologically by peripheral muscularization of the septum transversum. Hernias occur either through apertures resulting from imperfect development (congenital) or are acquired by increases in intra-abdominal pressure, rupturing weakened points, or enlargement of the preexistent apertures.

Congenital

Congenital diaphragmatic hernia (Fig. 27-7) is one of the true surgical emergencies of the newborn period of life; 80% occur through the left posterolateral foramen of Bochdalek, and 20% occur through a similar defect on the right side—presumably the tamponade effect of the liver on the right side accounts for this difference in incidence. Most Bochdalek hernias have no sac. Since the aperture in the diaphragm occurs early during intrauterine life, before rotation of the midgut has occurred, it is commonly associated with malrotation; for the same reason, the involved lung is frequently immature and incapable

of immediate normal expansion after surgical correction.

Rapid respiratory decompensation demands urgency in diagnosis and treatment of congenital diaphragmatic hernia. The sequential pathophysiology is as follows: the intestine rapidly fills with swallowed air postnatally, which expands the size of the herniated viscera in the chest, producing progressive mediastinal shift to the contralateral side with interference in respiratory exchange in the normal lung and impedance of venous return to the heart. The diagnosis is established by a plain upright roentgenogram demonstrating gas-filled loops of bowel in the chest with a contralateral mediastinal shift. Emergency endotracheal intubation and assisted respiration temporarily stabilize the child. Nasogastric suction halts the lethal ingress of swallowed air before early laparotomy with reduction of the abdominal viscera from the chest and suture approximation of the edges of the defect in the diaphragm.

Even with early diagnosis and proper management, less than half the babies with Bochdalek hernia *who become symptomatic within the first 24 hours of life* survive. In sharp distinction are afflicted infants diagnosed after 24 hours of age, virtually all of whom survive surgical correction. Factors that adversely affect survival in the symptomatic neonate include severe preoperative hypoxemia, hypoplasia and immaturity of the lungs, persistent fetal circulatory shunts, postoperative contralateral pneumothorax, and elevated intra-abdominal pressure.

Hiatal

Acquired diaphragmatic hernias (Fig. 27-8) generally involve the stomach, herniating either through an enlarged esophageal hiatus (the sliding type of esophageal hiatal hernia) or through a defect in the diaphragm just lateral to the diaphragmatic crura encircling the esophagus (paraesophageal or parahiatal type). The sliding hiatal hernia is many times more common than the paraesophageal; since it increases the acute esophagogastric angle, there is free reflux of stomach contents into the esophagus to produce the outstanding symptoms of esophagitis: regurgitation, heartburn, mild bleeding, and later scarring with stricture formation and dysphagia. Hiatal hernias are seen either in infants or in middle-aged to elderly patients with obesity and increased intra-abdominal pressure for one reason or another. The symptoms are aggravated when one lies down and are improved when one sits up. Often an acid-peptic diathesis is associated.

Treatment is tailored to the severity of symptoms and the patients' general operative risk status.

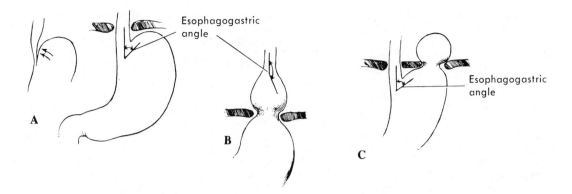

Fig. 27-8. A, Normal relationship of stomach and esophagus to diaphragm; acute esophagogastric angle helps prevent reflux from stomach into esophagus *(inset).* **B,** "Sliding" type of esophageal hiatal hernia; esophagogastric junction above diaphragm; obtuse esophagogastric angle favors reflux. **C,** Paraesophageal hiatal hernia; esophagogastric angle is normal, and no reflux into esophagus occurs.

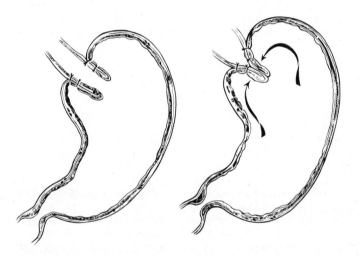

Fig. 27-9. Fundoplication. *Left,* Gastric fundus is wrapped around lower esophagus. *Right,* When stomach fills, pressure closes gastroesophageal junction, preventing reflux.

Hiatal hernias that are small and only mildly symptomatic or that occur in very poor-risk patients can be satisfactorily managed by restriction of the patient to an upright position postprandially, elevation of the head of the bed while sleeping, and introduction of an antacid medical regimen. Reduction of body weight and other factors that reduce intra-abdominal pressure also assist in the treatment program. Hiatal hernias that are large, progressively more symptomatic, or associated with complications of ulceration, bleeding, or stenosis should be treated surgically: the stomach is pulled down below the diaphragm, and usually the hiatal aperture is closed around the esophagus. Usually some sort of antireflux operation is then performed (Fig. 27-9) to further discourage gastroesophageal reflux. If an acid-peptic diathesis is present or the patient has an actual peptic ulcer, truncal vagotomy and an appropriate gastric drainage procedure are commonly added. The poor-risk patient who must be treated surgically because of complications can be improved by simple suture fixation of the reduced stomach to the anterior abdominal wall.

The less common parahiatal diaphragmatic hernias produce symptoms of vague epigastric and lower anterior chest pain aggravated by increases in intra-abdominal pressure and recumbency. Since the esophagogastric junction is undisturbed, none of the symptoms of esophagitis is present. Complications include ulceration and bleeding within the herniated stomach, incarceration and strangulation, and progressive enlargement until most of the stomach is intrathoracic (giving an "upside-down" radiographic appearance to the stomach).

Treatment principles are similar to those of the sliding type of hiatal hernia: surgical reduction and repair of the aperture in the diaphragm.

Indirect or direct trauma to the diaphragm may produce tears or weaknesses through which hernias develop. These are almost always on the left side because of the protection afforded by the liver to the right side of the diaphragm. Respiratory and gastrointestinal symptoms coexist, and the diagnosis is confirmed by plain films of the chest and by barium studies of the upper and lower intestine demonstrating loops of intestine within the thorax. Surgical reduction and closure of the diaphragmatic rent will prevent complications (intestinal obstruction, strangulation, atelectasis).

INTERNAL HERNIA

Internal hernia is the name given to the herniation of intestine through an aperture (natural or acquired) within the abdominal cavity. Thus small bowel herniation through the foramen of Winslow into the lesser sac would be termed an internal hernia. There are recesses in the paraduodenal and paracecal areas in which internal hernias may occur. Postoperative adhesions may form an aperture through which an internal hernia occurs.

Internal hernias are dangerous because they may remain undiagnosed until complications of intestinal obstruction or strangulation occur that necessitate emergency surgical exploration. Treatment is

directed at relieving the obstruction or strangulation by appropriate means and then closing the aperture through which the herniation occurred.

RARE EXTERNAL HERNIAS
Obturator hernia

A hernia may accompany the obturator vessels and nerve into the thigh through the obturator foramen. Obturator hernias are uncommon at any age but more often occur in elderly women. Obturator hernias can be diagnosed by a swelling in the upper and medial aspect of the thigh associated with pain radiating to the medial aspect of the knee, aggravated by sudden increases in intra-abdominal pressure but not by hip or knee movements. Hypesthesia in the area of pain radiation indicates irritation of the sensory component of the obturator nerve. The neck of the sac may be palpable on vaginal or rectal pelvic examination. Strangulation and incarceration are common, and morbidity and mortality remain high because of delay in diagnosis. Treatment is reduction of the viscera at the time of exploratory laparotomy with closure of the peritoneum over the aperture.

Sciatic hernia

Sciatic hernias can occur either through the greater or the lesser sciatic notches as bulges inferior to the gluteus maximus muscle. They become symptomatic either by producing intestinal obstruction or by pain that has a sciatic nerve distribution.

Spigelian hernia

A spigelian hernia sac, by definition, originates at the junction of the semilunar and semicircular lines just lateral to the rectus muscle in its lower fourth. As the hernia sac enlarges, it may track from this location interstitially in almost any direction to present a most puzzling clinical picture. Strangulation may occur.

28
Pediatric Surgery

Robert T. Soper
Kevin C. Pringle

Twenty-five years ago, medical (infectious) disorders accounted for most hospitalizations and deaths of children. However, today in industrialized countries more than half of hospitalized children have diseases with surgical overtones and, of all surgical patients, one fourth are children. Since there are approximately 70 million people under 14 years of age in the United States, these figures have staggering logistical and professional implications. Surgical disease in children is becoming more important for two reasons: (1) antibiotics, immunizations, and good medical care have dramatically decreased the infectious diseases that were responsible for most hospitalizations and deaths of children a quarter-century ago and (2) new drugs, instruments, and better training now allow routine correction of abnormalities hitherto considered inoperable, with open-heart surgery being a prime example.

Ill infants and children cannot be treated as small adults. There are enough differences in the etiology, course, and pathophysiology of disease in the very young to adequately justify special consideration and training. The obvious problems imposed by the small size of the patient, his different maintenance requirements, inability to give a history, and the magnitude of certain corrective operations all add to the need for a chapter devoted to the very young surgical patient.

THE NEONATAL SURGICAL PATIENT

The newborn infant epitomizes the profound differences that exist between the adult and the very young surgical patient. These differences become less striking and important as the baby grows into childhood and adolescence. About 0.5% (1 out of 200) of live-born babies require emergency neonatal surgery, generally because of congenital anomalies obstructing flow through one of the vital body conduits (food through the gastrointestinal tract, cerebrospinal fluid through the central nervous system, blood through the heart or major vessels).

In the following ways newborns tolerate operations surprisingly well:

1. The body systems that have developed correctly function remarkably well, despite measurable anatomical and physiological evidence of immaturity. The cardiovascular system is perhaps the outstanding example: the heart muscle is hypertrophied at birth because during gestation it pumps 20% to 30% more blood (through the placental circuit) than the postnatal circulatory volume. The heart therefore possesses relatively more functional reserve at birth than it will have later.

2. The newborn infant enjoys a higher relative circulating blood volume than he will have subsequently because (a) of return of extra blood to the baby from the placenta at the time of delivery and (b) relative to weight, the newborn has 50% more extracellular fluid, part of which is blood, than the adult does.

3. The newborn's blood has a higher oxygen-carrying capacity than it will have later, with hemoglobin and hematocrit levels often 50%

higher than those in adults. A relative hypoxemia in the fetus (from inefficient transport of oxygen across the placental barrier) stimulates fetal blood production. Increased tolerance to hypoxemia is carried over into the neonatal period.

A strong heart pump, hypervolemia, and the high oxygen-carrying capacity of the blood combine to make the newborn a relatively good operative risk.

Fluid therapy. The newborn has 10% to 15% more total body water relative to weight than the older child or adult does. This excess fluid is soon lost as urine. It dictates the low maintenance fluid requirement of 50 ml./kg. for the first day, which progressively rises to 100 ml./kg./day by the end of the first week of life. Thus the daily maintenance fluid of the week-old infant is three to four times that of the adult when calculated per unit of body weight. These requirements must be computed carefully on the basis of body weight, surface area, or calories expended.

One of the simpler methods for calculating daily maintenance fluid requirements for children is as follows: about 100 ml./day is needed for each of the first 10 kg. of body weight, about 50 ml./day for each of the second 10 kg. (from 10 to 20 kg. of body weight), and about 20 ml./day for each kilogram above 20 kg. of body weight. The average adult requires about 30 ml./kg./day.

Another method of calculating daily maintenance fluid is on the basis of body surface area. Surface area is expressed in square meters (m.^{2}) and is calculated from a nomogram with the patient's body length (height) in centimeters and body weight in kilograms. Daily fluid for maintenance normally is 1,500 ml./m.^{2} of body surface area, a figure that does not vary with age. Representative body surface areas for babies of given body weights are as follows:

Body weight (kg.)	Body surface area (m.^{2})
1.8	0.15
2.7	0.2
4	0.25
5	0.29
8	0.4
10	0.5
20	0.8
30	1

When a patient cannot be nourished enterally, the intravenous fluid that we prefer for maintenance purposes is N/5 saline in 5% dextrose solution. This solution contains 30 mEq./L. of NaCl. To this is added KCl, 20 mEq./L., after adequate urinary output is assured.

Parenteral (intravenous) fluids must be calculated precisely for volume and content and should be given at a rather steady rate over the entire 24-hour period. Unusual body fluid loss such as vomiting, diarrhea, nasogastric suction, and sequestered body fluids must be measured or estimated accurately and added to maintenance requirements. Hyperthermia or exposure to a dry environment increases fluid requirements. Oral feedings are self-regulated.

A newborn infant weighing 3 kg. has a total circulating blood volume of roughly 250 ml. Blood loss in the relatively modest amount of 25 ml. (less than 1 ounce) constitutes a significant hemorrhage that proportionately in the adult would approach 600 ml.

Environment. The newborn infant is much more sensitive to environmental temperature and humidity than the adult is because (1) he has almost three times the amount of skin exposed to the environment in relation to weight and (2) he has a meager insulating blanket of subcutaneous fat. The neonatal surgical patient must be nursed in an incubator. Advantages gained from the incubator include:

1. Humidification of the air to nearly 100% to reduce insensible fluid loss
2. Oxygenation of air breathed to 30% to 35% concentration to facilitate adequate oxygenation of tissue
3. Control of air temperature at about 85° F. (29.5° C) that will allow easy maintenance of normal body temperature; lower air temperature will induce body heat loss and require expenditure of energy to generate more body heat

The lack of subcutaneous fat in the neonate (in contrast to the adult) is significant for one other reason: fat provides calories when oral caloric intake is insufficient. Thus correcting factors that preclude oral intake of food in the newborn is vital, since adequate calories cannot be supplied by conventional parenteral fluids.

Respiration. Four factors, unique to the newborn, influence respiration:

1. Air exchange in the lungs and blood flow through the pulmonary circuit have just been initiated, and commonly a few days elapse before lung function becomes optimal.
2. The right upper lung lobe is predisposed to atelectasis for anatomical reasons (a dependent position of its bronchus).
3. The newborn depends entirely on diaphragmatic descent for lung expansion, because the ribs are horizontal and cannot "lift" on inspiration as in the adult. Anything impeding free motion of the diaphragm jeopardizes respiration: congenital diaphragmatic hernia, faulty

innervation of the diaphragm muscles, and increase in intra-abdominal pressure (intestinal obstruction).

4. The newborn breathes by preference through the nose rather than the mouth, and anything narrowing or occluding the nasal passages (choanal atresia, mucus plugs, nasogastric tubes) impairs respiratory exchange.

These factors of inefficient early lung function, atelectasis, inhibition of diaphragmatic motion, and obstruction of nasal passages must all be diagnosed and managed promptly to assure normal respiratory function.

Types of operations (newborn versus adults). Congenital anomalies are the most frequent indication for operations on the newborn, in distinction to infection, trauma, and degenerative and neoplastic diseases in the adult. Thus neonatal intestinal obstruction is generally caused by webs, bands, membranes, faulty innervation, or other abnormalities of development. On the other hand, intestinal obstruction in the adult is generally caused by hernias, postoperative adhesions, and neoplasms.

Surgical disease—rapid progression. The speed at which surgical disease progresses is often dramatically accelerated in the newborn patient and may result in death in just a few hours. Small actual volume of body fluids, low energy and nutritional reserves, and poor defenses against infection contribute to this rapid progression. Furthermore, the newborn must communicate his illness by indirect and often subtle signs such as changes in color and rates of pulse and respiration, inability to feed, irritability, and lethargy. The good pediatric nurse or physician must be an astute observer, for the baby is a poor historian. Time is truly of the essence in the newborn surgical patient.

THE NEWBORN AND THE OPERATING ROOM

Temperature. Body temperature must be monitored continuously. Body heat of the infant is conserved when the operating room air is warmed, the time periods out of the incubator before and after operation are shortened, large volumes of rapidly evaporating fluids to prepare the skin are avoided, and a heat exchange blanket on top of the operating table mattress is used. Infrared lamps also may be used to deliver radiant heat to the baby during operation.

During operation, body heat is lost rapidly when major body cavities such as the thorax or abdomen are opened, and this loss must be countered by lavages of normal saline solution heated to just above body temperature. Clear plastic adhesive drapes reduce convection loss of heat, provide a sterile barrier impervious to water, allow better visualization of the entire patient by the operating room team, and are therefore highly recommended.

Technique. Placing a plastic catheter in a vein by "cutdown" or percutaneous insertion must precede all major operations performed on infants, as a dependable route for administration of fluids and blood. Good surgical principles are never more important than in the neonate: precision (magnification is sometimes helpful), gentleness, protection of exposed viscera, miniaturized instruments, and fine suture material are essential. Gastrostomy tubes are preferable to irritating nasogastric tubes if lengthy suction or tube feeding is anticipated. Subcuticular closure of the skin incision will avoid the need for later suture removal, and clear plastic sprayed on the wound obviates the use of restricting conventional dressings that prevent observation and easy examination of the area. Above all, the *proper* operation must be performed *correctly.* The margin for error in neonatal surgery is narrow.

Postoperative care. Postoperative convalescence of the newborn surgical patient is generally gratifyingly rapid. Sedative and analgesic drugs are seldom required because of an apparently high pain threshold. The infant should be checked frequently visually through the transparent incubator, but manipulations should be held to a minimum, e.g., at regular 2-hour intervals.

Postoperative complications in the newborn patient are mainly those of the operation itself plus infection and aspiration of vomitus. The postoperative complications common in the adult patient (paralytic ileus, pneumonia, urinary retention, deep vein thrombophlebitis) are almost unheard of in the newborn surgical patient. Aspiration of vomitus, anastomotic leaks, adhesive postoperative intestinal obstruction, and wound infections are poorly tolerated by the infant; they are best prevented, or diagnosed and treated early.

The results of surgical treatment are very gratifying when the anomaly is completely corrected, no other anomalies are present, and no complications ensue. Multiple anomalies, incomplete surgical correction, prematurity, and postoperative complications are discouraging features that favor morbidity and mortality. There is no greater satisfaction to the surgeon or nurse than a newborn patient who has been given a normal life expectancy, surgically cured of an otherwise lethal anomaly.

CONGENITAL ANOMALIES

Congenital anomalies are simply abnormalities of development that are present at birth. Location, magnitude, and mode of origin differ. They constitute the most important single type of surgical problem in the newborn.

Cause. Congenital anomalies are the result of three basic causes:

1. Abnormal genes or chromosomes of the sperm or egg
2. Abnormalities that develop in previously normal genes or chromosomes (mutations) often because of noxious environmental influences
3. Unfavorable environment that prevents normal development of the fetus without any detectable chromosome or gene alteration

Abnormal genes or chromosomes. Some congenital disorders are caused by gross chromosomal abnormalities that can now be verified microscopically (Down's syndrome, Turner's syndrome, Klinefelter's syndrome, and intersex problems). These are characterized by multiple, widespread, and often severe changes in the developing fetus.

Other congenital anomalies are believed to result from an abnormality of a single autosomal gene (congenital cataract, achondroplasia, and syndactylism). Some of these are *dominant* (polydactylism, familial polyposis coli) and are expressed in the patient regardless of the fact that the other gene for this trait is normal. If the gene abnormalities are *recessive,* both members of the genic pair must be abnormal (albinism, cystic fibrosis) before it is expressed in the offspring. Some of the genetically determined abnormalities are sex-linked (such as hemophilia), are exhibited only in the male offspring, and are merely carried or transmitted without expression in the female.

Environment. Far more common than these are congenital abnormalities induced by exposure of the developing fetus to harmful stimuli, usually in early gestation. Vulnerability is directly proportional to the rapidity with which the body systems are developing; therefore the first trimester of pregnancy is the time when these harmful stimuli have their greatest effect. Some of the noxious environmental stimuli that have been identified are the following:

1. *Chemical:* alcohol, cyclophosphamide, diethylstilbestrol, phenytoin, tetracyclines, thalidomide, valproic acid.
2. *Maternal metabolic disturbances:* diabetes, hyperthermia, phenylketonuria, virilizing tumors.
3. *Infection:* viruses, rickettsia and bacteria; especially, cytomegalovirus, herpesvirus, rubella, toxoplasmosis, *Treponema pallidum.*
4. *Irradiation:* x rays, atomic fallout, radium (alpha particles), radioactive iodine, natural background irradiation.
5. *Mechanical:* malposition of the fetus (ex-tended knees, ankylosis), mechanical pressure (atrophic single extremities), hydraulic pressure (all four extremities atrophic).
6. *Defective fertilization and implantation:* tubal pregnancy.
7. *Parental age:* Down's syndrome, more frequent when parents are older.
8. *Anoxia:* possible ultimate pathway in many of the above conditions.
9. *Accidents of timing of embryological events:* During the first 8 weeks of gestation, the embryo progresses from a single fertilized cell to a recognizable fetus in whom the foundations of all organ systems have been laid. This phenomenal growth demands dovetailing of an infinite number of events that must occur precisely on time in order to achieve normal development. Misadventures in timing of these events may cause some congenital anomalies. For example, congenital diaphragmatic hernia seems to occur either when closure of the pleuroperitoneal canals is delayed or when the midgut returns early to the abdomen from its extracoelomic umbilical hernia.

Incidence. Over 25% of stillborn babies have congenital anomalies that caused the stillbirth; 3% of live babies will be found to have congenital anomalies on immediate careful examination, though an additional 4% harbor occult abnormalities. Fortunately, most of these are minor and do not significantly affect growth, development, or life expectancy; 75% are single, but 25% are multiple—thus when one congenital anomaly is discovered in a baby, others must be anticipated. Anomalies are about 15% higher in males than in females. The incidence is 2.5 times higher in multiple than in single births. When one anomalous child is born into a family, there is a 25 times greater chance that subsequent children will have anomalies than if previous siblings were normally developed. With two malformed siblings in a family, there is about a 50% chance that the anomalies will be similar in location and severity. The central nervous system, cardiovascular, skeletal, and intestinal systems appear to be most commonly involved in abnormal development.

History. The history is most important in diagnosing congenital anomalies, with the preceding causes being kept in mind. Questions should be directed to anomalies in previous generations and the maternal health and habits during the pregnancy.

Abnormalities of amniotic fluid volume (polyhydramnios is excessive volume; oligohydramnios is too little fluid) are frequently associated with fetal

Text continued on p. 280.

Table 28-1. Important aspects of the more common congenital anomalies

Type	Anatomical deformity	Clinical characteristics	Treatment, age	Prognosis
Central nervous system				
Myelomeningocele	Defect in bony and soft-tissue coverings of neural canal, generally lumbar level	Protrusion of cord coverings in back; paralysis and no sensation in lower extremities, anus, and bladder; about 75% will later develop hydrocephalus; meningitis a constant threat	Cover exposed nerve elements with tissue and skin in infancy	No improvement in nerve function
Hydrocephalus	Obstruction to flow or absorption of cerebrospinal fluid with increasing pressure of fluid	Enlarging head, deterioration of cerebral function, tense fontanelles	Shunt cerebrospinal fluid from brain to bloodstream or body cavity through plastic tubing and valve system; done in infancy	Malfunction of shunt may require revisions
Craniosynostosis	Premature closure of skull sutures (growth lines)	Small head, progressive cerebral deterioration	Osteotomy of suture lines to prevent closure; done in infancy	Good; repeat operations may be necessary
Cardiovascular system				
Interatrial septal defect	Hole in wall between left and right atrium	Systolic precordial murmur, some decrease in growth and exercise tolerance	Closure by suture or patch during heart-lung bypass; done in childhood; some close spontaneously	Excellent
Ventricular septal defect	Hole in wall between left and right ventricle	Systolic precordial murmur; if neglected, cyanosis and serious lung complications	Closure by suture or patch during heart-lung bypass; done in childhood; some close spontaneously	Excellent if repaired early
Tetralogy of Fallot	Interventricular septal defect, stenosis of pulmonary outflow tract, and takeoff of aorta from both ventricles	Cyanosis and breathlessness with exercise, stunted growth, systolic precordial murmur	Closure of septum to right of aorta, enlargement of pulmonary valve during heart-lung bypass; done in childhood	Higher risk operation, results good if complete correction can be achieved early
Malformation of heart valves	Stenosis or imperfect valves that allow regurgitation of blood	Systolic or disastolic murmur; dilatation, hypertrophy, and failure of heart with edema and breathlessness	Enlargement of stenotic valve, suture correction or replacement of deformed valve during heart-lung bypass; done in childhood	Good if complete correction can be achieved, guarded if not

Continued.

Table 28-1. Important aspects of the more common congenital anomalies — cont'd

Type	Anatomical deformity	Clinical characteristics	Treatment, age	Prognosis
Cardiovascular system—cont'd				
Coarctation of aorta	Narrowing of descending aorta	Headache, heart enlargement, hypertension in upper body, hypotension in lower body, absent femoral pulses	Excision under hypothermia or during heart-lung bypass; done in childhood	Excellent
Patent ductus arteriosus	Retention of fetal vessel joining pulmonary artery to aorta (to bypass lungs in utero)	"Machinery" type of continuous murmur heard in chest and back; bounding pulses, left atrial enlargement, congestive heart failure in premature infants	Suture closure or ligation; in infancy or childhood	Excellent
Otolaryngological system				
Cleft lip or palate, or both	Cleft, or opening, in lip or palate; often seen together	Obvious cosmetic defects, difficulty in feeding, speech, and dentition	Plastic surgical closure of lip in infancy, palate in young childhood	Good; generally requires large team of surgeons, dentists, speech and hearing experts for complete rehabilitation
Branchial cleft abnormalities	Retention of part, or all, of the embryonic branchial structure	Cysts, sinus, or fistula of lateral part of neck	Complete excision at time of election	Excellent
Thyroglossal abnormalities	Retention of embryonic thyroid tract from base of tongue to low anterior neck	Cyst or tract in anterior midline of neck	Complete excision at time of election	Excellent
Gastrointestinal system				
Atresia: complete closure of intestinal lumen; rare in stomach and colon	Esophagus: generally has blind proximal pouch, plus fistula connecting distal esophagus to distal trachea	Blind pouch: saliva and feedings vomited. Fistula: air distending bowel, stomach; HCl bathing lungs to cause pneumonia	Division and closure of fistula, anastomosis of ends of esophagus in neonatal period	Good; often correctable stricture of anastomosis; frequent gastroesophageal reflux
	Anorectal: no anal opening, closed rectum; 70% have narrow fistula connecting rectum to vagina and perineum in females, or to bladder, urethra, and perineum in males	Abdominal distension, bilious vomiting; either no meconium passed, or—females: meconium through vagina or on perineum; males: meconium in urine or on perineum	Division and closure fistula, pullthrough of end of rectum to perineum through anal muscles; may need preliminary colostomy in neonatal period	Good early results; ultimate fecal control is variable

	Ileum, jejunum: complete closure of lumen by membrane, or with loss of continuity of bowel	Abdominal distension, bilious vomiting, scanty meconium rectally	Excision and end-to-end anastomosis; in neonatal period	Excellent if enough bowel remains to support nutritional needs
	Duodenum: complete closure by membrane beyond ampulla of Vater (where bile and pancreatic juice enter); 30% have Down's syndrome	Scaphoid abdomen, copious bilious vomiting, scanty meconium rectally	Surgical bypass of membrane by side-to-side anastomosis of duodenum above the block to duodenum below the block; done in neonatal period	Excellent
Stenosis: narrowing of intestinal lumen; rare in esophagus, stomach, or colon	Duodenum: partial obstruction by membrane with a hole in it; 30% have Down's syndrome	No distension, bilious vomiting of feedings, some diminution in stools	Surgical bypass of membrane by side-to-side anastomosis when discovered	Excellent
	Jejunum, ileum: partial obstruction by membrane with a hole in it	Moderate abdominal distension, bilious vomiting of feedings, some diminution in stools	Excision and end-to-end anastomosis when discovered	Excellent
Malrotation of midgut	Abnormal embryological rotation of gut with extrinsic band across duodenum, small bowel in right side abdomen and colon in left; 50% have volvulus, or twisting, of gut around vessels	Bilious vomiting when duodenum obstructed by band; symptoms may be vague, intermittent, or absent; volvulus produces pain, strangulation, and shock	Lysis of extrinsic duodenal band; derotation of volvulus, resection if bowel dead; operate whenever discovered or symptomatic	Excellent if no volvulus; strangulating volvulus may require massive small bowel resection resulting in short gut syndrome
Meckel's diverticulum	Outpocketing on the surface of distal ileum, vestige of embryonic tract, seen in 2% of people; 15% contain stomach mucosa, secrete HCl acid, and produce symptoms of ulceration, inflammation, or bleeding	Many are asymptomatic; intermittent abdominal pain, distension, vomiting, and melena are characteristic symptoms	Excision and closure when diagnosed or symptomatic	Excellent
Hirschsprung's disease (congenital megacolon, or aganglionosis)	Absent autonomic nerve cells in wall of distal part of colon causing obstruction at this point because peristaltic waves not propagated	Abdominal distension, constipation since birth	Excision or bypass of involved colon; may require preliminary colostomy	Good

Continued.

Table 28-1. Important aspects of the more common congenital anomalies — cont'd

Type	Anatomical deformity	Clinical characteristics	Treatment, age	Prognosis
Gastrointestinal system—cont'd				
Meconium ileus	Seen in 8% of babies with mucoviscidosis (fibrocystic disease of pancreas); undigested meconium obstructing small bowel	Abdominal distension, bilious vomiting, scanty meconium passed	Irrigation or bypass of obstructing meconium block; administration of pancreatic digestive enzymes; done in neonatal period	Poor because of generalized mucoviscidosis and pneumonia
Genitourinary system				
Congenital obstruction	Ureteropelvic junction (at kidney outlet): caused by extrinsic band or vessel, or intrinsic narrowing; may be unilateral or bilateral; results in hydronephrosis and often infection	Flank pain or mass, fever, pus in urine; uremia if bilateral	Plastic revision to relieve obstruction if kidney good; done whenever diagnosed	Good
	Ureterocystic junction (where ureter joins bladder): intrinsic or extrinsic narrowing, poor peristalsis; unilateral or bilateral; produces hydroureter, hydronephrosis, and often infection	Flank pain or mass, fever, pus in urine; uremia if bilateral	Excision of obstructed area, reimplantation of ureter into bladder; done whenever diagnosed	Good
	Bladder neck (outlet): intrinsic valve or membrane; produces enlarged bladder and often bilateral reflux and infection to both kidneys	Lower abdominal mass, flank pain, fever, pus in urine, uremia if neglected	Resection of valve or membrane, plastic widening of stenosis	Good
Undescended testes	One or both testes in or above inguinal canal, often associated with hernia	Empty scrotal sac on one or both sides with groin swelling	Surgical placement in scrotum; in young childhood	Good; fertility likely to be impaired when bilateral
Lymphatic and vascular systems				
Cutaneous capillary hemangioma "strawberry"	Pink-red, slightly raised skin lesion	Cosmetic deformity mainly; occasionally ulcerates and bleeds	None; 95% thrombose and disappear in early childhood after infant growth spurt	Excellent

Cavernous hemangioma	Large venous channels with abnormal lymphatic and arterial connections	Enlarged, bulky, blue-red lesions with discomfort or dysfunction if extremity involved; occasionally ulcerates, bleeds, or becomes infected; gigantism may occur	Injection of sclerosing agents, partial excision with skin grafts or, rarely, amputation as symptoms necessitate	Poor; recurrence and progression common
Cystic hygroma	Enlarged lymphatic spaces that cannot empty watery tissue fluid	Cystic, soft, indentable mass of neck or axilla that transilluminates; rarely produces tracheal deviation and airway obstruction	Conservative excision at age of election	Excellent
Skeletal system				
Congenital dislocation of hip	Dislocation of femoral head out of shallow hip joint	Asymmetry of fat folds of leg and buttock; palpable "click" on passive abduction and external rotation of hip	Reduction by manipulation, plaster cast in neonatal period	Excellent
Clubfoot (talipes equinovarus)	Foot points downward and is twisted inward	Inability to elevate foot	Manipulation and plaster casts in increasing degrees of dorsiflexion in neonatal period	Excellent if begun early
Abdominal wall				
Umbilical hernia	Enlarged umbilical fascial ring with protrusion of intestines into sac covered by skin	Umbilical swelling, larger with straining; asymptomatic	None; almost all spontaneously disappear by the age of 7 years	Excellent
Omphalocele	Enlarged umbilical fascial ring with protrusion of intestines into thin translucent amniotic sac not covered by skin	Grayish sac bulging around base of umbilical cord at birth filled with viscera	If small, immediate excision and repair of abdominal wall; if large, prosthetic "silo" to house viscera 7 to 10 days until abdominal wall can be closed	Good
Gastroschisis	Small aperture in abdominal wall to right of umbilicus through which protrudes midgut: thickened, covered with exudate, aperistaltic	Grossly altered intestine protruding from abdominal wall defect; no covering whatsoever	Immediate reduction and closure of abdominal wall, if feasible; if not, temporary prosthetic "silo"	Good

anomalies and should be investigated carefully by midtrimester prenatal amniocentesis and fetal ultrasound studies.

Normally the fetus continually swallows amniotic fluid from the fifth gestational month until delivery. This fluid is absorbed from the proximal small intestine to circulate as tissue fluid, plasma, and cerebrospinal fluid. It is then partially excreted through the placental circuit into the maternal circulation and partially excreted by the fetal kidneys back into the amniotic sac. Interruption of this cyclic flow at any point in the fetus (proximal small bowel: atresia; central nervous system: anencephaly, hydrocephaly, myelomeningocele; urinary tract: atresia, renal aplasia) may upset the delicate balance of amniotic fluid to produce volume abnormalities (oligohydramnios or polyhydramnios).

Physical examination. Physical examination must be meticulous and detailed. It should include inspection of the freshly cut umbilical cord to see if one of the umbilical arteries is missing; this often is a clue to the presence of a hidden anomaly in the body. Small catheters passed into both ends of the gastrointestinal tract can allow rapid diagnosis of obstruction. Special tests are listed under specific congenital anomalies.

Treatment. The treatment of congenital anomalies must be individualized. No treatment is possible if the anomaly is so serious as to be immediately lethal or incorrectable, and none is necessary if the anomaly is so minor as to produce no significant change in function. Important aspects of the more common congenital anomalies are summarized in Table 28-1.

TRAUMA

A person is probably subjected to more trauma during childhood than at any later period of life. Some is self-occasioned by poor judgment and imperfect muscular and nervous coordination during the toddler years, and some results from poor parental supervision. Thanks to the resiliency of young tissue, most of the trauma is well tolerated, and few of the scars are carried into adulthood.

However, accidents are still the most common cause of death in the United States during the first half of life. In the United States in 1978, an estimated 19 million children were injured, of which 12,500 died. Motor vehicle accidents, drownings, and burns accounted for three fourths of these deaths. The general heading of accidents includes (roughly in decreasing frequency) lacerations; contusions and abrasions; fractures; ingestion of poisons, drugs, and foreign bodies; bites; sprains; head injuries; puncture wounds; eye trauma; and burns.

Approximately two thirds of accidents occur in or near the home and can be prevented by intelligent parental supervision and removal of the more common hazards. Safer playthings, supervised playgrounds, less accessible and tasty medications, and the manufacture of nonflammable clothing are public health measures that can diminish this toll. Automobile and bicycle accidents injure or kill thousands of children. Improved automobile safety engineering (seat belts, accident-proof door locks) and education of the adult driver and the child pedestrian or bicycle rider are worthwhile efforts to lower the number of children injured in this manner.

Surgical treatment of all the traumatic wounds mentioned varies according to the type and location of the trauma.

CHILD ABUSE

It has been estimated that approximately 1% of children in the United States are deliberately physically abused each year. Nearly 80% of child abuse is seen in children under 3 years of age (too young to communicate the cause of injury) and fully 90% is inflicted by caretakers of the child (parents, step-parents, babysitters, etc.). Often the abuse occurs in a family that is deprived socially, economically, and emotionally. The history of injury as given by the abuser is often vague and discrepant with the multiplicity and seriousness of the observed injury. Multiplicity of injuries is the rule: there are many fractures in different phases of healing and many ecchymoses and hematomas in various stages of resolution. The eyes, genitalia, and back are common targets for this kind of deliberate abuse. Occasionally fatalities occur. Almost all states in this country have enacted legislation to remove the threat of litigation (for false accusation) to the attending physician who reports a suspected case of child abuse to the proper authorities. In many states the physician who fails to report a suspected case of child abuse may be prosecuted.

CANCER

During the past 25 years, cancer has risen from twelfth to second place among the causes of death in young children in the United States. There is little to indicate an actual increase in the frequency of childhood malignancies, but rather a decline in other causes of death as described in the introduction to this chapter.

Comparison of adult and childhood cancer

Many basic differences distinguish adult from childhood cancer. Cancer in the adult generally arises from epithelial tissue lining glands, external surfaces, or hollow organs of the body. In contrast, childhood cancer emerges most often from mesenchymal tissue or cells of very primitive embryological origin. The organ systems involved are different; the adult has a high incidence of cancer arising from skin, breast, lung, prostrate, and intestinal epithelium. Cancer of these structures is almost unheard of in the child. About half the malignancies of children arise from lymphoid tissue in the form of leukemias and lymphomas. Another 15% to 20% are located within the central nervous system, and 10% arise from the adrenal glands and 10% from the kidneys.

Causes of cancer

A few tumors of childhood seem to have hereditary implications, including retinoblastoma, familial polyposis, and Hodgkin's disease. The incidence of cancer within the first decade of life exceeds that of the second decade, indicating that some of the malignancies may be congenital. Leukemia in the mother has been transmitted across the placenta to her fetus; cancers of the adrenal glands and kidney occur in newborns. Irradiation delivered to children for other causes has been incriminated in later development of some cancers, particularly of the thyroid gland and lymphoma family.

Treatment of cancer

Until the past decade the results of treating childhood malignancies were discouraging, partly because of their rapid growth rate, early spread, and a delay in diagnosis occasioned by either absence of symptoms or the inability of the child to communicate such symptoms. However, there is no room for a "defeatist" attitude in the treatment of childhood malignancy. The resiliency of the young and the occasional striking response to therapy in the face of seemingly hopeless odds justify an aggressive, confident approach to treatment. Recent cooperative studies and new chemotherapy drugs have spectacularly improved the prognosis of certain childhood cancers.

All the treatment modalities employed in adult cancer are used in children; chemotherapy shows particular promise in this age group. Combinations of therapy are the rule rather than the exception. This improvement has been so dramatic in some tumors (i.e., Wilms' tumor) that now the thrust of treatment is to select those patients with a good prognosis and give them as little treatment as possible. The more aggressive treatment protocols are reserved for those patients with a poor prognosis, based on histological appearance and extent of disease.

Specific types of childhood cancer
Lymphoma-leukemia family

Leukemia is the single most common malignant neoplasm seen in children. About 90% are of the acute lymphogenous type, with the peak incidence at about 4 years of age. Prognosis is guarded, though new drug and treatment protocols have remarkably increased remissions and cures. Chemotherapy is the treatment of choice at present; the surgeon is restricted to an occasional diagnostic node or bone marrow biopsy. The surgeon's role is more prominent in lymphoma, where he confirms diagnosis by biopsy, accurately maps the extent of involvement by "staging" operations that allow the radiotherapist to better tailor his treatment, and occasionally "debulks" large non-Hodgkin's lymphomas.

Neuroblastoma

Neuroblastoma is a malignancy arising in primitive elements of the sympathetic nervous system. Two thirds originate in or near the adrenal gland, about 20% in the posterior mediastinum, and about 5% each from the neck and pelvic areas. The average age at diagnosis is 18 months, and the growth rate is typically rapid.

Symptoms of neuroblastoma are nonspecific; bone pain and fever frequently herald bone marrow metastases. Diarrhea, weight loss, anemia, and irritability are often seen. About 80% of patients have an abdominal mass that often extends across the midline, occasionally associated with metastases palpable within the liver. Diagnosis is confirmed by plain roentgenograms showing the mass (which often contains calcium stippling) displacing hollow viscera, and intravenous pyelograms that show kidney displacement. Ultrasound and CT scans pinpoint location and extent of the primary tumor, as well as liver metastases. Metastases to bone occur in about 30% and to the lungs in 10%.

The surest diagnostic test of neuroblastoma is the presence of specific catecholamine hormones (vanillylmandelic acid and homovanillic acid) in the urine or blood, representing metabolic end products of tumor origin. Treatment consists of surgical removal of as much tumor as possible, generally followed by low-dosage irradiation. Chemotherapy in the form of vincristine and cyclophosphamide combinations may palliate neuroblastoma.

Onset within the first year of life or tumors primary in the neck, pelvis, or mediastinum command a favorable prognosis. Curiously, about 5% of neuroblastomas spontaneously transform into benign ganglioneuromas. Tumor antibodies have been demonstrated in some cured patients. Unfortunately, more than half of patients with neuroblastoma will die of their disease. Treatment has not significantly improved prognosis during the past decade.

Wilms' tumor

Wilms' tumor, or nephroblastoma, is a cancer arising in embryonal kidney cells that grows rapidly to destroy the normal kidney tissue. Again, the symptoms are nonspecific and include vague abdominal discomfort, fever, and occasionally hematuria. Early direct spread to perirenal tissues is the rule, with metastases to lung and liver in one third of the patients by the time a diagnosis is established; 90% of patients have a mass in the abdomen on physical examination, and intravenous pyelograms, ultrasound studies, and CT scans will differentiate from neuroblastoma. Regrettably, about 5% of patients develop Wilms' tumors of both kidneys. Treatment is combined surgical removal, x-ray therapy, and chemotherapy with actinomycin D and vincristine. Recent reports indicate a long-term survival of 75% of these patients.

Central nervous system tumors

Most central nervous system tumors arise below the membrane, or tentorium, which separates the cerebrum from the lower centers. Most of these cancers stem from supporting tissues within the brain and produce symptoms by disturbing balance and motor activity or by blocking the flow of cerebrospinal fluid to increase intracranial pressure. Surgical excision is the most effective treatment at this time. In keeping with central nervous system tumors of all ages, no distant metastases are seen.

Connective tissue tumors

Osteosarcomas have a peak incidence later in childhood, probably because of increasing bone growth rates at this time of life. Striated muscle cancers (*rhabdomyosarcoma*) in infancy are most commonly located in the bladder or genital tracts; in older children they are chiefly seen in the head and neck, but they may occur in any striated muscle. Surgical excision, x-ray therapy, and a number of therapeutic drugs are used in combination for treatment of these less common childhood malignancies. Prognosis is guarded, with salvage of the patient in less than one half of all cases. A notable exception is children with Ewing's sarcoma of bone in whom conservative surgical resection, x-ray therapy, and new chemotherapeutic drugs have remarkably improved the prognosis.

NEONATAL GASTROINTESTINAL OBSTRUCTION

Obstruction of the gastrointestinal tract in the newborn is both unique and serious enough to justify special consideration. Obstruction may occur anywhere from esophagus to anus, having a curious numerical predilection for both ends of the tract. All neonatal gastrointestinal obstructions are secondary to congenital anomalies that, however, arise from a host of different influences. Together they constitute by far the most common surgical emergency of the neonatal period of life.

Neonatal gastrointestinal obstructions are no exception to the rule that anomalies are often multiple. Two causes for intestinal obstruction may coexist at different levels, as exemplified by the association of esophageal atresia with duodenal atresia or anorectal atresia—or the associated anomaly may involve a totally different system, such as the major congenital heart defects that accompany esophageal or anorectal atresia. The intestine may be obstructed simultaneously by two different mechanisms at the same level (extrinsic duodenal obstruction resulting from malrotation, and intrinsic obstruction from duodenal membrane) or at different levels by the same mechanism (about 15% of patients with intestinal atresia have additional atretic areas downstream from the most proximal one). About one fourth of babies with neonatal gastrointestinal obstruction have other anomalies, which must be diagnosed and managed along with the primary obstructing lesion.

Prematurity (birth weight below 2,500 gm.) is associated in about one third of babies with congenital gastrointestinal obstruction. Both prematurity and serious associated congenital anomalies greatly worsen prognosis. The mortality for full-term newborns with obstruction who have no other major anomalies is about 10%, contrasting unfavorably with an 80% to 90% mortality expected in the obstructed premature baby with other major anomalies. If the obstruction is complicated by peritonitis, the mortality is 50%. If the intestine must be opened to relieve the obstruction, the mortality (40%) is much higher than it is when the obstruction is extrinsic (5%). Overall, the salvage rate for neonatal gastrointestinal obstruction is about 75%.

Family and pregnancy history. Some causes for neonatal gastrointestinal obstruction are familial or inheritable, and therefore a carefully taken history of the genealogy is helpful. Fibrocystic disease of the pancreas (with meconium ileus), congenital aganglionosis of the colon (Hirschsprung's disease), and hypertrophic pyloric stenosis are all examples of this tendency. Down's syndrome has a familial tendency and a predilection for duodenal atresia (about 7%).

The maternal pregnancy history is important in terms of illnesses, ingestion of drugs, and exposure to irradiation or other noxious environmental influences associated with congenital anomalies. Polyhydramnios, the presence of excessive amounts of maternal amniotic fluid, has a high association with obstructions of the proximal gastrointestinal tract, as explained on pp. 274 and 280.

Patient history. Bile vomiting, abdominal distension, and obstipation are the three cardinal signs of obstruction of the gastrointestinal tract at any age. However, exceptions to this rule occur frequently enough in the obstructed newborn baby to justify special attention. Thus esophageal atresia with tracheoesophageal fistula produces regurgitation of feedings and saliva unstained with bile; the abdominal distension is profound but is associated with free passage of meconium. The newborn with duodenal obstruction will indeed have copious bile vomiting but only mild epigastric distension and may pass one or two normal meconium stools. Paradoxically, the functional (nonmechanical) type of colonic obstruction produced by congenital aganglionosis (Hirschsprung's disease) is sometimes associated with diarrhea and only late and infrequent vomiting, although abdominal distension is conspicuous. Notwithstanding these exceptions, any newborn baby who (1) fails to pass meconium rectally within 24 hours after birth, or (2) vomits bile, or (3) exhibits abdominal distension should have a plain roentgenogram of the abdomen taken in the supine and erect (or decubitus) positions as a minimal initial step to investigate intestinal obstruction.

Relative incidence. Atresias of the esophagus and anorectal area are numerically the most common causes for neonatal gastrointestinal tract obstruction, each constituting roughly 25% of cases. An additional 20% are caused by atresia and stenosis of the small intestine, and another 25% will be about equally divided among midgut malrotation, meconium ileus, and congenital aganglionosis; 5% of cases comprise a miscellaneous group of very diverse causes.

Diagnosis. The diagnosis of gastrointestinal obstruction may often be made in the newborn baby before symptoms occur, by gentle passage of a small, soft, plastic catheter into both ends of the gastrointestinal tract. If the tube passes into the stomach, esophageal and choanal atresia can be ruled out; if 10 ml. or less of clear fluid is aspirated from the stomach, congenital obstruction of the small bowel is extremely unlikely. However, if more than 20 ml. of bile-stained material is present in the stomach, the diagnosis of obstruction should be entertained seriously, and an upright roentgenogram of the abdomen should be taken. Passage of the catheter through the anus and into the rectum rules out anorectal atresia.

Plain roentgeograms of the abdomen and chest in the supine and upright (or cross-table lateral) positions are the first step in diagnosis. Abnormal distribution or amounts of intestinal gas often allow a specific enough diagnosis that no additional radiographic procedures are necessary. Occasionally contrast enema is indicated, especially for showing the size and position of the colon. Upper gastrointestinal contrast studies are rarely needed—they are sometimes dangerous from the standpoint of aspiration of the contrast material used.

Differential diagnosis. There are many nonsurgical conditions that can simulate intestinal obstruction in the newborn baby. Some are very serious diseases in their own right, and it is tragic to compound an already grave medical problem by laparotomy undertaken with a mistaken diagnosis of intestinal obstruction. Examples of these nonsurgical conditions follow:

1. *Feeding problems:* Underfeeding, overfeeding, or improperly administered feedings are probably the most common cause for neonatal vomiting. Generally the material vomited consists simply of the feeding material itself or nonbile-stained material. Observation of a feeding or a carefully taken history of the feeding program should allow a proper diagnosis to be made.

2. *Infections:* Septicemia in the newborn can produce vomiting and abdominal distension, whether the infection is primary within the gstrointestinal tract or elsewhere. Cultures of the blood, pharynx, cerebrospinal fluid, urine, and stool plus detection of a source for the infection establish the correct diagnosis.

3. *Increased intracranial pressure:* Cerebral edema, hemorrhage caused by birth trauma, or hydrocephalus often cause vomiting in the newborn. Evaluation of fontanelle pressure and careful neurological examination should rule out these causes for neonatal vomiting.

4. *Obstructive uropathy:* Congenital obstruction of the urinary tract producing azotemia is associated with vomiting and difficult feeding of the baby. Observation of the urinary output, blood urea nitrogen determinations, and ultrasound studies are helpful clues in diagnosis.

5. *Endocrine and metabolic:* Congenital adrenal hyperplasia (adrenogenital syndrome), abnormalities of glucose metabolism (hypoglycemia, galactosemia, glycogenosis), maternal opiate addiction, and tetany from hypocalcemia can be associated with vomiting or ab-

dominal distension in the newborn. Appropriate maternal history or studies of the serum and urine electrolyte and glucose levels establish the appropriate diagnosis.

6. *Chalasia:* Chalasia, or congenital incompetence of the esophagogastric sphincter, allows easy regurgitation of gastric contents and feedings and is occasionally confused with obstructive causes for vomiting. The non–bile stained character of the regurgitated material and its relationship to the supine position are clues to the diagnosis, which is confirmed by upper gastrointestinal tract barium studies. Competence of the sphincter develops within a few weeks to months, and interim treatment consists in positioning the baby either prone or in the upright position in an appropriately constructed seat and offering thick feedings.

Embryology of the gastrointestinal tract

Misadventures that occur to the fetus resulting in abnormal development of the gastrointestinal tract are the most frequent cause for neonatal obstruction. This section reviews briefly the major stages of gastrointestinal tract development and some of the more common anomalies that occur.

For convenience and better understanding of its embryological development, the gastrointestinal tract is divided into three subdivisions: (1) the foregut, which embraces the esophagus, stomach, and proximal duodenum (including the bile ducts, liver, and pancreas), vascularized largely by the celiac axis, (2) the midgut, running from the ampulla of Vater in the second portion of the duodenum to the splenic flexure of the colon and supplied with blood by the superior mesenteric artery, and (3) the hindgut, extending from the splenic flexure of the colon to the rectum and having as its major blood vessel the inferior mesenteric artery. The venous return from all three embryological gut subdivisions is largely through the portal system to the liver.

In the early embryo the gastrointestinal tract is a straight tube running in the midline from the oral cavity to the anus, suspended by both a dorsal and a ventral mesentery. The ventral mesentery is lost early, but the dorsal mesentery is retained with the blood supply to the developing gastrointestinal tract. By the fourth gestational week the lung anlage separates from the proximal end of the foregut; incompleteness of this splitting mechanism results in the various forms of esophageal atresia and tracheoesophageal fistula.

Beginning at the fifth week of intrauterine life, the stomach sacculates and the midgut begins to proliferate, enlarge, and elongate in a very accelerated manner. Epithelial proliferation tends to narrow the intestinal lumen; in lower animals the proliferation continues until the lumen is obliterated to form the so-called *solid cord stage*. In the human embryo the solid cord stage develops rarely and only in the duodenum; vacuolization and coalescence of vacuoles rapidly reestablish the internal lumen of the tract.

Linear growth of the midgut rapidly outstrips the volume of the peritoneal cavity, resulting in elongation of the mesentery and herniation of the entire midgut into the base of the umbilical cord. The resulting *extracoelomic phase* (Fig. 28-1) of midgut development occurs from the sixth to the tenth weeks of intrauterine life.

As one views the fetus from the front, the midgut rotates 270 degrees in a counterclockwise direction around its vascular axis (the superior mesenteric artery) (Fig. 28-1, *A* to *D*) during this extracoelomic phase of development, after which an orderly return of the midgut to the enlarged peritoneal cavity occurs during the tenth to twelfth weeks of intrauterine life. Return of the midgut occurs in an aboral manner from proximal to distal, the duodenum returning to the right upper abdominal quadrant after the first 90 degrees of rotation (Fig. 28-1, *B*), where it is fixed retroperitoneally. This forces the stomach to rotate 90 degrees, so that its original left side is now anterior and its right side the definitive posterior wall. This is correlated with elongation of its dorsal mesenteric surface into what we refer to as the greater curvature of the stomach.

As the proximal jejunum returns, the 270-degree counterclockwise rotation is completed (Fig. 28-1, *C* and *D*) so as to carry the distal portion of the duodenum inferior (caudad) to the superior mesenteric artery and across the midline, where the duodenojejunal junction is fixed in a nearly retroperitoneal manner by the ligament of Treitz. The hindgut is pushed to the left by the returning small bowel (Fig. 28-1, *C*), and the cecum and the right colon are directed above (cephalad to) the superior mesenteric artery with the cecum ending in the right upper abdominal quadrant (Fig. 28-1, *D*). The embryological changes in the midgut are completed leisurely during the succeeding months of gestation and on into the first few weeks of postnatal life by the gradual descent of the cecum to the right lower abdominal quadrant (Fig. 28-1, *E*), where it becomes attached to the right posterior parietes in the normal adult position.

Two pathological states involving the midgut are attributable to misadventures occurring during these critical fifth to twelfth weeks of gestational life. *Omphalocele* (exomphalos) (Fig. 28-2) may be thought of as a retention of the extracoelomic phase of midgut development, with failure of both

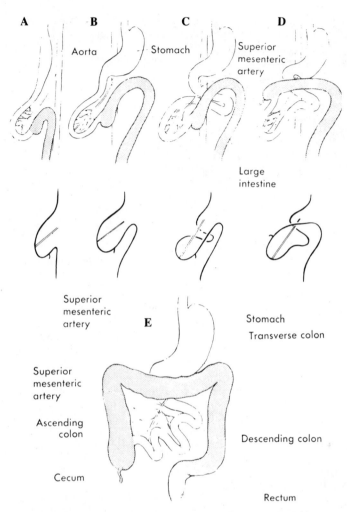

Fig. 28-1. Normal embryological rotation of midgut. (See text.)

normal rotation and return of the midgut. It complicates about 1:4,000 live births. The midgut is
contained extraperitoneally at the umbilicus in a
sac composed of amniotic membranes devoid of
skin. It is characterized by abnormalities of intestinal rotation and invariably is associated with a
small peritoneal cavity, which has not been
stimualted to enlarge by a normal return of the
midgut viscera.

The omphalocele sac is friable and poorly vascularized; 10% rupture during intrauterine life to
provoke a chronic peritonitis reaction of the bowel,
which is bathed in amniotic fluid (foreshortening,
matting of loops, lusterless serosal exudate). The
sac ruptures in an additional few during or shortly

after labor and delivery. In either event the exposed viscera must be covered immediately.

Treatment of omphalocele is individualized:
1. *Sac ruptured:* Emergent surgical protection of
   exposed bowel by either total repair of the
   abdominal wall defect (if the herniated viscera
   can be easily reduced back into the abdominal
   cavity) or coverage of viscera by synthetic
   material (usually Dacron-reinforced Silastic)
   that is sutured to the edges of the defect and
   then over the exposed viscera; in 7 to 10 days
   the viscera can usually be easily reduced, so
   that removal of the prosthetic "silo" and
   suture closure of the abdominal wall can be
   carried out.

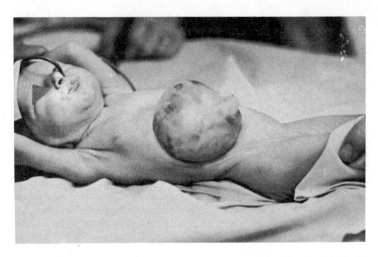

Fig. 28-2. Omphalocele—lusterless, semiopaque sac that contains herniated midgut.

2. *Sac intact:*
   a. *Nonsurgical* (generally restricted to poor-risk babies). Paint the sac with an astringent (0.5%) merbromin [Mercurochrome]) to thicken and toughen it as the abdominal wall skin gradually overgrows and replaces the sac during the ensuing weeks.
   b. *Surgical.* Excise sac, and either close the abdominal wall in layers or cover exposed viscera with a prosthetic "silo."

A principal vital to the surgial treatment of all omphaloceles is to avoid an excessively high intra-abdominal pressure when the bowel is being returned to the abnormally small peritoneal cavity. Elevated intra-abdominal pressure is tolerated poorly by the newborn because of (1) reduced respiratory exchange from restricted motion of the diaphragm, and (2) impedance of venous return to the heart from the lower compartment by compression of the inferior vena cava. Effective decompression of the gastrointestinal tract and intraoperative manual stretching of the abdominal wall help avoid this disaster. When reduction of the viscera is impossible or dangerous, the aforementioned prosthetic "silos" are sutured to the edges of the abdominal wall defect to allow slow, progressive reduction of bowel back into the gradually enlarging abdominal cavity. Total parenteral feeding avoids early postoperative oral feedings, which are poorly tolerated in the crowded abdominal cavity, especially by bowel that is temporarily aperistaltic from having been bathed in amniotic fluid throughout gestation.

Gastroschisis is an anomaly clinically similar to the antenatally ruptured omphalocele in that midgut protrudes through a small paraumbilical aperture in the abdominal wall, generally on the right side, throughout gestation. The bowel suffers the same chronic, aseptic, chemical peritonitis that characterizes the antenatally ruptured omphalocele, and treatment principles are the same. The embryopathy that results in gastroschisis is not clear.

Malrotation of the midgut is the second major problem resulting from faulty embryological development of the midgut. It is characterized by various degrees of incompleteness of the rotation and fixation mechanism. Most commonly, rotation occurs only through the first 90-degree arc (Fig. 28-1, *B*) with a normal position of the stomach and the proximal duodenum. The duodenojejunum descends to the right of the superior mesenteric artery, and in general the entire small intestine lies in the right hemiabdomen whereas the large bowel occupies the left hemiabdomen. The base or root of the midgut mesentery is invariably narrow.

With normal midgut rotation (Fig. 28-1, *E*), the base or root of the mesentery in the adult measures about 20 cm. in length and extends from the ligament of Treitz (to the left of the second lumbar vertebra) obliquely downward to the ileocecal area in the right lower abdominal quadrant. With failure of normal midgut rotation, the mesenteric root or base is very narrow, measuring only the width of the superior mesenteric artery and vein (Fig. 28-1, *B*). The combination of a narrow mesenteric vascular axis and a very lengthy fan-shaped periphery (along which the midgut itself courses) provides the setting for the most significant and lethal complication of midgut malrotation, namely, twist-

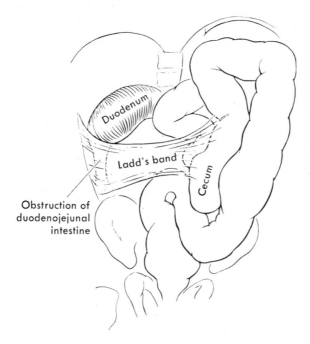

Fig. 28-3. Malrotation of midgut—entire colon in left hemiabdomen and Ladd's band running from cecum to right posterior parietes to cross and obstruct duodenojejunal intestine.

ing or *volvulus of the midgut*. Volvulus occurs in about 50% of patients with midgut malrotation. It involves a clockwise twist of the midgut around the very narrow vascular base or axis to produce varying degrees of occlusion of the lymphatic, venous, and arterial vessels of the mesentery. The volvulus always occurs in a clockwise direction for an unknown reason (perhaps because the liver developing in the right upper quadrant prevents an initial counterclockwise thrust) and may involve twisting through three or four complete turns.

Two potentially lethal conditions occur, then, with volvulus of the midgut: the twist (1) closes off the midgut on both ends to produce *closed-loop intestinal obstruction* and (2) results in varying degrees of mesenteric vascular stagnation as venous outflow and later arterial inflow are occluded. These two features set the stage for midgut perforation and infarction, either of which can be fatal.

Midgut malrotation without volvulus is generally symptomatic because of some degree of duodenal obstruction. Extrinsic duodenal obstruction occurs from peritoneal bands *(Ladd's bands)* (Fig. 28-3) stretching from the right posterior parietes across the duodenum to the cecum and ascending colon in the left upper abdominal quadrant; they can be thought of as bands that would have fixed the

cecum and ascending colon in the right gutter had normal rotation occurred. Approximately 15% of patients with extrinsic duodenal obstruction on this basis also have an intrinsic obstruction caused by a duodenal membrane. The duodenal obstruction is generally intermittent and partial, reflected by bouts of bile-stained vomiting associated with epigastric distension. If volvulus ensues, the morbidity is sharply increased by trapping of fluid within the closed midgut loop, thereby producing more abdominal distension and obstipation, and perhaps less vomiting. Strangulation will precipitate signs of peritoneal irritation progressing to shock and a critically ill patient within a matter of hours.

The diagnosis of midgut malrotation often must be made in the operating room, since it is difficult to distinguish duodenal obstruction occurring in young patients on this basis from other causes, such as duodenal stenosis, atresia, and annular pancreas. Plain abdominal roentgenograms show a dilated stomach and duodenum without clear differentiation as to cause. Upper gastrointestinal contrast study performed with pressure on the stomach often will force barium past the Ladd's bands and reveal the beaklike cutoff diagnostic of volvulus. When signs of intestinal strangulation are associated with duodenal obstruction in an infant or child, malrotation with midgut volvulus becomes the most likely cause and demands early laparotomy.

Surgical treatment of uncomplicated midgut malrotation involves (1) complete division of Ladd's bands, thereby allowing the cecum to lie freely within the left upper abdominal quadrant with the duodenum and jejunum proceeding down the right posterior parietes in an unobstructed manner, (2) prophylactic appendectomy so that left upper quadrant appendicitis will not later be a confusing clinical entity to diagnose, and (3) proof of intrinsic patency of the duodenum. If volvulus has occurred, the twist must be derotated completely in a counterclockwise direction, and necrotic bowel must be resected. Recurrent volvulus virtually never occurs, probably because of intestinal fixation from adhesions generated during the operation.

Origin of intestinal atresia and stenosis

Gastrointestinal atresia implies total closure of the bowel lumen. It may be composed simply of a membrane or diaphragm stretched across the lumen (Fig. 28-4), or it may be extensive with total loss of continuity and may even be multiple (Fig. 28-5). Stenosis results in a narrowing of the lumen

without complete obstruction, often represented by a diaphragm or membrane with a small aperture; it never involves loss of continuity of the intestine or complete obstruction.

Some dispute exists as to the embryogenesis of atresias and stenoses of the gastrointestinal tract. The traditional concept is that they represent a failure of canalization (vacuolization and coalescence of vacuoles) after the so-called solid core stage at about the fifth week of embryonic life, wherein the lumen of the developing intestine is occluded by hyperplasia of the mucosal epithelial cells. The basis for this solid core theory stems largely from embryological studies done on lower animal forms. More sophisticated and recent studies of the human embryo demonstrate a somewhat abortive epithelial cell hyperplasia that produces total obliteration of the lumen (only rarely) in the duodenum. Therefore this mechanism is a logical explanation for congenital atresia and stenosis of the human duodenum only. The solid core theory does not explain many of the features of jejunal and ileal atresia: loss of bowel continuity, defects in the adjacent mesentery and visible remnants of volvulus, intussusception, and meconium peritonitis.

A more attractive explanation for congenital

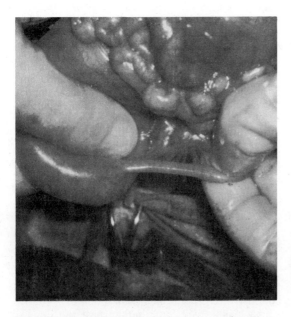

Fig. 28-4. Intestinal atresia with intrinsic membrane occluding lumen. Dilated and obstructed small intestine on left, and unused but patent "wormlike" bowel distal to membrane on right.

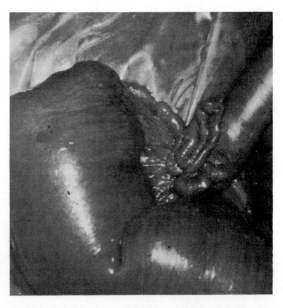

Fig. 28-5. Intestinal atresia with loss of intestinal continuity. Dilated and obstructed proximal bowel on left and below, and unused distal bowel on right.

stenosis and atresia of the of the jejunum, ileum, and colon implicates occlusion of the mesenteric vessels sometime during gestation, which provokes a sterile infarction of that segment of developing intestine supplied by the vessels. Thrombosis of a small terminal artery (Fig. 28-6) would infarct only a short segment of gut, with the resulting granulation and scar tissue forming a membrane characteristic of stenosis or the minor forms of atresia. Occlusion of major vessels (Figs. 28-7 and 28-8) nourishing longer segments of developing intestine would better explain the more gross and extensive degrees of atresia. Spontaneous thrombosis or strangulating misadventures, such as intussusception or volvulus, might be the basic origin of the mesenteric vascular occlusion.

Deliberate experimental production of mesenteric vascular occlusion in unborn animal fetuses has successfully reproduced all degrees of stenosis and atresia of the intestine, lending experimental credence to this thesis of origin. Because of the short dorsal mesentery nourishing the esophagus and duodenum and the nonmesenteric collateral circulation to the developing rectum, this seems to be a less attractive and plausible explanation for the embryogenesis of atresia of the esophagus, duodenum, and rectum.

Esophageal atresia with tracheoesophageal fistula

There are many anatomical variations of congenital esophageal stenosis and atresia, but approximately 80% have a blind proximal esophageal

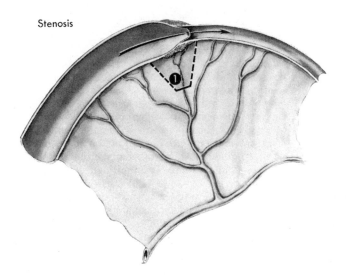

Stenosis

Fig. 28-6. Diagram of thrombosis of small mesenteric "end artery" of developing fetal intestine, producing sterile infarction of short segment of bowel nourished by this vessel. Resulting phagocytosis and repair reaction produce intrinsic diaphragm, which in diagram has small aperture through which some of intestinal content may pass.

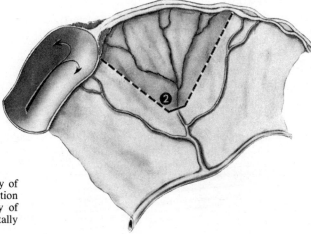

Fig. 28-7. Thrombosis of larger mesenteric artery of developing fetal intestine, producing sterile infarction of longer segment of bowel. External continuity of bowel is retained, but intrinsic membrane totally obstructs lumen. (See Fig. 28-4.)

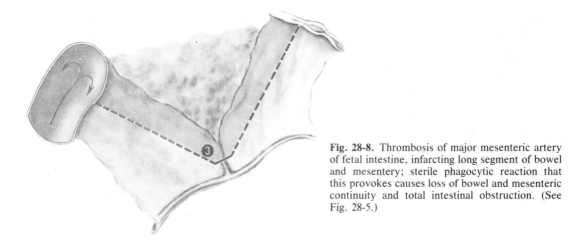

Fig. 28-8. Thrombosis of major mesenteric artery of fetal intestine, infarcting long segment of bowel and mesentery; sterile phagocytic reaction that this provokes causes loss of bowel and mesenteric continuity and total intestinal obstruction. (See Fig. 28-5.)

pouch extending to the upper thoracic level, with the distal esophagus connected to the tracheobronchial tree near the carina (Fig. 28-9). Because of its frequency, this is the only type that is discussed here.

A glance at Fig. 28-9 allows the student to predict the symptoms produced by this anatomical arrangement. Polyhydramnios is the earliest sign of esophageal atresia, which begins during the midtrimester of gestation. Postnatally, the blind proximal esophagus fills with saliva, which is then regurgitated back into the mouth, producing a seemingly "mucusy" baby who salivates excessively. The first feeding provokes gagging and immediate regurgitation, with explosive coughing and cyanosis if any spills over into the trachea. The fistula between the trachea and the stomach through the distal part of the esophagus is a "two-way" street. Some of the inspired air is diverted into the stomach and on downstream to produce unusual degrees of abdominal distension and tympany. When the infant is recumbent, hydrochloric acid from the stomach flows up into the lungs through the distal part of the esophagus to produce the most serious complication of this variety of esophageal atresia, namely, a severe chemical pneumonitis.

Diagnosis is quickly made when one can pass a soft, small, plastic catheter through the nose and find that it meets an obstruction within 10 cm. A single upright roentgenogram outlines the blind proximal pouch and reveals pneumonitis and the unusually large accumulation of intestinal gas characteristic of this disorder. Until further treatment can be carried out, the infant should be positioned upright, and continuous suction should be applied to the nasoesophageal tube to retrieve saliva.

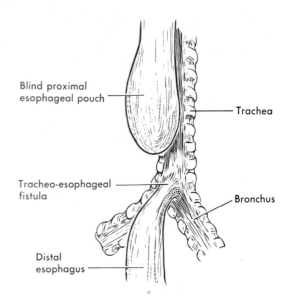

Blind proximal esophageal pouch

Trachea

Tracheo-esophageal fistula

Bronchus

Distal esophagus

Fig. 28-9. Esophageal atresia with tracheoesophageal fistula.

Definitive treatment of esophageal atresia must be individualized according to the degree of pneumonitis, the weight of the baby, and the precise anatomical form of the anomaly. In good-risk babies, primary repair may be carried out either transthoracically or retropleurally, with ligation and division of the fistula and end-to-end anastomosis of the two esophageal ends. If the infant is premature and has other major anomalies or a severe pneumonitis, preliminary gastrostomy is carried out under local anesthesia to remove the

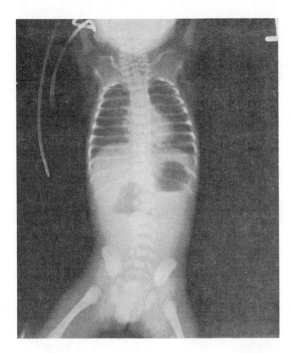

Fig. 28-10. "Double bubble" roentgenographic sign of complete duodenal obstruction in newborn. Air-fluid level in left upper quadrant is in dilated stomach; that to right of midline is in dilated and obstructed duodenum.

threat of further chemical pneumonitis; the baby is then nourished parenterally until repair can be safely undertaken. If the proximal pouch is short, it may be elongated by daily dilatations during this waiting period to facilitate primary anastomosis later.

Neonatal duodenal obstruction

Most neonatal obstructions of the duodenum occur distal to the ampulla of Vater, with bilious vomiting the outstanding clinical feature. If the obstruction is complete, plain roentgenograms of the abdomen taken in the upright position show the classical "double-bubble" sign (Fig. 28-10), which results from air-fluid levels in the stomach and proximal part of the duodenum.

Duodenal atresia is the most common cause for complete duodenal obstruction with about one third of the babies also suffering from Down's syndrome. Malrotation of the midgut with or without volvulus can cause total neonatal duodenal obstruction but also is capable of producing intermittent obstruction at various times during infancy and young childhood. Duodenal stenosis is the most common cause for partial obstruction, and

the most rare cause of all is annular pancreas. Diagnosis of partial or intermittent duodenal obstruction often requires an upper gastrointestinal tract barium series.

Duodenal atresia, stenosis, and annular pancreas are treated by surgical bypass; a side-to-side anastomosis is created between the duodenum proximal to the obstruction and the duodenum immediately beyond the obstruction. The treatment of malrotation with duodenal obstruction is discussed in detail on p. 286.

Jejunal and ileal obstruction

Neonatal obstruction of the jejunum and ileum is generally caused by congenital atresia or stenosis and less commonly by meconium ileus. Clinically the obstruction is manifested by bilious vomiting with abdominal distension proportionate to the level of the obstruction, its degree of completeness, and the time elapsed since delivery. Plain roentgenograms of the abdomen taken in the upright position will diagnose the level and completeness of the obstruction but will not label the cause precisely.

Atresia is a much more common cause of complete ileal or jejunal obstruction than meconium ileus, with stenosis the most likely cause of partial obstruction. Resection and anastomosis is the preferred treatment of atresia and stenosis.

Meconium ileus complicates about 8% of children with generalized mucoviscidosis or fibrocystic disease of the pancreas. The obstruction is caused by extremely inspissated and tenacious meconium occluding the lumen because of insufficient digestive enzymes of pancreatic origin. A specific diagnosis is possibly indicated by a family history of cystic fibrosis of the pancreas and palpation of cordlike masses of meconium within the abdomen. Plain abdominal roentgenograms show variable-sized small bowel loops and a "soap-bubble" appearance of gas dispersed within tenacious meconium.

Because of the systemic (largely pulmonary) complications of cystic fibrosis, it is best to first try to relieve the obstruction of meconium ileus by nonsurgical means. This is best achieved by instillation of hypertonic, water-soluble contrast material (gastrografin) into the rectum and under direct vision (by cinefluoroscopy) controlling the progress of the contrast material retrogradely throughout the colon and on past the ileocecal valve into the obstructed terminal ileum. Fluids must be running intravenously while this is done because the hypertonic material draws fluids into the bowel to liquify and break up the tenacious meconium enough to allow its expulsion rectally. Of course, this method of treatment can be undertaken only in uncomplicated cases (with no perforation), and reports indicate its success in only about two thirds of the cases. If this method of therapy is unsuccessful, prompt surgical intervention must follow.

Surgical treatment consists in disimpacting the undigested meconium by irrigation with mucolytic agents, when possible. Alternate methods include temporary ileostomy through which proteolytic enzymes are directly instilled into the obstructed distal small bowel. The complicated forms of meconium ileus require appropriate resection and anastomosis or exteriorization of the perforated bowel. The prognosis is guarded from the standpoint of the intestinal obstruction itself, let alone problems with atelectasis and pneumonia to which the tenacious bronchial mucus predisposes the patient.

NEONATAL OBSTRUCTION OF THE COLON

Early in embryonic development, the hindgut and allantois are joined as the cloaca. Division into a urogenital sinus anteriorly and rectum posteriorly occurs during the sixth to eighth weeks of gestation by descent of the urorectal septum. Shortly thereafter, rupture of the cloacal membrane in the proctodeum produces separate genital and intestinal orifices. Defects in these mechanisms produce

the many anatomical variations that characterize rectal atresia and imperforate anus.

The most common cause for congenital obstruction of the colon is the various forms of *anorectal atresia;* additional causes are the *meconium plug syndrome, congenital aganglionosis (Hirschsprung's disease),* and *congenital atresia* of the colon, in descending order of frequency.

There are many anatomical variations of *imperforate anus* and *rectal atresia,* but the common type consists of an absent anus with a dilated and obstructed rectum terminating somewhere in the pelvis. In *high rectal atresia* the rectum ends above the levator sling (the muscular pelvic diaphragm through which the rectum normally courses and that contributes most to fecal control), and in *low rectal atresia* the rectum passes through the sling (anterior to the puborectalis muscle) before terminating. In 70% to 80% there will be a fistula that, in the male, connects the rectum to the bladder neck, urethra, or perineal skin. In the female the fistula opens into the vagina or perineum.

Obstipation with progressive abdominal distension and late bilious vomiting characterize the disorder clinically. Diagnosis can generally be made by inspection alone (Fig. 28-11). A plain roentgenogram of the abdomen taken after the

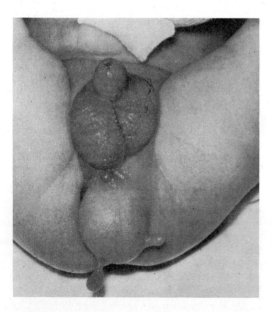

Fig. 28-11. Anorectal atresia, with abortive attempt at formation of perineal fistula marked by bluish, meconium-filled tract in scrotal raphe. Large lipoma occupies intergluteal cleft.

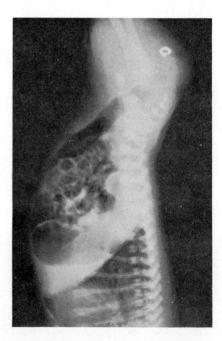

Fig. 28-12. Lateral roentgenogram taken after baby was inverted for several minutes, showing distance from perineum (radiopaque marker) to end of atretic, air-filled rectum.

infant has been inverted for several minutes (Fig. 28-12) gives a clue as to the distance between the end of the rectum and the perineum. Much more precise documentation of the abnormality is afforded when radiocontrast material can outline the atretic rectum after colostomy.

Probes are helpful in locating perineal and vaginal fistulas, and meconium or air in urine is diagnostic of rectourethral or rectovesical fistula in male infants.

Relief of the colonic obstruction is the first aim of treatment and can occasionally be satisfied by dilatation of the larger perineal and vaginal fistulous tracts. In good-risk patients primary perineal anoplasty (Fig. 28-13) is carried out as definitive treatment of the low-lying rectal atresia. Colostomy is necessary with the higher rectal atresias or in poor-risk newborns to allow temporary relief of the obstruction. Later, the rectum is "pulled through" to the perineum by a posterior or transabdominal approach. The most crucial aim of the operation is to draw the rectum in front of the puborectalis muscle and inside of the external sphincter muscles to provide effective fecal continence.

Congenital aganglionosis of the colon (Hirschsprung's disease) may produce an acute obstruc-

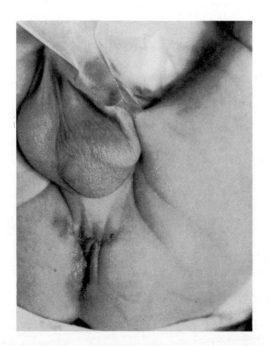

Fig. 28-13. Photograph taken 2 weeks after anoplasty repair of anorectal atresia in baby shown preoperatively in Fig. 28-11.

tion in the neonatal period of life. It is characterized by abdominal distension with the passage of little or no meconium rectally and late bilious vomiting. Occasionally, paradoxical diarrhea may occur to confuse the diagnosis of obstruction. This diagnosis may be indicated by rectal digital examination that reveals a narrow rectal ampulla and often provokes explosive passage of gas and meconium when the finger is withdrawn. Barium enema reveals a narrow rectum that enlarges at some point proximally, with poor evacuation of barium. Anorectal manometry reveals that the internal anal sphincter does not relax when the rectum is distended. Absolute confirmation rests with biopsy demonstration of absent ganglia in the autonomic nerve plexuses in the submucosal and intermuscular planes on rectal wall biopsy.

Initial treatment consists in relieving the intestinal obstruction. Usually colostomy (within ganglionated bowel) is necessary. Definitive corrective operation can occasionally be carried out primarily on a good-risk baby; it is best delayed in small or otherwise compromised babies until later in infancy or young childhood.

The *meconium plug syndrome* consists of obstruction generally of the rectum or sigmoid colon by a long, pale, and stringy plug of inspissated meconium. Delayed passage of meconium rectally, gross and progressive abdominal distension, and late bilious vomiting are the clinical signs and symptoms. Plain roentgenograms show nonspecific dilatation of multiple bowel loops with air and fluid.

Both diagnosis and treatment rest on barium enema examination, which reveals a long *filling defect* of the plug of meconium, proximal to which the colon is dilated and obstructed. Dissection of the barium around the plug commonly dislodges and allows passage of the obstructing bolus of meconium. Signs of obstruction are relieved promptly. A few of these babies later are found to have Hirschsprung's disease or cystic fibrosis. The cause of the inspissated meconium is unknown.

Besides the stomach, the colon is the least likely site for atresia or stenosis of the gastrointestinal tract to occur. It will produce complete (atresia) or partial (stenosis) obstruction at the site of the membrane, which must be distinguished from other causes of colonic obstruction by barium enema examination. Excision and anastomosis constitute proper surgical treatment.

NECK MASSES IN INFANTS AND CHILDREN

Cervical masses in infants and children are extremely common; a careful examiner is able to find neck nodules in virtually every youngster from 2 to 10 years of age. Fortunately, most of these are innocent lymph nodes that are simply residua of previous upper respiratory infections.

Lymph nodes

Acute cervical lymphadenitis arises from a primary infection (usually in the pharynx) and in itself justifies no specific therapy other than that directed to the inciting primary inflammation. Less commonly, acute lymphadenitis becomes suppurative, manifested as a fluctuant, tender neck mass. Specific treatment in the form of warm soaks followed by surgical incision and drainage should be undertaken at this point, and cultures usually show *Staphylococcus* as the causative organism. The use of antibiotics depends on the organism, the status and site of the primary infection, and the general condition of the patient.

Chronic cervical lymphadenitis is less common than acute or subacute forms. In this country chronic cervical adenitis is rarely attributed to tuberculosis and is generally caused by atypical *Mycobacterium,* cat-scratch disease, or fungal infections.

Neoplasm

Cervical adenopathy in children can also herald a malignancy, generally primary and belonging to the lymphoma family and less commonly cervical neuroblastoma or rhabdomyosarcoma. Metastatic carcinoma to cervical lymph nodes is much less common in the child than in the adult and is most likely to originate from a primary thyroid neoplasm.

The surgeon is frequently asked to perform a biopsy on a persistently enlarged cervical lymph node for histological confirmation of diagnosis. Neck dissection for therapy of cervical malignancy is limited to localized cervical neuroblastoma or rhabdomyosarcoma and for the surgical treatment of thyroid carcinoma, commonly adjunctive to x-ray therapy and chemotherapy.

Branchial remnants

Embryological *remnants* of the *branchial arch system* produce *sinuses, cysts,* and *fistulas* that occur from the external pinna to the clavicular insertion of the sternocleidomastoid muscle in infants and children. Only the first two branchial arch systems are usually involved in these vestigial remnants.

The very common preauricular sinuses and skin tabs arise simply from misadventures occuring when the epithelial precursors of the external pinna merge together. They usually produce only cosmetic defects, but the sinuses can become infected. Either of these represents a valid indication for surgical excision.

First branchial remnants are only one tenth as common as second branchial remnants. They present as sinuses or fistulas, which commonly

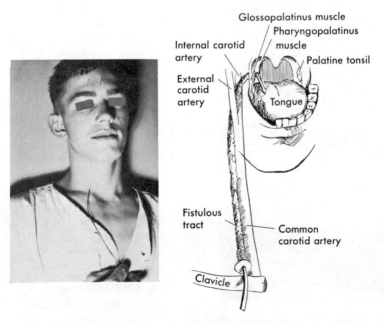

Fig. 28-14. Branchial fistula. Ureteral catheter passes from external ostium on up tract to tonsillar fossa.

become infected, below or behind the ear or in the upper lateral part of the neck. Proper treatment requires complete excision, preferably performed when inflammation is quiescent and always in the operating room with proper anesthesia, light, and exposure, to avoid recurrences and injury to the facial nerve (cranial nerve VII).

Second branchial arch remnants present as cysts, sinuses, or fistulas in the anterior triangle of the neck. The cysts generally arise later in childhood as fluctuant swellings just anterior to the upper half of the sternocleidomastoid muscle. They represent approximately 10% of all branchial abnormalities. The cysts are prone to recurrent bouts of infection, thus justifying prophylactic complete excision.

Cervical fistulas and sinuses constitute the bulk of branchial remnants and in about 15% of patients are bilateral. The external ostia always open on the skin along the anterior border of the sternocleidomastoid muscle, usually in its lower one third (Fig. 28-14). The sinuses extend cephalad for varying distances to terminate blindly. The fistulas extend completely cephalad to empty into the pharynx at the tonsillar fossa; the tract invariably passes behind the posterior belly of the digastric muscle and between the branches of the carotid artery (in keeping with its second branchial arch derivation). Both cysts and fistulas are lined by epithelium and are prone to infection. Prophylactic total excision is the treatment of choice; long fistulas often require two parallel neck-crease incisions (stepladder incisions) to allow the exposure necessary for their safe and total removal. Recurrence is certain with incomplete excision.

Cystic hygroma

Cystic hygroma (cavernous lymphangioma) is the classical developmental abnormality of the lymphatic system. It consists of multiloculated cysts filled with watery tissue fluid that may appear as relatively asymptomatic masses anywhere on the body; however, 85% are confined to the lateral neck and face area (Fig. 28-15) (the left side is slightly more common than the right side); 2% to 3% of the cervical cystic hygromas have extensions into the mediastinum. The axilla is the second most common location of cystic hygroma.

Cystic hygromas are generally present at birth and commonly enlarge rapidly during infancy. They tend to invade or displace surrounding structures, thereby producing their only serious symptoms: interference with deglutition and the airway. Pathologically, they are considered hamartomas rather than neoplasms. Cystic hygromas seem to represent lymphatic spaces that receive tissue fluid through afferent channels but do not establish the proper efferent connections to the venous system, resulting in accumulation of lymph. Correct diagnosis is made by palpation of a soft, cystic mass that does not change the color of the overlying skin, which is nontender and transilluminates brilliantly (Fig. 28-15).

Treatment by aspiration of cystic hygromas has largely been abandoned: (1) the needle cannot penetrate into all the multiple cysts, and (2) it carries the risk of introducing infection, which can be acute and fulminant. The most commonly accepted treatment of cystic hygroma is excision of as much of the lesion as possible without damaging vital neurovascular structures. Excision is carried out at an elective age, except in the rare instance when the airway is threatened by displacement or involvement.

Thyroglossal duct remnants

Thyroglossal duct remnants (Fig. 28-16) produce masses in the anterior midline of the neck, generally at about the level of the hyoid bone. They

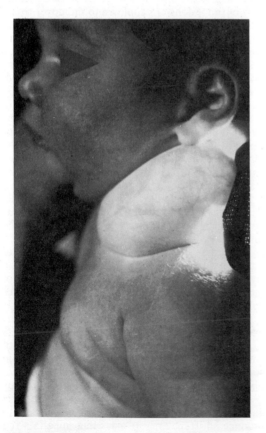

Fig. 28-15. Cystic hygroma of neck. Notice how brilliantly it transilluminates.

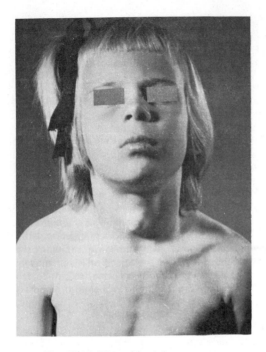

Fig. 28-16. Thyroglossal duct remnant.

represent cystic dilatation of remnants of the thyroglossal duct, the embryological anlage of the thyroid gland that normally involutes and disappears. The thyroglossal tract arises as a midline diverticulum from the back of the tongue (*foramen cecum*) and moves caudally through the midportion of the hyoid bone before splitting into the two definitive lateral thyroid lobes in their normal position low in the anterior cervical area.

Thyroglossal cysts may appear anywhere along this tract but are most common in and around the hyoid bone. They must be differentiated from these other midline neck masses in children:

1. *Submental lymph nodes* are generally multiple, movable in a lateral plane, and not cystic in consistency.
2. *Dermoid cysts* are generally lower in the anterior midline of the neck than thyroglossal duct cysts, are more superficial, sometimes actually attaching to the skin, and are not elevated by protruding the tongue.
3. *Ectopic thyroid tissue* can arise anywhere along the thyroglossal tract, is solid rather than cystic, and concentrates iodine on diagnostic radioactive iodine uptake studies. Ectopic thyroid tissue should *not* be removed if it is the *only* thyroid tissue that the patient possesses.

Thyroglossal duct cysts are fairly deep seated, are cystic in consistency, are not tender unless secondarily infected, and move cephalad on protrusion of the tongue. Treatment is surgical excision of the cyst and the remnant of the thyroglossal tract that connects the cyst to the foramen cecum of the tongue; this obligates the removal of a 1 cm. block of midline hyoid bone and the entire tract up to the base of the tongue.

VASCULAR ANOMALIES
Hemangiomas

The *capillary hemangioma (strawberry mark, raspberry mark)* is the most common peripheral vascular abnormality in infants and children. It is generally present at birth but can appear after a few weeks or even months of life. Histologically it is composed of numerous tiny vascular channels. Grossly the capillary hemangioma is a bright red mass that may be small and flat or quite elevated and nodular but that retains the characteristics of blanching with compression, best observed when a glass slide is pressed firmly over the lesion. About 70% of the lesions are confined to the upper torso, head, and neck.

Although initially small, capillary hemangiomas almost uniformly display a growth spurt for the first 6 to 12 months of life, often at an alarming rate, with a slowing of growth during young childhood. Well over 90% begin to regress spontaneously during the middle childhood years, with progressive diminution in size by thrombosis of the vascular channels. The thrombosis typically begins centrally as whitish areas that appear within the pink-red lesion; these whitish areas then coalesce and spread peripherally to encompass the entire lesion.

Because of their tendency to regress spontaneously, active treatment of capillary hemangiomas is not recommended unless they compromise a vital function by virtue of their location, or if their growth rate is continuous and entirely out of proportion to body growth rate. Surgical excision is often more disfiguring than the ultimate result of the untreated lesion. Systemic steroids sometimes will control a lesion that is growing rapidly.

Cavernous hemangioma (Fig. 28-17) is numerically only about one tenth as common as its capillary counterpart. It consists principally of larger-sized vascular channels that often contain some lymphatic elements and abnormal connections with the arterial vascular tree. Cavernous hemangiomas most commonly involve the dermis and subcutaneous tissues of the extremities to produce an irregular, soft mass that imparts a red to blue discoloration to the overlying skin. They may diminish in size on compression, reverting

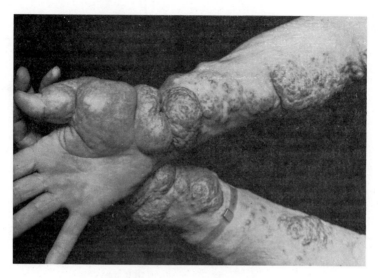

Fig. 28-17. Cavernous hemangiomas.

quickly to their former size on release of pressure and enlarging during periods of increased venous pressure (Valsalva effect, crying, or straining).

Cavernous hemangiomas are much more serious than the capillary type because (1) they infrequently involute, (2) they are cosmetically more disfiguring, and (3) local gigantism results when the member is extensively involved, probably because of the increase in blood flow to the tissue. Treatment is generally unsatisfactory, whether by injection of sclerosing agents, excision and skin grafting, or irradiation. Complete surgical excision is performed safely only on small cavernous hemangiomas. Extensive lesions must be approached cautiously and conservatively, with therapy individually tailored to forestall or treat ulceration, infection, and hemorrhage and to ablate gigantism.

OTHER COMMON PEDIATRIC SURGICAL DISEASES
Tonsils and adenoids

Tonsils and adenoids are part of the lymphatic system of the body. The tonsils are paired clumps of lymphoid tissue lying on each side of the pharynx at the base of the tongue, and the adenoid tissue is in the nasopharynx behind and above the uvula. As with lymphoid tissue elsewhere in the body, they enlarge with infections as mechanisms of defense. Because of the frequency of upper respiratory tract infections in children, they are commonly enlarged at this age.

Tonsils are not removed because of their size alone. Untreated tonsillitis can result in peritonsil-

lar abscesses or bloodstream infections. Enlargement of the adenoids blocks nasal respiration and obstructs drainage of the eustachian tube connecting the middle ear with the pharynx to produce recurrent bouts of otitis media. Chronic adenoid enlargement encourages a mouth-breathing habit, poor humidification of inspired air, and resultant episodes of bronchitis and cough.

Tonsillectomy and adenoidectomy are performed if tonsil and adenoid enlargement are associated with repeated middle ear infections, recurrent bouts of bronchitis or pneumonia, or a chronic habit of breathing through the mouth. Introduction of antibiotics has reduced the number of tonsillectomies and adenoidectomies performed in recent years.

Appendicitis

Appendicitis is the most common cause for emergency abdominal operation in the child though its actual incidence appears to be declining. Extremely rare in the infant and unusual under the age of 5 years, its incidence increases rapidly thereafter with the peak incidence at about 11 years of age.

Obstruction of the lumen initiates appendicitis (Fig. 28-18). This occurs either from enlargement of the lymphoid tissue underneath the lining mucosa of the appendix (generally in the younger child) or by a concretion of feces and undigested vegetable matter called a fecalith (Fig. 28-19) (generally in the older child or adult). The obstruction traps the mucoid secretions of the appendiceal

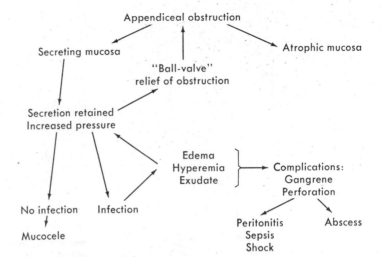

Fig. 28-18. Pathophysiology of appendicitis.

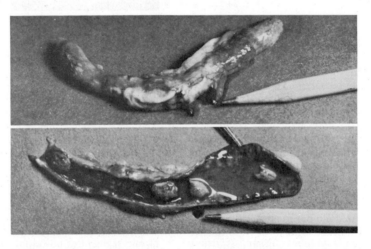

Fig. 28-19. Acute suppurative appendicitis. *Above,* Distended, injected, and edematous appendix. *Below,* Opened specimen shows obstructing fecalith to left and other fecaliths, pus, and debris filling lumen.

cells to progressively build up intraluminal pressure; intestinal organisms cause infection and abscess. Occasionally the obstruction relents and the attack of appendicitis is aborted; if it persists, the appendix becomes turgid, swollen, edematous, and inflamed, which then progresses by vascular thrombosis to gangrene and perforation. Perforation results in peritoneal contamination with rapid development of peritonitis with generalized abdominal pain, high fever, paralytic ileus, and abdominal rigidity (an acute surgical abdomen).

Very rare is the situation where there are no organisms resident in the appendix when its lumen

becomes obstructed. The sterile mucoid secretions then gradually increase in volume to produce the so-called *mucocele of the appendix.* Vague right lower quadrant abdominal discomfort and a mass clinically herald the mucocele; its rupture is one of the causes of the condition known as *pseudomyxoma peritonei.*

The speed of progression from obstruction to perforation is rapid in the very young since defense mechanisms are limited and the symptoms difficult to communicate. The complication rate of appendicitis in children under the age of 5 years is understandably high, approximately 80% by the

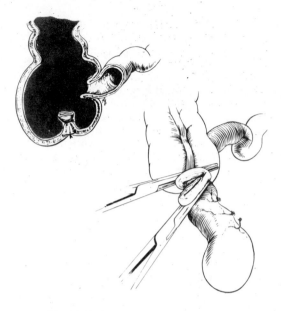

Fig. 28-20. Removal of inflamed appendix.

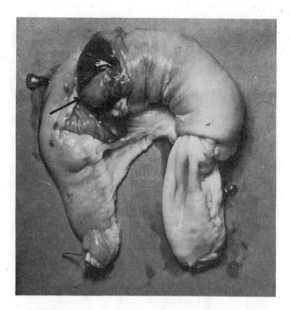

Fig. 28-21. Intussusception of small bowel. Notice telescoping of bowel toward left side of specimen, which has been opened in its midportion to disclose polyp *(arrow)* causing intussusception.

time operation is undertaken. The older the child, the slower the progression, the more accurate the history, and the lower the complication rate.

Symptoms begin with epigastric pain that gradually migrates to the umbilical area and then localizes to the right lower abdominal quadrant as the parietal peritoneum in this area becomes involved in the inflammatory process. Anorexia, nausea and vomiting, low-grade fever, leukocytosis to a range of 9,000 to 14,000 cells/cu. mm., and malaise are common findings. Diagnosis can be difficult because of early nonspecificity of symptoms and findings. Localized tenderness in the right lower abdomen is the most accurate sign. Occasionally plain abdominal x-ray studies show an opacified obstructing fecalith.

Many nonsurgical illnesses mimic appendicitis; right lower lobe pneumonia, mesenteric lymphadenitis, and enterocolitis to mention only a few. A carefully performed barium enema examination carried out by a radiologist who is experienced with this technique may help in diagnosis: an appendix that does not fill completely, indentation of the cecum, displacement of terminal ileum, and mucosal inflammation of periappendiceal bowel are radiographic signs of acute appendicitis. Because of the very serious potential complications of appendicitis, exploration is indicated whenever the possibility of appendicitis exists. The surgeon is

wrong in about 15% of cases, but he accepts this in order not to miss the "difficult-to-diagnose" case that, if untreated, would become complicated by perforation and peritonitis. Surgical treatment involves removal of the inflamed appendix, closure of the base of the appendix leading into the cecum, and drainage of localized pus (Fig. 28-20).

Intussusception

Intussusception is an invagination or telescoping of one segment of bowel into another (Fig. 28-21); its cause is often not known. Intussusception results in intestinal obstruction with the threat of strangulation of the involved bowel as its blood supply becomes compromised. The majority involve the distal ileum telescoping into the cecum with propagation around the colon to varying levels. Intussusception is characteristically seen in the 6-month-old to 18-month-old well-nourished child. Abdominal pain occurs every 5 to 10 minutes (intestinal colic), during which the child cries and doubles up, followed by a period of disarming quiet. Vomiting of bile and the passage of bloody stools resembling currant jelly are classical features. The intussuscepted bowel can often be palpated as a tubular mass across the upper abdomen when the child relaxes between episodes of intestinal colic.

Barium enema (Fig. 28-22) confirms diagnosis

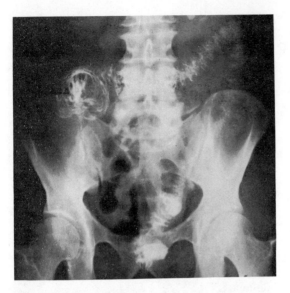

Fig. 28-22. Barium enema showing diagnostic "coil-spring" appearance of ileocolic intussusception at about hepatic flexure of colon in patient's right upper abdomen.

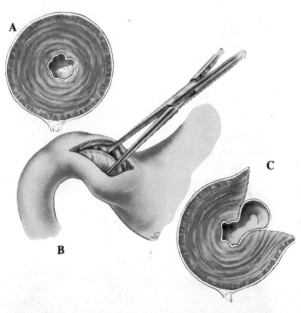

Fig. 28-23. Hypertrophic pyloric stenosis. **A,** Cross section of thickened pyloric muscle and narrow channel. **B,** Ramstedt pyloromyotomy showing instrument spreading muscle apart after it has been incised longitudinally, allowing intact mucosa to bulge outward as in **C** to greatly enlarge lumen of pyloric channel and relieve obstruction of stomach.

and also can be used to reduce the intussusception safely (in about two thirds of the patients). This reduction is observed by fluoroscopy; the barium column is elevated no higher than 30 to 36 inches above the table to avoid perforation of the bowel or reduction of strangulated bowel. Signs of *intestinal obstruction* or *peritonitis* are related to bowel strangulation and mandate operative reduction. These signs contraindicate attempted barium enema reduction, since they are associated with an unacceptably high rate of perforation when hydrostatic reduction has been attempted. Surgical reduction (and sometimes bowel resection) is also required when barium reduction is ineffective.

Hypertrophic pyloric stenosis

Hypertrophic pyloric stenosis is the most common cause for intestinal obstruction in the baby 2 to 6 weeks of age (occurring once in 400 births). It occurs in males twice as often as in females. Forceful vomiting of gastric contents not discolored by bile is the outstanding feature of the history. Prominent waves travel from left to right across the epigastrium; these represent forceful peristaltic contractions of the stomach attempting to squeeze gastric material through the narrowed pyloric channel. The pylorus, the muscle surrounding the outlet of the stomach, becomes thickened (Fig. 28-23, *A*). Its lumen (the pyloric channel) narrows, obstructing the outflow of material from the stomach. The basic cause for this hypertrophy is unknown.

The diagnosis is confirmed in about 80% of the patients by palpation of the thickened muscle, the "olive" mass, in the right upper abdominal quadrant. If the age, history, or findings are atypical, an upper gastrointestinal series establishes the diagnosis by outlining the narrow pyloric channel. Acute pyelonephritis, increased intracranial pressure, and the adrenogenital syndrome occasionally mimic the symptoms of pyloric stenosis.

Operative treatment is simple; the thickened pyloric muscle is incised and spread apart (Fig. 28-23, *B* and *C*), thereby enlarging the channel and relieving the obstruction. Pyloromyotomy (Ramstedt procedure) has perhaps the highest success rate and the lowest morbidity and mortality of any common operative procedure.

Inguinal hernia, hydrocele

Inguinal hernia in the male child results from retention of an embryological outpocketing of peritoneum known as the *processus vaginalis,* which precedes testicular descent into the scrotum. The walls of this structure normally adhere to obliterate the sac (Fig. 28-24, *A*), but if obliteration fails, the sac will remain and allow bowel to enter as a hernia (Fig. 28-24, *B* and *C*).

Surgical correction is carried out when the diagnosis is made because of possible complications of incarceration or strangulation of the herniated bowel; this occurs in 5% to 15% of babies with a hernia. Hernia repair requires division and closure of the neck of the sac to remove the connection with the peritoneal cavity.

A hydrocele is embryologically related to the hernia (Fig. 28-24, *D* and *E*), the difference resting in the size of the connection of the patent *processus vaginalis* with the peritoneal cavity. In a hydrocele the connection is large enough to allow fluid to gravitate into the unobliterated sac but not large enough to allow bowel to enter. The majority of hydroceles spontaneously disappear when the small peritoneal connection becomes obliterated, allowing no further peritoneal fluid to enter. Only rarely is surgical closure of this connection necessary. About 15% of hernias are preceded by a hydrocele, the peritoneal connection having enlarged sufficiently to allow bowel to enter the sac.

Hirschsprung's disease of the older child (congenital aganglionosis of the colon, congenital megacolon)

Hirschsprung's disease is the most common functional congenital obstruction of the colon. The colonic obstruction is caused by absence of peristalsis within that segment of colon in which the autonomic ganglion cells (both intermuscular and submucosal) are congenitally absent. Proximal to the aganglionic segment, the colon dilates and hypertrophies to warrant the descriptive term "megacolon." The obstruction may be acute and relatively complete immediately after birth (discussed in the section on neonatal obstruction of the colon, p. 292). Bouts of distension, vomiting, and paradoxical diarrhea interspersed with constipation characterize the disease during the first year of life. As the child grows older, chronic constipation emerges as the dominant complaint. Life-threatening complications of bowel perforation, enterocolitis, and sepsis accordingly bear an inverse relationship to age.

In about 80% of children aganglionosis is limited to the rectum and rectosigmoid but occasionally

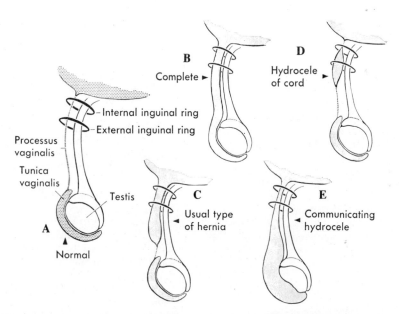

Fig. 28-24. A, Normally obliterated processus vaginalis. **B,** Complete failure of obliteration of processus vaginalis, with large opening into peritoneal cavity allowing bowel to enter as complete, or scrotal, hernia. **C,** Proximal part of processus vaginalis does not obliterate, allowing bowel to enter as usual type of indirect inguinal hernia. **D,** Hydrocele of cord. **E,** Communicating hydrocele; connection with peritoneal cavity is large enough to allow peritoneal fluid to enter sac, but not large enough for bowel to enter.

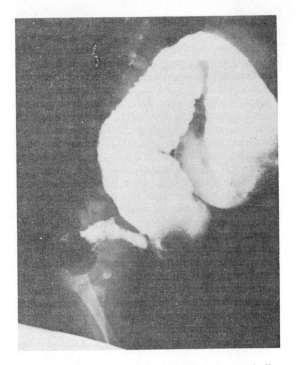

Fig. 28-25. Congenital aganglionosis (Hirschsprung's disease). Barium enema shows narrow, spastic rectum and rectosigmoid (aganglionic) flaring into megacolon (ganglionated bowel) at sigmoid colon.

extends higher in the colon, and in nearly 5% of cases involves the entire colon. There are reported cases of aganglionosis of the entire gastrointestinal tract. Regardless of its proximal point of origin, the aganglionosis invariably extends from that point on down to include the internal anal sphincter, therefore allowing completely reliable diagnosis by the simple expedient of rectal wall biopsy carried out transanally. Abdominal distension and evidence of poor nutrition parallel the degree of obstruction. Children with Hirschsprung's disease are predisposed to acute necrotizing enterocolitis (Chapter 24), a complication that carries approximately a 20% mortality.

The history given by children with congenital aganglionosis may be extremely varied, though abnormal bowel function of some degree is present from the day of birth. There often is a delay of 24 to 48 hours in the passage of meconium rectally after delivery, with varying degrees of constipation or explosive diarrhea thereafter. Abdominal distension, vomiting of feedings, and poor weight gain are common complaints. Invariably changes in formula and the use of laxatives, enemas, and suppositories have all been attempted for symptomatic control.

Physical examination reveals a somewhat pale and malnourished infant or child with soft abdominal distension. Loops of colon are often palpable, distended by gas and hard feces. Rectal digital examination reveals a small rectal ampulla. If the aganglionosis extends only to the rectosigmoid, the examining finger may reach the dilated and stool-filled sigmoid colon and provoke an explosive escape of liquid stool and gas on withdrawal of the finger.

Barium enema is helpful in diagnosis, characteristically showing a narrow or normal-sized rectum that flares into a megacolon above the point of obstruction (Fig. 28-25); only small amounts of barium should be used, with no effort made to fill the entire colon, since tardy expulsion of the barium is a second feature of the roentgenographic diagnosis. Confirmation of diagnosis rests on rectal wall biopsy.

The treatment of Hirschsprung's disease is surgical, except in rare instances of a very short aganglionic segment that can be easily controlled by conservative methods (stool softeners and enemas). One initially directs one's efforts toward relief of the intestinal obstruction generally by performing a colostomy; the proximal extent of aganglionosis is histologically determined by seromuscular biopsy of the colon obtained at appropriate levels. The colostomy must be placed within an area of normal ganglion cells.

Definitive treatment consists of resection of the aganglionic colon to within 1 to 3 cm. of the anus. Anastomosis of the ganglionated colon to the rectal pouch is achieved by one of a variety of abdominoperineal techniques. Prognosis is good.

Intensive Care

J. Scott Millikan
John F. Hansbrough

Intensive care is a manner of treating patients with serious and often life-threatening trauma or illness by use of special resources, manpower, and technology. The intensive care unit (ICU) is an *area* where patients requiring this specialized care are concentrated and where these resources, technology, and expertise are developed and maintained. Here the physician's knowledge, judgment, and skills are often tested, and critical decisions are frequently made. In this context, the ICU also provides an excellent forum for the medical student to study physiological principles in the treatment of surgical disease (Fig. 29-1).

HISTORY

Centralization of health care is an old concept. The so-called Nightengale wards of the early 1900s allowed a single nurse to simultaneously care for many patients. This style of hospital care set the stage for specialized treatment centers. During World War II, "shock units" were developed to handle increasing numbers of injured patients brought about by improved methods of medical evacuation. These units grouped specialized equipment and staff with those patients who were most seriously injured.

Stimulated by reports of increasing numbers of postanesthesia deaths, many hospitals in the 1940s designated postoperative observation areas where patients were closely monitored until the effects of anesthesia had dissipated. Before 1950, these "recovery rooms" were usually the only specialized care areas in hospitals. However, subsequent technological advances led to increasingly complex operations requiring prolonged recovery and extensive monitoring that could not safely be carried out on regular wards. The solution to this problem was a natural extension of the recovery room concept—the intensive care unit.

Once principles of intensive care proved successful, ICU's became subspecialized. Surgical intensive care in some medical centers diversified into burn, trauma, cardiovascular, neurosurgical, pediatric, and general surgical units. Medical ICU's have similarly specialized into pulmonary, general medical, and coronary care units.

PROS AND CONS

Advantages of this type of care are numerous. The ICU allows for placement of a patient into an environment containing the most expertise in dealing with his particular problems. In addition, when patients with similar problems are concentrated in one area, the experience of a few highly trained staff members, both medical and nursing, is enhanced. The ICU also provides for efficient utilization of the technology and equipment available to a hospital. Several studies have demonstrated improved survival among patients treated in an intensive care setting.

Disadvantages of ICU care include increased risk of cross contamination and subsequent infection. ICU patients, often immunosuppressed, are more susceptible to infection, sources of which include mechanical ventilators, open and contaminated wounds, and indwelling catheters. Cross contamination is all too frequent, and miniepidemics have on occasion nearly wiped out entire ICU

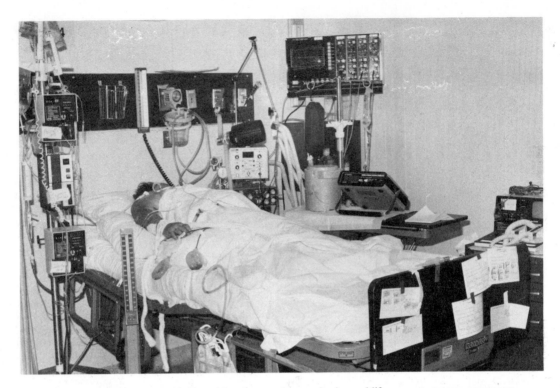

Fig. 29-1. Intensive care unit illustrating the complex monitoring and life-support systems necessary for moment-to-moment care.

populations. Sleep deprivation and lack of privacy are also notable problems.

MAINTENANCE OF CELLULAR AND ORGAN SYSTEM FUNCTION

Perhaps the most important purpose of the intensive care unit is to monitor, correct, and maintain normal cellular and organ system function throughout a patient's illness. This demands a thorough knowledge of basic physiological principles. Cellular homeostasis requires adequate delivery of oxygen and nutrients, normal removal of waste products, and correction of metabolic abnormalities.

Oxygen-substrate delivery

Optimum delivery of oxygen to tissues requires adequate pulmonary, cardiac, and vascular function. Enough oxygen must be presented to the patient and delivered to the alveoli for diffusion across the pulmonary-capillary membrane. Sufficient hemoglobin should then be available for oxygen binding. In addition, effective cardiac function is required to transport blood to the tissues.

Finally, resistance to arterial flow must allow delivery of blood to the capillaries. There, after oxyhemoglobin dissociation, oxygen and metabolic substrates diffuse into tissues.

Waste product removal

Removal of carbon dioxide and acid metabolites also requires proper pulmonary, cardiac, and vascular function. Delivery of these metabolites to the lungs, liver, and kidneys, critically important in maintaining normal cellular physiology, requires normal venous and arterial vascular function.

Although these pathways seem simple, any defect along the way may result in end-organ dysfunction, which often triggers a vicious cycle eventually leading to death. Numerous variables in this framework of oxygen-substrate delivery and by-product removal must be monitored and controlled by the ICU physician in order to optimize end-organ function.

The pulmonary system

The initial step in ensuring normal cellular physiology is evaluation and correction of abnormalities in pulmonary function. Pulmonary failure results from defects in gas exchange and is manifest initially as irregularities in arterial blood gases and later as organ and tissue failure. Pulmonary failure is heralded by an arterial P_{O_2} below 50 mm. Hg or an arterial P_{CO_2} above 50 mm. Hg. Ventilation and oxygenation are the two principle components of pulmonary function. These may fail separately or together and must be individually evaluated when pulmonary abnormalities are suspected.

Ventilatory failure results when an inadequate amount of gas is actively exchanged with pulmonary venous blood. The degree of ventilation at the alveolar level is inversely proportional to the partial pressure of carbon dioxide (P_{CO_2}) in arterial blood. Ventilatory failure is present when the P_{CO_2} is greater than 50 mm Hg. Alveolar ventilation can be increased and the P_{CO_2} decreased by improvement in minute ventilation, which is directly proportional to respiratory rate and tidal volume of each breath.

Hypoventilation may be attributable to alterations in central nervous system function (narcotics, anesthetics, stroke, head or spinal cord injury), defects in neuromuscular activity (tetanus, aminoglycoside antibiotics, Guillain-Barré syndrome), or ineffective diaphragm and chest well motion (pain after abdominal or thoracic surgery, hemopneumothorax, flail chest, scoliosis). Impairment in ventilation may also result from defects within the pulmonary airways (asthma, foreign body, mucus plug, laryngospasm) or lung parenchyma (atelectasis, aspiration, fluid overload). On the other hand, hyperventilation most often results from improper management of the mechanical ventilator but may also be secondary to central nervous system dysfunction.

Oxygenation failure is manifest by a decrease in partial pressure of oxygen in arterial blood (P_{O_2} < 50 mm. Hg) and an abnormally low percentage of oxygen saturation of hemoglobin. Causes of hypoxemia include (1) decreased inspired oxygen fraction (F_{IO_2}), (2) alveolar hypoventilation, (3) abnormalities of oxygen diffusion across the alveolar capillary membrane, and (4) regional mismatching of pulmonary ventilation and blood flow, the most frequent cause of hypoxemia among intensive care patients. Mismatching occurs when pulmonary blood flows across nonventilated alveoli. Unoxygenated blood then mixes with normally oxygenated blood, and the overall oxygen content of systemic arterial blood diminishes. The percentage of blood that shunts through the pulmonary vascular circuit without being oxygenated (shunt fraction) can be calculated and is normally less than 5%. Hypoxemia from pulmonary shunting is often poorly responsive to increases in F_{IO_2}.

Treatment usually involves correction of underlying causes, which may include atelectasis, pneumonia, aspiration, and adult respiratory distress syndrome (ARDS). Another, though infrequent, cause of hypoxemia is a right-to-left central vascular shunt in which desaturated systemic venous blood flows directly into the systemic arterial circuit, usually subsequent to congenital anomalies of the heart or great vessels. This type of hypoxemia is unresponsive to oxygen therapy and generally requires operative correction.

Depending on the clinical situation, oxygenation may be improved by augmentation of the percentage of oxygen in the inspired air (F_{IO_2}), or by an increase in the ventilation (respiratory rate × tidal volume). Oxygenation can also be improved by maximization of the number of open and functioning alveoli, thus limiting pulmonary vascular shunting. In most patients, vigorous pulmonary toilet and deep breathing exercises will achieve this. However, the patient on a mechanical ventilator may have alveolar collapse, particularly after expiration. When one increases the amount of air remaining in the lungs at the end of a breath (i.e., the functional residual capacity, FRC), alveolar collapse may be limited resulting in less ventilation-perfusion mismatching and improved oxygenation.

This result is attained clinically by use of positive end-expiratory pressure (PEEP), which maintains positive airway pressure throughout the respiratory cycle, thereby increasing the functional residual capacity. Usual amounts of PEEP range from 5 to 20 cm. H_2O. Although PEEP improves oxygenation, this maneuver can reduce cardiac output because increased intrathoracic pressure can lead to decreased venous return to the heart and myocardial dysfunction. The net result may be an actual *decrease* in total oxygen delivery to the tissues.

Pulmonary support

Most ICU patients adequately ventilate, oxygenate, and clear tracheobronchial secretions spontaneously. Effective respiratory therapy including incentive spirometry exercises, chest physiotherapy, and sufficient hydration often prevent major pulmonary problems. Many patients also benefit from supplemental oxygen (given by nasal cannula or face mask).

Critically ill patients, however, often require endotracheal intubation. Indications for artificial airway placement include (1) relief of airway obstruction, (2) protection from aspiration, (3) control of tracheal secretions, and (4) pulmonary failure with the need for mechanical ventilation. The first three goals are achieved with a "T-piece" system whereby humidified and heated gas of preset oxygen concentration flows across the end of an endotracheal tube. The fourth indication, pulmonary failure, requires endotracheal intubation and mechanical ventilation.

The indications for intubation and mechanical ventilation are listed as follows:

1. Decompensation of chronic lung disease
2. Central nervous system disorders
3. Chest wall or diaphragm dysfunction
4. Adult respiratory distress syndrome (ARDS)
5. Pulmonary aspiration
6. Severe pneumonia

Ventilators open airways, improve oxygenation, increase alveolar ventilation, and reduce the work of breathing. There are two basic types of ventilators: pressure and volume cycle.

Pressure cycle. A pressure cycle ventilator delivers gas to the patient until a preset airway pressure is obtained. The amount of gas given is difficult to control, varying with the compliance of the lungs and the airway resistance to gas flow. Inaccuracy of ventilation management has led many centers to abandon its use.

Volume cycle. A volume cycle machine delivers a fixed volume of gas to the lungs with each breath. Pressure subsequently generated within the tracheobronchial tree and alveoli varies depending on the compliance (distensibility) of the lungs and chest wall. Low peak inspiratory pressures imply easily distensible (highly compliant) lungs, whereas high peak inspiratory pressures imply poor compliance and "stiff lungs." Poor chest wall compliance, mucous plugging of the ventilatory circuit, and PEEP may also increase peak inspiratory pressures.

Abnormally elevated airway pressure during mechanical ventilation is potentially dangerous. Increased pressure may overinflate alveoli causing rupture. Gas may then dissect the visceral pleura from the contiguous tissues and move into the mediastinum, abdominal cavity, and subcutaneous tissues of the chest and neck causing crepitus on palpation. Gas can also migrate into the pericardial space. Tension pneumopericardium, seen most often in infants, may precipitate cardiovascular collapse. In addition, gas escaping from ruptured alveoli may penetrate the visceral pleura and enter the pleural space causing pneumothorax with complete or partial collapse of the lung. If a "flap valve" effect in the lung occurs, whereby gas is forced into the pleural space but cannot escape, pressure increases in that hemithorax causing complete collapse of the lung and eventual shift of the mediastinum away from the affected side (tension pneumothorax). Severe mediastinal shift may cause a sudden decrease in venous return to the heart and cardiovascular collapse. Pneumothorax or tension pneumothorax, a surgical emergency, must be treated immediately by evacuation of the air from the pleural space, thus allowing the lung to reexpand and the mediastinum to resume normal position. This is achieved by placement of a chest tube through the thoracic wall and into the pleural space. The tube is then attached to a suction-drainage system (Fig. 29-2).

Because of the potential dangers, volume cycle ventilators are equipped with a pop-off valve, which limits peak inspiratory pressure by diverting additional tidal volume away from the patient. Activation of this valve should sound an alarm and receive prompt attention. If excessive volume is shunted away from the patient, hypoventilation and hypoxemia may occur.

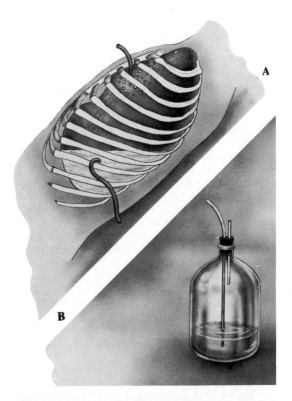

Fig. 29-2. Intercostal chest tubes with underwater-seal drainage. **A,** Tube to remove air from pleural space is introduced through second intercostal space at midclavicular line; tube to remove liquid (blood, pus, and postoperative fluid collection) is introduced through eighth intercostal space at anterior axillary line. **B,** Tubing is connected to glass rod on bottle that is covered with sterile water; pleural air bubbles into bottle and escapes to outside, while fluid collects in bottle.

Ventilator mode

The type of mechanical support required by patients in pulmonary failure varies, depending on the clinical setting. Most ventilators are equipped to deliver several types or modes of ventilatory assistance as listed below.

Continuous mandatory ventilation delivers gas at a set tidal volume and rate regardless of the patient's respiratory activity. Patients who lack functional respiratory drive and require total support need this mode of ventilation.

Intermittent mandatory ventilation (IMV) allows the patient to breathe at his own rate and volume but also delivers additional breaths of fixed volume and rate. This mode can be adjusted to deliver the mandatory breaths synchronously with the patient's own inspirations (synchronous IMV, or SIMV). This type of ventilation permits the patient to exercise his own respiratory muscles. The amount of support may be varied according to the patient's needs, and as the number of machine-delivered breaths is decreased, the patient can increase his own respiratory activity and be slowly weaned off the ventilator.

Assist control delivers a fixed volume of gas each time the patient initiates an inspiratory effort. This mode is used in patients with an intact respiratory drive and virtually eliminates any work of breathing. Patients, however, can hyperventilate and develop respiratory alkalosis if not carefully monitored.

Ventilator adjustments

All the parameters previously discussed including tidal volume, respiratory rate, FIO_2, PEEP, and peak inspiratory pressure are adjustable on mechanical ventilators. The ratio of inspiratory to expiratory phases, as well as inspiratory and expiratory patterns, may also be adjusted on newer models. By properly modulating these variables the ICU physician in most cases ensures effective oxygen delivery and carbon dioxide removal at the alveolar level. Careful monitoring including chest roentgenography and arterial blood gas analysis should detect most abnormalities in pulmonary function and guide any necessary corrections.

Ventilator weaning

Once the underlying cause of pulmonary failure is diagnosed and successfully treated, the ventilator patient can be weaned from mechanical support. If the patient tolerates this and fulfills the following criteria for extubation, the endotracheal tube can be removed:

1. Vital capacity greater than 10 cc./kg.
2. Tidal volume greater than 3 to 5 cc./kg.
3. Inspiratory force greater than 25 cm. H_2O
4. Respiratory rate less than 25 breaths per minute
5. Intrapulmonary shunt measurements less than 20%
6. Stable "T-piece" trial for 30 minutes
   a. Normal or usual arterial blood gases
   b. FIO_2 at 40%
   c. No PEEP
   d. Hemodynamic stability: normal pulse and blood pressure
7. Patient can protect his own airway

Arterial gases and close monitoring are essential after extubation. If the patient fails weaning, mechanical support is reinstituted until the patient's condition improves.

Cardiovascular system

The cardiovascular system also requires frequent evaluation and correction of abnormalities to assure adequate oxygen-substrate delivery along with carbon dioxide–metabolite removal at the tissue level.

Hemoglobin

Efficient oxygen transport requires adequate amounts of hemoglobin, which should be maintained at greater than 10 gm./dl. Hematocrit should be kept greater than 30%. These values may fluctuate depending on the the patient's state of hydration. An abnormally elevated hematocrit may increase blood viscosity and cause capillary sludging and decreased oxygen delivery.

Cardiac function

Cardiac output, the amount of blood pumped by the heart and theoretically delivered to the tissues each minute, depends on two parameters: heart rate and stroke volume. Heart rate is easily monitored and can be manipulated to improve cardiac output; usually with pharmacological agents that have a chronotropic effect or with pacemakers that stimulate the myocardium. Stroke volume, the other determinant of cardiac output, is less easily measured and depends on numerous variables including (1) the amount of left ventricular filling and subsequent myocardial fiber stretching (preload) as described by the Frank-Starling hypothesis, (2) the degree of impedence to left ventricular ejection (afterload), which is related to arterial vascular resistance, and (3) the performance of the heart independent of preload and afterload (i.e., contractility). Preload, afterload, and cardiac contractility along with heart rate are the parameters that the intensive care physician must monitor and vary to achieve optimum cardiovascular function.

Preload. Cardiac preload is best approximated by measurement of left ventricular volume at the

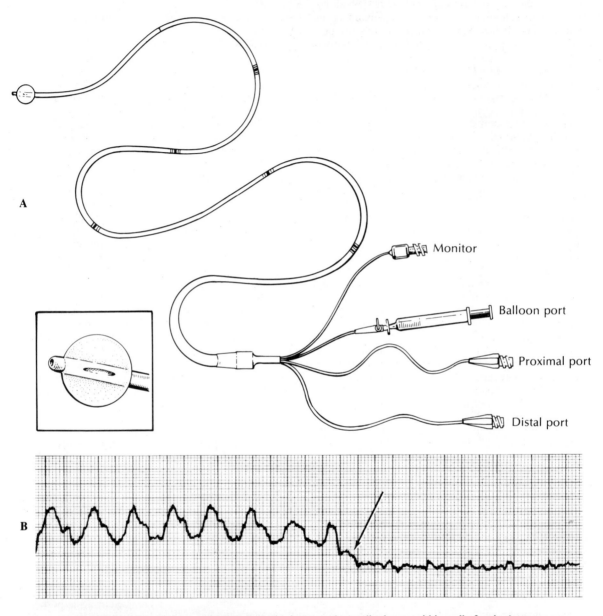

Fig. 29-3. A, Swan-Ganz catheter has a major lumen and a smaller lumen within wall of major lumen. Latex balloon at top of catheter contains a side hole that enters minor lumen. Proximal lumen terminates about 30 cm from catheter tip so that its lumen is in right atrium when distal lumen is in pulmonary artery. Proximal lumen can be used to obtain central venous pressure measurements and right atrial pressures. Major lumen is attached to pressure transducer. **B,** Pulmonary artery pressure becomes wedge pressure with inflation of balloon *(arrow)*. With deflation one should see return of pulmonary artery pressure tracing. (From Moore, E.E., Eiseman, B., and Van Way, C.W.: Critical decisions in trauma, St. Louis, 1983, The C.V. Mosby Co.)

end of diastole, just before systolic ejection. Direct measurement of this volume is not currently feasible in clinical practice. However, given certain assumptions, left ventricular *volume* is directly related to left ventricular diastolic *pressure,* which, at the end of diastole with the mitral valve open, is directly related to left atrial pressure. Therefore, measurement of left atrial pressure approximates measurement of preload, or end-diastolic left ventricular filling.

Indirect measurement of left atrial pressure was also difficult until 1970 when Drs. Swan, Ganz, and Forrester developed a flow-directed pulmonary artery catheter. This catheter (Fig. 29-3) is introduced into the central venous system. An inflated balloon near its tip carries the cathether by venous flow into the right atrium and then through the right ventricle and into the pulmonary artery. As it advances, pressures are recorded from the aforementioned vascular spaces. As the catheter moves along the pulmonary artery, the inflated balloon eventually "wedges" into and occludes the arterial segment. The "pulmonary wedge pressure" is that recorded just beyond the occluded pulmonary artery and reflects pulmonary capillary pressure, which in turn approximates left atrial pressure. The Swan-Ganz catheter thus allows for bedside estimates of cardiac preload. In addition, these devices contain various blood-drawing ports for evaluation of venous blood gases. They are also equipped with thermistors that allow direct calculation of cardiac output by temperature-dilution curves, often vital in caring for the critically ill patient.

Normal "pulmonary capillary wedge pressure" or "ventricular filling pressure" is 5 to 10 mm. Hg. However, a damaged or sick heart may require greater filling pressures (10 to 15 mm. Hg) to generate an optimum cardiac output. Ventricular filling pressure is augmented by intravenous fluid (or blood) infusion. Abnormally elevated wedge pressure (over 20 mm. Hg) indicates fluid overload and impending pulmonary edema. In addition, excessive ventricular filling may overstretch myocardial sarcomeres and decrease stroke volume and cardiac output. For fluid overload, diuretics remain the key treatment. However, nitroglycerin dilates venous capacitance vessels and decreases ventricular filling as well.

Afterload. Decreased stroke volume may be related to abnormally elevated peripheral vascular resistance (afterload). Although only infrequently required in clinical situations, afterload reduction by arterial vasodilatation may dramatically improve stroke volume and cardiac output. Pharmacological agents most frequently used include chlorpromazine, trimethaphan camsylate, and so-dium nitroprusside. Blood pressure must be closely monitored during vasodilator therapy because hypotension is a frequent and often serious sequela.

Contractility. Stroke volume is also directly related to the contractility state of the heart at any given end-diastolic volume and afterload. Contractility is affected by numerous commonly used drugs. Myocardial depressants include lidocaine, barbiturates, and local or general anesthetics. Myocardial ischemia, acidosis, and myocardial depressant factors that probably occur in certain disease states, such as sepsis, also decrease contractility. Myocardial infarction also hinders the effectiveness of cardiac contraction and must be considered when poor cardiac output is evident. Cardiac contractility is augmented by many pharmacological agents. Cardiac glycosides (digoxin), ionized calcium, catecholamines, and xanthines (theophylline) have a positive inotropic effect on heart muscle.

Treatment plan

Inadequate cardiovascular function may become clinically manifest in numerous ways, including hypotension, acidosis, poor peripheral perfusion, or abnormal end-organ function such as low urine output and confusion. All clinical signs, unfortunately, are nonspecific; thus accurate evaluation of cardiac output requires direct measurement with a Swan-Ganz catheter. As mentioned previously, skilled physicians can insert this device at the bedside with little morbidity.

If measured cardiac output is normal (over 3.5 L./min./m.²), other causes of end-organ dysfunction should be actively sought out. Potential sources include pulmonary dysfunction, low hemoglobin, sepsis, and other metabolic abnormalities.

If cardiac output is low, optimize preload by fluid administration. If cardiac dysfunction continues, measure peripheral vascular resistance. If vascular resistance is abnormal, pharmacological correction may be warranted. After preload and afterload are optimized, continuing poor cardiac output then requires inotropic agents to improve cardiac contractility.

Oxyhemoglobin dissociation

The final checkpoint in the oxygen-substrate delivery scheme is transfer of oxygen from the hemoglobin molecule to tissues. Metabolic abnormalities that impair oxygen delivery at the cellular level including hypothermia and alkalosis should be frequently monitored and corrected.

Once pulmonary and hemodynamic functions are optimized, end-organ dysfunction can safely be evaluated and treated on a system-by-system basis.

DAILY CARE OF THE ICU PATIENT

The critically ill patient is often in a state of flux. Changes occur rapidly and delay in the diagnosis of developing problems often can lead to a tragic outcome. The ICU physician must continually know his patient's status. This requires frequent bedside *examination* and *evaluation* of the patient by the physician, as well as intensive care nurses, respiratory therapists, and consultants.

ICU monitoring

The critically ill patient requires close attention to vital signs and organ-system function, often on a second-to-second basis. Advances in technology have engendered numerous monitoring systems that, when combined with frequent physical examination, help one to recognize physiological instability.

Vital signs

Temperature is recorded at regular intervals, depending on the patient's condition. The most accurate measure of core temperature is obtained by use of a central venous thermistor on a Swan-Ganz catheter, though rectal probes are also satisfactory. Oral temperatures, often inaccurate, should not be used. Both hypothermia and fever are important findings requiring careful appraisal.

Respiratory rate is calculated by observation of chest well motion. Not only rate but also quality of respiratory effort should be noted. As discussed previously, hyperventilation and hypoventilation must be evaluated promptly. Physical exam and chest roentgenography, as well as blood gas analysis, are helpful in sorting out pulmonary problems.

Pulse and rhythm pattern are usually recorded continuously on an ECG monitor. Normal pulse and rhythm pattern displayed on a monitor must, however, be properly interpreted. It does *not* necessarily imply normal cardiovascular function. The patient with electromechanical dissociation may have a normal-appearing monitor but no stroke volume or cardiac output. An effective pulse is best verified by both precordial auscultation and confirmation of peripheral blood pressure transmission (established by palpation, or a monitored indwelling arterial pressure catheter).

Cardiac rhythm disturbances are frequent in ill patients. Dysrhythmias are often secondary to easily treated underlying conditions such as electrolyte abnormalities (hypokalemia), acid-base disorders, volume problems (fluid overload), or hypoxia. Some dysrhythmias require specific drug therapy. All rhythm disturbances demand immediate diagnosis and appropriate treatment because many benign dysrhythmias may, if uncorrected, degenerate into life-threatening rhythm patterns. Once diagnosed, malignant dysrhythmias require aggressive therapy, often pharmacological, and correction of the underlying cause. Dysrhythmias can be categorized into atrial or ventricular, depending on the source of the abnormal impulse. Ventricular dysrhythmias are generally more serious. The categorization and treatment of the numerous dysrhythmias, however, is beyond the scope of this chapter.

On occasion, a patient with a severe cardiac conduction defect may require a *temporary pacemaker* to support a rhythm and pulse. These devices consist of an electrical current generator and a conduction cable (lead) to the myocardium. The pacemaker leads can be placed percutaneously into a large central vein and maneuvered into the right ventricle, which can then be stimulated to produce regular cardiac contractions. These leads can also be placed under emergency conditions directly through the anterior chest wall into the epicardium. Temporary pacemaker cables are often placed during cardiac surgery, since rhythm disturbances may arise both intraoperatively and postoperatively. Patients who remain pacemaker dependent require conversion to a permanent pacemaker (Chapter 31).

Blood pressure is also measured frequently, depending on the patient's condition. The sphygmomanometer is most accurate but cumbersome and time consuming. The seriously ill patient requiring potent cardiovascular agents or demonstrating unstable blood pressure needs continuous monitoring by having a pressure line placed into a peripheral artery. The pressure wave form is transmitted through fluid-filled tubing to a transducer that converts pressure changes to electrical signals. These signals are displayed as an arterial wave form on a monitor with continuous systolic and diastolic pressure readings (Fig. 29-4). The radial artery is most frequently utilized followed by brachial or femoral arteries. Catheter sepsis and ischemia distal to the arterial catheter are potential serious complications. Arterial catheters also provide access for blood samples, including arterial blood gas analysis.

Volume status

The injured or postoperative patient often experiences major changes in intravascular, intracellular, and interstitial fluid volumes (Chapter 3). *Total body fluid status* must be calculated at least on a shift-to-shift (8-hour) basis. Physical exam including evaluation of skin turgor, mucous membranes, and the presence or absence of edema, pulmonary rales, or perspiration gives a rough estimate of

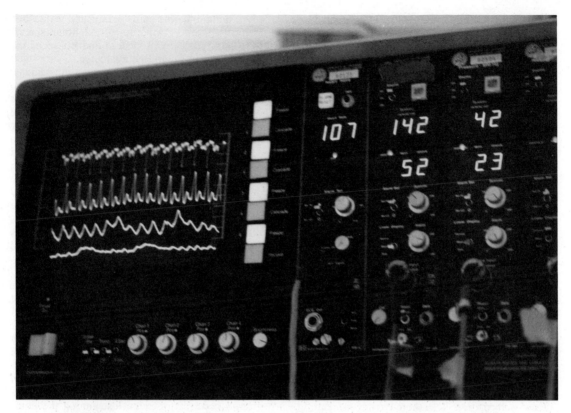

Fig. 29-4. Monitor showing, *top to bottom,* electrocardiographic pattern, systemic arterial pressure, pulmonary arterial pressure, and central venous pressure wave forms. Digital readout of pulse, systemic arterial pressure, and pulmonary arterial pressure is illustrated on right side of monitor.

hydration status. Careful recording of all fluid given to the patient (the "ins") and all fluid removed (the "outs"), including urine output and drainage from all tubes, is mandatory. In addition, one must estimate unmeasured or insensible losses, taking into account increased losses with fever or other hypermetabolic states and decreased losses among patients on mechanical ventilators. Body weight measured daily on the same scale gives an accurate estimation of total body fluid changes.

Intravascular fluid status, as previously discussed, is an important element in maintaining hemodynamic stability and adequate organ function. Inadequate intravascular volume may lead to tachycardia, hypotension, and poor tissue perfusion (hypovolemic shock). Intravascular fluid overload may cause pulmonary edema and myocardial dysfunction. The most readily available ways to monitor intravascular volume include physical exam (e.g., jugular-venous distension) and end-organ evaluation (e.g., mental status, urine

output). Other methods include measurement of pulmonary wedge pressure or central venous pressures.

Central venous pressure (CVP), obtained by placement of a catheter in the superior vena cava near its junction with the right atrium, measures filling pressure of the right ventricle (just as the pulmonary wedge pressure reflects the filling pressure and volume of the left ventricle). If pulmonary vascular resistance and cardiac ventricular function remain stable, changes in central venous pressure generally reflect variations in intravascular volume. CVP measurements are reliable, safe, and easy to obtain.

Intracellular and interstitial fluid status is clinically less significant and rarely measured. An exception occurs when so-called third-space interstitial fluid accumulation is large and must be considered in the patient's overall fluid status evaluation. Examples of "third-space" losses include abdominal ascites, pleural effusion, fluid sequestration in the gastrointestinal tract, and massive tissue swelling.

Diagnostics

Information generated from the hospital laboratory, nuclear medicine, and radiology departments is important in evaluation of the ICU patient. Unfortunately, these services are often overutilized, representing a common source of mismanagement of health care funds. Each patient should be evaluated daily. Laboratory and radiologic tests are then carefully ordered, as needed. The "shotgun monitoring" of a patient with unnecessary lab data and roentgenograms is wasteful.

The ICU flow sheet

Data collected by the nurses and technicians are recorded on a flow sheet. Data include vital signs, fluid "ins" and "outs," hemodynamic measurements, and mechanical ventilator parameters. The flow sheet can thus be easily read, the patient's status evaluated, and further therapy adjusted. These sheets are not to replace frequent physical exam of the patient by the physician, or close communication between the physician and nursing staff.

Systems management

Once information is gathered from (1) careful questioning of the patient, (2) communication with the ICU nurses and technicians, (3) physical examination of the patient, (4) evaluation of flow sheet data including vital signs, ins and outs, fluid status, hemodynamic and pulmonary data, and (5) consideration of laboratory and other special test results, each organ system and phase of the patient's support should be evaluated.

The central nervous, pulmonary, and cardiovascular systems and as well the renal, gastrointestinal, musculoskeletal, and hematological systems should be individually assessed and the appropriate therapeutic interventions taken to ensure ongoing recovery. In addition, daily attention must be given to the patient's nutritional and infection status (Chapters 6 and 7). Metabolic problems, including endocrine derangements, fluid and electrolyte disorders, and acid-base abnormalities must similarly be evaluated and treated. By dealing with the patient on a system-to-system basis, one is less likely to overlook details regarding the patient's care. In the intensive care unit attention to detail best ensures a successful outcome.

SUMMARY

The intensive care unit is unique in the hospital environment. Its main concern (and that of this chapter) often leads to dissociation of the patient into groups of cells and systems that ultimately integrate into a functioning organism. Care in this somewhat dehumanized environment should, however, go beyond treating kidneys, hearts, and lungs. The concept of the patient as a complete person, a concept too often lost among the data, numbers, and measurements, must be kept at the forefront of the ICU physician's thoughts if the best care is to be delivered.

30

Thoracic and Pulmonary Surgery

Nicholas P. Rossi
Wade C. Lamberth, Jr.

Thoracic surgery deals with some of the most important organ systems of the body. Their integrated function is vital to life. To this end, the thoracic surgeon operates on these structures to correct abnormalities of development, relieve obstruction, drain and contain infections, and extirpate tumors. Adequate function of the heart and lungs must be maintained during operation, which often requires highly sophisticated techniques and instruments.

Diseases of the chest are among the most common and important in man. Most of them have become amenable to surgery within this century, mute testimony to great advances in understanding the pathophysiology of the thoracic viscera. This chapter summarizes the most important surgical diseases of the thorax.

SPECIAL PROCEDURES

Certain procedures are commonly used for diagnosis and treatment of patients with thoracic and pulmonary disorders that every student should understand. Since they will be referred to often on the succeeding pages of this section, their principles are discussed here.

Thoracentesis

Thoracentesis is simply needle aspiration of the pleural cavity. It is performed both for diagnosis and for treatment of disorders causing abnormal accumulations of gas or fluid within the pleural space. The accumulations may consist of air (pneumothorax), blood (hemothorax), serum (pleural effusion), chyle (chylothorax), pus (empyema), or varying combinations thereof (hemopneumothorax, pyopneumothorax).

Normally, the pleural cavity is simply a *potential* space that is under negative pressure (-5 to -10 cm. H_2O) during inspiration (expansion of the rib cage and depression of the diaphragm) and under positive pressure (up to $+5$ cm. H_2O) during expiration. The space is bounded by *parietal pleura* lining the inside of the chest wall and *visceral pleura* covering the surface of the lungs. Normally, the pleural cavity contains only a few milliliters of lubricating serum to allow frictionless gliding of the apposed pleural surfaces during respiratory excursion.

Since the chest wall is relatively unyielding, accumulations within the pleural space first collapse the ipsilateral lung to impair its expansion and aeration, proportionate to the volume accumulated. Progressively greater volumes shift the mobile mediastinal structures to the other side, impairing expansion of the contralateral lung and diminishing the return of venous blood to the heart. There results a cardiopulmonary dysfunction that is proportionate to the volume and speed with which the gas or fluid accumulates within the pleural space.

The technical details of thoracentesis are sketched in Fig. 30-1. Thoracentesis is performed aseptically after shaving, scrubbing, and painting the skin with an antiseptic solution. The operator is gloved and often wears a mask and gown. The needle is introduced just *above* an appropriate rib

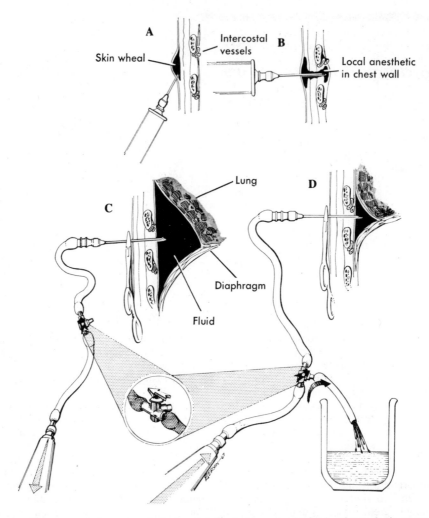

Fig. 30-1. Thoracentesis for removal of pleural fluid. **A,** Skin wheal with local anesthetic agent. **B,** Infiltration of chest wall with local anesthetic agent. **C,** Thoracentesis needle introduced above superior surface of appropriate rib so that its tip just enters pleural space; needle clamped by hemostat at skin level to prevent further advancement; fluid aspirated into syringe. **D,** Stopcock changed to allow delivery of fluid from syringe into side arm and container; system is not disconnected until needle is withdrawn, to avoid air entering pleural space.

to avoid the intercostal vessels that travel along the *inferior* rib surface. The patient with pneumothorax is supine, and the needle is introduced parasternally in the second or third intercostal space, since air gravitates upward. When fluid is to be removed, the needle is introduced into the seventh or eighth intercostal space in the midaxillary line while the patient is in an upright position, since fluid gravitates inferiorly (Fig. 30-1, *C*). If the fluid is loculated or localized, radiographic examination of the chest or fluoroscopy should guide placement of the needle.

Diagnostic thoracentesis is performed when physical examination and radiographic examination of the chest disclose pleural collections (generally fluid) of an unknown type. Generally, only a few milliliters of the fluid are aspirated, with no attempt being made to tap the pleural space dry. The aspirate can be inspected, cultured, stained, examined cytologically, and tested for clotting properties, specific gravity, pH, and chemical constituents. Definitive treatment is facilitated when one knows the precise nature of the pleural effusion.

An attempt is made to evacuate the pleural fluid or air totally in a thoracentesis performed for *therapeutic* purposes. The visceral and parietal pleural surfaces are thereby apposed to one another and help seal off the source of leakage of air or blood. Removal of large amounts of pus aids in the supportive treatment of empyema and thins the fibrous "peel" that subsequently forms. Occasionally, drugs are injected into the pleural space (fibrinolytic enzymes, antibiotics) before withdrawal of the needle. Diagnostic and therapeutic thoracenteses are often combined.

Complications of thoracentesis are few: (1) bacteria may be introduced if the needle is dirty, if the skin is inadequately prepared, or if the needle is inserted through a contaminated area of the chest wall, (2) air is sucked into the pleural space if the needle, tubing, or syringe becomes disconnected, because of the negative intrapleural pressure, and (3) the lung may be punctured by the needle tip, provoking a pneumothorax or hemothorax. These complications are minimized by careful attention to the technique illustrated in Fig. 30-1.

Pleural space drainage

Underwater-seal drainage is the standard technique of *closed tube drainage* of the pleural space to remove pleural space air or fluid aseptically and encourage lung expansion. It is selected in preference to thoracentesis when the leakage is expected to continue for some time (hours or days), with rapid reaccumulation likely after simple needle aspiration.

In keeping with the principles outlined for thoracentesis, the chest tubes are introduced aseptically high anteriorly for the removal of air, and low and laterally when fluid is removed. They may be inserted through a trochar under local anesthesia, but more commonly they are left indwelling at the conclusion of thoracotomy operations in which functioning lung tissue remains in that hemithorax. Tube drainage is *not* used after total pneumonectomy because the risk of postoperative air leak or infection is low, and the serum that fills the empty hemithorax obliterates the space created by the removal of the lung. The process is completed by the organization of the fluid mainly through the action of fibroblasts to produce a fibrothorax.

Fig. 30-2 diagrams the principles of underwater-seal drainage. The fluid or blood enters the bottle under the surface of the water, with the length of glass tubing immersed determining the positive pressure that must be exerted by the patient before drainage occurs. Air bubbles off through the vent in the top of the bottle while fluid accumulates in the bottle. The fluid cannot backtrack up the tubing to reenter the pleural space. If the tubes are not

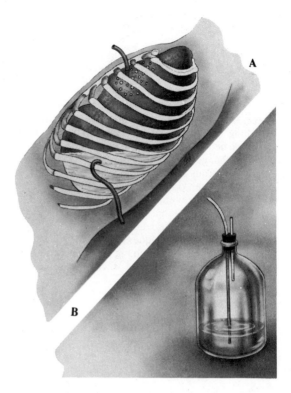

Fig. 30-2. Intercostal chest tubes with underwater-seal drainage. **A,** Tube to remove air from pleural space is introduced through second intercostal space at midclavicular line; tube to remove liquid (blood, pus, and postoperative fluid collection) is introduced through eighth intercostal space at anterior axillary line. **B,** Tubing is connected to glass rod on bottle that is covered with sterile water; pleural air bubbles into bottle and escapes to outside, while fluid collects in bottle.

plugged, one can tell that an air leak has sealed when bubbling ceases and that pleural fluid has disappeared when the fluid level in the bottle becomes stabilized. The tubes are generally removed at this time.

Open tube drainage of the pleural space simply communicates the pleural space directly to the outside, generally through one or two hard rubber tubes. The tubes are introduced through an appropriate intercostal space, or (preferably) through the bed of a short segment of resected rib. Open tube drainge is simpler and quicker than closed tube (underwater-seal) drainage, but it can be used only under the following circumstances: (1) when contamination is already present (empyema), (2) when the negative intrapleural pressure has been lost, and (3) when the lungs and mediastinal structures are fairly fixed, or stabilized, so that they cannot be dislocated. With these limitations, the open tube method is usually restricted to the drainage of chronic empyema.

Tracheobronchial toilet

Good tracheobronchial toilet is essential at all times and is automatically carried out by all of us as we periodically change position, sigh, breathe deeply, clear our throats, or cough. Maintenance of a clear airway is especially important in patients with lung disease or postoperative patients. It is accomplished best by the patient himself with frequent changes in position, periodic deep breathing, and vigorous coughing. In most instances such measures insisted on by nursing and physiotherapy personnel will prevent atelectasis and encourage expansion of the lung, the two main goals of postpulmonary resectional care. *Endotracheal suction* is one of the techniques to facilitate tracheobronchial toilet, as outlined in Fig. 30-3. The irritation that the tube provokes in the trachea itself gener-

ally induces uncontrollably vigorous coughing, raising sputum and dislodging mucus plugs that are then sucked out. Saline and mucolytic agents can be injected through the tube to liquefy secretions and improve cleansing of the respiratory tree. A "trap" in the tubing allows collection of the aspirate for examination and culture. The apparatus must be sterilized before being used.

Periodic assisted ventilation bronchoscopy and *tracheostomy* are more extreme measures used without delay if simpler methods fail. Ventilation can be assisted by bag and mask but is administered more effectively when one passes an endotracheal tube and ventilates with a bag. Irrigation and aspiration can be performed through the tube, and poorly aerated or atelectatic areas of lung are expanded to improve respiratory exchange. If ventilation is impaired because of an obstructing mucus plug or thick secretions the patient cannot raise, bedside bronchoscopy may be required. This

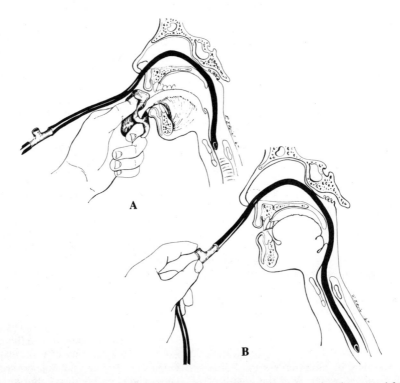

Fig. 30-3. Endotracheal suction. **A,** Patient in sitting position, tongue grasped and retracted forward to enlarge hypopharynx; suction catheter introduced through nose curves around posterior pharynx to enter larynx and upper trachea. **B,** Suction applied to remove secretions brought to catheter tip by violent coughing that catheter provokes; suction is intermittently broken by removal of finger from adapter, to prevent mucosa from being sucked into catheter tip and to minimize arterial hypoxemia that accompanies aspiration of gas from airway. Administration of oxygen before, during, and after endotracheal suction reduces hypoxic complications.

is most easily accomplished with a flexible fiberoptic bronchoscope.

Tracheostomy allows irrigation, aspiration, and assisted ventilation to be performed by a nurse or technician and, in addition, reduces respiratory "dead space." However, it is accomplished at the expense of increased nursing care, desiccation of inspired air, loss of phonation, and occasionally misadventures such as erosion of the trachea and bleeding.

Bronchoscopy

Bronchoscopy allows visualization of the interior of the trachea and main bronchi through an illuminated, rigid, tubelike instrument. The bronchoscope is introduced with topical anesthesia in the cooperative and sedated adult but requires general anesthesia in children and uncooperative adults. Mucosal ulceration, inflammation, or tumors can be seen at bronchoscopy, as well as deviation, distortion, and narrowing of the trachea and bronchi. Secretions can be aspirated, foreign bodies removed, and suspicious mucosal lesions biopsied through the bronchoscope. The rigid bronchoscope complemented by the use of telescope lens systems allows visualization of the airway to segmental bronchi and is therefore of greatest use in centrally located proximal lesions.

Direct examination of subsegmental bronchi is possible by means of the flexible bronchofiberscope, which utilizes the fiberoptic principle allowing the visual image to be transmitted along a curved pathway. Because of this unique property and a relatively small diameter, the device can be manipulated into subsegmental bronchi, thereby expanding direct airway visualization. In addition, the instrument provides access to distal bronchi for the passage of brush catheters and small biopsy forceps. These devices can be guided under fluoroscopic control into peripheral lung lesions, allowing diagnosis in 80% of cases.

Bronchography

Bronchography allows roentgenographic visualization of the smaller ramifications of the tracheobronchial tree. Roentgenograms are taken in different projections after a rather viscid radiopaque material has been injected endobronchially through a nasotracheal catheter. The patient is positioned appropriately to allow filling of any or all of the lung segments. Bronchography outlines filling defects caused by tumors or foreign bodies, localizes endobronchial obstruction, and diagnoses bronchiectasis and abnormalities of position of the various lung segments. Once widely used, it is now of limited use.

Prescalene lymph node biopsy

Occasionally a diagnosis of known pulmonary disease cannot be made by roentgenographic examination of the chest, bronchoscopy, bronchography, sputum analyses, and other routine measures. In such patients biopsy of the prescalene lymph nodes is sometimes helpful in diagnosis. The procedure is done under local anesthesia for all but children and uncooperative adults, with a supraclavicular transverse incision preferred. The incision is made on the side of palpable nodes, and a diagnosis is nearly always secured. If the nodes are not palpable, a diagnosis is provided in only 10% to 15% of cases, and lymph node pathological changes are nonspecific in the remainder. With nonpalpable nodes, the left prescalene nodes are biopsied if the pulmonary disease involves the left upper lobe (which drains to this side), but the right prescalene nodes are biopsied if the disease predominantly involves the right lung or the left lower lobe. This choice of sides is made to avoid the thoracic duct, which is on the left side at the junction of the jugular and subclavian veins, and also because of the known crossover of the lymphatic drainage of the left lower lung to the right prescalene lymph node chain.

Prescalene lymph node biopsy is especially helpful in the diagnosis of Boeck's sarcoid, obscure lung carcinoma, hilar masses, and diffuse bilateral pulmonary infiltrates, but there is a low yield in tuberculosis, pulmonary mycoses, solitary peripheral lung lesions, bronchopneumonia, and pleurisy.

Mediastinoscopy and anterior mediastinotomy

Biopsy of mediastinal lymph nodes is more likely to yield a diagnosis in patients with pulmonary disease than biopsy of more distant regional lymph nodes. These procedures require general anesthesia. Mediastinoscopy is performed by insertion of a lighted scope through a small cervical incision in the suprasternal notch. The instrument is passed along the anterior surface of the trachea deep to the pretracheal fascia to the level of the bifurcation of the trachea. Lymph nodes adjacent to the trachea, proximal right and left bronchi, and subcarinal area are visualized and biopsied. Anterior mediastinotomy is an extrapleural mediastinal exploration through the bed of the second or third costal cartilages. These procedures are nearly always diagnostic in sarcoidosis or lymphoma with hilar adenopathy and are of great value in assessment of mediastinal spread of bronchogenic carcinoma.

Lung biopsy

For diffuse disease of the pulmonary parenchyma it may be necessary to obtain a specimen of the lung for analysis. A trephine air drill or cutting needle may be used percutaneously to allow biopsy of the lung but carries the hazard of pneumohemothorax. Open biopsy of lung through small anterior thoracotomy is usually the best means of obtaining adequate, representative tissue.

LUNGS
Pulmonary function tests

Pulmonary function tests are as much a part of medicine as the tests for hepatic, renal, or cardiac function are. They are valuable in determining the location or type of process causing respiratory impairment and in serially documenting changes that occur during therapy. Table 30-1 outlines commonly used pulmonary function tests. For more elaborate tests the student should consult other references.

Blood gases

When the lungs cannot maintain arterial O_2 pressures and saturation at normal levels, pulmonary insufficiency for oxygenation (hypoxemia) results. When they cannot prevent the increase of arterial CO_2 tension, insufficiency exists for CO_2 elimination (hypercapnia, or hypercarbia).

Hypercapnia is always caused by alveolar hypoventilation that is secondary to severe impairment of the mechanics of breathing. The trouble may be in the lungs (pneumonitis), the airways (mucus plug), the pleural space (pleural effusion), respiratory muscles (tetanus), or respiratory center (cerebrovascular accident). Impairment of diffusion does *not* cause hypercapnia because the tissue CO_2 solubility quotient is 20 times that of O_2. Arteriovenous shunting also is not an important cause. Hypercapnia is almost always associated with hypoxemia, but hypoxemia can coexist with a normal CO_2 arterial pressure and saturation.

Hypoxemia, unlike hypercapnia, may be caused by several mechanisms and may exist with no measurable impairment of the mechanics of breathing. The most important causes of hypoxemia are venoarterial shunts (as seen with congenital intracardiac shunts, or in areas of lung atelectasis), underventilation, poor diffusion (thickened alveolar-capillary membrane), and breathing air of low O_2 content (high altitudes).

Congenital malformations
Congenital lobar emphysema

Congenital lobar emphysema is an important cause of respiratory distress in the newborn and at times is life threatening. The involved lobe (usually the left upper and right middle lobes) is overdistended because of a ball valve effect of a partially obstructed bronchus; air readily enters the lobe but

Table 30-1. Pulmonary function tests*

Test	Definition	Normal value	Explanation and remarks
Vital capacity (VC)†	The volume of gas exhaled by maximum voluntary effort after maximum inspiration	Depends on age, weight, sex, nutrition, height	The VC alone is of very limited value; it is useless in evaluation of obstructive disease and correlates poorly with dyspnea; it is reduced in the restrictive lung diseases
Timed vital capacity (TVC)†	The amount of the vital capacity exhaled in a given time interval: 1, 2, or 3 seconds; in 1 second it is called the forced expiratory volume, or FEV 1	About 85% of VC is normally exhaled in 1 second	This test relates much better to the overall evaluation of ventilatory function and to dyspnea than the VC does; the shortest 1-second volume correlates best with symptoms
Air-velocity index	$\dfrac{\text{% predicted MBC}}{\text{% predicted VC}}$	A value below 0.8 is indicative of airway obstructive disease; a value greater than 1 indicates restrictive airway disease	The actual value of the two components must be considered first

Test	Description	Normal value	Remarks
Maximal voluntary ventilation (MVV)	The amount of gas exchanged per unit of time during maximum voluntary hyperventilation; usually done over 10 to 15 seconds, or to 1 minute if possible	Formulas based on age and surface area	Unlike single-breath tests, it reflects the integrity of the respiratory bellows as a whole, including fatigue, muscular strength, blood supply, and air trapping; better correlates with dyspnea
Mean maximal inspiratory flow (MMIF)	The mean maximal flow measured between 200 and 1,200 ml. on the inspiratory spirogram	400 to 600 L./min.	Normally is a straight line throughout
Mean maximal expiratory flow*	The mean maximal expiratory flow rate for that portion of the VC between 200 and 1,200 ml.	From formulas: 400 to 600 L./min., average adult	A reduction indicates that a mechanical problem exists; this is serious because it decreases the patient's ability to cough and remove secretions from his airway because of excessive air trapping
Dyspnea index	The percentage of the MBC required for a standard exercise	8% to 15% walking at 2 m.p.h.	An increase in the dyspnea index is most commonly the result of a decreased ventilatory capacity and rarely the result of increased respiratory requirement
Transfer factor for carbon monoxide (D_{CO})	A test for evaluation of the diffusion capacity of the lungs; several techniques; the simplest is a single breath test in which the amount of CO entering the blood is measured after one inspires a gas mixture of known CO concentration and holds the breath after one preliminary breath	25 ml./min./mm. Hg; frequently reported as a percentage of a predicted value based on known dependent factors	Depends on many factors—position, body size, hematocrit, and alveolar P_{O_2}; normal value indicates normally functioning pulmonary capillary membranes; does not require patient cooperation
Single-breath nitrogen test	Another test to evaluate diffusion capacity	Less than 1.5% N_2	Used to determine uneven distribution of the inspirated air; may be normal in obstructive and restrictive lung disease but means serious lung disease when abnormal

*These tests are readily available and require minimal instructions; all are used in screening.

†Part of the routine physical examination.

cannot escape. The lesion may be associated with insufficient blood supply to the involved portion of the lung, or the bronchus may have faulty cartilaginous support, but frequently the cause is obscure. In cases in which careful pathological study has been carried out, a cause can be found in no more than half. Progressive respiratory distress (tachypnea, dyspnea, cyanosis) is the chief clinical problem. Serial plain chest roentgenograms show an enlarging, airfilled cyst. Resection of the involved lobe gives excellent results.

Pulmonary intralobar sequestration

Pulmonary sequestration is a bronchovascular anomaly produced when the bronchus supplying a part of the lung (usually the lower lobes) develops abnormally and loses its connection with the tracheobronchial tree and receives its arterial supply from the lower thoracic or abdominal aorta. The involved lung contains many cysts lined by ciliated or mucus-producing columnar epithelium. Recurrent infection is common. The chest roentgenogram may simulate the changes of bronchiectasis, abscess, localized empyema, and occasionally a tumorlike form. Aortography showing the abnormal vessel may be diagnostic. The lesion is four times more common in males. Excision of the sequestered lesion is the treatment of choice.

Arteriovenous fistulas

Congenital connections between a pulmonary artery and vein occasionally occur. This anomaly, in a diffuse form, may be related to hereditary hemorrhagic telangiectasia. Congenital arteriovenous fistulas are multiple in more than 50% of the cases and vary from miliary proportions to large communications occurring peripherally in all lobes. Symptoms include dyspnea, cyanosis, clubbing, hemoptysis, and easy fatigability. Central nervous system manifestations are related to the associated polycythemia or to intracranial vascular abnormalities. Bruits may be heard on auscultation of the chest. In the localized form the disorder is very rarely recognized during childhood, but when widespread, it causes severe respiratory disorders in the newborn. In longstanding cases severe complications, such as hemoptysis, cerebrovascular accident, and brain abscess, have occurred.

Single lesions are excised. In the miliary form surgical therapy has little value. Ligation of the supplying vessels is worthless.

Agenesis, hypoplasia, aplasia of the lungs

The lesions of agenesis, hypoplasia, and aplasia of the lungs are rare. They may be bilateral or unilateral and may involve a lobe or an entire lung. Bilateral pulmonary agenesis is the rarest and

severest form, is associated with cardiac defects, and, of course, is incompatible with life. Unilateral agenesis of the lung also causes a high toll in infant mortality but is in itself compatible with life. There is usually a history of some respiratory difficulties, and the chest film shows a homogeneous density. An incorrect diagnosis of massive atelectasis may be made, as with foreign body inhalation.

In hypoplasia the lung is underdeveloped, as the corresponding artery and bronchus are, and this is sometimes associated with congenital diaphragmatic hernia. In aplasia no aerated lung tissue is present in the involved segment, and the bronchus is rudimentary. Recurrent infection is common. Surgical excision is the usual therapy of both hypoplastic and aplastic lung segments.

Congenital bronchogenic cysts

Congenital bronchogenic cysts are usually found in the midmediastinum near (but not communicating with) the tracheal bifurcation and main bronchus. They are usually single but may be multilocular. They are lined by respiratory epithelium, and the walls often contain smooth muscle and cartilage. Infection may destroy the epithelium to make specific histological identification difficult. Symptoms depend on the size, location, and the presence of infection: wheezing, pain, cough, atelectasis, and nonspecific symptoms of infection are all possible. Excision should be performed.

Acquired disease
Chylothorax

Chylothorax, an uncommon clinical entity, is associated with tumor, trauma, or tuberculosis. By far the most common is trauma (about half the cases). It also occurs after operations, especially after dissections around the subclavian artery for patent ductus, coarctation of the aorta, Blalock shunts, and esophagogastrectomy. It may follow some abdominal operations, such as vagotomy and gastric resections. It may be the first sign of an unrecognized lymphoma.

Spontaneous chylothorax occurs in the newborn and causes symptoms of tachypnea, cyanosis, and chest wall retractions. In older children chylothorax with symptoms of respiratory difficulty, cough, or recurrent pneumonias indicate an intrathoracic anomaly.

Aspiration alone is effective therapy in children. It will usually be successful in benign cases but is frequently ineffective for chylothorax caused by tumors. The cause should always be sought.

Inflammatory bronchiectasis

Inflammatory bronchiectasis is a chronic suppurative disease of lung segments resulting from pulmonary infections, asthma, and bronchial obstruction (i.e., aspirated foreign body). In the group derived from infections, bronchiectasis begins in the first 5 years of life. The pathogenesis is now generally believed to be a necrotizing infection around the branches of segmental bronchi. The smaller bronchi become obliterated, and the larger proximal bronchi undergo dilatation and widening during the healing, fibrotic phase of the inflammatory process. Sinusitis and allergy are common.

Bronchiectasis is described according to anatomical type: cylindric, saccular, fusiform, or cystic. Mild cylindric bronchiectasis is reversible, but otherwise anatomical classification is not clinically significant. In children bronchiectasis is commonly associated with aspiration of foreign bodies, chronic upper and lower respiratory tract infections, and cystic fibrosis of the pancreas. Bronchiectasis is a disease of the lower lobes, except when found in conjunction with tuberculosis.

The symptoms are those of recurrent pulmonary infection: fever, morning cough, production of foul-smelling sputum, hemoptysis, chest pain, and retarded physical development. Socioeconomic problems are common. Bronchography is the most important diagnostic examination, also documenting the extent and location of the disease. Bronchoscopy rules out tumor or foreign body. Complications of the disease are hemorrhage, empyema, and metastic spread of the infection (brain abscess).

Treatment of bronchiectasis consists of rest, adequate nutrition, antibiotics, and postural drainage. Operative removal of the involved segments is carried out during a quiescent phase in selected patients with adequate pulmonary function and with appropriate antibiotic coverage. In bilateral cases the operations are staged, with the more advanced areas in one lung resected first.

Empyema

Empyema, or infection of the pleural space, is a complication of lung disease and not a primary disease in itself. The diagnosis is suspected by signs of fluid within the pleural cavity on physical examination (absence of breath sounds, dullness to percussion, tracheal deviation to the other side) and roentgenographic examination of the chest (Fig. 30-4) and is confirmed by diagnostic thoracentesis with smear and culture of the purulent fluid. The physician's first duty is to rule out underlying obstructive lung disease by bronchoscopy. Then he must consider if the infection is coming from the lung (lobar pneumonia), from the esophagus or the mediastinum, or from below the diaphragm.

The aim of treatment is the restoration of normal respiratory function. This demands full expansion of the lungs with obliteration of the empyema space, as well as restoration of normal mobility of the lungs, diaphragm, and chest wall. In the acute phase, when the pus is thin and no organizing exudate has formed over the lungs, one or more thoracenteses may accomplish these ends. In the chronic phase closed tube drainage of the pleural space may suffice; the most common mistake is premature removal of the tube, which should remain in place with periodic shortening until the lung has fully expanded. Decortication is necessary in chronic forms when a fibrous peel encases the collapsed lung (captive lung); the operation is excision of the peel to allow reexpansion of lung.

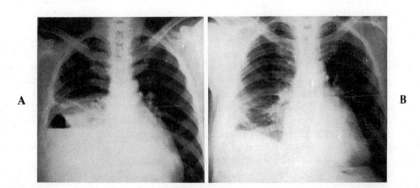

Fig. 30-4. Empyema. **A,** Air-fluid level in right pleural space in patient with pneumonia; indeterminate nature of fluid (blood, pus, serum) by roentgenogram, but thoracentesis yielded pus. **B,** Same patient after 2 weeks of closed pleural drainage through intercostal tube; pus virtually gone and lung expanded.

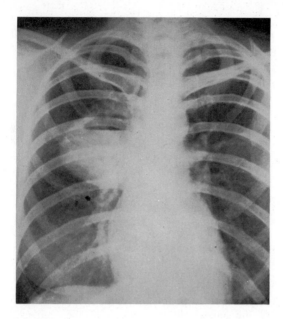

Fig. 30-5. Lung abscess. Underlying cause was carcinoma of lung; air-fluid level indicates connection with bronchus.

Lung abscess

Lung abscess is a destructive, suppurative process in the lung caused by microorganisms (Fig. 30-5). The infection is usually polymicrobic. Unlike bronchiectasis, which follows an anatomical segment of the lung, the destructive process of lung abscess crosses segmental lines. Several underlying causes must be considered:

1. *Aspiration of vomitus:* Probably the most common cause of lung abscess, it happens especially in alcoholics, epileptics, patients with central nervous system diseases, and patients who have been unconscious for long periods of time.
2. *Bronchial obstruction with infection distal to the point of obstruction:* Carcinoma, bronchial adenoma, and foreign body are causes.
3. *Pneumonia:* The type of organism determines the pattern of resulting lung abscess. The pneumococcus (type III) and *Klebsiella* produce multilocular cavities, usually in the upper lobes. *Staphylococcus,* the most common cause of lung abscess in infants and children, produces a necrotizing bronchopneumonia leading to multiple abscesses, which can become huge from bronchial obstruction and air trapping.
4. *Abscess from infected cysts or from breakdown of a bronchial carcinoma:* Infection destroys the lining of a cyst, making it very difficult to determine its true nature. The "carcinomatous abscess" is one of the many faces of lung carcinoma (Fig. 30-5).
5. *Abscess caused by trauma:* Infection of a hematoma or embedded foreign material.
6. *Extension from abdominal infection:* Subdiaphragmatic abscess and amebic infection of the liver are the usual precursors.
7. *Metastatic septic abscess:* Seeding of the bloodstream from a distant focus (prostate, soft tissue, liver, etc.) is the method of spread of the infected material to the lungs. The abscesses are usually small and multiple.

Complications of lung abscess include brain abscess, empyema, septicemia, and endotoxic shock.

Clinical signs of lung abscess are fever, cough, production of purulent sputum, anemia, and clubbing of the fingers. Roentgenographic examination of the chest generally confirms the diagnosis of lung abscess, but bronchoscopy and bronchography are often helpful.

The treatment of acute lung abscess is conservative: postural drainage, bronchoscopic aspiration, bed rest, high caloric diet, blood transfusions, and antibiotics. Resection of involved lung is indicated when stenosis of the bronchus is present, empyema is associated, localized lung damage is extensive, and conservative therapy has failed.

Middle lobe syndrome

Middle lobe syndrome refers to intermittent or chronic collapse of the middle lobe of the right lung (Fig. 30-6). The cause is obscure and variously ascribed to pressure from lymph nodes surrounding the middle lobe bronchus or to its acute angle of entry into the main bronchus. Tuberculosis is one of the known causes for lymph node enlargement leading to this syndrome, but often no specific infection is found.

The three predominant symptoms are recurrent pneumonia, hemoptysis, and dull chest pain aggravated by breathing. Cystic bronchiectasis is commonly present in the atelectatic lobe. Bronchoscopy and bronchograms rule out carcinoma, tuberculosis, and foreign body. Resected specimens may reveal congenital bronchial stenosis, cysts, specific infections (coccidioidomycosis or histoplasmosis), chronic nonspecific pneumonia, or granuloma.

Characteristically, roentgenographic examination of the chest shows a triangular density best seen on the lateral projection (Fig. 30-6).

Some cases can be treated conservatively by postural drainage and specific antibiotic therapy. If this is not successful, the middle lobe should be resected.

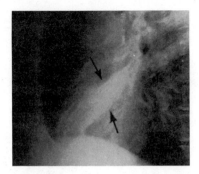

Fig. 30-6. Middle lobe syndrome. Triangular density of collapsed middle lobe is best seen between arrows on lateral chest roentgenogram.

Pulmonary tuberculosis

Pulmonary tuberculosis has long been a scourge of mankind, but with epidemiological methods and modern drug therapy it can be controlled, if not eradicated. Despite this control, the incidence of new cases in the United States currently is in the range of 28.7 per 100,000 population, with a death rate of about 5 per 100,000. These figures indicate that tuberculosis is still a health problem of major proportion.

The surgical treatment of pulmonary tuberculosis has changed radically since the introduction of streptomycin and para-aminosalicylic acid in the late 1940s, isoniazid in 1952, and rifampin in the late 1960s. Those who lived through this era recall the "old days" with the same terror invoked by other infectious diseases. Records show that 70% of patients who had a persistent tuberculous cavity died within 5 years. Total cure was impossible, and methods of treatment, such as induced pneumothorax, often produced more harm than good. Sanatoriums were crowded to overflowing, since each patient required an average of 2 years of confinement. All of this has changed for the better, and now the indications for surgical treatment or institutional care are few.

Pathogenesis. Clinically, an initial primary or "childhood" type of tuberculous infection occurs in the lungs that requires about 2 years to develop into the adult type of disease, in those few whose disease progresses. In children pulmonary tuberculosis is frequently accompanied by pleural effusion and by mediastinal and cervical adenopathy. A conservative approach of combined drug therapy is most rewarding in this group. The adult disease is caused by reinfection from a previous tuberculous focus, or a new infection from without. Reactivation is seen more commonly in untreated patients or in those who were inadequately treated with drugs.

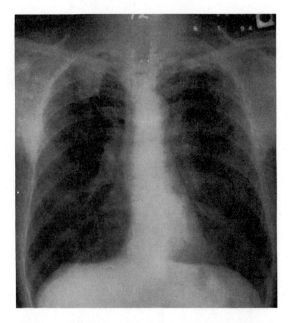

Fig. 30-7. Pulmonary tuberculosis. Bilateral apical fibronodular densities, upward retraction of both lung hila, and compensatory emphysema of both lower lobes.

Types of pulmonary tuberculosis. Types of pulmonary tuberculosis are tuberculoma, cavities, bronchitis and bronchostenosis, empyema, bronchiectasis, tuberculous lymphadenitis, and pericarditis.

Tuberculoma. Tuberculoma is a somewhat confusing term, since it has been applied to a first infection focus in the lung. It should be restricted to describe a focus of reinfection or to a cavity filled with caseous material. Without treatment, about 25% of tuberculomas break into a bronchus and cause endobronchial spread.

Cavities. Tuberculous cavities are lung abscesses that cross segmental barriers between lobes. The cavities may attain a large size, sometimes because of the tension produced by air trapped within them. Some become inspissated with caseous material to form tuberculomas. Sometimes they are small and multiple, and as healing progresses with increasing fibrous tissue reaction, a honeycomb or bronchiectatic appearance is produced.

Bronchitis and bronchostenosis. Tubercles in bronchi produce bronchitis. The resultant scarring may so narrow the bronchus as to cause bronchostenosis, which may lead to tension cavities, tuberculomas, persistent cavities, or heavy scar formation in the involved segment or segments.

Empyema. Tuberculous empyema results from tuberculous pleurisy or may follow induced pneu-

Table 30-2. Fungus diseases of the lungs

Disease	Agent	Endemic geographic distribution	Transmission	Roentgenographic findings	Laboratory diagnosis	Symptoms	Treatment
Sporotrichosis	*Sporotrichum schenckii*	Worldwide	Direct inoculation into skin from puncture wound	Pleural effusion and fibrocavitary appearance similar to tuberculosis; variable degree of infiltration, cavitary miliary disease (in the disseminated form)	Fusiform organism on biopsy or form sputum or exudate	Involves all organs	KI; amphotericin; hydroxystilbamidine
Aspergillosis	*Aspergillus*	Worldwide	May be normal saprophyte in sputum; usually found in sick patients with lymphoma, carcinoma, tuberculosis	Pneumonic abscess, intracavitary fungus ball	Only dependably established by tissue biopsy	Bronchitis, acute or chronic pneumonia, allergic form; hemorrhage a serious threat	KI value limited; amphotericin B; resection
Candidiasis (candidosis)	*Candida albicans*	Worldwide	Invasion under conditions of reduced resistance, prolonged antibiotic or steroid therapy	Pneumonia or miliary spread	Only when organism is found in blood or seen in tissue	Those of a severe bronchopneumonia	Amphotericin B
Actinomycosis	*Actinomyces bovis*	Worldwide	Aspiration from mouth to lower respiratory tract; not a contagious disease	Dense, progressive infiltrates; abscess	Organism seen as sulfur granules in pus or sputum; gram-positive, anaerobic; skin or serology tests no good	Seldom acute cough, purulent sputum, weight loss, low-grade fever; occasionally constrictive pericarditis	Sulfa drugs, penicillin, drainage of abscesses or empyema
Nocardiosis	*Nocardia asteroides*	Worldwide	Saprophytes in soil also found in respiratory tract associated with tuberculosis, lupus erythematosus, leukemia, pulmonary alveolar proteinosis	Dense infiltrates; abscess or cavity formation common	Acid-fast gram-positive, cultured early from pus, sputum	Acute or chronic cough, hemoptysis, night sweats, weight loss, pleural involvement, brain abscess and meningitis, mycetoma on foot (Madura foot)	Sulfadiazine, drainage of pus and abscess; pulmonary resection only occasionally

Disease	Organism	Geography	Source	Radiographic findings	Diagnosis	Clinical features	Treatment
Histoplasmosis (Fig. 30-8)	*Histoplasma capsulatum*	Most common in Mississippi River basin	From soil contaminated by excreta of birds, bats, and rodents	Variable pneumonia; dense infiltrates, miliary patterns, coin lesion, Ghon type of complex, sclerosing mediastinitis	Demonstration of organism in sputum or lung tissue; complement fixation test 1:8 is regarded as significant	Primary infection is transient; heavy infiltration results in acute pneumonia, protean symptoms in the disseminated form	Amphotericin B; resection of localized disease, otherwise biopsy and drug therapy
Coccidioidomycosis	*Coccidioides immitis*	Southwestern United States	Airborne, highly infectious but not contagious; can be passed on by fomites	Variable: thin-walled cavity, solitary lesion, infiltrates; pneumonitis, pleural effusion, adenopathy	PAS stain of biopsy material; organisms grow readily on Sabouraud's agar; any complement fixation titer significant	Primary infection, "flu-like," erythema nodosum (20% in females); 1:1,000 clinically ill; small number hematogenous spread with meningitis	Amphotericin B, but not for most cases that are self-limited; surgery for persistent cavities
Cryptococcosis	*Cryptococcus neoformans*	Worldwide; soil especially contaminated by pigeon excreta	Common in leukemia, Hodgkin's disease, diabetes, sarcoid, prolonged steroid therapy; lung principal portal of entry	Solitary or multiple nodules, pneumonitis, mediastinal adenopathy; cavitation rare	Organisms in tissue, C.S.F., or sputum; no skin or complement-fixation test available	Human infection usually subclinical; meningitis common; diagnosis is made in only half of patients before operation	Amphotericin B is only agent of value; localized pulmonary disease; resection and drug coverage
North American blastomycosis	*Blastomyces dermatitidis*	United States and Canada	Inhalation of spores, not contagious, common in persons in contact with soil	Variable, usually dense pneumonitis or infiltration; may resemble bronchogenic carcinoma	Budding yeast found in sputum, pus, gastric juice, prostatic secretion; treated with potassium hydroxide without staining; skin test not reliable	Similar to those of tuberculosis: suspect with lesions in skin, bone, and lung	Amphotericin B; pulmonary resection rarely indicated

mothorax, spontaneous pneumothorax, or resection. Pyogenic organisms may also be present, usually after bronchopleural fistulization.

Bronchiectasis. Bronchiectasis results from bronchostenosis caused by healing endobronchial disease, or by compression of the bronchus by tuberculous lymph nodes. Fistulous connection between the bronchiectatic sacs differentiates it from nontuberculous bronchiectasis. Differentiation, however, may be difficult.

Tuberculous lymphadenitis. Tuberculous lymphadenitis may have serious sequelae: bronchostenosis, erosion into a bronchus with endobronchial spread, or spread to the esophagus, pleura, or pericardium. Many of these problems are seen in children with untreated disease.

Pericarditis. In the past, constrictive pericarditis was most often caused by tuberculosis. Recently, viral and other forms of pericarditis have become more important clinically.

Diagnosis. The protean clinical manifestations of pulmonary tuberculosis indicate that the diagnosis is difficult to establish. Ordinarily this is not so. Most cases are diagnosed correctly by skin tests, roentgenographic examination of the chest (Fig. 30-7), and multiple examinations of sputum or gastric washings (swallowed sputum) for acid-fast organisms on smears, culture, and guinea pig inoculations. Thoracentesis, bronchoscopy, bronchography, and prescalene lymph node biopsies are occasionally necessary for diagnostic confirmation. A few obscure cases defy diagnosis by all conventional methods.

Surgical treatment of pulmonary tuberculosis. The aim of treatment in pulmonary tuberculosis is to inactivate the disease permanently (sputum negative for tubercle bacilli). The disease can be prevented by chemoprophylaxis in persons known to be high risks: people (especially children) who are exposed to patients with active pulmonary infection, patients with inactive tuberculosis who have never been treated with drugs, especially if they are diabetics, receiving steroids, or have had gastrectomy.

Operations used in the surgical treatment of pulmonary tuberculosis fall into two groups:

1. *Relaxant procedures* designed to collapse the involved lung to promote healing
2. *Resectional therapy:* the trend in the last two decades has been toward this group, but the need for all operative procedures is decreasing

The *relaxant procedures* are as follows:

1. Induced pneumothorax and pneumoperitoneum
2. Creation of an extrapleural space by stripping the parietal pleura from the chest wall

3. Extraperiosteal plombage, filling the space between the lung and ribs with poly(methyl methacrylate) balls or some other inert material
4. Thoracoplasty, removal of the ribs and section of bands of deep cervical fascia attached to the apex of the lung (apicolysis); extensive thoracoplasty is used to close bronchopleural fistulas

Resectional therapy is indicated for the following:

1. Tuberculosis bronchiectasis
2. Destroyed lung
3. Thick-walled cavity unsuitable for collapse
4. Tuberculoma
5. Giant cavity
6. After a thoracoplasty that has not rendered the patient sputum-negative
7. Suspicion of carcinoma—the incidence of carcinoma of the lung is three times greater in tuberculosis patients than in the general population; any patient receiving adequate antituberculous drug therapy whose disease has been stable but who shows a change in his x-ray studies becomes highly suspect for carcinoma

Pulmonary infections caused by atypical mycobacteria

In recent years atypical mycobacteria (*Mycobacterium kansasii* and *M. intracellulare*—the Battey bacillus) have caused pulmonary lesions that are amenable to treatment. In properly selected patients the chance of obtaining negative status has been three to four time greater in surgically treated patients than in medically treated ones.

Fungus diseases

Table 30-2 includes the agent, endemic geographic distribution, transmission, roentgenographic examination, laboratory diagnosis, symptoms, and treatment of fungus diseases of the lungs.

Pulmonary neoplasms
Bronchial carcinoma

Fifty years ago lung cancer was an infrequent disease. Today it kills more men than any other type of cancer, and its incidence is still rising (Chapter 11). Several environmental materials are known to be related causally: asbestos, arsenic, nickel, chromium, and uranium. Average male smokers of cigarettes are 10 times more likely to develop lung cancer than nonsmokers are, and for heavy smokers the risk is 20 times greater than for nonsmokers. Carcinomas arise from surface epithelium of the bronchus, progressing from squamous metaplasia to carcinoma in situ and on to invasive cancer.

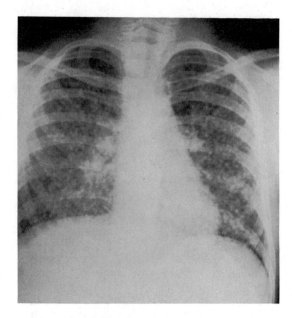

Fig. 30-8. Histoplasmosis. Innumerable tiny calcific nodules scattered diffusely throughout both lungs.

Histologically, lung carcinoma is classified as squamous (epidermoid) cell carcinoma, adenocarcinoma, alveolar carcinoma, and undifferentiated carcinoma.

Squamous (epidermoid) cell carcinoma is slow growing, involves lymph nodes by direct extension, and tends to be central (toward the hilum) in origin.

Adenocarcinoma is more common in young women than in men, but in women it is still less common than epidermoid carcinoma. It tends to be peripheral in location and spreads rapidly by vascular and lymph node involvement.

Alveolar carcinoma (bronchial carcinoma, pulmonary adenomatosis, bronchoalveolar carcinoma) occurs diffusely or as an area of consolidation. It spread endobronchially through the lung. A multicentric origin is suspected but not definitely established. Histologically the picture is one of well-differentiated, full columnar mucosa. It is usually asymptomatic until it becomes diffuse.

Undifferentiated carcinoma consists of small cells (oat cells, polygonal cells) or large cells. Oat cell carcinoma begins in the main bronchi but rapidly involves the hilar lymph nodes to form a collar of neoplastic tissue around the bronchus. Early metastasis is common, and the prognosis is poor.

Symptoms. The symptoms of bronchial carcinoma are cough, weight loss, recurrent or unresolving pneumonia, hemoptysis, chest pain, weakness, fever, and wheezing. Extrapulmonary manifestations are clubbing (usually seen in epidermoid carcinoma), Cushing's syndrome (undifferentiated neoplasm), hypercalcemia, carcinomatous neuropathy, phlebitis, osteoarthropathy, and connective tissue disorders.

Diagnosis. Lung carcinoma presents many faces roentgenographically: hilar mass (Fig. 30-9), atelectasis, single nodule (Fig. 30-10), abscess (Fig. 30-5), pleural effusion, and parenchymal infiltrate.

The big three in the diagnosis are chest roentgenograms, bronchoscopy and biopsy (positive in only 20% to 30% of cases), and sputum cytology. Prescalene lymph node biopsy is helpful if the nodes are enlarged. Additional diagnostic measures that are useful in selected cases are mediastinoscopy, mediastinal biopsy, intraosseous azygography, pulmonary angiography, needle biopsy, thoracentesis, and bronchography. The biggest advance in diagnosis in recent years has been the bronchial brush biopsy. In this technique undiagnosed peripheral lesions can be identified histologically in a much greater number of patients. We have been able to make the diagnosis by the brushing method in 70% of those patients in whom the standard methods have failed.

The treatment is surgical extirpation (segmental resection, lobectomy, or pneumonectomy). Preoperative irradiation is helpful in treating apical thoracic tumors (Pancoast's disease), but its place in the treatment of cancer elsewhere in the lung has not been clearly established. Prognosis is poor, with those who survive 5 years ranging from 5% to 20%.

Sarcoma

Lymphosarcoma may originate in the lung without involvement of lymph nodes in other areas of the body. Primary thoracic lymphosarcoma is rare but has a slow rate of growth, making it a suitable lesion for surgical excision. X-ray therapy is also frequently employed. Roentgenographic examination of the chest reveals an area of consolidation around a patent bronchus, giving an air-bronchogram effect.

Primary sarcomas arising in the lung parenchyma are rare. They occur in young patients as solitary lesions, large masses, or atelectasis. A radiolucent meniscus is sometimes seen over the mass on the chest film. Few symptoms occur unless atelectasis is produced by bronchial obstruction. Leiomyosarcoma has the best prognosis, rhabdomyosarcoma has the worst, and angiosarcomas with spindle cell sarcoma are intermediate.

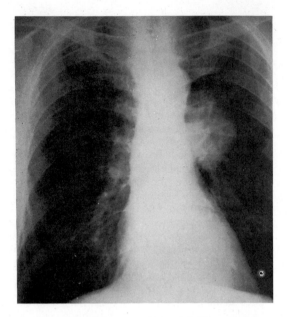

Fig. 30-9. Carcinoma of lung; left hilar mass.

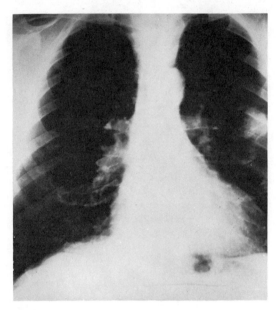

Fig. 30-10. Carcinoma of lung; nodule in left midlung field.

Bronchial adenoma

Two types of bronchial adenoma occur, the carcinoid and the cylindromatous. They account for about 5% of all pulmonary neoplasms. These two types are morphologically and histologically different but are usually separated from carcinoma (Table 30-3).

Bronchoscopy is diagnostic in 90% of patients with bronchial adenoma, but bronchoscopic removal should never be attempted. Bronchotomy with local excision may be used in some of the smaller lesions, but if any doubt remains as to the completeness of removal, appropriate excision (lobectomy, pneumonectomy) is required.

Hamartoma

Hamartoma is a developmental error that produces an abnormal arrangement and mixture of normal tissue and is the most common benign tumor of the lung. It must be considered in the differential diagnosis of solitary lesions in the lung. Generally this is not difficult because of the extreme peripheral location of the hamartoma, increased radiodensity, and characteristic eccentric, lobular, or "popcorn" type of calcification. Hamartomas of the lung contain cartilage, fibrous connective tissue, cubical or columnar epithelium, fat, and smooth muscle. They are not encapsulated but readily shell out. If their characteristic pattern of

calcification is not present (which is quite often), they must be distinguished from other peripheral lesions by thoracotomy.

Other benign tumors of the lung are mesothelioma, pseudotumors, lipoma, leiomyoma, hemangioma, mixed tumors, intrapulmonary teratomas, and thymomas.

Tumors of the trachea are rare. The most common is the squamous cell carcinoma of the distal trachea. Cylindromas are next most common but usually occur in the upper third. Reconstruction of the trachea after partial excision is generally unsatisfactory, and direct suture approximation must be done. The prognosis for carcinoma of the trachea is very poor, but the prognosis is very good for cylindroma.

Metastatic lung cancers

After the liver, the lungs are the most common site of visceral metastases of cancer. All the circulating blood must pass through the pulmonary capillary bed on each circuit, as lymph does after it enters the venous system at the jugular-subclavian confluence in the root of the neck. Thus tumor emboli from neoplasms that spread either through the venous or lymphatic systems ultimately pass into the rich lung capillary bed. If conditions (which we do not understand) are right, the tumor emboli filter out and begin growing as pulmonary

Table 30-3. Types of bronchial adenoma

	Carcinoid	*Cylindroma*
Location	Proximal bronchus	Primary bronchi and trachea
Comparative incidence	85%	15%
Histological features	Squamous metaplasia, small uniform cell with acidophilic neoplasm; mitosis and argentaffin granules rare	Cells less uniform, smaller, occasionally oncocytic
Lymph node metastasis	Uncommon	Twice as common (30%), also distant metastases more common
Bronchoscopic appearance	Smooth, rounded protrusion into lumen, mucosa intact, bleeds freely	Extends along the bronchus wall; paler and firmer
Invasiveness	Local iceberg effect common: small intraluminal component with rather large endobronchial or extrabronchial component	Recurrence rate seven times that of carcinoid
Symptoms	Obstruction, infection, bleeding, wheezing	Same

metastases. Undoubtedly, many more tumor emboli die, or remain dormant in, or pass on through the pulmonary capillary system, then lodge there and grow as metastases.

Usually, lung metastases produce multiple, rounded, discrete nodules in the periphery of both lungs, which gradually enlarge in size. Plain chest roentgenograms are generally diagnostic. Carcinomas can secondarily metastasize to hilar lymph nodes, but sarcomas do not. Pulmonary complaints are often nonspecific and include vague chest discomfort, cough, breathlessness, and pulmonary osteoarthropathy, tending to mimic symptoms of primary lung cancer. Rarely, biopsy is necessary to distinguish metastatic from primary cancer of the lung.

Treatment of metastatic lung cancer is generally palliative (chemotherapy, x-ray therapy) if the patient's general condition is good enough to justify any treatment at all. Surgical resection of cancer that is metastatic to lung is restricted to the occasional patient who has (1) no recurrence of the primary cancer, (2) no metastases elsewhere, and (3) lung metastases confined to one area, making surgical resection of that area possible.

The slower the doubling time of the tumor, the better the prognosis. Disease-free interval, bilateralism or location of the tumor, and multiplicity of lesions are less important in survival than the nature of the primary. Melanoma as a primary tumor carries a much worse prognosis than osteogenic sarcoma in this setting.

Resection of metastases is mainly carried out to determine the nature of the lesion, obtain tumor markers, establish the presence of the disease to determine whether adjuvant therapy should be continued, and to provide tumor for in vitro sensitivity studies.

Pulmonary embolism

Pulmonary embolic disease is a major problem. Intriguing new methods of diagnosis and treatment have been developed, but the clinical diagnosis is often difficult to make, and the efficacy of treatment is difficult to judge.

The true incidence of this disease is unknown. Pulmonary emboli are much more commonly found at autopsy than are diagnosed clinically. This dichotomy exists because of the subtle and variable clinical manifestations of pulmonary emboli. This variability occurs because of the following:

1. *Size of the occluding thrombus:* Small emboli that do not involve the visceral pleura frequently produce no symptoms because of the enormous reserve of the pulmonary vascular bed and because of natural mechanisms of clot lysis that are present in the lungs.

2. *Extent of the occlusion:* A single massive embolus produces the catastrophic picture characteristic of pulmonary embolism, but repeated small emboli produce a picture of respiratory insufficiency of obscure cause.

3. *Infarction:* Pulmonary emboli need not produce lung infarction. Infarction depends on other factors, such as collateral bronchial artery supply, infection, and the degree of ventilation of the involved segment.

4. *Condition of the lung:* Other diseases can

influence the symptoms greatly—if congestive heart failure exists or the pulmonary vascular bed has been reduced by previous emboli, a small embolus may produce severe effects.

Predisposing factors. Pulmonary emboli most commonly arise as thrombi within veins of the legs and pelvis that become detached and travel through the vena cava and right side of the heart to become lodged in the narrow pulmonary artery branches. Many patients with pulmonary emboli have no history of previous venous disease or evidence of thrombophlebitis on examination. Certain patients are predisposed to peripheral vein thrombosis: patients *immobilized* for long periods of time, the *elderly,* the *obese,* those with *malignancies, congestive heart failure,* previous emboli, and other serious medical disease (the incidence is three times higher in medical than in surgical patients). Prevention of peripheral thrombophlebitis and phlebothrombosis will obviate the problem of pulmonary emboli. (See Chapter 33.)

Diagnosis. Massive pulmonary emboli produce a catastrophic picture of collapse, shock, cyanosis, extreme dyspnea, restlessness, and chest pain followed by cough and blood-tinged sputum. The time from onset to death may be minutes to days. Small emboli produce only minimal symptoms of pleuritis, pain, and hemoptysis, and in many instances no symptoms at all. Nonspecific effects are low-grade fever, leukocytosis, and elevation in the serum lactic dehydrogenase. Signs of lower extremity thrombophlebitis are helpful, but inconstant.

Dyspnea and *tachypnea* are seen with pulmonary emboli, and the lungs demonstrate a *loss of compliance.* The second cardiac sound is exaggerated, and the *electrocardiogram* shows signs of right ventricular strain or bundle branch block. Roentgenographic examination of the chest often shows a prominent *pulmonary artery shadow.* Hypoxemia is mild in minor episodes of embolization but is increased with activity. Major emboli produce *cyanosis* and *pulmonary edema.* In either case oxygen does not alleviate the hypoxemia. *Arterial CO_2 tensions* are higher than expected because increased hypercapnia from the poorly perfused lung (dead space) offsets the hypocapnic effect of tachypnea.

Lung scanning and pulmonary angiography are sophisticated studies that have been developed recently to aid in diagnosing pulmonary embolus. The lungs are scanned after infusion of macromolecular particles of ^{131}I-tagged serum albumin; poor uptake of ^{131}I is seen in areas of the lung that are perfused by vessels plugged with emboli. This method is still in developmental stages. Pulmonary angiography allows roentgenographic visualization of the pulmonary artery tree, outlining clearly which branches are occluded by clot, and is the most reliable diagnostic test of pulmonary embolism.

Treatment. Treatment of pulmonary emboli consists of rest, oxygen, allaying of anxiety, and anticoagulation. Vena caval ligation is required with repeated episodes of embolization. When to perform pulmonary embolectomy is an agonizing decision, since the operative mortality is 50% to 60%. Complicating the problem is the fact that even massive emboli may resolve spontaneously. In several instances patients have been operated on only to find that the diagnosis was incorrect. The procedure should be used when all else fails in a deteriorating patient in whom the diagnosis has been definitely established.

Intravenous heparin is the most reliable anticoagulant drug for treating pulmonary embolus. It possesses the distinct advantage of rapid onset, short period of activity (6 to 8 hours) to allow good control, with anti-inflammatory and some fibrinolytic activity, and has a specific antidote (protamine sulfate). Initial dosage is 10,000 units every 8 hours, with subsequent size and frequency of administration depending on the response to treatment as reflected by coagulation times, which should be two to three times the patient's control levels. Fibrinolytic drugs (streptokinase and urokinase), which effectively lyse clot already present, currently are being evaluated and may well be added to treatment in the near future.

Fat pulmonary embolism

Fat embolism is a most common and important cause of complication and death after fracture. It affects many organs, the most important being the lung, brain, and kidneys, but the lung is such a good filter that in 75% of autopsied cases fat embolism can be found only there. The heart is secondarily involved when the fat emboli elevate pulmonary resistance to produce cardiac dilatation, tachycardia, hypotension, and increased central venous pressure. The physician may ascribe shock entirely to the injury, forgetting that fat embolism may be the basic cause. When shock coexists, a smaller fat pulmonary embolus produces serious consequences earlier, with a higher death rate.

The patient develops tachypnea, dyspnea, and cyanosis. There may be a lag of 24 to 48 hours between injury and the clinical appearance of symptoms, with this "latent" period representing the time taken for the lung to filter out enough fat to be symptomatic. Confusion, disorientation, acute psychosis progressing to coma, and stupor may exist. Their significance must be evaluated in light of whether the patient has suffered a head injury or was intoxicated.

Other variable clinical signs are bubbling rales; white, fluffy, patchy retinal exudates; and petechial hemorrhages on the neck, shoulders, chest, soft palate, and conjunctiva but rarely over the abdomen.

The chest x-ray examination shows diffuse, small, nodular infiltrates, enlarged pulmonary arteries, and perhaps cardiomegaly. In the absence of bleeding, a sharp drop in the hemoglobin is also suggestive. In the first few days after injury fat droplets appear in the urine. Sputum examination for fat is of no value. Later an elevated serum lipase is of diagnostic and prognostic (the higher, the better) value.

Treatment. Treatment consists of respiratory support, immobilization of the fracture, heparin (increases lipase activity), dextran, and steroids.

Spontaneous pneumothorax

Acute collapse of the lung caused by the sudden escape of air from the lung into the pleural space is known as spontaneous pneumothorax (Fig. 30-11). It occurs typically in young robust males about three times more frequently than in females and is caused by rupture of a subpleural bleb (Fig. 30-12). The pneumothorax occasionally coincides with a period of physical exertion, but generally it develops when the patient is engaged in routine activities. Pain, commonly referred to the shoulder, can be excruciating and is associated with some degree of dyspnea. Other conditions occasionally associated with spontaneous pneumothorax are tuber-

culosis, emphysema, chronic bronchitis, giant bullae, and obstructive emphysema.

In infants and children, tension pneumothorax is caused more often by staphylococcal pneumonia than by rupture of true congenital blebs. Sometimes no predisposing lung disease is identified. Spontaneous pneumothorax occurs often in the newborn period; 15% of newborns have asymp-

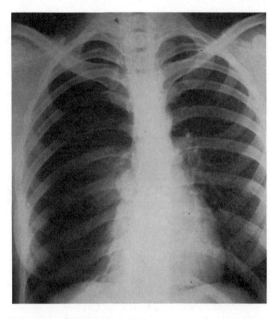

Fig. 30-11. Spontaneous right pneumothorax; lung about 60% collapsed by pleural air.

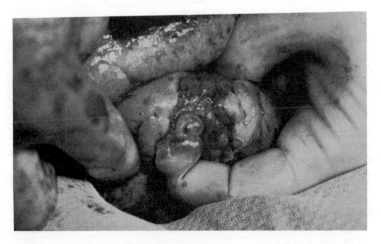

Fig. 30-12. Subpleural bleb, rupture of which produces spontaneous pneumothorax.

tomatic pneumothorax. In symptomatic neonates pneumothorax is frequently accompanied by pneumomediastinum and is usually related to the aspiration of blood, meconium, or squamous debris during delivery, with resulting obstruction in the bronchial tree. The pneumothorax occurs after the increased respiratory effort of these patients and the frequent resuscitative measures they receive. The condition may be missed if only an anteroposterior chest roentgenogram is taken, but there is almost 100% accuracy of diagnosis with a cross-table lateral roentgenogram. Persistence or recurrence of pneumothorax in infants and children is suggestive of another abnormality (e.g., cystic fibrosis or multiple lung cysts).

Physical examination reveals decreased vocal and tactile fremitus, tympany to percussion, tracheal shift to the opposite side, and perhaps cyano-sis. Occasionally tearing of a vascular adhesion leads to serious intrapleural bleeding. Roentgenographic examination of the chest is diagnostic.

Treatment. *Bed rest* and *anterior thoracentesis* are usually tried in lesser degrees of collapse during the first or perhaps the second episode.

Intercostal drainage with a chest tube (Fig. 30-2) inserted in the second intercostal space parasternally is the preferred treatment. The tube is connected to underwater-seal drainage, allowing the egress of air and encouraging reexpansion of the lung by restoration of negative intrapleural pressure. Pleural adhesions seal the leak.

Thoracotomy is employed after multiple recurrences, when blebs or bullae are seen on the chest film, and for chronic states of collapse. The blebs are oversewed or excised, and the parietal pleura is abraded to stimulate the formation of adhesions

Table 30-4. Mediastinitis

Method of contamination	Symptoms and signs	Etiology	Roentgenographic findings	Treatment
Acute				
1. Direct penetrating trauma 2. Hematogenous, or spread from thoracic viscera (heart, lungs, esophagus, or from chest wall) 3. From the neck along fascial planes 4. Direct extension from the lungs or pleura	High fever, pain under the sternum; highly toxic state; dysphagia; hacking cough; mediastinal and subcutaneous emphysema; edema of chest wall; prominence of veins on chest wall	1. 60% caused by ruptured esoph-agus (carcinoma, from endo-scopy) 2. Spread by blood or lymphatic drainage from thoracic viscera 3. Spread from neck along the vis-ceral fascial planes from in-fection in neck 4. Extension from empyema or lung abscess	Widening of medias-tinum, displace-ment of trachea; interstitial emphy-sema; fluid level of abscess; extrava-sation of swal-lowed contrast material	Drainage is most im-portant; antibiot-ics are only a help-ful adjunct
Chronic Same as acute	Usually insidious in onset; weakness; weight loss; chronic cough; anemia; chest pain; low-grade fever; symptoms of superior vena caval obstruction; swelling of face and neck; esoph-ageal obstruc-tion; occasionally esophagobronchial fistula with lithop-tysis	A granulomatous in-fection, often not specifically identi-fied; histoplasmo-sis is the most common cause, tu-berculosis only oc-casionally in the United States	Paratracheal mass, subcarinal or paresophageal; 50% not calcified, one third heavily calcified	Largely nonsurgical; treatment for spe-cific infection if found (tuberculo-sis, actinomyco-sis, histoplasmo-sis); mediastinal granulomas should be removed if heavily calcified

between the parietal and visceral pleura. Parietal pleurectomy accomplishes a similar end. Chemical irritants are seldom employed to produce pleural abrasion.

MEDIASTINUM
Inflammation

Mediastinitis is uncommon. Once uniformly fatal, it can now (in most cases) be treated successfully (Table 30-4).

Mediastinal neoplasms

Mediastinal tumors arise from (1) the mediastinum proper, (2) adjacent structures, and (3) outside the thoracic cavity. In general, they produce symptoms by compression or interference with function of mediastinal organs, or by the development of infection or malignant change in the tumor itself.

Extraneous lesions *simulating* primary mediastinal neoplasms are the following:

1. *Thyroid:* extension of a cervical goiter through the thoracic inlet, or truly aberrant thyroid tissue (very rare)
2. *Chest wall neoplasms:* they may have no palpable external component: chondroma, chondrosarcoma, chordoma, Ewing's sarcoma
3. Congenital or acquired *herniations* through the *diaphragm*
4. *Aneurysms* of the great vessels
5. Mediastinal *meningoceles:* 70% have stigmas of neurofibromatosis
6. *Achalasia* of the esophagus

Neurogenic tumors make up about 30% of all mediastinal tumors, teratomas about 15%, cysts 15%, thymomas 10%, goiter 10%, and all others 20%; about 15% are malignant. Each of the different types of mediastinal tumor tends to occur in a characteristic part of the mediastinum, making an important clue to diagnosis (Fig. 30-13).

Anterior mediastinum

Intrathoracic goiters are almost always extensions of cervical goiters. The trachea is displaced and the neck veins are prominent because of compression, which accounts for symptoms of dyspnea, stridor, dysphagia, and facial swelling. Plain roentgenograms show a lobulated shadow high in the anterior mediastinum with displacement of the trachea, and barium swallow proves the mass moves with deglutition; failure of the mass to move with deglutition indicates either that the goiter may be malignant or that some other diagnosis must be entertained. Removal is recommended, generally with cervical thyroidectomy.

Thymomas are composed of the normal cellular elements of the thymus, except usually lacking Hassall's corpuscles. Initially encapsulated, they later invade locally as low-grade malignancies,

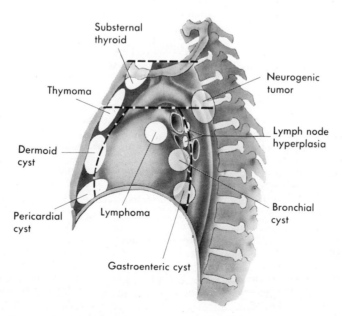

Fig. 30-13. Diagram of mediastinum, indicating typical location of different mediastinal tumors.

especially when accompanied by *myasthenia gravis*. The degree of malignancy depends on its behavior (i.e., gross findings) and not on histological appearance. Calcification is sometimes seen, but this is not a sign of benignity. They are slow growing, with as long as 10 years elapsing with little enlargement seen. Thymomas often are totally asymptomatic, but when large, they produce pain, venous obstruction, stridor, cough, and dyspnea. Surgical excision is recommended, with postoperative irradiation if the thymoma is malignant clinically.

The relationship of the thymus to myasthenia gravis has long been recognized: about 85% of patients with myasthenia have a normal thymus, and about 50% of thymomas are associated with myasthenia. The role of thymectomy for myasthenia gravis is still unsettled because results are variable. In most instances anticipated benefits outweigh the operative risk. The best results of thymectomy for myasthenia are obtained in women with symptoms of short duration. Thymomas have been reported to occur with red blood cell aplasia, Cushing's syndrome, megaesophagus, and hypogammaglobulinemia. Steroids may be helpful in patients who are not benefited by thymectomy or anticholinesterase drugs.

Dermoids (benign teratomas) histologically contain only tissue of ectodermal origin. They are usually large and unilocular and are found in middle-aged patients.

True *teratomas* contain elements of all three germ layers, commonly with hemorrhagic or polycystic areas; 70% ultimately become malignant. The usual symptoms of mediastinal teratoma are cough, pain, and dyspnea, but they may rupture into the pleura, pericardium, and blood vessels. Expectoration of hair is pathognomonic; hemorrhage may be severe. Roentgenographic examination is diagnostic if cartilage, bone, or teeth are seen in a tumor high in the anterior mediastinum. The preferred treatment is surgical removal.

Pericardial cysts are fairly common, arising from a pinched-off portion of the pleuroperitoneal membrane, which occurs during the formation of the diaphragm. They are always anterior (usually on the right side) and close to the cardiophrenic angle. They contain fluid similar to pericardial fluid, prompting the descriptive term "springwater" cysts. They sometimes have a pedicle attached to the pericardium. Pericardial cysts are always benign and usually are asymptomatic.

Posterior mediastinum

Neurogenic tumors comprise over 90% of posterior mediastinal tumors. The main histological types are the ganglioneuroma, neurofibroma, neurilemoma, and the highly malignant neuroblastoma. Neurofibromas and neurilemomas are frequently associated with intercostal nerves, ganglioneuromas with the sympathetic chain. Neurofibromas are least common, and ganglioneuromas are quite common. Immature elements indicate a potentially malignant ganglioneuroma. In some instances the syndromes of diarrhea and abdominal distension or of hypertension, flushing, and sweating occur with ganglioneuroma. Urinary levels of vanillylmandelic acid may also be elevated.

Neurogenic mediastinal tumors are often asymptomatic, discovered on incidental roentgenographic examination of the chest as a "cannonball" lesion; spreading of the involved intercostal space and rib erosion are highly suggestive of neurogenic tumor. Occasionally a tumor will proceed dumbbell fashion through an intervertebral foramen to cause paraplegia. Mediastinal neurofibromas are associated with general neurofibromatosis. Neuroblastomas occur in children high in the posterior mediastinum and are highly malignant; calcific stippling characteristically is seen on roentgenographic examination. Treatment is surgical removal followed by irradiation.

In general, treatment for mediastinal tumors of neurogenic origin is thoracotomy and excision. Those tumors with intraspinal projections require preliminary laminectomy.

Enterogenous cysts are generally seen lying along the right side of the esophagus in infants and young children, probably because of displacement by the aorta. They often are associated with abnormally formed vertebral bodies, to which they may attach, and occasionally extend through the diaphragm juxtaposed to stomach or intestine. Enterogenous cysts have walls of smooth muscle with an inner lining of mucosa. If the mucosa actively secretes, expansion and perforation may occur, but these cysts are asymptomatic if the lining is inactive. Large cysts cause obstructive symptoms (cough, dyspnea). Total surgical removal is the recommended treatment.

Middle mediastinum

The *lymphoma* family of mediastinal tumors includes leukemia, Hodgkin's disease, and lymphosarcoma, the latter accounting for 60% of the total. The disease occurs characteristically in males in the fourth and fifth decades of life. Hepatosplenomegaly, lymphadenopathy, and fever are well-known systemic manifestations of lymphoma. Lymphosarcoma and Hodgkin's disease occasionally are localized to the mediastinum and may then be cured by excision, irradiation, or a combination of the two.

Bronchogenic cysts sometimes occur in the mid-mediastinum; they have been discussed in the section on congenital malformations of the lungs.

CHEST WALL
Congenital malformations of the chest wall
Pectus excavatum

The most common anterior chest wall deformity is pectus excavatum (Fig. 30-14). Although opinions differ as to cause, it is most likely caused by a congenitally foreshortened central tendon of the diaphragm, sometimes associated with anomalous attachments to the lower ribs anteriorly. Mechanical factors are mainly responsible for the progression of the deformity during growth of the thoracic cage. The point of fixation at the lower end of the sternum prevents proper respiratory excursion by maintaining the thoracic cage in a position of semiexpiration. As the lower portion of the rib cage and cartilages becomes fixed, the rib cage is forced to expand in a lateral direction. The mediastinal structures are usually displaced to the left as the midline anteroposterior dimension of the thorax foreshortens. Although initially symmetrical, growth produces asymmetry during childhood. It occurs three times oftener in males than in females.

Mild, nonprogressive deformities require no treatment. Operative correction is indicated for cosmetic and psychological reasons or if the deformity progresses in early childhood (Fig. 30-15). In adolescents and adults, physiological changes (detected by pulmonary function studies and cardiac catheterization) are occasionally cogent indications for repair.

The operative technique consists in "turning over" the involved area of sternum after severance of all attachments, molding the segment by appropriate osteotomies, and securing it in its reversed position.

Pectus carinatum

The rare deformity pectus carinatum produces anterior displacement and bulging of the sternum. It seems to be a counterpart of pectus excavatum, with a fixation point at the lower end of the anteriorly tilted sternum and secondary changes in the rib cartilages.

Neoplasms of the chest wall
Chondroma

Chondromas occur as painless swellings anteriorly near the costochondral junction, or in the sternum. They are benign and cause no symptoms. Roentgenographic examination reveals bony expansion without bony destruction and occasionally calcification.

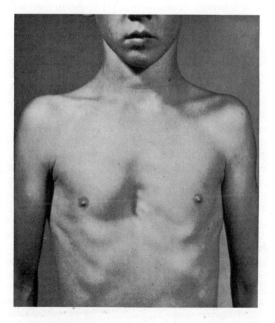

Fig. 30-14. Pectus excavatum, preoperative.

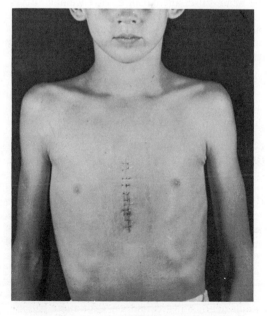

Fig. 30-15. Pectus excavatum, postoperative.

Chondrosarcoma

Chondrosarcomas, on the contrary, occur in the posterior portion of the bony thorax and may involve vertebra and transverse processes. With inward growth they resemble mediastinal tumors on chest roentgenographs. They are usually hard, locally painful external swellings that enlarge slowly and progressively invade surrounding structures. Chondrosarcomas have a great propensity to recur locally after excision, and metastases appear after several recurrences. The differential diagnosis includes osteomyelitis of the ribs, bony tuberculosis, and nonunited rib fracture. Total early excision is curative.

Myeloma

Solitary myelomas occur in thoracic vertebrae. They tend to take a benign course, though their osteolytic appearance on roentgenographic examination always produces concern. The chief symptom is pain.

The ribs are the most common site of solitary *fibrous dysplasia* of bone. They are multilocular and sometimes cystic. A typical "soap-bubble" pattern is seen on the roentgenograph. If several ribs are involved, biopsy is required to distinguish fibrous dysplasia from neoplasm.

Eosinophilic granuloma

Eosinophilic granuloma is another benign destructive process of the ribs, most common in children and young adults. The typical history is the acute onset of a painful rib swelling. Fever, fracture, and a history of trauma may confuse the picture. The roentgenographic appearance is that of a rounded osteolytic lesion. Biopsy is generally needed to rule out malignancy.

Sarcoma

Sarcomas of the chest wall require wide excision and reconstruction of the chest wall with a prosthetic material, such as Marlex mesh.

Chest wall and lung injuries
Chest trauma

Next to cardiovascular disease and cancer, trauma is the most common cause of death in the United States. Urban violence and automobile accidents are in large measure responsible for this. Trauma to the chest is the chief cause of 25% of deaths from auto accidents, and another 50% of patients who die have significant chest trauma.

Multiple rib fractures, often seen after steering-wheel injuries (Fig. 30-16), produce an unstable segment of the chest wall that on inspiration moves paradoxically inward and on expiration balloons outward (flail chest). The inspiratory concavity in

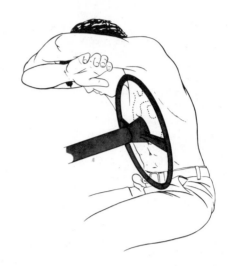

Fig. 30-16. Chest trauma. Chest wall impact with steering wheel may fracture multiple ribs and sternum, resulting in paradoxical motion of chest wall (flail chest). Contusion of underlying heart and lungs causes reduced cardiac output and arterial hypoxemia.

the chest wall compresses the underlying lung, shifts the mediastinum to the opposite side, impairs venous return to the heart, and limits expansion of the good lung. Tachypnea increases the movement of the chest wall (mediastinal flutter) to aggravate these changes. Contusion of the underlying lung (traumatic wet lung), however, is the most important factor because of associated severe arterial hypoxia. Interstitial and intra-alveolar hemorrhage accompanying contusive injury to the lung results in pronounced ventilation/perfusion abnormalities such that deoxygenated blood passes through the lung without proper gas exchange (physiological shunt). Admixture of desaturated blood to pulmonary venous return produces arterial hypoxemia. In addition, blood and debris entering the airway from the area of injury may be aspirated to uninvolved areas of the lung to compound the problem. Splinting of the cough mechanism from pain and chest wall instability prevents adequate clearing of the airway.

Traumatic asphyxia is the term applied to a striking syndrome of petechiae and edema of the face, neck, and upper extremities that occurs after sudden, severe compression of the chest. It is caused by forceful retrograde pulsion into the superior vena cava of blood in the heart reservoir on the right side, producing disruption of small blood vessels and extravasation of blood into the tissues drained by this system.

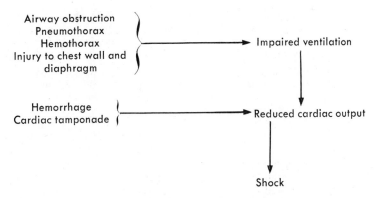

Fig. 30-17. Physiological effects of penetrating thoracic trauma. (After Creech, O., and Pearce, C.W.: Am. J. Surg. **105:**496, 1963.)

The physiological derangements accompanying traumatic wet lung and flail chest are best treated by clearing and maintaining an open airway and positive pressure ventilation with a mechanical respirator. The respirator assures adequate alveolar ventilation and also stabilizes the chest wall.

Wounds of the chest caused by penetration of a sharp object or missile may cause pneumothorax or hemothorax. Blood or air entering the pleural space causes collapse of the lung because of compression. If the air or blood accumulates rapidly, the mediastinum is shifted toward the uninvolved side so that the opposite lung is compressed (tension pneumothorax or hemothorax). The combined effects of these changes are decreased ventilation, increased pulmonary vascular resistance, and reduced venous return to the heart; cardiac output falls, and circulatory shock results.

When there is loss of continuity of the chest wall, there is a similar chain of events as just described except that outside air enters the pleural space through the "sucking wound."

The physiological effects of penetrating thoracic trauma are summarized in Fig. 30-17. Each of these factors must be evaluated and corrected, with maintenance of the airway and restoration of blood volume taking the first and second priority.

Pneumothorax of 20% or less of the volume of the pleural space is often treated expectantly, but if larger than this or if under tension, it requires tube thoracostomy in the second interspace anteriorly and underwater-seal drainage (Fig. 30-2). If blood is present in the pleural space, it is removed by repeated thoracenteses (Fig. 30-1) or by closed chest tube drainage instituted low in the chest (Fig. 30-2). The patient is kept in a semiupright position to facilitate drainage. Persistent bleeding demands

thoracostomy to stop the bleeding, expand the lung, and obliterate the pleural space. Failure to remove blood may necessitate decortication later on.

Rupture of a major airway (trachea, larynx, or bronchus)

Most of these injuries are produced by blunt trauma that tears the large airway structures, producing severe air leaks. Dyspnea, cough, hemoptysis, tension pneumothorax, and subcutaneous emphysema are promptly produced, which immediately place the patient in grave jeopardy. Bronchoscopy often confirms the diagnosis. Early thoracostomy and repair are most desirable, since bronchial stenosis, infection, and a destroyed lung may otherwise result. Late repair occasionally improves lung function but does not restore the respiratory tree to normal. Occasionally the esophagus will also be injured; an esophagobronchial fistula may result.

Cardiac trauma

Cardiac trauma may be classified into penetrating and nonpenetrating injuries. The penetrating types involve injury to the heart by a sharp object or missile. If the patient survives the immediate penetrating injury to the heart, he often quickly develops cardiac tamponade. A relatively small amount of blood within the closed pericardial space is sufficient to interfere with cardiac filling, thereby reducing cardiac output. The patient is restless and has air hunger. Heart tones are distant, and there may be a pericardial friction rub; blood pressure is reduced, and pulse pressure is narrow. Venous pressure is elevated and neck veins are distended. Chest films show a normal-sized heart, and the electrocardiogram is helpful in diagnosis only when there is coronary artery injury.

Immediate treatment is pericardiocentesis. A needle is passed into the pericardial space (with electrocardiographic monitoring) to remove accumulated blood. A large-bore needle is inserted alongside the sternum at the left sternocostal angle and directed cephalad and posteriorly toward the heart at a 45-degree angle to the sternum. As the needle passes through the chest wall to the pericardial sac, the electrocardiogram is similar to lead V_2. If the needle contacts the myocardium, a current of injury similar to multiple premature ventricular contractions will be noted on the electrocardiogram. The needle is then withdrawn slightly, and the contents of the pericardial sac are aspirated. Blood extracted from the pericardium does not clot, because clotting has already occurred within the pericardium; the substance that is removed is serum and cells, and the fibrin clot is left behind. If blood pressure improves and central venous pressure falls after pericardiocentesis, the patient may be safely observed and closely monitored. Should signs of cardiac tamponade return, immediate operation is indicated to remove blood from the pericardial sac and repair the myocardial injury.

Nonpenetrating injury of the myocardium caused by blunt trauma to the chest wall is probably more frequent than clinically recognized. Steering-wheel injury in an automobile accident (Fig. 30-16) and other forms of trauma to the anterior chest wall can produce this injury. The physiological consequences of this injury are cardiac arrhythmia and reduced cardiac output, which are directly related to amount of contused myocardium. Despite these two complications, it is remarkable that patients often survive tremendous trauma to the myocardium. The diagnosis of cardiac contusion is difficult because of a low index of suspicion of the injury and a nonspecific electrocardiographic and serum enzyme pattern. New radioisotope techniques involving technetium-labeled phosphate complexes are useful in demonstrating injured myocardium. Treatment of this condition is similar to treatment of myocardial infarction and involves rhythm monitoring and aggressive treatment of cardiac arrhythmia, inotropic agents to support cardiac output, and bed rest while the myocardium heals.

Aortic injuries

Of patients with thoracic aortic injuries, 85% die at the time of the injury. The most common site of rupture is in the proximal descending aorta just beyond the origin of the left subclavian artery, and the next most common is in the ascending aorta just above the aortic valve. The tears are usually transverse and may involve the entire circumference, with the aorta being held together by thin adventitia in those who survive. The diagnosis is frequently missed because it is not considered. Roentgenographic examination of the chest shows widening of the mediastinum, and angiography confirms the diagnosis. Other suggestive signs are cervical hematoma, tracheal deviation, hemothorax, asymmetry of radial pulses, and a paralyzed left vocal cord. Immediate repair should be carried out. In the ascending aorta, total cardiopulmonary bypass is required for repair, but a left-sided bypass (left atriofemoral bypass) suffices for injuries distal to the brachiocephalic vessels.

Ruptured diaphragm

Blunt trauma and crushing injuries are the usual cause of a ruptured diaphragm. Diaphragmatic rupture most commonly occurs on the left side adjacent to the esophageal hiatus, but injury to every part of the diaphragm has been described. The symptoms are not specific, and if there is no evidence of external trauma, the diagnosis can be missed. Progressive cardiorespiratory distress is seen as more and more viscera enter the chest to collapse the lung, push the mediastinal structures to the opposite side, and impede venous return to the heart and expansion of the good lung. Suggestive signs of ruptured diaphragm are bowel sounds heard in the chest and difficulty in passing a nasogastric tube. A chest film is extremely valuable in diagnosis, especially the lateral view, showing bowel loops within the chest. Patients in cardiorespiratory distress must be explored either through the chest or abdomen to allow reduction of the viscera and closure of the diaphragm laceration. Some patients with diaphragmatic rupture are asymptomatic, and the rent is repaired electively after other injuries are treated.

Esophageal lacerations and ruptures

Lacerations of the esophagus, usually caused by instrumentation or by penetrating objects, occur most frequently in the upper third. Any cervical wound penetrating the platysma should be explored. Within a few hours after injury, the rent may be repaired; otherwise drainage, prevention of pleural complications, and antibiotic therapy are required. Chemical injury followed by bacterial infection rapidly produces a life-threatening mediastinitis and empyema.

Injuries of the thoracic esophagus from blunt trauma are rare, and the trauma need not be severe to cause disruption. Penetrating esophageal injuries are accompanied frequently by injuries to the heart and great vessels. In all such cases repair of the injury should be carried out immediately, if possible.

Spontaneous rupture of the esophagus (Boerhaave's disease) occurs usually after large meals and strenuous vomiting. Occasionally it is seen after lifting, seizures, and childbirth. On several occasions we have seen it in newborns.

Perforations and lacerations of the esophagus usually cause dysphagia, vomiting, and subcutaneous emphysema. Movement and inspiration aggravate the pain. Air bubbles, an air fluid level, or widening of the mediastinum on roentgenographic examination are suggestive of esophageal injury. Pleural effusion (which is potentially an empyema) frequently accompanies esophageal trauma.

If recognized early, the rent should be repaired regardless of location except for small cervical perforations, which may be treated by drainage and antibiotic coverage.

Foreign bodies

Foreign bodies in the chest are not in themselves an indication for emergency removal. They are removed when (1) associated with a nearby infection, (2) very large, or (3) adjacent to the heart, aorta, or some other important structure.

ESOPHAGUS
Benign tumors of the esophagus

Benign tumors are uncommon and may arise from any layer of the esophagus. The majority are leiomyomas, originating in the muscle coats. On plain roentgenographs they appear as lobulated densities in the posterior mediastinum that on fluoroscopy move with swallowing. Esophagoscopy is often negative. These tumors are usually easily enucleated.

Tumors originating in the mucosa or submucosa project into the lumen and are pedunculated from peristaltic activity. Polyps, adenoma, fibroma, and lipoma are examples. They are more likely to produce dysphagia than the leiomyomas and also may ulcerate and bleed. Excision of the lesions without resection of the esophagus can usually be done.

Carcinoma of the esophagus

Carcinoma is the most important disease of the esophagus and represents about 5% of all gastrointestinal malignancies. About 90% are epidermoid carcinomas, and the remainder, adenocarcinomas. Therapy is usually only palliative because (1) the prime symptom, *dysphagia,* is delayed (at least a year's tumor growth precedes its onset), (2) most are poorly differentiated histologically (Broders' class III and IV), (3) the tumor extends submucosally both upward and downward, (4) absence of a serosal coat in the esophagus permits early mediastinal invasion, and (5) many of the patients are first seen after severe weight loss and debilitation.

Cancer of the esophagus is more common in men than in women (8:1). In men it occurs more commonly (80%) in the middle and lower thirds, and in women it tends to arise proximally. It spreads mainly by lymphatics.

Dysphagia is generally the first symptom, though unfortunately a very late one. On close questioning, one obtains a history of progressive difficulty in swallowing, first with solids, then with semisolids, and finally with liquids. Weight loss is often severe. Pain and hoarseness are grave signs.

The diagnosis of esophageal cancer is established by barium swallow (Fig. 30-18), esophagoscopy, and biopsy. The differential diagnosis includes those diseases in which dysphagia is also a prominent symptom: achalasia, peptic esophagitis, foreign body, and diverticulum.

Carcinoma of the esophagus is inoperable if there is also present (1) fistulation into the bronchial tree, (2) vocal cord paralysis, or (3) distant metastasis (liver, lungs, vertebrae, or cervical nodes). Bronchoscopy should always be done to rule out invasion of the bronchial tree.

Curative treatment is total extirpation of the

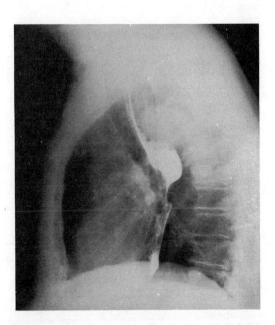

Fig. 30-18. Barium swallow showing carcinoma of middle third of esophagus producing abrupt narrowing of dye column.

tumor, which is rarely possible. About 50% of patients with cancer of the middle and lower third of the esophagus have metastases to the nodes along the left gastric artery, and removal of these nodes is a necessary part of a curative resection. Palliative treatment is directed at the relief of the esophageal obstruction, if possible. Gastrostomy rarely affords satisfactory palliation. Upper third lesions are usually best treated by irradiation, since the cure rate is extremely low after resection (which usually requires laryngectomy and complicated plastic reconstruction). Middle and lower third lesions are often resected for palliation, with restoration of continuity by esophagogastric anastomosis. Critically ill or debilitated patients are occasionally treated by the insertion of plastic tubes through the tumor and into the stomach, to allow the patient to swallow.

Treatment of esophageal carcinoma is mainly palliative. X-ray treatment is often chosen for its expediency. However, a high incidence of restenosis within a few months and of serious morbidity such as fistulation into the airway has prompted the resurgence of surgical methods to circumvent the near total dysphagia, which is the most distressing symptom to the patient. This can be accomplished with a low mortality by use of colon interposition, esophagogastrostomy or an isoperistaltic gastric tube.

Barrett's esophagus, anomalously columnar cell lined, is of unknown cause, with evidence being equally convincing for a congenital or an acquired origin. It occurs most often in men and is accompanied by weight loss, dysphagia, hiatal hernia, and esophagitis. Adenocarcinoma is prone to develop so that the physician's main responsibility in management is close surveillance.

Peptic esophagitis

Esophageal mucosa is very susceptible to injury from gastric juice. The source of acid-peptic irritation may be exogenous or endogenous. Endogenous peptic esophagitis is rare; it results from ectopic islands of gastric mucosa in the esophagus, generally toward either end. Esophagitis from reflux of acid gastric juice is far more common and is generally caused by a sliding hiatal hernia (Chapter 27). Rare additional causes of reflux peptic esophagitis are a congenitally short esophagus and operations that destroy the esophagogastric junction or its sphincteric mechanism.

The principal early symptoms of peptic esophagitis from sliding hiatal hernia are "heartburn" and regurgitation of bitter-tasting material, worse when the patient lies down. The regurgitated material may be bloody, and the stools will then contain gross or occult blood. Long-standing, recurrent peptic esophagitis leads to *stricture* by scar formation, at which time dysphagia and weight loss occur. Barium studies of the upper gastrointestinal tract and esophagoscopy are diagnostic.

Treatment should at first be conservative, consisting of rest, antacids, bland diet, abstinence from tobacco, spices, and alcohol, and avoiding the supine position after eating. Dilatation of a stricture by bougienage is helpful unless scar formation is dense. Surgical treatment should return the stomach to the abdominal cavity and restore the obliquity of the esophagogastric angle and greatly ameliorate the symptoms. A number of procedures have been proposed to treat advanced esophageal strictures: esophagogastrostomy (using the fundus), or resection with intestinal interposition. No uniformly acceptable solution to this problem has been found.

Achalasia

Achalasia is an intrinsic disorder of the esophagus characterized by failure of the lower esophageal sphincter mechanism to relax. The esophagus gradually hypertrophies, dilates, becomes tortuous, and loses effective peristalsis. In the early stages motility is normal or hyperactive, but later the esophagus "decompensates" to a saccular, atonic structure. Etiology is unknown; degeneration of Auerbach's plexus is seen on micro-

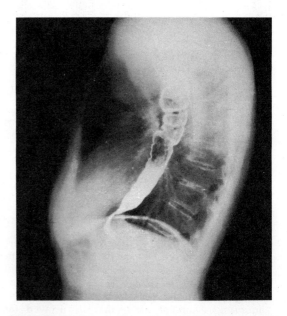

Fig. 30-19. Barium swallow of achalasia. Dilatation and some tortuosity of esophagus, narrowing of esophagogastric junction.

scopic study of the lower esophagus, but these changes could be secondary; 20% of patients with dysphagia from intrinsic esophageal disease have achalasia, and 10% of patients with achalasia have pulmonary complications.

The classical triad of symptoms of achalasia is dysphagia, regurgitation, and weight loss. The sex distribution is equal. The disease is found at the extremes of age, but the median age at operation is about 55 years. Barium swallow is diagnostic (Fig. 30-19), showing concentric or sigmoid dilatation of the esophagus with abrupt narrowing at its entrance into the stomach. Currently a "modified Heller" procedure is most widely used for both the concentric and the sigmoid types of achalasia, in which the constricting muscle at the esophagogastric junction is divided without the mucosa being opened. It gives satisfactory results in 85% of the cases.

Esophageal diverticula

The three most common locations for esophageal diverticula are (1) at the pharyngoesophageal junction (Zenker's diverticulum), (2) in the midthoracic esophagus adjacent to the lung hilum, and (3) in the epiphrenic esophagus just above the diaphragm. They differ enough in origin, symptoms, and treatment to justify individual discussion, though all are diagnosed by barium swallow.

The pharyngoesophageal or Zenker's diverticulum arises in the posterior midline of the esophagus just above the cricopharyngeus muscle, where the pharynx and esophagus join. At this point a triangular area of the inferior pharyngeal constrictor muscle is relatively devoid of muscular support (Killian's triangle), through which the mucosa herniates. Spasm of the cricopharyngeal muscle may be causally related. Collection and stagnation of food occur, elongating the sac generally to the left of the esophagus, with large diverticula descending into the mediastinum. Dysphagia, regurgitation, and aspiration are the chief symptoms, and the patient may be aware of a "gurgling" sound in his neck after drinking fluids. These diverticula should be excised if symptomatic or larger than 1.5 cm. Division of the cricopharyngeal muscle also is performed.

Thoracic diverticula are produced by traction on the esophagus by mediastinal tissue, usually inflammatory lymph nodes. The fundus of the diverticulum is higher than the ostium, so that pocketing of food is unlikely and symptoms are rare. Operation is required only in the unlikely instance of fistula formation with the airway.

Epiphrenic diverticula are associated with difficulty in emptying the esophagus at its lower end, with achalasia the most common predisposing cause. Impaction of food, ulceration, and infection with periesophagitis can result. Excision of the diverticulum and esophagomyotomy are required.

31
Cardiac Surgery

Donald B. Doty

Operations on the heart and use of cardiopulmonary bypass techniques have provided increased knowledge of the normal and abnormal function of the circulatory system.

It is the purpose of this chapter to provide a working knowledge of the facts peculiar to surgery of the heart, with the assumption that the reader will pursue textbooks of cardiology for details of etiology, pathology, diagnosis, and treatment of heart disease.

CARDIAC ANATOMY
Cardiac chambers

The business of the heart is to pump blood. In the heart there are two ventricles (pumping chambers) and two atria (filling chambers). The heart is divided by a septum so that chambers on the right side pump to the lungs and those on the left pump blood to all the rest of the body. The left ventricle, a conical chamber surrounded by a thick-walled muscle (Fig. 31-1), is the focal point of the circulation. As the ventricular muscle mass shortens, blood is compressed and ejected into the aorta and through the arterial system to the cells of the body.

The anatomical relations of the cardiac chambers have been confused by nomenclature and textbook illustrations. The right atrium and ventricle are not only to the right side anatomically, but are also *anterior* to the left atrium and ventricle, which occupy a position to the left and posterior. The dividing septa lie in an oblique plane. The pulmonary artery, which receives blood from the right ventricle, is actually located to the *left* of the aorta because of the complex embryological rotation of the heart.

Valves

The aortic and pulmonary valves have *semilunar* valve cups. The cuplike configuration of the sinus of Valsalva allows competence when the valve cusps are approximated during cardiac diastole. The atrioventricular (A-V) valves (mitral and tricuspid) that separate the atria and ventricles are more complex. Valve competence depends on approximation and support of leaflets maintained by the dynamic adjustment of tension on the leaflet by the papillary muscles and chordae tendineae. Hence abnormal function of ventricular

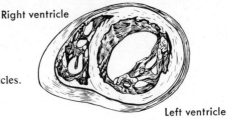

Right ventricle

Left ventricle

Fig. 31-1. Cross section of heart, midportion of ventricles.

myocardium and papillary muscles may produce malfunction of an otherwise structurally normal valve.

Conduction system

The specialized conduction system of the heart is important because nearly every intracardiac procedure involves manipulation of the sinus node, intra-atrial conduction pathways, the atrioventricular node, or the His bundle and its branches. A special surgical landmark is the papillary muscle of the conus, located on the septum below the crista supraventricularis (Fig. 31-2). The bundle of His has divided into bundle branches beyond the base of this muscle in its course through the septum. The first septal branch of the anterior descending coronary artery—which often provides important blood supply to the conduction system—is located in the septum somewhat anterior to the papillary muscle of the conus.

The conus

The crista supraventricularis and its septal and parietal muscle bands separate the body of the right ventricle from the infundibular or conal portion. The conus consists of the crista supraventricularis, the infundibular chamber below the pulmonary valve, the pulmonary anulus, valve, and proximal portions of the pulmonary artery. Abnormalities in the embryological development or rotation of the conus explain many cyanotic congenital cardiac anomalies.

Coronary vessels

The anterior descending and circumflex branches of the left coronary artery and the right coronary artery are the three vessels that distribute blood to the heart. The coronary artery giving origin to the posterior descending coronary artery supplying the posterior one third of the intraventricular septum is termed the *dominant* coronary artery because it provides important blood supply to the posterior left ventricle. The nutrient branches of the coronary arteries originate at right angles from the primary coronary arteries and course straight through the myocardium, so that the distant point most vulnerable to ischemia is the endocardial surface. Since these arteries course through contracting muscle, most flow occurs during diastole when the myocardium is relaxed. At the capillary level the vascular channels are sinusoidal and capable of immense dilatation, and they have the remarkable ability to form new flow pathways (collaterals).

CARDIAC PHYSIOLOGY

The heart pumps blood to deliver nutrients to the cells of the body. Oxygen is a critical nutrient, since nearly all metabolic processes require the oxidative pathway. Reduction in oxygen supply to the cell because of reduced blood flow (low cardiac output) or abnormality of oxygen transfer has the same measurable end result: reduced total body oxygen consumption. If this process develops acutely (minutes to hours), usually accompanied by reduced arterial blood pressure, the condition is called *circulatory shock*. When the time course is measured in days to months modified by complex, autoregulatory, mechanisms, the condition is called chronic *heart failure*. So, with most cardiac conditions, therapy is directed at improving oxygen consumption and cardiac output.

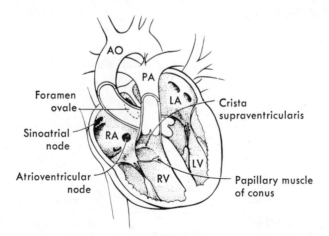

Fig. 31-2. Normal heart. Some important surgical landmarks are demonstrated. *AO*, Aorta; *PA*, pulmonary artery; *RA*, *LA*, right and left atria; *RV*, *LV*, right and left ventricles.

Determinants of stroke volume

Cardiac output is the product of heart rate and ventricular stroke volume. Heart rate is the major reserve mechanism for increasing cardiac output and is regulated by neurohumoral mechanisms. Stroke volume is determined by three factors:

1. *Preload* (end-diastolic stretch of myocardial sarcomeres, or Frank-Starling mechanism)
2. *Contractility* (contractile state of myocardium)
3. *Afterload* (load resisting shortening of sarcomeres during systole)

The first two factors are related in a positive fashion, whereas the last has an inverse relationship (Fig. 31-3). In practice, *preload* in the intact ventricle is taken to mean the end diastolic pressure of the ventricle, provided that the A-V valve is normal. *Afterload* is the systolic intraventricular pressure, which is identical to aortic systolic pressure if the aortic valve is normal. Aortic pressure is related to systemic or peripheral vascular resistance, which determines afterload.

Separate performance of the ventricles

There are separate determinants of stroke volume for the right and left ventricles. Obviously, a steady state must be reached in which the output of the systemic and pulmonary ventricles is equal, or all the blood would end up in the lungs or the feet. Inequality of ventricular stroke volume can exist transiently, which explains differences in right and left atrial pressures as they reflect conditions in the ventricle during diastole. As a practical consideration, the highest pressure will be observed in the atrium that fills the ventricle, which governs or limits total blood flow. Under normal conditions and in most disease states, this is the left ventricle so that left atrial pressure is greater than right atrial pressure. Great variability can occur, however, so that it is virtually impossible to predict the levels of atrial pressure. It is best to measure simultaneously in both atria. Left atrial pressure may be measured indirectly from the right side as the pulmonary wedge pressure.

MANAGEMENT OF THE CARDIOVASCULAR SYSTEM
General principles

The goal of successful management of the cardiovascular system is to develop *cardiac output* adequate for the metabolic demands of the situation with a *minimum* of pharmacological intervention (because of possible deleterious side effects of drugs). To improve cardiac output, *heart rate, preload, afterload,* and *contractility* may be manipulated. Cardiac output should be measured directly because of inaccuracy of clinical signs used to estimate the cardiac output. Arterial blood pressure, urine flow, cerebral function, appearance of the extremities, and blood gas analysis and pH estimate the *adequacy* of cardiac performance related to perfusion of individual capillary beds.

Monitoring
Arterial pressure

An indwelling Teflon catheter is placed in a systemic artery. In addition to the absolute values for systolic, diastolic, and mean arterial pressure, study of the pulse contour and upstroke relative to time (dp/dt) assists in the estimation of stroke volume.

Atrial pressure

Small tubes are placed directly in the right and left atria during cardiac surgery. In other patients a

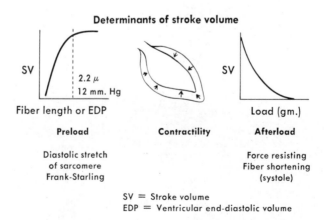

Determinants of stroke volume

Preload	Contractility	Afterload
Fiber length or EDP		Load (gm.)
Diastolic stretch of sarcomere Frank-Starling		Force resisting Fiber shortening (systole)

2.2 μ
12 mm. Hg

SV = Stroke volume
EDP = Ventricular end-diastolic volume

Fig. 31-3. Factors affecting cardiac output.

catheter passed from a peripheral vein into the right atrium plus a Swan-Ganz flow-directed balloon catheter placed in the pulmonary wedge position will accomplish the same goal. In the normal heart at rest, mean pressure in the right atrium is 4 to 8 mm. Hg and pressure in the left atrium is 8 to 12 mm. Hg; these values reflect ventricular end diastolic pressure. Atrial pressure above the normal range generally means diminished ventricular performance and represents the *preload* on the ventricle at that moment.

Electrocardiogram

Continuous monitoring is essential to document cardiac rhythm and rate. Ventricular arrhythmia is important because it not only is suggestive of myocardial ischemia but also may lead to cardiac arrest. Atrial arrhythmia is important because rapid rate may reduce cardiac output. Abnormally slow ventricular rate may also diminish cardiac output. Temporary pacing wires are often placed on the atrium or the ventricle at operation or passed from a peripheral vein to control heart rate and augment cardiac output or suppress arrhythmia.

Cardiac output

Cardiac output may be measured at the bedside by the thermal dilution technique. A thermistor catheter is placed in the pulmonary artery at operation or through a peripheral vein with a Swan-Ganz catheter. This is the sampling site to detect changes in temperature of the blood caused by injection of a bolus of fluid at a predetermined temperature into the right atrium. Although more cumbersome, measurement of oxygen consumption and the content of oxygen in pulmonary and systemic arteries allows calculation of cardiac output by the Fick principle. The result in liters per minute corrected for surface area of the patient is expressed as the cardiac index (L./min./m.^{2}).

Practical aspects of management
Normal cardiac output (>3.5 L./min./m.^{2})

No intervention is necessary. Fluid losses are replaced in addition to maintenance fluids.

Suboptimal cardiac output (2.2 to 3.5 L./min./m.^{2})

Manipulate *preload.* Blood or other fluid is infused to raise atrial pressure. End diastolic pressure of 12 mm. Hg achieves an optimal 2.2 μ stretch of the sarcomere (Fig. 31-3). Atrial pressures above 12 to 14 mm. Hg probably do not increase stroke volume appreciably, but in practice atrial pressure may be taken somewhat higher. Hydrostatic pressure exceeds oncotic pressure at 25 mm. Hg, and a net flux of fluid out of the vascular space (edema) may occur.

Manipulate *afterload.* Occasionally, decreased stroke volume is related to increased peripheral arteriolar resistance. Sodium nitroprusside or nitroglycerin are administered intravenously to reduce afterload.

Manipulate *contractility.* Digoxin, 0.9 mg./m.^{2} given intravenously in divided doses, should be spaced as determined by urgency. Evidence indicates that toxicity may occur at half expected doses during the first 24 hours after cardiopulmonary bypass.

Poor cardiac output (<2.2 L./min./m.^{2})

The patient is seriously ill. Manipulation of preload and afterload may help, but usually improvement of myocardial contractility is necessary. Catecholamines are indicated. Epinephrine, 5 to 10 mg./500 ml. of D5W, is given by continuous intravenous infusion. At low dose levels the effect of the drug is primarily to increase myocardial contractility, and few peripheral effects are observed. Other pharmacological agents may be equally effective depending on the clinical situation. Isoproterenol may be used if the heart rate is slow and arterial blood pressure is not too low. If there is oliguria, dopamine may be indicated to increase renal blood flow.

CARDIAC ARREST
Diagnosis

Ventricular *asystole* or *fibrillation* results in cessation of cardiac output. At normal body temperature, loss of consciousness from absence of cerebral blood flow occurs in a matter of seconds, and irreversible brain damage follows in 3 to 4 minutes. Cardiac arrest is diagnosed by absence of pulsation over the carotid or femoral artery, pallor or cyanosis, and loss of consciousness. Gasping agonal respiration or grand mal seizure is also common. Treatment should be instituted immediately. One should not waste precious time listening for heart tones or obtaining an electrocardiogram if circulatory collapse is evident. As treatment is established, however, electrocardiographic diagnosis is a helpful guide to the resuscitative effort.

Treatment
Ventilation

Adequate ventilation of the lungs is the primary step. Initially, this may be established by mouth-to-mouth ventilation. Later, a tight-fitting mask and resuscitation bag may be used. If a laryngoscope and endotracheal tube are available, a tube should be placed accurately and expeditiously in the trachea. Time lost during a difficult intubation or inadvertent, unrecognized intubation of the esophagus can be fatal. Oxygen should be administered to the airway if available.

Cardiac massage

Closed chest cardiac massage should be instituted as soon as possible. With the patient supine on a hard surface (floor or board), the heel of the hand is placed over the lower third of the sternum, and pressure is applied so as to depress the sternum 3 to 4 cm. Pressure is applied intermittently at a rate of about 60 compressions per minute. The heart is compressed between the sternum and spine, with lateral motion limited by the pericardium. Effectiveness of massage is measured by restoration of pulsation over the carotid or femoral artery. With effective massage and ventilation, patients have survived cardiac arrest periods of over an hour without irreversible damage to brain or other organs. Fatigability of the person performing the massage is minimized by positioning well above the patient's chest so that pressure may be transferred from the back and shoulders through the arms, locked in full extension at the elbows, to the heel of the hand over the sternum.

Infusion and medications

If no intravenous access is available, a needle catheter may be readily inserted into the common femoral vein or medications may be injected through a needle penetrating the heart through the chest wall. *Epinephrine* (1 ml. of 1:10,000 solution) may improve quality of fibrillation or restore forceful contraction of the ineffectively beating heart. *Calcium chloride* (5 to 10 ml. of 1% solution) is also helpful as a cardiac stimulant. *Sodium bicarbonate* (44 mEq. every 10 minutes) should be administered to combat metabolic acidosis, which always accompanies cardiac arrest. *Lidocaine (Xylocaine)* (50 to 100 mg. bolus doses) may stabilize ventricular dysrhythmia. *Propranolol, procaine amide,* and *potassium chloride* are occasionally useful in treating cardiac dysrhythmia.

Electrical defibrillation

Ventricular contraction may be synchronized by application of 20 to 200 watt/sec. of a direct current to the chest wall. A defibrillator unit equipped with special paddle electrodes applies the current through the chest wall between the base and apex of the heart. Vigorous closed chest massage and medications right before the countershock are often helpful. Nearly all fibrillating hearts can be defibrillated, but effective cardiac output may not be established if myocardial contraction produces insufficient stroke volume.

CARDIOPULMONARY BYPASS AND ASSISTED CIRCULATION

The purpose of cardiopulmonary bypass is to maintain circulation and respiration while the heart is emptied of blood during an operative procedure. Cardiopulmonary bypass involves placement of venous cannulas to drain the blood from the body to the pump-oxygenator (heart-lung machine). Gas exchange occurs within the oxygenator, and the blood is pumped through the arterial cannula back to the body, as shown in Fig. 31-4. The driving force for the circulation during cardiopulmonary bypass is the single arterial roller pump. The flow characteristic is essentially nonpulsatile, but depending on the size of the tubing being compressed and the occlusiveness of the rollers, pulse pressures of approximately 15 to 20 mm. Hg can be developed. As the pump head rotates, blood is forced through the entire circulatory system. Return to the venous side is therefore accomplished by displacement of the blood, using energy supplied by the arterial pump. Venous return to the oxygenator drains by gravity to the reservoir of the oxygenator.

The principles of this simple system help one understand how the left ventricle functions as the driving force of the entire circulation during normal cardiac action. The left ventricle expels blood through the arterial circulation to the capillaries. Each contraction of the left ventricle displaces blood through the capillaries into the venous system, where it is returned to the heart (again by displacement) for recirculation. The *vis a tergo* (push from behind) is a concept defined by cardiac physiologists. As such, the left ventricle by its own stroke volume becomes a determinant of venous return to the right side of the heart. Although this may seem a rather simplistic explanation of venous return, it is reasonable that some source of energy for moving blood through the veins must be supplied. The left ventricle is that energy source for venous return. Trivial sources of energy such as thoracic negative pressure or sucking action of the right ventricle confuse the straightforward nature of the circulation, which can be readily observed during cardiopulmonary bypass when a single pump drives the entire circulation.

Nearly all the blood is excluded from the heart when venous blood is diverted to the pump oxygenator through cannulas placed in the superior and inferior vanae cavae. Oxygenated blood that is returned to the aorta does not enter the heart if there is competence of the aortic valve. Blood returning to the cardiac chambers through the coronary circulation may be excluded by occlusion of the aorta between the aortic perfusion cannula and origin of the coronary arteries. Venous drainage of the bronchial circulation to the pulmonary veins and left atrium is continuous and requires aspiration by vent catheter into the left atrium or left ventricle during operations on the left side of

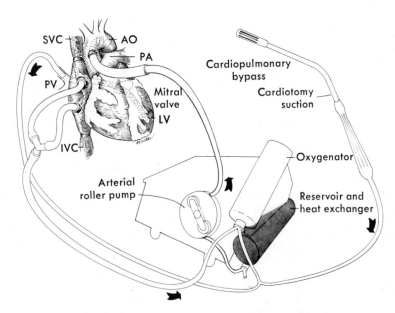

Fig. 31-4. Cardiopulmonary bypass. Blood drains by gravity from patient to oxygenator where gas exchange occurs. Single roller pump returns blood to patient and is driving force of circulation.

the heart. This source of blood returning to the heart is especially important in the fibrillating heart and in patients with cyanotic congenital cardiac disease who develop a noticeable increase of the bronchial circulation as a collateral pathway for pulmonary circulation.

Oxygenators

Two types of devices are used for exchange of gases during cardiopulmonary bypass, as follows:

Bubble oxygenator. Microbubbles of oxygen diffuse through a column of blood, and gas exchange occurs on the surface of the bubbles. Microbubbles and foam are removed in a special chamber of the oxygenator system. This oxygenator is available as a disposable device and is used most frequently in clinical practice at the present time.

Membrane oxygenator. A thin membrane of Silastic, Teflon, or polypropylene is placed between the blood and the gas. Gas exchange occurs across the membrane, with no direct contact between blood and gas. The membrane may be supplied in sheets that separate blood and oxygen or as tiny tubes through which the blood passes. This system mimics lung and is the least traumatic to the blood elements. Oxygenator size is directly proportional to the size of the patient because enough membrane surface area must be available for appropriate gas exchange. These systems are gaining popularity and more frequent use.

Hypothermia

The metabolic needs of tissues are directly proportional to the temperature at which metabolism is taking place. At *normothermia* conditions (34° to 37° C.), total body perfusion must exceed 2.5 L./min./m.^{2} to prevent accumulation of products of anaerobic metabolism. As body temperature is lowered, the metabolic requirement is reduced about 10% for each two Celsius degrees of temperature drop so that many intracardiac procedures are performed under *moderate hypothermia* conditions (28° to 32° C.), at which total body flow rates of 1.8 to 2.2 L./min./m.^{2} are adequate for periods of cardiopulmonary bypass up to 3 hours. As the body temperature is reduced to *deep hypothermia* levels (20° to 24° C.), cardiopulmonary bypass flow rates are reduced proportionally and circulation may be totally arrested for limited periods either to enhance the operating conditions or to reduce the period of cardiopulmonary bypass. This is especially important for intracardiac surgery in infants and small children, in whom deleterious effects of cardiopulmonary bypass are most often observed. Clinical practice has shown that if the body temperature is at 20° C., total circulatory arrest up to 60 minutes is well tolerated in children under the age of 2 years. Adults may tolerate circulatory arrest somewhat less well, but limited periods of circulatory arrest at temperatures between 18° and 20° C. have been successfully utilized in adults for various intracardiac and extracardiac operations.

Consequences of cardiopulmonary bypass and open-heart surgery

Cardiopulmonary bypass and intracardiac operation require a large incision, considerable tissue manipulation, and direct trauma to blood elements in the pump oxygenator. Activation of complement, denaturation of protein, abnormalities in platelet function, and destruction of the cellular elements of blood with the liberation of free hemoglobin, aggregates of white cells and platelets, and other microparticles in the blood such as microgas bubbles are consequences of this procedure and will be manifest in the postoperative period as typical physiological response to trauma. Elevation of the body temperature, respiratory insufficiency, mild renal insufficiency, and some observable dysfunction of most other organ systems are also present. Fortunately, the body has good reserve for this type of trauma, and the effects of cardiopulmonary bypass are self-limiting within a few days.

CONGENITAL CARDIAC ANOMALIES
General principles

Abnormalities of embryological development of the heart and great vessels involve about 8 babies out of 1,000 live births. These defects represent a spectrum of disease from simple errors to complex malformations producing gross deformity of the heart or great vessels and severe physiological impairment. As a general principle, complete surgical correction of these abnormalities is the therapeutic goal. Operative mortality and long-term functional results are directly related to the completeness with which the defect is corrected. When total correction of the defect is not possible, temporary or palliative operations are occasionally performed, but the results are not so good as those for total repairs.

Congestive cardiac failure caused by excessive pulmonary blood flow associated with intracardiac or extracardiac shunt or some obstruction to flow of blood is an indication for surgery. Arterial hypoxemia in patients with cyanotic congenital cardiac disease with increasing polycythemia or loss of consciousness (hypoxic spells) is another common indication for surgery.

Palliative operations
Aortopulmonary shunts

Aortopulmonary shunt is used in patients with defects reducing pulmonary blood flow, such as tetralogy of Fallot or pulmonary atresia with ventricular septal defect, transposition of the great arteries with pulmonary stenosis, and tricuspid atresia.

Three types of aortopulmonary anastomoses are commonly performed to shunt blood between the aortic systemic circulation and the pulmonary circulation (Fig. 31-5).

Blalock-Taussig shunt. In the Blalock-Taussig shunt the subclavian artery is anastomosed end-to-side to the pulmonary artery. A modification in which prosthetic polytetrafluoroethylene graft material is used to carry blood between the subclavian artery and pulmonary artery has also gained popularity. This is the most widely used and perhaps best shunt because the size of the subclavian artery allows optimal controlled increase of pulmonary blood flow.

Waterston shunt. The ascending aorta is anastomosed side-to-side to the right pulmonary artery. The connection is 3 to 4 mm. in diameter, but occasionally the shunt flow is too great, and pulmonary arteriolar hypertension develops. The Waterston shunt is used only in tiny babies.

Potts shunt. The Potts shunt is a side-to-side anastomosis of descending thoracic aorta and left pulmonary artery. The size of the shunt is difficult to control, and it is the most difficult of the shunt procedures to take down at the time of total repair of the intracardiac defect. This shunt is described for historical purposes because it is seldom used in current practice.

Systemic venous-pulmonary artery shunts

Glenn shunt. An anastomosis of the superior vena cava to the right pulmonary artery, the Glenn shunt is used in selected older patients with tricuspid atresia. Ordinarily it is a permanent anastomosis because it is most difficult to revise or take down later.

Atrial septectomy

Rashkind procedure. A defect in the atrial septum is created at cardiac catheterization. A balloon-tip catheter is passed through the femoral vein across the foramen ovale into the left atrium. The balloon is inflated, and the catheter is forcefully withdrawn, rupturing the membrane of the foramen ovale (Fig. 31-6) to produce a large interatrial communication. The Rashkind procedure is used in patients with transposition of the great arteries, total anomalous pulmonary venous connection, tricuspid or mitral valve atresia, and hypoplastic right-sided heart syndrome.

Blalock-Hanlon procedure. In the Blalock-Hanlon procedure, the right lateral portion of the interatrial septum is resected (Fig. 31-6); a side-biting clamp excludes a portion of the right and left atria and septum so that some of the septum can be excised without interruption of the blood flow. This procedure is used in patients with transposition of the great arteries who are very young or otherwise

Aorta-pulmonary shunts

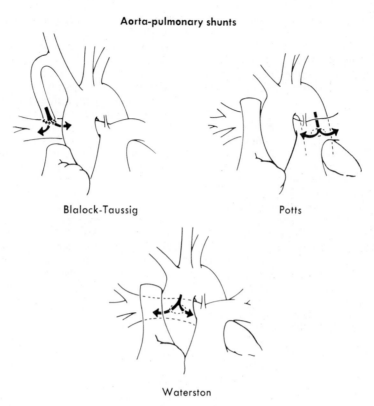

Blalock-Taussig

Potts

Waterston

Fig. 31-5. Palliative operations. Three common types of procedures to shunt blood from systemic to pulmonary circulation.

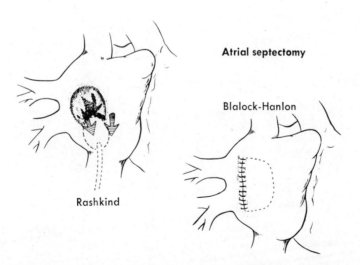

Atrial septectomy

Blalock-Hanlon

Rashkind

Fig. 31-6. Two methods of producing defects in atrial septum. Rashkind procedure is rupture of foramen ovale with balloon catheter. Blalock-Hanlon procedure is surgical excision of portion of atrial septum.

not candidates for total intracardiac repair of the defect.

Pulmonary artery banding

The pulmonary artery is narrowed when a band is tightened around its external circumference. Blood flow to the lung is reduced when the pulmonary outflow resistance is increased. The operation is used in defects such as common ventricle with excessive pulmonary blood flow when there is no means of complete repair.

Total repair—extracardiac anomalies
Patent ductus arteriosus

The ductus arteriosus, which joins the thoracic aorta and the pulmonary artery, closes shortly after birth under the stimulus of air in the lungs and the presence of blood with high oxygen tension in the ductus. If these normal physiological stimuli fail to close the ductus arteriosus, a shunt remains between the aorta and the pulmonary artery so that the pulmonary blood flow is increased (Fig. 31-7). Patent ductus arteriosus is common in premature infants and is associated with the idiopathic respiratory distress syndrome. Surgery to close the ductus arteriosus may be lifesaving in these tiny patients. If the shunt is small, the patient may be asymptomatic, with the diagnosis being made by the presence of a continuous heart murmur. In these patients the ductus is surgically closed electively because of the threat of congestive cardiac failure developing later in life. The operation consists of either ligation or division of the ductus arteriosus. The risk of operation in small, even in premature infants who require ligation of ductus arteriosus for respiratory distress syndrome.

Coarctation of the thoracic aorta

Coarctation of the thoracic aorta is a pronounced narrowing of the upper portion of the descending thoracic aorta (Fig. 31-7). Circulation to the lower half of the body is maintained by collateral circulation. The diagnosis is made by absence of normal femoral pulsation and hypertension in the upper extremities. Heart failure may occur during infancy, and operative correction has high risk because of associated cardiac anomalies. If the child survives the first year of life, elective operation is

Extracardiac anomalies

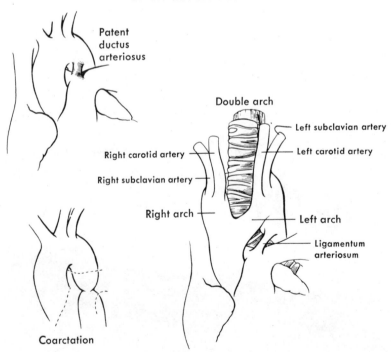

Fig. 31-7. Anomalies of great vessels subject to complete repair.

performed between 5 and 10 years of age to prevent complications of the anomaly that occur later in life. Operation consists in resecting the coarcted segment and end-to-end anastomosis of the aorta. Sometimes bypass graft or enlargement of the aorta by patch angioplasty, using the turned-down left subclavian artery or prosthetic material, is performed. The risk of the operation is mostly related to hemorrhage from the enlarged collateral circulation. Complications of intestinal or spinal cord ischemia are rare.

Vascular ring

A number of aortic arch malformations may obstruct the esophagus or trachea by compression within a ringlike vascular anomaly. Most commonly the ring is caused by a double aortic arch (Fig. 31-7) or other arch abnormality with compressing ligamentum arteriosum. Symptoms are those of airway obstruction or difficulty in swallowing (*dysphagia lusoria*). Posterior indentation of the barium-filled esophagus by the vascular ring is seen on x-ray examination. One performs the operation through a left thoracotomy incision with complete dissection of the aortic arch and branch vessels before dividing the ring at an appropriate point. Postoperative complications are related to the loss of airway support because of tracheal malacia at the area of tracheal compression by the vascular ring.

Complete repair—intracardiac anomalies
Anomalies with left-to-right shunts

Anomalies with left-to-right shunts include atrial and ventricular septal defects, which are the most common forms of congenital intracardiac anomalies, the less common anomalies of the atrioventricular canal, and anomalous pulmonary venous connection (Fig. 31-8). The anatomical abnormality is increased pulmonary blood flow caused by shunting of blood from the left cardiac chambers back to the right heart chambers because of higher pressure on the left side of the heart. Recirculation of the blood through the pulmonary circuit increases cardiac work and leads to congestive cardiac failure if the shunt is large. In addition to dyspnea, heart failure often produces growth failure in children. Late complication of the increased pulmonary blood flow at high pressure is the development of obstructive changes in pulmonary arterioles leading to increased pulmonary vascular resistance. In extreme forms pulmonary resistance may exceed systemic resistance with reversal of shunt flow from right to left (Eisenmenger complex). When the patient reaches this stage, correction of the defect is not possible. With heart failure or increased pulmonary vascular resistance, complete repair is elected regardless of age of the patient. Asymptomatic children are repaired and surgery is performed just prior to school age to avoid heart failure later in life. Defects of the septum are closed by direct suture or by patch material. Pericardium is used to repair atrial septal defects, whereas Dacron cloth is employed to close ventricular septal defects because it is more resistant to the high ventricular pressures. Repair of atrioventricular canal anomalies involves reconstruction of the A-V valve as well as closing of the septal defect. Anomalous pulmonary venous connection is reconnected to the left atrium by direct anastomosis or by conduit through the atrial septum. In all these, sutures must not be placed in the cardiac conduction system because atrial arrhythmia or complete heart block may occur.

Anomalies with right-to-left shunts

The *tetralogy of Fallot* group of anomalies is associated with pulmonary outflow obstruction, which reduces pulmonary blood flow (Fig. 31-9). There may be severe pulmonary stenosis or total

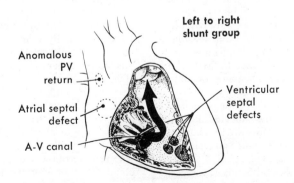

Fig. 31-8. Anomalies producing left-to-right shunt flow. Increased pulmonary blood flow may cause congestive heart failure or increased pulmonary vascular resistance, or both.

Tetralogy of Fallot

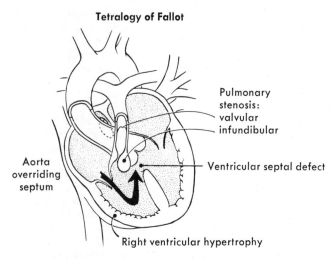

Pulmonary
stenosis:
valvular
infundibular

Aorta
overriding
septum

Ventricular septal defect

Right ventricular hypertrophy

Fig. 31-9. Four defects of tetralogy of Fallot. Decreased pulmonary blood flow and direct ejection of right ventricle to aorta (right-to-left shunt) cause arterial hypoxia.

interruption of the connection between the heart and the pulmonary artery (pulmonary atresia) with severe cyanosis. On the other hand, the mildest form will involve little outflow tract obstruction, and the patient will not be cyanotic. There is always a ventricular septal defect and the aorta is positioned to the right, overriding the septum so that the right ventricle ejects deoxygenated blood directly to the aorta. Hypertrophy of the right ventricle is compensatory. The defect results from hypoplasia of the conus portion of the heart with the degree of hypoplasia correlated with severity of the condition. Polycythemia, which follows, is a compensatory response to arterial desaturation. A peculiar manifestation of this condition is the "hypoxic spell." This is related to acute change in right ventricular outflow obstruction resulting from spasm of the hypertrophied obstructing muscle bands of the crista supraventricularis, causing acute reduction of pulmonary blood flow with loss of consciousness. These patients often assume a squatting position as an adaptive mechanism to increase systemic arterial resistance to favor blood flow to the pulmonary circuit by acute angulation of the arteries of the lower extremities.

The diagnosis of tetralogy of Fallot is made by angiography. Contrast material injected into the right ventricle simultaneously fills the aorta and the narrowed outflow tract of the right ventricle. Typically, the outflow tract is obstructed by hypertrophy of the septal and parietal bands of the crista supraventricularis.

Operative repair consists in relieving right ventricular outflow obstruction and closing the ventricular septal defect so that the overriding of the aorta

is corrected by placement of the patch to the right side of the aorta. When the pulmonary valve anulus is larger than one third the diameter of the aortic valve anulus, excision of the obstructing septal and parietal bands of the crista supraventricularis and pulmonary valvotomy relieve outflow obstruction. If the pulmonary valve anulus is greatly stenosed, it is widened by placement of a Dacron patch extending from the right ventricle across the pulmonary valve anulus into the pulmonary artery. When the pulmonary valve is absent (pulmonary atresia), a new connection is created between the right ventricle and the pulmonary artery by means of an external valved conduit (Rastelli procedure). This procedure is also used in patients with common truncus arteriosus, a condition in which the aorta is the only exit of blood from the heart and the pulmonary arteries originate from the aorta.

The risk of surgical correction of tetralogy of Fallot is directly related to the complexity of the abnormality. When standard repair can be accomplished, the operative mortality is between 5% and 10%. If the anatomy is more complex and the right ventricular outflow tract requires major revision, the operative risk increases. Long-term functional improvement in these patients is remarkable. Patients with a standard tetralogy of Fallot repair enjoy essentially normal exercise tolerance; those who require outflow tract revision may have slight compromise of exercise ability.

Transposition of the great arteries

The attachment of the great vessels to the heart is reversed so that the right ventricle is in con-

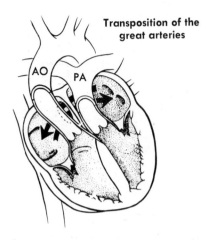

Transposition of the great arteries

AO PA

Fig. 31-10. Transposition of the great arteries. Position of great vessels reversed. Defect in atrial or ventricular septum allows mixing of systemic and pulmonary circulation.

tinuity with the aorta and the left ventricle empties into the pulmonary artery (Fig. 31-10). Deoxygenated blood returning from the body is recirculated through the systemic circulation without passing through the lungs, and pulmonary venous blood (fully saturated with oxygen) is recirculated through the pulmonary artery (*parallel* circulation). Survival is possible in transposition of the great arteries because of connections that provide mixing between the systemic and the pulmonary circulations, usually at the atrial level through a patent foramen ovale. If a large ventricular septal defect coexists, admixture of the systemic and pulmonary venous blood may bring systemic arterial oxygen saturation to near-normal levels.

The diagnosis is made by angiography in a cyanotic infant. Contrast medium injected into the right ventricle fills the aorta; when injected into the left ventricle, it enters the pulmonary artery. There are a number of variations of this anomaly, and the details of the complex anatomy must be clearly defined by angiography.

A severely cyanotic newborn infant with transposition of the great arteries is treated by Rashkind balloon atrial septostomy. This usually allows adequate oxygenation of blood so that operative intervention may be postponed for several months. If the Rashkind procedure fails to relieve hypoxia, a palliative operation (Blalock-Hanlon procedure) or total repair is performed. If the child is over 4 months of age, an intra-atrial redirection of venous return operation is usually selected. In the Mustard operation the atrial septum is excised, and a new

partition of the atrium is made by means of a pericardial patch (Fig. 31-11). A related operation in which the atrial septum and flaps of the right atrium are used to redirect blood flow within the atrium (Senning procedure) has recently found favor in treatment by transposition of the great arteries. In both these operations the systemic venous blood returning through the venae cavae is brought into communication with the mitral valve, left ventricle, and pulmonary artery while pulmonary venous blood is brought into continuity with the tricuspid valve, right ventricle, and aorta (Fig. 31-12). The circulation is then in *series,* physiologically correcting the defect even though it is not a true anatomical correction because the right ventricle remains the systemic pumping chamber. The risk of the operation depends on a number of complex factors, including age and associated anomalies. Functional results are good, and the right ventricle is capable of supporting systemic circulation in patients followed over 10 years. Anatomic correction of the defect in which the transposed great arteries are actually switched to "normal" position has also been used in selected patients.

Other congenital cardiac anomalies
Valvular lesions

Pulmonary valve stenosis is a common valvular lesion producing outflow obstruction and right ventricular enlargement and hypertrophy. Stenosis of the aortic valve causes obstruction of systemic flow. Children having these valvular lesions are usually asymptomatic but have a loud heart murmur. If the stenosis is severe, however, heart failure may occur within the first few hours or days of life. Severe stenosis of the aortic valve may be associated with scarring of the subendocardial layers of the left ventricle (endocardial fibroelastosis), which impairs left ventricular performance. Operation to relieve valve stenosis consists in incising the valve commissures (valvotomy). Hemodynamics are improved, but blood flow through the abnormal valve may be turbulent so that residual murmur is typical and replacement of the aortic valve is eventually required.

Complex lesions with absence of major intracardiac structure

When atrioventricular valves are stenosed, the stenosis is usually complete (atresia), and so there is no communication between the atrium and the ventricle (Fig. 31-13). These complex lesions are associated with hypoplasia of the ventricle and outflow tract distal to the atretic atrioventricular valve. Patients with tricuspid valve atresia and reduced pulmonary blood flow require an aortopulmonary shunt or the Glenn procedure. The right

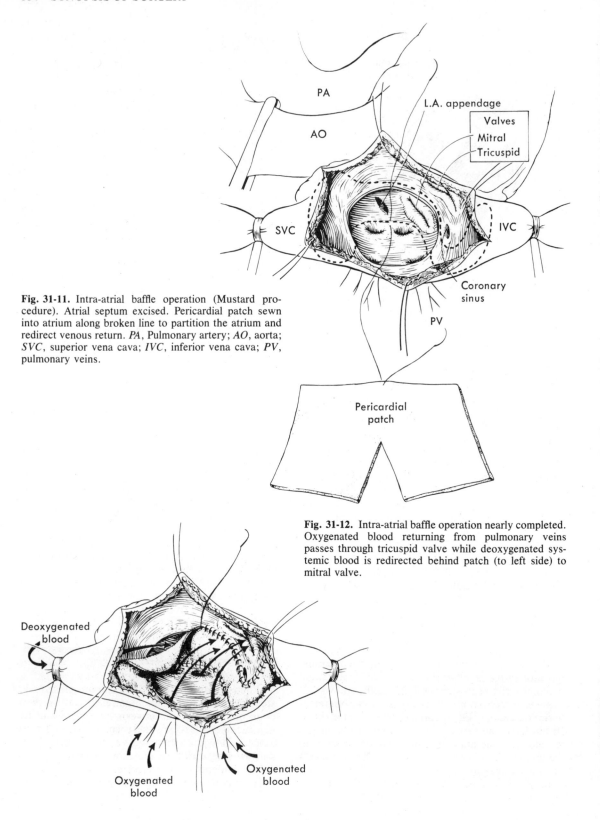

Fig. 31-11. Intra-atrial baffle operation (Mustard procedure). Atrial septum excised. Pericardial patch sewn into atrium along broken line to partition the atrium and redirect venous return. *PA,* Pulmonary artery; *AO,* aorta; *SVC,* superior vena cava; *IVC,* inferior vena cava; *PV,* pulmonary veins.

Fig. 31-12. Intra-atrial baffle operation nearly completed. Oxygenated blood returning from pulmonary veins passes through tricuspid valve while deoxygenated systemic blood is redirected behind patch (to left side) to mitral valve.

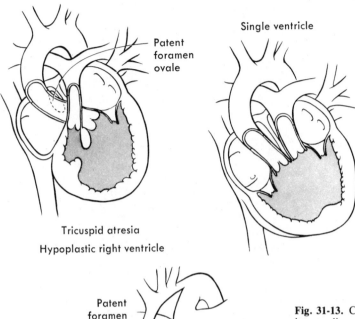

Patent
foramen
ovale

Single ventricle

Tricuspid atresia
Hypoplastic right ventricle

Patent
foramen
ovale

Mitral atresia
Hypoplastic left ventricle

Fig. 31-13. Complex anomalies with absence of major intracardiac structure. Septal defects and mixing of systemic and pulmonary circulation often allow survival.

atrium may be connected directly to the pulmonary artery with closure of the atrial septal defect (Fontan procedure). Blood then flows through the lung by left ventricular *vis a tergo* and a small contribution of right atrial contraction. There is no corrective operation for mitral atresia and other forms of hypoplastic left heart syndrome, though some progress with palliative operations has been reported recently.

Single ventricle, caused by absence of the ventricular septum or hypoplasia of one ventricle with large ventricular septal defect, may require surgery to alter the amount of pulmonary blood flow. Operations for this condition are usually palliative, though some cases have had total correction when a ventricular septum was created with a Dacron

partition. The Fontan procedure has been used in most cases to create physiological correction.

ACQUIRED HEART DISEASE
Coronary artery disease

Coronary atherosclerosis with myocardial ischemia is a significant public health problem. It is estimated that approximately 4 million people in the United States have coronary artery disease, accounting for 675,000 deaths per year. Surgical treatment of coronary atherosclerosis was made possible by perfection of selective coronary arteriography and the development of surgical procedures that directly revascularize the coronary arteries. About 90% of patients with coronary atherosclerosis will have the major atherosclerotic

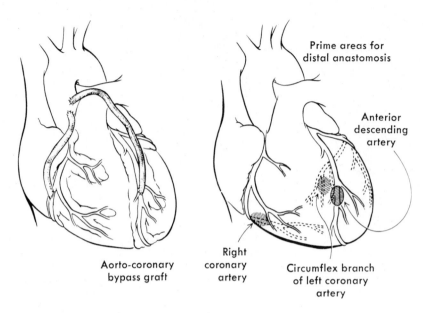

Fig. 31-14. Surgery for coronary artery disease. Segments of saphenous vein used to bypass obstructed portions of coronary arteries. Grafts attached directly to branches of coronary arteries in areas shown on right.

narrowing confined to the proximal portions of the coronary arteries with the distal portions sufficiently normal to accept revascularization procedures. Using microsurgical techniques, direct vascular anastomosis is possible on vessels as small as 1 mm. in diameter.

The most common operation is the aorto-coronary bypass graft utilizing saphenous vein (Fig. 31-14). The saphenous vein is removed from the leg and used to join the ascending aorta and the coronary artery distal to the area of obstruction. The internal mammary artery, freed from its anatomical position along the sternal margin, may also be sutured directly into branches of either the right or left coronary artery. Cardiopulmonary bypass quiets the heart while the anastomosis to the coronary artery is made. Usual sites for distal anastomosis to the coronary arteries are shown in Fig. 31-14.

The most common indication for coronary revascularization is in patients with chronic, stable angina pectoris that is intractable to usual forms of medical management. These patients have recurrent attacks of angina pectoris, usually with exercise or emotion, which are not abolished by therapeutic doses of short- and long-acting nitrates, beta adrenergic blocking agents (propranolol) in doses sufficient to reduce resting pulse below 60 beats per minute) or calcium channel–blocking agents to reduce coronary artery spasm. When angina pec-

toris is sufficient to impair quality of life or capability of gainful occupation, surgery is recommended. In young patients (less than 50 years) or patients with extensive involvement (three-vessel) or critical location (left main coronary artery), the indications are liberalized, because it is known that these patients are at highest risk of early death. Similarly, a more aggressive surgical approach is taken in patients who continue to have notable abnormalities in the graded exercise test (treadmill stress test) while receiving optimal medical management. About 75% of patients are relieved of angina pectoris after coronary revascularization, 20% will have continued but less frequent angina, and about 5% will remain the same or worse. There is a general correlation between symptomatic improvement and the graft patency; 66% to 75% of saphenous veins are patent 1 year after the operation, depending on location of the graft. Long-term patency rates approaching 90% have been reported using the internal mammary artery. The mortality for aortocoronary bypass graft operations in patients with chronic angina pectoris is about 2%.

Patients with unstable angina pectoris (preinfarction syndrome) require a coronary care facility to monitor cardiac rhythm and intensively treat myocardial ischemia. Enthusiasm for aggressive diagnostic and surgical interventions to prevent myocardial infarction should be tempered by knowledge that infarction in this clinical setting is usually not fatal and that the risk of the operation is slightly higher because of the possibility of completed myocardial infarction at the time of surgery. For patients with completed acute myocardial infarction, the place of aortocoronary bypass operations is questionable because of the high mortality (over 40%) and the short time after coronary occlusion in which irreversible myocardial damage occurs. For operative intervention to be successful in preserving myocardium and to have a reasonable risk, it must be performed within 4 hours after onset of chest pain. A similar time frame is required for pharmacological revascularization with use of a catheter or systemically infused streptokinase.

Patients who have congestive cardiac failure resulting from coronary artery disease also are not often helped by aortocoronary bypass operations. Improving myocardial blood flow does not significantly improve ventricular function under these conditions. Congestive heart failure, caused by an infarcted area that subsequently thins out and becomes aneurysmal (ventricular aneurysm), is benefited by excision of the aneurysmal portion of the ventricle. This may be complemented by aortocoronary bypass graft. Similarly, patients with heart failure caused by postinfarction ventricular septal defect or mitral valve incompetence associated with papillary muscle dysfunction may respond to surgical intervention. Results are best when the operation can be delayed for 30 days after infarction.

Valvular heart disease
Aortic valve

Stenosis or incompetence of the aortic valve results from degenerative changes of a congenitally abnormal valve or from rheumatic pathological changes. Aortic valve stenosis causes muscular hypertrophy of the ventricle, which encroaches on the ventricular cavity, making it effectively smaller. Aortic valve insufficiency, on the other hand, produces diastolic overload and dilatation of the ventricle. Unfortunately, symptoms of aortic valve disease do not appear until relatively late in the natural course. Once symptoms of angina pectoris or syncope appear, threat of sudden death is imminent. Heart failure is a late sign and is accompanied by some irreversible changes in left ventricular performance.

Children and teenagers with aortic valve stenosis are treated by aortic valvotomy, but adults and all patients with aortic valve incompetence require valve replacement. Risk of operation is about 5% for aortic valve replacement. Functional improvement is often dramatic even in patients with poorly functioning left ventricles.

Mitral valve

Stenosis or incompetence of the mitral valve is usually related to rheumatic degenerative changes with fibrosis and thickening of the leaflets and chordae tendineae and ultimate deposition of calcium to produce rigidity of the valve. Pure mitral valve incompetence may result from rupture of chordae tendineae or myxomatous degeneration of the valve. Symptoms of heart failure, especially those related to pulmonary venous hypertension and fluid accumulation, appear gradually. The lengthy course of the disease gives adequate time for diagnostic confirmation and thoughtful timing of surgical intervention. There may be exacerbation of symptoms with change in cardiac rhythm to atrial fibrillation or rupture of chordae tendineae. The decision to operate is usually based on symptoms sufficient to interfere with quality of life that are not adequately controlled medically.

Patients less than 40 years of age with pure mitral valve stenosis having an otherwise pliable, noncalcified valve (with a good opening snap on auscultation) may often be treated by mitral valvotomy. In this operation the fused commissures are incised to increase to the size of the mitral valve orifice. Older patients and those with calcareous valves or mitral valve incompetence usually require replacement of the valve with a prosthesis, but in a few patients, especially those with ruptured chordae tendineae, the valve may be reconstructed with appropriately placed plication or anuloplasty sutures. Replacement of the valve with a prosthesis has 5% to 10% mortality and 5% to 10% risk of later thromboembolic complications. Functional improvement is good, but patients with mitral valve disease often require continued medical treatment for fluid retention.

Tricuspid valve

Stenosis of the tricuspid valve caused by rheumatic degeneration is unusual; incompetence with dilated, pulsating neck veins, enlarged pulsatile liver, and immense fluid retention generally follows pulmonary hypertension and right ventricular dilatation associated with severe mitral valve disease. Surgical intervention is based primarily on symptoms similar to the criteria for mitral valve surgery.

Operations on the tricuspid valve are always performed with the cardiopulmonary bypass. A stenosed tricuspid valve must be replaced. When the tricuspid valve is incompetent because of dilatation of the anulus, the configuration of the anulus may be restored with a special ring prosthesis or nearly circumferential sutures that narrow the anulus (anuloplasty), or the valve may be replaced with a prosthesis. If mitral valve disease coexists, operative risk is highest of all surgery for valvular heart disease (10% to 20%).

Prosthetic valves

A variety of valve prostheses are used in the surgical treatment of valvular heart disease (Fig. 31-15). The valve that has been used for the longest time is the ball-in-cage prosthesis of the Starr-Edwards design. This prosthesis has a high cage and the round poppet is bulky, and so it occupies a considerable portion of the left ventricular volume when used in the mitral position. In contrast, the disk-in-cage prosthesis offers a low profile, which is more suitable for mitral valve replacement in the small left ventricle. The disk valve, however, creates more turbulent blood flow and sometimes obstructs, impeding blood flow causing pressure gradients, and so it is seldom used in current practice. The tilting-disk prosthesis has more central flow with favorable hemodynamic properties, especially in replacement of valves with a small anulus. Several types of tilting-disk prostheses are available and are the most extensively used types of mechanical prosthetic valves.

Several tissue prostheses have been devised. The aortic valve taken from cadavers (homograft) is implanted in the aortic position either as a free-hand graft or on a metal stent. Favorable experience with porcine heterograft prostheses is accumulating; the pig aortic valve is mounted on a flexible stent generously covered with Dacron and stabilized in glutaraldehyde. Similar valves using calf pericardium are widely employed. Tissue valves are desirable because of improved hemodynamic properties and low incidence of thromboembolic complications even without anticoagulant prophylaxis. Long-term durability of the preserved biological material is still unknown.

Common types of valve prostheses

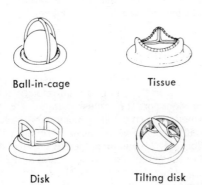

Ball-in-cage   Tissue

Disk   Tilting disk

Fig. 31-15. Examples of various devices for replacing damaged heart valves.

Bacterial endocarditis

There is a constant threat of infection occurring in any abnormal heart valve or valvular prosthesis. Antibiotics usually control acute or subacute bacterial endocarditis, but irreversible damage with acute valvular insufficiency may accompany the infection. Severely damaged heart valves should be replaced before cardiac decompensation occurs. Risk of operation is increased with associated heart failure and sepsis. A period of 4 to 6 weeks of intravenous antibiotics is recommended because bacterial infection of a prosthetic valve is very difficult to cure and sometimes progresses to fungal infection, which is nearly always fatal.

Cardiac tumors

Tumors of the myocardium are rare. The most common tumor found within the cardiac chambers is the atrial myxoma. This benign tumor is generally attached to the atrial septum; it is most common on the left side, and the patient has either peripheral arterial embolization of the myxomatous tumor or symptoms of mitral valve stenosis from obstruction of the mitral valve orifice by the tumor mass. Operation involves removal of the tumor and the portion of the atrial septum to which it is attached. The only malignant tumor of significance is the rhabdomyosarcoma, which may involve atrium or ventricle and by its anatomical location is often impossible to remove. This highly malignant tumor is generally fatal.

Pericardial disease
Tumors

Benign cyst of the pericardium is a mediastinal mass usually located on the right side of the pericardium. It is filled with yellowish-brown, clear fluid and the term "springwater cyst" aptly describes the contents. The lesion is important in the differential diagnosis of mediastinal masses and is usually removed surgically.

Pericarditis

Inflammation of the pericardium resulting from tuberculosis, viral disease (idiopathic pericarditis), or uremia may produce effusion into the pericardium sufficient to cause cardiac tamponade. Pericardiocentesis relieves the symptoms of cardiac tamponade, after which definitive treatment of the disease process is administered. Rapid fluid reaccumulation requires operative intervention. The operation may excise nearly all of the pericardium (pericardiectomy) or remove a portion of the pericardium on the left side so that pericardial fluid can drain into the left pleural space (pericardial window). This operation is usually both diagnostic and therapeutic.

Some cases of the idiopathic variety may fibrose the pericardium with subsequent scar contraction; this constrictive process in the pericardium also causes symptoms of cardiac tamponade. Operation is indicated to remove the contracted pericardium and involved epicardium.

Heart block and pacemakers

Acquired or congenital disease of the specialized conduction system in the heart may disturb cardiac rhythm. Complete heart block caused by a lesion in the bundle of His produces a slow idioventricular rhythm that may not provide adequate cardiac output, resulting in temporary loss of consciousness (Adams-Stokes syndrome). These patients are initially treated with a temporary electrode catheter passed through a peripheral vein and lodged in the right ventricle under fluoroscopic control. The electrode wire is connected to an external pulse generator, which provides electrical stimulation to the myocardium at an appropriate rate. Permanent pacing devices are inserted later.

Electrodes for permanent pacing are placed either transvenously on the endocardium or directly onto the myocardium (Fig. 31-16). The transvenous electrode is passed through a peripheral vein under fluoroscopic control to lodge on the endocardial surface of the right ventricle. Local

anesthesia suffices, simplifying the procedure in the high-risk elderly patient, but the electrode is occasionally dislodged in the postoperative period. Dislodgement does not occur when the electrode is attached directly to the myocardium during an open operation in which the heart is exposed. Durability of the myocardial electrode is probably enhanced so that this type of electrode is chosen for younger, better risk patients.

The most commonly used type of pacemaker at the present time is the ventricular inhibited demand type of pulse generator, in which electrical stimuli at the rate of approximately 70 per minute are passed through the electrodes. A sensing circuit recognizes spontaneous ventricular depolarization and suppresses the subsequent pacemaker stimulus. Ventricular fibrillation caused by an inappropriate stimulus during the refractory period of the heart should not occur with this type of pacing unit.

New pulse generators that sequentially stimulate the atrium and the ventricle through two electrodes are gaining popularity because the natural contractile nature of the heart is utilized. These devices are more complex and thus more expensive.

The pulse generator units rarely fail primarily, but the batteries that provide the energy for the pacemaking stimulus deteriorate with time. It is a

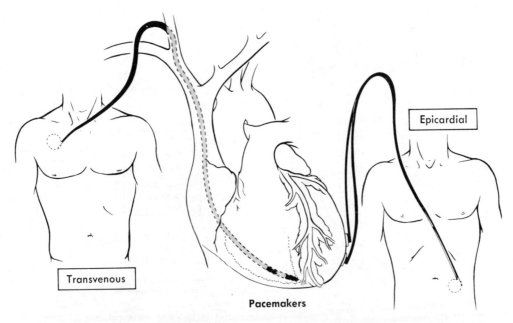

Pacemakers

Fig. 31-16. Cardiac pacemakers. Electrodes may be placed through peripheral vein to contact endocardial surface of right ventricle or attached directly to epicardial surface of left ventricle. Pulse generator (pacemaker) is attached to electrode and placed in subcutaneous pouch.

simple operation, however, to replace a subcutaneous pulse generator. Most units have a predicted life of approximately 5 to 10 years with lithium energy sources. Atrioventricular pacemakers have shorter useful time because batteries are depleted more rapidly by the two electrical discharges required to separately stimulate the atria and ventricles.

CARDIAC TRANSPLANTATION, ARTIFICIAL HEARTS, AND ASSISTED CIRCULATION
Cardiac transplantation

Complete removal of the heart with replacement of a cadaver organ has been successfully accomplished for patients with terminal heart failure in many centers throughout the world. Interest in cardiac transplantation has been steadily increasing so that the procedure is no longer considered experimental. The operation consists of removal of most of the patient's heart, with a portion of the atria being retained to simplify implantation of the donor heart. The donor heart is taken from a patient in whom cerebral death has occurred but myocardial function is normal. The donor organ is placed in the recipient by anastomosis of the atria and great vessels. Technically the operation is not difficult, but control of the rejection phenomenon is a major problem. New agents, such as cyclosporin, that control the immune response have greatly reduced the frequency of uncontrollable rejection. Survival of over 75% of patients for a year or more has been reported.

Another approach utilizes a transplanted auxiliary heart for severe heart failure. In this operation the left atria of the donor and recipient hearts are joined, and the aorta of the donor and recipient vessels are joined such that part of the cardiac output may be taken over by the auxiliary heart to reduce left ventricular load in the patient. Competing heart rates require control by pacemaking. Success of this concept again depends on control of the autoimmune mechanism.

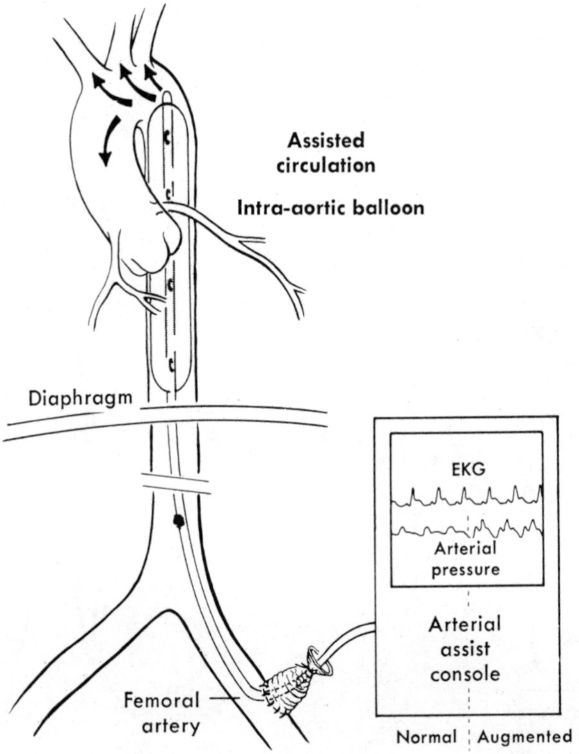

Fig. 31-17. Assisted circulation. Balloon catheter placed in thoracic aorta via femoral artery is attached to assist device that inflates balloon during diastole and deflates just before systole. Displacement of blood produces increased diastolic pressure and better blood flow in coronary and cerebral arteries.

The artificial heart

Implantation of an artificial heart has been successfully accomplished with survival of animals in excess of many months. The devices consist of polyurethane ventricles that are compressed by insufflation of air from an external high pressure pulsatile system. The valves utilized in the artificial heart are typically those of the aortic or mitral prosthesis type. Control of attendant pulmonary hemorrhagic disorders, thromboembolism, and inflow obstruction have been solved sufficiently to allow the planned implantation of such a device in man with temporary survival. On the horizon, of course, is the problem of supplying an energy source that will allow total implantation of the device.

Assisted circulation
Intra-aortic balloon assist

Intra-aortic balloon devices to improve blood flow to critical organs are currently used in patients who have continuing cardiac action but inadequate cardiac output. A balloon catheter is passed into the upper portion of the descending thoracic aorta (Fig. 31-17). The catheter is passed into the common femoral artery by percutaneous technique in adults or by cutdown and use of a prosthetic device as a side arm on the artery in children. The balloon is forcefully inflated and deflated in a pulsatile fashion by an external compressed gas source. Blood pressure and coronary blood flow are enhanced during diastole as the balloon is inflated and blood is displaced from the thoracic aorta. Afterload on the ventricle is decreased as the balloon rapidly deflates just before systole. Complex electrical gating devices ensure proper timing of inflation and deflation relative to the cardiac cycle. These devices have been used mostly in patients with myocardial infarction and reduced left ventricular performance and in patients after cardiac surgery who have inadequate cardiac output.

32
Peripheral Arteries

Howard P. Greisler
William H. Baker

The four basic phenomena (obstruction, erosion, perforation, and a mass) that are so important in other surgical diseases are frequently and often dramatically evidenced in diseases of the arteries. Obstruction from arteriosclerosis is one of the most common of all vascular ailments. Aneurysms may erode or appear as pulsating masses. Perforation of a major artery may dramatically result from degenerative arterial diseases or trauma. In addition, there are a variety of rarer but interesting vascular syndromes.

DIAGNOSIS

The most important facet of the vascular examination remains the history and physical examination. Despite the recent development of various new laboratory and roentgenographic diagnostic modalities, arterial disease and its clinical significance are best evaluated at the bedside by the examining physician. The other tests (Table 32-1), however, are very useful in quantitating the suspected disease, localizing arterial lesions, and often planning surgical procedures.

Plain roentgenograms may demonstrate arterial calcification (Fig. 32-1). Although this finding demonstrates the presence of arterial disease, it is not informative regarding arterial patency and it has an excessive incidence of false-negative results. An enlarged artery demonstrated by ultrasound or computerized tomographic (CT) techniques is more accurate for the diagnosis of aneurysm.

In the noninvasive vascular laboratory, physiological data are collected by Doppler ultrasound and plethysmographic techniques, and anatomic information is collected by other ultrasound studies. Ultrasonic waves are reflected by moving red blood cells. The reflected energy may be made audible or recorded on hard copy. The presence of a Doppler signal indicates that flow is present, and analysis of that signal may indicate reduced or abnormal flow. The Doppler signal can be detected in all major arteries in the extremities. When used in concert with ordinary blood pressure cuffs, the pressure in different segments of the arterial tree can be determined and the segment containing a significant obstruction to flow can often be localized. Analysis of the pitch of the Doppler signal and of the contour of the wave generated by the arterial pulse is often useful for further definition of the extent of the obstruction to flow. Doppler signals can be similarly detected in the extracranial carotid arteries. The response of the Doppler-detected supraorbital arterial flow to certain compressive maneuvers is an important part of the cerebrovascular examination. Analysis of the frequency of the Doppler signals from the common, internal, and external carotid arteries is useful in determining the degree of obstructive flow in these vessels. Because of their noninvasive quality, such studies are especially useful when the course of arterial disease is followed over time. In addition, a sterile Doppler probe may be used in the operating room to verify patency of a vascular anastomosis and to help assess the immediate effect of a vascular procedure.

Plethysmography measures volume changes. Various-sized sensors are available to measure

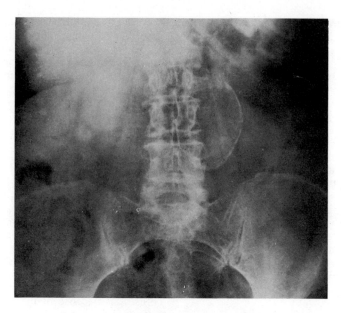

Fig. 32-1. Calcified abdominal aortic aneurysm.

Table 32-1. Diagnostic aids in arterial disease

Diagnostic method	Technique	Results
Plain x-ray studies	Usual	Shows calcification in vessel or aneurysm (Fig. 32-1)
Arteriography	Injection of contrast dye in artery	Shows intraluminal contour and abnormalities of flow (Fig. 32-7)
Ultrasound velocity detector (Doppler)	Listen over the arterial tree to detect flow characteristics	Locates altered flow characteristics; can be used with a blood pressure cuff to accurately measure the arterial pressure at different levels of the extremity
Plethysmography	Gauge placed around extremity: cup placed on eyeball	Additive to Doppler
Ultrasound examination of the abdomen	Noninvasive scan of abdomen	Can measure accurately the size of aneurysms

changes in the volume of the finger, arm, toe, calf, thigh, or penis with the cardiac cycle to quantitate flow or, when used with blood pressure cuffs, to measure pressure. Specially designed suction cups are used with either an air- or fluid-filled system to measure eyeball-volume changes as a reflection of the flow through the internal carotid and ophthalmic arteries.

Contrast angiography most precisely identifies the anatomy of occlusive arterial disease. Newer iodinated agents are relatively risk free, and sophisticated catheter techniques make virtually every artery in the body available for study. Although this invasive technique is uncomfortable, even the cerebrovascular examination has only a 1% morbidity and mortality. Computerized digital subtraction angiography (DSA) is currently clinically used as a screening test in high-risk patients and perhaps as a substitute for conventional arteriography in assessment of certain lesions. The DSA technique may utilize either the intra-arterial or intravenous injection of contrast depending on the indication for examination and the area to be studied. Radionuclide angiography is also of value in assessment of arterial anatomy in patients with a strong history of dye allergy, though the resolution of this technique does not yet rival that of conventional angiography.

TYPES OF ARTERIAL DISEASE
Congenital lesions

Congenital arteriovenous fistulas occur as café-au-lait spots, cirsoid aneurysms, or racemose connections between major arteries and veins. Even though the subcutaneous lesions may be disfiguring, nonoperative therapy is usually indicated initially, since they may disappear spontaneously or regress in size. Excision or irradiation is indicated if venous lakes or multiple arteriovenous fistulas enlarge or produce changes in cardiovascular dynamics. If they are localized, excellent palliation may be afforded by the occlusion of major "feeder vessels" surgically or by embolization. However if there is widespread involvement, amputation is indicated (Fig. 32-2).

Arterial injuries

Both blunt and penetrating trauma can result in any of three major types of injuries to blood vessels: laceration (incision), perforation (ice-pick injury, needle injury after arteriography or cardiac catheterization), or contusion (Fig. 32-3). After complete transection of an artery the ends retract and contract to assist in hemostasis. After partial transection this retraction is impossible and hemorrhage is often greater than with complete transection. Contusion of an artery may injure the intima and promote local thrombosis.

These lesions are usually obvious on examination. However, occasionally even a complete transection is difficult to detect if hemorrhage is arrested by tamponade within a fascial compartment and distal pulses are present because of collateralization. Arterial injury will threaten life or limb if not corrected promptly. Consequently, if there is any question, emergency arteriography is indicated. Hemorrhage must be controlled, blood loss replaced, and in most cases the artery reconstructed. Autogenous tissue (vein grafts, arterial grafts, arterioplasties) is preferred over a synthetic prosthesis because of the threat of infection. An infected graft produces septic emboli, thrombosis, or disruption of the graft with the threat of false aneurysm or exsanguination. The physician should never attribute peripheral ischemia after injury to "arterial spasm"; such patients should have either

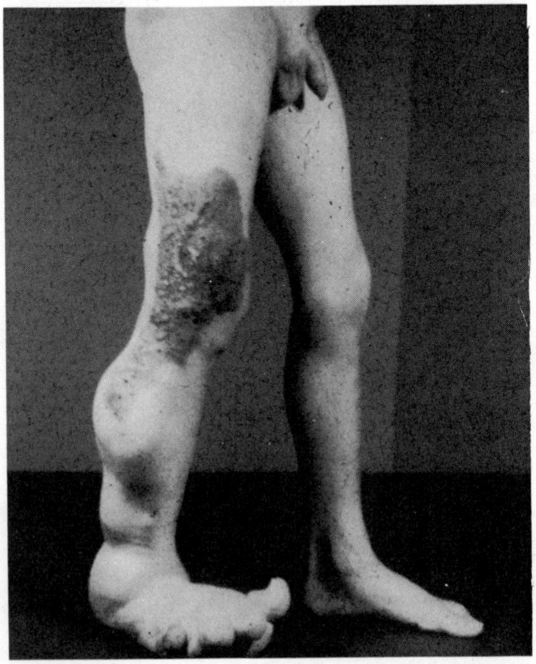

Fig. 32-2. Multiple arteriovenous fistulas in right leg associated with hemolymphangioma. Partial amputation was required.

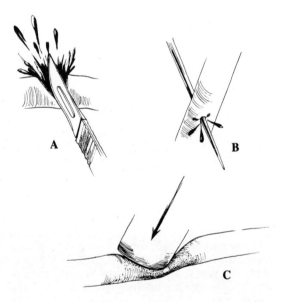

Fig. 32-3. Arterial injuries. **A,** Laceration. **B,** Perforation. **C,** Contusion. *Note:* Partial lacerations usually result in brisk bleeding because severed ends cannot retract. Complete transections permit severed ends to retract; spasm and thrombosis often limit bleeding.

immediate arteriography for diagnosis or emergency exploration for treatment of a suspected arterial injury.

Delayed complications of arterial injury include arterial occlusion with intermittent claudication, rest pain or limb loss, false aneurysm (Fig. 32-4), or traumatic arteriovenous fistulas. False aneurysms have a predilection for sudden expansion and rupture with massive hemorrhage and can often be detected by palpation and auscultation. Traumatic arteriovenous fistulas may become manifest as congestive heart failure (the fistula increases venous return, dilating the cardiac chambers and producing high-output cardiac failure), pulsating veins, or typical bruits, heard over the involved vessels. Resection or ligation of the fistula often with reconstruction of the vascular system is the reparative procedure of choice.

Arterial emboli

Acute arterial occlusion is most commonly caused either by embolization of thrombus or atherosclerotic plaques from more proximally in the cardiovascular system or from in situ thrombosis of previously diseased arteries. Most arterial emboli arise from within the heart. Atrial fibrillation, aortic and mitral valvular disease, recent myocardial infarction with a mural thrombus, or rarely myxomas of the heart are antecedent causes. Another less common source is arteriosclerotic plaques that break off from more proximal arterial walls and embolize. The common sites of embolic obstruction are at the bifurcations of the major vessels: popliteal, femoral, iliac, aortic, and occasionally brachial, carotid, or mesenteric arteries. The lower extremities are the site of approximately 80% of embolic occlusions.

Peripheral arterial emboli appear as an abrupt onset of ischemia. The classical "five *P*'s" of acute arterial occlusion are *p*ain, *p*allor, *p*ulseless, *p*aresthesia, and *p*aralysis. The sudden onset of ischemic pain allows the majority of patients to accurately recount the precise timing of the occlusion. Paresthesia and paralysis are suggestive of limb nonviability and indicate ischemia severe enough to cause nerve or muscle damage. Despite prompt, excellent treatment, morbidity and mortality in this group will be increased because of neuromuscular ischemia, which eventually becomes irreversible.

When the diagnosis of an arterial embolus is made, intravenous heparin is immediately administered (usually in the emergency room). This will not dissolve the embolus but will prevent propagation of the thrombus in the involved vessels.

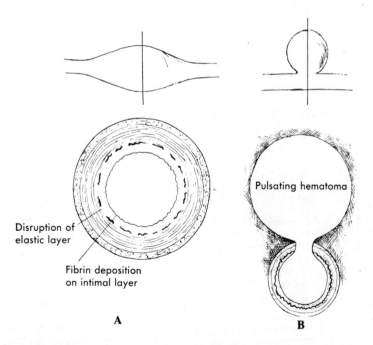

Disruption of
elastic layer

Fibrin deposition
on intimal layer

Pulsating hematoma

A

B

Fig. 32-4. Types of aneurysms in cross section. **A,** True aneurysm. **B,** False aneurysm usually caused by trauma; pulsating hematoma results; intimal layer grows into aneurysm that is covered by clot and later by fibrous tissue.

Embolectomy is performed as soon as possible, preferably within 12 hours. The balloon catheter technique of embolectomy accomplished through a peripheral artery (e.g., an aortic saddle embolus is removed through the femoral arteries) can be done under general, regional, or even local anesthesia. Although delayed embolectomy (duration of occlusion greater than 12 hours) is sometimes successful, it is fraught with lower success rates and with increased mortality in patients with nonviable limbs. The source of the emboli is treated to prevent recurrent embolization (i.e., anticoagulants, valvuloplasty, valve replacement, ventricular aneurysmectomy, or cardioversion). Occlusion of arteriosclerotic vessels may require combining embolectomy with endarterectomy or bypass grafting. In patients with acute occlusions from thrombus, an alternative therapy is the intra-arterial infusion of fibrinolytic agents. However, this treatment is also best performed in the immediate postocclusion period. Thrombolytic therapy must be combined with surgery or transluminal angioplasty in patients with atherosclerotic or other underlying arterial pathosis. Because of the longer time required to reestablish arterial patency, it should not be used in patients with severely threatened limb loss.

Aneurysms

Aneurysms are localized dilatations of arteries. They may be true (containing all three layers of the arterial wall) or false (containing only adventitia) (Table 32-2 and Fig. 32-4). Most aneurysms are atherosclerotic in origin, but a few result from trauma or infection.

The gross pathological condition of aneurysms includes degenerative dilatation with deposition of fibrin and clot within the lumen. Microscopically the tunica intima is thickened with fatty deposits and calcifications and the tunica media is disrupted (Fig. 32-4). Many patients (60% to 70%) are unaware of the pulsating mass unless it occurs in a superficial location, such as the extremities.

Most aneurysms are discovered while still asymptomatic. However with progression they may rupture, thrombose, embolize, or erode into adjacent structures. The diagnosis of aneurysm is usually made by discerning palpation or by plain roentgenograms that show calcification within the wall of the aneurysm (Fig. 32-1). Accurate measurement of the dimensions of the aneurysm is best accomplished with either ultrasound scanning or computerized tomography. Arterial visualization (arteriogram) is not mandatory unless the proximal and distal extent of the aneurysmal dilatation must be known before operation (thoracic aortic aneurysm and aneurysms believed to involve the renal arteries) or the distal arterial tree is of questionable quality (femoral and popliteal aneurysms). Most aortic aneurysms are asymptomatic, but since their rupture is such a threat to life, the treatment of choice is surgical excision and replacement with a

Table 32-2. Aneurysms

Location	Cause	Relative incidence	Treatment	Prognosis
Thoracic aorta	Arteriosclerotic, infection, trauma	Occasional	Medical or surgical (depending on anatomical site and patient)	Fair
Abdominal aorta	Arteriosclerotic	Frequent	Resection	Good
Femoral and popliteal	Arteriosclerotic, trauma, infection	Occasional	Resection or exclusion bypass graft	Good
Carotid	Arteriosclerotic	Rare	Resection	Good
Upper extremities	Trauma, arteriosclerotic, infection	Rare	Resection	Good
Splenic	Arteriosclerotic	Occasional	Resection if symptomatic or in females under 40 years	Good
Renal	Arteriosclerotic	Occasional	Aneurysm resection or nephrectomy, sometimes nonoperative	Good

synthetic prosthesis (Fig. 32-5). All extremity aneurysms should be treated surgically because of the risk of thrombosis or distal embolization, or both. Because the thoracic and suprarenal aorta supply organs that do not tolerate prolonged anoxia (spinal cord, kidneys), aneurysms in these areas may require temporary bypass (with the pump oxygenator, atriofemoral bypass, or tube shunts) during repairs.

Occlusive disease
Lower extremities

Atherosclerosis is the almost universal cause of chronic occlusive disease of the legs. The characteristic pathological features of atherosclerosis are intimal thickening and degeneration. Loss of the endothelial surface with lipid and calcium deposits in the intima are followed by progressive obstruction, which may be partial (stenosis) or complete (occlusion).

Clinically atherosclerosis is characterized by slowly progressive arterial insufficiency. It occurs most commonly in older men but affects both sexes and sometimes emerges as early as the third decade of life. It is common in diabetics, in whom it affects both the larger, surgically accessible arteries and the smaller arteries of the foot and leg.

History. Pain is the most common symptom of arteriosclerosis obliterans. Intermittent claudication, a specific symptom of arterial insufficiency, is a cramping pain in muscles that occurs after a period of exercise and is relieved by a few minutes of rest. This pain is repetitive with precisely the same amount of exercise. Accumulation of acid waste products from anoxic muscle probably causes the pain. Calf claudication means that the obstruction is at or proximal to the popliteal artery, whereas hip claudication indicates aortoiliac disease. Aortoiliac atherosclerosis may produce not only claudication, but also impotence (Leriche's syndrome) (Fig. 32-6).

Pain at rest in the foot occurs from inadequate perfusion in the horizontal position (i.e., sleeping) in the patient with severe occlusive arterial disease. Pain at rest is often alleviated when the foot is placed in a dependent position and must be differentiated from calf cramps from other causes.

Nonoperatively treated intermittent claudicants uncommonly come to amputation, whereas patients exhibiting ischemic pain at rest have a more advanced disease and, unless treated, face a major amputation.

Physical examination. Careful evaluation of the pulses is the most important part of examining a patient with peripheral artery disease. The pulse (arterial pressure) is directly related to the inflow of blood and the resistance to flow. Diminished, absent, or asymmetrical pulses often pinpoint the exact site of arterial obstruction. Auscultation of the pulses may demonstrate a bruit denoting turbulent flow past a stenotic lesion or through an arteriovenous fistula.

Chronic occlusive disease is characterized by skin coolness, atrophic shiny skin, absent hair, and thickened toenails. A later more grave sign is ulceration of the distal extremity. Inadequate perfusion is suggested by slow capillary and venous refilling times. The skin blanches with pressure and the color returns slowly after releasing pressure. In acute obstructions the affected extremity appears suddenly and persistently cadaveric because of the absence of collateralization. Elevation of the

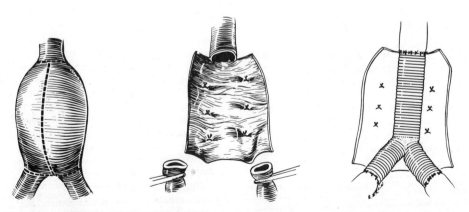

Fig. 32-5. Abdominal aortic aneurysm is incised after proximal and distal control is obtained. Bleeding lumbar arteries are controlled from within aneurysm. Anterior wall of aneurysm is resected, but posterior wall is left intact. Vascular integrity is reestablished with Dacron graft.

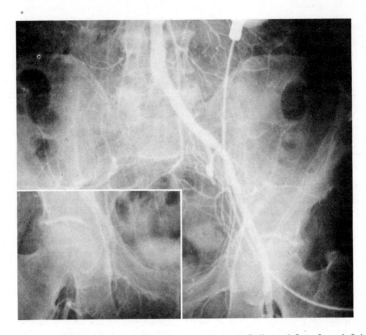

Fig. 32-6. Occlusion of right common and external iliac artery. Collateral flow from left internal iliac system supplies right profunda femoris artery through obturator and gluteal branches of right internal iliac artery.

ischemic extremity produces pallor, and dependency produces cyanosis. This results from the following chain of events: (1) elevation lowers the perfusion pressure, producing pallor; (2) local anoxia and metabolic acidosis result; (3) capillary dilatation occurs, causing (4) slowing of an already inadequate blood flow, and (5) cyanosis with dependency.

The presence of leg complaints, diminished pulses, and deformed, arthritic joints makes a diagnosis difficult. In other patients typical complaints of intermittent claudication will be combined with satisfactory pulses. It is imperative that the physician exercise the problem patient to produce symptoms and reexamine him at that time. Is the pain really calf pain, or is it joint pain? Have the pulses changed? Are the bruits louder? Is the symptomatic foot paler? Many difficult problems can be solved in the astute clinician's office.

Vascular laboratory examination. A normal patient has the same systolic blood pressure in the arm and ankle (ankle/arm $\cong 1$). A reduction in this ratio indicates arterial disease; the more extensive the occlusive disease, the lower the ankle-to-arm ratio. Segmental pressures obtained with either the Doppler technique or plethysmography or analysis of pulse wave velocity contours are used to localize the level(s) of disease. Any abnormalities can be exaggerated with stress (treadmill, inflow occlusion) testing, which decreases pressures and wave amplitudes in the ischemic extremity.

Arteriography. Contrast angiography is required, not to diagnose the level of obstruction (this is done on physical examination and in the vascular laboratory examination) but to aid in the planning of surgical intervention. All methods give excellent details and have low morbidity ratios. Translumbar aortography is always associated with some bleeding, but transfusion is a rarity. Thrombotic and embolic complications are more common after the transfemoral approach. Bleeding after the transaxillary approach may lead to brachial plexus injury from compression unless the hematoma is promptly recognized and drained. Computerized digital subtraction angiographic techniques following intra-arterial dye injection can often enhance the visualization of the smaller more distal arteries, which occasionally may not be adequately seen with conventional angiography.

Extracranial cerebrovascular disease

Although arteriosclerosis may involve any neck vessel, typically it causes a localized stenosis at the origin of the internal carotid artery. Symptoms arising from this lesion may result from embolization of atherosclerotic debris or platelet emboli

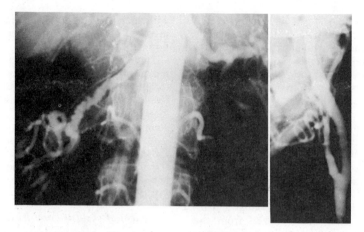

Fig. 32-7. These arteriograms represent fibromuscular hyperplasia. Notice "chain of lakes" present in right renal artery and septa present in carotid artery.

distally, or from low flow past the lesion. In younger female patients fibromuscular hyperplasia may involve a major portion of the extracranial internal carotid artery. Microscopically in this lesion the media is alternately thinned (areas of aneurysmal dilatation) and thickened (areas of stenosis), producing a "chain of lakes" arteriographically (Fig. 32-7); this is the same picture seen in similar renal artery lesions. Fibromuscular hyperplasia is frequently associated with intracranial aneurysms.

Patients with cerebrovascular disease may be classified into at least three neurological categories: (1) a transient ischemic attack (TIA) is a neurological deficit that lasts less than 24 hours; (2) a reversible ischemic neurological deficit (RIND) lasts longer than 24 hours but neurological recovery is complete; (3) a permanent neurological deficit (either an acute or chronic stroke) may occur.

The patient's neurological complaints and findings can be further categorized into hemispheric, vertebrobasilar, and nonspecific, as follows:

Hemispheric
Contralateral motor and sensory
Ipsilateral visual symptoms—amaurosis fugax
Dysphasias
Vertebrobasilar
Vertigo (true)
Ataxia
Diplopia
Bilateral visual aberrations
Shifting paresis or paresthesias
Drop attacks
Dysarthrias
Syncope

Nonspecific
Dizziness
Light-headedness
Decreased mentation
Headache
Confusion
Personality change
Tinnitis
Decreased visual acuity
Seizures

Occlusive disease of the subclavian artery proximal to the vertebral artery can lead to the subclavian steal syndrome. Classically exercise of the ipsilateral arm leads to a reversal or exacerbation of reversed flow in the ipsilateral vertebral artery as blood from the circle of Willis and contralateral vertebral artery is redirected from the brain to the ischemic arm, resulting in neurological symptoms.

On physical examination diminished carotid or subclavian pulses with overlying bruits may be found. It is important to differentiate these more distal carotid bruits from murmurs transmitted to the neck from aortic valvular disease. The blood pressure in each arm must also be compared.

Vascular laboratory examination. Periorbital Doppler examination detecting flow in the supraorbital artery should normally be unaffected by superficial temporal or facial artery compression and be reduced by common carotid artery compression. An abnormal examination indicates collateral blood flow because of at least 75% stenosis of the internal carotid artery. A carotid phonoangiogram (CPA) is a pictorial display of the neck bruit. Oculoplethysmography (OPG) compares the volume expansion of each eyeball. The globe on the side of a carotid stenosis will expand at a slower rate than the contralateral globe supplied by normal arteries. The Gee modification of the OPG indirectly measures ophthalmic artery pressure, which reflects internal carotid artery pressure. Frequency analysis of Doppler-detected carotid velocity aids in quantitating the degree of stenosis. Real-time B-mode ultrasound can noninvasively provide anatomic information. The extent of noninvasive testing and its exact interplay with contrast studies has not been definitely decided and varies between institutions.

Arteriography and treatment modalities. Transfemoral cerebral angiography is preferred over direct carotid punctures. The extracranial and intracranial arteries must be visualized from the aortic arch for diagnosis of all lesions and formulation of a comprehensive treatment plan that may include anticoagulation therapy, surgery on the extracranial carotid or vertebral arteries, or extracranial-intracranial bypass. Most patients with acute strokes are not immediate operative candidates, in contrast to patients with transient ischemic attacks. Patients who are asymptomatic but have a severe stenosis and access to a reliable surgeon are now frequently being surgically treated to lessen the chance of stroke. Stenosis in the internal carotid artery is typically suited for endarterectomy. The details of the operative procedure (use of an internal shunt, patch angioplasty, and hypercapnia or hypocapnia) remain controversial, but the reported results are excellent with a variety of techniques (combined mortality and morbidity of 1% to 3%).

Visceral arterial stenosis

Atherosclerotic stenosis of any or all of the visceral arteries (celiac axis, superior mesenteric artery, inferior mesenteric artery) may cause symptoms, as may external compression (by the median arcuate ligament). See Chapters 21 and 24 and Table 32-3 for clinical details.

Renal artery stenosis

Renal artery stenosis is becoming more commonly recognized as a cause of arterial hypertension. In patients in their fifth to seventh decades, atherosclerosis is the most common cause, but in younger women fibromuscular hyperplasia is more common. Rarely renal artery aneurysms cause hypertension.

On physical examination an abdominal bruit is heard in a hypertensive patient. Intravenous pyelography reveals a small kidney with delayed function. Renal vein renin is elevated on the affected side and often suppressed on the contralateral side. Split renal-function studies show a diminished urine volume and sodium concentration with increased creatinine concentration from the involved kidney. The arteriogram reveals the nature and extent of the lesion.

Surgical treatment is directed toward the removal or bypass of the responsible lesion. More rarely nephrectomy is required for removal of a Goldblatt kidney. Percutaneous passage of a balloon catheter for dilatation of the responsible stenosis is an alternative therapy in some cases and has its best results in fibromuscular hyperplasia. Indications for surgical therapy or percutaneous transluminal angioplasty are uncontrollable hypertension and preservation of deteriorating renal function.

Treatment of occlusive arterial disease

There are three levels of treatment in vascular disease: (1) maintenance of life, (2) maintenance of limb form, and (3) maintenance or restoration of limb function. The vascular surgeon often resects an abdominal aortic aneurysm in a poor-risk patient, since this is a life-threatening lesion. A reconstructive procedure is indicated in less than ideal situations if limb loss is imminent. Operations designed to alleviate intermittent claudication alone must be accomplished by low-risk surgery.

Direct reparative arterial surgery is possible for localized segments of occlusive disease in medium to large arteries. When arterial disease is diffuse or involves small arteries, the only treatment option is nonoperative therapy or sympathectomy or amputation.

Reconstructive arterial surgery. Reconstructive arterial surgery depends on the following fundamentals: (1) an accessible lesion is responsible for the patient's symptoms or is life or limb threatening, (2) there is adequate inflow and outflow of the proposed reconstructed segment (a superficial femoral artery stenosis is not bypassed with significant aortoiliac obstructive disease), and (3) the choice of operation must be tailored to the patient (a subcutaneous axillofemoral artery bypass is done in an extremely poor-risk patient).

There are several methods of arterial revascularization, as follows.

Endarterectomy. The diseased intima is dissected from the media by the open (Fig. 32-8) or closed (loop endarterectomy) method. This is applicable in the aortoiliac system, the proximal profunda femoris artery (profundoplasty, which is often done along with a patch angioplasty), and carotid bifurcation and visceral arteries, but this method has met with high recurrence rates in the superficial femoral and more distal arteries of the lower extremities.

Bypass graft. A graft (either a prosthesis or autogenous tissue) shunts blood around the diseased segment (Fig. 32-9). Dacron and poly-

Table 32-3. Chronic occlusive disease

Site	Clinical findings	Diagnosis	Treatment	Comment
Aortoiliac	Men, fifth to seventh decade, pain, intermittent claudication, impotence	Decreased or absent femoral and distal pulses, bruits over stenotic arteries; aortography shows diseased areas	Thromboendarterectomy, bypass graft, sympathectomy, amputation	Results good if outflow adequate
Femoral	Men, fifth to seventh decade, intermittent claudication, skin changes	Decreased or absent distal pulses, evidence of ischemia in foot or leg	Bypass graft, patch angioplasty, sympathectomy, amputation	Results good if outflow adequate
Renal	Hypertension, males and females	Bruit over abdomen, renal arteriogram, intravenous pyelogram—small kidney with delayed function, differential renal function, renal vein renin assay	Bypass graft, endarterectomy, patch angioplasty, nephrectomy	Good results if case selection is strict, saves kidney function
Cerebrovascular	Hemispheric vertebrobasilar, nonspecific	Carotid pulse decrease, bruit over carotid, arteriography shows stenosis or ulceration	Endarterectomy	Good results
Celiomesenteric	Visceral angina: pain after eating, weight loss, diarrhea (constipation), abdominal bruit, infarction	Angiography, difficult diagnosis in acute occlusion	Bypass graft, endarterectomy, bowel resection	Good results if done before infarction
Upper extremities	Claudication, skin changes, sensory disturbances	Absent pulses, bruit over involved vessel, arteriogram	Endarterectomy, bypass vein graft, resection of first rib, cervical sympathectomy, amputation	Fair

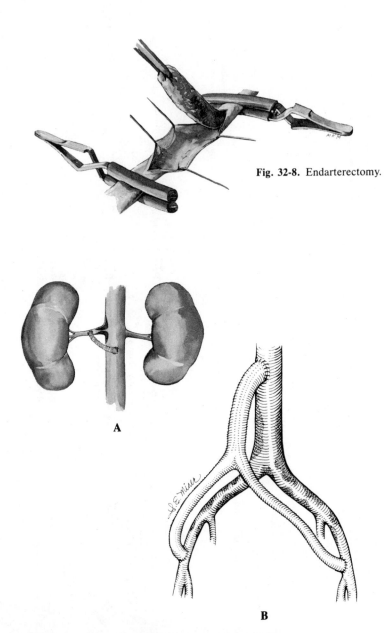

Fig. 32-8. Endarterectomy.

A

B

Fig. 32-9. Bypass grafts. **A,** Bypass of stenotic renal artery. **B,** Aortofemoral bypass of iliac atherosclerosis.

tetrafluoroethylene (PTFE) aortofemoral bypass grafts have largely supplanted endarterectomy as the treatment of choice for aortoiliac atherosclerosis. Excellent long-term results are expected even in patients with a distal superficial femoral artery stenosis, provided that the deep femoral artery is patent. Reversed autogenous vein or in situ saphenous vein after valve obliteration are the preferred grafting techniques in femoral-popliteal-tibial disease, but synthetic material can be used in patients without suitable or available veins.

Replacement grafts. The diseased arterial segment is resected and replaced by a prosthesis or autogenous tissue (usually vein but sometimes another artery).

Patch graft (angioplasty). Either autogenous tissue or prosthetic material is used to enlarge stenotic arteries (Fig. 32-10).

Percutaneous transluminal angioplasty. In this newer technique a balloon-tipped catheter is percutaneously passed under fluoroscopic control to a stenotic arterial segment, and the balloon is inflated to dilate the vessel lumen. This method has produced good early success rates in short stenosis of the renal, aortoiliac, and femoral arteries with less success more distally in the lower extremities. It provides an alternative to open surgical intervention for patients with suitable highly localized obstructive disease, particularly those considered to be high anesthesia risks.

Nonoperative treatment of ischemic lower extremity. If the arteriosclerosis is diffuse, direct surgical correction is impossible. Nonoperative treatment involves the following:

1. Stop smoking!
2. Avoid trauma: corns and calluses should not be cut.
3. Avoid pressure by using soft mattresses and adequate-sized shoes.
4. The feet are washed carefully and dried daily, followed by bland ointments.

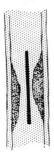 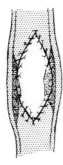

Fig. 32-10. Vein patch graft.

5. We believe that vasodilator drugs have little value in generalized arteriosclerosis. (Theoretically, they dilate only pliable arteries and any pliable small arteries in ischemic beds are already vasodilated from high levels of tissue carbon dioxide.)
6. Ulcers are cleaned by sharp débridement and intermittent saline soaks, and grafted with skin, if possible.
7. Local medications are contraindicated, since the ischemic skin is sensitive to chemical agents; antibiotic ointments are used only against specific organisms resistant to other treatment.
8. Exercise daily and frequently to tolerance to develop collateral circulation optimally.

Sympathectomy. Destruction of the sympathetic ganglia in the lumbar chain may dilate small and medium-sized arteries. If sufficient collateral arterial supply exists around obstructed arterial segments, sympathectomy may somewhat improve a marginal blood supply primarily to the skin. The duration of its effectiveness and its value in improving the blood supply to the muscles are controversial. Usually at least one of the first lumbar ganglia is preserved in males to prevent impotence. Plethysmography and skin temperatures before and after sympathetic nerve block may help predict the efficacy of sympathectomy, but a negative result does not necessarily rule out a positive clinical result. Sympathectomy is less commonly of value in diabetics in whom autosympathectomy is commonplace. Sympathectomy alone will rarely heal large ulcerations or alleviate rest pain and is seldom recommended in modern practice.

Amputation. Gangrene, advancing infection, recalcitrant ulceration and unremitting pain at rest necessitate amputation. Amputation is a last resort after all nonoperative and direct attempts to treat ischemia have failed. The level of amputation depends on a blood supply sufficient to heal the incision. Despite an absent popliteal pulse, a below-knee stump can often thrive on collateral circulation. The adequacy of blood supply to the proposed level of amputation is estimated by physical examination and by vascular laboratory examination. If pressure is below 50 mm. Hg at the ankle, local digital or forefoot amputations are usually doomed to failure. Excellent results with below-knee amputations and early physical rehabilitation on prostheses are being obtained by use of plaster dressings postoperatively.

The effects of amputation need not be disastrous. With a proper prosthesis the patient may reenter society in a productive role. It is the surgeon's duty to encourage this goal.

Inflammatory and miscellaneous àrterial diseases
Buerger's disease

Buerger's disease is an inflammatory disease of unknown cause that involves both arteries and veins. Also known as thromboangiitis obliterans, it was previously frequently diagnosed. However, newer diagnostic modalities have shown that its true incidence is quite rare. It usually occurs in young men (onset at 20 to 35 years) and involves small and medium-sized arteries (posterior tibial, anterior tibial) in the lower extremities. Besides sex and age, tobacco is the only other important etiological factor.

Pathologically the arteries show an early panarteritis with chronic inflammatory cells and a relatively diffuse scattering of multinucleated giant cells. The internal elastic lamina remains intact. Fibrosis of the entire artery with small discontinuous recanalized channels occurs in late stages.

Clinical examination. Lower extremity pain from inflammation and ischemia, with appearance of small segments of migratory superficial phlebitis, keynotes the symptoms. Migrating phlebitis (with no other cause) is suggestive of Buerger's disease. Raynaud's phenomenon is common. Arteriography usually shows sharply demarcated obstruction of involved arteries, with the remaining arteries appearing suprisingly normal.

The course of this disease is variable. In some it smolders for years with minor sequelae. In contrast, we have been forced to amputate the lower extremity in a 19-year-old man after less than 6 months of symptoms.

Treatment. Abstinence from tobacco is probably the most important factor. Bed rest with protection of the extremity is the only other available treatment measure. Antibiotics are used only to treat secondary infections. Sympathectomy may delay or prevent amputation after subsidence of the acute process. Because of its distal nature, direct surgical revascularization procedures are often impossible but must be considered. Amputation is done only after all other treatment has failed.

Angiospastic diseases

The blood flow to surface areas of the body constantly fluctuates in response to tissue demands, temperature variations, and emotions. Vasomotor control is greater in the hand and feet, and these areas consequently reflect, most noticeably, abnormalities in vasomotor response. With exaggerated response the skin becomes white (with spasm), cyanotic (from anoxic capillary dilatation), and then intensely red (from reactive hyperemia) before becoming normal.

Raynaud's phenomenon, an intermittent, cold-induced peripheral ischemia, generally involves the upper extremities. It may become chronic with eventual loss of tissue. The phenomenon is associated with the following numerous conditions, with symptoms fluctuating with progression of the underlying disease:

1. Obliterative arterial disease
   a. Arteriosclerosis
   b. Buerger's disease
   c. Arterial emboli
2. Trauma
   a. After injury or operation
   b. Occupational
      (1) Pneumatic hammer operators
      (2) Pianists, typists
3. Neurogenic
   a. Thoracic outlet syndromes
   b. Primary neurological diseases
4. Hematological diseases
   a. Cold agglutinins
   b. Cryoglobulins
   c. Hemoglobinopathies (such as sickle cell anemia)
   d. Polycythemia
5. Systemic diseases
   a. Scleroderma
   b. Systemic lupus erythematosus
   c. Polyarteritis nodosa
   d. Rheumatoid arthritis
   e. Malignant disease
6. Drugs
   a. Ergots
   b. Heavy metals

If no underlying conditions causing Raynaud's phenomenon become evident, a diagnosis of Raynaud's disease is made. These patients, usually young females (less than 40 years old), develop numbness or a burning pain in the fingers and hands with the typical color changes on exposure to cold. These changes are bilateral and tissue loss is limited.

A modified Allen's test helps in the diagnosis of vascular disease distal to the wrist. Pressure is maintained over the radial and ulnar arteries by the examiner while the patient clenches his fist to empty blood from the hand. Release of either artery should produce a rapidly spreading erythema of the dependent hand and fingers, thereby demonstrating patency of that artery. Release of an occluded (radial or ulnar) artery will not produce erythema. If a distal or palmar artery is diseased, the portion of the hand it supplies will become erythematous later than the rest of the hand.

The diagnosis of Raynaud's disease is made clinically. Arteriography is not indicated unless the physical examination indicates major proximal artery disease. All efforts are made to diagnose an underlying condition.

Treatment includes avoiding cold and wearing warm clothing. Vasodilators and pharmacological sympathectomy are occasionally beneficial. Surgical sympathectomy is reserved for patients with tissue necrosis but is usually only temporarily helpful. Recent trials using the calcium channel–blocking agent nifedipine have been promising.

Vasculogenic impotence

Impotence has numerous vasculogenic, neurogenic, and psychogenic causes, and it has long been recognized as a symptom of aortoiliac occlusive disease (Leriche's syndrome). Newer diagnostic modalities have identified many cases secondary to disease within the hypogastric arteries and its branches supplying the penis. The diagnosis of vasculogenic impotence rests on noninvasive penile plethysmography and Doppler ultrasound penile artery pressures along with arteriography. Other psychogenic and neurogenic causes must be carefully considered. Direct arterial reconstructive procedures on select patients are currently producing good results.

Erythromelalgia

Erythromelalgia is a rare condition of unknown cause. Clinically the patient complains of a red, warm, painful area on the lower extremities precipitated by excess heat and dependency. Sympathectomy is contraindicated in these patients.

Thoracic outlet syndrome

The thoracic outlet syndrome is a clinical syndrome of pain in the arm and numbness and sometimes coldness in the hand, secondary to compression of the neurovascular bundle as it leaves the chest. The most frequent symptom patterns refer to ulnar or median nerve involvement, but vascular compression often accompanies the brachial plexus compression. The neurovascular bundle is entrapped between a cervical rib and the first rib, the scalenus anticus muscle and the first rib, or the clavicle and the first rib. Clinically, hyperabduction of the shoulders (military position) or tensing the scalenus anticus muscle (Adson maneuver) will diminish the radial pulse. This clinical test will be abnormal in at least half the population without thoracic outlet syndrome. Nerve compression, either at the vertebral bodies or distal to the shoulder (i.e., carpal tunnel syndrome) must be differentiated. Treatment is the surgical removal (either transaxillary, transpleural,

or transcervical) of the first rib beneath the neurovascular bundle. The surgeon must be aware that a poststenotic dilatation (aneurysm) may harbor thrombus leading to distal embolization. If present, this is repaired in order to ensure a successful therapeutic effort.

Arteritis

Although Buerger's disease is the most widely discussed inflammation of the arteries, there are numerous other causes of arteritis, as listed below:

Infective
  Pyogenic arteritis
  Fungal arteritis
  Tuberculous arteritis
  Mycotic aneurysm
  Syphilitic arteritis
Noninfective
  Systemic lupus erythematosus
  Polyarteritis nodosa
  Rheumatoid arthritis
  Pulseless disease (Takayasu's arteritis)
  Necrotizing arteritis after coarctation repair
  Buerger's disease

Specific infections are caused by direct bacterial invasion (i.e., from the retroperitoneal lymph nodes into the aorta), infection occurring after trauma or surgery, and septic emboli.

The causes of noninfective arteritis are many. Most are manifestations of a "collagen vascular disease." The necrotizing arteritis that occasionally complicates successful repair of an aortic coarctation is allegedly secondary to mechanical stretching of the artery. Giant cell (temporal) arteritis causes headaches and visual disturbances. Physical examination discloses a tender, enlarged superficial temporal artery. Pulseless disease (Takayasu's disease, aortic arch syndrome) occurs in young women. Symptoms and findings depend on which arteries of the aortic arch are involved. Pathologically, the artery is thickened with a panarteritis, degeneration of the elastic fibers, and round cell infiltrations in all layers.

Specific infective arteritis responds to appropriate antibiotic determined by cultures. Surgical therapy is reserved for resistant cases, complications, or mycotic aneurysms. Autogenous tissue is employed rather than synthetic material. Treatment (usually steroids) of a noninfective arteritis is directed toward the underlying disease. Steroids have also successfully ameliorated pulseless disease and temporal arteritis. Reserpine improves the necrotizing arteritis that sometimes occurs after repair of aortic coarctation.

33
Peripheral Veins

William H. Baker
Howard P. Greisler
Robert T. Soper

Veins return blood to the heart from the vast capillary system, and in contrast to their arterial counterparts, flow rates are low and intermittent. Physiologically the veins return blood to the right side of the heart so that the cardiac output of the right and left ventricles is equal. Venous pathological conditions, however, rarely interfere significantly with the filling pressure of the right heart but clinically cause increased venous pressure distal to the point of the pathological entity. Increased peripheral venous pressure increases the egress of fluid out of the capillary bed causing clinical edema and poor nutrition of the limb. Additionally, emboli within the venous system may travel through the right side of the heart to the pulmonary tree and be associated with sudden death. This chapter deals with the prevention, recognition, and treatment of these problems.

ANATOMY

Since most venous surgical diseases involve the lower extremities, the discussion of venous anatomy is limited to these members. The normal venous drainage of the lower extremity includes (1) a *superficial* network of veins traveling in the subcutaneous areolar tissue above the deep fascia of the leg and (2) the *deep* venous system, which lies among the muscle groups in the lower extremity deep to the fascia.

Normally the superficial veins carry approximately 10% of the venous return from the legs, with deep veins carrying the rest. These two systems are interconnected segmentally by per-

forating or communicating channels, with flow normally being from superficial to deep.

The normal direction of flow in both the superficial and deep venous systems is always from peripheral to central and from higher pressure to lower pressure areas.

The propulsive force generated by the left ventricles is mostly dissipated through the arterial and capillary systems, leaving inadequate pressure in the distal veins to overcome gravity in returning blood to the heart in the standing position. This problem is normally overcome by the milking action of the muscles, which generates flow in the deep system in the legs, and by humoral and sympathetic stimuli as well. There are several unidirectional bicuspid valves in both the superficial and deep set of veins as well as in the communicating (perforating) veins. When competent, the valves prevent retrograde flow with its resultant elevation of tissue pressure distally (Fig. 33-1, *A*).

The *greater* and *lesser saphenous veins* form the superficial set of veins of the lower extremity. The greater saphenous vein arises at the dorsal venous arch of the foot and ascends anterior to the medial malleolus, passing anteromedially up the thigh to empty into the deep venous system (the *common femoral vein*) in the groin via a fascial aperture known as the *fossa ovalis*. The greater saphenous system drains blood from the skin and subcutaneous tissues of the entire circumference of the thigh and the medial and anterior aspect of the leg and foot. The other component of the superficial

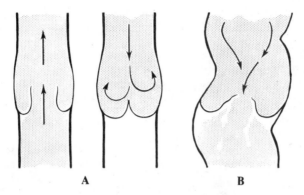

Fig. 33-1. A, Competent vein valve opens to allow forward blood flow but closes snugly to prevent retrograde flow. **B,** Incompetent vein valve cusps cannot close; retrograde flow of blood results.

saphenous system (the lesser saphenous vein) begins behind the external malleolus and ascends posterolaterally in the calf to empty into the deep system (the popliteal vein) in the upper portion of the popliteal space. The physiologically more important deep set of veins are often paired with and run along the like-named arteries.

DEEP VENOUS THROMBOSIS (DVT)

Thrombosis of the deep veins of the lower extremity is a debilitating, sometimes lethal entity. Phlebothrombosis, an older descriptive term, implies less inflammation than thrombophlebitis, but this differentiation is moot. In general, stasis in the veins of the calf or stasis behind any valve cusp leads to thrombus formation, which then propagates proximally into the tibial, popliteal, or larger veins. Virchow's triad of stasis, endothelial injury, and hypercoagulability is still considered central in the pathogenesis of deep venous thrombosis with platelets in sluggish blood adhering to subendothelial tissue. Initially the thrombus is almost free floating but soon attaches to the adjacent vein wall. The thrombus often propagates proximally until the next major tributary where blood flow increases. If vein wall and coagulation conditions permit, the thrombus may continue to propagate and occlude the tributary as well. If a portion of the thrombus becomes detached, pulmonary embolism is the result. Pulmonary emboli from the tibial veins are small enough to be well tolerated by most patients, but thrombus from the popliteal or large veins may produce sudden right-sided heart failure and death. Eventually the DVT may be cleared by the body's thrombinolysins, but scarred valves or obstructed, fibrotic veins are often sequelae. DVT is associated with reduced blood flow and inactivity as in the postoperative state, obesity, age greater

than 60 years, malignancy, trauma, elevated estrogen levels secondary to birth control pills or pregnancy, ulcerative colitis, and a previous history of deep venous thrombosis and varicose veins.

Signs and symptoms. The classical patient with acute deep venous thrombosis has calf tenderness and edema. Dorsiflexion of the foot (Homans' or dorsiflexion sign) produces calf pain, and a palpable cord may be present in the popliteal space. As the thrombus progresses proximally and venous obstruction is increased, the entire lower extremity becomes painful, edematous, and pale (phlegmasia alba dolens).

With further progression and arterial compromise from tissue compression, the limb takes on a bluish hue (phlegmasia cerulea dolens). Massive thrombosis leading to venous gangrene is fortunately rare (Fig. 33-2).

These classical findings are present in approximately 50% of the patients. That is, at least half of the patients with some element of deep venous thrombosis will be entirely asymptomatic, whereas half of the patients with calf pain or swelling may not have deep venous thrombosis. Prophylactic treatment is therefore advocated in high-risk patients. However, any patient suspected of having deep venous thrombosis requires a more elaborate work-up before long-term, potentially dangerous anticoagulation is prescribed.

The differential diagnosis of deep venous thrombosis includes superficial thrombophlebitis; ailments of the knee and in particular ruptured Baker's cysts; spontaneous or trauma-related rupture of the muscles of the calf (especially the plantaris muscles), which produces sudden pain in the calf and is followed some days later by ecchymosis of the calf; acute arterial occlusion that may produce pain and blanching, but swelling is rare

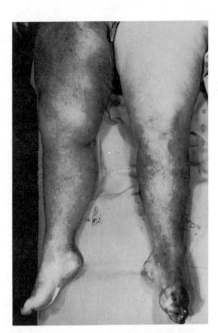

Fig. 33-2. Bilateral phlegmasia cerulea dolens. Notice swelling and mottling of both legs and necrosis of skin of left foot.

and of course the absence of pulses should be an excellent clue; and edema from any cause (i.e., congestive heart failure, etc.).

Diagnosis. When carefully performed, noninvasive laboratory studies can allow accurate diagnosis of acute iliofemoral vein thrombosis in greater than 90% of affected patients. *Doppler ultrasound* detects flow in the major veins. When one is listening over any vein, compression distally in the extremity should produce a proximal rush of blood past the probe. Proximal compression should obliterate the flow unless there are incompetent valves between the compressing hand and the listening probe. Release of the proximal compression produces a release augmentation of flow beneath the probe. These maneuvers can be used to test the venous sounds at the ankle, behind the knee, in the midthigh, and over the common femoral vein in the groin. Although the accuracy of the test varies, 90% accuracy can be expected in good laboratories.

A *plethysmograph* measures volume; i.e., a gauge placed around the calf measures the volume of the calf. When a blood pressure cuff placed proximally is inflated to between arterial and venous pressures, the calf plethysmograph records a volume increase (venous capacitance). When the cuff is suddenly deflated, blood flows from the calf and the calf volume is thereby reduced. The rate of volume change is calculated in terms of venous outflow. The overall results parallel those of the Doppler ultrasound, with both tests less accurate in diagnosing DVT of the calf than in finding more proximal disease.

[125]I-labeled fibrinogen is injected intravenously, and both legs are scanned hours and days later. Since active ongoing thrombosis incorporates fibrinogen at the site of thrombosis, any increase in radioactivity indicates that thrombosis is occurring. This test is extremely accurate for diagnosing small, less clinically important calf vein thrombosis but is less accurate for the upper thigh and pelvis because of background radiation from the bones and bladder. We do not use the test to diagnose acute DVT because there is a waiting period (hours and sometimes days) between injection and the time of results. This is an excellent tool for studying the pathophysiology of deep venous thrombosis, prospectively monitoring high-risk patients, assessing therapeutic measures, and differentiating acute and chronic venous disease.

Isotope venography requires injection of an isotope into the dorsum of the foot and observation of its course up the leg with a scanning device. It is not accurate in the diagnosis of calf vein thrombosis, but it allows reliable diagnosis of thrombosis of the veins of the thigh and pelvis.

Contrast venography is the "gold standard" of venous diagnosis. Iodinated contrast material is injected into a foot vein with the patient in a reverse Trendelenburg position. All the veins of the deep and superficial system should become visualized. When the contrast medium reaches the groin, the legs are quickly elevated to fill the veins of the pelvis. A partially occluding thrombus will be outlined by the contrast material (Fig. 33-3), whereas no contrast medium will be seen in totally occluded veins, i.e., only collateral channels will be visualized.

A patient suspected of having deep venous thrombosis should have this diagnosis confirmed by one of the previously mentioned tests (Table 33-1). If the testing procedures are necessarily delayed, treatment is started immediately to prevent the complications of pulmonary embolism. However, diagnostic confirmation is always obtained before treatment is continued on a long-term basis to avoid anticoagulating patients who have complaints from other causes. If one of the noninvasive tests is nondiagnostic or does not correlate well with the clinical picture, contrast venography is obtained.

Treatment. The treatment of deep venous thrombosis is anticoagulation. An initial dose of between

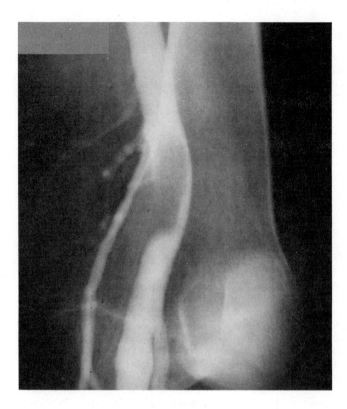

Fig. 33-3. Contrast venogram showing popliteal vein thrombosis.

Table 33-1. Diagnosis of deep venous thrombosis

| | Sensitivity | | |
Method	Calf	Thigh	Pelvis
History and physical examination	±	±	±
Doppler ultrasound	±	+	+
Plethysmograph	±	+	+
^{125}I fibrinogen scan	+	±	−
Radionuclide venogram	−	+	+
Contrast venogram	+	+	+

5,000 and 10,000 units of heparin is given intravenously followed by 1,000 to 2,000 units hourly on a continuous basis using an infusion pump. The exact dose of heparin is that which maintains the partial thromboplastin time (PTT) between 60 and 80 seconds. Either the activated partial thromboplastin time (APTT) or the activated coagulation time (ACT) can also be used to monitor heparin dosage. Continuous intravenous heparin has an advantage over intermittent heparin in that there are no wide swings of the measured clotting times and so bleeding complications are kept at a minimum. Intermittent subcutaneous heparin does not ordinarily achieve adequate levels of anticoagulation, and intramuscular heparin may produce significant bleeding complications. The heparin itself is not considered to be a thrombolytic agent, but it protects against the propagation of thrombus, thus reducing the risk from pulmonary embolism. The patient usually requires bed rest for as long as the leg is symptomatic. Ambulation is then cautiously begun with the leg supported in elastic bandages or stockings.

Warfarin (Coumadin) is overlapped with heparin for 5 to 7 days and continued for 3 to 6 months to protect against late pulmonary embolism. Thrombolytic therapy for massive acute iliofemoral DVT can be of value in select cases, but bleeding complications are high, and this therapy should be used only with extreme caution. It has produced good results in some difficult cases of phlegmasia cerulea dolens.

The surgical extraction of venous thrombi is rarely performed. This operation is reserved for those patients who have threatened limb loss and who do not respond immediately to heparin therapy. Past published series have shown that the incidence of rethrombosis is high and, in addition, the late results of surgery are not superior.

Interruption of the inferior vena cava (IVC) to prevent pulmonary embolism is indicated in the patient who has recurrent pulmonary embolism on therapy or who has an absolute contraindication to anticoagulation (recent gastrointestinal bleeding or intracranial hemorrhage). The IVC may be approached retroperitoneally through a flank or subcostal incision. The transperitoneal approach has the advantage of allowing ligation of the left ovarian vein in female patients. The ligature is placed directly beneath the renal vein so that there is no blind cul-de-sac in which a thrombus may form between the ligature and the renal veins. In ill patients either a balloon or a filter is inserted under local anesthesia through the jugular vein into the IVC under fluoroscopic control. Newer filters have a lower incidence of venous stasis complications in the lower extremity because they are designed to not totally occlude caval flow. They have the disadvantage of not interrupting the left ovarian vein through which pelvic vein thrombi can travel.

Prophylaxis. Prevention of DVT in hospitalized patients is currently in a state of flux. Early postoperative ambulation reduces stasis, as do newer intermittent calf compression devices, which also appear to activate the fibrinolytic system. Elastic stockings increase femoral vein velocity flow, but their clinical value is debated. Low-dose heparin administered subcutaneously (5000 units per 12 hours) has been shown to reduce DVT, pulmonary embolism, and death in general surgical patients. This effect is based upon heparin's ability to activate antithrombin III, an effect not detected by partial thromboplastin time determinations. No elevation of the partial thromboplastin time is desired. However, some reports have indicated increased operation transfusion requirements in patients receiving heparin prophylaxis. High-risk patients should, however, be considered for perioperative intermittent calf compression devices or low-dose heparin therapy and should be closely monitored for DVT with noninvasive studies to avoid the grave complications of pulmonary emboli.

SUPERFICIAL THROMBOPHLEBITIS

Thrombosis and inflammation involving the superficial veins immediately underneath the skin is a very troublesome but not medically serious disorder in most patients. Pulmonary embolism and leg ulceration are distinctly unusual from isolated superficial thrombophlebitis. The involved vein is tender, has overlying erythema, and may form a palpable cord. Lymphangitis mimics superficial thrombophlebitis, but the patient's temperature is usually elevated and a site of distal infection is evident.

Superficial thrombophlebitis may be associated with a deep venous thrombosis; thus these patients are noninvasively evaluated to rule out DVT. Treatment is symptomatic and consists of bed rest, heat, and analgesics including aspirin. Phenylbutazone is reserved for refractory patients. In recurrent or resistant cases, warfarin (Coumadin) anticoagulation or surgical excision and ligation of the involved veins may be indicated. If the thrombophlebitis is septic in origin (associated with prolonged intravenous cannulation, etc.), excision of the infected vein is required.

VARICOSE VEINS

Primary varicosities form without any evidence of prior deep venous thrombosis. A specific cause in these patients is often difficult to pinpoint, but in about 40% of the patients there is a family history of varicose veins, often with the onset early in adult life. Varicose veins have a pronounced female sex incidence (2 or 3:1), presumably related to the smooth muscle–relaxing effect of female sex hormones manifest by cyclic dilatation of veins and increase in tissue fluids premenstrually. Commonly, pregnancy is associated with the onset of worsening of varicose veins. Perhaps the upright position of *Homo sapiens* is important.

Patients with *secondary* varicosities have had a prior episode of deep venous thrombosis, which either has destroyed valvular competency or has created venous obstruction. Incompetent deep veins lead to a reflux of blood pedally with the resultant dilatation of distal veins, which itself causes valvular incompetence, setting up a vicious cycle. Patients with primary and secondary varicosities are differentiated by history, by the previously mentioned noninvasive tests, and by the Trendelenburg test (Figs. 33-4 and 33-5). With the leg elevated and the veins emptied, digital pressure or a tourniquet is placed over the saphenofemoral junction. The leg is quickly placed in the dependent position. No filling of the varicosities is seen if the communicating or perforating veins are competent. Rapid filling of the varicosities with the tourniquet in place indicates incompetent perforating veins (secondary varicosities). Release of the tourniquet leads to retrograde filling of the saphenous vein in patients with an incompetent saphenofemoral function (primary varicosities). Any patient whose

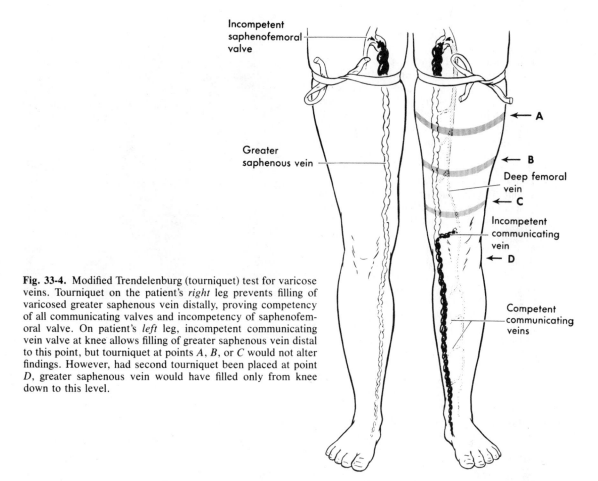

Incompetent
saphenofemoral
valve

← A

← B

Deep femoral
vein

← C

Incompetent
communicating
vein

← D

Greater
saphenous vein

Competent
communicating
veins

Fig. 33-4. Modified Trendelenburg (tourniquet) test for varicose veins. Tourniquet on the patient's *right* leg prevents filling of varicosed greater saphenous vein distally, proving competency of all communicating valves and incompetency of saphenofemoral valve. On patient's *left* leg, incompetent communicating vein valve at knee allows filling of greater saphenous vein distal to this point, but tourniquet at points *A*, *B*, or *C* would not alter findings. However, had second tourniquet been placed at point *D*, greater saphenous vein would have filled only from knee down to this level.

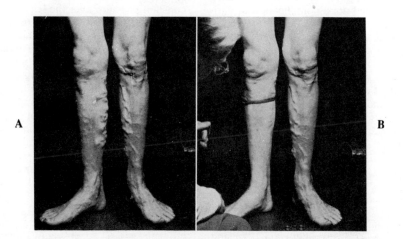

A   B

Fig. 33-5. A, Bilateral greater saphenous varicosities; veins fill promptly on standing. **B,** Vein does not fill distal to tourniquet; communicating vein valves are competent below this point.

varicosities are filled through incompetent perforators is assumed to have had previous deep venous disease.

Clinical features. The most common reason women bring their varicose veins to the attention of the physician is purely cosmetic. Occasionally, however, the varicose veins cause a dull nagging ache or discomfort in the calf and ankles, which is worsened with prolonged standing or a day of activity. This sensation of heaviness and fullness is not usually associated with significant ankle edema. Excessive bleeding may occur if these superficially located veins are traumatized.

Treatment. The treatment for most varicosities is expectant. Some patients feel much better wearing elastic stockings and should be encouraged to do so. Sheer suport hose, though not being ideally compressive, are usually preferred for cosmetic reasons. There are some patients, however, who wish to have the varices excised. Ligation and stripping of primary varicosities can be expected to give an excellent cosmetic and functional result. The patient with secondary varicosities may initially be improved, but the varicosities and symptoms are likely to recur because of the deep venous disease; thus stockings are recommended for this group of patients. Sclerotherapy is usually reserved for small varicosities that involve veins other than those of the greater or lesser saphenous system. Although this treatment is very popular on the European continent and in England it is less frequently employed in the United States.

POSTPHLEBITIC SYNDROME

The patient with postphlebitic syndrome and superficial varicosities (Fig. 33-6) should be recognized as having a complication of extensive deep venous thrombosis and not a complication of varicose veins. A patient with an ankle ulceration rarely has isolated varicosities but almost always has valvular incompetence or occlusion of the deep veins of the legs.

The hallmark of treatment is effective external compression. Most patients do not wrap an elastic bandage evenly, and in addition the bandage may become dislodged several times during the day. A fitted elastic stocking is applied on arising. The patient should not stand or sit for prolonged periods of time; activity that encourages the pumping action of the soleus muscle (walking) is prescribed. Resting with legs elevated several times daily is advised. Some patients find that the swelling goes down spontaneously at night, but others require elevation of the foot of the bed. Most importantly the patient should have excellent skin care and avoid irritation to the skin. Any skin breakdown along the medial aspect of the ankle, regardless of the cause, should be promptly treated.

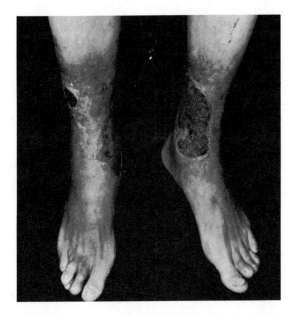

Fig. 33-6. Stasis dermatitis with skin ulcers. Although this patient may have secondary varicosities, ulcers are attributable to old deep venous disease.

Skin ulcerations are managed initially by bed rest to reduce the edema and dressing changes to clean the ulceration. Sometimes antibiotics are necessary to combat deep infection. Once edema and infection have been controlled, a medicated compressive dressing is applied and changed as required, usually weekly. These dressings have the advantages of being bacteriostatic, maintaining a constant pressure over the leg and thus assisting in venous hemodynamics, and keeping the patient's irritating hands away from the ulceration. Some patients wear them for many months before the ulceration has finally healed, but during this time, they maintain an active life-style.

Patients may also be hospitalized to have the ulceration excised surgically and skin grafted. This treatment has the advantage of healing the ulcer in a relatively short period of time (weeks) but has the disadvantage of requiring an expensive hospitalization.

Although advocated by some surgeons, extensive excision of ulcerations, with ligation of perforating veins and excisions of all superficial varicosities, is infrequently carried out. This method of treatment does not treat the cause of the patient's problem, namely, deep venous incompetence. Despite this extensive operation, compressive stockings are still required on a lifetime basis.

New methods of surgical therapy for selected

patients with chronic venous insufficiency are being used in some centers. Patients with isolated unilateral iliofemoral vein thromboses can benefit from anastomosis of the distal end of the divided contralateral greater saphenous vein to the deep venous system on the affected side. Patients with incompetent valves in the deep veins occasionally benefit from transplantation of a segment of brachial or greater saphenous vein containing a competent valve into the deep venous system. However, the selection of suitable candidates for these procedures must be scrupulous and the long-term benefits are still unknown.

PULMONARY EMBOLISM

Each year approximately 400,000 patients suffer fatal pulmonary embolism and 560,000 patients suffer nonfatal pulmonary embolism in the United States, making this the most dreaded complication of deep venous thrombosis.

Minor pulmonary emboli may go undetected and estimates of the true incidence are as high as 25 patients per 100 hospital admissions, of which five are fatal. The pathophysiology reflects pulmonary hypertension and bronchoconstriction. The clinical diagnosis at times is difficult to make and a high index of suspicion is required. The common symptoms of pulmonary embolism are dyspnea, cough, apprehension, chest pain, sweating, and syncope. The most reliable physical finding is tachypnea followed by rales, accentuated pulmonary second sound, tachycardia, and fever. An accentuated S_3 and S_4 gallop sound may be present in more massive pulmonary emboli.

The "classic" signs of pleural friction rub and hemoptysis reflect pulmonary infarction and are present in less than 25% of cases. The white blood cell count is most often below 15,000 and the so-called diagnostic triad of elevated LDH and serum bilirubin with a normal SGOT is seldom found. The chest x-ray study is normal early, but in severe and late pulmonary embolism, pulmonary consolidation, effusion, and a high diaphragm on the side of the embolus are common findings. The electrocardiogram may show some right-sided heart strain, but more commonly the tracing remains unchanged.

Since clots within the pulmonary arterial tree will cause decreased absorption of oxygen, a P_{O_2} greater than 90 mm. Hg virtually rules out pulmonary embolism. Patients should be evaluated noninvasively for the presence of deep vein thrombosis because 95% of patients with proved pulmonary emboli will have demonstrable deep venous thrombosis. Other emboli may derive from the pelvic veins. A ventilation-perfusion lung scan should show a diminished perfusion in the area of pulmonary embolism with normal ventilation.

Later, as the lung consolidates, ventilation may also be decreased. In equivocal cases a pulmonary angiogram is performed. The contrast material will either outline partially occluding thrombi or show decreased perfusion in certain areas.

The treatment of established pulmonary embolism is intravenous heparin. If repeated embolism occurs or there is a contraindication to anticoagulation, interruption of the inferior vena cava, as outlined previously, should be performed. Pulmonary embolectomy is performed on patients with massive pulmonary embolism with refractory hypotension. Thrombolytic therapy is considered in massive pulmonary embolus as an alternative to pulmonary embolectomy. Although less invasive, this method is slower in its effect and may produce hemorrhages and immunological complications.

SPECIFIC LARGE VEIN THROMBOSIS

Acute occlusion or thrombosis of any major vein will produce a syndrome of signs and symptoms specific to the vein, the region drained by it, and the adequacy of collateral venous circulation. Two recognized clinical syndromes are associated with obstruction of the superior vena cava and the axillary (subclavian) vein, respectively.

Acute superior vena caval obstruction occurs with extrinsic compression of the vein by tumor or enlarged lymph nodes or by thrombosis associated with direct trauma and infection (Fig. 33-7). Clinically, the *superior vena caval syndrome* consists of a plethora or cyanosis of the skin of the head and neck associated with varying degrees of venous distension and edema of the upper torso and extremities. This is attended by headache, vertigo, tinnitus, epistaxis, and sometimes fainting. Elevated upper extremity venous pressure and delayed arm-to-lung circulation times support the diagnosis; venography confirms the level and length of obstruction. Treatment is directed at the cause of the original obstruction, including surgical resection of the extrinsically compressing tumor or nodes or simply anticoagulation. Rarely the obstruction is bypassed by use of a vein graft.

Acute axillary (subclavian) vein thrombosis, often termed "effort thrombosis," is seen in younger men who strenuously use their upper extremities in sports or occupation, particularly those activities requiring frequent and violent abduction of the arm on the shoulder. Progressive trauma to the vein probably initiates the thrombosis, which then propagates to totally occlude the vessel. Since the venous collaterals are poor at this point, insidious swelling and cyanosis of the upper extremity occur with distension of the superficial veins. Elevated venous pressure, delayed arm-to-lung circulation times, and venography again are useful in diagnosis. Anticoagulation is indicated

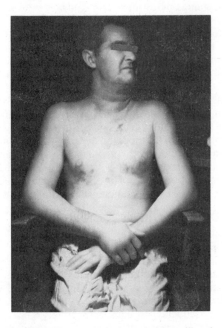

Fig. 33-7. Superior vena caval syndrome—dilated veins on chest wall, swelling of neck and upper extremities caused by lung cancer obstructing vena cava.

acutely; mechanical causes such as thoracic outlet syndrome, cervical rib, and lymph node enlargement must be looked for and appropriately treated.

Thrombolytic therapy and venous thrombectomy have been successfully used in effort thrombosis.

LYMPHEDEMA

The remarkable appearance of lymphedema (excessive lymph in the tissue spaces) caused Caesar's legions to coin the term *elephantiasis* to describe the afflicted lower limbs of their North African opponents, whose lymphatics were obstructed by filariasis.

Primary lymphedema occurs early in life as a result of developmental defects of the lymphatics of a specific site. It may be hereditary or simple (nonhereditary). More frequently the lower limbs and less frequently the upper limbs, genitals, or facial features are affected. Under the microscope the diseased tissue shows any of three patterns: aplasia, hypoplasia, or dilatation and tortuosity of the lymphatics. Injected vital dyes diffuse randomly through the subcutaneous tissues and are not picked up by the defective lymphatic system. *Congenital* (primary) *lymphedema* (10%) is obvious at birth. (Milroy's disease is congenital lymphedema limited to one or both lower limbs and characterized by permanence, steady progress, increasing severity, and absence of constitutional symptoms.) *Lymphedema praecox* (71%) has the characteristics of congenital lymphedema except

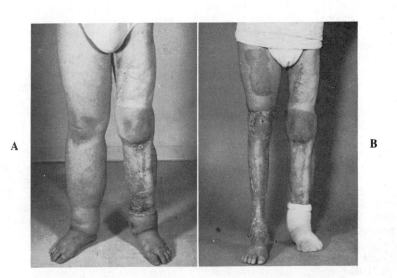

Fig. 33-8. A, Lymphedema praecox in 21-year-old patient; left leg was treated surgically 10 years before; right leg developed recent edema. **B,** Same patient 3 weeks after surgical treatment of right leg.

that it becomes obvious in the patient 10 to 30 years old (Fig. 33-8). (The rare cause of primary lymphedema arising in later years is the *forme tardive,* 19%.)

Secondary lymphedema characteristically occurs later in life and results from obstruction, destruction, or overload of the lymphatics from any of a number of causes, such as (1) repeated lymphangitis or chronic bacterial (commonly streptococcal) infections, (2) neoplastic invasion of lymphatics, (3) circulatory changes occurring after thrombophlebitis (postphlebitic syndrome), (4) filariasis (Fig. 33-9), (5) extensive fibrosis and scarring from radiation, burns, or other trauma, and (6) repeated allergic reactions. Lymphedema of the lower limbs beginning after 40 years of age should raise suspicions of intrapelvic carcinoma in women, or carcinoma of the prostate in men, or lymphoma. Lymphedema of the upper limb after radical mastectomy may signal the presence of lymphatic metastases of breast carcinoma, but more frequently it results merely from fibrosis, thrombosis, and localized infections in the postoperative period. A rare malignancy, *lymphangiosarcoma,* appears in a chronically lymphedematous arm (Stewart-Treves syndrome) or leg decades after the onset of the lymphedema.

Unlike venous edema, lymphedema rarely causes brown (hemosiderin) discoloration or ulceration.

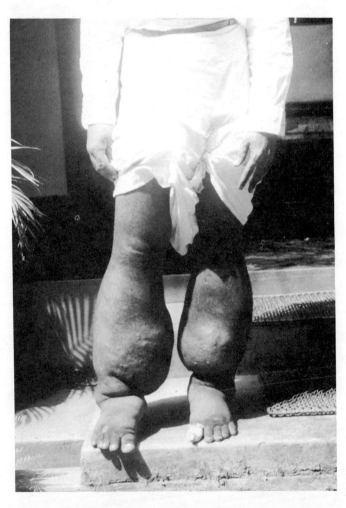

Fig. 33-9. Patient with lower extremity edema secondary to filariasis.

Treatment. Search out and eliminate the cause if possible. History, genealogy, physical examination, cultures, venograms, and lymphangiograms are helpful. Elimination of infections or parasitic infestations or excision of neoplasms may be required. Long-term prophylactic antibiotic treatment is sometimes necessary to prevent repeated episodes of acute lymphangitis. Well-fitted elastic supportive stockings or garments, intermittent pressure devices, elevation of the affected part, massage, exercises, and protection of areas of vulnerable skin from injury are helpful.

Lymphedema uncontrolled by these measures may be relieved by direct surgical attack (Fig. 33-8, *B*). The defective lymphatics and therefore the lymphedema are chiefly limited to the tissues lying between the superficial $\frac{1}{50}$ of an inch of skin (epidermis has no lymphatics, uppermost dermis has very few) and the lymphatics superficial to the deep fascia.

In severe, long-standing cases the afflicted skin, often including the investing fascia, is completely excised and split-thickness skin grafts are placed directly on the investing fasciae or muscles. The grafts may be cut from the excised specimen or from unaffected areas.

A currently popular surgical approach is to supply an escape route for the trapped lymph with a pedicle. One pedicle consists of skin and subcutaneous tissue from the affected leg, which is denuded of its epidermis. The denuded skin is passed through a long incision in the deep fascia and is attached intimately to the underlying muscles, which always have normal lymphatics. The lymph exits from the skin across this bridge to the muscle (Noel Thompson procedure). A novel pedicle consists of omentum tunneled subcutaneously from the abdominal cavity to the limb; lymph is returned from the limb to the abdominal cavity.

Other surgical approaches have included lymphaticovenous anastomoses and direct microvascular lymphatic reconstructions. However, the long-term success of surgical therapy in relieving lymphedema is not encouraging and these methods should be applied only to carefully selected patients.

34
Plastic and Reconstructive Surgery

David W. Furnas
Ivan M. Turpin

PLASTIC SURGERY

The word "plastic" stems from the Greek word *plassein,* which means "to form." *Plastic operation* refers to a procedure that "forms" by means of *shifting* or *transplanting tissues.*

The branch of general surgery that is the specialty of *plastic surgery* deals particularly with the facial features (Fig. 34-1), the jaws and oral cavity, the hand, and the body surface in general, including the breasts and the external genitals. The plastic surgeon attempts to *restore a patient to his original state* after injuries, after removal of tumors, or after changes from aging; he attempts to *improve on the patient's original state* when there are congenital defects or body features that are believed to fall too short of ideal. The "four C's" of plastic surgery are congenital deformities, calamities, cancer, and cosmesis. *Wound care, free grafts,* and *pedicles* are the foundation of the plastic surgeon's art and are fundamental to the craft of surgery in general. Craniofacial surgery and microvascular surgery are areas of recent rapid advances (Fig. 34-2).

Free grafts

A *free graft* is a piece of living tissue that is detached from one site and transplanted to another site where it survives as living tissue. It is termed *autograft* (self), *isograft* (identical twin), *allograft* (same species), or *heterograft* (different species), depending on the relationship of the donor to the recipient.

Mechanisms of graft survival or "take"

Skin graft. A skin graft appears white when first placed on a raw defect. It is nourished entirely by the host tissue fluids that bathe its deep surface *(plasmatic circulation).* After a few hours it becomes quite adherent, cemented in place by the formation of a fibrin coagulum. In less than a day the white graft becomes pink by *inosculation* or linking up of the graft capillaries with host capillaries. After 1 or 2 days the graft is *penetrated* by new capillary buds that grow out from the host. As these develop, the graft's original vessels degenerate. The new vessels assume the entire circulatory load and the graft "takes" firmly. Final healing occurs by the same processes seen in other wounds.

Other free grafts. The "take" of grafts of other tissues (dermis, tendon, bone, fascia) is in some ways similar to that of skin; however, the process is much slower in bone, and fewer of the bone graft's cells remain alive; in cartilage a type of plasmatic circulation is the final form of nutrition.

Failure to "take"

The three chief causes of failure of a skin graft to "take" are (1) *bleeding* beneath the graft (Fig. 34-3), (2) *infection,* or (3) *movement* of the graft. If a hematoma forms, the graft is lifted from its bed and dies. *Beta hemolytic streptococci* form exotoxins that lyse the skin graft from its bed and destroy it. *Pseudomonas, Proteus,* and *Staphylococcus aureus* form pus that lifts the graft from the

Text continued on p. 392.

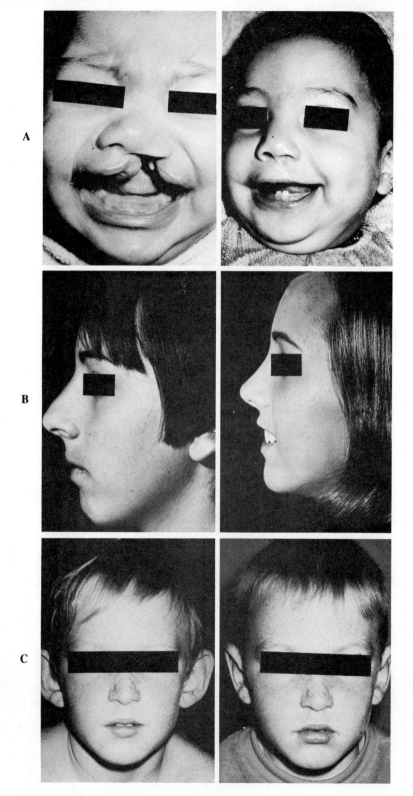

Fig. 34-1. For legend see opposite page.

Fig. 34-1. A, Cleft lip. *Left,* Unilateral cleft lip in infant. *Right,* Lip closure several months postoperatively (scar minics left column of philtrum and will be scarcely noticeable in several years). **B,** Nasal hump and receding chin. *Left,* Preoperative. *Right,* Postoperative rhinoplasty and mentoplasty using cartilage and bone from nasal hump and septum. **C,** Prominent ears. *Left,* Preoperative. *Right,* Postoperative otoplasty.

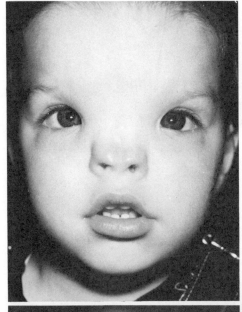

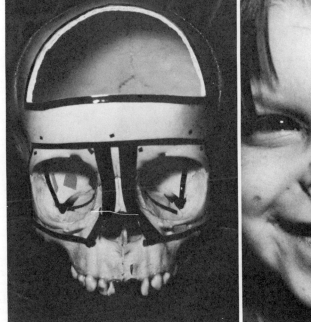

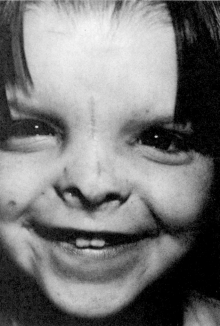

Fig. 34-2. A, Child with hypertelorism. **B,** Mock-up of bone cuts and bone removal for Tessier procedure. **C,** Postoperative status.

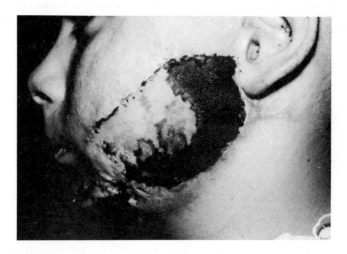

Fig. 34-3. Necrosis of skin graft from hematoma. Bleeding beneath this graft resulted after severe post-operative vomiting. Dark portion of graft is dead and must be replaced with another skin graft.

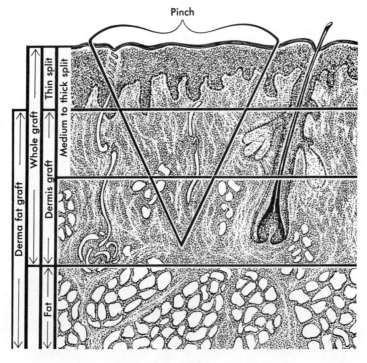

Fig. 34-4. Types of grafts taken from skin and subcutaneous tissue.

Table 34-1. Commonly used free skin grafts

Type	Common donor site	Uses	Comment
Split skin graft (thin, medium, or thick)	Thighs, abdomen, buttocks, back, and elsewhere	To close defects of integument almost anywhere on body	Donor sites epithelialize
Full-thickness skin graft (Wolfe or whole skin graft)	Retroauricular area, supraclavicular area, antecubital fossa	To close skin defects of limited size, particularly on face	Superior appearance and function; donor sites must be closed surgically
Dermis graft (whole graft with a thin graft removed from surface)	Abdomen or elsewhere	To fill out defects in contour or to bolster fascial defects	Buried beneath the skin surface
Dermafat graft (dermis graft with fat attached)	Abdomen, buttocks, or elsewhere	To fill out larger defects in contour	Loses ¼ to ½ of bulk after implantation
Hair follicle–bearing skin grafts	Scalp, eyebrow	To repair scalp, eyebrow, or lashes	Usually applied in small patches or strips
Composite skin grafts (whole skin + cartilage; skin + fibrofat or bone)	Helix, anthelix, lobe of external ear	To repair defects of nose, ear, eyelid	Only small grafts will survive
	Fingertip (accident)	To replace finger part	Works best for children

Other composite grafts finding occasional use are *nipple-areolar grafts* and *nailbed-nail grafts*

Table 34-2. Commonly used autografts of tissues other than skin

Tissue	Common donor site	Uses	Comment
Fat + dermis	Buttock, abdomen	To fill out defects in contour	Easily reabsorbed; dermafat grafts are much better
Fascia	Fascia lata of thigh and elsewhere	To repair fascia, dura, or tendons; to lash or support other structures	May be used in sheets or strips
Tendon	Palmaris longus, plantaris, extensors of toes	To replace or elongate tendons; to bind other structures	Congenital absence of palmaris longus or plantaris is not infrequent
Bone	Ilium, ribs (especially in children), and sites on long bones	To replace missing bone and correct nonunion of fractures and skeletal contour defects	New ribs regenerate from donor defects in children if periosteum is left
Cartilage	Costal cartilage, nasal septum	To replace missing cartilage or bone; to correct contour defects	Tends to warp if not cut with a symmetrical section
Vessels	Greater saphenous vein	To replace absent or occluded arteries; to patch arterial incisions	Valves must be placed in correct direction
Nerves	Sural, saphenous, greater auricular nerves	To replace absent or damaged nerve segments	The more peripheral the site of injury, the better the results

recipient bed. Excessive movement of graft shears the capillary connections between the graft and host, and the graft dies. Therefore meticulous hemostasis, aseptic technique, and adequate immobilization of the graft are important for success.

Clinical use of autologous grafts

The factotum among skin grafts is the *split skin graft* (Tables 34-1 and 34-2 and Fig. 34-4). It can furnish viable cover for fresh wounds, granulating wounds, mucosal defects (mouth, vagina, nose), fascia, paratenon, periosteum, and even exposed lung, brain or pericardium. Split skin grafts do poorly if the vascularity of the recipient bed is poor, as in heavily scarred or radiated wounds, or on bare bone, bare cartilage, or bare tendon. Large split skin grafts are cut with special knives or *dermatomes,* small ones with ordinary scalpels. The donor sites heal by *epithelialization* in 1 to 4 weeks, depending on the thickness of the graft.

Thin split grafts are more likely to "take" in unfavorable circumstances, but they tend to contract and develop inferior appearance and durability (Fig. 34-5).

Thick split grafts are more likely to perish from excessive movement or from bacterial activity than are thinner grafts, but on surviving they furnish a more durable surface (Fig. 34-6).

Full-thickness grafts furnish a better quality coverage, but "take" is less reliable; the size of the graft is limited by the need to suture or graft (with split-thickness skin) the donor site (Fig. 34-7).

Split skin grafts may be cut in sheets, in strips, or in "postage stamps" (small squares). Sheet grafts furnish a superior surface; the smaller grafts are used to expand the area of coverage when donor sites are limited or to improve survival in the presence of infection, movement, or irregular contours.

Composite graft is skin plus other attached tissue. Only small blocks of composite tissue will survive (Fig. 34-8).

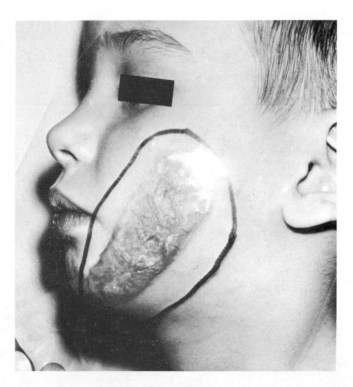

Fig. 34-5. Contraction of thin skin graft. Dark circle represents original granulating wound that resulted from full thickness burn. Very thin skin graft was the same size as this inked pattern, but over period of 3 months it has contracted to half the original size. Graft was later excised and replaced by advancement flap.

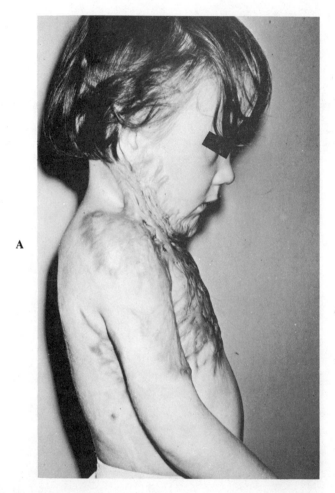

Fig. 34-6. Medium thickness split skin graft. **A,** Flaming nightgown caused burn scars that have contracted mandible tightly against sternum. *Continued.*

Fig. 34-6, cont'd. B, Raw surface is covered with single sheet of medium thickness split skin taken from abdomen. **C,** Graft has matured. Even though texture and color are not exact match, neck-chin angle has been restored and potential for deformity of skeletal growth has been greatly reduced.

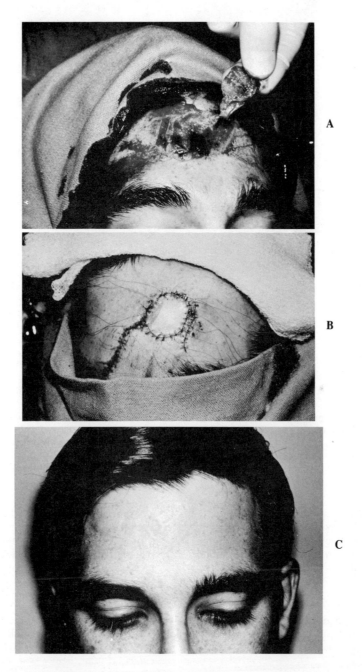

Fig. 34-7. Salvage of doomed flap by conversion into graft. **A,** Windshield injury to forehead has elevated a flap of skin. Pedicle attachment is too narrow for survival, and flap is rapidly becoming congested as blood flows in but fails to flow out. **B,** Flap is detached, trimmed, and replaced as full thickness skin graft. **C,** When mature, replaced graft is inconspicuous and gives perfect color match.

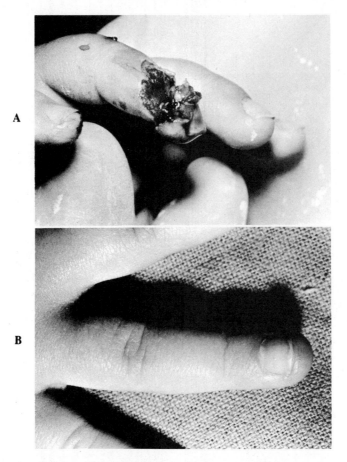

A

B

Fig. 34-8. Composite graft. **A,** Tip of ring finger of 3-year-old child was avulsed when caught in car door. It is held in place by tiny dermoepidermal remnant, but no active circulation is present and thus no congestion occurs. Fingertip was immediately sutured back into place with meticulous care. **B,** Survival of graft is complete. Results of this procedure are generally better in children than in adults.

Replantation of traumatically amputated parts are the most complex clinical autograft in current surgical practice. These grafts, of course, depend on blood flow through major vascular anastomoses for their survival.

Recently advances have been made in allograft transplantation surgery using cyclosporine to prevent rejection of skin and composite tissues. Dramatic results have been achieved with allograft leg transplantation in rats and allotransplantation of skin in humans as well.

Pedicles

Pedicle, flap, pedicled graft, and *pedicled flap* are synonyms for tissue (usually skin with attached subcutaneous tissue) that is transferred to a different site with an intact blood supply. A pedicle is nourished by blood circulating through its own capillaries via a bridge of intact tissue, the base of the pedicle (Figs. 34-9 and 34-10), or circulation is reestablished by microvascular anastomoses (Fig. 34-11).

Use of pedicles

Pedicles commonly surpass free grafts as the best procedure in the following instances: (1) where the defect to be treated is *poorly vascularized* (e.g., heavy scar, radiation changes), (2) where *bare tendons, bare cartilage,* or *bare cortical bone* is exposed, (3) where *padding* is needed over the defect (e.g., pressure sores), (4) where *bulk* is required (e.g., replacement of a missing

Text continued on p. 404.

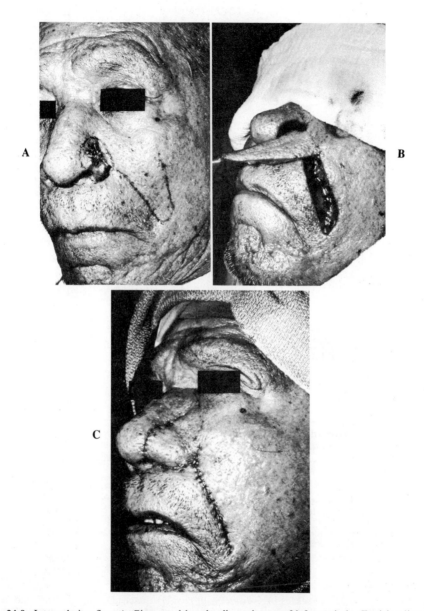

Fig. 34-9. Interpolation flap. **A,** Pigmented basal cell carcinoma of left nasal ala. Excision line and labial interpolation flap have been plotted with ink. **B,** Tumor has been excised. Frozen sections show that margins of specimen are free of tumor, and flap has been incised, undermined, and moved to nasal defect. **C,** Flap has been trimmed and doubled over to furnish interior lining for defect. Defect and donor site are closed.

LOCAL FLAPS

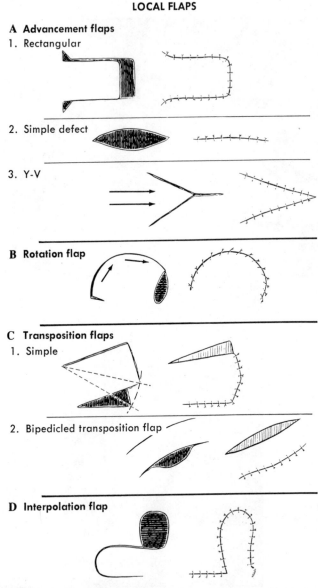

A Advancement flaps
1. Rectangular

2. Simple defect

3. Y-V

B Rotation flap

C Transposition flaps
1. Simple

2. Bipedicled transposition flap

D Interpolation flap

Fig. 34-10. Types of local pedicles. **A,** *Advancement flap:* (1) stretched directly forward into defect aided by excision of Burow's triangles; (2) advancement of edges of simple defect; (3) Y-V advancement flap. **B,** *Rotation flap:* stretched in arc toward defect; donor site closed without skin graft is four to five times bigger than defect; if ratio is smaller, split-skin graft may be required for defect. **C,** *Transposition flap:* (1) moved laterally into adjacent defect; split-skin graft may be required for donor site; (2) bipedicled transposition flap. **D,** *Interpolation flap:* moved over intervening tissue to reach defect, donor site closed with secondary flap or split-skin graft.

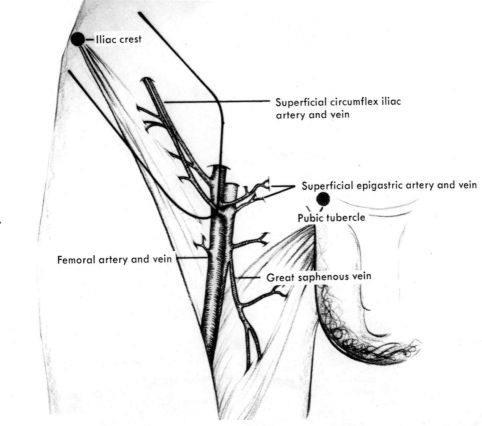

Fig. 34-11. A, Outline of groin flap and axial blood supply.
Continued.

Fig. 34-11, cont'd. B, Free flap transferred to recipient area; inset shows microvascular anastomosis of 1.5 mm. artery. **C,** Completed free flap transfer.

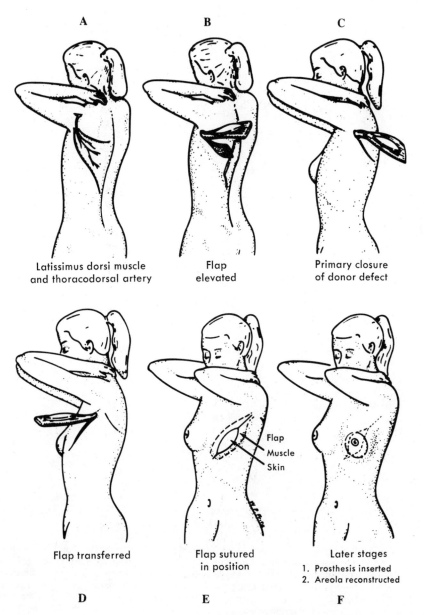

A

B

C

Latissimus dorsi muscle
and thoracodorsal artery

Flap
elevated

Primary closure
of donor defect

Flap
Muscle
Skin

Flap transferred

Flap sutured
in position

Later stages
1. Prosthesis inserted
2. Areola reconstructed

D

E

F

Fig. 34-12. Latissimus dorsi myocutaneous flap for breast reconstruction after mastectomy.

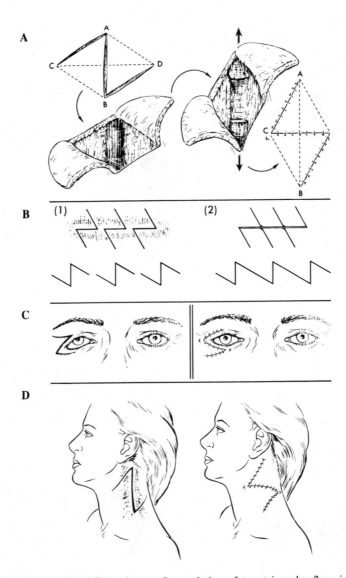

Fig. 34-13. Four functions of Z-plasties. **A,** Interpolation of two triangular flaps increases length along path *AB* at the expense of width along path *CD*. (In effect, dimensions are exchanged between *AB* and *CD*.) **B,** Interpolation of series of disconnected, *1*, or connected, *2*, series of Z's breaks up a straight line and also gives it increased length. **C,** Shift of topographic mark. Correction of contracted lateral canthus effected by Z-plasty; corner of mouth, eyebrow, or nasal ala may be similarly managed. **D,** Obliteration of secondary webbed scar contractures with a Z-plasty shifts the two planes of web so that they form planes of depression at base of neck.

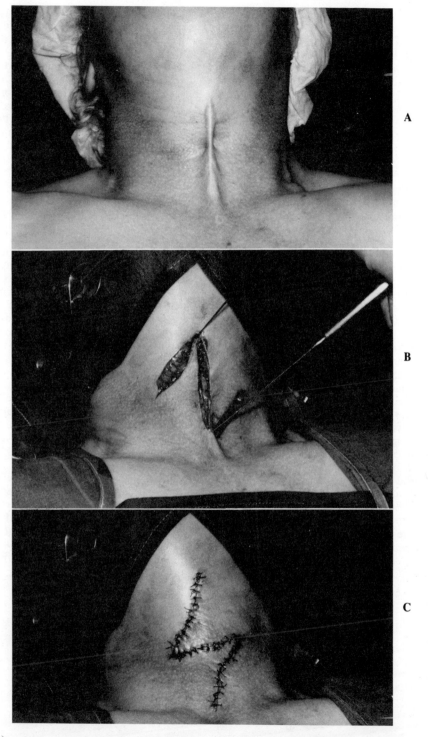

Fig. 34-14. A, Posttraumatic webbed-scar contracture of the anterior neck. **B,** Scar has been excised, and the flaps have been elevated. **C,** The flaps have been rotated into position and the vertical tension has been relieved.

nose, filling out a sunken wound), (5) *where exact match of color, texture, and resilience* is desired (e.g., correction of a check defect with a pedicle from neighboring cheek and neck tissue), (6) where a *double facing* is required (e.g., replacement of full-thickness defect of the cheek or mouth), (7) or where there is likelihood that the new surface will have to be temporarily elevated at a future time to permit further reconstructive surgery (e.g., in anticipation of secondary tendon grafts, tendon transfers, bone grafts, or nerve repairs).

Types of flaps according to blood supply

Random blood supply. No named blood vessels are included in the flap. For hundred of years this has been the most common type of flap. Flaps can be created from tissue adjacent to the defect (local flaps). Terms such as rotation, advancement, transposition, or interpolation are added to describe the manner of movement (Fig. 34-9). Flaps may be brought from remote areas and applied directly to a defect (distant, *direct*) or *migrated* in stages.

Axial blood supply. A specific artery and vein are included in the flap and provide its circulation. Examples are the deltopectoral flap (internal mammary perforators) and the groin flap (superficial circumflex iliac vessels). Unfortunately, most vessels to the skin arise at right angles to vessels within the underlying muscles.

Myocutaneous flap. A whole new family of axial flaps has now been described in which an entire muscle with its overlying skin is transferred (myocutaneous) (Fig. 34-12). Examples include the pectoralis, gluteus, tensor fasciae latae, gracilis, and gastrocnemius muscles. Of course the muscle can be transferred without the skin and can then be skin grafted *(muscle flap)*.

Island flap. A complete island of skin is excised and elevated, but its subcutaneous connections with blood vessels are maintained. The artery is dissected free, and the island is burrowed subcutaneously to reach the recipient site with its arterial umbilicus trailing after. An eyebrow may be replaced with a temporal scalp island supported by the superficial temporal artery, or a thumb may be given an area of normal sensation with an island of skin from the ring finger supported by a digital neurovascular bundle *(sensory island flap).*

Free flap. It is now possible to completely detach a flap, transfer it to its new location, and then, using microsurgery, anastomose the 1 to 2 mm. vessels, reestablishing the circulation. Thus what used to take many operations and several months can be accomplished in one day (Fig. 34-11).

Complications of pedicle surgery

Pedicle procedures are subject to the same problems as any other wound (e.g., hematoma, infection, etc.), plus special problems that can threaten the precarious circulation. If a pedicle is too narrow, if it is detached too early, if the blood flow is obstructed by external pressure (the patient's own weight, tight dressings, heavy bedding), or if it is kinked or twisted, the pedicle may die. If the newly incised free end of a pedicle is placed at a lower level than the base of the pedicle, the pedicle may become congested *(gravitational congestion)* and die from circulatory stasis.

Z-plasty

The Z-plasty is a useful surgical technique that may perform any of four basic functions: (1) *increase length along a specific path* (Fig. 34-13, A), (2) *break up and reorient a straight line scar* (Fig. 34-13, B), (3) *shift topographical landmarks* (Fig. 34-13, C), and (4) *deepen webs or obliterate clefts* (Fig. 34-13, D).

The Z-plasty is performed by elevation of two triangular flaps in the form of a Z and *interpolating* them so that the final figure is a reversed Z. The incisions should be of approximately equal lengths. The angles may be unequal, but the most common form of a Z-plasty has two 60-degree angles. Z-plasties may be single or serial (Fig. 34-14).

Care of the Acutely Injured Patient

John F. Hansbrough
Ben Eiseman

The most important environmental health problem this nation faces is accidental injuries. Deaths by accident lead all causes of death in the first half of man's life-span. In the United States accidents afflict 50 million people each year, killing 120,000 and disabling at least 14 million others. The overall cost (including medical expenses, property loss, insurance claims, working hours lost, etc.) totals more than $40 billion yearly. Even though the general public tends to forget the enormity of this problem, the medical profession cannot, because accident victims occupy one of every eight beds in a typical general hospital.

This chapter introduces the student to the acutely injured patient and the early, lifesaving procedures in the emergency room. Other chapters discuss the later, specialized care of these patients.

THE EMERGENCY ROOM

Every modern hospital provides emergency rooms equipped to receive and treat the injured. Readily accessible to ambulances and automobiles, some emergency services feature heliports as well. Probably more important, special centers train paramedics who travel to the accident site and begin immediate treatment. Programs in many areas have reaffirmed the worth of these ultra-modern, regional emergency centers that initiate treatment on the spot.

Emergency room physicians must become expert at triage—*sorting first things first*. They rapidly scan patients for life-threatening conditions: (1) airway and respiration, (2) heart and circulation, (3) active bleeding, (4) state of consciousness,

and (5) obvious threatening injuries (i.e., sucking chest wound, flail chest, sharp bone fragments near major vessels). They know the conditions that threaten life, and they attack these problems rapidly and systematically, the most urgent ones first.

Airway and respiration

The airway is the first consideration in all emergency situations; the physician must determine immediately if the patient is breathing adequately. Cyanosis with gasping chest movement's and upper airway noise (stridor) indicates airway obstruction. The most common cause of obstruction in injured patients is posterior displacement of the tongue; the physician should force the mouth open and thrust the mandible forward. Any foreign matter should be removed with the finger or with suctioning. If there is any suspicion of a neck injury, the neck should not be extended but kept in a neutral position. An oral airway may be placed in the comatose patient but will not be tolerated if the patient is awake. If these procedures fail to relieve the obstructed breathing, tracheal intubation (orally, nasally, or through a tracheostomy) will bypass an obstructed larynx and assure an open upper airway.

Continuing cyanosis indicates lower respiratory problems; *pneumothorax,* usually resulting from fractured ribs, heads the list. Any fractured rib can puncture a lung, often without gross chest wall deformity. Characterized by a tympanitic hemothorax, absent breath sounds, tracheal displacement (to the opposite side), and subcutaneous emphysema, pneumothorax can become *tension pneumo-*

thorax from a flutter-valve defect in the puncture site that forces air into the intrapleural space with each inspiration. As the air builds up, it compresses the opposite lung, sometimes fatally. Aspiration of the entrapped air by needle or thoracostomy tube reverses this process.

Crushing chest trauma that fractures several ribs at multiple sites results in *flail chest*. The shattered chest wall, lacking normal rigidity, moves paradoxically (in with inspiration and out with expiration). Although external bracing helps somewhat, intubation and mechanical ventilation continued until the chest wall solidifies (10 to 20 days) have proved most effective. Simple tamponade with an occlusive dressing temporarily repairs open "sucking" wounds of the chest wall while thoracostomy tubes drain out the entrapped air.

Acute gastric dilatation (from ileus and swallowed air) may impede diaphragmatic movement and thus hinder ventilation. Nasogastric suction provides instant relief and also helps prevent vomiting and aspiration pneumonitis. Removing gastric juice also decreases stress ulceration.

Circulation

Once assured that the patient has an adequate airway, the physician checks circulation. He should tamponade any serious bleeding sites at once, insert a large intravenous catheter, and start crystalloid solutions (after removing a blood sample for typing and matching blood).

Many patients in shock respond to this treatment alone, but if shock (cold clammy skin, weak rapid pulse) persists despite adequate fluid and blood replacement, one of the following causes is likely: cardiac tamponade, tension pneumothorax, internal bleeding (chest, abdomen, or fracture sites), bowel rupture, aortic tear, or, rarely, adrenal failure. At this point a central venous catheter immensely aids further evaluation.

Cardiac tamponade

In patients with chest trauma, distant, muted heart sounds, low pulse pressure, and a high central venous pressure (CVP) (and often a paradoxical pulse) indicate cardiac tamponade. Echocardiography, if available, can rapidly confirm these clinical signs. Needle aspiration of the pericardial blood, repeated if necessary, will usually reestablish normal heart action. (See Chapter 31.) Unresponsive cases may require thoracotomy and direct repair of any bleeding site.

Hemothorax

Because of two factors (collapsible lung tissue and low pulmonary blood pressure), bleeding from lung parenchyma rarely persists. Continued intrapleural bleeding usually comes from severed intercostal or internal mammary vessels. Needle aspiration or insertion of a thoracotomy tube (with suction) removes the blood and allows the lung to expand. Tube drainage provides a constant monitor to assess continued bleeding. (See Chapter 30.) Less than 10% of these patients will require thoracotomy.

Hemoperitoneum

The neophyte physician can easily be misled by the relatively normal appearing abdomen that contains 2,000 ml. of blood or more. Thus he should always suspect the abdomen as a likely source of continuing bleeding and persistent shock. Although four-quadrant, intraperitoneal aspiration with an 18-gauge needle serves as a rapid indicator of bleeding, a negative tap means nothing. Peritoneal lavage yields more reliable results. We instill 500 to 1,000 ml. of lactated Ringer's solution through a peritoneal dialysis catheter that enters the abdomen through a tiny skin incision in the lower midline. The bottle, placed on the floor, siphons the fluid from the abdomen. A pink tinge indicates bleeding. More than 100,000 RBC's/ml. indicate significant bleeding. Bacteria, fecal material, or amylase indicates visceral perforation. Any one of these indicators signals the need for laparotomy. (See Chapter 25.)

Aortic tears

Severe chest trauma may shear the aortic arch, causing dissection along the wall. A widening mediastinum on x-ray examination or absent or unequal peripheral pulses justify emergency arteriography. (See Chapter 30.)

Adrenal failure

Long-term steroid therapy suppresses normal adrenal response to stress. The physician should suspect adrenal failure in patients who give a history of steroid intake or in comatose patients with stigma of arthritis, asthma, or chronic dermatoses.

Coma

Head trauma rarely causes shock. In fact, a patient whose skull and brain sustain the shattering impact necessary to produce hemorrhagic shock seldom reaches the emergency room alive. But shock itself produces coma by depriving brain cells of oxygen. Thus our initial efforts to restore airway and circulation aim most urgently at getting more oxygen to brain cells because cerebral cells, unlike other tissues, die rapidly (within minutes) from hypoxia. These efforts alone often restore consciousness as the brain receives its vital oxygen.

Brain cells suffer hypoxia from a second major cause after trauma—edema or hemorrhage within the skull depresses local cerebral circulation. Although slowing pulse and respiration, fever, and dilated pupils indicate increased intracranial pressure, the *level of consciousness* remains the most reliable sign. The physician must record his early neurological findings, especially noting state of consciousness, and immediately call for neurosurgical consultation. (See Chapter 40.) He should also note other possible causes of coma (alcohol, drugs, diabetes, epilepsy). The most important early treatment in minimizing brain edema is hyperventilation of the patient.

Other injuries

After he has stabilized the patient's cardiorespiratory function, the physician should systematically review other areas. He should question the patient or those who accompany him for pertinent information concerning the accident and the patient's health (diabetes, cardiac status, renal status, etc.) while surveying the patient for pulses, bony abnormalities, hematuria (after catheterization), and other defects.

The conscious patient can move his digits and respond to pain stimuli from extremities, but the unconscious patient withdraws from these stimuli. These responses indicate an intact spinal cord. To lessen the chance of vertebral fractures or dislocations injuring the spinal cord, the patient must be moved cautiously and only when necessary.

Treatment priorities

One person, usually a general surgeon or traumatologist, must take charge, coordinate his consultants, and assign immediate priorities throughout this critical period. He arranges priorities as follows: (1) restore cardiorespiratory function (stop bleeding, visible and hidden), (2) repair hollow viscera injuries (intestine, bladder), (3) repair vascular injuries, (4) treat head and spinal injuries, (5) repair open fractures, and (6) treat lacerations and closed fractures. For example, a patient sustains a skull fracture, femoral fracture, colon rupture, lacerations, and shock. The admitting surgeon treats the shock, stops external bleeding by pressure or ligation, and places a simple splint on the fractured femur. As soon as the patient's vital signs stabilize, the surgeon repairs the colonic tear in the operating room and thus interrupts lethal peritonitis at an early, curable stage. Other surgeons meanwhile clean and close the patient's lacerations. Skull films, taken en route to the operating room, show no displaced bone fragments, and echoencephalography reveals no midline shift; thus craniotomy can be deferred. Although the patient is unconscious before and during the operation, his coma does not interdict the lifesaving laparotomy.

The team captain must oversee the total care of acutely injured patients. He uses consultants for specialized problems and coordinates their diagnostic and treatment recommendations. Studies have proved that acutely injured patients treated in efficient emergency centers have the best chance of surviving.

SUMMARY

All emergency room personnel must keep clearly in mind the following steps for the care of acutely injured patients:

1. Assure airway and respiratory exchange
2. Assure circulation
   a. Stop bleeding
   b. Treat shock
   c. Prepare to treat cardiac arrest at any moment
3. Determine need for operative control of internal bleeding or bowel rupture
4. Determine need to restore peripheral circulation
5. Determine need for operative decompression of spinal cord or brain
6. Treat open fractures first, then repair lacerations, then treat closed fractures

Because severe injury disrupts many vital functions, critically ill patients require a variety of conduits that connect them to outside supports. Life-sustaining substances flow in through some tubes; displaced bodily fluids (or gases) drain out through others. Some catheters serve mainly as monitors to help us alter, as necessary, this artificial flux. As a rapid reminder of these lifesaving priorities, the student should picture a patient with five tubes in place, each serving a vital function.

Tube	*Reason*
Oral airway or endotracheal tube	Assure adequate ventilation
Intravenous catheter	Restore fluids; treat shock
Central venous catheter	Monitor fluid load, hemopericardium, heart failure
Urinary catheter	Monitor renal perfusion; detect blood from urinary tract
Nasogastric tube	Prevent vomiting and aspiration pneumonia; prevent stress ulcers

Other tubes sometimes indicated	*Reason*
Arterial catheter	Blood gas analyses
Thoracotomy tube	Treat pneumothorax or hemothorax

Transplantation

Richard Weil, III

The sixteenth-century Italian surgeon Tagliacozzi, often considered the father of plastic surgery, developed detailed techniques for rotating soft-tissue pedicles for reconstruction of nasal mutilation caused by disease or trauma; however, the free transfer of even skin was not considered feasible until the nineteenth-century. The distinctions between autografts (grafts from one part of an individual to another part of the same individual), allografts or homografts (grafts from one individual to another individual of the same species), and heterografts or xenografts (cross-species grafts) were not clearly appreciated until well into the twentieth century. The technique for suturing together small blood vessels with reliable patency was developed by Alexis Carrel in the first decade of this century and in part won him the 1912 Nobel Prize in Physiology and Medicine; this technique was a prerequisite for successful organ transplantation. The immunological basis for graft rejection was established in the 1940s by Sir Peter Medawar, who also received the Nobel Prize in Physiology and Medicine in 1960 for his contributions to transplantation immunology.

Although there were sporadic earlier efforts, the first systematic attempts at human organ transplantation were the kidney transplants carried out at the Peter Bent Brigham Hospital in Boston in the 1950s. In 1954 a transplant between identical twins (isograft), in whom immunological rejection of the transplanted organ was not biologically operative, was chronically successful. In the late 1950s, in Boston and in Paris, total body irradiation of the recipient was tried in an effort to prevent rejection of the transplant, but this form of immunosuppression was dangerous and was replaced in the early 1960s by pharmacological immunosuppression, which has remained the principal immunosuppressive tool for preventing and treating rejection of all allografts. In 1963 the human liver was replaced by Dr. Thomas Starzl in Denver, Colorado. In 1967, the human heart was replaced by Dr. Christiaan Barnard in Capetown, South Africa.

A considerable number of human-tissue allotransplants are carried out: cornea transplants to restore vision, skin grafts to cover burn wounds, bone-marrow infusions to restore hematopoietic function (in aplastic anemia or leukemia treated with massive cytotoxic agents), bone chips for spine fusion, and others. However, this chapter focuses mainly on transplantation of solid internal organs.

BIOLOGY OF REJECTION

The immune system is a protection against foreign substances or nonself. The strength of the immune response to transplants increases with the genetic disparity between the donor and recipient, but violent immune responses can occur even when donor and recipient species are the same, as in human-cadaver kidney transplantation.

Graft rejection is initiated by foreign histocompatibility antigens on cell surfaces or free within the graft. Mismatched ABO blood group antigens can elicit strong graft rejections in recipients with natural isoantibodies. Vertebrate species have a major histocompatibility complex (MHC) that is primarily responsible for allograft rejection. The human MHC, located on chromosome 6, is the human leukocyte antigen (HLA) complex; it governs the production of cell-surface antigens of major and minor strengths. The HLA complex, which has been divided into class I and class II, can be identified on cell surfaces by monospecific typing antisera (HLA typing). The class I antigens, such as HLA-A and HLA-B, are recognizable by cytotoxic allogeneic T-lymphocytes but usually cannot initiate proliferation of allogeneic lymphocytes. The class II antigens, such as HLA-DR, can initiate allogeneic helper T-lymphocyte proliferation.

When an allograft is revascularized in a patient, the donor histocompatibility antigens initiate an immune response in the recipient. Strong allograft-specific responses result from the direct presentation of donor antigens on the surfaces of "macrophage type" of cells in the graft. Donor antigens may also be processed by recipient macrophages, monocytes, or dendritic cells, which activate helper T-lymphocytes and B-lymphocytes in the recipient's spleen and lymph nodes. The multiple steps in this activation process are incompletely understood, but the lymphokines interleuken-1 and interleuken-2 are almost certainly important intercellular activation messengers.

The T-lymphocytes (thymus dependent) primarily mediate cellular immune responses. T-lymphocyte subclasses can be defined by antigenic markers (e.g., T_4 and T_8) that purport to identify functionally distinct subsets (T_4 helper and T_8 cytotoxic); however, such absolute functional distinctions are questionable.

The B-lymphocytes are named after the avian "bursa of Fabricius," the human functional analog of which is probably bone marrow and gut lymphoid tissue. B-lymphocytes produce antibodies against donor antigens. These antibodies are not required for graft rejection, which can occur without antibody; however, alloantibodies against donor antigens participate in some forms of rejection.

PATTERNS OF REJECTION

The patterns of rejection vary among different tissues and solid organs. The clinical and corresponding histopathological characteristics have been most fully described for kidney allografts. The histopathology of liver, heart, lung, and pancreas rejection is less clearly defined. The physiological and microscopic characteristics of rejection are most clearly expressed in experimental animals that have received no immunosuppression; however, the clinician must work with immunosuppressed patients in whom the characteristics of rejection are less clear.

Hyperacute rejection

When a kidney is transplanted into a patient who has circulating preformed cytotoxic antibodies against the histocompatibility antigens of the donor, there is a high probability of a violent early rejection within a few minutes to a few hours after revascularization of the kidney. The cause of these antibodies in the recipient may be prior pregnancies, transplants, or blood transfusions, but such antibodies also occur without a history of preexposure to foreign histocompatibility antigens.

In hyperacute rejection the reaction between preformed IgG antibody and the vascular endothelial antigens of the graft, in the presence of complement, results in irreversible activation of the clotting system and rapid thrombosis of the microcirculation of the graft, which infarcts.

Hyperacute rejection has been observed many times in human kidney transplants. Eleven human livers were transplanted despite preformed recipient cytotoxic antibodies against the donor, but hyperacute rejection was not observed in any case; the liver appears resistant to hyperacute rejection.

Acute rejection

Many human kidney transplants undergo at least one acute rejection episode after transplantation, mediated primarily by T-lymphocytes that infiltrate the graft. Acute rejection is usually not detected until at least a few days after transplantation; acute rejection episodes may occur months or occasionally years after transplantation. T-lymphocytes are often visible by light microscopy in biopsied kidney allografts, but these round cell infiltrates do not always impair renal function. In some grafts, the infiltrating lymphocytes and other round cells, by direct cellular contact or by release of cytotoxic factors, physically damage the cells of the graft and thereby interfere with function.

Chronic rejection

Months or years after kidney transplantation, some degree of slow rejection, mediated primarily but not exclusively by humoral antibody, usually leads to the destruction of graft function. The host immune system almost never fully accepts the graft, even though chronic low-dose immunosuppression is continued. It is unusual for kidney transplants to survive this process for more than 10 years; grafts seldom last for a lifetime, even if initial function is excellent. In kidney transplants, chronic rejection is histologically manifested by thickening of glomerular basement membrane and damage to the intima of arterioles with resultant narrowing of the arteriolar lumen and eventually tissue ischemia. This process in almost all cases eventually causes cellular damage and loss of graft function.

DIAGNOSIS OF REJECTION

Even after more than 30 years of study of graft rejection, the precise events of rejection are not clearly understood and methods for diagnosis are inexact. No single test can reliably establish a diagnosis of rejection of a kidney, liver, heart, lung, or pancreas. Biopsy information is often helpful but also difficult to interpret. When a transplant does not function well, the physician initially attempts to rule out problems other than rejection, such as insufficient circulation to the graft or obstruction of excretory drainage (urine in kidney transplants, bile in liver transplants, exocrine fluid and enzymes in pancreas transplants) before making a working diagnosis of rejection. The clinical diagnosis of rejection remains to some extent a diagnosis of exclusion.

PREVENTION OR CONTROL OF REJECTION
Matching of recipient with donor
(immunological testing)

ABO blood group. As with blood transfusions, group O is a universal donor, and group AB is a universal recipient in organ transplantation. Persons with blood group A or B should not donate kidneys to blood group O patients because of the high probability that recipient isoantibodies would result in violent early rejection of the transplant. Breech of ABO blood group barriers is less dangerous in liver transplantation. The Rh system appears to be unimportant in organ transplantation.

Direct cross-match. The most predictive and therefore most important of the histocompatibility matching tests is the direct cytotoxic cross-match test to look for the presence of preformed cytotoxic antibodies in the recipient against cells of the potential donor. If the recipient has IgG antibodies that in the presence of complement are cytotoxic to the lymphocytes of the donor, hyperacute rejection is very likely to occur if a kidney is transplanted. Hyperacute liver rejection has not been observed even after transplantation in the presence of preformed cytotoxic antibodies.

Human leukocyte antigens (HLA). Each person inherits from each parent one chromosome 6 and one haplotype of HLA. Siblings may therefore be perfectly matched or completely mismatched for HLA (Fig. 36-1). HLA's are present on all nucleated human cells. Clinical HLA testing is done by microcytotoxicity methods using monospecific typing sera, which then allow one to infer the antigen specificities of the person being tested. The force of the rejection response in kidney transplants from living relatives is to some extent governed by the degree of mismatch of donor and recipient HLA, but even nonidentical twin kidney transplants or kidney transplants from siblings perfectly matched for HLA antigens can be violently rejected. Table 36-1 depicts a patient (recipient) and five potential donors, all with ABO blood group and direct cytotoxic cross-match compatible with the recipient, who have 0-4 HLA-A and HLA-B matches.

For cadaver kidney transplantation, matching of

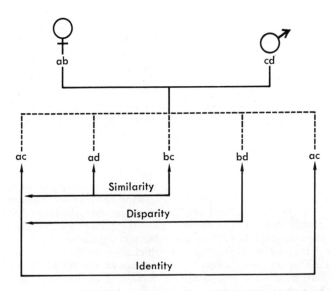

Fig. 36-1. Possible genetic relationships in a family. Since siblings inherit one haplotype from each parent, there is 1 in 4 chance of identity, 2 in 4 chance of similarity, and 1 in 4 chance of disparity.

Table 36-1. Simplified scheme of HLA-A and HLA-B typing showing some of the antigens*

Donor or recipient	ABO	HLA A2	HLA A3	HLA A10	HLA A11	HLA A29	HLA AW33	HLA B8	HLA B13	HLA B16	HLA BW22	HLA BW35	HLA BW40	Cross-match
Recipient	A	+	+	−	−	−	−	+	−	+	−	−	−	
Donor 1	O	+	+	−	−	+	−	+	−	+	−	−	−	Neg.
Donor 2	A	+	−	−	+	−	−	+	−	+	−	−	+	Neg.
Donor 3	A	−	+	−	+	+	−	−	+	+	−	−	−	Neg.
Donor 4	O	−	−	−	+	+	+	−	+	−	+	−	−	Neg.
Donor 5	A	−	−	−	−	−	+	−	−	−	+	+	−	Neg.

*Varying degrees of match and mismatch between recipient and donors 1 to 5 are present. Donor 1 is completely matched, whereas donor 5 is completely mismatched.

the HLA-A, HLA-B, and HLA-DR antigens has not been a powerful predictor of graft success, especially in the United States where the population is genetically heterogeneous. The HLA system has not been extensively evaluated in nonrenal solid organ transplantation but appears to exert only a minor influence on the outcome of these grafts.

Mixed lymphocyte culture (MLC). For kidney transplantation (in contrast to bone marrow transplantation), the mixed lymphocyte culture tests the unidirectional reactivity of recipient lymphocytes against donor lymphocytes. This test correlates to some extent with HLA-DR matching. The MLC test generally requires 5 days of tissue culture for completion and can allow identification of the immunologically optimal living related donor among a group of relatives who are equally well matched to the recipient at the HLA-A and HLA-B loci.

Immunological modification of donor or donor organ

If it were possible to modify the donor organ before transplantation so that it did not elicit a strong immune response in the recipient, immunosuppression of the recipient could be reduced. Attempts at pretransplant treatment of the donor organ have mainly been directed at decreasing antigen outflow from the graft by pharmacological agents such as cyclophosphamide or corticosteroids, by radiotherapy, and by long-term perfusion of the graft. These techniques have been partly intended to eliminate passenger leukocytes of donor origin that remain within any transplanted graft. Another means of removing these donor-origin passenger leukocytes from small grafts such as pancreatic islet fragments is temporary storage of the grafts in vitro in organ culture, particularly with a high ambient oxygen atmosphere. Such storage is more toxic to donor-origin passenger leukocytes than to donor endocrine tissue. Reduction of passenger leukocytes by any of these techniques reduces the immunogenicity of the transplant.

Recipient immunosuppression

The goal of immunosuppression is to render the recipient specifically tolerant of the transplant without lowering defenses against infection or cancer and without any side effects. This goal has not yet been attained.

Immunological preparation of recipient

Splenectomy and total lymphoid irradiation decrease central lymphoid tissue and increase the success rate of cadaver kidney transplantation.

Although splenectomy has been done in association with liver transplantation, neither splenectomy nor total lymphoid irradiation has been systematically evaluated in nonrenal organ transplantation. Splenectomy may be carried out a few weeks before kidney transplantation or concurrently; total lymphoid irradiation, originally developed for treatment of Hodgkin's disease, requires a few weeks for completion and has been carried out before transplantation. Splenectomy, a major operation with perioperative risks, carries the late postoperative risk of overwhelming sepsis from encapsulated bacteria such as *Diplococcus pneumoniae* or *Haemophilus influenzae*. Total lymphoid irradiation has been associated with radiation sickness.

A third method of immunological preparation, thoracic duct drainage, removes billions of lymphocytes from the circulation each day through a catheter inserted into the root of the left side of the neck, where the thoracic duct enters the confluence of internal jugular and subclavian veins. Thoracic duct drainage is most effective when done continuously for at least 4 weeks before transplantation, but this form of therapy is cumbersome and expensive.

A fourth, simpler but not entirely risk-free, method of immunological preparation is the use of pretransplant blood transfusions. For many years blood transfusions were withheld from potential transplant patients on chronic dialysis, even very anemic patients, for fear of generating cytotoxic antibodies, which would decrease the probability of finding a safe kidney donor. In the early 1970s, Dr. Paul Terasaki's UCLA kidney transplant registry showed that patients who had received at least a few blood transfusions in fact had less kidney transplant rejections than patients who had never received transfusions. Most patients waiting for cadaver kidney transplants are now immunologically prepared for transplantation by several transfusions from random donors, and many patients who receive living related kidney transplants are immunologically prepared by the administration of pretransplant donor-specific blood transfusions from the living relative who subsequently provides the related kidney transplant. The administration of immunologically nonspecific blood transfusions from blood banks carries a small risk of transmission of non-A, non-B hepatitis and an exceedingly small risk of transmission of acute immunodeficiency syndrome (AIDS), but the potential benefit of reducing graft rejection outweighs these small risks. A few patients who receive transfusions (approximately 10% to 15%) become so highly sensitized by the transfusions that a safe donor cannot easily be found, and the opportunity for kidney transplantation may thereby be lost, but the patients who develop such strong antibodies might violently reject a kidney transplant without antecedent transfusions.

Pharmacological immunosuppression

Azathioprine (Imuran) and adrenal corticosteroids were the pharmacological agents most commonly used for all organ transplants during the 1960s and 1970s. In the early 1980s cyclosporine began to replace azathioprine. Heterologous antilymphocyte serum or globulin, produced in animals, was widely used in the 1960s and 1970s as an adjunct to azathioprine and corticosteroids; in the 1980s monoclonal antilymphocyte antibodies made by cell hybridization techniques began to replace less precise antilymphocyte preparations.

Azathioprine. The active portion of azathioprine is 6-mercaptopurine, which is liberated from the larger molecule by the liver. 6-Mercaptopurine is a purine-analog antimetabolite that, in the form of 6-mercaptopurine ribonucleotide, interferes with intracellular purine metabolism in host cells that are actively dividing in response to donor antigen stimulation. Its main side effect is bone marrow toxicity.

Adrenal corticosteroids. The exact mechanism of corticosteroid immunosuppression is not known, but lymphocytolysis, particularly of T-lymphocytes, is almost certainly one mechanism. Steroids have less effect on B-lymphocyte function than on T-lymphocyte function. Steroids also reduce the inflammatory activity of many cells, including macrophages and polymorphonuclear leukocytes, by stabilization of their lysosomal membranes. Adrenal corticosteroid toxicities are multiple and can be very debilitating: hypertension, moon facies, acne, peptic ulcer, pancreatitis, ocular cataract, aseptic necrosis of bone, diabetes mellitus, psychosis, and interference with growth in children.

Cyclosporine. This relatively new polypeptide extracted from fungus is a potent immunosuppressive agent that is not a bone-marrow depressant. It probably inhibits T-lymphocytes from secreting interleukin-2, which is necessary for full activation of the T-lymphocyte immune response. Cyclosporine inhibits the generation of cytotoxic T-lymphocytes, but once cytotoxic T-cells have been activated, cyclosporine will not inhibit expression of their cytotoxic activity. Its major side effect is nephrotoxicity; it has additional mild side effects of hirsutism, gastrointestinal disturbance, central nervous system toxicity, and hepatotoxicity. Cyclosporine is very hydrophobic and is orally administered in oil; its intestinal absorption is often erratic.

Antilymphocyte preparations. Antilymphocyte

(or antithymocyte) sera or globulins can be generated in animals against human T-lymphocytes, B-lymphocytes, lymphocyte subpopulations, or cultured lymphoblasts, by injection of these cells into animals and subsequent harvesting of serum from the responding animal. If human lymphocytes are injected into a mouse, the sensitized mouse spleen cells can be fused with mouse myeloma cells to form hybridomas capable of producing a continuous supply of monoclonal mouse anti–human lymphocyte antibodies. Heterologous antilymphocyte preparations are often highly cytotoxic to circulating lymphocytes, but such lymphocytotoxicity is not necessarily associated with improved graft survival. Allergic reactions are not uncommon with these agents and occasionally take the form of life-threatening anaphylaxis.

Disadvantages

The chief disadvantages of all the preceding methods of recipient immunosuppression are increased risks of infection and malignancy. The goal of immunosuppressive therapy is to provide just enough immunosuppression to permit graft acceptance without interfering with the patient's ability to resist infection or malignancy. Unfortunately this objective is not always attainable with current immunosuppressive tools. Immunological monitoring techniques designed to guard against both underimmunosuppression and overimmunosuppression of the patient have generally been ineffective.

Infection is the main cause of death after transplantation; it reflects the imperfection of available immunosuppressive agents. The infections observed after transplantation are caused by bacteria, viruses, protozoa, and fungi, including saprophytes incapable of causing infection in nonimmunodepressed hosts. Posttransplant infection can to some extent be reduced by elimination of all sites of infection before transplantation. One can partially reduce the consequences of infection by promptly decreasing or discontinuing immunosuppression in patients who develop signs of life-threatening infection, even though the grafts may be rejected.

Malignancy occurs 60 to 100 times more frequently in kidney transplant patients than in age-matched normal controls. Malignancy also afflicts recipients of nonrenal transplants. Squamous cell carcinoma of the skin, the commonest malignancy in kidney transplant patients, is usually highly curable. Lymphoproliferative tumors, some of which are truly malignant, also occur and often involve the brain. Malignancy, like infection, probably reflects excessive immunosuppression. The precise mechanisms of tumor induction or facilitation in transplant patients are unclear, but depressed immune surveillance and increased propensity for virus-induced malignancy are two possible pathways.

CLINICAL TRANSPLANTATION

Tissue and organ autotransplants are common: skin, hair, teeth, digits, tendons, blood vessels, pericardium, nerves, bone, cartilage, parathyroid fragments, and intestinal segments are not infrequently transferred from one part of a patient's body to another part for reconstitution of appearance or function. Allotransplants of these structures have been attempted less frequently than autotransplants because of the probability of rejection in the absence of immunosuppression; however, allografts or even xenografts of skin serve as temporary coverage for large burn wounds, and allografts of blood (blood transfusions) are used extensively all over the world. Corneal allografts are not rejected unless the cornea, which normally is nourished by diffusion, develops an ingrowth of capillaries carrying host cells capable of rejecting the graft. Bone marrow allografts (infusions) are sometimes provided to patients with primary or secondary bone marrow failure; the bone marrow allografts are not only subject to rejection by the host but are also capable of attacking the host (graft-versus-host disease). Allograft or xenograft (porcine) heart valve replacements, in some ways superior to synthetic artificial heart valves, tend to deteriorate slowly, perhaps partly because of rejection.

Immunosuppression, invariably administered to recipients of bone marrow allografts, is occasionally appropriate for persons who have rejected multiple corneal grafts or for burn patients receiving skin grafts from living relatives. However, most tissue allografts or xenografts are not considered vulnerable enough to rejection to justify the risks of immunosuppression.

For patients who have vascularized organ allografts such as kidney, liver, pancreas, heart, heart-lung, or intestine, immunosuppression is initiated prophylactically at or before the time of transplantation to prevent rejection before it starts. For recipients of identical-twin kidney transplants or identical-twin partial pancreas transplants, immunosuppression is unnecessary (rejection does not occur between monozygotic twins), but immunosuppression in low doses is sometimes used to suppress recurrence of the original disease (glomerulonephritis or type I diabetes).

Kidney transplantation

Patients with irreversible end-stage renal disease (ESRD) have two potential ways of replacing the lost kidney function: chronic dialysis or kidney transplantation. A pretransplant period of peritoneal dialysis or hemodialysis is usually advisable to treat uremia and optimize the patient's general health before transplantation. Either a peritoneal dialysis catheter is inserted or an arteriovenous vascular access is established to carry out dialysis. Peritoneal dialysis, a slower exchange process than hemodialysis, can be carried out on a continuous ambulatory basis (CAPD) with three or four fluid exchanges per day or by a stationary mechanical pump for approximately 8 hours per night while the patient sleeps (IPD). The main difficulty with peritoneal dialysis is peritonitis; some patients' peritoneal cavities are so scarred from previous operations or previous intraperitoneal infections that peritoneal dialysis is impossible. Patients undergo hemodialysis for 4 to 5 hours three times per week, either in a dialysis facility or at home. The main difficulty with hemodialysis is thrombosis of vascular access, which occurs more often with synthetic arteriovenous vascular grafts than with autogenous arteriovenous fistulas.

In the early 1960s when kidney transplantation was just starting to be developed, there were very strict criteria for acceptance into transplant programs. In the 1980s kidney transplantations became a realistic option for most patients with irreversible end-stage renal disease, but patients older than a range of 55 to 60 years of age, less able to tolerate immunosuppression, are less frequently candidates than younger patients are. A history of recent malignancy is a contraindication to transplantation because of the risk that immunosuppression will foster the growth and spread of any residual foci of cancer. In the United States in the early 1980s, less than 10% (5000 to 5500) of the chronic dialysis population (approximately 60,000) received kidney transplants each year; one third of the kidneys were provided by living relatives and two thirds by cadaver donors.

The kidney-transplant operation (Fig. 36-2) consists in performing three anastomoses: artery, vein, and ureter. Any of these anastomoses can become stenotic or occluded, but technical anastomotic complications occur in less than 10% of kidney-transplant recipients.

In the early 1980s when donor and recipient were ABO compatible and the recipient did not have preformed cytotoxic antibodies (IgG) against donor T-lymphocytes (negative direct cross-match test), the 1-year cadaver graft survival rate in some transplant centers rose to a range of 80% to 85% and the 1-year patient survival rose to a range of 90% to 95%. The main cause of graft failure was still rejection, and the main cause of patient mortality was still infection. These results with cadaver

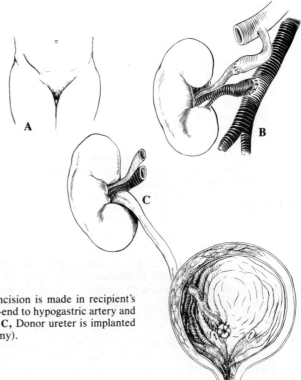

Fig. 36-2. Renal homotransplantation. **A,** Incision is made in recipient's groin. **B,** Renal artery is anastomosed end-to-end to hypogastric artery and renal vein end-to-side to external iliac vein. **C,** Donor ureter is implanted into recipient's bladder (ureteroneocystostomy).

kidneys were only very slightly inferior to the results with living related transplants.

The majority of irreversible rejections of kidney transplants and of patient deaths occur within the first 3 to 6 months after transplantation. A recipient's immune system almost never fully accepts a transplanted organ, and even a kidney transplant that is initially accepted is likely to be chronically rejected over a period of years. After the first year after transplantation, the rate of graft loss from rejection is approximately 5% per year. Infection continues to be a major cause of patient mortality, but atherosclerotic heart disease and other causes of death in the general population also take their toll.

Liver transplantation

Liver transplantation is recommended for some patients with irreversible end-stage liver disease. The timing of liver transplantation is more critical than the timing of kidney transplantation because there is no mechanical support system for patients with liver failure, in contrast to dialysis for patients with kidney failure. A patient with fulminant irreversible liver failure rarely survives for more than a few days. Liver transplantation, seldom recommended until a patient's predicted survival is less than a few months, should be carried out before the patient becomes moribund.

Congenital biliary atresia, cirrhosis caused by hepatitis, and cirrhosis caused by inborn errors of metabolism are indications for liver transplantation. Alcoholic cirrhosis, a more common problem, is less amenable to treatment by liver transplantation because of the high probability of persistent alcoholism and resultant sequelae. Primary liver cancer has been treated by liver replacement, but the cancer is likely to recur and metastasize widely under the influence of immunosuppression.

For nonmalignant liver disease, the heterotopic auxiliary liver transplant (Fig. 36-3) is an appealing concept because it spares the patient the risk of

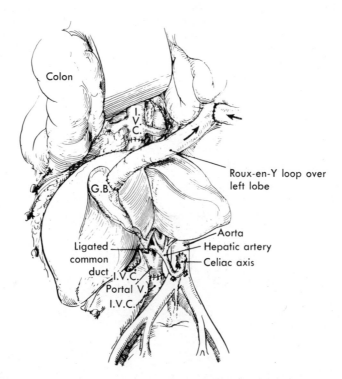

Fig. 36-3. Heterotopic liver transplantation. Patient's own liver is under retractor at top of illustration. Recipient's vena cava was transected below level of renal veins and donor liver was revascularized as follows: Donor portal vein was anastomosed to recipient's distal inferior vena cava; donor's suprahepatic vena cava was joined to recipient's proximal inferior vena cava; donor celiac axis was anastomosed to recipient's aorta. Donor subhepatic vena cava was closed with suture. Common bile duct was ligated below its junction with cystic duct, and biliary drainage was provided by anastomosis of gallbladder to Roux-en-Y loop of small bowel. (From Starzl, T.E.: Experience in hepatic transplantation, Philadelphia, 1969, W.B. Saunders Co.)

removal of the cirrhotic liver and provides the advantage of retaining potential functional hepatic reserve in the cirrhotic liver. However, the few attempted human auxiliary liver transplants were not chronically successful, partly because the old liver competes with the transplant for hepatotrophic substances such as insulin.

The majority of human liver transplants have been orthotopic liver replacements (Fig. 36-4). This operation is extremely difficult in patients with advanced cirrhosis because of massive intraoperative hemorrhage attributable to portal hypertension and impaired blood-coagulation mechanisms. Autotransfusion by means of a venovenous shunt without heparin has recently been developed to reduce the risk of hemorrhage during the procedure. The liver replacement operation usually requires four vascular anastomoses: suprahepatic inferior vena cava, infrahepatic inferior vena cava, portal vein, and hepatic artery. The fifth anastomosis, for bile drainage, has been the least reliable of the five anastomoses because of bile leakage and biliary obstruction. If the recipient's common bile duct is patent, choledocho-choledochostomy over a T-tube stent is the preferred method of bile drainage. If the recipient's common bile duct is not usable, as in congenital biliary atresia, choledocho-

jejunostomy or cholecystojejunostomy are alternatives.

With an experienced surgical team, using cyclosporine and prednisone immunosuppression, the 1-year survival after liver replacement in the early 1980s rose to more than 70%, in contrast to 30% to 50% during the 1970s. The longest current survivor is a 16-year-old girl who underwent liver transplantation more than 14 years ago.

Heart transplantation

At Stanford University, which has the largest experience with this procedure, heart transplantation has become highly therapeutic. Three parts of the operative technique are illustrated in Fig. 36-5. The recipients have usually been young adults with intractable heart failure from cardiomyopathy caused by severe coronary artery disease, viruses, or unknown agents. Severe pulmonary hypertension interdicts orthotopic cardiac replacement because of the inability of the donor right ventricle to pump effectively against high resistance. Percutaneous transjugular endomyocardial biopsy specimens of the right ventricle have been valuable guides to early rejection. In the early 1980s at Stanford University the 1-year patient survival after orthotopic heart transplantation (replace-

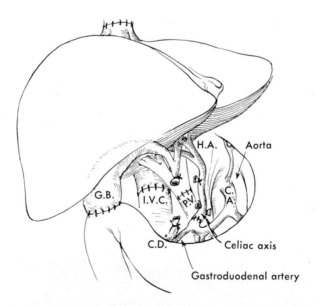

Fig. 36-4. Orthotopic liver transplantation. Host's diseased liver and related segment of inferior vena cava have been removed. Donor liver and related segment of inferior vena cava have been placed in position with anastomoses of vena cava above and below liver, portal veins, and hepatic arteries. Donor common bile duct was ligated and biliary drainage provided by anastomosis of gallbladder to duodenum. This method of biliary drainage (cholecystoduodenostomy) has been replaced by choledocho-choledochostomy over a T-tube stent or by choledochojejunostomy (Roux en Y). (From Starzl, T.E.: Experience in hepatic transplantation, Philadelphia, 1969, W.B. Saunders Co.)

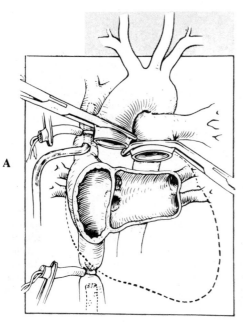

Fig. 36-5. Transplantation of heart. **A,** Using cardiopulmonary bypass recipient's heart has been excised with transected posterior portions of both atria, ascending aorta, and pulmonary artery being left behind. **B,** Entire donor heart has been removed. Superior vena cava has been ligated. Right atrium has been opened by incision from inferior vena cava opening extending toward atrial appendage, with care being taken to preserve sinus node and sinoauricular pathways. Left atrium has been opened by incision joining orifices of the four pulmonary veins. **C,** Donor heart is sewn into recipient. Left and then right atrial anastomoses are completed, followed by anastomosis of pulmonary artery and aorta. (From Cooley, D.A.: J.A.M.A. **205:**479-486, 1968.)

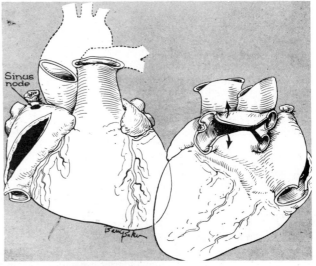

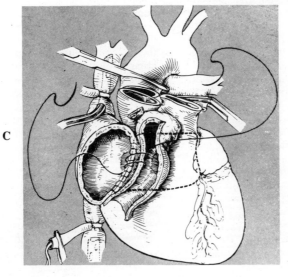

ment) rose to approximately 70%, with a 5-year survival of approximately 50%. Immunosuppression for most of these patients was cyclosporine and prednisone. Recurrence of coronary artery disease was decreased by dietary measures and antilipidemia medications. Most patients surviving heart transplantation, whose life expectancies were only a few months without transplantation, have been successfully rehabilitated.

Auxiliary (heterotopic) heart transplantation is an appealing alternative to heart replacement in patients with protracted but reversible heart failure, who cannot be maintained by intra-aortic balloon assist pumps. Auxiliary heart transplantation may also apply to patients with end-stage heart disease whose pulmonary hypertension precludes heart replacement; however as with auxiliary liver transplantation, the therapeutic value of the auxiliary graft remains uncertain.

Lung and heart-lung transplantation

Between 1963 and 1980, approximately 25 patients had one lung replaced, and a few patients had transplantation of one pulmonary lobe. One patient in 1970 had transplantation of both lungs. The longest survivor, 10 months, was a patient who had a single lung transplant in 1968 for silicosis. Most of the other patients died soon after transplantation.

The three main problems for these patients were suboptimal quality of donor lung, disruption of bronchial anastomoses, and graft rejection. All brain-dead cadaver organ donors are ventilated mechanically, and their lungs are often abnormal by the time of death. Bronchial anastomotic healing was often impaired by ischemia of the graft bronchus because of interruption of bronchial arteries. In these patients, lung allograft rejection was difficult to distinguish from pulmonary problems of nonimmunological origin.

Combined heart-lung transplantation was initially undertaken at Stanford University in 1981 for patients with end-stage pulmonary hypertension secondary to Eisenmenger's syndrome or unknown cause. Of the first 13 patients to have this procedure at Stanford between 1981 and 1983, three died during the first month after operation, but the longest survivor was doing well 22 months after operation. The combined heart-lung transplant, in addition to its applicability for patients with pulmonary hypertension, may prove to be a better procedure than isolated lung transplantation for patients with end-stage parenchymal lung disease.

Pancreas transplantation

The pancreas is not essential for life. Transplantation of this organ is undertaken to improve quality of life by alleviating the vascular complications of type I diabetes mellitus, which may at an early age result in blindness from retinopathy, loss of limb from peripheral arterial disease, or renal failure from glomerulopathy. The discovery of insulin in 1921 and its subsequent widespread use has usually prevented death from diabetic coma, but even constant infusion of insulin from portable pumps connected to subcutaneous delivery systems has not convincingly prevented the vascular complications of diabetes.

Although the precise cause of the vascular complications of diabetes is not known, experimental work in animals indicates that these complications can be prevented or arrested by transplantation of the endocrine part of the pancreas (the islets of Langerhans). It is mechanically difficult to separate adult human pancreatic islets from the surrounding exocrine pancreas tissue without damage to the islets, but islet transplantation is an attractive concept because of its simplicity: islets can be injected into a vein or implanted in tissue without a complex operation. Fetal human islet tissue is more immunogenic than adult islets but is also easier to isolate than adult human islet tissue; it is therefore a potentially reliable source of transplantable islet tissue. Up to now no human islet transplant has been chronically successful.

A second more complex method of pancreas transplantation is revascularization of the whole pancreas (with or without duodenum) or the body-and-tail segment of pancreas. Such large grafts are revascularized by use of donor celiac axis and superior mesenteric artery in pancreaticoduodenal grafts, or by donor splenic artery in segmental body-and-tail grafts. The proteolytic proenzymes in the exocrine pancreas can become activated by inflammation, causing serious intra-abdominal complications. In order to avoid such complications, the pancreatic exocrine output has been blocked by injection of quick-setting polymers into the pancreatic duct system; alternatively the exocrine output has been drained into the free peritoneal cavity, Roux-en-Y–jejunal limb, ureter, or bladder. None of these techniques has been an entirely safe or effective method for handling the exocrine secretions of large pancreas grafts. This unresolved mechanical problem of the exocrine pancreatic output has been a major reason for the unsatisfactory results of pancreas transplantation (approximately 25% successful). Recurrent diabetes in the graft (manifested by beta cell destruction in the islets) and graft rejection appear to have been less important causes of failure, though the relative importance of these processes might increase if the mechanical exocrine drainage problem could be solved.

Intestinal transplantation

There are a small number of children with intestinal atresia and a small number of adults with midgut infarction or extensive inflammatory bowel disease who could benefit from small-bowel transplantation, if bowel rejection (with anastomotic disruption) and if graft-versus-host disease from intestinal lymphoid tissue could be prevented. Intestinal transplantation is still highly experimental.

Retransplantation

When a transplant fails, retransplantation is a potential option. Patients with renal failure sometimes undergo multiple retransplantations if they desire this form of therapy rather than chronic dialysis. Patients with end-stage heart, lung, or liver failure whose transplants fail have no way of surviving other than retransplantation; however such patients are usually very ill and retransplantation of these organs has been less successful than primary transplantation.

ORGAN PRESERVATION

Organ preservation, a vital component of transplantation technology, allows time for transport of the organ from donor to recipient. In kidney transplantation, the preservation also allows time for histocompatibility matching.

The most important aspect of organ preservation is cooling, to reduce metabolism and to reduce oxygen demand. Balanced intracellular type of electrolyte solution containing potassium ion at approximately 115 mEq./L. and sodium ion at 10 mEq./L. is used for preservation of most cadaveric kidneys, heart, and livers. At 4° to 8° C, kidneys can be stored in this solution for 24 to 48 hours; longer storage periods are associated with greater than 50% initial nonfunction. Initial nonfunction, even for weeks, is acceptable in kidney transplantation because dialysis can support the patient until adequate function begins. In liver transplantation, where early function after transplantation is essential for survival, the safe cold storage time is currently 8 to 10 hours. In heart transplantation,

where immediate function after transplantation is essential for survival, the safe cold storage time is currently less than 6 hours. Heart-lung grafts are performed with donor and recipient in adjacent operating rooms to reduce transfer time to an absolute minimum.

Organ preservation can also be accomplished by a pulsatile perfusion machine, which cools the organ to 4° to 8° C and at the same time pumps through it cryoprecipitated (to remove lipoproteins) plasma, or a plasma substitute, as well as oxygen. Pulsatile perfusion currently appears to have little advantage over simple cold storage for most purposes.

Whichever of the two methods for organ preservation is used, the organ must be well perfused and well oxygenated in the brain-dead cadaver donor until the moment the organ is removed from the donor, so that irreversible warm ischemic damage is avoided.

ORGAN DONOR ISSUES

In the United States the concept of brain death is now well accepted, as reflected in brain-death legislation presently in force in most states. Federally controlled organ-sharing programs may replace the less controlled but effective regional organ-sharing arrangements developed during the 1960s and 1970s. As the availability of cadaver kidneys for transplantation increases and the results of cadaver kidney transplantation approach the results of living related kidney transplantation, families can ethically be spared the trauma and risks of living related kidney donation.

CONCLUSIONS

More than 50,000 kidney transplants, 500 liver transplants, and 500 heart transplants have been carried out during the last 20 years. Despite imperfections in immunosuppression and in other aspects of transplantation medicine and surgery, many of these grafts have improved the quality of life and increased the length of life of the patients who received them.

Thermal Injuries

Charles E. Hartford
Albert E. Cram

Each year in industrialized Western nations approximately 250 people per million population are admitted to hospitals for the care of burns. More than half of these patients are less than 20 years of age. In the United States there are about 6,500 fire-related deaths each year. Among survivors, morbidity is often prolonged because of scarring and disfigurement. In addition, property loss from fire is considerable. The burn injury and fire problem is a silent epidemic.

Most burns occur in and around the home, particularly in the kitchen, utility room, garage, and yard. Those at highest risk for burns are the young, the aged, and the mentally and physically infirm. Altered mentation from drugs, alcohol, and disease frequently contribute to burn injury. Many of these persons have neither the physical capability nor the presence of mind to protect themselves from scalding liquids or to extinguish or remove burning clothing. Furthermore, when clothing burns, an injury of lethal extent can easily occur within 1 minute.

Many who treat burns believe the next important advance in this field lies in prevention. In the United States, federal legislation requires that flame-retardant material be used for the manufacture of night-wear size 12 and smaller. Although this is an important advance, it is clearly not enough. There is federal legislation pending that would mandate self-extinguishing properties for cigarettes. It is estimated that this alone would reduce fire deaths in the United States by one half.

PATHOPHYSIOLOGY
The wound

Heat from many sources can cause burns. Although pain from heat is perceived at 47.5° C., injury to cells will occur at 45° C. The damage done depends on the intensity and duration of exposure. Protein coagulates instantly at 65° C., and instantaneous exposure at 72° C. produces a blister (a burn of second degree or partial thickness of skin).

The gross appearance of thermally injured tissue ranges from erythema and blisters of more superficial burns to the charred black, leathery brown, or cadaveric white of deep burns. Coagulated veins usually signify full-thickness skin injury. Intense and prolonged exposure may cause the skin to split, exposing subcutaneous fat.

The skin is the major organ injured in a burn; an appreciation of its basic anatomy, physiology, and reaction to thermal injury is essential to understand depth of injury and healing.

Skin is composed of squamous epithelium on the surface, beneath which are several layers of maturing cells originating from the stratum germinativum. These layers and the epidermal appendages are supported by interwoven collagen fibers of the dermis (Fig. 37-1). The epidermal appendages are derived from ectoderm and include hair follicles, sebaceous glands, and sweat ducts and their glands. The lining cells of these appendages retain the ability to transform to squamous epithelium, a process known as *squamous metaplasia*. Therefore, if viable epidermal appendages remain after injury and their viability can be preserved, the wound will reepithelialize by squamous metaplasia.

Very superficial burns (commonly known as first degree) are characterized by erythema. Only the upper portion of the surface epithelium is destroyed, and rapid healing without scarring occurs.

In superficial partial-thickness burns (superficial dermal burns or superficial second-degree burns) the injury extends deeper into the skin, but the

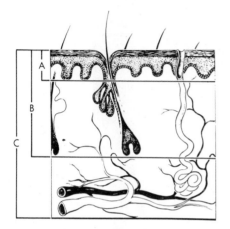

Fig. 37-1. Diagram of skin showing a practical classification of depth of injury. Injury down to level *A* is known as superficial partial-thickness burn; to level *B*, deep partial-thickness; and to level *C*, full-thickness burn.

stratum germinativum and the major portion of each epidermal appendage is preserved. Therefore spontaneous reepithelialization or healing occurs rapidly and usually within 3 weeks. Because there is virtually no disturbance of the collagen in the dermis, there is rapid return of skin tone and texture, and scarring is minimal.

In deep partial-thickness burns (deep dermal burns or deep second-degree burns) the injury extends below the level of the stratum germinativum, but, depending on the depth, varying portions of epidermal appendages remain viable. Cells of viable portions of these appendages undergo squamous metaplasia and appear in granulation tissue as islands of epithelium that expand and coalesce to resurface the wound (Fig. 37-2). When the entirety of the pyelosebaceous unit and a large portion of the sweat duct are destroyed, and only the deep-seated sweat glands, which may lie in the superficial portion of the subcutaneous tissue, are preserved, healing takes much longer and may occur as late as 120 days after injury.

The existence of these sweat glands is tenuous. Their destruction by infection may be a frequent occurrence and is a mechanism by which partial-thickness burn is converted to full-thickness injury. In deep partial-thickness burns there is also extensive disturbance of dermal collagen fibers. As healing progresses, the reformed collagen fibers are often in disarray and irregular whorls are seen histologically. A *hypertrophic scar* forms. This kind of scar is erythematous, raised, and indurated

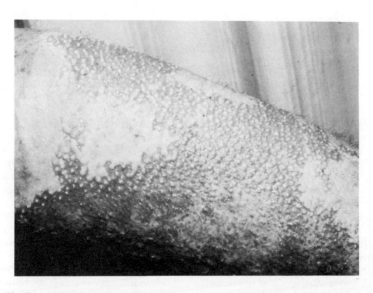

Fig. 37-2. Healing partial-thickness burn showing islands of squamous epithelium that have emerged from epidermal appendages. Epithelium will expand to resurface wound.

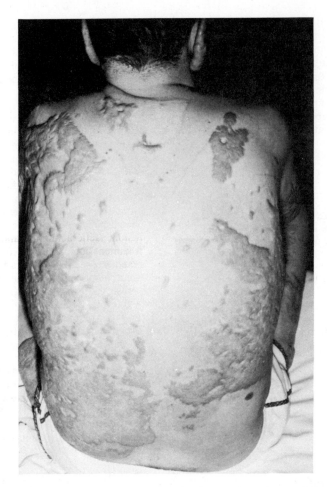

Fig. 37-3. Most of this patient's back was burned, but it all healed without skin grafting. Adjacent to unburned skin (outlined by straps of overalls) are unscarred areas intermixed with irregular raised areas, which constitute hypertrophic scarring. Superficial partial thickness burns usually heal with minimal scarring, but the deeper the partial thickness burn, the more likely the chance of hypertrophic scarring. Hypertrophic scarring rarely occurs when burns heal spontaneously within 3 weeks.

(Fig. 37-3). The longer it takes for a wound to heal and the more extensive the granulation tissue, the greater will be the tendency to form hypertrophic scars. For this reason, it may be better to close a deep partial-thickness wound by skin graft rather than to allow it to heal spontaneously, provided that donor skin is available. A hypertrophic scar is not to be confused with a *keloid,* which is a neoplasm.

In full-thickness (third-degree) burns, surface epithelium and all epidermal appendages as well are destroyed. Spontaneous healing from the depth of the wound is impossible. Coverage of the wound occurs only by epithelial ingrowth from the edges or by autogenous skin grafting.

Identification of burn depth by gross inspection is unreliable. Depth can be determined with certainty only by biopsy. To await spontaneous healing is not accurate because partial-thickness burns may be converted to full thickness. However, recent experiences with perfusion and photographic fluorometry have been helpful in distinguishing partial- from full-thickness level of injury. These techniques quantify fluorescence of tissues after intravenous injection of small quantities of fluorescein.

Necrotic tissue caused by heat is known as *eschar* and acts as a foreign body. At the interface between eschar and viable tissue inflammation initiates removal of eschar by autolysis, digestion,

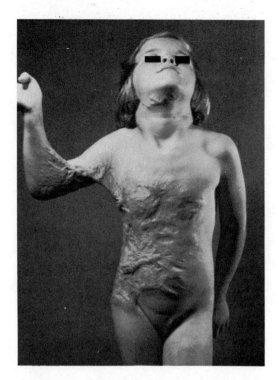

Fig. 37-4. Burn contracture of axilla and antecubital fossa, severely limiting motion of right upper extremity.

and liquefaction. These processes also effect separation of eschar, which cause it to be cast off as a sequestrum.

Eschar is invariably colonized by bacteria. As a consequence, several devastating events can occur. By virtue of unimpeded access to the body through the wound, these microorganisms may initiate bacteremia or septicemia or both. Price and co-workers showed that bacteria implanted on an experimental burn could be recovered from regional lymph nodes as early after injury as 8 hours. Many bacteria, both gram negative and gram positive, fungi, and even viruses can cause invasive infection of burns.

Contraction plays an important role in the healing of all burns and contributes to much of the deformity after a burn has healed. The resulting *contracture* is defined as epithelized scar that inhibits normal range of motion (Fig. 37-4).

Fluid shifts and burn shock

Thermal injury causes translocation of body fluids, the net result of which is hypovolemia. If the burn is large enough and the patient is not properly treated, circulatory and renal failure occur; that is known as *burn shock*. There is a decrease in peripheral vascular resistance with a lesion in the microcirculation where capillaries become abnormally permeable, initiating the shift in body fluids. This lesion may arise from hypoxia, direct thermal injury, biologically active substances produced in heated tissues, released intracellular enzymes, or a combination of these factors. Obligatory sequestration of fluid, containing an ultrafiltrate of plasma, occurs into the extravascular space in both injured and uninjured tissues. This produces edema, which at times is massive (Fig. 37-5). The shift of fluid from the intravascular space progressively diminishes plasma volume, blood volume, and cardiac output and leads to hemoconcentration, hypotension, poor tissue perfusion, lactic acidemia, and metabolic acidosis. If treatment is inadequate or the patient does not respond to the resuscitative effort, acute renal failure supervenes and intravascular thrombi form as blood flow slows. Death ensues.

The rate of obligatory sequestration of fluid, maximal soon after injury, follows a descending parabolic curve. Sometime between 18 and 30 hours after injury microcirculatory integrity is restored. At this point edema is maximal. Then there is gradual resorption of edema concurrent with an increase in the intravascular volume, cardiac output, and urine production; during this phase of recovery, congestive heart failure and pulmonary edema may occur. The diuresis continues at a steady pace until the patient returns to water balance, which occurs in 4 to 14 days depending on the size of the burn. Fluid is also lost at an obligatory rate through the wound and insensibly through the lung.

Urinary output is an important index of the adequacy of fluid resuscitation. Patients with biologically significant burns become oliguric unless they receive adequate fluid. Even with clinically acceptable urine flows, there is depression of renal plasma flow and a slight decrease in the glomerular filtration rate.

Although some of the red cell mass is destroyed during the injury, the hematocrit level and hemoglobin concentration are elevated because of the aforementioned hemoconcentration. Hemoglobinuria may occur. The serum potassium and sodium levels are usually normal. The serum bicarbonate and pH and PCO_2 of arterial blood are usually low, reflecting metabolic acidosis. If the $PaCO_2$ is normal or elevated, it may indicate either an associated inhalation injury or preexisting pulmonary insufficiency, and the prognosis is worse. The $PaCO_2$ is usually low to normal. The serum levels of BUN and creatinine are usually normal; an elevation may indicate preexisting renal

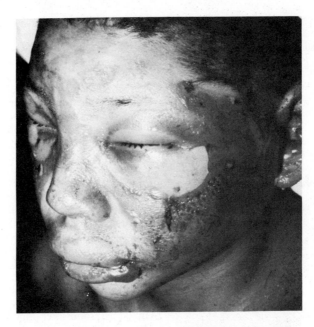

Fig. 37-5. Swelling caused by burn that healed without scar.

disease or a delay in treatment, implying a poorer prognosis.

Many systemic effects are associated with large surface and deep burns; for example, a circulating myocardial depressant factor, alterations in clotting mechanisms, suppression of leukocyte function, and alterations in immunological mechanisms have been reported. Some of these systemic effects are a consequence of released intracellular enzymes or "toxins" produced in heated tissues.

KINDS OF BURN
Solar (sunburn)

Sunburn is the result of a complex photochemical reaction caused by exposure to sunlight or an ultraviolet lamp. The burn is superficial and usually not biologically significant. An occasional patient will need to be admitted to the hospital for control of pain with analgesics and cool dressings. The largest number of patients requiring this kind of treatment are injured by sunlamps, especially when the victim falls asleep during exposure.

Flame

Approximately 75% of those treated in a burn care facility receive their injury from flame. When clothing burns, the exposure to heat is prolonged. This enhances the extent of injury, depth of injury, amount of skin grafting required, and mortality.

The pattern of burn sustained from a clothing fire is predictable and depends on the flammability of cloth and style of clothing worn. For instance, the burn from a dress or nightgown classically extends from midthigh to the midportion of the face, whereas the major damage from a fire involving pants is below the level of the belt.

Scald

Patients with scalds have the same mortality risk as those with flame burns of the same extent. However, in most instances the surface area involved by a scald is less than one third of the body.

There are patterns of scalding that are easily recognized. Infants intentionally or unintentionally placed in scalding bathwater sustain a burn of the lower portion of the body (Fig. 37-6). When this kind of injury is found, one should investigate for child abuse or neglect. Toddlers who spill scalding liquids on themselves sustain a unilateral burn. Occasionally, scalding liquids are thrown maliciously; if they are laced with chemicals, the injury is enhanced. Devastating injury to the eye may result by this mechanism.

Heat contact

Except for immersion in molten metals, burns from heat contact are usually limited in extent and therefore are not an important cause of death. However, these burns are usually deep and often require skin grafting.

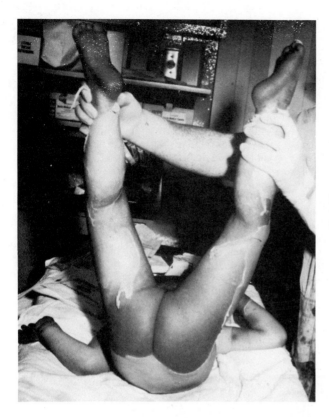

Fig. 37-6. Deep burn sustained while patient was seated in bathtub when sibling turned on hot water tap.

Chemical

The list of potentially injurious chemicals appears infinite. Each year in the United States there are an estimated 3,000 deaths from enteric ingestion and topical contact from chemicals. An additional 60,000 persons seek medical attention for nonlethal chemical burns. The majority of serious chemical injuries occur in industrial accidents.

Chemicals do not burn in the classical sense, i.e., by hyperthermic activity. They damage tissue by coagulation of protein in a variety of ways: reduction, oxidation, salt formation, corrosion, protoplasmic poisoning, metabolic competition or inhibition, desiccation, or ischemia. The injury depends on the nature of the chemical, its concentration, duration of contact, penetrability into tissues, and systemic effect, if any.

As long as the chemical is active and in contact with tissues, injury continues. Therefore, as soon as practical, it is important to either wash the chemical away or neutralize it. Except in rare instances, the most efficacious first-aid treatment is lavage with copious volumes of water. If lavage can be started within 15 seconds, damage is minimized. Although it is not known how long the lavage should be continued, most authorities rec-

ommend 20 to 30 minutes. Beyond these principles, management of wounds that result from chemicals is the same as for any burn.

Electrical

Tissue damage from electricity is caused by heat. The typical injury is a deep necrotic wound often involving skeletal muscle and other tissues far beyond the injury to the skin (Fig. 37-7). In the pathogenesis of electrical injury, two physical laws apply: Ohm's law, $I = \dfrac{V}{R}$, and Joules' law, Calories $= 0.24\ (I)^2 \times R$. Since the voltage is usually constant, the amperage generated is inversely proportional to the resistance of tissues. Bone has the greatest resistance, nerve tissue has the least, and skin is between. The tissues that have the least resistance are the most heat sensitive (e.g., nerve) and vice versa.

As the current passes through the body, several sequelae are possible. A cardiac arrest or life-threatening cardiac arrhythmia may occur from passage of the current through the heart or middle of the brain. Sixty-cycle alternating current, which generates 300 milliamperes of current as it passes through the torso, is the most dangerous to the heart. Effective cardiopulmonary resuscitation is lifesaving because, even in the presence of massive tissue injury, the prognosis for life is excellent once the patient reaches a hospital. When electrical current passes through the brain, unconsciousness commonly occurs. This is usually temporary, followed by a period of incoherent behavior and agitation before the patient becomes lucid again. In a small percentage of cases there are permanent neurological sequelae. As current passes through the torso, the large cross-sectional area dissipates the energy and therefore necrosis of any internal organ, though possible, rarely occurs. If an internal organ is injured, it is usually adjacent to the site of electrical entrance or a contact grounding point. When the current passes through the head, the patient is at risk for developing traumatic cataracts, which occur within 3 years in about 5% of cases. The current leaves the body in contact grounding sites or accumulates in the subcutaneous tissue and bursts through the skin leaving characteristic punctate necrotic wounds known as current marks.

Electrical accidents can conveniently be divided into three categories, those caused by low voltage (less than 1,000 volts), high voltage (1,000 volts or greater), and lightning.

In low-voltage injury, usually caused by house current, tissue damage is usually small. However, when children chew on defective electrical cords, an unsightly deformity of the mouth may occur. Death from cardiac arrhythmia is not unusual from 60-cycle alternating house current, even without visible tissue damage.

Young adult males at work are those most frequently involved in high-voltage accidents. Tissue damage is usually extensive, especially at the site of electrical entrance. Underlying muscle damage may be extensive and extend far beyond the skin injury; therefore a major amputation is often necessary (Fig. 37-7). Electrical accidents are accompanied by arcing of electrical current. When high voltages are involved, the temperatures generated may exceed 2,400° C., causing either a burn of the skin or ignition of the victim's clothing.

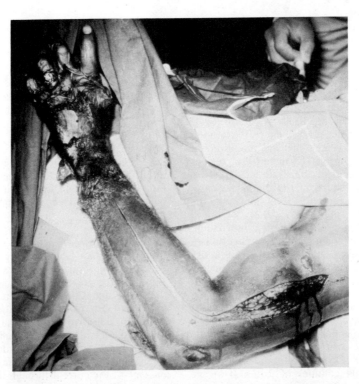

Fig. 37-7. High-voltage electrical injury. Obvious charring of hand and wrist. Incision through skin caused bleeding only in mid-arm. Muscle in both arm and forearm was necrotic; shoulder disarticulation was necessary. Patient survived.

Patients with extensive tissue damage from electricity may require prodigious volumes of fluid to successfully restore circulation. In addition, two chromogens, myoglobin from destroyed muscle and hemoglobin from injured red blood cells, together with acidosis from poor perfusion and hypovolemia, all increase the possibility of acute renal failure. High-volume urine flows should be maintained until these pigments (chromogens) are cleared from the plasma.

The proper time to debride patients with deep necrosis is a matter of controversy. We believe the risk of and the sequelae from bacterial infection and clostridial myonecrosis are too great to treat these wounds expectantly. We advocate the following plan. Soon after admission the wounds are incised and the underlying muscle examined (Fig. 37-7). If the muscle is viable, the wound is managed as any thermal burn. If the muscle is necrotic, plans are made for débridement in the operating room. We usually do not debride until the danger of acute renal failure is past. It may take several procedures to remove all the dead tissue.

FACTORS THAT INFLUENCE PROGNOSIS
Depth of burn

Classification of burn depth was discussed in the section on pathophysiology of the burn wound. The deeper the burn, the greater the mortality. If partial-thickness burns are converted to full thickness by infection, the prognosis is much worse because of the increased risk associated with septicemia.

Age of patient

Fig. 37-8 emphasizes the importance of age as a function of survival for burned patients. Burns are poorly tolerated by infants because of immature organ and immunological systems. Among the aged, the prognosis is poor because of associated degenerative disease and diminished properties of healing inherent in the aging process.

Percent burn	Age (years)				
	0-<2	2-9	10-39	40-59	60+
0-9	0% 0 80	0% 0 93	0% 0 284	0% 0 83	4% 2 49
10-29	0% 0 64	1% 1 96	<1% 2 349	3.5% 4 115	26.5% 27 102
30-59	0% 0 15	0% 0 40	4% 7 159	17% 10 59	67% 33 49
60-79	50% 1 2	50% 4 8	25% 12 48	60% 9 15	100% 17 17
80-100	100% 2 2	100% 7 7	62.5% 15 24	100% 13 13	100% 14 14

Fig. 37-8. Burn mortality for 1,787 patients at the University of Iowa between September 1969 and July 1984. In each block the number of patients is in the lower right corner, the number of deaths is in the lower left corner, and the mortality percentage is in the center.

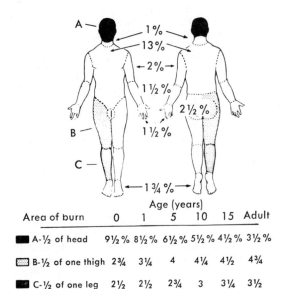

Area of burn	Age (years)					
	0	1	5	10	15	Adult
■ A-½ of head	9½%	8½%	6½%	5½%	4½%	3½%
▨ B-½ of one thigh	2¾	3¼	4	4¼	4½	4¾
■ C-½ of one leg	2½	2½	2¾	3	3¼	3½

Fig. 37-9. Modified from Lund and Browder. This is an accepted method to calculate surface area involved by burn. It takes into account that as one grows from infancy to adulthood, surface area of head becomes relatively less and surface area of lower extremities becomes relatively greater.

Sex of patient

Reports encompassing large numbers of burn patients suggest that the human female tolerates thermal injury less well than the human male. Although this is true at virtually every age, the cause of this statistically significant difference is unknown.

Surface area involved by burn

The greater the body surface area burned, the greater the mortality.

A rapid estimate of the surface area burned can be obtained when the "rule of nines" is applied,* but this rule is not accurate. The method of Lund and Browder (Fig. 37-9) gives a more accurate assessment.

Fig. 37-8 clearly illustrates the relationship between percentage of burn and mortality. To aid in discussing results, the figure is divided into three areas: unshaded, cross-hatched, and shaded.

The unshaded area represents those patients who were virtually assured of survival, based on the size of burn, age, and treatment rendered. This group consists of 1,483 of the 1,787 patients treated (83%). However, 26 of these patients died, most from unusual causes of death for burned patients:

direct thermal injury to the brain, trauma from an automobile accident, serious intercurrent illness, or, among the elderly, degenerative diseases. Smoke inhalation may cause death in a patient with a small surface area burn.

The 248 patients (14% of the total) in the cross-hatched area of Fig. 37-8 had a mortality ranging from 25% to 67%. Although this mortality compares favorably with those in other burn care facilities, some patients who were potentially salvageable died. The burns of these patients were neither large enough nor distributed in such a way to cause early death, but the metabolic reserve or the treatment rendered, or both, were not good enough to allow survival. Most of the deaths were attributable to sepsis, still the most frequent cause of death in burned patients.

The 53 patients (3% of the 1,787) in the shaded area of Fig. 37-8 had virtually no chance of survival because of extremely large and deep burns or advanced age. These patients could not be effectively resuscitated and died within several days of injury. Survival is being reported increasingly in patients with greater than 80% body surface area burn, particularly among young adults and children.

To try to improve survival, new techniques are being investigated. These include early and staged excision of the burn with closure of the wound either permanently with autograft skin or temporarily with viable cadaver homograft skin or with one of several synthetic skin substitutes under

---

*Rule of nines: The body is divided into areas, each representing 9% or 18% (twice 9) of the body surface area; head and each upper extremity are 9%; anterior torso, back, and each lower extremity are 18%.

development or clinical trial; new drugs to control infection caused by gram-negative bacteria, fungi, and viruses; and improvements in nutritional and supportive care.

Preexisting medical conditions

Although patients with advanced degenerative, neoplastic, and other serious medical conditions have been successfully treated for burns, these conditions generally indicate a poorer prognosis. Burned patients with chronic renal disease or those who develop renal impairment from whatever cause have a poor prognosis. Burns are also poorly tolerated by the morbidly obese, primarily because of their diminished pulmonary reserve and the fact that obese people are often not well nourished.

Respiratory tract damage

It is well recognized that respiratory tract damage from smoke and carbon monoxide poisoning have a detrimental effect on outcome from flame burns. Many authorities identify inhalation injury and advanced age as the current most important limiting factors in survival. This is reflected in mortality data from the Crozer-Chester Medical Center, Chester, Pennsylvania, for 1977. During that year, there were 30 burn deaths. Twenty-six of those patients had, as a component of their injury, respiratory tract damage. Inhalation injury will be discussed further later in this chapter.

TREATMENT OF BURN SHOCK

Prevention of, or resuscitation from, burn shock is the most important item in the early management of a seriously burned patient. The timely administration of fluids to patients with large surface burns prevents death from burn shock. These fluids must contain sodium, but whether colloids are needed or even desirable is controversial.

Several formulas have been devised for calculating fluid requirements of the burned patient. These formulas are only guides, and each patient's response to treatment must be assessed repeatedly and adjustments made in fluid therapy.

The Brooke formula, published in 1953, is a modification of the Evans formula, which was described in 1952. According to the Brooke formula, the volume of fluid recommended for each of the first two 24-hour postburn periods is calculated from the body weight and the percent surface area of burn. A percentage of this fluid is given as crystalloid and a percentage as colloid.

Brooke formula

FIRST 24 HOURS:
    Crystalloid: 1.5 ml./kg. body weight/% burn as lactated Ringer's solution

Colloid: 0.5 ml./kg. body weight/% burn as plasma, Plasmanate, or dextran
    Maintenance: 2,000 ml. as 5% dextrose in water
    Half the calculated volume is given during the first 8 hours, the other half during the next 16 hours
SECOND 24 HOURS:
    Half of the first 24 hours of calculated colloid and crystalloid
    Maintenance: 2,000 ml. as 5% dextrose in water

To avoid fluid overload, the authors of these two formulas recommended that the initial estimate should not exceed the volume estimated for a 50% surface area burn. However, in actual practice the calculation accurately predicts the fluid requirement for a burn of up to 50% of the body surface; above that the volumes increase linearly as the extent of burn increases.

Many patients are successfully resuscitated with balanced salt solution alone. This technique is based on the premise that the amount of sodium needed is the common denominator for successful resuscitation and that colloid given during the first 18 to 24 hours after injury does not augment the plasma volume. However, after the leaky capillaries seal, colloid then augments the plasma volume by the amount of colloid given. The original technique of using balanced crystalloid developed by Moyer and co-workers has been modified by Baxter. The latter recommends 4 ml. lactated Ringer's solution/kg. body weight/% body surface burn, half of the calculated volume to be given in the first 8 hours and the rest over the next 16 hours. After all the calculated fluid has been given, the patient is evaluated for adequacy of resuscitation; if signs are less than optimal, the patient is cautiously given colloid (plasma) to expand the plasma volume.

By prospective study, we have found that adding albumin to lactated Ringer's solution to make a 2.3% solution of albumin reduced by one third the amount of fluid and sodium needed for successful resuscitation when compared with the lactated Ringer's solution alone (Table 37-1). Children require more fluid than adults with the same percentage of body surface burn. We did not find a difference in mortality among patients treated with the two solutions. However, there was a statistically significant reduction in complications of fluid therapy among those treated with the albumin in lactated Ringer's solution.

Most previously healthy young adults with burns of less than two thirds of the body surface are successfully resuscitated by a variety of regimens. However, the following circumstances make treatment difficult: burns in excess of two thirds of the body surface, extremes of age, premorbid impairment of the cardiovascular, respiratory, and renal

Table 37-1. Average volumes of fluid given in first 24 hours*

Age (years)	LR† ml./kg./% burn	LR + A‡ ml./kg./% burn
2-12	5.2	3.4
13-59	2.9	2.0

*Fluid volume data derived from 29 patients with burns in excess of 30% of the body surface who were successfully resuscitated and whose urinary output was maintained between 30 and 50 ml. an hour.
†Lactated Ringer's solution.
‡2.3% albumin in lactated Ringer's solution.

systems, and delay in treatment. *Since fluid resuscitation is actually a clinical problem those physicians who attend their patients with frequent, careful, and knowledgeable assessment, making the necessary adjustments in therapy, have the best results.*

Our technique of fluid resuscitation

As soon as the patient is admitted, the extent of injury and the patient's overall condition are rapidly assessed. Children with burns of greater than 10% of the body surface and adults with burns of greater than 15% of the body surface receive intravenous fluids to prevent burn shock.

Immediately, a large-bore cannula is placed in a vein. If no practical unburned site is available, the cannula is inserted through burned tissue. Venous blood is obtained for laboratory studies and cross matching of blood. Arterial blood is obtained for measurement of pH and blood gases.

The urinary bladder is catheterized and the hourly urine volume is recorded. Because many burn patients develop paralytic ileus, a nasogastric tube is inserted to decompress the stomach and prevent vomiting and aspiration.

The fluid given intravenously is lactated Ringer's solution, to each liter of which is added 25 gm. of albumin. Sodium bicarbonate is used to correct metabolic acidosis if it exists.

Fluid is administered rapidly until urine flow is established and then is adjusted to maintain a urine flow of 30 to 50 ml./hour, with corresponding but lesser amounts for children. The amount of fluid required to maintain circulation and the desired urine flow decrease gradually during the first day after injury. Our data on the volumes of fluid required during the first 24 hours are given in Table 37-1. These are averages; the actual amount needed varies with the individual.

Hourly assessments are made of urinary output, pH, and specific gravity; blood pressure; pulse rate and rhythm; respiratory rate; ease or difficulty of breathing; and the level of consciousness. From these observations and reexamination of the patient, the physician adjusts the rate of fluid administration and determines whether additional kinds of therapy or laboratory tests are needed.

A practical way to reduce the amount of fluid administered is to decrease the rate of intravenous fluid by 50 ml./hour when the urine flow exceeds 50 ml./hour for 2 consecutive hours. This method will prevent the recurrence of shock, which often occurs when the rate of fluid administration is too rapidly curtailed. This often happens when there is a good initial urinary output response to fluid volume replacement.

Between 18 and 30 hours after injury the patient should be satisfactorily resuscitated. Shock persisting beyond this time is usually not the result of the burn, and other causes should be sought, e.g., heart failure or renal failure. When the need for the intravenous cannula and urinary bladder catheter has been met, these should be removed to prevent infection. When the patient regains gastrointestinal function, enteral alimentation is instituted.

COMMON EARLY BURN COMPLICATIONS
Edema

The accumulation of edema in extremities with circumferential burns of either partial- or full-thickness depth may trigger a rise in tissue pressure. The circumferential burn prevents underlying tissues from expanding as fluid sequesters into the tissues, progressive obstruction of lymphatic and venous outflow ensues, and eventually arterial perfusion of the extremity shuts off. Even modest but sustained elevations of tissue pressure of 40 mm. Hg can cause permanent injury to nerve and muscle. Severe ischemia is easily detected clinically by cool, pale, painful and immobile digits without capillary refill, by the absence of pulse or by altered flow characteristics on Doppler flowmeter examination. However, modest elevations of tissue pressure cannot be detected accurately by physical diagnosis and require direct tissue-pressure measurement. The needle technique described by Whitesides et al., using relatively inexpensive materials readily available in any hospital, is sufficiently accurate. Escharotomy, an incision through the burn, effectively relieves the pressure and restores circulation. Escharotomy is performed whenever the tissue pressure exceeds 40 mm. Hg. The incisions begin at the proximal extent of the burn and are made along the medial and lateral aspects of the limb, with care being taken not to cross flexion creases. As the tissues are released, the incision separates widely and the subcutaneous fat bulges through, tissue tension is reduced, and blood flow is restored.

A dense eschar surrounding the abdomen and chest may compromise ventilation as underlying edema increases. Relief of respiratory distress often follows release of the chest by escharotomy, permitting full respiratory excursions.

As a consequence of edema beneath a burn involving the neck, obstruction of the upper airway may occur. The symptoms are inspiratory stridor, intercostal retraction, tachypnea, and hypoxia. Although this may be treated successfully by escharotomy of the neck, an endotracheal tube or tracheostomy is usually necessary. When the edema resolves in 3 or 4 days, the tube is removed.

Respiratory tract complications

In the early postburn period, there are three complications related to the respiratory tract: upper airway obstruction from edema, carbon monoxide poisoning, and smoke inhalation syndrome. These are devastating complications that increase mortality from burns.

Upper airway obstruction from edema is caused either by inhaled irritating fumes that injure the mucosa of the upper respiratory tract or by transmural edema from burns of the neck. Although inspiratory stridor, inspiratory wheezing, and intercostal retraction herald far advanced upper airway obstruction, lesser degrees of obstruction can be identified by fiberoptic bronchoscopy. The flow-volume loop, a noninvasive bedside test, detects even small degrees of upper airway impairment and is used as a screening procedure.

Endotracheal intubation preserves the airway until the edema resolves. Among patients with rapidly developing edema from burns of the face and neck, it may be prudent to anticipate upper airway obstruction from massive edema and intubate the trachea early. It can be exceedingly difficult to do this later when intubation might be urgently needed.

When an endotracheal tube (a foreign body) lies in an injured upper airway, necrotizing infection of the larynx may occur. Therefore tracheostomy should be seriously considered if the patient has sustained an airway injury by smoke inhalation or burn and if the trachea needs to be intubated beyond 4 or 5 days. If there is no injury to the upper airway, the endotracheal tube may, as advocated by some, be left in for a longer period. Although we often extend this period, we recognize the danger to the larynx of prolonged use of a nasotracheal or orotracheal tube.

Carbon monoxide (CO) poisoning must be considered in those injured by flame in a closed space or when smoke is inhaled. CO is a component of virtually all smoke and has an affinity for hemoglobin over 100 times that of oxygen. Although it is not toxic to tissues, it displaces the oxygen-dissociation curve to the left causing low tissue oxygen tension. These effects are enhanced by metabolic acidosis and low flow states from hypovolemia or cardiac arrhythmias. Patients afflicted with CO poisoning have cherry red mucous membranes and blood, low normal Pao_2, low levels of arterial oxygen saturation, and elevated levels of CO in the blood. Clinical manifestations include headache, dizziness, nausea, angina, and central nervous symptoms of hypoxia. Anoxic encephalopathy may occur.

Patients at risk for CO poisoning should receive 100% inspired oxygen until the level of CO in the blood is below 5 vol. %. With 100% inspired oxygen, the half-life of CO in the blood is 40 to 50 minutes. If the patient has neurological symptoms, such as abnormal motor activity or prolonged unconsciousness, other modalities of therapy should be considered, such as hyperbaric oxygen, controlled ventilation, and systemic hypothermia.

When smoke is inhaled, the irritating noxious gases may cause a clinical illness known as *smoke inhalation syndrome*. This syndrome occurs most frequently among those injured in closed spaces. There is a high incidence of burns of the face, singed nasal vibrissae, superficial burns of the cornea, and burns of the oral mucosa. The condition is identified when one finds soot in the sputum; soot, erythema, and ulcerations in the lower airway on fiberoptic bronchoscopy; abnormalities on xenon-133 ventilation-perfusion scanning of the lungs; and changes of respiratory acidosis and hypoxia on arterial blood gas analysis.

There may be a symptom-free interval, but clinical manifestations occur within 72 hours of the accident. Early signs include tachypnea, dyspnea, and wheezing caused by bronchospasms or debris in the lower airway. Initially the chest x-ray studies may be normal, but in the full-blown syndrome noncardiogenic pulmonary edema occurs. Pulmonary edema may occur early and among those who die in fires from the inhalation of smoke. Pulmonary edema is often found at autopsy.

Treatment in the early stages and of milder forms consists in the use of humidified and warmed air. Large doses of steroids, once believed to have a salutary effect, are now known to be of no benefit and actually increase mortality.

If exposure is severe, progressive pulmonary insufficiency may occur. If indicated, positive pressure ventilation is instituted. It may be 3 weeks or longer before the patient can be weaned from the ventilator. Meticulous tracheal toilet is essential to a successful outcome. The principal complication of smoke inhalation syndrome is superimposed bacterial pneumonia.

TREATMENT OF THE BURN

After fluid resuscitation is begun and a complete history and physical examination is completed, attention is directed to the burn. The burn is gently cleansed, with removal of debris and dead skin. Topical therapy is then started.

Topical antibacterial therapy

Generation after generation of physicians have believed that something should be applied on the burn wound to try to control or alter its microbial flora. Currently, there are several agents that improve survival by favorably modifying bacterial growth on wounds without doing appreciable damage to viable tissue. These agents include 0.5% silver nitrate soaks, mafenide, silver sulfadiazine, silver sulfadiazine with cerium nitrate, and povidone-iodine. There are no data that prove superiority of one agent over the others. Silver sulfadiazine is currently in widest use because of its low incidence of side effects. Although these topical agents do modify wound microbial flora, none perpetually sterilizes all burn wounds. In many instances, a new topical agent will temporarily delay colonization and decrease bacterial counts on or in wounds. However, in time, organisms not affected by topical agents are selected out or find their way to the wound. Furthermore, there is no convincing evidence that changing topical antibacterials will alter the clinical course of a patient with systemic sepsis originating in the wound, without at least systemic antibiotic therapy being employed.

Silver sulfadiazine

Silver sulfadiazine was approved by the Food and Drug Administration for topical burn therapy in 1974. Currently it is the most widely used topical antibacterial agent. The active component is the silver ion, which binds with bacterial DNA to release the sulfonamide moiety.

Silver sulfadiazine has wide antibacterial activity. Although the current major pathogens—*Pseudomonas aeruginosa, Enterobacter aerogenes, Escherichia coli,* and *Proteus* species—can be cultured from biopsy samples of wounds treated with this agent, it is as effective in inhibiting bacterial growth and invasive infection as the other topical agents in use. Early colonization of wounds with penicillinase-producing *Staphylococcus aureus* requires systemic treatment with a penicillinase-resistant antibiotic.

Silver sulfadiazine can be used by the semiopen or closed technique. The agent is usually applied twice a day. The major advantage of silver sulfadiazine is absence of the biological dangers that exist with 0.5% silver nitrate and mafenide.

Surgical care of the burn

Topical antibacterial agents are adjuncts in the therapy of burns and are not substitutes for care of the wound based on well-established surgical principles.

Necrotic tissue produced by the burn must be removed. This not only reduces the possibility of invasive wound and systemic infection but also is a necessary step in preparing the wound for closure by skin graft.

There are two commonly employed methods of removing eschar: (1) épluchage (French, 'picking, cleaning')—piecemeal removal of necrotic tissue that has spontaneously separated and (2) excision, either tangentially—an excision in which necrotic tissue is shaved sequentially until viable tissue is exposed—or directly to fascia. Although each of these two widely divergent methods of removing eschar have strong advocates, neither side can prove superiority based on prospective clinical trials. Épluchage implies that when the wounds are inspected daily the necrotic tissue that has separated and loosened is gently cut away (Fig. 37-10). This should not produce pain or bleeding. It usually takes 3 to 5 weeks for the eschar to separate completely, but the process may be expedited when the débridement is completed in the operating room with the patient anesthetized. Separation of eschar is delayed among the elderly and when there is effective bacteriological control of the wound; it occurs rapidly with infection. When the eschar is removed, there remains a base of granulation tissue, which is an excellent barrier to invasive infection. A decision is now made as to whether a particular area will reepithelialize from epidermal appendages or it requires autogenous skin grafting. This decision requires judgment based on experience. Some burn surgeons use a biological dressing to protect surfaces that will epitheliali spontaneously or to prepare a surface for skin grafting.

Accumulated evidence during the past two decades indicates that the principal adjunct responsible for improvement in survival may have been earlier wound closure. Therefore many burn surgeons, disappointed with the épluchage method, have "rediscovered" excision of the burn in an effort to remove sepsis-generating burn eschar and attain earlier healing of the burn.

Excision is done as soon as is practical and is started within several days of injury. Experience shows that only 15% to 20% of the body surface can safely be excised in one operation. Therefore, when there is a large burn, multiple procedures are required. The excised wound is immediately covered with autograft, a biological dressing, or a synthetic skin substitute. Viable cadaver allograft is preferred if a biological dressing is used.

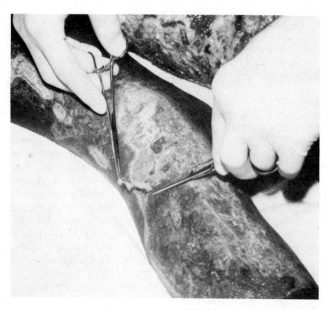

Fig. 37-10. Débridement of loose eschar should not produce pain or bleeding. Wound is debrided daily until all necrotic material is removed, with clean granulation tissue surface being left, as shown in Fig. 37-11.

Excision has been used successfully among children with large burns whose predicted mortality would have been nearly 100% if treated by conventional methods. The data concerning adults treated by the excision method have not been so convincing. Advocates of excision contend that this method will reduce the incidence of infection, enhance survival rates, and shorten hospital stay. Except for shortened hospital stay these contentions are not supported by controlled studies.

There are several disadvantages of excision. First, because it is difficult to identify accurately the depth of the burn soon after injury, a partial-thickness burn may unnecessarily be excised. Second, the cosmetic and functional result of grafted split-thickness skin on muscle or fascia, particularly over joints, may be less than desired. Third, the blood loss may be prodigious.

We use the following generalizations for planning wound closure of each patient. Planning is considerably hampered by no currently reliable noninvasive method of accurately determining depth of injury. Wounds that will heal spontaneously within 3 to 4 weeks after injury are allowed to do so. Among those patients whose wounds will not heal spontaneously within 1 month, the residual necrotic debris and granulation tissue are tangentially excised and the excised area is closed with autogenous split-thickness skin grafts. In many instances,

the debrided area is first covered with a biological dressing or a synthetic skin substitute and the skin graft is applied during a second anesthetic several days later. This delay in autografting ensures precise control of bleeding and avoids disastrous loss of skin graft when exposed fat becomes devitalized. This sequence of tangential excision followed by skin graft is repeated until all wounds are healed. Areas of full-thickness burns are closed first.

When donor skin is available and unless spontaneous closure is imminent, wounds of partial-thickness depth are also skin grafted. We believe this produces a better quality of skin covering with less hypertrophic scarring. In most instances, burns of the dorsum of the hands and fingers are grafted first, usually by the end of the second week. Closure of face and neck burns takes next priority. Patients with a great risk of dying from large deep partial- and full-thickness burns who have limited donor skin available undergo one or two staged excisions down to fascia as soon as practical after admission. Blood loss is less with excision to fascia than with tangential excision. Each excision is limited to about 15% of the body surface. These wounds are closed with either expanded meshed or postage-stamp autogenous split-thickness skin grafts, intermingled autograft and viable cadaver homograft skin, or, when autogenous donor skin is not available, cadaver homograft skin alone or a synthetic skin substitute. At times, the excised area is initially covered with a biological dressing or synthetic skin substitute and the skin graft is applied during a second anesthetic several days later.

Daily bathing in a tub of water, with débridement done at the same time, once the hallmark of burn care, has no known benefit for the wound or the patient's metabolism.

Biological dressings

Biological dressings consist of allograft or xenograft and are used to cover wounds temporarily in place of conventional dressings. Commonly employed materials are human cadaver skin, human fetal membranes, and pigskin.

Viable allograft of split-thickness skin has been used for many years in treating burn patients. The skin, usually from a cadaver, is placed on a wound prepared as for skin grafting. Adherence and "take" of biological dressings require the same wound conditions that are necessary for adherence and take of autogenous skin grafts. This in effect closes the wound and improves the patient's overall condition.

Advantages of a biological dressing include the following:

1. It reduces fluid and protein loss from the wound to improve the patient's nutritional condition.
2. Wounds become pain free.
3. It inhibits bacterial growth.

4. It enhances healing of partial-thickness burns.
5. Adherence of the biological dressing ensures a favorable wound for autografting.

If the allograft skin is allowed to adhere, it will then become vascularized, followed by rejection in 1 to 3 weeks. At that point not only must the wound be prepared again for skin grafting, but the patient's overall condition worsens because of the physiological sequelae of rejection. However, if the allograft skin is used only as a temporary dressing, all the benefits derived from closing the wound can be realized without any of the adverse effects of rejection. The technique is as follows. After removal of the eschar, allograft skin is placed on the wound. The allograft is changed every 4 to 5 days until it becomes feasible to use autogenous skin grafts (Fig. 37-11). The allograft is allowed to remain on a partial-thickness burn, since it protects the viable epidermal appendages; as epithelialization occurs, the allograft will slough.

The demand for allograft skin is great, and at times the supply is limited. An effective alternate is porcine xenograft skin. This material in the nonviable form is available commercially and is in wide use. Fetal membrane is a readily available material used by some burn surgeons as a temporary biological dressing. Fetal membrane is believed to be superior to nonviable porcine skin and as efficacious as viable cadaver skin.

Synthetic skin substitutes

Recently a number of synthetic membranes that are excellent and possibly superior substitutes for

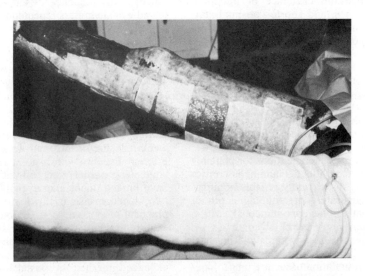

Fig. 37-11. Clean granulation tissue on posterior medial aspect of right thigh and leg covered with biological dressing of pigskin. Left leg shows completed dressing used for 0.5% silver nitrate.

biological dressings have been developed. They have in common a porous collagen layer into which grows granulation tissue fixing it to the wound and a covering layer of rubberized silicone, which is impervious to liquids and bacteria but allows diffusion of gases. The porous layer of one of these synthetic skin substitutes is composed of shark collagen, which is biodegradable, leaving a "neodermis." After 10 days the silicone layer is removed, and a thin skin graft is applied. To use synthetic skin substitutes as biological dressings, wound conditions must be equivalent to that used for successful take of skin grafts. We have allowed synthetic skin substitutes to remain on wounds for as long as 3 weeks; after their removal, there remains a wound upon which skin grafts can be applied without further preparation other than the control of fine capillary bleeding.

Synthetic skin substitutes may be much more practical to use than biological dressings. The former can be stored in a sterile state on the shelf without refrigeration, can be made in large sizes, and, since they are pliable, conform more easily to irregular surfaces and contours than dressings.

Considerations for operations on burn patients

Hypothermia is a major factor limiting the duration of operations done on burn patients. To prevent this complication a warm operating room or heat shield is employed, parts of the body not being operated on are covered, blood is given through a warmer, and every effort is made to limit the operation to 2 hours.

Most seriously ill burn patients require blood replacement during operation.

Failure of skin graft to "take" is disastrous. Not only does the grafted wound remain open, but also the partial-thickness skin injury created in the donor site adds to the area of open wound. Skin grafts fail because of (1) slippage of the graft, (2) foreign material under the graft (blood, serum, necrotic tissue, suture material), or (3) infection: (a) streptolysin produced by the group A beta hemolytic streptococcus dissolves skin grafts, or (b) 100,000 organisms or greater per gram of tissue usually signifies invasive infection.

Donor sites must be properly healed and free of foreign material. Donor sites can be treated in a variety of ways but are best managed the same way the patient's burns are being treated. Currently the most popular dermatomes used to obtain split-thickness skin grafts are those driven by air or electricity. Grafts are cut as thin as possible, yet thick enough so as not to tear with careful handling. There are several methods to expand available skin to cover large surfaces. The most popular instrument for this purpose is the Tanner-Vandeput

mesh machine, which makes a series of cuts in the donor skin so that it is stretched out as lace.

COMMON LATE BURN COMPLICATIONS
Infection

Infection is the most frequent cause of death in burn patients; pneumonia and septicemia account for over half the deaths.

The responsible organism causing death in burn victims has changed in recent decades. Before the 1940s, the *group A beta hemolytic streptococcus* was the primary offender. This organism colonized the edematous tissues within a few days after injury, and death rapidly ensued. Death from this organism has been virtually eliminated by penicillin.

In the 1950s, hemolytic *Staphylococcus aureus,* especially those producing penicillinase, emerged as the most dangerous organisms to the burn patient. However, penicillinase-resistant antibiotics have greatly reduced this threat.

During the 1960s, organisms once believed to be of low-grade pathogenicity emerged as serious threats to burned patients. The most important group was the gram-negative bacilli, especially *Pseudomonas aeruginosa*. During the 1970s, topical antibacterials and newer antibiotics have been responsible for bringing *Pseudomonas aeruginosa* and other gram-negative organisms under control. As a result, *Staphylococcus aureus* organisms, particularly those with methicillin resistance, are becoming increasingly important again. However, any bacterium, fungus, or virus can gain a foothold in a burned patient to produce clinical infection. As a matter of fact, since more effective measures against the gram-negative bacilli have been developed, fungi (particularly *Candida albicans*) have become a threat.

The risk of invasive infection varies with the extent of burn and the age of the patient. That is to say, each patient has the immunological capability and metabolic reserve to tolerate a certain amount of thermal injury, and when the limit is exceeded, the patient is at high risk for infection. When the burn is less than 30% of the body surface, the risk of septicemia is small; but when the burn exceeds 30% of the body surface, the risk is great and increases exponentially thereafter. The aged and infants are at much greater risk for septicemia than older children and young adults are.

Within several days of injury, pathogens can be cultured from the wounds of patients who are not treated with effective topical chemotherapeutic agents. However, if effective agents are used, colonization of the wound is delayed, colony counts are reduced, and different organisms are recovered.

Serious infection occurs much earlier and in a more insidious fashion than is generally appreciated. Among burn patients who eventually die of septicemia, bacteremia is common during the first week. The clinical manifestations of the septicemia are at first subtle but then become over-whelming during the second week. If treatment is ineffective, death will likely ensue during the third week.

It is crucial to recognize the early, subtle manifestations of septicemia because if one waits for overt signs before obtaining blood cultures and then waits for positive bacteriological proof before starting appropriate therapy, the patient's life will be irretrievable. Therefore treatment is instituted on the clinical suspicion of septicemia and a reasonable prediction of the most likely offending organism or organisms.

Important early manifestations of septicemia are as follows:

1. Core temperature greater than 39° C., or hypothermia
2. Leukocyte count of greater than 20,000 cells/mm.[3], or leukopenia
3. Persistent thrombocytopenia
4. Gastroduodenal bleeding or perforation
5. Azotemia with blood urea nitrogen level greater than 30 mg./dl.
6. Anemia, or failure to maintain a normal hemoglobin
7. Change in sensorium
8. Ileus, often heralded by anorexia
9. Gain of body weight along with a decrease in caloric intake
10. Deterioration in blood gases, especially unexplained reduction in PaO_2 or metabolic acidosis

Presence of two of these manifestations provides enough suspicion of septicemia to justify obtaining the necessary cultures and beginning appropriate therapy.

The common sources of burn sepsis are the wound (e.g., sepsis from pathogenic bacteria on or in the wound, invasive infection), veins (e.g., septic thrombophlebitis), and lungs (e.g., aspiration pneumonia, hypostatic pneumonia, bronchopneumonia as a sequel to smoke inhalation injury).

Prevention and treatment of burn infection

Burns are tetanus-prone wounds; burned patients should be immunized.

Most burn-care physicians advocate use of one of the topical antibacterial agents to reduce the incidence of invasive infection. There is no statistical evidence that one agent is superior to another.

A major contributing factor to burn sepsis is the large volume of necrotic tissue on the wound. As discussed previously in the section on "Surgical care of the burn," two techniques are advocated for removal of nonviable tissue—excision and piecemeal débridement (épluchage). Which method is superior is not known, but each may be advantageously employed in a given case.

Many burn-care physicians give penicillin for several days to prevent infection from *group A beta hemolytic streptococcus*. Beyond that most authorities advocate systemic antibiotics only for the specific indication of infection. All agree that the majority of patients with burns in excess of 30% of the body surface area will require one or more antibiotics during treatment. Burn therapists must keep current with developments in the field of antibiotics and know the contemporary indigenous microorganisms of their burn unit or hospital.

Subeschar clysis of antibiotics has been advocated by some as a method to control invasive infection of burns. Proponents of this method do a biopsy of the burn with quantitative bacterial counts to determine when clysis should be used. If the bacterial count exceeds 10^4/gram of tissue, this signifies a dangerous level of organisms, and subeschar clysis is used. The proper place of this technique in burn care has yet to be determined.

Curling's ulcer

Hemorrhage from "stress," or Curling's ulcer, is a classical but now infrequent complication of a severely burned patient. The ulcers, located in either stomach or duodenum, are usually multiple, round, punched out, and often painless. Frequently ileus precedes massive bleeding; septicemia predisposes to stress ulcer. Often there is no prior history of acid-peptic disease. The most important preventive measure is to control systemic infection. The incidence of ulcers can further be reduced by use of antacids to maintain the pH of the gastric contents above 4.0. Perforation and excessive bleeding are indications for operative treatment.

Scars and contractures

The principal late complications of burns are hypertrophic scars and contractures. These entities are defined in the section on pathophysiology of the wound.

Hypertrophic scars (Fig. 37-3) are dynamic lesions. With time the disordered collagen tends to realign into a more orderly and linear pattern. The scar also gradually loses its erythema and becomes softer and more pliable and usually flat. This process is known as *maturation* of the scar. In some cases all the hypertrophic qualities do not disappear and the scar remains raised. Maturation is believed to be hastened by application of pressure, usually by a rubber elastic bandage or a custom-made elastic garment.

Recently healed or grafted burns often itch, frequently to an extremely annoying extent. The cause is not known. Symptoms are relieved by antipruritic medication, analgesics, and bland skin lubricants. In many instances itching gradually disappears within 18 months.

Contraction is a factor in the healing of all wounds, and burns are no exception. When preventive care is inadequate and at times even when preventive care seems adequate, contractures occur. The major sites of contracture are the neck, axilla, antecubital fossa (Fig. 37-4), and hand; however, any joint may be involved. Contractures of the face are particularly dangerous: eyelid contracture may expose the cornea with all its horrible sequelae; mouth contracture may produce microstomia, which makes eating, oral hygiene, and dental manipulations difficult and the delivery of an anesthetic excessively dangerous.

Prevention of contractures is the key. This includes proper splinting in the anticontracture position (e.g., elbows extended) and conscientious physical exercise until the danger of contracture is past. Splinting and physical therapy may reverse the contracture process. However, in some instances surgical relief of the contracture is necessary.

Among the severely and extensively burned, it takes about 2 years to complete scar-maturation and necessary reconstructive procedures.

A late and infrequent complication of burns is *Marjolin's ulcer*—a squamous cell carcinoma arising in an old scar.

Emotional problems

A severe burn is emotionally devastating. This is true not only for the patient but for his family as well.

Virtually all patients with burns manifest emotional symptoms, including depression, regression, anxiety, excessive sensitivity, emotional lability, insomnia, and phobias. The severity of symptoms depends on the patient's premorbid emotional maturity and the length of hospitalization; therefore the symptoms are worse among those with the larger burn and more immature personality. Delirium and frank psychosis are common among the severely burned, especially during septicemia. In most instances the psychosis abates as the patient's burns heal and his condition improves.

During fluid resuscitation, edema of the eyelids frequently prevents the patient from opening his eyelids, and the patient believes that he is blind. The patient must be reassured that in a few days he will be able to open his eyes and see again. Males with scrotal edema often believe themselves to be impotent; this of course is not true. The greatest fear among the burned is deformity and mutilation. In many instances this is justifiable, and professional psychiatric help may be needed.

The overall emotional prognosis for adults is not as poor as previously believed. For instance, if an adult is emotionally mature before his injury, he likely will reattain emotional maturity. The traumatic neurosis from the burn usually resolves by 1 year after injury. However, persons with pathological emotional symptoms before injury often develop a permanent traumatic neurosis, and their emotional problem is compounded. The prognosis among children is not good, especially among those with noticeable disfigurement. They do poorly because their emotional development is interrupted by the burn, and they must face life with the emotional problems that attend deformity.

In dealing with the burn patient's family it is essential that they be realistically appraised of the prognosis, both for life and for deformity. Unrealistic encouragement should not be given. We believe it important that the family visit the patient frequently and at times help with the nonprofessional aspects of the patient's care. This assures the patient that he has not been abandoned by his loved ones.

Nutrition

Recognizing the importance of nutrition in the care of burned patients has been one of the most important recent advances in the field. A large surface burn probably causes a greater catabolic stress than any other disease or injury. Tissue breakdown and exhaustion of body stores occur extremely rapidly unless measures are taken to preserve nutritional integrity. A patient with a large surface burn and with improper nutritional support can easily within 3 weeks reach a level of nutritional depletion from which he cannot be salvaged. The metabolic activity of a burned patient is reset at a higher level and does not return to normal until after the wounds are closed.

The catabolic process is augmented by a variety of stimuli, the most serious of which is infection. Cold, pain, anxiety, and hypovolemia are all potent catabolic stimuli mediated through augmented catecholamine response. Much has recently been written about vaporizational heat loss contributing to the metabolic demands of the burn patient. One can minimize this loss by nursing these patients in a temperature environment similar to that of the wound by using heat lamps or shields, and by dressing techniques similar to those described for 0.5% silver nitrate.

An adult with a large surface burn requires approximately 2,000 kcal./m.^{2} of body surface area each day. Infants and young children require proportionately more. Most patients refuse to eat this much food because of anorexia, making tube feedings necessary. If caloric needs cannot be met by enteral alimentation, central venous alimentation should be used, with recognition of an enhanced risk of infection with the latter technique.

In practice, the patient's nutritional situation must be repeatedly assessed. When the initial ileus has resolved, the proper number of calories is given by mouth. If the patient's body weight and nutritional integrity cannot be maintained on the prescribed diet, the diet or method of delivery or both should be altered.

An integral part of nutrition is maintenance of proper hydration. Otherwise, hyperosmolality may occur because of the obligatory loss of fluid from open wounds. The amount of water lost is linearly related to the size of the wound.

COLD INJURIES

Freezing induces tissue injury equally severe to that produced by burns. Exposure to cold induces vasoconstriction of arterioles and small arteries with consequent local tissue hypoxia. In addition, cold produces direct tissue injury. As with burns, frostbite injury can be quantitated by the degree of damage provoked: superficial damage (first degree), partial damage to the dermis (second degree), and complete damage to the dermis (third degree).

Frostbitten tissue initially feels numb and begins to ache in the rewarming process. The feet, nose, ears, and hands are most commonly involved because these parts are exposed most to cold and are located peripherally in the circulatory system. Initial redness of the skin is followed by a pale or waxy whiteness in a few hours. The area then becomes bluish red and swollen. Vesicle formation and areas of eschar indicate severe damage; a thick black eschar marks third-degree stages. Wetness of the area, as in immersion of the extremities, exaggerates the damage. However, since most civilian cold injuries occur in a dry atmosphere, actual freezing is uncommon, except in alcoholics who fall asleep in the cold.

Treatment

The emergency management requires removing all clothing, with rapid rewarming of the injured part by immersion in water at 34° to 40° C. Blisters are covered with a dry dressing to prevent contamination. Bed rest is mandatory until edema resolves and demarcation of tissues has occurred. Areas of gangrene undergo autoamputation, or the surgeon anticipates the demarcation line and amputates to save hospital time. During this period, necrotic tissue is debrided. Antibiotic therapy helps prevent massive infection.

38
Orthopedics

Reginald R. Cooper

Orthopedics encompasses the investigation, preservation, and restoration of form and function of the musculoskeletal system and related structures. Orthopedists employ medical, surgical, and physical methods of treatment.

Numerous conditions affect the musculoskeletal system, but I will discuss only the common ones that involve most orthopedic patients seen in clinical practice. These disorders can be categorized according to etiology as follows:

1. Congenital and developmental
2. Infectious and inflammatory
3. Traumatic
4. Metabolic
5. Neoplastic
6. Neuromuscular
7. Degenerative
8. Mechanical and postural
9. Idiopathic

Some disorders involve only one region, but others are not so restricted.

ORTHOPEDIC EVALUATION OF A PATIENT

Medical, emotional, social, and economic factors influence the patient with an orthopedic disorder. The astute physician considers each of these in its proper perspective.

The patient who seeks the advice of an orthopedist usually complains of one or more of the following: (1) something feels wrong (pain, numbness, tenderness), (2) something looks wrong (deformity, limp, bump), or (3) something moves wrong (limp, weakness, stiffness, instability).

If the disorder is localized, complaints often remain in the involved part; however, pain can be referred to a remote site (e.g., knee pain from hip disease). A lesion that irritates a peripheral nerve produces pain in the area supplied by the nerve (e.g., pain in the lower extremity from a herniated lumbar intervertebral disk). In the back and extremities, protective muscle contraction frequently produces symptoms at a distance from the disease.

With the doctor's guidance, the patient must relate a pertinent, integrated, chronological history of all complaints. Important questions about pain include the following: What are the circumstances surrounding its onset? What is its progression? Was the onset associated with injury? Was it sudden or gradual? Was this the first episode? Has the pain been continuous? Is it sharp or dull, superficial or deep? What relieves it? What makes it worse? Does it interfere with function or sleep?

A similar chronology must be documented for complaints other than pain.

A normal opposite part serves as a valuable comparison during an examination of a patient with a musculoskeletal problem. Depending on the involved region, the physician can modify the following physical examination outline:

Joints
Inspection: In what position is the joint held? Is this normal? What is the joint contour? Is it swollen? Is the overlying skin normal? Are there discolorations, venous distensions, cuts, scars?
Palpation: Is there tenderness? Does it feel hot or cold? Is there excessive joint fluid? Is a fluid wave ballotable? Is the synovium thickened? Are all the ligaments intact? Is there unstable, abnormal motion?

Range of motion:

Active: Is motion produced by the patient limited? If so, why? Is there pain, muscle spasm, contracture (fixed, spasm), bony block? In what direction is the limitation? Record range of motion in degrees.

Passive: Can you move the joint through a greater range than the patient can? If so, is muscle torn, paralyzed, or reflexly inhibited? Record range of motion in degrees.

Muscles

Does each one contract?

What is its strength?

Grade 5, normal, 100%—range of motion against full resistance

Grade 4, good, 75%—range of motion against some resistance

Grade 3, fair, 50%—range of motion against gravity

Grade 2, poor, 25%—range of motion with gravity eliminated

Grade 1, trace, 10%—slight contraction, no motion

Grade 0—no contraction

Is there measurable atrophy or enlargement?

Compare limb circumference with the opposite side.

Find the same level on two sides by measuring from a *fixed* part to a given site. *Example:* To find thigh circumference, measure 6 or 7 inches proximally to the tibial tubercle (a fixed part), not from the patella (a movable part).

Does the tendon glide freely? Is it tender? Is it intact?

Are there masses in muscle or tendon?

Bone

Is the integrity maintained? (stability, crepitus [grating of bone fragments on each other])

Is it obviously deformed? (angulated, curved)

Is it of normal size? (length, width)

Is it in proper relation to other bones?

Is it tender?

Is the overlying skin normal?

Are any masses present? If so, notice type, location, size, consistency, fixed or free, pulsatile, bruit, transillumination.

Neurological examination

Motor, sensory, reflexes

Vasculature

Skin changes of vascular insufficiency, pulses, veins, masses, bruit

Function

Put the part through voluntary motions of everyday activities

Gait: Is it normal? If not, what abnormal components are present? (short leg limp, hip abductor weakness—lurch to involved side, hip dislocation, waddle)

Roentgenographic studies are usually necessary, if not mandatory, for complete evaluation of a complaint related to the musculoskeletal system. Comparable views of the opposite normal side sometimes aid in making a diagnosis.

Table 38-1. Disorders of the neck

Age	Disorder	Cause
Birth to 2 years	Torticollis	Developmental
4-8 years	Acute wryneck	Traumatic or inflammatory
Adult	Stiff neck	Inflammatory (?)
	Degenerative joint disease (cervical spine arthritis, degenerative disk disease, cervical spondylosis)	Degenerative
	Acute sprain	Traumatic

REGIONAL ORTHOPEDICS

Neck (Table 38-1)

Torticollis (wryneck, congenital muscular torticollis)

A fibrotic, contracted sternocleidomastoid muscle tilts the head to the ipsilateral side and turns the face to the contralateral side (Fig. 38-1). The cause remains unknown. Theories include birth trauma, muscle fibrosis, and abnormal muscular development. Many involved babies were breech presentations. About 3 weeks after birth, the parents find a lump in the child's sternocleidomastoid muscle. The mass disappears in a few weeks, and some of these infants later develop torticollis. Some afflicted children had no noticeable mass. Asymmetry of face and skull bones accompanies torticollis.

The parents should stretch the tight muscle gently each day. They should position the bottle and toys so that the baby turns to them in a way that stretches the tight sternocleidomastoid muscle. Many cases correct spontaneously and do not develop a wryneck. Severe persistent deformity at 2 or 3 years of age warrants excision of a segment of the contracted muscle. Much of the asymmetry disappears with subsequent face and head growth.

Any of the following can produce torticollis: hemivertebra and other cervical spine abnormalities, visual disturbances in which the patient tilts the head to see better, or acute cervical lymphadenopathy that causes the patient to tilt the head to relieve pain.

Acute wryneck

Children develop acute wryneck because of inflammation and cervical lymphadenopathy associated with acute pharyngitis or because of rotatory subluxation of the cervical spine. A history of acute onset differentiates either from congenital muscular torticollis.

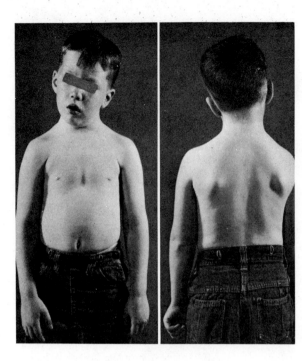

Fig. 38-1. Congenital torticollis. Head tilts to side to fibrotic sternocleidomastoid muscle, and face turns to opposite side.

At times during acute pharyngitis, hyperemia and inflammation around cervical spine ligaments allow rotatory subluxation of cervical spine facets. Treatment consists of appropriate therapy of the primary disorder, head halter traction to realign facets, and postreduction immobilization for 2 to 3 weeks in a cervical collar.

Occasionally a child suddenly twists the neck, hears a click, experiences sharp neck pain, and locks in a twisted position. An open mouth roentgenogram of C1-C2 vertebrae demonstrates a subluxated facet of C1 on C2. Head halter traction with the spine in neutral or slight flexion reduces the subluxation. The child should wear a collar or brace for 3 weeks.

Stiff neck

A person who has slept with the neck twisted or who has been in cold air often complains of a stiff neck. He or she holds the head rigidly inclined to the involved side and complains of sore, tender neck muscles. Neck motion produces pain. The cause is unknown. Some believe that an inflammatory myositis produces stiff neck. With heat, analgesics, rest, and support by a collar or traction, symptoms usually subside in 3 to 10 days. Transcutaneous electrical nerve stimulation (TENS) may be of value.

Degenerative joint disease (cervical spine arthritis, degenerative disk disease, cervical spondylosis)

In degenerative joint disease, intervertebral disks and cervical facets degenerate. Spurs of bone and inflammation adjacent to disks, intervertebral body joints, and facets impinge on cervical nerve roots at one or more levels. At times, degeneration occurs after trauma, but it can arise spontaneously. Symptoms vary from mild to severe. Frequently, pain radiates from the neck to the head or upper extremities. Pain and paresthesias can follow a nerve root distribution. Persistent nerve root irritation causes reflex sympathetic nerve stimulation with blurred vision, loss of balance, and headaches. Often, the patient inclines the head away from the painful side to get temporary relief. Neck motion decreases. Pressure over spinous tips and longitudinal compression of the spine produce pain. Reflexes and sensation decrease. Roentgenographic examinations help in localizing the level(s) of disk narrowing and spur formation (Fig. 38-2).

Periods of rest, pillows designed to support the cervical spine in neutral position or extension, moist heat, salicylates, intermittent head halter traction (7 lb./15 min., 3 times a day), and night head halter traction often relieve symptoms. If conservative measures fail, the patient might need surgery. Depending on the severity and location of

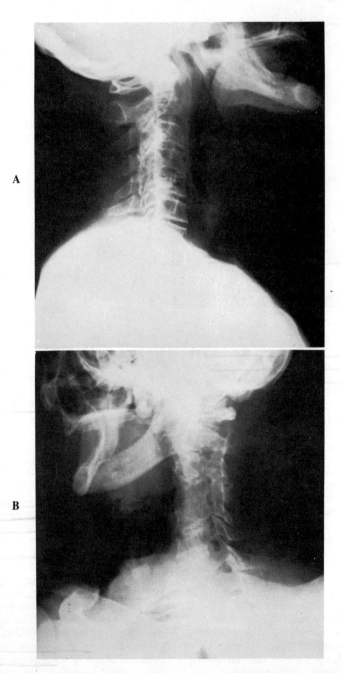

Fig. 38-2. Degenerative joint disease of cervical spine. **A,** Lateral view. Normal cervical curve is gone, and C4-C5 disk space is narrow. **B,** Oblique view. Degenerative spurs have narrowed intervertebral foramina.

the disorder, surgeons can remove the disk, enlarge the foramina, or fuse the cervical spine.

Cervical disk herniation can produce motor loss, decreased reflexes, and sensory loss that follows a definite nerve root pattern. Myelograms help confirm the diagnosis and localize the level.

Acute sprain

Cervical sprains concern the legal profession about as much as they concern the medical profession. The occupant of an automobile struck from the rear often sustains neck injury. Some patients have immediate neck pain, but others have none for 12 to 36 hours. Patients complain of diffuse pain over the posterior surface of the neck and head. Protective muscle contraction decreases neck motion in an attempt to prevent pain. At times, patients develop sore muscles, stiff neck, severe pain, vertigo, nausea, headache, and paresthesias. Symptoms tend to be intermittent and frequently persist for months but subside eventually in most instances.

Interspinous ligaments and neck and shoulder muscles are tender. Cervical spine motion decreases. Decreased sensation in the upper extremities usually does not follow a well-defined nerve distribution and varies from examination to examination. Definite, severe, and persistent neurological signs should lead one to suspect more than ligamentous or muscular damage. Roentgenograms are usually normal but *must be taken* to rule out fracture and dislocation.

Analgesics, heat, rest, massage, and mild head halter traction for 2 to 10 days often relieve acute symptoms. If so, the patient should gradually increase neck motion as symptoms decrease. The use of a neck support may be necessary in some instances. Transcutaneous electrical nerve stimulation (TENS) may help. Many patients with persistent symptoms have pending lawsuits. Doctors often speculate about the relation of symptoms to insurance settlements.

Shoulder (Table 38-2)
Fractured clavicle

The clavicle is the bone most frequently fractured during delivery. It begins ossification before other long bones, and the shoulders are the widest part of a newborn's body. When an examiner attempts to elicit a Moro reflex, the baby with a fractured clavicle does not move the arm on the involved side (pseudoparalysis). Brachial plexus injury, fracture of the humerus, and dislocated shoulder produce a similar sign.

No reduction is necessary. Strapping the baby's arm to the chest for 7 to 10 days relieves discomfort. A lump of callus appears within a few days

Table 38-2. Disorders of the shoulder

Age	Disorder	Cause
Birth to 2 years	Fractured clavicle	Traumatic
	Brachial palsy (obstetric palsy)	Traumatic
2-4 years	Pulled shoulder	Traumatic
Adult	Rotator cuff degeneration (acute bursitis, noncalcific or calcific; rotator cuff disease)	Degenerative
	Frozen shoulder (adhesive pericapsulitis)	Degenerative
	Acute rupture of the rotator cuff	Traumatic and degenerative
	Snapping scapula	Inflammatory (?) Degenerative (?)

and disappears during the ensuing weeks, and full function returns.

Brachial palsy (obstetric palsy)

Mechanical stretch of the brachial plexus during delivery paralyzes various muscles of the upper extremity and produces loss of sensation in the distribution of involved nerves. Nerves may remain intact but stretched, or they rupture completely. The infant does not move the involved arm or forearm. Signs depend on the anatomical location of the lesion. In the common upper arm type of Erb-Duchenne (caused by downward traction of the shoulder), an injury of C5-C6 nerve roots paralyzes deltoid, supraspinatus, infraspinatus, and biceps muscles. The arm adducts and internally rotates, and the forearm pronates. In the lower arm paralysis of Klumpke (caused by upward traction with the arm overhead), an injury of C8 and T1 paralyzes intrinsic muscles of the hand or the long finger flexors, or both. In the whole-arm type, various combinations of paralyses lead to severe dysfunction.

During the months after birth, the infant usually improves but seldom recovers completely. Prognosis is best in the upper-arm type. Treatment soon after birth prevents contractures. Each day the child's shoulder should be moved passively into abduction and external rotation and the forearm into supination. In older cases release of contractures, transfer of tendons, and osteotomies might improve function.

Pulled shoulder

Occasionally a parent grabs a child by the hand and pulls him or her onto a curb or in a given direction. The infant has immediate pain and refuses to move the arm. The shoulder is tender. If roentgenograms reveal no fracture, the child probably has a partial tear of the shoulder capsule and bleeding into the joint. Resting the part for a few days by strapping the arm to the body relieves symptoms. If left to his or her own devices, with pain as a guide, the child will regain motion in the arm. No physical therapy is needed.

Rotator cuff degeneration (acute bursitis, noncalcific or calcific; rotator cuff disease)

The rotator cuff, composed of the supraspinatus, infraspinatus, teres minor, and subscapularis muscles, holds the head of the humerus downward and medially against the glenoid, thereby producing a stable fulcrum for arm abduction. The floor of the subdeltoid (subacromial) bursa covers the superior surface of the rotator cuff, and a disorder of one involves the other. Frequently cuff degeneration of unknown cause produces pain and limits shoulder motion. The supraspinatus usually degenerates near its insertion into the greater tuberosity of the humerus. If the degenerated area and surrounding repair tissue extend to the external surface of the tendon, subacromial bursitis develops. If the degenerated tendon calcifies, this calcium can rupture into the bursa. Degeneration can partially rupture the rotator cuff. Symptoms vary with the following syndromes.

Acute degeneration and bursitis. With acute degeneration, the patient notices sudden, sharp, severe pain in the subacromial region. Pain radiates down the arm. Shoulder motion, especially abduction and external rotation, decreases. Examination discloses point tenderness over the greater tuberosity, and active and passive motions produce pain. As the greater tuberosity passes beneath the acromion during abduction from 30 to 80 degrees, the patient experiences the most severe pain (painful arc syndrome). Roentgenographic studies either reveal no abnormality or show calcification in the tendon or bursa.

The patient should rest and use analgesics and hot packs to relieve pain. Oral analgesics and anti-inflammatory drugs or local injection of an anesthetic or steroids into the bursa often helps. Pain should decrease in 48 to 72 hours. If it does not, the physician might wish to aspirate calcium or remove it by operative incision. When pain subsides, the patient must begin shoulder circumduction, abduction, and external rotation to prevent a frozen shoulder. (See "Frozen shoulder," this page.)

Chronic degeneration and bursitis. With or without a previous acute episode, the patient with rotator cuff disease complains of intermittent aching in the shoulder, tenderness over the cuff insertion, and pain on motion. If the cuff ruptures, shoulder abduction weakens. Patients with chronic and recurrent rotator cuff disease should use heat and analgesics to decrease pain. Between acute episodes, they should initiate active range-of-motion exercises. If calcium produces a mechanical obstruction to motion, it should be excised.

Tenosynovitis of the long head of the biceps. Tenosynovitis produces symptoms much the same as those of acute rotator cuff tendinitis except that tenderness is over the biceps groove. Supination of the forearm against resistance produces shoulder pain. Conservative treatment is the same as in acute bursitis. If the process continues and motion gradually decreases, the patient might need surgical release of the long head of the biceps.

Frozen shoulder (adhesive pericapsulitis)

Adhesions form in the gliding planes about the shoulder after trauma, shoulder disease, or any disorder that limits shoulder motion. Patients, usually 40 to 60 years old, complain of severe pain. Motion decreases greatly. Roentgenograms usually disclose no abnormalities. Occasionally they show signs of previous shoulder disease. Heat and active circumduction exercises help restore shoulder function. On rare occasions, if the range of motion is not improving, manipulation under anesthesia might be necessary. This disorder tends to subside in 12 to 18 months, and motion increases.

Acute rupture of the rotator cuff

A force applied during lifting or during a fall can rupture a normal rotator cuff or a previously degenerated one. With a complete tear, the patient experiences severe pain, feels a sharp snap, and loses active abduction and external rotation of the shoulder. If the arm is passively elevated above the head, the patient might be able to hold it there by use of the deltoid muscle. Immediate surgical repair of a complete tear produces a good chance for recovery of function. Partial tear is common. The patient complains of mild pain and moves the shoulder to a limited extent. With symptomatic treatment, the patient regains function.

Snapping scapula

The patient complains of grating, snapping, or pain as the scapula rotates over the chest wall. Persons in certain occupations have difficulty working. Although a subscapular exostosis can produce symptoms, snapping is usually caused by poor posture, an abnormally formed scapula, subscapular bursitis, or inflammation in fascial planes.

Table 38-3. Disorders of the elbow

Age	Disorder	Cause
2-4 years	Pulled elbow (nurse-maid's elbow)	Traumatic
Adult	Tennis elbow (lateral humeral epicondylitis tendinitis)	Degenerative, traumatic

Table 38-4. Disorders of the hand

Age	Disorder	Cause
Birth to 2 years	Syndactyly	Congenital and developmental
	Polydactyly	Congenital and developmental
	Congenital bands	Congenital and developmental
Adult	Dupuytren's contracture	Idiopathic
	de Quervain's disease	Developmental, inflammatory
	Trigger finger	Developmental, inflammatory

The physician should obtain roentgenograms to rule out lesions of the scapula. Usually attempts to correct poor posture, injection of tender areas with local anesthesia, and exercises to strengthen the scapular muscles relieve symptoms.

Elbow (Table 38-3)
Pulled elbow (nursemaid's elbow)

The history of a child with a pulled elbow is similar to that of one with a pulled shoulder. Pulled elbow is more common. The child holds the forearm pronated and the elbow flexed 30 to 40 degrees. Roentgenograms are normal. In this disorder the radial head probably subluxates through the annular ligament. In a child over 6 years of age the larger radial head does not subluxate. If the doctor quickly manipulates the child's forearm into supination and extension, a click occurs as the radial head reduces. To prevent recurrent subluxation, the physician should splint the forearm in supination and extension for 7 to 10 days. The patient then initiates motion. No physical therapy is needed.

Tennis elbow (lateral humeral epicondylitis, tendinitis)

The patient with tennis elbow complains of pain over the lateral humeral epicondyle. This often occurs after injury or activities wherein the forearm repeatedly supinates and extends (a backhand in tennis). The cause of symptoms is debatable. Some attribute complaints to a disrupted common extensor origin at or immediately distal to the lateral humeral epicondyle. Others believe that the radiohumeral bursa beneath the common extensor origin becomes irritated. In any case, the lateral humeral epicondyle is tender. The patient complains of pain during attempts at forearm supination or wrist extension against resistance. Warm, moist packs, rest, analgesics, and injections of local anesthetic and occasionally steroids usually relieve symptoms. Some patients have recurrence that again responds to conservative therapy. In these instances exercises to strengthen the wrist extensors may be of value. Some obtain relief with a strap around the forearm over the tender point.

In 5% to 10% of the cases, persistent symptoms warrant surgical exploration and excision of the degenerated and torn extensor tendon.

Hand

The age for and cause of disorders of the hand are given in Table 38-4 and are discussed in Chapter 39.

Spine (Table 38-5)
Spina bifida and meningomyelocele

In spina bifida, a developmental disorder, one or more vertebral arches fail to fuse in the posterior midline. At times the incomplete neural arch allows the contents of the spinal canal to herniate. Spina bifida occurs in about one out of every 1,000 births. It most frequently involves lumbar and sacral vertebrae but can affect others. In many children with meningomyelocele, extensive defects lead to death at birth or soon thereafter. Within the last few years medical teams have improved prospects for increasing the life-span of these children.

The several types of spina bifida depend on the anatomical defect. In spina bifida occulta the neural arch is defective, but neural contents do not herniate, or at least not enough to cause neurological symptoms. In some instances the overlying skin is pigmented, indented, or hairy. Later in life some of these children gradually develop incomplete paralysis, sensory loss, weakened intrinsic foot muscles, cockup toes, and cavus feet. In spina bifida with meningocele one or more layers of the meninges herniate through the neural arch defect. In spina bifida with meningomyelocele the hernial sac contains meninges, cerebrospinal fluid, spinal cord, or nerve roots. Frequently these children have extensive paralysis, sensory loss, lack of bowel and bladder control, and associated hydrocephalus.

Table 38-5. Disorders of the spine

Age	Disorder	Cause
Birth to 2 years	Spina bifida and meningomyelocele	Congenital and developmental
2-4 years	Scoliosis	Idiopathic, infantile, congenital
4-8 years	Scoliosis	Idiopathic and paralytic
8-14 years	Scoliosis	Idiopathic and paralytic
	Juvenile round back (vertebral epiphysitis, Scheuermann's disease)	Developmental— osteochondritis, epiphysitis (?)
Adult	Spondylolysis and spondylolisthesis	Developmental defect; traumatic (?)
	Acute back sprain	Traumatic
	Intervertebral disk degeneration, herniation, and spinal stenosis	Degenerative
	Coccygodynia	Traumatic (?), unknown(?)

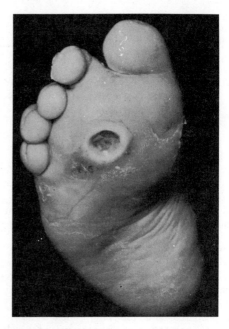

Fig. 38-3. Chronic foot ulcer in patient with spina bifida and meningomyelocele.

Symptoms and signs in spina bifida are produced by the protruding mass, neurological loss, and resulting deformities. Frequently the skin over the hernial sac ulcerates and becomes infected. Meningitis follows. Neurological defects vary with extent and location of the lesion. Sensory loss and skin ulcerations are common (Fig. 38-3). Paralyzed muscles are usually flaccid. Deformities depend on the level of nerve root involvement. Many children have hip flexion contractures, dislocated hips, knee contractures, and equinovarus feet.

The complex treatment of the child with spina bifida is best done by a team that includes parents, pediatrician, neurosurgeon, orthopedic surgeon, urologist, orthotist, physical therapist, and social worker. The neurosurgeon closes the hernial sac and treats hydrocephalus. Urologists prevent and treat urinary tract infections and provide proper emptying of the urinary collecting system. Orthopedic surgeons prevent and correct deformities by physical therapy, manipulation, splints, braces, and surgery. Therapists help in gait training and instruct the child in self-care. The child needs nursing care to prevent ulcers. Parents must understand the magnitude of the magnitude of the problem and be willing to help with therapeutic programs.

Scoliosis

Lateral curvature of the spine can result from neuromuscular disorders (polio, muscular dystrophy, spinal cord tumor, neurofibromatosis), congenital defects (wedge vertebra or failed segmentation), or any disorder producing muscle spasm (disk herniation). However, most cases of idiopathic scoliosis develop during rapid spine growth at adolescence.

Idiopathic scoliosis is more frequent in girls 8 to 14 years of age and often consists of one main thoracic or lumbar curve and one or two compensatory curves. In thoracic curves the spine and chest not only deviate laterally but also rotate. The chest protrudes anteriorly on the concave side of the curve and posteriorly on the convex side of the curve to produce a hunchback. In lumbar curves the hip and pelvis on the side of the concavity appear prominent.

Patients with scoliosis usually have no symptoms. The patient or the parents notice the curve, the high shoulder, or the prominent thorax or hip. The physician must rule out all known causes of scoliosis before classifying it as idiopathic. Spinal roentgenographic studies (Fig. 38-4) with the patient standing up and lying down and bending to

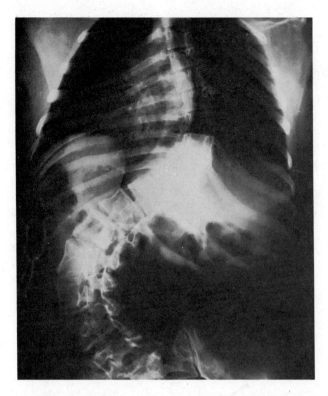

Fig. 38-4. Postpoliomyelitis scoliosis with right thoracic and left lumbar curve. Notice rotation of vertebral bodies.

each side indicate the amount of curve flexibility. From these, the orthopedist measures the angle of the curve. If it is over 20 or 30 degrees, treatment should start at once. If it is not, the physician might observe the patient carefully to see if the curve increases. If roentgenograms 3 months later show an increased curve, the patient needs treatment. In general, the thoracic curves progress rapidly, especially if the patient is young. After spine growth stops, curves progress slowly if at all.

A Milwaukee or another type of brace distracts the head from the pelvis and applies corrective lateral and rotatory forces to the spine by means of pads against the ribs. The orthopedist must check the brace frequently to be sure that it fits well. As the curve corrects and as the child grows, the orthotist must adjust and lengthen the brace. Some curves, if treated early by the brace, improve greatly or correct almost completely. If a curve progresses despite a brace or if a severe curve remains, the orthopedic surgeon can correct the curve and fuse the spine with or without internal fixation by rods. Even then, pseudarthrosis may

develop. This break in the fusion may produce no pain but might allow progression of the curve and necessitate refusion.

Juvenile round back (vertebral epiphysitis, Scheuermann's disease)

Occasionally the secondary ring epiphyses and the upper and lower margins of vertebral bodies ossify poorly. Boys between 12 and 16 years of age develop epiphysitis more often than girls. Thoracic vertebrae are most commonly involved. Anterior vertebral body growth is decreased. The patient at times has mild backache. Thoracic kyphosis increases to give a round back and stooped shoulders. X-ray examination discloses an irregular upper and lower vertebral surface and an anterior wedging of the vertebral body (Fig. 38-5). The patient should limit activities to the point where he or she is free of pain. In the case of rapid progression of dorsal kyphosis, a Milwaukee brace helps prevent and correct deformity. The disorder is self-limiting. Spine fusion is indicated in severe deformity.

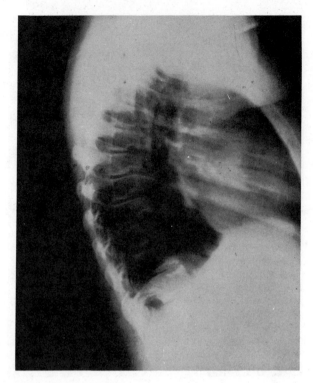

Fig. 38-5. Scheuermann's disease. Dorsal kyphosis is increased, vertebral bodies are wedged anteriorly, and epiphyseal rings are irregularly ossified.

Spondylolysis and spondylolisthesis

In spondylolysis the pars interarticularis of the neural arch is defective and the posterior portion of the arch has no bony continuity with the remainder of the vertebra. In spondylolisthesis the neural arch is defective, and one vertebral body, usually L5, slides forward upon another, S1 (Fig. 38-6). The defect may be congenital, but the actual slip tends to occur between 6 and 12 years of age. Once established, the slip usually does not progress; however, the intervertebral disk degenerates sooner than normal at the involved site. Spondylolisthesis is usually not so painful unless the disk degenerates. The patient might then have low back pain with radiation into the posterior aspect of the lower extremities. The patient must be taught to lift properly. He or she should stoop so that the spine does not bend but the hips and knees do. The patient builds up abdominal muscles by sit-up exercises with the hips and knees flexed. If pain persists, spinal fusion becomes necessary.

Acute back sprain

Acute flexion during a fall or while lifting frequently tears ligaments, fascia, and muscles of the low back. Patients experience sudden, sharp pain. On examination, muscle spasm and tenderness are found. Spine motion decreases. Roentgenograms may reveal no abnormalities. Rest, heat, and protection against extremes of motion relieve symptoms in 1 or 2 weeks.

After a sudden twist or bend, the spine at times locks in one position. Patients have severe pain. Based on the theory that facets lock in a subluxated position, doctors have called this a facet syndrome. Roentgenographic studies commonly show asymmetry of lumbosacral facets. Bed rest and sedation relieve acute symptoms.

Intervertebral disk degeneration and herniation and spinal stenosis

Because of its ability to retain fluid and its intradiskal tension, the intervertebral disk gives the spine both flexibility and stability. As persons age, intervertebral disks lose their elasticity and ability to retain fluid. Some disks then consist of nonelastic connective tissue, and others have clefts. Whether degeneration represents a variation of normal aging or is a disease is debatable. Disk degeneration often produces spine instability in the

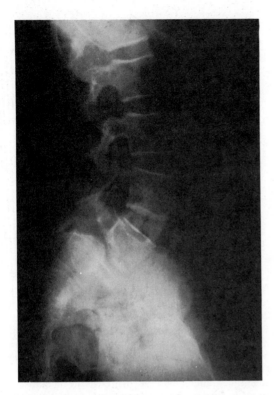

Fig. 38-6. Spondylolisthesis. L5 has slipped anteriorly on S1. Neural arch is defective.

involved segment. This places abnormal stresses on ligamentous structures and spinal facet joints. In an attempt to repair and stabilize the spine, the body produces bone spurs. The inflammatory process often involves nerve roots. Frequently the patient complains of back pain and pain radiating into the thigh along the sciatic nerve. Pain is usually mild and intermittent for several months. Lifting, bending, and twisting increase pain, and rest relieves it. In some, pain starts in the low back and later radiates into one lower extremity. Motion of the involved segment of the spine decreases. The doctor sees this best if he or she views the patient from the side and asks the patient to bend forward. Normally, motion starts at the neck and continues smoothly until the entire spine forms a continuous curve. In a patient with disk degeneration, involved segments remain flat. Hyperextension causes discomfort. Pressure over the spinous tip at the involved site produces pain. If the patient then hyperextends the back by lifting the head and shoulders off the table and pressure produces less pain, this is a positive instability test that helps localize the level of degeneration. The straight leg–raising test is positive when it reproduces

radiating pain or back pain. Reflex, sensory, and motor activity vary from patient to patient. Roentgenograms often reveal a narrowed interspace and degenerative changes, most often at L5-S1 or L4-L5. Flexion and extension lateral views of the spine at times show sliding of one vertebral body upon the other or tilting open of a disk space anteriorly on hyperextension.

During the acute stage of pain, bed rest usually relieves symptoms. The patient must then use the back properly. He or she should avoid bending, lift only by bending the knees, and avoid soft chairs and beds that allow the spine to sag. In the early stages of treatment, a low back brace reminds the patient of the proper position for the spine. Later, the patient should start on progressive resistance exercises (sit-ups) to build up the abdominal muscles and spine flexors. He or she should do sit-ups with the hips and knees flexed. Most patients improve with this therapy.

If the anulus tears, the nucleus pulposus can herniate and press on a nerve root. This causes radiating pain and often interferes with reflex, motor, and sensory function in the lower extremity. The patient usually gives a history much like one with a degenerated disk. In many instances the most recent episode is severe and unrelenting. On physical examination, the physician often finds changes similar to those in a person with degenerative disk disease. In addition, the patient's reflexes decrease (ankle or knee jerk), muscles lose strength (toe extensors), and sensation in the L5 or S1 dermatome decreases.

Bed rest and medication for relief of pain lead to improvement in most patients. If so, the patients are then treated as outlined for disk degeneration. Some patients need surgical removal of the intervertebral disk if (1) they fail to improve in 3 or 4 weeks on a conservative therapeutic regime, or (2) neurological loss progresses. The physician should do a myelogram if he or she is not sure of the level of herniation or if there is a question about the diagnosis. After disk removal, some surgeons fuse the involved level of the spine. Others do not. After surgery, the doctor should treat the patient as one with a degenerated disk until the intervertebral region stabilizes. Spinal fusion is probably indicated if the patient has a defect such as spondylolisthesis. Recently protolytic enzymes have been injected into intervertebral disks for treatment of acute disk symptoms.

Spinal stenosis, a narrow spinal canal, results from disk degeneration, osteophytes, or spondylolisthesis. In addition to the other symptoms of disk degeneration, this produces pain and paresthesias in the legs during walking (neurogenic claudication). Decompression of the spinal canal and foramina may be necessary.

Coccygodynia

Women develop a painful tailbone more often than men do. Some give a history of an acute injury to the coccyx. In others trauma seems to play no role. Sitting and motion of the coccyx increase the pain. The physician must rule out psychoneurosis, spine disease (bone tumors), and spinal cord and nerve lesions with pain referred to the coccyx. Rectal examination is mandatory. X-ray examination helps rule out bone lesions. Rest and heat often relieve acute coccygodynia. The patient is instructed to sit on a soft pillow or ring. Excision of the coccyx is rarely warranted since most patients continue to have pain despite surgery.

Hip (Table 38-6)
Congenital dislocation

The physician must diagnose congenital dislocation of the hip soon after birth of the affected infant. If the physician does not, he or she often commits the child to a life of disability. Hip joint capsule relaxation and acetabular dysplasia of unknown cause produce congenital dislocation of the hip. Girls are affected seven times oftener than boys are. The disorder is at times familial. The doctor should warn parents of an affected child to have all subsequent children examined carefully. The degree of involvement varies from mild dysplasia (shallow acetabulum) to complete dislocation. In some babies the hip is dislocated before birth. In others the femoral head slips out of the acetabulum after birth. For clinical purposes, the disorder is classified as a dysplastic hip, subluxation, or dislocation.

The doctor examining a newborn must look for signs of hip dislocation. The most common reliable sign is a slight jerk and snap as the femoral head slides in and out of the acetabulum (Ortolani's sign). This is produced when the thighs, in flexion and slight abduction, are alternately pushed posteriorly and pulled anteriorly (Fig. 38-7). Other signs include limited abduction while the hip is flexed, posterior and lateral displacement of the greater trochanter, an extra fold or asymmetrical gluteal folds, and telescoping (abnormal cephalocaudad motion of the femur with push and pull). If diagnosis and treatment are delayed until the child walks, she waddles. The involved leg is shorter. When the patient stands on the involved extremity, the pelvis drops toward the opposite side (positive Trendelenburg test).

Initial x-ray examination often reveals only lateral displacement of the proximal femur. Later roentgenograms (Fig. 38-8) show a shallow, sloping acetabular roof, a laterally displaced proximal femur (if the acetabular region is divided into quadrants by a line passing through the triradiate

Table 38-6. Disorders of the hip

Age	Disorder	Cause
Birth to 2 years	Congenital dislocation	Developmental
4-8 years	Legg-Calvé-Perthes disease (coxa plana)	Metabolic (?)
	Synovitis	Viral (?)
8-14 years	Slipped capital femoral epiphysis	Metabolic (?)
Adult	Snapping hip	Anatomical variation

cartilage of both acetabulums and a line dropped from the superior acetabular edge, the femoral head should lie in the lower inner quadrant), a delay in ossification of the femoral head, a break in Shenton's line (the normal continuous arch formed by a line drawn along the inferior border of the femoral neck and head and continued along the superior border of the obturator foramen), and an acetabular angle over 30 degrees (the acetabular angle is formed by one horizontal line that goes through the triradiate cartilages and another that goes from the superior acetabular edge to the triradiate cartilage on the involved side).

A child who remains undiagnosed has abnormal hip mechanics and develops early degenerative changes in the hip. To prevent crippling sequelae, the doctor must diagnose and treat congenital hip dislocation soon after birth. With the appropriate treatment, results are gratifying.

Treatment in the newborn depends on the degree of hip involvement. If the patient has a mild dysplastic hip, the mother should keep the child's legs abducted by pillows designed for this purpose. If the femoral head is well centered, a dysplastic acetabulum deepens and develops as the child grows. If the femoral head is subluxated or dislocated, the orthopedist can do a gentle, manipulative reduction after a few days of skin traction. Tight hip adductors might necessitate a subcutaneous adductor tenotomy. A plaster cast then holds the child's hips reduced. After this, the patient wears a brace to hold the hips in place. As the acetabulum deepens, the brace is gradually worn less, but it is worn at night for several years. If closed reduction is impossible, operative measures are needed. The doctor must follow a child with congenital dislocation during the growth years to be sure that the hip does not displace again.

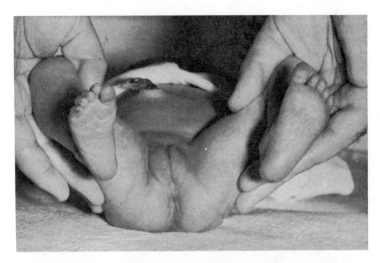

Fig. 38-7. Ortolani's test for congenital dislocation of hip. Examiner's thumb pushes posteriorly on baby's knee while examiner's fingers lift greater trochanter anteriorly and push medially to snap femoral head into acetabulum.

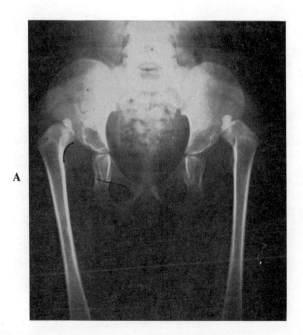

A

Fig. 38-8. Bilateral congenital dislocation of hips. **A,** Notice shallow, sloping acetabular roofs, superior lateral displacement of femoral heads, and broken Shenton's line. *Continued.*

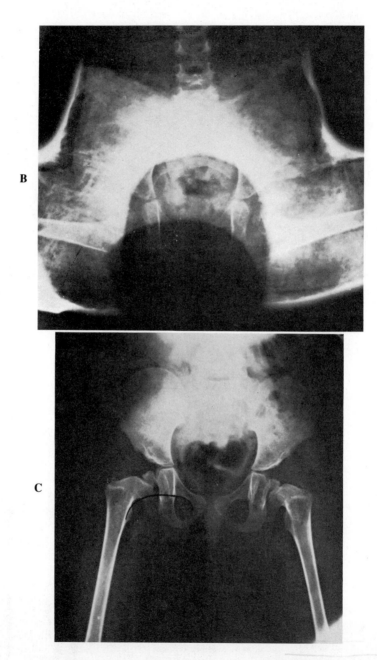

Fig. 38-8, cont'd. B, Roentgenogram through plaster after traction, adductor tenotomy, and closed reduction. **C,** Roentgenogram 8 months later. Femoral heads are centered in acetabulum, and Shenton's line is unbroken.

Legg-Calvé-Perthes disease (coxa plana)

Avascular necrosis of the femoral head of unknown cause is more common in boys 4 to 9 years of age than in girls. Biopsy of the epiphyseal plate shows derangement of chondrocytes and clefts in the cartilage. These probably interfere with blood vessels passing through the periphery of the epiphyseal plate and supplying the femoral head.

The child first complains of mild pain in the medial aspect of the knee and thigh or in the anterior part of the hip. The parents notice a limp. On examination, the physician finds limited motion of the child's hip. Abduction and internal rotation decrease greatly. The child complains of tenderness and pain on motion. Muscle spasm is frequently severe. In early stages of the disorder roentgenographic examination shows a distended joint capsule and slight flattening of the femoral head. Later the femoral metaphysis widens, and the epiphyseal plate becomes irregular. The necrotic portion of the femoral head is radiopaque as compared to surrounding bone that has undergone disuse atrophy (Fig. 38-9). If the child bears weight, the femoral head collapses, widens, and leads to joint incongruity that can produce degenerative joint disease.

Treatment does not always restore a normal hip joint. Early treatment includes rest or traction with the thighs in abduction to relieve the pain of muscle spasm and acute synovitis and to center the femoral head in the acetabulum. The child walks with crutches or a brace to limit weight bearing on the involved extremity until the new bone replaces necrotic bone. After this, the child gradually increases the amount of weight bearing. A differential diagnosis in Legg-Calvé-Perthes disease should include tuberculosis, rheumatoid arthritis, and idiopathic synovitis.

Synovitis

Occasionally children complain of hip or knee pain and limp to protect the involved extremity. Past history is noncontributory. Hip motion decreases. The child holds the hip flexed, externally rotated, and abducted. Pressure over the hip anteriorly produces discomfort. The doctor must do laboratory and roentgenographic studies to rule out pyogenic arthritis, osteomyelitis, and rheumatoid arthritis. By exclusion, he or she diagnoses idio-

A

B

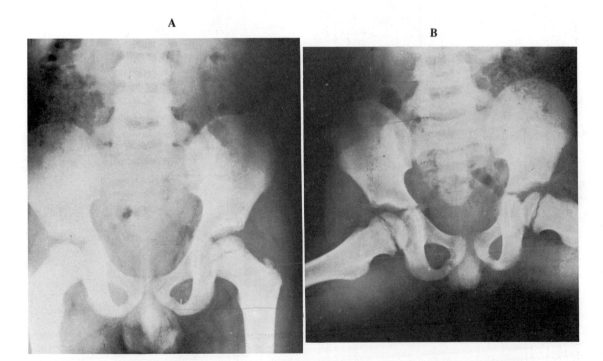

Fig. 38-9. Legg-Calvé-Perthes disease. **A** and **B,** Anteroposterior and lateral roentgenograms a few weeks after child limped and complained of mild right hip discomfort; right femoral head is somewhat irregular and smaller than left. *Continued.*

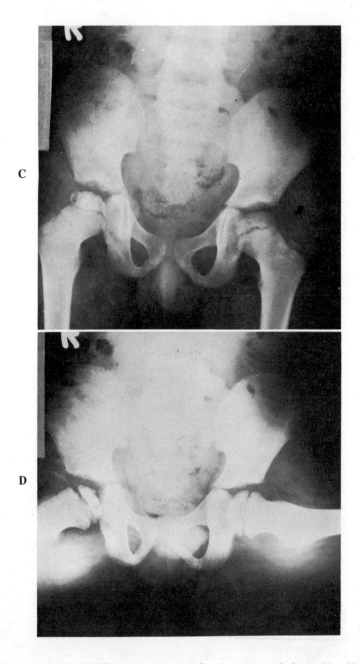

Fig. 38-9, cont'd. C and **D,** Six months later, the flat, dense, necrotic femoral head is obvious.

Fig. 38-9, cont'd. E and **F,** In another 6 months, new bone is replacing dense, dead bone; femoral head is still flat, and metaphysis is wide. *Continued.*

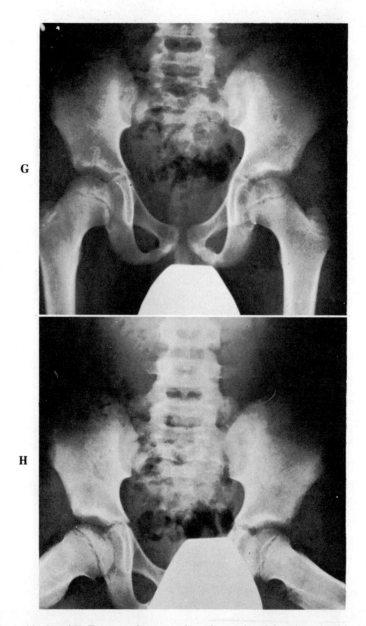

Fig. 38-9, cont'd. G and **H,** Two years later, new bone has replaced dead bone, and femoral head has only mild residual flattening.

pathic synovitis, treats the child by rest with traction, bed, or crutches, and follows the patient at frequent intervals. If, in fact, the child has idiopathic synovitis, he or she improves in 2 or 3 weeks and has no residual difficulty.

Slipped capital femoral epiphysis

Slipping of the capital femoral epiphysis is usually a gradually progressive displacement of the femoral neck anteriorly and superiorly in relation to the femoral head. The cause is unknown, but the disorder involves epiphyseal plate cells. The changes in the cartilage cells of the plate are similar to those in Legg-Calvé-Perthes disease. Slipped epiphysis develops between 10 and 16 years of age. The patient complains of discomfort in the knee, thigh, or hip. Discomfort, though mild and intermittent at first, usually persists and becomes more pronounced. The parents notice that the child limps. Slipped epiphysis commonly affects one of two types of children. The child is either fat and physically and sexually immature, or he is tall and thin. In the latter instance he has recently grown rapidly.

The patient holds the involved hip externally rotated and adducted. He or she complains of pain on motion and limits internal rotation and abduction as compared to the normal side. Characteristically the leg goes into external rotation on flexion of the hip with the knee flexed. Often anteroposterior roentgenographic studies show slight widening of the epiphyseal plate and metaphysis, but lateral views reveal anterior displacement of the femoral neck (Fig. 38-10). This varies from minimal displacement to complete separation of the femoral head from the femoral neck.

To prevent further displacement and serious hip disability, the child should bear no weight. A patient with a mild displacement should have the epiphysis fixed to the femoral neck by means of threaded pins. He or she then uses crutches until the femoral head unites by bone to the femoral neck. In a person with pronounced displacement, the physician applies skin or skeletal traction to the limb over a period of several days to abduct and internally rotate the leg in a manner that reduces displacement to the point where the head can be fixed to the femoral neck by pins. Vigorous manipulative reduction damages the blood supply to the femoral head and produces aseptic necrosis.

A few children with slipped capital femoral epiphysis develop one of the following complica-

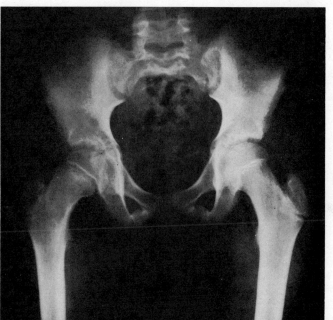

A

Fig. 38-10. Slipped capital femoral epiphysis. **A,** Anteroposterior roentgenogram showing early slip of right femoral epiphysis; epiphyseal plate is widened, and femoral neck is displaced superiorly and anteriorly in relation to femoral head. *Continued.*

Fig. 38-10, cont'd. B, Lateral view; slip is more obvious. **C,** Roentgenogram 6 months after internal fixation.

tions: acute arthritis of the hip, chondrolysis, residual joint incongruity, or aseptic necrosis. These can produce a degenerative joint that later needs reconstructive surgery.

Snapping hip

Flexion, abduction, or internal rotation of the hip produces an audible, palpable, or visible snap located over the greater trochanter of the femur. A thickened band of fascia snaps over the trochanter. Differential diagnosis includes loose bodies in the hip or subluxation of the hip. In case of a fascial band, pain is usually not severe enough to warrant treatment. Rest and anti-inflammatory drugs may give relief.

Knee (Table 38-7)
Bowlegs (genu varum)

Bowlegs are most often a variation of normal, but the doctor must be sure that the child does not have rickets or an epiphyseal plate disorder.

Most newborns have bowlegs. This physiological bowing persists for several years, but the majority correct spontaneously with growth. A few severe and persistent bowlegs need treatment with a long leg brace designed to apply pressure laterally at the knee and medially over the thigh and lower leg. An even fewer number persist to the point of needing osteotomy to correct the bowing.

In this country bowlegs caused by vitamin D–deficient rickets are infrequent. An occasional patient with vitamin D–resistant rickets may develop bowlegs. Roentgenograms of a child with

rickets show the widened epiphyseal plate and metaphysis wherein cartilage and bone matrix are produced but fail to mineralize. The physician must treat the primary disorder. Some of these children need osteotomies to straighten the legs.

Tibia vara (Blount's disease) produces bowlegs by delay in growth and irregular development of the medial and posterior portion of the epiphyseal plate of the proximal tibia. The deformity increases until the epiphyseal plate disturbance subsides. A child with severe deformity needs tibial osteotomy.

Knock-knees (genu valgum)

Knock-knees are usually a variation of normal. Probably because of their wider pelvis, girls have knock-knees more frequently than boys do. Most children need no treatment. The legs straighten as the child grows. The physician must rule out an underlying bone disorder. A few children with severe knock-knees need a long leg brace or an osteotomy.

Congenital pseudarthrosis of the tibia

The term *congenital pseudarthrosis* is a misnomer for this rare condition of unknown cause. Most children who develop this disorder are born with an intact tibia that is thin at the junction of its middle and distal one third and bowed anteriorly (Fig. 38-11). Some of the children have manifestations of neurofibromatosis. The bone breaks soon after birth and resists healing. Surgeons have used numerous operative procedures, most with bone grafts, to try to obtain union of these defects. Often pseudarthrosis remains and the leg is short and must be amputated. Recently, treatment with electric current shows some promise in obtaining union.

Osgood-Schlatter disease

In Osgood-Schlatter disease, common in boys 10 to 15 years of age, the tibial tubercle becomes fragmented. The patient complains of a tender bump and has pain if he kneels or jumps. On examination, the physician finds a swollen, hard, tender tibial tubercle. Extension of the knee against resistance produces pain. Roentgenograms show a dense fragmented portion of bone separated from the underlying tibia (Fig. 38-12). This process is similar to "osteochondritis" in other areas. In most cases the fragment ossifies normally and complaints subside. The child should limit activity during the acute painful stage to relieve strain on the tibial tubercle. A cylinder cast alleviates severe pain. The child resumes activity as symptoms subside. In a few children the fragment does not heal, and a small separate dense piece of bone remains surrounded by fibrous connec-

Table 38-7. Disorders of the knee

Age	Disorder	Cause
Birth to 2 years	Bowlegs (genu varum)	Developmental or metabolic
	Knock-knees (genu valgum)	Developmental
	Congenital pseudarthrosis of the tibia	Developmental (?)
8-14 years	Osgood-Schlatter disease	Traumatic (?)
	Recurrent dislocation of the patella	Developmental
	Osteochondritis dissecans	Traumatic (?)
	Baker's cyst (popliteal cyst)	Developmental or inflammatory
Adult	Bursitis	Bursal inflammation
	Chondromalacia	Degenerative(?)

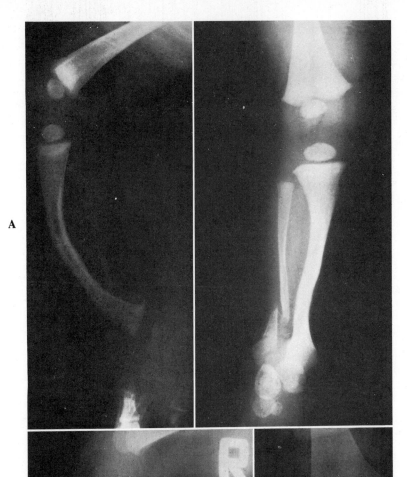

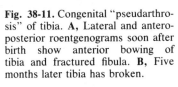

Fig. 38-11. Congenital "pseudarthrosis" of tibia. **A,** Lateral and anteroposterior roentgenograms soon after birth show anterior bowing of tibia and fractured fibula. **B,** Five months later tibia has broken.

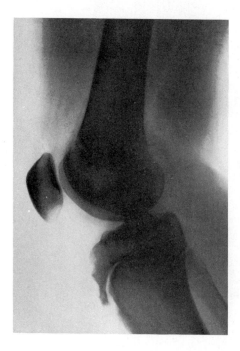

Fig. 38-12. Osgood-Schlatter disease. Tibial tubercle is irregular and fragmented. Small, dense piece of bone remains ununited.

tive tissue or a bursa, or both. These may remain symptomatic and necessitate removal of the fragment.

Recurrent dislocation of the patella

Recurrent dislocation of the patella is more likely to occur in girls 8 to 16 years of age than in boys. One or more of the following predisposing developmental defects cause this disorder: high-riding patella, knock-knees, flattened lateral femoral condyle, and lax medial patellar retinaculum. The patient gives a history that the leg gave way during vigorous physical activity while the knee was flexed. This produced severe knee pain, and the knee locked in flexion. Some astute observers tell the doctor that the kneecap slid to the outside of the knee, and the knee was swollen and tender for a week or so. Young girls with such a history often have subsequent episodes of subluxation wherein the kneecap slides over and back without locking in complete dislocation.

On examination, the physician often finds the patella higher than it should be, and it does not lock against the femur as it normally should when the knee is flexed 30 degrees. Often roentgenograms show no abnormalities, but they might disclose a high-riding patella, valgus knees, or an underdeveloped lateral femoral condyle. At times they show a chip fracture of the lateral femoral condyle produced by the patella sliding over the condyle. A patient who has repeated episodes of patellar dislocation usually wants treatment. The older the patient, the less is the likelihood of subsequent dislocation. The physician might advise girls 16 to 18 to wait and see if the frequency of dislocation decreases. In other instances he or she will advise surgical repair. The orthopedic surgeon reconstructs the extensor apparatus by transferring the patellar tendon insertion distally and medially on the tibia, reefing the medial patellar retinaculum, or releasing the lateral retinaculum, or all three. In some patients who have had multiple dislocations, patellar cartilage degenerates. In such cases the orthopedist might remove the patella and transfer the extensor apparatus to prevent it from dislocating.

Osteochondritis dissecans

In osteochondritis dissecans of the distal femur an osteochondral fragment, usually on the lateral surface of the medial femoral condyle, loses its blood supply and separates from the rest of the femur. No one knows the cause. The fragment can revascularize and be replaced by new bone but frequently detaches and becomes a "joint mouse." If the fragment is not detached, the patient usually complains of vague knee pain and swelling made worse by activity. If the fragment becomes a loose body, the knee frequently locks and gives way. At times the patient feels loose bodies sliding about in the joint.

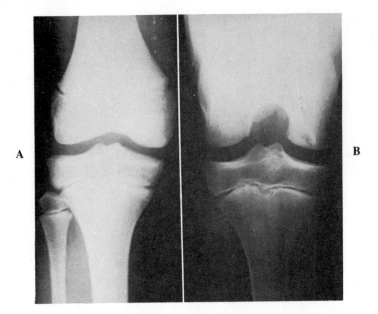

Fig. 38-13. Osteochondritis dissecans. **A,** Routine anteroposterior roentgenogram does not outline defect well. **B,** Anteroposterior roentgenogram with knee flexed shows fragment in its most common location on lateral surface of medial femoral condyle.

Roentgenograms show the fracture line with the overlying dense bone, if the fragment does, in fact, contain much bone (Fig. 38-13). Roentgenograms show a free fragment only if it contains bone or mineralized cartilage. The defect on the femoral condyle is often visible.

If the physician sees a patient with an intact fragment, he should advise no weight bearing and observation to see if the fragment revascularizes. If a free body produces symptoms, it should be removed.

Baker's cyst (popliteal cyst)

Baker's cyst is not unusual in children. The cysts result from enlargement of the semimembranous bursa or the bursa beneath the medial head of the gastrocnemius muscle. Herniation of knee joint synovium through the posterior capsule of the knee also produces popliteal cysts. Symptoms consist in dull aching, swelling that fluctuates in size, and at times, constant pain. If the patient has severe symptoms, the surgeon can excise the bursa and close any defect in the posterior knee capsule.

Bursitis

Bursas, synovial-lined sacs located between tendons, muscles, and fascia in gliding areas, reduce friction. Adventitious bursas are produced by constant friction or repeated trauma. There are many bursas about the knee. They can be acutely or chronically inflamed, infected, or involved by a systemic disorder such as rheumatoid disease or gout. Pain is the most prominent symptom, and swelling and tenderness are the prominent signs. Treatment depends on the underlying cause. Any systemic disorder must be treated. Locally, trauma and irritants should be eliminated. Rest, hot packs, elevation, and compression help relieve symptoms. In noninfected cases bursas can be aspirated. To avoid infection, the physician must use extreme care. If an aspiration is to be done, the skin must be prepared as if one were going to do an open operation. One should avoid injecting directly through the skin over the bursa. Instead of this, the needle should start at a distance from the bursa in normal skin and subcutaneous tissue and enter the bursal sac from its deep surface. In this way infection is less likely to be introduced. Incision and drainage and antibiotics usually cure an acutely infected bursa. Excision of a chronically infected bursa might be necessary.

Chondromalacia

Chondromalacia, of unknown cause, consists of softening, yellow discoloration, fraying, and degeneration of the articular surface of the kneecap. Women 14 to 28 years of age frequently acquire chondromalacia. They complain of knee discomfort that is mild at first but later is severe. Activities such as stair climbing that produce forcible knee flexion increase the pain. The joint swells, and patellar compression produces pain and crepitus. Joint fluid increases, and patellar margins become tender. Roentgenograms often show no abnormalities. Straight leg–raising exercises to increase quadriceps strength and avoidance of strenuous activities that aggravate symptoms usually relieve discomfort. In some patients conservative treatment does not control symptoms. In these instances the surgeon might explore the knee joint and either skive (pare) the diseased cartilage or remove the patella.

Foot (Table 38-8)
Clubfoot

Congenital defects or neurological disorders (myelodysplasia, cerebral palsy) produce clubfoot. The name of the most frequent congenital variety, talipes equinovarus, describes the position of the foot. The heel cord is tight, the ankle (talipes) is plantar-flexed (equinus), and the foot is inverted (varus) (Fig. 38-14). The forefoot is adducted. Talipes equinovarus affects boys much more frequently than it does girls. In most instances no one knows the cause of clubfoot. The heel cord and the structures on the medial side of the foot contract. This pulls the calcaneus into plantar flexion, the navicular medial to the talus, and the cuboid medial to the os calcis. Children do not outgrow talipes equinovarus, and in fact the older they get, the more the foot bones become deformed. The orthopedist must institute treatment soon after birth while contracted soft tissues are more easily stretched. Long leg casts are changed at 5- to 7-day intervals. Each cast produces a corrective force that slides the foot beneath the talus, thereby correcting forefoot adduction and inversion. The casts extend above the knee to prevent rotation of the cast. Some of the deformity corrects with each cast until the foot overcorrects except for the equinus. At this stage, subcutaneous section of the heel cord (Achilles tendon) corrects equinus immediately. After this, the child wears a cast in a corrected position for 5 weeks while the tendon heals. (Some physicians use casts to correct the equinus. Extreme caution is needed to avoid pressing up beneath the forefoot while the heel cord holds the os calcis in equinus. Such pressure "breaks" the foot and produces a rocker-bottom foot.) After correction of deformity, the infant should use night splints to hold the feet corrected until 5 to 7 years of age. Such treatment instituted

Table 38-8. Disorders of the foot

Age	Disorder	Cause
Birth to 2 years	Clubfoot	Developmental
	Metatarsus adductus (metatarsus varus)	Developmental
	Calcaneovalgus	Developmental
	Congenital bands (constriction rings)	Developmental
	Toeing in	Developmental
	Toeing out	Developmental
	Flatfoot (pes planus)	Developmental
2-4 years	Köhler's disease	Osteochondritis
8-14 years	Sever's disease	Osteochondritis
	Freiberg's disease	Osteochondritis
Adult	Bunions (hallux valgus)	Developmental (?)
	Hallux rigidus	Arthritic (?), developmental (?)
	Metatarsalgia	?
	Corns	Traumatic
	Heel spur	Traumatic (?)
	Ingrown toenail	Traumatic (?)
	Digital neuroma (Morton's neuroma)	Traumatic (?), developmental
	Cockup toes and hammer toes	Congenital, neuromuscular, arthritic

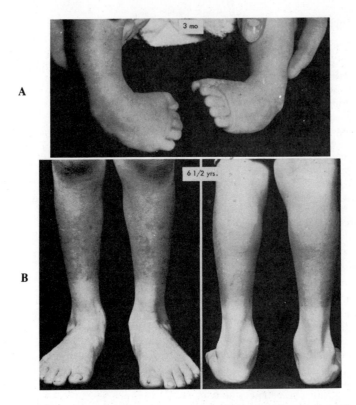

Fig. 38-14. Congenital talipes equinovarus. A, Feet at beginning of treatment when child was 3 months old. B, Feet at age 6½ after treatment with corrective casts and night splints.

soon after birth leads to satisfactory results in 90% of cases. However, the foot tends to redeform until maturity. The doctor must stress this point to parents. Frequently, resistant, neglected, or recurrent clubfoot require surgery of soft tissues or bones of the foot. Such surgery may leave the foot more rigid than normal.

Metatarsus adductus (metatarsus varus)

In the congenital disorder metatarsus adductus, the child's forefoot adducts (Fig. 38-15). On examination, the doctor might be able to correct passively the forefoot to neutral. If so, he or she advises the parents to hold the child's heel fixed in one hand and stretch the forefoot into a corrected position several times daily. If the infant is walking, he might also wear straight-last shoes. If, however, the doctor finds that a child's foot is too rigid to correct to neutral, he or she should apply a series of casts and obtain gradual correction. This should be done between 3 and 6 months of age. The child wears straight-last shoes to keep the feet out of a deformed position.

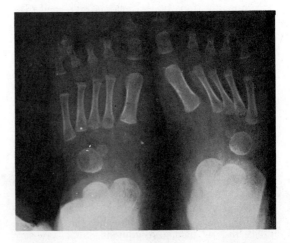

Fig. 38-15. Metatarsus adductus. Roentgenogram shows adduction of right forefoot.

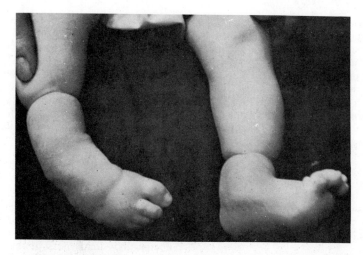

Fig. 38-16. Congenital bands (constriction rings) of both legs. (Fron Kenney, W.E., and Larson, C.B.: Orthopedics for the general practitioner, St. Louis, 1957, The C.V. Mosby Co., p. 27.)

Calcaneovalgus

Occasionally newborn babies' feet dorsiflex in front of the tibia and evert (valgus). In contrast to talipes equinovarus, these feet improve with time and need only gentle daily stretching. Calcaneovalgus must be differentiated from vertical talus, a rare disorder in which the foot is rigid and must be corrected surgically.

Congenital bands (constriction rings)

Tight fibrous connective tissue bands that surround a digit or extremity involve the skin and subcutaneous tissues and constrict underlying muscle and vessels (Fig. 38-16). Occasionally edema and vascular insufficiency distal to the band produce gangrene. These bands, once believed to be amniotic remnants, probably represent developmental defects. Frequently, the patient has associated congenital anomalies (syndactyly and polydactyly). The surgeon should excise the bands by multiple Z-plasties several weeks apart to avoid interruption of circulation to the extremities. Z-plasties prevent circumferential scarring with subsequent recontracture. (See Chapter 34.)

Toeing in

Parents frequently bring pigeon-toed children to the doctor. Usually toeing in results from one of three disorders: (1) metatarsus adductus, (2) internal tibial torsion, or (3) medial femoral torsion or femoral neck anteversion. The physician often obtains a clue as to which of these is present by observing the child walk. He or she diagnoses metatarsus adductus when the forefoot adducts in relation to the hindfoot. If the child has no foot deformity and the kneecaps point straight ahead during gait, the problem is probably internal tibial torsion. Normally, the lateral malleolus is 15 to 20 degrees posterior to the medial malleolus. In internal tibial torsion this angle may decrease or reverse. If, on the other hand, the kneecaps point medially when the child walks, femoral torsion or anteversion of the femoral neck is likely. Sitting and sleeping with the feet turned in aggravates tibial and femoral torsion. As the child grows and sitting and sleeping positions change, femoral and tibial torsion usually correct. Although thousands of dollars are spent each year on shoe corrections, they probably do not influence toeing in caused by bone torsion. The physician should follow the patient, and if the disorder is not correcting, the child should wear a night splint to hold the feet externally rotated. This splint consists of a metal bar fixed to the shoe soles in a manner that holds them rotated to the desired position. A few persons with severe residual torsion need corrective rotational osteotomy.

Toeing out

Toeing out, too, is produced by intrinsic foot deformity, external tibial torsion, or external femoral torsion. A child just learning to walk frequently toes out to obtain a wider base for balance. External femoral or tibial torsion tends to correct with growth.

Flatfoot (pes planus)

The physician should exercise caution in diagnosing flatfoot in a child under 2 or 3 years of age. Before this age a fat pad in the foot obscures any arch that might be present. Flatfeet in children are either flexible or rigid. In the common, flexible type the arch flattens and the heel goes into valgus during weight bearing. These correct when body weight is removed. These feet are not painful in childhood, and most of them correct as the child gets older and foot ligaments tighten. Even if a flexible flatfoot does not correct, the child has no functional handicap. Shoe corrections probably do nothing to help these feet. Medial heel wedges and arch pads keep shoes from running over and wearing out rapidly. These inexpensive corrections save the parents the cost of buying new shoes at frequent intervals.

Bone defects such as congenital fusion of tarsal bones (tarsal coalition) produce most rigid flatfeet. These feet are not passively correctable. If the child has foot and leg pain, an orthopedic surgeon should see him or her. Surgery might be necessary to relieve pain and deformity.

Köhler's disease

Aseptic necrosis of the tarsal scaphoid usually affects children 6 to 11 years of age. Activity accentuates foot pain and rest relieves it. The physician finds tenderness in the medial side of the foot arch. Roentgenographic studies show a dense, narrow scaphoid. Limiting the child's activity controls discomfort. Osteochondritis is self-limiting, and the scaphoid usually revascularizes.

Sever's disease

A child 7 to 12 years of age with fragmented ossification of the os calcis apophysis complains of pain over the posterior aspect of the heel. The doctor finds tenderness in this area. Roentgenograms show a dense fragmented os calcis apophysis. Shoes that raise the heel and relieve pressure over the tender area and limitation of activity decrease symptoms. The disease is self-limiting.

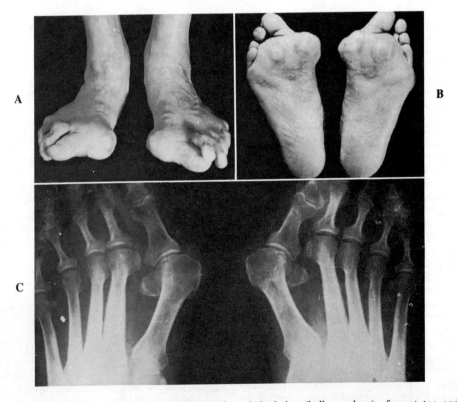

Fig. 38-17. Bunions. **A,** Dorsal view, showing lateral deviation (hallux valgus) of great toe and overlapping second toes. **B,** Plantar views showing callosities beneath prominent metatarsal heads. **C,** Roentgenogram showing bilateral hallux valgus.

Freiberg's disease

Osteochondritis of the second metatarsal head affects girls 10 to 15 years of age more often than it does boys. Symptomatic treatment is instituted until the area revascularizes. Occasionally the articular surface of the metatarsophalangeal joint collapses, and pain continues. In such an instance excision of the metatarsal head or arthroplasty might be necessary.

Bunions (hallux valgus)

A painful bunion results when the great toe deviates laterally at the metatarsophalangeal joint (hallux valgus), the head of the first metatarsal bone becomes prominent medially, and a callus or bursa, or both, develop over the metatarsal head (Fig. 38-17). Congenital adduction of the first metatarsal bone or lax ligaments produce deviation of the great toe. Perhaps aggravated by some of the ridiculous shoes they tolerate, bunions in women develop much more often than in men. Some bunions produce slight discomfort. In such an instance shoes fitted to relieve pressure or cut out over the bunion relieve pain. The patient with severe pain often needs surgical correction including arthroplasty to remove overgrowth on the metatarsal head, decompression of the metatarsophalangeal joint, and correction of angulation between the great toe and first metatarsal bone.

Hallux rigidus

In hallux rigidus the great toe fails to dorsiflex normally at the metatarsophalangeal joint. A bunion of long duration or any process that destroys the metatarsophalangeal joint can cause hallux rigidus. The patient who lacks dorsiflexion at the first metatarsophalangeal joint develops pain and walks in a protective manner to relieve this pain. Surgical treatment is by resection of the bunion and decompression of the metatarsophalangeal joint by removal of the proximal half of the proximal phalanx of the great toe.

Metatarsalgia

Pain beneath metatarsal heads is common. Weight bearing increases pain. Painful calluses develop over a prominent metatarsal head. Proper shoes and a pad in the shoes decrease pain. The pad must support weight in the region posterior to the metatarsal heads. Removal of a prominent metatarsal head beneath a persistent callus might be necessary.

Corns

Pressure on the skin against an underlying bony prominence produces corns that frequently become exquisitely painful. Treatment consists in the use of proper shoes, pads and cutouts to relieve pressure, and gentle trimming of the superficial dead skin. If conservative measures fail, the underlying bony spike can be removed.

Heel spur

A heel spur per se is not a disease but is a manifestation of bone repair reaction at the site of degeneration of the plantar ligaments near the os calcis. The patient may give a history of a recent change from one type of shoe to another or of walking a prolonged distance. The doctor should treat the heel spur with a pad cutout to relieve pressure. This disorder tends to repair itself after several months. In general, excision of the spur does not hasten repair time.

Ingrown toenail

An abnormal shape of the great toenail, an infected area along the toenail, pressure from tight shoes or socks, and trimming the nail too close at its corners all contribute to an ingrown toenail. The patient develops intermittent acute inflammation of soft tissues at the medial side of the great toenail (Fig. 38-18). During the acute stage, warm soaks, elevation, and antibiotics help control infection. After the acute episode, the patient should let the nail grow out, trim it straight across and not back at the corners, and avoid shoes and socks that cause pressure on the toe. At times elevating the nail edge and packing sterile cotton beneath it help the nail to grow out. If a deformed nail causes

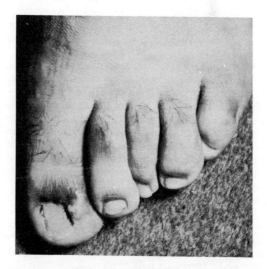

Fig. 38-18. Ingrown toenail. Soft tissues at lateral edge of great toenail are hypertrophied and infected.

continued symptoms, the patient might want surgical treatment. The surgeon can remove the medial one third of the nail, curet the nail base, and suture the skin beneath the nail bed to close the defect and create a new nail groove. If this fails, he can remove the entire nail, nail bed, and distal portion of the phalanx.

Digital neuroma (Morton's neuroma)

The patient, usually a women, with a neuroma of the common digital nerve to the contiguous sides of the third and fourth toe gives a classical history of episodes of severe, sharp, knifelike pain and paresthesias radiating into the adjacent sides of two toes. She removes the shoe and rubs the foot to relieve discomfort. Metatarsal pads may relieve pressure. If symptoms are severe enough, surgical excision of the neuroma may be necessary.

Cockup toes and hammer toes

Cockup toes hyperextend at the metatarsophalangeal joints and flex at the proximal interphalangeal joints. A variety of disorders (congenital, neuromuscular, arthritic) cause them. Any muscle imbalance that produces relatively strong extrinsic toe extensors and weak intrinsic toe extensors might produce cockup toes. These toes correct passively in contrast to hammer toes, which are fixed in their deformed position. Painful callosities develop over the proximal interphalangeal joints of hammer toes or cockup toes. During the flexible stage, deformity is corrected when the muscle balance is restored through the use of intrinsoplasties—the restoration of intrinsic muscle function by transplantation of the extrinsic toe flexors into the extensor hood. If deformities are fixed, excision or fusion of the proximal interphalangeal joint relieves symptoms.

INFECTION

In osteomyelitis, an infection of bone, offending organisms migrate through the bloodstream from a remote soft-tissue infection to the bone (acute hematogenous osteomyelitis), or they invade bone directly through an open wound or extend from an adjacent infection. Pyogenic bacteria induce the majority of bone infections. *Mycobacterium tuberculosis, Treponema pallidum,* and fungi infect bone infrequently.

Acute hematogenous osteomyelitis

Acute hematogenous osteomyelitis is one of the few orthopedic emergencies. Bacteria invade the bloodstream from a boil, a cellulitis, a sore throat, etc. They travel to bone and lodge in the metaphysis where the bone blood flow is greatest but where the *rate* of flow is slow and capillaries are open. The bacteria invoke an inflammatory reaction, suppuration, bone erosion, and bone death. A piece of dead bone surrounded by pus or infected granulation tissue is a *sequestrum*. If phagocytosis, body defense mechanisms, and antibiotics do not destroy the bacteria, the abscess takes one or more of the following routes:

1. Pus extends into the medullary cavity of the bone, and its pressure compromises the blood flow in nutrient vessels that enter the endosteal surface of the cortex and supply its inner half to two thirds. Much of the bone shaft becomes sequestrated.
2. The abscess perforates the cortex, dissects beneath the periosteum, strips it from the bone, destroys the periosteal blood supply, and sequestrates the outer third of the cortex. Subperiosteal and endosteal new bone form around the sequestrums. This new bone is an *involucrum*. If the infection subsides, granulation tissue erodes the sequestrums and replaces them with new bone.
3. The infection perforates the periosteum and forms a soft-tissue abscess.
4. Pus enters the adjacent joint, especially if the metaphysis is intracapsular as in the hip.
5. Although the epiphyseal plate acts as a barrier to infection, granulation tissue occasionally destroys it and alters growth.

Occasionally bacteria reenter the bloodstream, perpetuate septicemia, and establish metastatic foci in other sites including bone.

Acute hematogenous osteomyelitis usually affects children, boys more than girls, and most commonly attacks the upper tibia or the distal femur. The most common offending organism varies somewhat with the patient's age. In the child under 1 month of age, a gram-negative rod enters the bloodstream from an infected umbilicus and produces osteomyelitis. In the infant *Streptococcus* is common, but in the older child and adult *Staphylococcus* causes most bone infections.

In most instances the child has an infected cut, a boil, or a sore throat; 2 to 10 days later, he or she suddenly develops bone pain and loses function of the involved part. Generalized symptoms vary with the severity of the septicemia. If the organism is of low virulence or antibiotics have been used, the temperature often increases only slightly. At times, antibiotics suppress clinical symptoms while underlying bone destruction continues. In an infant with severe septicemia the temperature frequently rises to 104° or 105° F. The child is warm, dry, restless, and sometimes develops toxic myocarditis and pericarditis.

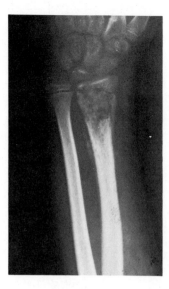

Fig. 38-19. Acute hematogenous osteomyelitis of radius 3 weeks after onset of symptoms. Infection has destroyed metaphyseal bone. Periosteal new bone is forming.

On examination, the physician finds heat, redness, and well-localized tenderness. By using a small object such as a pencil eraser to press on various parts of the bone, one can demonstrate circumscribed point tenderness in the infected portion of the bone. A fluctuant mass indicates subperiosteal or soft-tissue abscess. If the infection involves only bone, the child moves adjacent joints slowly without pain. Usually the sedimentation rate and white blood count rise, and the differential count shifts to the left. During septicemia, offending organisms can be grown from a blood culture.

The doctor *must* make the diagnosis clinically because during the first several days roentgenographic studies show nothing but soft-tissue swelling. Only after 8 to 10 days do roentgenograms disclose periosteal new bone (Fig. 38-19). To avoid disastrous sequelae, the physician *must make the diagnosis before this,* while the infection remains confined in metaphyseal bone. The orthopedist should treat the child with acute hematogenous osteomyelitis by general supportive measures, correct dehydration, restore an adequate hemoglobin level, start antibiotics, surgically drain bone abscesses, culture the pus, obtain sensitivities, and institute appropriate antibiotic treatment. The patient improves dramatically within a few hours. Postoperatively, rest with a cast or plaster splint prevents pathological fracture until new bone replaces dead bone and areas of bone destruction. The patient takes antibiotics for 4 to 6 weeks after all symptoms and signs have disappeared. With this treatment, the child has the best chance to control the infection and avoid chronic osteomyelitis.

Chronic osteomyelitis

Chronic osteomyelitis is difficult to cure. It follows one of several courses. Some patients develop intermittent acute exacerbations. In some the infection remains dormant only to flare up years later, whereas in others draining sinuses persist. After years of drainage, a few of these patients develop epidermoid carcinoma in sinus tracts.

Unresorbed sequestrums and unobliterated cavities surrounded by sclerotic bone perpetuate chronic infection (Fig. 38-20). Patients with acute exacerbations need appropriate antibiotics and drainage of abscesses. In those with chronic draining areas, surgeons remove underlying diseased bone, collapse cavities, and use appropriate antibiotics in an attempt to close wounds.

Osteomyelitis associated with open wounds

Open-wound osteomyelitis usually localizes and gives fewer generalized symptoms than acute hematogenous osteomyelitis does. Surgeons can prevent most of it by thoroughly debriding wounds and using antibiotics if indicated. A patient with this type of infection needs drainage of abscesses, removal of diseased bone and dead tissues, and antibiotics.

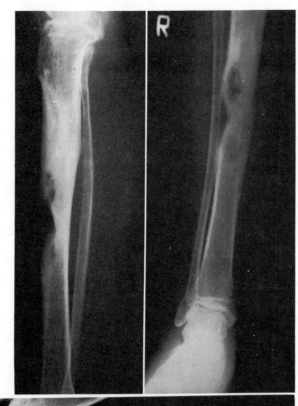

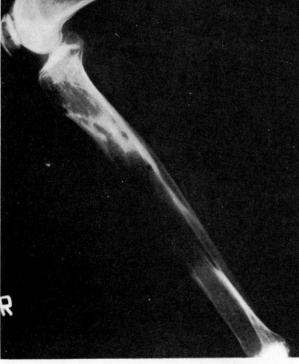

Fig. 38-20. Chronic osteomyelitis. **A,** Seventy years prior to this roentgenogram, patient had acute hematogenous osteomyelitis. Since then, recurrent chronic infection has drained intermittently. For 2 years, drainage had been continuous. Multiple lytic areas are surrounded by sclerotic bone. **B,** Eight months later, patient had increased drainage and pain and foul-smelling wound. Roentgenograms reveal extensive destruction from epidermoid carcinoma that developed in draining sinus.

Acute pyogenic arthritis

Bacteria enter a joint from underlying osteomyelitis, from an open wound, or directly from the bloodstream. Infected synovium and purulent joint exudate interfere with proper nutrition of articular cartilage by synovial fluid. This, and perhaps proteolytic enzymes, destroys cartilage in the weight-bearing area. The infection extends to subchondral bone. Capsular and intra-articular adhesions combined with incongruous joint surfaces limit joint motion.

The patient with acute pyogenic arthritis develops acute joint pain. The joint swells, and the part loses function. Often generalized symptoms of infection prevail. On examination, the doctor finds a swollen joint with excessive joint fluid. Joint motion triggers pain.

Roentgenograms reveal a distended capsular outline. After several days, the joint space narrows. If uncontrolled, infection destroys bone. In many instances, at 8 to 10 days a focus of osteomyelitis becomes evident.

The physician confirms the diagnosis by aspirating purulent, synovial fluid and finding bacteria on microscopic examination. The patient should have (1) general supportive measures, much the same as in acute hematogenous osteomyelitis, (2) surgical drainage of the joint and underlying bone infection, and (3) appropriate antibiotics. To avoid permanent joint damage, *treatment must be started at once.*

Acute idiopathic synovitis of children presents one of the most confusing differential diagnostic problems. The child holds the joint, usually the hip, immobile, complains of tenderness, and cries with pain on motion. He usually has no generalized symptoms. The patient often gives no history of prior infection; joint fluid contains no bacteria; roentgenograms show no abnormalities; and the condition subsides spontaneously with rest.

Cellulitis overlying the metaphysis of a child must be considered osteomyelitis until proved otherwise. The patient with cellulitis has fewer generalized symptoms, less pain, and more diffuse tenderness than one with osteomyelitis.

Acute rheumatic processes often begin gradually. The patient gives no history of prior infection. He or she has fewer generalized symptoms and no bone tenderness. The process involves many joints. The white blood count and sedimentation rate rise less than in patients with osteomyelitis.

At times neoplasm, especially Ewing's tumor, simulates an acute infection even to the extent of demonstrating heat and tenderness, generalized symptoms, fever, and sedimentation rate and white blood count elevation. X-ray studies usually reveal the bone involvement.

Tuberculosis

At times tuberculosis involves bone without entering a joint, but more often it infects both. The bacteria from a pulmonary lesion (less often from an enteric lesion) travel through the bloodstream to subarticular bone or synovium. Synovium proliferates with a tuberculous, granulomatous pannus that grows across and erodes beneath articular cartilage. The pannus from opposing joint surfaces bridges the joint with fibrous tissue that limits joint motion. Sometimes this ossifies and fuses the joint. The infection frequently destroys the joint capsule and forms a soft-tissue abscess (cold abscess) of caseous material. This can penetrate skin and form sinuses that become secondarily infected with pyogenic organisms.

Bone tuberculosis often attacks the hip and spine of children. The patient notices gradual onset of pain, joint swelling, and loss of motion. Later, contractures ensue. Children with tuberculosis commonly perspire and cry at night. The temperature rises in the afternoon, and the white count increases. In early stages of the disease x-ray examination shows distension of capsular outlines and bone atrophy, especially of subchondral cortex. Later, marginal notching is visible. In advanced lesions bone and joint are destroyed.

Pulmonary tuberculosis and a positive skin test support the diagnosis. Isolation of bacteria by culture or guinea pig inoculation proves the diagnosis.

The doctor should treat the patient with general supportive measures, continue appropriate antituberculous drugs for 12 to 18 months, and immobilize the part by a cast, splint, or traction. When the patient is in a good general condition, the orthopedist can excise localized lesions and attempt to restore function of the part, drain abscesses, excise advanced lesions, and fuse the involved joint.

TRAUMA
Fractures

A *fracture* is a break in continuity of bone or articular cartilage (Fig. 38-21).

Etiology. Fractures result from (1) a direct force at the site of fracture, or (2) an indirect force transmitted from a distance, i.e., fracture of the humerus from a fall on the outstretched hand.

Types

Closed: No communication between the external surface of the body and bone

Open: Communication between the external surface of the body and bone through an open wound

Pathological: A break, usually produced by less force than that required to break a normal

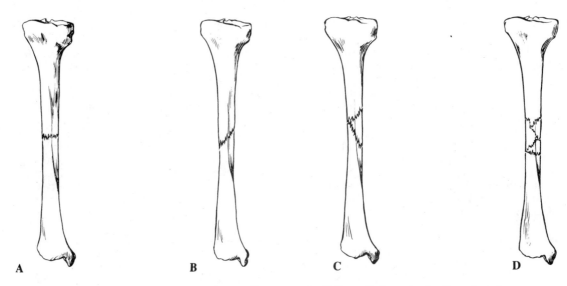

Fig. 38-21. Fracture configuration. **A,** Transverse. **B,** Oblique. **C,** Butterfly. **D,** Comminuted.

bone, through a bone weakened by disease (infection, neoplasm, osteoporosis)

Avulsion: A fragment of bone pulled off by ligament or tendon at its attachment

Epiphyseal separation: A break in the region of a child's epiphyseal plate (Fig. 38-22); most involve subepiphyseal spongy bone, but some cross the epiphyseal plate or crush epiphyseal cells and result in subsequent growth disturbance (angulation or length discrepancy) (Fig. 38-23)

Greenstick: One side of a child's bone "bends," and the other side breaks (Fig. 38-24)

Comminuted: A break with three or more fragments (Fig. 38-21)

Diagnosis. The physician should suspect a fracture in a patient who gives a history of injury and complains of pain, swelling, and loss of function. Displaced fragments produce obvious deformity. Point tenderness at the fracture line is demonstrable, and gentle motion produces crepitus—one bone fragment grates on the other. Roentgenographic studies in at least two planes at right angles to each other are mandatory, and views of the opposite normal counterpart are valuable, especially in children where epiphyseal plates, nutrient arteries, and irregular ossification centers might be confused with a fracture.

Before he or she treats a fracture, the doctor must examine and record the neurovascular status of the extremity distal to the fracture. He or she

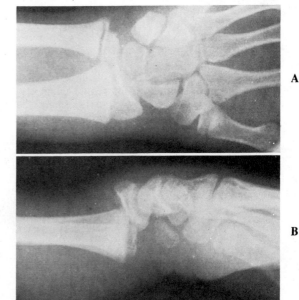

Fig. 38-22. A, Epiphyseal separation of distal radial epiphysis. Lateral view, **B,** shows triangular fragment of metaphysis that remained with dorsally displaced epiphysis. (From Cooper, R.R.: J. Iowa Med. Soc. **54:**689, 1964.)

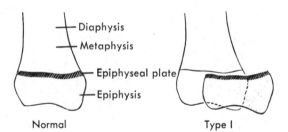

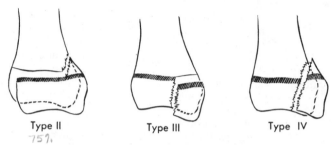

757,

Fig. 38-23. Four types of epiphyseal fractures.

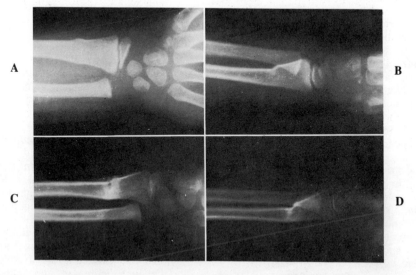

Fig. 38-24. Greenstick fracture. **A,** Anteroposterior view shows expanded cortex at site of fracture. **B,** Lateral view shows "buckle" of dorsal cortex of radius. **C,** Anteroposterior view after 3 weeks of treatment in long arm cast; repair has made fracture more obvious. **D,** Lateral view at 3 weeks. (From Cooper, R.R.: J. Iowa Med. Soc. **54:**689, 1964.)

must document associated nerve, artery, ligament, or other soft-tissue injuries.

Treatment. By applying certain basic principles, the physician can treat the great majority of fractures satisfactorily, especially in children. Deviation from these principles frequently produces disastrous sequelae. Many fracture complications result from poorly indicated and improperly applied therapy, usually in the form of overtreatment with nuts, bolts, rods, and various pieces of hardware. Before treating a fracture, the physician must diagnose and treat associated injuries that threaten life and that demand priority (airway obstruction, hemorrhage, shock, perforated viscus).

Goals in treatment of fractures are to (1) prevent further damage, (2) gain satisfactory position of involved bones, (3) obtain union as rapidly as possible, (4) use the safest method, and (5) preserve or restore function of the involved part. Stages in fracture treatment are as follows.

First aid. Prevent further damage and relieve the patient's discomfort until institution of definitive therapy. The following two actions usually accomplish first aid of extremity injuries:

1. Cover wounds with a pressure dressing of the cleanest bandage available to prevent further contamination and control hemorrhage. As a general rule, tourniquets are unnecessary and can be dangerous.
2. Immobilize the involved part to relieve pain and prevent further damage—penetration of nerves, arteries, and muscles by bone ends and penetration of skin, thereby converting a closed fracture to an open one. One can immobilize the part effectively with simple splints of magazines, pillows, boards, and strips of cloth.

Reduction. Place bone fragments in proper relationship to each other. Before this can be done, the doctor must relieve the patient's pain by:

1. Local injection of an anesthetic into the fracture hematoma—two precautions are necessary: use strict sterile techniques since a tract is established between a closed fracture and the body surface with the risk of subsequent infection; to obtain satisfactory anesthesia, insert the needle into the hematoma as evidenced by aspiration of blood
2. Regional anesthesia (axillary block, sciatic block, etc.)
3. General anesthesia; to minimize the risk of vomiting and aspiration, allow sufficient time to elapse after the patient eats or drinks (±6 hours)

Thoroughly and carefully debride (i.e., remove all devitalized tissue and foreign bodies) all open wounds. Decide whether to close the skin depending on time since injury, amount of contamination, site of injury, and degree of tissue damage. To make this decision, one needs clinical judgment that comes only with experience. If an open wound accompanies a fracture, tetanus prophylaxis must be instituted, and "prophylactic" antibodies are warranted.

Three considerations in the reduction of a fracture are listed in order of importance as follows:

1. *Alignment:* Malalignment of a fracture resolves into two components (Fig. 38-25):
   a. *Rotary malalignment:* Malposition of one fragment in relation to the other because of turning about an axis parallel to the long axis of the bone; e.g., if a patient fractures his tibia and his toes point posteriorly, one may reasonably assume that rotatory malalignment exists. A fracture unites in a malrotated position and does not correct with time in either a child or an adult.
   b. *Angulation:* Malposition of one fragment in relation to another because of rotation about an axis at 90 degrees to the long axis of the bone (Fig. 38-26). In certain instances angulation is acceptable. In children growth corrects angulation in some locations depending on the child's age and the degree and direction of angulation. In general, the younger the child and the nearer the fracture to the end of a long bone, the more angulation is permissible, provided that the apex of the angle points in the direction of the plane of greatest motion of the adjacent joint (anteriorly or posteriorly in a fracture) near the knee. In no case should more than 25 degrees of angulation remain. Even in adults, in a bone deeply buried in muscle, some angulation does not mean an unsatisfactory result.
2. *Length restoration:* In completely displaced fractures, fragments override because of muscle spasm. The physician must restore appropriate length. Anatomical reduction is not always necessary. In certain instances some overriding is not only acceptable but even desirable. In a child with a completely displaced long bone shaft fracture, one can accept 1 cm. of overriding with side-to-side union. After such a fracture, blood supply to the limb increases and causes increased growth of the involved extremity. In an adult, side-to-side union of a deeply buried bone is permissible. One should err on the side of overriding rather than distracting the fracture, since distraction predisposes to delayed union or nonunion.

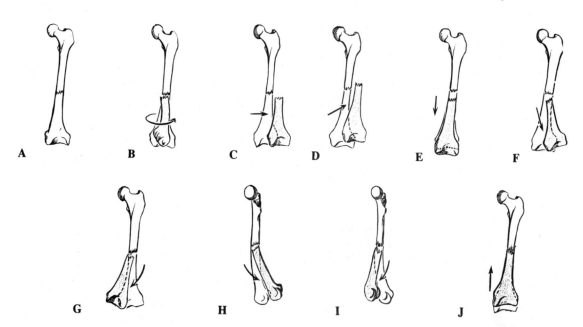

Fig. 38-25. Fracture deformities. **A,** No deformity. **B,** Rotation. **C,** Apposition loss. **D,** Overriding. **E,** Distraction. **F,** Angulation: valgus. **G,** Angulation: varus. **H,** Angulation: anterior apex. **I,** Angulation: posterior apex. **J,** Impaction.

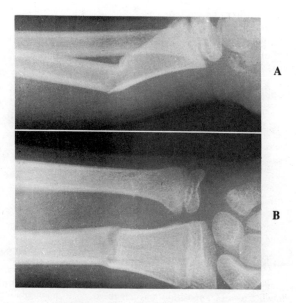

Fig. 38-26. Angulated fracture of distal third of child's forearm. Lateral view, **A,** shows angulation. Anteroposterior view, **B,** shows no loss of length or apposition. (From Cooper, R.R.: J. Iowa Med. Soc. **54:**689, 1964.)

3. *Apposition:* The amount of end-to-end contact of fragments ranks least important of the three factors, unless the fracture involves a joint surface or unless the bone is subcutaneous where the "stepoff" produced by appositional loss would be cosmetically undersirable. In side-to-side union, complete loss of cross-sectional apposition exists (Fig. 38-27).

When the preceding factors have been corrected, the fracture is reduced. In obtaining a reduction, the physician should always think in the following sequence:

"Can I manipulate the fracture and apply a plaster cast?"

If so, this is the best method yet devised for treatment of a fracture. If he cannot do this or if he knows from past experience that he cannot, he should next think:

"Can I apply traction either to the skin, by attaching adherent tapes to the skin, or to the skeleton, by placing a pin through bone distal to the fracture?"

Traction is retained until fracture fragments adhere sufficiently to go without immobilization or to maintain position in a cast. Both methods of traction have advantages and disadvantages. Skin traction is easily applied and does not open a bone. In some patients the skin reacts to tape. The amount of traction and the length of time it can be maintained are limited with skin tapes. Skeletal traction is comfortable and tolerates more weight for a longer time than skin traction does. It can be applied under local anesthesia, but strict sterile technique and a threaded pin must be used to decrease the risk of infecting the bone.

A physician should use no other methods in treating children's fractures except for a few rare articular fractures and the following three common elbow fractures: (1) most fractures of the lateral condyle of the humerus require open reduction; (2) fractures of the medial epicondyle need open reduction if the bone fragment is entrapped in the elbow joint or the ulnar nerve is impinged; (3) a few fractures of the radial neck cannot undergo closed reduction.

"Must I do an open reduction?"

Only in instances in which the first two methods do not work. Fractures must have a blood supply in order to heal. Any open reduction destroys some vessels. Open reduction must definitely be indicated and used only by one aware of all risks and technically competent to do open reductions.

Fixation. Hold the fragments reduced by plaster, traction, or in certain instances internal devices.

Immobilization. The fracture must be as free of motion as possible until the fracture unites as determined by clinical examination (lack of tenderness and motion) and x-ray examination (obliteration of the fracture line by new bone). Union usually occurs more rapidly in children than in adults.

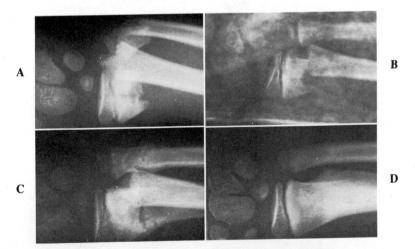

Fig. 38-27. Loss of apposition in fracture of distal third of child's forearm. **A,** Anteroposterior roentgenograms showing loss of apposition and length. **B,** With manipulative reduction, length is restored; 50% loss of apposition remains. **C,** Four weeks later, new bone has united fragments. **D,** Six months later, loss of apposition is being corrected by resorption of bone on medial side and bone deposition on lateral side. (From Cooper, R.R.: J. Iowa Med. Soc. **54:**689, 1964.)

Preserve or restore function to the involved part. The physician must constantly remember the goal of preservation or restoration of function. It is useless to obtain a perfectly united fracture if, in so doing, function is lost. Children restore function well if left to their own devices with pain as their guide to activity. Some adults need physical therapy to help restore function during and after fracture treatment. After an epiphyseal injury, the doctor must follow the child to see if the bone becomes deformed.

Specific fractures

Clavicle. Children and young adults frequently fracture the clavicle, usually by indirect force transmitted up the arm from a fall on the outstretched hand or through the acromion from a fall on the shoulder. Less frequently, a direct blow breaks the clavicle. After fracture, the weight of the upper extremity displaces the distal fragment caudad and the sternocleidomastoid displaces the proximal fragment cephalad (Fig. 38-28). Despite its subcutaneous location, the fractured clavicle usually fails to perforate the skin.

Children commonly sustain a greenstick fracture of the clavicle. In adults, brachial plexus, vessel, rib, and pulmonary injuries infrequently accompany clavicle fractures.

A figure-of-eight dressing relieves pain, lifts the distal fragment, and pulls it posteriorly to appose the proximal fragment (Fig. 38-29). In children the dressing consists of a stockinette filled with padding. In adults plaster over padding effectively holds the clavicle.

Clavicle fractures nearly always unite, and excellent function returns even if moderate displace-

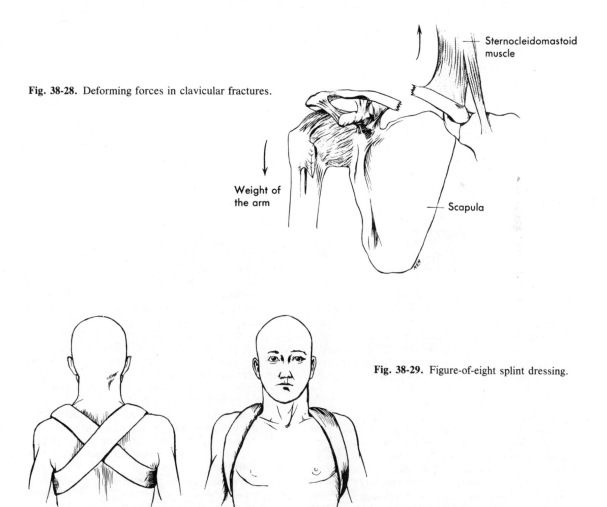

Fig. 38-28. Deforming forces in clavicular fractures.

Fig. 38-29. Figure-of-eight splint dressing.

ment remains. Anatomical reduction becomes a goal only if cosmesis is the primary concern.

Humerus. Usually a force transmitted upward through the hand and forearm fractures the humerus. Although shaft, lateral condyle, and medial epicondyle fractures and proximal epiphyseal separations are not uncommon in children, the bone breaks most often at the supracondylar level. In adults the shaft or surgical neck fractures most frequently.

Humerus fractures usually remain closed. Associated injuries include radial nerve injuries, either at the time of fracture or by entrapment in callus during healing. In adults arterial damage is uncommon. Brachial artery injury must always be considered during treatment of supracondylar fractures in children.

A supracondylar fracture of the humerus constitutes perhaps the most dangerous common fracture in a child's extremity. The distal fragment usually displaces posteriorly and proximally and compresses the brachial artery and median nerve between swollen soft tissues and the sharp distal end of the proximal fragment. Most children with this fracture should be hospitalized and the fracture reduced as soon as possible with skin traction applied to the forearm or with skeletal traction by a pin in the proximal ulna. The hand must be observed carefully and frequently for signs of neurovascular compression (pain, pallor, paresthesias, paralysis, lack of capillary refill, and disappearance of a radial pulse). Progression of any of these signs may necessitate surgical exploration of the brachial artery to prevent the dread complication of Volkmann's ischemic contracture. (See "Complications of fractures," p. 484.) After 5 to 10 days in traction, the elbow can be held safely in flexion during immobilization in a posterior splint or Velpeau dressing for 3 or 4 weeks.

Treatment of humeral shaft and surgical neck fractures usually is by a long arm hanging cast. The latter acts as a weight on the arm to prevent overriding and to align fragments during healing. The hanging cast allows early shoulder joint motion, an important consideration in the elderly. Most humeral fractures unite readily. Radial nerve defects occurring at the time of fracture usually resolve. Late entrapment of the radial nerve by callus may require neurolysis.

A lateral humeral condyle fracture in a child extends into the articular surface. Usually, the common extensor muscle origin rotates the fragment 180 degrees so that the articular surface of the distal humerus contacts the fractured surface of the proximal fragment. These fractures fail to reduce by closed methods and if left alone become nonunited, with a subsequent progressive cubitus valgus deformity. This produces delayed ulnar nerve paralysis from stretching the ulnar nerve around the increased valgus angle of the elbow. Appropriate treament is by open reduction of the fragment and fixation with one or two pins in an anatomically reduced position. Care must be taken not to strip the common extensor origin from the fragment since this constitutes its only blood supply. After reduction, the child remains in a posterior splint or cast for 5 or 6 weeks, at which time the pins are removed.

A medial humeral epicondyle fracture in a child results when the common flexor muscle origin avulses the epicondyle. The fracture remains extraarticular. It requires open reduction if (1) the fragment displaces and becomes entrapped in the joint, or (2) signs of ulnar nerve compression exist. Open reduction may also be indicated if there is noticeable displacement, since a fibrous union or a lack of union might weaken forearm muscles. The fragment is fixed to its original position either with sutures or a wire.

Forearm. Radial neck fractures in children ordinarily angulate only mildly and reduce by pressure applied directly over the radial head as the forearm is rotated into pronation and supination. Occasionally a radial neck fracture angulates nearly 90 degrees and fails to reduce by closed methods. In this instance open reduction and replacement of the radial head onto the radial shaft become necessary. Postoperatively, the part is immobilized for 3 or 4 weeks until the fracture unites firmly.

Unlike children, adults frequently fracture the radial head. This at times is severely comminuted and, if left in place, leads to degenerative changes in the radiohumeral joint. In adults an injured radial head can be safely excised.

Olecranon fractures in adults frequently result from a fall on the elbow with application of direct force to the proximal ulna. If the proximal fragment includes less than one third of the ulnar articular surface, the fragment may be excised and the triceps tendon attached to the remaining portion of the ulna. If the olecranon fragment is larger, it can be replaced and fixed to the ulnar shaft by means of an intramedullary screw or with wires. Postoperatively, the elbow is immobilized in a posterior plaster splint for 3 to 6 weeks and then progressive active motion begins.

A direct blow or a fall on the outstretched hand may fracture the radius or ulna, or both. In children forearm fractures are commonly greenstick. In older children distal radial epiphyseal separations are not unusual. Older adults frequently fracture the distal 3 cm. of the radius and the ulnar styloid (Colles' fracture). The mechanism of injury, a fall on the outstretched hand, displaces the distal fragment dorsally, proximally, and ra-

Fig. 38-30. Distal radial fracture. **A,** Anteroposterior. **B,** Lateral.

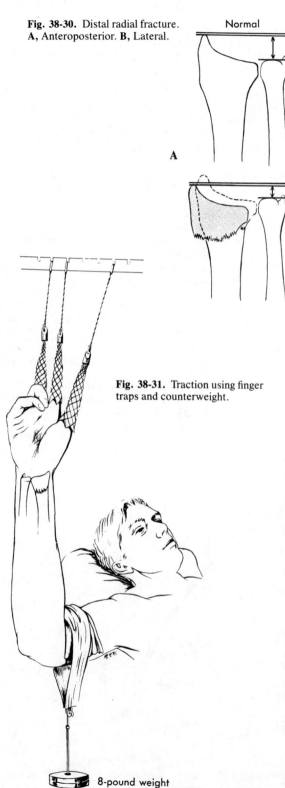

Fig. 38-31. Traction using finger traps and counterweight.

8-pound weight

dially (Fig. 38-30). Surrounding tissues usually remain uninjured.

Local anesthesia affords satisfactory relief of pain for closed reduction of many forearm fractures in adults and children. After the fracture hematoma is injected, distraction accomplished by finger traps and a counterweight on the upper arm (Fig. 38-31) often corrects angulation, overriding, and displacement. In children a long arm cast then holds the fracture until it unites. In the older patient with Colles' fracture, a plaster cast from metacarpophalangeal joints to elbow for 3 to 4 weeks often suffices. This allows elbow, shoulder, and finger motion so necessary to avoid crippling stiffness of the arm and hand.

In adults with a radial and ulnar shaft fracture, closed reduction may be impossible, thereby necessitating open reduction and internal fixation.

Hand. See Chapter 39.

Vertebra. Vertebral fractures may be classified into (1) vertebral body fractures, usually with anterior wedging and compression, and (2) fractures that involve the neural arch, often with a shift of one vertebral body upon the other. The mechanism of injury in the first type is usually compression of the vertebral body as in a fall from a height onto the legs or buttocks or from striking the top of the head as in diving into shallow water. The second type of fracture may also occur by these mechanisms but often follows severe rotational and displacement forces such as those produced in an automobile accident.

Vertebral fractures usually remain closed. Frequently spinal cord or nerve injuries accompany these fractures. Usually no external deformity is seen in vertebral fractures, though with great compression there may be visible angulation. Roentgenograms show anterior wedging of the vertebral body or fractures of the neural arch with displacement of one vertebral body upon the other. Treatment is aimed at preventing spinal cord damage or further cord damage in patients demonstrating initial neurological deficit.

Fracture dislocations of the cervical spine require reduction by tongs placed in the skull followed by further immobilization in plaster or by operative fusion of the involved vertebral bodies, or by both methods. Mild dorsal and lumbar compression fractures may be treated by bed rest with walking as soon as pain disappears. Residual deformities do not usually limit function, and late results often depend on the degree of spinal cord injury.

Fractures with spinal cord or nerve injury, especially if the loss progresses, require early neurosurgical or orthopedic care.

Pelvis. Pelvic fractures result from direct trauma or from forces transmitted to the pelvis through the femur. Some fractures pass through weight-bearing portions of the pelvis, and some do not (Fig. 38-32). Pelvic fractures usually remain closed. Associated bladder, urethral, or rectal injuries must be suspected. Sacral fractures may lacerate nerves emerging through sacral foramina. Displacement in pelvic fractures is often minimal. Displaced fractures in one part of the bony pelvic ring usually signify fractures through opposite portions of the ring. In some fractures the hemipelvis displaces cranially (Fig. 38-33). Treatment in this situation is by the use of traction through the corresponding leg to attempt restoration of alignment. Nondisplaced fractures warrant ambulation as early as symptoms permit.

Acetabular fractures that involve displacement with incongruity between the femoral head and the weight-bearing acetabular dome often require open reduction and fixation. These frequently result in subsequent degenerative joint changes and hip pain.

Other pelvic fractures usually produce no residual severe deformity. Appreciable displacement in women of childbearing age may mitigate against future vaginal delivery.

Hip (femoral neck and intertrochanteric). Hip injuries usually occur from minor trauma in aged patients with osteoporosis. Pathological fractures from metastatic carcinoma often involve these locations. The deformity in both femoral neck and intertrochanteric fractures consist in shortening and external rotation of the extremity, a deformity usually obvious clinically and roentgenographically.

Treatment of femoral neck fractures consists in closed reduction by traction, internal rotation, and abduction of the limb followed by internal fixation with multiple threaded pins or a nail or screw through the femoral neck and head (Fig. 38-34).

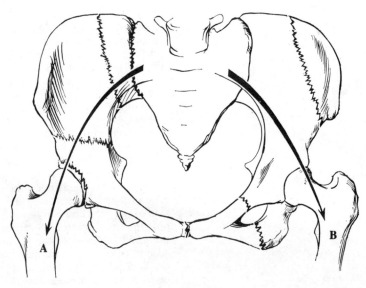

Fig. 38-32. Pelvic fractures. **A,** Fractures through weight-bearing line. **B,** Fractures not through weight-bearing line.

Fig. 38-33. Double vertical fracture of pelvis.

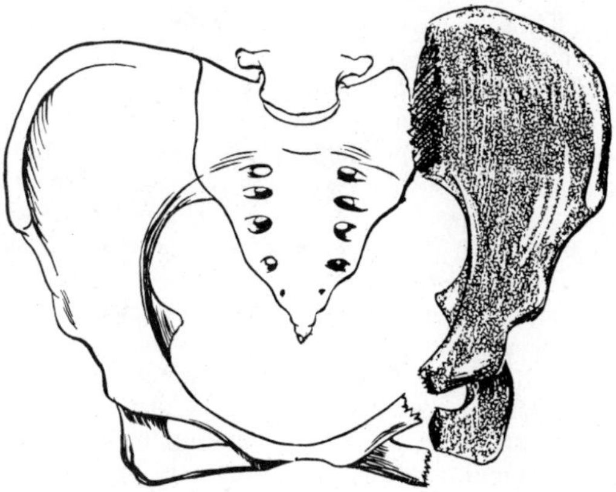

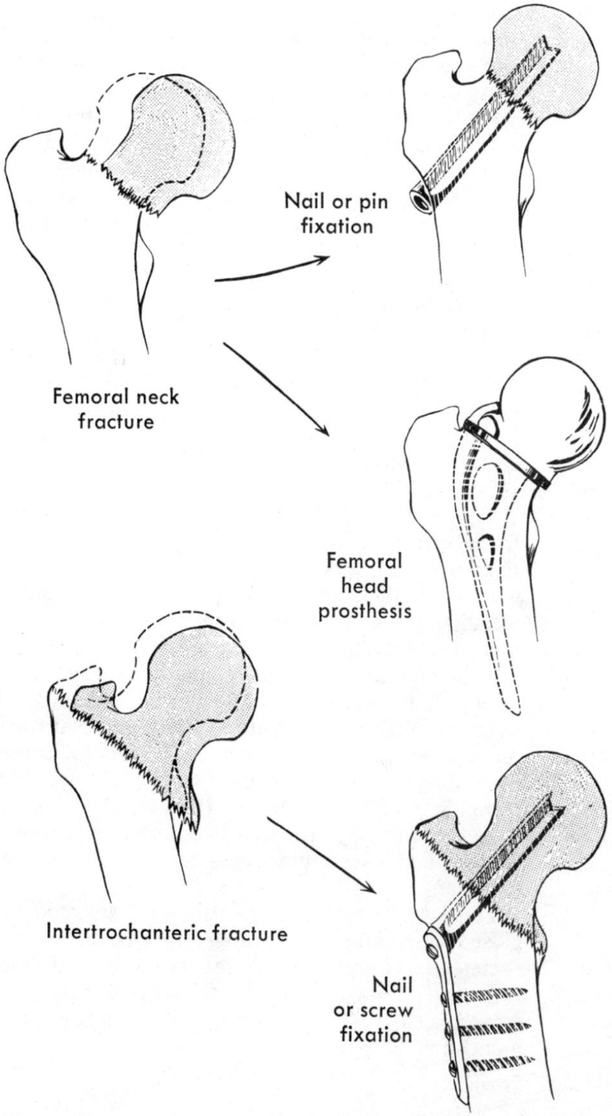

Femoral neck
fracture

Nail or pin
fixation

Femoral
head
prosthesis

Intertrochanteric fracture

Nail
or screw
fixation

Fig. 38-34. Hip fractures and their treatment.

The femoral head is replaced by a prosthesis in selected cases. Intertrochanteric fractures are treated by closed reduction and internal fixation with a nail or screw and side plate (Fig. 38-34). Fixation permits patients to sit by 1 or 2 days postoperatively and walk in a walker or on crutches without bearing weight if they have sufficient strength. This prevents a multitude of complications (thrombophlebitis, pulmonary emboli, pneumonia, renal stones, pressure ulcers) that often lead to death.

Results in hip fractures leave much to be desired. Many patients die during the first year after treatment. Intertrochanteric fractures usually heal, but nonunion with aseptic necrosis may follow femoral neck fractures. Replacement prostheses eliminate nonunion but introduce unique problems of their own.

Femoral shaft. The injuring force to the femoral shaft may be a direct blow or transmission of stress upward through the foot and tibia. Most femoral shaft fractures remain closed. Considerable blood loss (up to 3 L.) accompanies femoral shaft fractures. Varying degrees of muscle injury, especially to the quadriceps, may produce fibrosis with subsequent functional loss.

The clinical examination usually reveals shortening of the extremity and swelling of the thigh, both from the fracture hematoma and the shortened musculature. The fracture fragments almost always override, angulate, and rotate. Distraction, because of excessive traction, greatly increases chances of nonunion. A small amount of overriding is desirable, especially in the growing child since the stimulus of increased blood supply to epiphyseal plates increases linear bone growth. Rotational deformities must be avoided, since even the child's growing bone will not correct rotational malalignments spontaneously.

Femoral shaft fractures in adults may be treated with 8 to 20 pounds of traction through a skeletal traction pin followed by the use of a cast brace. This is designed to permit knee motion and to take partial weight bearing through the fractured bone and partial weight bearing on the ischial tuberosity and through the soft tissues of the thigh. This method has the advantage of allowing healing to be stimulated by some forces being transmitted through the bone, and it allows earlier walking. In children skin traction often suffices. Toddlers may bear full weight with solid bony union in about 4 weeks. Certain femur shaft fractures in adults can be treated by an intramedullary rod. This shortens hospitalization but adds risks of an operation.

Patella. Fracture of the patella includes two general types that often differ in mechanism of injury, associated damage to surrounding structures, and treatment.

Transverse fractures occur with violent sudden contraction of the quadriceps muscle (when one slips and attempts to prevent a fall). Less often, a direct blow produces a transverse fracture. The two fragments may be equal or the fracture line can occur toward either pole of the patella, producing dissimilar fragments. If the fragments retain opposition, physical examination shows only mild local swelling and tenderness with pain on knee extension. Wide separation of the fragments produces a palpable sulcus. This also indicates medial and lateral tearing of the quadriceps expansion and the joint capsule.

If the fragments do not separate, treatment is by use of a posterior plaster splint or cylinder cast with graduated quadriceps exercise started at 2 to 3 weeks and with progressive weight bearing soon thereafter. Wide separation of fragments demands operative realignment, suture of the torn quadriceps expansion, and 6 to 10 weeks of plaster immobilization. Great disparity in fragment size justifies removal of the smaller one and repair of tendon or muscle attachments to the retained fragment.

Comminuted patellar fractures generally result from a direct blow. Associated lacerations of the joint capsule or quadriceps expansion are less severe; however, damage of the articular surfaces of femur and patella is frequently extensive. Treatment is then by patellectomy and suture of the patellar tendon to the quadriceps tendon. A plaster cast immobilizes the extremity in extension for 6 to 10 weeks.

Tibia. Tibial shaft fractures result from torsional force or from a direct blow (bumper fracture), and tibial plateau fractures result from a force transmitted up the tibia and to the femoral condyles (body weight). Bone fragments from the subcutaneous tibia frequently protrude through skin lacerations. Tibial fractures may injure the posterior tibial artery. Skin injuries often result in difficulty of obtaining soft tissue closure over open tibial fractures. Lateral displacement sufficient to cause overriding is uncommon in transverse fractures but common in oblique fractures. Rotational deformity must be suspected in displaced tibial fractures. Tibial plateau fractures angulate into varus or valgus.

Tibial shaft fractures can usually be treated by closed reduction and a long leg plaster or by skeletal traction distal to the fracture until the fragments unite sufficiently to prevent displacement in a cast. Solid union may not occur for 3 to 8 months.

Tibial plateau fractures may be comminuted and require splinting with subsequent early motion, or they may consist of one large fragment that can be openly reduced and fixed to the remaining tibia.

Ankle (medial and lateral malleoli and ankle ligaments). The medial malleolus (tibia), posterior malleolus (posterior lip of the distal articular surface of the tibia), and lateral malleolus (fibula) fracture alone or in various combinations. Ligament injuries may accompany one or more of these fractures and often demand as much or more attention than the fracture itself. The mechanism of injury is excessive movement of the mobile leg upon the fixed foot or of the mobile foot upon the fixed leg. The injuring force frequently externally rotates or abducts the foot, talus, and distal tibia and fibula. Certain combinations of forces produce characteristic fracture patterns. Ankle fractures remain closed unless a direct injury lacerates the skin or the injuring force dislocates the talus from

the tibia with resulting skin loss or subsequent necrosis.

The deformity of a fracture dislocation of the ankle is obvious on inspection (gross loss of the relationship between the foot and leg). Without dislocation, the injury produces swelling and tenderness over the injured malleoli. Final distinction between bony and ligamentous injuries requires roentgenographic studies in the anterior, posterior, lateral, and oblique projections.

Adequate reduction demands reconstitution of the forklike configuration of the medial and lateral malleolus (closing the ankle mortise). Interposition of a flap of soft tissues (deltoid ligament) between the medial malleolus and talus may necessitate open reduction to restore normal congruity between the articular surfaces of the talus and tibia (Fig. 38-35). Many ankle fractures can be reduced closed and immobilized 6 to 8 weeks in a short leg walking cast. More complicated fractures and frac-

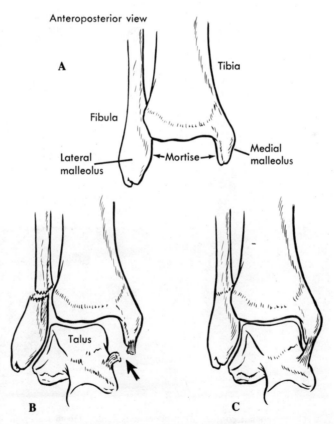

Fig. 38-35. Ankle mortise. **A,** Normal. **B,** Fracture of lateral malleolus and tear of deltoid ligament *(arrow)* opens mortise. **C,** Mortise closed with restored congruity of talus and tibia.

ture dislocations may require a long leg cast and no weight bearing for varying periods or open reduction with ligament repair and internal fixation of the fracture.

The results of treatment are usually good if (1) tibiotalar congruity is restored (the ankle mortise is closed) and (2) ligamentous injuries are recognized and treated adequately. Delayed union or nonunion occasionally occurs in medial malleolar fractures.

Foot

Talus. Fractures often involve the neck of the talus and are frequently accompanied by ankle or subtalar dislocation. These fractures reduce with difficulty and may require surgical reduction. Because of the source of blood supply, aseptic necrosis of the body of the talus frequently develops and adds to morbidity and produces long-term complications.

Calcaneus. Fractures of the calcaneus usually occur during a fall from a height. These falls crush the bone and frequently extend into the subtalar joint. The foot becomes extremely swollen. Initial treatment is by rest, elevation, and compression. After swelling decreases, many fractures can be managed with a short leg cast and weight bearing as tolerated. Several operations are designed to attempt reconstruction of various calcaneal fractures. After treatment, subtalar joint motion often remains decreased.

Metatarsus and phalanges. Metatarsal and phalangeal fractures usually require closed reduction and plaster immobilization for 3 to 4 weeks. Some, with great displacement, demand open reduction and internal fixation.

Complications of fractures
Complications of casts—compartment syndrome

Improperly applied plaster or subsequent swelling produces pressure of the cast against underlying soft tissues over bone prominences. Skin circulation decreases, and necrosis results. In applying a cast the physician should expose the tips of the patient's toes or fingers in order to observe the parts for signs of neurovascular compression. Pressure from a tight cast or padding, or hemorrhage and swelling into a muscular compartment compromise circulation to the extremity. Persistent neurovascular interference invokes the dreaded Compartment Syndrome which, if ignored, leads to Volkmann's ischemic paralysis, especially after humeral supracondylar fractures and fractures or dislocations near the knee. In this syndrome muscular circulation decreases, necrotic and fibrotic scar replaces muscles, and permanent contractures ensue (Fig. 38-36). Associated sensory loss further impairs function.

Because of these disastrous sequelae, the doctor must investigate and correct complaints of pain and numbness beneath a cast. Pain, pallor, swelling, discoloration, and lack of capillary refill indicate circulatory embarrassment. The doctor must treat a patient with any of these immediately by splitting the cast and the underlying padding, elevating the part, and observing the patient carefully to see if surgical exploration of the involved compartment is indicated. Intracompartmental pressure can be measured by insertion of a wick catheter. A persistent pressure of 35 to 40 mm. H_2O is an indication to open the tight osteofascial compartment.

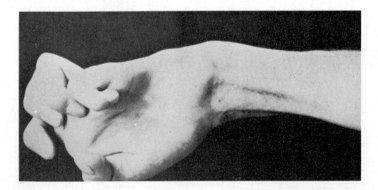

Fig. 38-36. Volkmann's ischemic contracture. Clawhand is rigid and useless. (From Steindler, A.: The traumatic deformities and disabilities of the upper extremity, Springfield, Ill., 1956, Charles C Thomas, Publisher, p. 296.)

Malunion

If a fractured bone is improperly reduced or loses reduction as swelling decreases, the bone unites in an unsatisfactory position. To avoid this complication, the doctor must reduce the fracture properly and follow the patient to be certain that reduction is *maintained*. If a malunion is cosmetically or functionally unacceptable to the patient, an orthopedic surgeon can rebreak the bone (osteotomy) and restore satisfactory position.

Delayed union

At times a bone fails to heal solidly after a reasonable period as determined by location of the fracture, type of fracture, and method of treatment. Continued adequate immobilization corrects most delayed unions.

Nonunion

Some bones fail to unite. Gross motion is generally demonstrable. X-ray examination reveals sclerosis of adjacent bone ends and obliteration of the medullary canal. Fibrous scar tissue or a false joint (pseudarthrosis) fills the gap between bone ends. Bone grafting stimulates repair at these sites.

The causes of delayed and nonunion are not always immediately apparent and usually include a combination of inadequate reduction, inadequate fixation, inadequate immobilization, severe trauma to soft parts, improper operative treatment, distraction of fragments, infection, and fracture location. The femoral neck, carpal scaphoid, and junction of the distal one third and middle one third of the tibia unite slowly.

Shock

Bone is extremely vascular. At the time of fracture large volumes of blood escape from the circulating blood into soft tissues or externally through an open wound. Neurogenic shock from pain aggravates shock from blood loss. For the patient in shock, the physician must provide an adequate airway and oxygen, control hemorrhage and pain, and restore blood volume.

Fat embolism

Patients who sustain massive trauma occasionally develop clinical signs and symptoms of fat embolism. This syndrome results from vascular impaction by fat, especially in the lungs, brain, and kidney. After massive trauma to long bones, marrow fat may contribute to intravascular aggregation of lipoproteins.

Classically, the patient begins to recover from the initial acute trauma and then regresses clinically. Regression occurs on the average of 24 hours after the acute injury and appears as an increase in the pulse, temperature, and respiration. The patient becomes apprehensive, delirious, may eventually exhibit focal neurological signs, convulse, and lapse into stupor and coma. Cyanosis may accompany these signs and symptoms. Frequently, petechiae at or before the development of other signs and symptoms appear, especially over the upper chest wall and in the conjunctivae. Chest roentgenograms often reveal diffuse cloudlike densities in the lungs. Fat may be demonstrated in the urine of some patients. Blood gas studies are of critical importance in monitoring the status of a patient with fat emboli. Therapy must be instituted promptly if the patient's life is to be saved. Further manipulation of injured extremities should be avoided. The patients need appropriate blood, fluid, and electrolyte replacement therapy. They should be digitalized if they develop cardiac failure. Blood gases serve as a guide to the need for and the use of oxygen therapy. The degree of pulmonary damage may necessitate positive pressure oxygen by means of tracheotomy and a respirator.

Some have advocated the use of steroids, alcohol, and heparin in management of fat embolism, but their status is more debatable than that of the critical need of oxygen by the patient with this syndrome.

Peripheral nerve injuries

At the time of fracture or during reduction, bone ends might injure nerves. Before attempts at reduction, the physician must evaluate motor and sensory nerve function distal to the fracture and record these observations. Closed fractures occasionally contuse nerves. These usually recover fully. Immediate open exploration is not warranted. In open fractures with nerve injuries, the surgeon inspects the nerve at the time of wound débridement and, if it is severed, plans appropriate surgical repair.

Infection

Bacteria can enter bone from an open fracture or from implantation during surgery. (See discussion on treatment of osteomyelitis, p. 469.)

Posttraumatic degenerative joint disease

After articular fractures, incongruous joint surfaces can subsequently develop degenerative joint changes. At times the physician can minimize this by adequate apposition of fragments. If trauma is extensive, subsequent degenerative changes cannot be prevented. Patients with degenerative changes must be treated with appropriate measures depending on the severity of their symptoms. (See the discussion of degenerative joint disease on p. 497.)

Acute atrophy (reflex dystrophy, postimmobilization atrophy, Sudeck's atrophy)

In certain patients, a part that remains immobile undergoes acute atrophy, including bone atrophy (Sudeck's atrophy). Patients who do not use portions of the extremity that are free of a cast develop atrophy more frequently than others. They complain of pain, motion decreases, edema develops, and the skin atrophies and becomes shiny. If the disorder progresses, contractures develop, adhesions limit joint function, and a useless part results. To prevent or treat this disorder, patients must use the part actively and institute range-of-motion exercises.

Aseptic necrosis

When a fracture isolates bone from its blood supply, the bone dies. Necrosis most often develops after fracture of the femoral neck, carpal navicular, and neck of talus. Dead bone appears radiopaque in contrast to surrounding normal bone that atrophies from disuse. Dead bone is slowly destroyed by granulation tissue and replaced by new bone. If force is transmitted before repair is complete, the bone fractures in the zone of replacement at the junction of dead and new bone. Bone grafting hastens repair of necrotic areas and, by supporting bone, prevents collapse.

Joint injuries
Sprains

A sprain is a tear in ligament and capsule fibers. Without proper treatment, ligaments heal in an elongated position with residual laxity that predisposes to further episodes of injury and the eventual need for surgical reconstruction. Sprains are classified clinically and treated as follows.

Mild (first degree). In the mild sprain, a few fibers separate. The region is tender, swollen, and bruised. The joint retains stability. The patient is treated with analgesics, rest, elevation, and cold packs for the first 12 to 24 hours. He or she then needs warm packs, a compression wrap or taping, and rest of the part for 7 to 10 days.

Moderate (second degree). In the moderate sprain, several fibers tear. The patient complains of more tenderness and the part swells and becomes ecchymotic. On examination, the doctor notices some effusion and slight instability of the joint. Immobilization in a plaster cast for 3 to 6 weeks, depending on the joint involved, permits healing.

Severe (third degree). In the severe sprain, the ligaments disrupt completely, and the joint loses stability. An orthopedic surgeon should repair these ligaments.

Dislocations

During a dislocation, articular surfaces of opposing bones completely and persistently separate. During subluxation, opposing articular surfaces partially and temporarily separate. A dislocation damages joint capsule and ligaments. Prior to reduction of a dislocation, the physician should obtain roentgenograms for diagnostic and legal purposes. Fractures accompany many dislocations, and if a fracture is found after reduction, some might assume that the doctor produced it. Only if dislocation compromises vascular supply must reduction be done on an emergency basis before roentgenograms are obtained.

Before a dislocation is reduced, the patient needs proper anesthesia or analgesia. Complicated maneuvers are unnecessary to reduce most dislocations. Simple traction reduces many of them. Some must be reduced surgically.

The physician must obtain postreduction roentgenograms to be sure that he or she has reduced the dislocation. The physician then immobilizes the part for 3 to 6 weeks so that the ligaments heal properly. The patient restores function by using the part.

Torn ligaments that are not well protected heal in an elongated position with predisposition to recurrent dislocation that must often be treated by surgery.

Intra-articular derangement

Knee joint menisci are particularly prone to injuries. Medial menisci tear 10 to 12 times more frequently than lateral menisci. The patient usually has the foot fixed and the knee partly flexed. He or she then forcibly rotates the body to the opposite side and feels sudden pain over the joint line. The joint *locks* (the knee will not fully extend or fully flex). An effusion develops over the next few hours. At times, traction unlocks the knee. Most meniscal tears do not heal but result in subsequent episodes of locking and giving way. Surgical removal of a torn meniscus alleviates these symptoms. Differential diagnosis includes osteochondral fractures and osteochondritis dissecans. During an osteochondral fracture, a piece of articular cartilage and subchondral bone breaks free from the underlying bone. In osteochondritis dissecans, common in teen-agers, a piece of articular cartilage and underlying bone separates from the remainder of the bone. The bone fragments and dies. This disorder is usually located on the lateral surface of

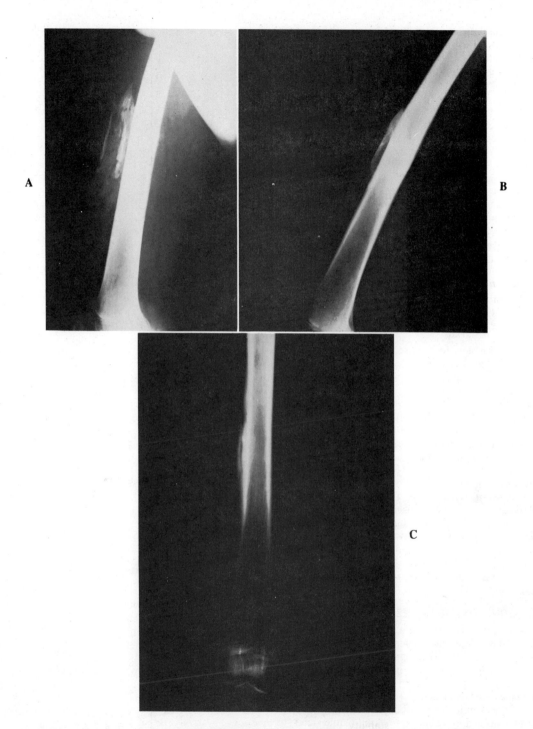

Fig. 38-37. Myositis ossificans. **A,** Roentgenogram of thigh 1 month after injury showing ossification in quadriceps muscle and beneath periosteum of femoral shaft. **B,** Twelve months later myositis ossificans is resorbing. **C,** Two and one-half years after injury, some periosteal bone remains.

the medial femoral condyle. Frequently the fragment revascularizes and heals, but it sometimes drops into the joint. In either of these disorders a free fragment in the joint gives symptoms like those of a torn meniscus. Roentgenograms often reveal a defect in the femoral condyle where the fragment separated. If the fragment contains bone, a roentgenogram shows it. These free fragments should be removed.

Injuries of muscles and tendons

Excessive force produces separation of musculotendinous units at the junction of muscle and tendon, through the tendon, or at the site of tendon insertion into bone. The patient notices immediate pain, swelling, ecchymosis, and loss of function. Soon after disruption, the muscle or tendon should be restored surgically, especially if it is an important functional unit. If treatment is neglected, many units regenerate sufficiently to give adequate function. If not, surgical reconstruction is indicated.

Myositis ossificans

A direct blow to a muscle causes intramuscular hemorrhage that usually resorbs but on occasion ossifies. Several days or even weeks after injury, the patient notices a lump. The mass enlarges and becomes firm during the next 5 to 10 weeks. In some instances it is mildly tender and interferes with muscle function. Usually the mass then decreases in size and disappears after 6 to 8 months. Roentgenograms reveal increased ossification while the mass grows (Fig. 38-37). The bone becomes mature and usually resorbs. In a few instances it remains. A thorough history helps differentiate myositis ossificans from a bone-forming tumor. Despite this, the doctor must observe the patient carefully. Excision of the mass soon after it develops leads to more hemorrhage and greater ossification. If after a year or 18 months the mass persists, the physician can safely excise it.

BENIGN BONE TUMORS

To diagnose bone tumors, the physician must use a correlative approach wherein he or she integrates clinical facts, roentgenographic appearance, and histopathology, each in its proper perspective. Doing so is especially important in the diagnosis of a malignant tumor and perhaps even more important in prevention of misdiagnosis of malignancy in a benign lesion. Such an error would lead to unwarranted, mutilating overtreatment. Table 38-9 describes in detail benign lesions that are frequently misdiagnosed as malignancies.

Table 38-9. Benign lesions often diagnosed as malignancies

Lesion	Common age (years)	Sex distribution	Common location	Symptoms	Roentgenographic appearance	Treatment
Osteocartilaginous exostosis: A cartilage-capped projection of bone; enchondral ossification continues at the cartilage-bone junction until growth stops; developmental defect	6-10	Equal	Metaphysis, distal femur, proximal tibia	Mass; pain if: (1) bursa, (2) fracture, (3) nerve irritation	Sessile or pedunculated bony prominence projects from the metaphyseal cortex (Fig. 38-38)	Less than 1% become malignant (chondrosarcoma from the cartilage cap); remove for pain, neurological symptoms, or rapid growth especially after the epiphyseal plates close
Metaphyseal fibrous defect: A developmental defect that consists of fibrous connective tissue, giant cells, and foam cells in the cortical and subcortical bone	4-10	Equal	Metaphysis, distal femur, proximal tibia	None; incidental x-ray finding	Eccentric metaphyseal lytic lesion surrounded by scalloped edge of reactive new bone (Fig. 38-39)	*DO NOT* ascribe pain to them; find the true cause of limb pain in a child

Lesion	Age	Sex	Location	Symptoms	Radiographic findings	Treatment
Bone cyst: A juxtaepiphyseal cavity lined by a thin layer of connective tissue and filled with yellow serum	4-14	Males	Metaphysis, proximal humerus, proximal femur	Pathological fracture	Metaphyseal central lytic and trabeculated cyst; the cortex expands on either side (Fig. 38-40)	Some heal after one or more fractures; others need treatment by curettage and bone grafting, preferably after 10 years of age
Osteoid osteoma: A reactive lesion consisting of a central nidus of osteoid and new bone in a fibrovascular stroma	10-25	Males	Femur and tibia	Severe pain, worse at night; relieved by aspirin	Lytic lesion less than 1 cm. in diameter; a dense, central nidus surrounded by reactive new bone	Excision
Osteoblastoma: A reactive lesion similar to but larger than osteoid osteoma	15-35	Equal	Vertebra, metacarpus, femur	Pain that is less severe than in osteoid osteoma	Central lytic lesion over 1 cm. in diameter surrounded by reactive new bone	Excision if possible
Aneurysmal bone cyst: A reactive "blowout" of the cortex by a lesion composed of vascular lakes surrounded by fibrous connective tissue, foam cells, and giant cells	12-25	Females	Femoral metaphysis and vertebra	Pain and expanding mass	Lytic lesion with a "blownout" distension of the cortex; frequently a thin layer of periosteal new bone surrounds the cyst	Curettage and bone grafting
Enchondroma: A mass of hyaline cartilage within the confines of bone	10-50	Equal	Diaphysis, phalanx of hand, metacarpus, humerus, femur	Swelling, pain, fracture	Oval lytic area with "expanded" cortex, stippled calcifications	Curet and pack bone chips if fracture, rapid growth, or symptomatic; long bone enchondromas can become malignant (chondrosarcoma)
Fibrous dysplasia: A developmental error; certain regions of bone are replaced by a dense, fibrous connective tissue stroma from which trabeculae of new bone arise	5-25	Males	Diaphysis, ribs, femur, humerus	Incidental finding; fractures or deformity	Lytic, ground glass–appearing lesions; cortex expands and bones deform	Curet and pack if symptomatic
Giant cell tumor: A lesion of polyhedral stromal cells and many multinucleated giant cells within the confines of bone	20-50	Females	Epiphyseal, distal radius, distal femur, proximal tibia	Pain and mass	Central or eccentric epiphyseal destructive or trabeculated area surrounded by an expanded cortex	Excise if compatible with function of the part; if not, curet and graft; on recurrence, do a wide local excision or amputation since a strong potential for malignancy exists

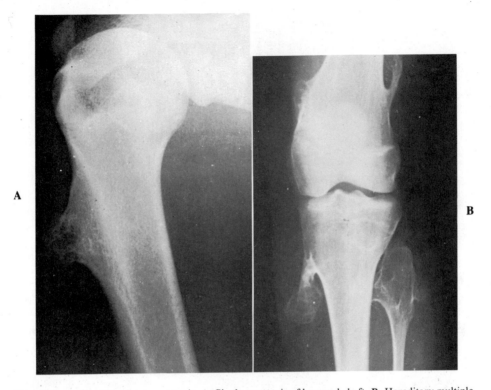

Fig. 38-38. Osteocartilaginous exostosis. **A,** Single exostosis of humeral shaft. **B,** Hereditary multiple exostoses.

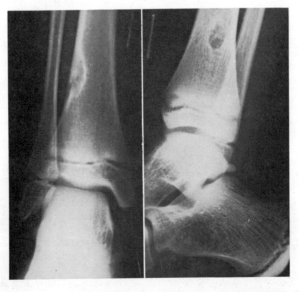

Fig. 38-39. Metaphyseal fibrous defect of tibia. Reactive new bone surrounds radiolucent defect.

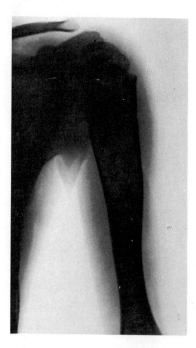

Fig. 38-40. Solitary bone cyst. Humeral metaphysis is expanded, and cortex is thin. Ridges of bone on cyst walls produce trabeculated appearance.

MALIGNANT BONE TUMORS
Tumors primary in bone

Malignant bone tumors produce the same symptoms regardless of their histological type. Patients complain of pain, often mild and intermittent at first, but increasing to become severe and constant, especially at night. On examination the physician finds a mass, local tenderness, and warm skin with dilated subcutaneous veins. In more advanced cases generalized symptoms include weakness and weight loss. Anemia is common. If a patient's complaints are suggestive of a malignancy, the physician must make the diagnosis. This usually involves a biopsy. The orthopedist, radiologist, and pathologist must maintain close liaison to make the correct diagnosis and outline the plan of treatment. Table 38-10 gives the characteristics of malignant tumors primary in bone.

Tumors metastatic to bone

Carcinoma commonly spreads to bone. In extensive autopsy studies of patients dying from carcinomatosis, pathologists find as many as 70% with bone metastases. Metastases most frequently involve the vertebral column, pelvis, skull, humerus, and femur. They rarely spread to bones distal to the elbow and knee. Carcinomas of the prostate, breast, kidney, lung, and thyroid produce most bone metastases. Lesions can lyse bone (hypernephroma, thyroid), provoke an osteoblastic reaction (prostate), or be a mixture of these two (breast, lung).

Some metastases produce no symptoms. With others, the patient complains of pain and swelling. Frequently the involved bone fractures. At times the bone lesion causes symptoms before the primary tumor does. If in such a case the history, physical examination, and routine roentgenograms do not readily reveal the primary lesion, the orthopedist can biopsy a bone. This not only rules out a primary bone tumor, but in certain instances the histology of a metastatic lesion provides a clue to the primary site. Pathological fracture through a metastatic tumor usually heals. Orthopedists treat these fractures with internal fixation so that the patient is free of pain and can be ambulatory. Depending on the type of tumor, its size, and its location, treatment of the bone lesion is by radiotherapy, chemotherapy, and hormonal therapy, or a combination of these. The physician strives to prolong life and to make the patient as comfortable and functional as possible.

Table 38-10. Malignant tumors primary in bone

Lesion	Age (years)	Sex	Common location	Roentgenographic appearance	Treatment	Prognosis
Osteosarcoma: A connective tissue tumor composed of malignant stromal cells that have osteogenic potential as manifested by the ability to produce tumor osteoid and bone	10-25	Male	Metaphysis, distal femur, proximal tibia	Metaphyseal osteolytic or osteoblastic, or both; a triangle of subperiosteal reactive new bone, a sunburst appearance from striae of new bone, cortical destruction in a jagged manner (Fig. 38-41)	Amputation or disarticulation; chemotherapy	30% to 50% 5-year survival; tends to spread rapidly through the bloodstream
Juxtacortical sarcoma: An uncommon lesion that arises in relation to the periosteum or adjacent tissue; tends to form a deceptively benign-appearing fibrous stroma from which tumor bone arises; some areas contain clumps of cartilage	30-40		Distal femoral metaphysis	A sclerotic, lobulated mass extending from the cortex; tends to invade the underlying bone	Wide, local excision or amputation	30% to 50% 5-year survival
Chondrosarcoma: A tumor of malignant cartilage cells; *primary,* a chondrosarcoma arising at the site of no known preexisting defect; *secondary,* a chondrosarcoma arising from an osteocartilaginous exostosis or enchondroma; microscopically, chondrosarcoma is difficult to differentiate from a benign enchondroma; evidence for malignancy includes history, roentgenographic evidence of destruction, microscopic hypercellularity, plump nuclei, and double nuclei	30-50	Female	Diaphysis, ribs and pelvis, proximal femur and humerus	Mottled osseous destruction with fusiform expansion of the shaft; mottled calcification	Wide excision or amputation	40% to 60% 5-year survival; tends to spread locally and along veins; metastasizes through the bloodstream

Fibrosarcoma: A tumor composed of malignant stromal cells that produce a fibrous, non-ossifying matrix	Male	10-40	Distal femur, proximal tibia	A lytic, destructive, non-bone producing defect	Amputation	20% to 30% 5-year survival
Ewing's tumor: A highly malignant round cell tumor probably derived from primitive reticular cells of the bone marrow	Male	10-25	Diaphysis of femur or tibia, pelvis	A lytic, destructive process, reactive periosteal new bone in layers and occasionally through reactive new bone much like osteogenic sarcoma	Irradiation, chemotherapy	30% to 40% 5-year survival
Reticulum cell sarcoma: A round cell tumor composed of reticulum cells of the bone marrow	Male	20-40	Pelvis, femur	A lytic, destructive lesion with little tendency to produce reactive new bone	Irradiation or amputation	60% 5-year survival
Multiple myeloma: A round cell tumor arising from primitive reticulum cells that have the capacity to differentiate into plasma cells	Male	50-70	Multiple sites, vertebra, skull, ribs, long bones	Multifocal lytic lesions without much tendency to reactive new bone; osteoporosis (Fig. 38-42)	Irradiation, urethan, and antimetabolites	In many cases, eventually fatal

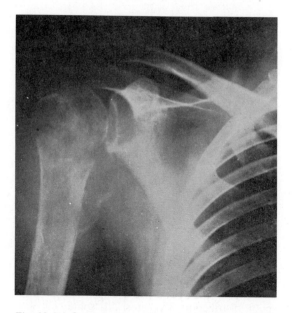

Fig. 38-41. Osteosarcoma of proximal humerus. Bone destruction is extensive. Thin layer of new bone outlines soft tissue extension of neoplasm. There is pathological fracture of neck humerus.

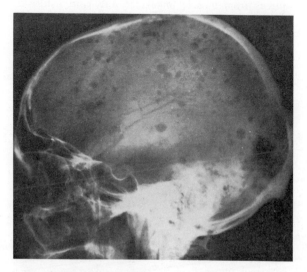

Fig. 38-42. Multiple myeloma. Roentgenogram shows multiple radiolucent lesions.

Secondary invasion of bone by adjacent soft-tissue tumors

Fibrosarcoma, synovial sarcoma, neurosarcoma, liposarcoma, and hemangioendothelioma at times erode adjacent bone. They produce symptoms like those of a malignant bone tumor. Roentgenograms reveal the soft-tissue mass and an underlying lytic defect in the outer surface of the bone cortex. At times the tumor destroys the entire cortex and invades the medullary canal. The physician uses the same diagnostic methods and treats the patient much the same as one with a primary malignant bone tumor.

NEUROMUSCULAR DISORDERS
Poliomyelitis

Poliomyelitis has disappeared as a major cause of neuromuscular disability in children. Vaccines have precipitously reduced the incidence of the disease. The poliovirus attacks brainstem motor nuclei and spinal cord anterior horn cells in a spotty distribution. The virus kills some cells and temporarily inactivates others. The localization and severity of muscular paralysis vary from person to person. If motor neurons recover, weakened muscles regain function. Many patients improve for 1 or 2 years after their acute attack of poliomyelitis. However, about 70% of muscle strength returns within 3 or 4 months.

Paralysis and deformity produce loss of function in patients who have poliomyelitis. Various factors result in deformity: (1) muscle imbalance, (2) decreased growth of a severely paralyzed extremity, and (3) abnormal bone growth caused by irregular forces from muscle imbalance and gait disturbances.

Depending on the extent and location of postpoliomyelitis residuals, orthopedists treat patients with a variety of measures:

1. Bracing to:
   a. Support body weight
   b. Stabilize a joint—limit abnormal motion
   c. Counteract muscle imbalance—prevent a strong muscle from stretching a weak antagonist and deforming the part
   d. Assist a weak muscle—a spring-loaded brace
   e. Prevent deformity—distribute forces in muscle imbalance or gait disturbances
2. Tendon transfers—restore muscle balance by moving one or more strong musculotendon units to replace function in a paralyzed muscle group
3. Tendon lengthening—if a contracture develops
4. Arthrodesis (fusion)—to control a frail, unstable joint

5. Osteotomy—to correct bone deformities
6. Leg length equalizations—an extremity with loss of muscle function grows slower than normal; significant leg length discrepancy produces deformity and disordered gait mechanics, which strain the hips and spine and result in pain and further deformity.

Leg lengths are measured from the anterosuperior iliac spine to the tip of the medial malleolus. Orthoradiographs (roentgenograms of both lower extremities against a centimeter scale) (Fig. 38-43) disclose the exact discrepancy. Orthopedic surgeons correct discrepancy in one of three ways:

1. Lengthen the short limb; osteotomy and gradual traction with extreme caution because of the distinct chance of neurovascular complications.
2. Stop growth of the normal limb. Charts based on studies of normal children show predicted growth from each epiphyseal plate at a given age. When a child with unequal leg lengths reaches an age where his expected leg growth equals his length discrepancy, orthopedists arrest growth of the normal limb by curetting the epiphyseal plate or by placing staples across the plate. The shorter limb continues to grow, and leg lengths equalize.
3. Shorten the normal limb.

Cerebral palsy

The term *cerebral palsy* denotes various syndromes that have in common nonprogressive neuromuscular dysfunction from brain damage. Causes are prenatal (fetal anoxia, German measles, developmental defects of the brain), associated with birth (prematurity and anoxia from drugs, prolonged labor), or postnatal (encephalitis).

Cerebral palsy is classified according to the type of neuromuscular dysfunction:

1. Spastic—stretch reflex, increased deep tendon reflexes, clonus
2. Athetoid—involuntary, writhing movements
3. Ataxia—poor coordination, nystagmus, adiadochokinesis
4. Rigidity—"lead pipe" resistance, absence of stretch reflex
5. Tremor—intention or nonintention tremor
6. Mixed—two or more of the preceding

Cerebral palsy is also classified as to site involved.

1. Monoplegia—one limb
2. Hemiplegia—one arm and one leg
3. Paraplegia—both legs
4. Triplegia—three limbs
5. Quadriplegia—all four limbs

Many patients with muscular manifestations of cerebral palsy have associated defects of hearing,

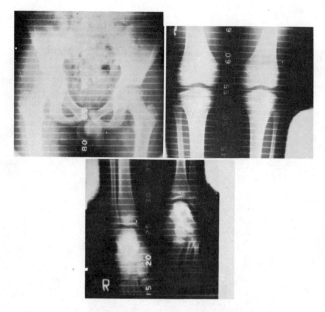

Fig. 38-43. Orthoroentgenograms showing that left leg is 6.5 cm. shorter than right.

speech, and mentality. A team of physicians, physical therapists, occupational therapists, vocational counselors, speech therapists, and social workers should evaluate all aspects of the patient, establish realistic medical, social, and vocational goals based on motor and mental ability, and treat the patient with the proper modality:

1. Physical therapy—to aid in gait training, stretching tight muscles, sitting and standing balance, and muscle control
2. Occupational therapy—to teach self-care
3. Bracing—to prevent deformity, prevent a spastic muscle from stretching a weak or normal muscle, give stability, help control involuntary motion, and give a solid base for walking.
4. Surgery:
   a. To release or lengthen spastic muscle contractures.
   b. Neurectomy—to decrease spasticity
   c. Arthrodesis—to stabilize deformed and uncontrolled joints in functional positions
   d. Tendon transfer—to restore muscle balance

Myopathies and neuropathies

In certain stages of their disease, some patients with muscular dystrophy or Charcot-Marie-Tooth disease and Friedreich's ataxia need orthopedic treatment. In early stages of a slowly progressive

neuromuscular disorder, bracing relieves deformity and increases function. Tendon transfers and bone-stabilizing procedures are sometimes useful.

IDIOPATHIC DISORDERS
Rheumatoid arthritis

Rheumatoid arthritis, one of our great cripplers, is a part of a generalized disease that can involve almost any organ in the body. No one knows the cause of rheumatoid disease, nor can its course be predicted in any individual. Rheumatoid arthritis attacks persons of all ages but is most common in women 25 to 40 years of age. Arthritis usually begins as a synovial inflammation in smaller joints, is migratory, and can involve any joint. Synovitis often subsides without residual damage. If the disease continues, inflamed synovium extends as a pannus across the joint, destroys cartilage, and erodes underlying bone. The joint loses stability and motion and becomes deformed.

The afflicted patient complains of pain, deformity, or loss of function. Early in the disease, roentgenograms reveal soft tissue swelling and marginal destruction of the joint. Later progressive disease narrows and destroys the joint.

Rheumatologists and orthopedic surgeons, working together, should manage the rheumatoid patient with medical and surgical therapy used at the proper time for optimum results. The rheumatologist initiates appropriate drug therapy. The

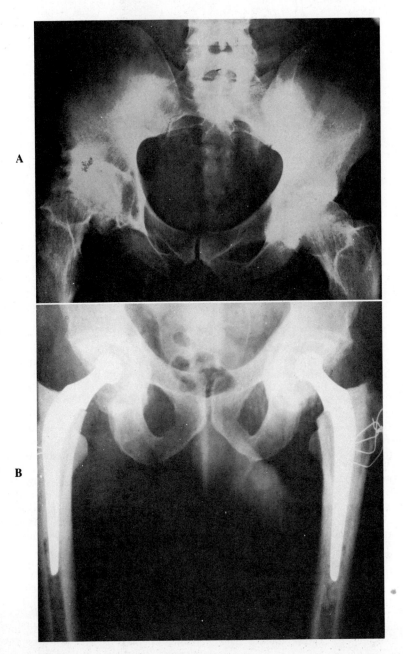

Fig. 38-44. Degenerative joint disease. **A,** Right femoral head has moved laterally, and joint space is narrow; notice osteophytic overgrowth of bone on inferior margin of femoral head and inferior acetabulum; acetabular cysts are surrounded by sclerotic bone. **B,** Recent method of treatment is total hip replacement with metal femoral component and polyethylene acetabulum.

orthopedist aids in treatment by splinting involved joints in a position that avoids undesirable contractures. He or she also directs the active exercise program and passive stretching of contractures. If a particular joint does not respond and synovitis and joint effusion persist, a synovectomy may prevent further joint destruction. After synovectomy, the synovium regrows and at times resists rheumatoid disease. At various stages of the disorder the surgeon might help the patient with one of several surgical procedures: release tight muscles and fascia, transfer muscles, perform arthroplasties (remolding of distorted joint surfaces with or without interposing metal or fascia over the reshaped bone surfaces), perform arthrodeses (fusion of painful and destroyed joints), and replace joints with prostheses and total joint replacements (Fig. 38-44, *B*).

Degenerative joint disease

The term *degenerative joint disease* denotes changes wherein articular cartilage loses fluid, becomes less resilient, loses normal color, fragments, and thins. Weight-bearing portions of larger joints degenerate most often. The underlying bone contains cysts filled with fluid or granulation tissue. New bone production results in sclerosis of bone ends and spurs at joint margins. Free pieces of cartilage and bone frequently displace into the joint.

Degenerative joint disease can arise after processes that produce incongruity of opposing joint surfaces (infection, trauma) with resultant abnormal joint mechanics. In most instances, however, no one knows the cause. Some view degenerative joint disease as part of normal aging, and others believe that it is a disease. Degenerative changes in the knees, hips, and spine are common in persons over 65. A person with clinical and roentgenographic signs of degenerative joint disease is not necessarily symptomatic.

Patients often relieve joint stiffness and discomfort with rest, heat, antiinflammatory drugs, and analgesics. Severe pain and loss of function necessitate one of the following surgical measures: joint débridement (excision of loose bodies and rough areas on the joint surface); release of tight muscles, fascia, and joint capsule; arthroplasty (Fig. 38-44); arthrodesis; prosthetic replacement; or total joint replacement.

Paget's disease (osteitis deformans)

Paget's disease, a disorder of unknown cause, usually affects men over 55 years of age. Bone is destroyed and produced in an irregular manner. Microscopic examination shows many fragments of bone fitted together in a mosaic with blue "cement lines" between the pieces. A fibrovascular stroma fills spaces between bone trabeculas. Paget's disease commonly affects the spine, pelvis, and proximal femora. Roentgenographically, increased density from new bone production accentuates the major trabecular pattern. Bone destruction produces radiolucent areas. The involved bones often deform. At times patients with Paget's disease have aches and pains. Often, however, the physician discovers the disorder when he obtains roentgenograms for other reasons. Some patients obtain relief of discomfort by the use of aspirin and other medications. They occasionally develop osteosarcoma superimposed on Paget's disease, and the doctor should follow them closely with this possibility in mind.

METABOLIC DISORDERS
Rickets

In rickets, a disorder of growing children, skeletal manifestations develop from a continued production of bone matrix and epiphyseal cartilage matrix that fails to mineralize properly. A deficiency of sunlight or vitamin D or a lack of response to vitamin D produces this lack of mineralization. In the absence of vitamin D the intestinal tract mucosa does not absorb calcium and phosphorus normally. In this country lack of vitamin D intake combined with lack of exposure to sunlight occurs only rarely and in lower economic groups. Patients with fat absorption disorders (celiac disease, sprue, and obstructive jaundice) lose vitamin D in the stool.

Children with rickets are restless and irritable. Their legs bow. The long bone metaphysis enlarges (trumpeting), the frontal and parietal bones protrude (craniotabes), costochondral junctions enlarge (rosary of rickets), the ribs sink in at the attachment of the diaphragm (Harrison's grooves), the pelvis collapses inward, and the spine curves. X-ray examination reveals a wide, cupped metaphysis, a wide, irregular epiphyseal plate, an irregular hazy zone of provisional calcification, and bowing of the long weight-bearing bones. Serum phosphorus decreases, serum calcium remains normal, and serum alkaline phosphatase increases. Urine calcium decreases, and phosphorus remains normal or increases.

Vitamin D–deficient children heal rickets in 3 or 4 weeks if they take 3,000 to 6,000 units of vitamin D daily. If they are positioned properly during the active stage of the disease, they will not deform soft bones. The surgeon corrects severe, persistent deformities by osteotomy.

Vitamin D–resistant rickets

In some children active rickets fail to respond to the usual doses of vitamin D. No one knows the exact cause of this disorder, which is often familial. An affected child often requires 10,000 to 1,000,000 units of vitamin D for treatment and 3,000 to 500,000 units for maintenance. The physician should use 24-hour urine calcium studies to determine the correct dosage of vitamin D.

Renal rickets

Patients who lose phosphorus or calcium because of renal defects frequently acquire rickets. Defective kidney tubules lose protein. If the glomeruli are defective, the patient frequently retains urea and sometimes becomes acidotic. The prognosis is not good in renal rickets. The physician must treat the associated defects.

Osteomalacia

Osteomalacia, the adult counterpart of rickets, is characterized by increased bone matrix and lack of mineralization. The bones soften and bend. In this country physicians rarely see this disorder on a vitamin D deficiency basis. Steatorrhea or renal disease causes osteomalacia most frequently. The patients complain of weakness and deformity. Their bones fracture easily. Roentgenograms reveal a decrease in bone density, deformities, and Looser's zones (a fracture line surrounded by relatively dense bone). Serum and urine changes are similar to those in rickets. The physician must correct the underlying defect and use orthopedic measures to correct deformities.

Scurvy

Vitamin C deficiency is uncommon. Patients with scurvy do not produce normal connective tissue. Increased capillary fragility produces painful subperiosteal hemorrhage with resultant pseudoparalysis. Roentgenograms reveal osteoporosis produced by a lack of bone matrix. The zone of provisional calcification increases; a lytic zone (scorbutic band) crosses the metaphysis; a dense ring of bone surrounds the epiphysis; spurs form at metaphyseal edges; and periosteal new bone is produced. Occasionally an epiphysis separates from the metaphysis. Ascorbic acid, 100 to 120 mg. daily, corrects the disorder.

Hyperparathyroidism

Parathyroid hormone acts on kidney and bone to maintain normal serum calcium and phosphorus levels. Parathyroid adenoma or parathyroid hyperplasia produces hyperparathyroidism most frequently in women 25 to 45 years of age.

The following cause symptoms in hyperparathyroidism:

1. Increased serum calcium—lethargy, weakness, anorexia, constipation
2. Bone destruction—pain or fractures
3. Calcium increase in the urine—renal stones, renal insufficiency

Serum phosphorus decreases, serum calcium increases, and serum alkaline phosphatase increases. Urinary phosphorus and calcium increase. Roentgenographically, bones demineralize, the cortex thins, the lamina dura of the teeth disappears, subperiosteal bone of the midphalanx of the fingers is resorbed, and the outer table of the skull thins and becomes indistinct. "Brown tumors" composed of fibrous connective tissue, hemorrhage, and giant cells appear as bone cysts.

After the offending portion of the parathyroid gland has been removed, the surgeon must observe the patient carefully for postoperative tetany and must treat it promptly.

Osteoporosis

In a patient with osteoporosis, the total mass of bone matrix and mineral decreases. Osteoporosis results from one or more of the following:

1. Disuse—normal stress is needed to prevent loss of bone mass
2. Endocrine:
   a. Cushing's disease—increased steroids and increased catabolism
   b. Postmenopausal—decreased stress and decreased sex hormones
   c. Hyperthyroidism
   d. Acromegaly
3. Scurvy
4. Protein deficiency caused by decreased intake or excessive loss
5. Multiple myeloma and carcinomatosis
6. Idiopathic, senile, or postmenopausal states

No one knows exactly why the bone mass decreases. Most patients remain in the idiopathic group. Osteoporosis is most common in women over 60 in whom diet, disuse, and endocrine changes probably play a role.

The patients complain of bone pain and tenderness. Vertebral bodies and femoral necks frequently break. Calcium, phosphorus, and alkaline phosphatase usually remain normal. Some patients are in negative nitrogen and calcium balance. X-ray studies disclose relatively radiolucent bone, thin cortices, and widened medullary canals. The vertebral bodies often collapse. Vertebral subchondral cortices curve, and vertebral bodies become biconcave.

Physicians diagnose idiopathic osteoporosis by excluding other disorders that give similar roentgenographic findings (osteomalacia, multiple myeloma, hyperparathyroidism, metastatic malignancies, Cushing's disease, and hyperthyroidism). Since one cannot determine the cause in most instances, treatment is difficult. The patient should consume at least one quart of milk and 70 gm. of protein each day. In addition to this regime, some physicians add vitamin D, 5,000 units a day for the first 3 months and then 1,000 units a day. The patient remains as active as possible. Estrogens may be of value in certain patients. Some physicians use sodium fluoride to try to increase bone deposition. Physical therapy and spine supports sometimes provide symptomatic relief.

Gout

In gout, a metabolic disorder, the body produces excessive uric acid. Blood uric acid increases. Ureate crystals form deposits (tophi) in joints and para-articular structures. These crystals destroy the joint surface and erode underlying bone. During an acute attack, patients complain of severe pain in a joint or bursa. Uricosuric agents alleviate symptoms during the acute episode. Patients then use drugs to maintain a decrease in the blood uric acid. In some patients with gout, orthopedists excise tophi and perform arthroplasties or arthrodeses on destroyed joints.

39
The Hand

David W. Furnas
Adrian E. Flatt
Ivan M. Turpin

Man's hands have allowed him to put human thought into action, exerting control over his environment. Sensation in the hand (an organ containing one fourth of all pacinian [touch] corpuscles of the body) is the only sense among five in which man is clearly superior to animals. Pictures gained from earliest tactile and kinesthetic activities of the hand lay the groundwork for one's self-image and feelings of individuality. The hand also serves as a means of expression.

Thus afflictions of the hand are of great significance to the patient and his physician; moreover, they are very common: approximately one third of all industrial accidents and one third of injuries seen in the emergency departments of metropolitan hospitals involve the hand.

NORMAL ARCHITECTURE

Everyday use of the hand demands a structure that has stability and power, combined with mobility, dexterity, and precision. *Stability* is furnished by the rigid *central pillar* of the hand (Fig. 39-1), formed by the firmly united carpal bones and the second and third metacarpal bones. Around this central pillar, in the manner of twin loading booms, rotate the two mobile units of the hand: (1) the extremely mobile first metacarpal invested with thenar structures and (2) the less mobile fourth and fifth metacarpals invested with hypothenar structures.

The *digits* with their two or three joints represent other highly mobile units. The *metacarpophalangeal joints* of the fingers have lateral *mobility* when

they are *extended,* but lateral *stability* when they are *flexed* into grasp (where stability is required) because of the arrangement of their collateral ligaments (Fig. 39-2). All the *interphalangeal joints* have lateral *stability throughout* flexion and extension.

Three arches are formed by these units of the hand (Fig. 39-3): a *proximal transverse arch,* which is rigid, a *distal transverse arch,* which is flexible, and a *longitudinal arch* (the digital rays), which is rigid proximally and flexible distally.

Power to the wrist and hand is supplied by *five* groups of muscles (Fig. 39-4): two *extrinsic* (muscle bellies in the forearm) and three *intrinsic* (muscle bellies in the hand). The muscles are innervated by three nerves: median, radial, and ulnar.

Extrinsic muscle groups

The *flexor-pronator muscles* pronate the hand and flex the wrist and digits. The flexor-pronator group (the three flexors of the wrist, the nine flexors of the digits, and the pronators teres and quadratus) is supplied by the *median nerve (except for the ulnar half of the flexor digitorum profundus,* which is supplied by the ulnar nerve). The *extensor-supinator group* supinates the hand and extends the wrist and digits. The extensor-supinator muscles (the three extensors of the wrist, the four common and two proper extensors of the fingers, the two extensors and the long abductor to the thumb, and the supinator) are supplied by the *radial nerve.*

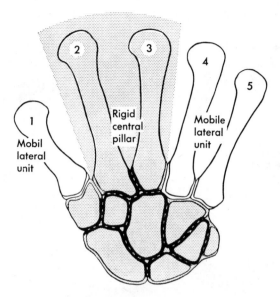

Fig. 39-1. Central pillar and lateral units of hand. Shafts of second and third metacarpals are firmly united to carpal bones, forming stable central pillar. Two lateral units of hand articulate freely with carpal bones and are mobile.

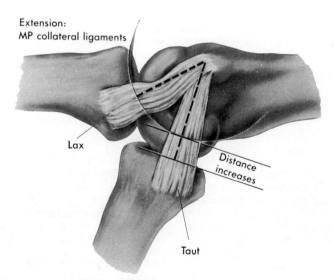

Fig. 39-2. Stability of metacarpophalangeal (MP) joints. In flexion, collateral ligaments are placed under tension because of eccentric profile and lateral bulges of metacarpal head; this prevents lateral motion of joints. In extension, ligaments are flaccid, and lateral movements are possible. Position of flexion is usually chosen when immobilizing this joint, to prevent shortening of ligament and deformity.

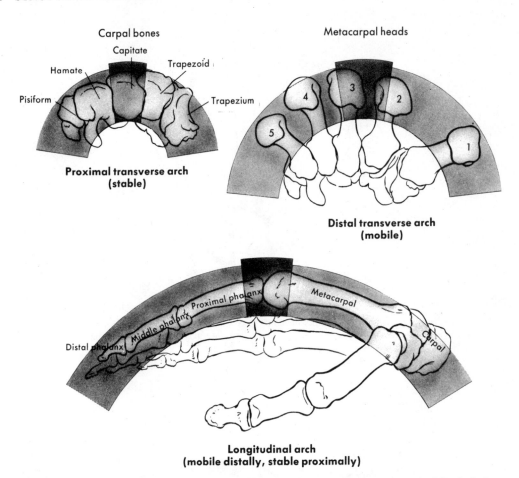

Fig. 39-3. Arches of hand. Stable, immobile proximal transverse arch is composed of firmly knit carpal bones. Mobile distal transverse arch is made up of metacarpal heads and intervening tissues. Longitudinal arches, which are extremely mobile distally and stable proximally, are made up of digital rays.

Intrinsic muscle groups

The *thenar muscles* (short flexor, short abductor, and opposing muscles of the thumb) are supplied by the *median nerve,* and the *hypothenar muscles* (abductor, short flexor, and opposing muscles of the little finger) are supplied by the *ulnar nerve.* These two groups work together to cup the palm and to oppose the thumb to the fingers. The *lumbricals, interossei,* and *adductor pollicis* are supplied by the *ulnar nerve* (*except* for the first two lumbricals, which are median innervated). They furnish digital *adduction-abduction* movements, *flexion* at the metacarpophalangeal joints, and *extension* at the interphalangeal joints. (The *extrinsic flexors* are *also* able to flex the metacarpophalangeal joints, and the *extrinsic extensors* are *also* able to extend the interphalangeal joints.) The tendons of the intrinsic muscles interweave with the tendons and aponeuroses of the extrinsic muscles, forming a coordinated network (Fig. 39-5). This system of motors, superbly linked with input from the eyes and the sensory organs of the hand, lends precision and dexterity to movements of the hand.

CLINICAL ASSESSMENT OF THE HAND

History. Intelligent assessment necessitates understanding the patient, including his personality, occupation, hobbies, and life expectations. Specific history relating to the hand should generate a clear understanding and documentation of the duration, nature, and onset of the complaint, as well as the patient's definition of his disability.

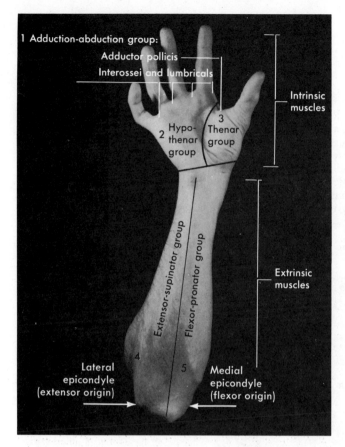

Fig. 39-4. Muscle power to hand. Three groups of intrinsic muscles: *1* and *2* supplied by *ulnar nerve* and *3* supplied by *median nerve*. Two groups of extrinsic muscles: *4* supplied by *radial nerve* and *5* supplied by median nerve and *ulnar half of flexor digitorum profundus* supplied by ulnar nerve.

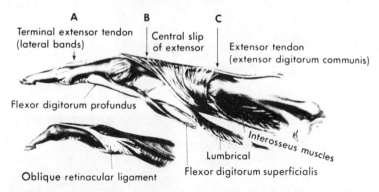

Fig. 39-5. Intrinsic and extrinsic networks for flexion and extension of fingers. Distal interphalangeal joint is flexed by *flexor digitorum profundus;* proximal interphalangeal joint is flexed by *flexor digitorum superficialis* (plus transmitted increment from *flexor digitorum profundus*); metacarpophalangeal joint is flexed by *interosseus muscles* through their direct osseous insertions and through their insertions into wings of dorsal aponeurosis. (This flexion force is augmented by transmitted increment from *flexor digitorum profundus* and *flexor digitorum superficialis.*) Distal interphalangeal joint is extended through insertion of lateral bands of dorsal aponeurosis, powered by extrinsic extensors and intrinsics (*interossei* and *lumbricals*) (either or both may act); proximal interphalangeal joint is extended by central slip of dorsal aponeurosis, powered in same way as distal phalanx; metacarpophalangeal joint is extended by extrinsic extensor tendons alone, acting through dorsal aponeurosis. *Oblique retinacular ligaments* assist in coordination of these movements. For injuries at levels *A, B,* and *C,* see Fig. 39-18.

Exclusion of causes of hand ʼdisability arising proximally in the upper limb or higher, neurologically, should be routine.

Physical examination. As a part of hand examination, consider the entire upper limb and a comparison of right and left sides at a minimum. *Look at, feel,* and *move* the hand to assess the five essential elements of function: *cover, mobility, stability, sensibility,* and *circulation.* Initially look for abnormal postures. These occur because of an imbalance of forces with loss, exaggeration, or disruption of normal arches. Common patterns of pathological postures include claw deformity (intrinsic minus hand) (Fig. 39-6), dropped wrist and

hand (Fig. 39-7), and intrinsic plus hand (Fig. 39-8). Assessing cover implies checking the skin for unstable scars or contractures and its color, temperature, and mobility as well. Mobility must be determined actively and passively. During active motion, ask the patient to put his wrist through a full range of motion, to extend the wrist and fingers completely, and then to flex all the digits fully. The normal thumb can describe a cone, oppose, flex, and extend, as well as pinch and grasp (Fig. 39-9).

Active and passive motion must be compared and documented quantitatively, and any discrepancies between the two must be explained. Loss of passive motion is associated with a corresponding

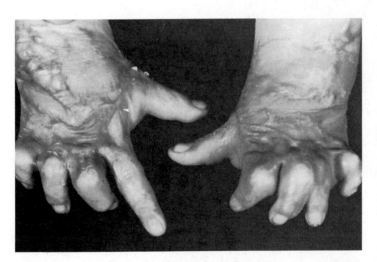

Fig. 39-6. *"Intrinsic-minus"* deformity or clawhand. Distal transverse arches are flattened. Metacarpophalangeal joints are hyperextended, proximal interphalangeal joints are hyperflexed (distal interphalangeal joints are sometimes flexed, sometimes hyperextended), thumb is held parallel to palm. Cause in this patient is scarring and skin destruction from scald of dorsum of hands, but in others paralysis of intrinsic muscles will result in same posture. (See Fig. 39-24.)

Fig. 39-7. *Wristdrop.* Ability to extend wrist against gravity is lost because of denervation of extensor-supinator group of muscles from resection of basal cell carcinoma of forearm that invaded *radial nerve.* Notice pale semicircle of skin, which is flap covering resected area.

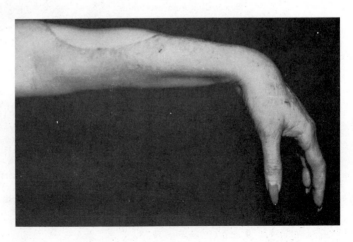

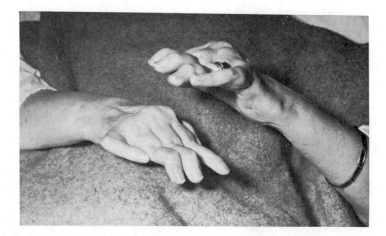

Fig. 39-8. *"Intrinsic-plus"* deformity. Arches are exaggerated. Metacarpophalangeal joints are flexed, and interphalangeal joints are in "swan-neck" position (proximal interphalangeal joint hyperextended [recurvatum], distal interphalangeal joint locked in flexion). Sometimes both interphalangeal joints are extended (accoucheur's hand). (From Flatt, A.E.: The care of the rheumatoid hand, ed. 3, St. Louis, 1974, The C.V. Mosby Co.)

A

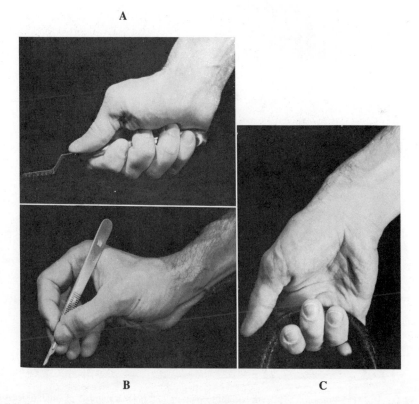

B   **C**

Fig. 39-9. Power grip. Object is clamped securely between flexed fingers and palm, counterpressure being applied by thumb. **B,** Precision grip (or "handling"). Object is pinched between flexor pads of opposing thumb and fingers. **C,** Hook grip. Only fingers are used, as a primitive hook.

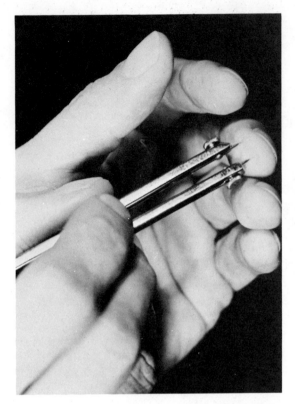

Fig. 39-10. *Two-point discrimination.* Two points are simultaneously pressed against skin; distance between points is varied to determine narrowest spread that can be distinguished as two separate points rather than one. Fingertips can usually distinguish two points spread as little as 2 to 4 mm. Proximal dorsal part of digit can only distinguish two points if spread is 10 mm. Two-point discrimination is one of the best means of detecting partial nerve injuries and in following nerve repairs.

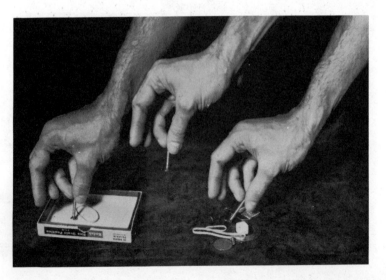

Fig. 39-11. *Moberg's "pickup" test.* Ask patient to pick up and place a number of small objects at top speed. This serves to reveal deficiencies in critical sensation and fine coordination that might be missed with cruder tests. Incomplete return of median sensation indicated by patient's preference of ulnar-innervated ring finger.

loss of active motion, but the converse does not hold. Before active motion can occur, any encumbrances of normal passive mobility such as joint, tendon, and skin contractures or adhesions must be eliminated. Stability requires normal functional integrity of the bones and joints of the hand. Disturbances of this integrity are particularly common after trauma, whether recent or remote, and in rheumatoid arthritis. Sensibility is determined by the usual pin and wisp of cotton, two-point discrimination (Fig. 39-10), a pickup test (Fig. 39-11), and stereognosis. Normally two points that are as close together as 2 to 4 mm. can be distinguished with the tips and flexor surfaces of the digits, whereas on the dorsal skin two points closer than 10 to 12 mm. are interpreted as one. Color and temperature are clues to adequacy of circulation. Normal perfusion requires adequacy of arterial supply, the capillary bed, and venous drainge. Loss of any of these three will compromise viability. Aberrations may be focal, as in an unstable scar or crushed skin, or involve the hand as a whole, as in combined radial and ulnar arterial injuries. Palpation of the pulses, Allen's test (Fig. 39-21), and examination with the Doppler flow detector are useful procedures. Injection with fluorescein and observation with a Wood's light shows viable tissue.

Roentgenological examination. Roentgenological examination is an integral part of routine hand assessment. There is no therapeutic benefit conferred by diagnostic radiation. Careful examination will guide inquiry to an appropriate area. For example, the whole hand need not be examined if the terminal phalanx of the thumb has been injured, nor is it diagnostically accurate to assess the scaphoid without special scaphoid views. In short, request appropriate films and reduce needless exposures.

PRINCIPLES OF MANAGEMENT OF HAND PROBLEMS

Restoration of grasp (both power and precision), fine tactile sense, dexterity, and normal appearance are the sometimes elusive goals of surgery of the hand. These are achieved by restoring cover and stability, mobility, sensibility, and circulation to the hand. Skin grafts and pedicles restore missing or contracted skin cover. Fracture fixation, bone grafts, and joint fusions may be required for bone and joint stability. Tendon repairs, grafts, or transfers restore transmission of power for active mobility. Loss of passive mobility is best managed conservatively. Motor nerve deficits may be corrected by nerve repairs, nerve grafts, or tendon transfers. Repairs or grafts of sensory nerves (or occasionally transferring sensory island flaps [see Chapter 24]) may provide some restoration of functional sensibility. Finally, vascular repair may be essential.

Mobilization is a necessary element in managing trauma, accidental or surgical. The hand reacts badly to prolonged immobilization, worse to swelling, and worst of all to both. Elevation and earliest feasible motion are immutable priorities.

CONGENITAL DEFORMITIES

Congenital deformities of the hand are relatively common and present a diverse array and range of disorders. Polydactyly or excessive number of digits is the most common, occurring in 0.5% of live births. It is frequently bilateral and commonly

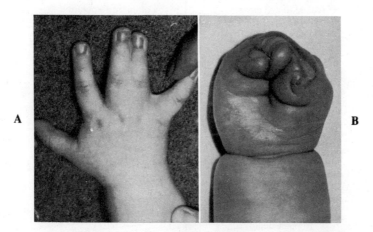

Fig. 39-12. Syndactyly. **A,** Simple syndactyly of ring and long fingers. **B,** Complex syndactyly causing mittenlike hand in patient with acrocephalosyndactyly, or Apert's syndrome.

the extra digit is the ulnarmost or radialmost of the hand.

Syndactyly (Fig. 39-12), failure of digits to separate from one another, is the second most common hand anomaly, occurring in 0.2% of live births. The long and ring fingers are the most commonly adherent, often bilaterally. Syndactyly ranges in complexity from a single slight obliterated web space to complete fusion of all the digits into a tight mitten.

Brachydactyly (shortened fingers), symphalangia (end-to-end fusion of phalangeal bones), ectrodactyly (absence of a part of one or more digits), and clinodactyly (lateral deviation of the fingers) are some of the less common congenital disorders.

In most instances the safest guiding principle is early referral to a surgeon with special interest in this field. Early operative treatment is mandatory if there is any distortion of growth or progression of deformity.

ACQUIRED DISORDERS
Traumatic (Table 39-1)
Laceration

Skin lacerations or wounds may be tidy or untidy. The tidy wound has clean incised margins that heal promptly after simple cleansing and clo-

sure. It is, however, essential to maintain a high index of suspicion of hidden problems. Severed tendons, nerves, arteries, and buried splinters of glass or metal can be present in the most innocent appearing wounds (Fig. 39-13). Untidy wounds are ragged, crushed, or torn at the margins and are more widely damaged in the depths. Missing or nonviable skin must be replaced. Dirt, foreign material, and devitalized tissue must be debrided. Complications of infection, excessive swelling, and necrosis are more likely to occur in an untidy wound.

No wound, tidy or untidy, should ever be considered for closure until the full extent of the injury is identified. If any uncertainty exists, formal exploration is mandatory.

Flexor tendon. The diagnosis of digital flexor tendon severance is confirmed by loss of the position of rest (Fig. 39-14) and the inability to perform the test for superficialis action (Fig. 39-15) or the test for profundus action (Fig. 39-16). If the patient performs these tests but shows pain and weakness, suspect *partial division of the tendon.*

The level of severance determines the therapeutic approach. Tendons divided distally to "no-man's-land" (Fig. 39-17) (near bony insertion) may have their proximal end advanced and sutured into

Table 39-1. Common injuries of the integument and digits.

Injury	Treatment	Injury	Treatment
Laceration	Cleansing, irrigation, and simple surgical closure	Partial amputation	Replace severed part if circulation appears adequate
Flaplike laceration	Suture into place if viable		Repair vessels microsurgically if needed
	If not viable, remove skin and close defect directly or with skin graft	Complete amputation	Microvascular replant if digit is important
Amputated skin	Defat the skin and replace as a skin graft, or		Closure with preservation of length
	Take grafts from elsewhere	Crushed fingertip	Meticulous reassembly using magnification
Digital pulp	Cross finger flap, palmar flap, triangular island flaps, or skin graft	Avulsion of nail or nail bed	Trim nail and replace as a splint to wound; carefully repair nail bed
Degloving injury (skin peeled back from digit as if it were a glove, e.g., ring caught in machinery)	Repair injured vessels with vein grafts and close skin, or		Replace any missing areas of nail bed with split-skin graft
	Amputate ring finger or unimportant digit, or	Subungual hematoma	Perforate overlying nail with heated paper clip or needle and evacuate hematoma
	Replace degloved skin with flap		

Fig. 39-13. "Tidy" injury of hand. This clean, penetrating wound of palm was caused by broken thermometer. Despite its innocuous appearance, examination revealed area of anesthesia (crosshatches in ink on ring finger), inability to abduct-adduct fingers, and positive Froment's sign (Fig. 39-20, *B*). Transection of motor branch of ulnar nerve, transection of part of sensory branch of ulnar nerve, transection of deep palmar arterial arch, and partial transection of flexor digitorum profundus tendon to ring finger were found at operation.

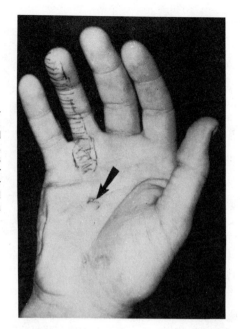

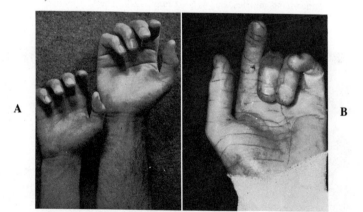

A   B

Fig. 39-14. *Position of rest.* **A,** Normal position of rest. With hand lying palm upward on flat surface, muscle tone of flexors causes slight flexion of thumb and orderly gradation of flexion of fingers, which increases from index to little finger. **B,** *Loss of position of rest.* Razor slash of flexor compartment of wrist has caused loss of position of rest of thumb and index finger because of complete severance of associated flexor tendons; small strand of intact profundus tendon prevents complete loss of position of rest in little finger; all sublimis tendons were divided, as median nerve and radial artery were; areas of sensory loss from transection of median nerve are crosshatched with inked lines; notice that *much of damage to wrist is readily assessed without removal of dressings,* (**A,** From Flatt, A.E.: The care of minor hand injuries, ed. 4, St. Louis, 1979, The C.V. Mosby Co.)

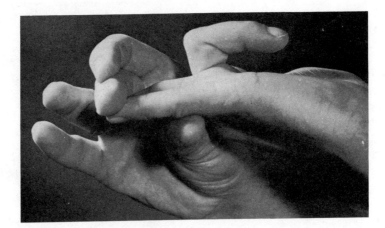

Fig. 39-15. Test for *flexor superficialis* action. Flexor digitorum profundus muscles and tendons form more or less solid sheet in forearm, dividing only quite distally into separate tendons that have little or no independence of action, i.e., the four tendons tend to act as one unit. Therefore, if three of the four digits are forcefully held in extension, flexor digitorum profundus to remaining digit is carried into extended position with its fellows and is unable to act as flexor. However, flexor digitorum superficialis, which has distinct and independent muscle belly for each of the four tendons, can still act as flexor; flexion takes place only at proximal interphalangeal joint, not at distal interphalangeal joint. Flexor digitorum superficialis to long finger shows normal function in photograph (From Flatt, A.E.: The care of minor hand injuries, ed. 4, St. Louis, 1979, The C.V. Mosby Co.)

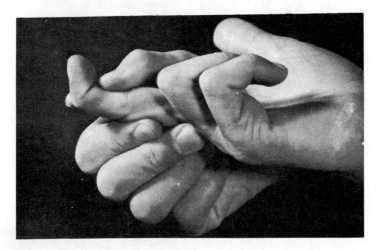

Fig. 39-16. Test for *flexor digitorum profundus* action. Finger is held forcefully in passive extension at metacarpophalangeal and proximal interphalangeal joints. Ability to flex distal interphalangeal joint indicates normal action of flexor digitorum profundus. (From Flatt, A.E.: The care of minor hand injuries, ed. 4, St. Louis, 1979, The C.V. Mosby Co.)

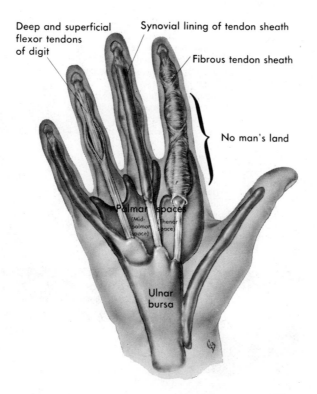

Deep and superficial flexor tendons of digit

Synovial lining of tendon sheath

Fibrous tendon sheath

No man's land

Palmar spaces (Midpalmar space) (Thenar space)

Ulnar bursa

Fig. 39-17. *No man's land:* here the two flexor tendons of each finger of right hand are tightly enclosed in synovium-lined fibrous sheath made up of unyielding cruciate and annular ligaments; tendon anastomoses in this region tend to fail because of massive adherence to surrounding structures. *Palmar spaces:* these two fascial clefts are located behind digital flexor tendons; midpalmar space is separated from thenar space by septum that connects bursa or flexor tendons (ulnar bursa) to third metacarpal bone.

the distal phalanx. Tendons severed proximally to "no-man's-land" are anastomosed immediately with nonabsorbable suture material.

Flexor tendon injuries in "no-man's-land" (where the flexor digitorum profundus and superficialis cross through the fibrous digital sheath) yield notoriously poor results in anything but optimal circumstances. If divided tendons are sutured primarily, the exuberant fibroblastic outgrowth causes dense adherence between the tendon and sheath with loss of function. The best course of action for the primary physician is to clean the wound, close the skin, and send the patient promptly to an experienced hand surgeon. The surgeon may choose to perform immediate repair of one or both tendons. If the circumstances are less than ideal, the surgeon will postpone definitive surgery and instruct the patient in exercises to maintain joint suppleness. A silicon rubber rod may be placed to maintain a patent tendon sheath. When reaction to the initial injury has

subsided sufficiently (weeks or months later), elective tendon grafting can be carried out.

In flexor tendon injuries of the wrist (Fig. 39-14, *B*) it is best to assume injuries to major nerves and arteries. If this is confirmed clinically, hemorrhage should be controlled by pressure and the patient should be transported to a surgeon competent to perform multiple nerve, artery, and tendon repairs. Circumstances such as transport over a distance may demand exploration and ligation of bleeders, irrigation of the wound, and closure of the skin. *Accurate repair* of tendons and nerves is more important than immediate repair.

Extensor tendon. The extensor tendons are flat, fine structures that are interwoven with tendons of the intrinsic muscles forming the intricate extensor aponeuroses. They do not hold sutures well, and surgical restoration is frequently difficult. Diagnostically, the most frequent error is overlooking closed injuries to this extensor apparatus. The most common closed extensor injuries (cited in

Table 39-2. Extensor tendon injuries

Entity	Mechanisms and level of severance	Treatment
Drop finger (Fig. 39-18, *D*); (injury at level C, Fig. 39-5)	Laceration or rupture of extensor tendon on dorsum of hand or wrist or at metacarpophalangeal joint	Direct suture
Boutonnière deformity (develops several weeks after injury) (Fig. 39-18, *B* and *C*); (injury at level B, Fig. 39-5)	Laceration, rupture, or erosion of extensor tendon at proximal phalanx or proximal interphalangeal (PIP) joint	Immobilization in extension with cast extending to forearm for 3 weeks; if chip fracture present, direct suture; late treatment requires complex operation
Mallet finger (or baseball finger) (Fig. 39-18, *A*); (injury at level A, Fig. 39-5)	Avulsion or laceration of insertion of tendon into distal phalanx (fragment of distal phalanx frequently avulsed with tendon insertion)	Immobilize in plaster with distal interphalangeal (DIP) joint in hyperextension and PIP joint in flexion; if wound is open, suture tendon ends and place intramedullary wire through DIP joint

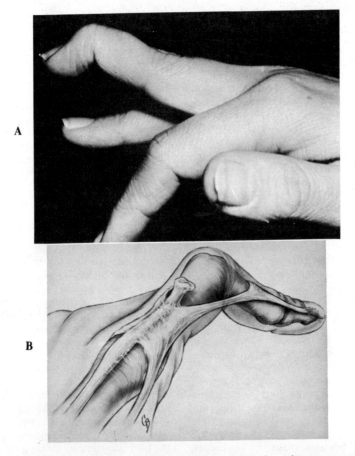

Fig. 39-18. A, *Mallet finger* (baseball finger): disruption of insertion of extensor tendon at distal phalanx. (Injury near level **A,** Fig. 39-5.) **B** and **C,** *Boutonnière deformity:* after disruption of central slip of the extensor tendon where it inserts on middle phalanx, lateral bands of extensor apparatus tend to migrate in palmar direction causing flexion of proximal interphalangeal joint and extension of distal interphalangeal joint. (Injury near level **B,** Fig. 39-5.) **D,** *Drop finger:* long, ring, and little fingers cannot be extended against gravity (see level *C* of Fig. 39-5) because of tendon rupture at wrist; patient has rheumatoid disease and attrition of tendons on bony projection. (Injury proximal to level *C,* Fig. 39-5.)

Table 39-2) must be excluded when assessing a "sprained finger."

The boutonnière deformity (Fig. 39-18, *B*) is caused by loss of restraint of the lateral bands of the extensor mechanism. After the central slip has been divided, these lateral bands become attenuated and migrate volarward, allowing the proximal interphalangeal joint to protrude dorsally as if through a buttonhole. Extensor tendons are prone to attrition injuries. Drop finger (Fig. 39-18, *D*) is seen in rheumatoid arthritis when slips of the extensor digitorum communis rupture because of tendon disease or erosion from a rough bony prominence at the level of the distal radius and ulna. Drummer's palsy, or drop thumb, is caused by rupture associated with avascular necrosis of the extensor pollicis longus near the lower end of the radius. Open disruption of an extensor tendon

is treated by direct suture unless delay, contamination, or other circumstances contraindicate primary repair. Immobilization for 4 or 5 weeks is customary after suture of extensor tendons, whether open or closed.

Nerve injuries. Compulsive care must be taken to rule out nerve injuries in hand lacerations. For example, a child falling with outstretched hand onto broken glass must be assumed to have significant nerve injury. This assumption is essential because of the difficult and frustrating task of attempting accurate clinical asessment of a frightened, agitated child.

If the median nerve is divided (Fig. 39-14, *B*), the hand is blinded from loss of critical sensibility in the most important parts of the thumb and index, long, and ring fingers, and motor power is lost in the thenar muscles. Ulnar nerve transection crip-

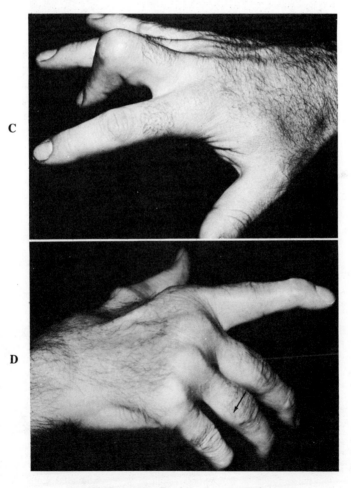

Fig. 39-18, cont'd. For legend see opposite page.

ples the greater part of the intrinsic musculature, depriving the hand of dexterity; it also numbs sensation to the ulnar side of the fourth and the entire fifth digit. Accurate testing of the motor and sensory branches of these nerves is mandatory in any hand injury. Even an inconspicuous nick can mark the entry point of glass or steel slivers that may have selectively divided a significant sensory or motor branch (Fig. 39-13).

In addition to the baseline assessment outlined earlier, the characteristic silky, dry texture of denervated skin should be sought. This texture is caused by disrupted sympathetic fibers that accompany sensory nerve injury. The most reliable tests for isolated motor function of the median nerve in the hand are the abductor pollicis brevis test and the opponens pollicis test (Fig. 39-19). For motor function of the ulnar nerve (Fig. 39-20, A) the most reliable test is adduction and abduction of the long finger. Froment's sign (Fig. 39-20, B) is useful in detection of paralysis of the adductor pollicis.

Distal nerve transections, transections of pure motor or sensory nerves, and nerve transections in children have the best prognosis after surgical repair. Immediate repair of cleanly cut nerve ends gives superior results to delayed repair. If a branch 1 mm. or smaller in diameter is divided, it can be anastamosed accurately by use of an operating microscope or loupes.

Vessel injuries. The hand can usually survive with only one of its two major arteries intact and occasionally with neither. However, arterial anas-

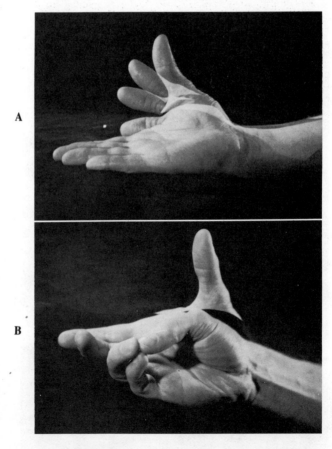

A

B

Fig. 39-19. Tests for motor function of median nerve. **A,** Abductor pollicis brevis raises thumb forward, perpendicular to plane of palm; ability to perform this movement against resistance is best single test of median nerve function. **B,** Opponens pollicis sweeps abducted thumb across palm so that flexor pad of thumb meets flexor pad of ring or little finger face-to-face and parallel.

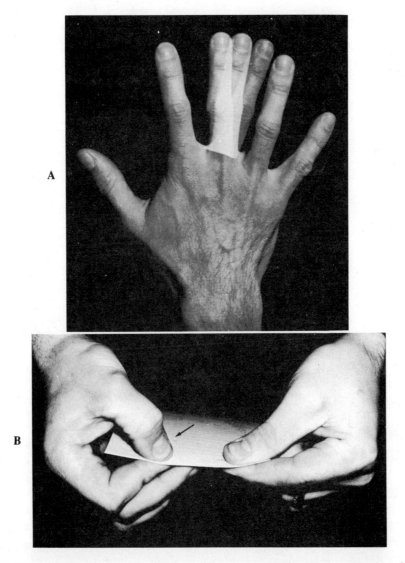

Fig. 39-20. Tests for motor function of ulnar nerve. **A,** Independent adduction-abduction of fingers, against resistance, and adduction of thumb with hand extended on flat surface demonstrates action of interossei and adductor-pollicis muscles, which are supplied by ulnar nerve; each muscle should be tested separately for localization of nerve damage. **B,** Froment's sign. Patient pinches piece of paper forcefully; examiner then pulls paper away, or patient pulls paper taut with both hands as if to tear it; to prevent paper from slipping away from weak adductor pollicis, patient must bring flexor pollicis longus into play causing flexion of interphalangeal joint of thumb; patient's right thumb shows Froment's sign because of transection of motor branch of ulnar nerve (same patient as shown in Fig. 39-13).

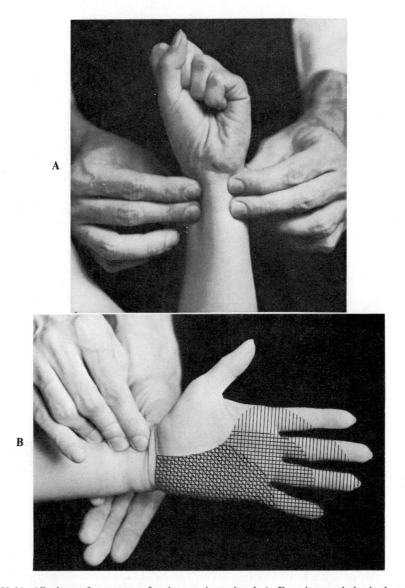

Fig. 39-21. Allen's test for patency of major arteries to hand. **A,** Examiner occludes both radial and ulnar arteries with his fingertips while patient holds his hand aloft and milks out any residual blood by repeatedly flexing digits into tight fist and extending them; hand is then lowered to dependent position, with arteries still occluded by digital pressure and digits extended. **B,** Artery in question is then released; rapid, bright, pink blush beginning near point of release signifies patent artery; slow or absent blush denotes occlusion or absence of artery. If blush does not occur after releasing one artery, remaining artery is released after pause of 1 to 2 minutes; patency of second artery is demonstrated by blush. Digital Allen's test uses same means for testing digital arteries.

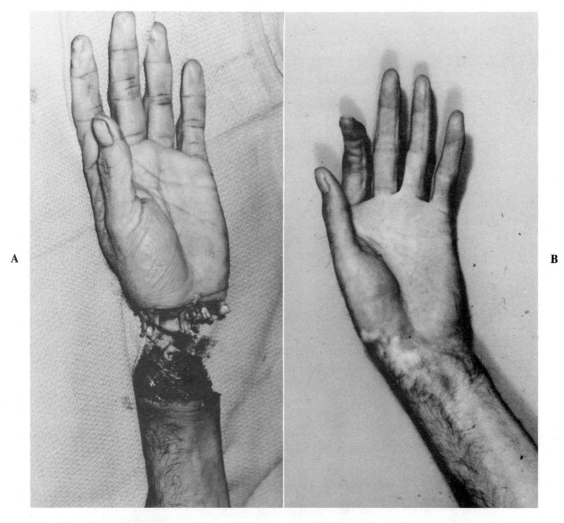

Fig. 39-22. A, Hand amputation. **B,** Successful replantation can usually be achieved in 90% of cases.

tomosis or grafts should be carried out if the blood supply is in question. Clinically, the Allen test (Fig. 39-21) is useful in determining patency of the radial or ulnar arteries. Operatively, viability is best assessed by bright red bleeding occurring at freshly cut edges of muscle or skin. If a tourniquet is used, one may assess viability by the "blush test," i.e., noting the color that develops in the questionable area after the tourniquet is released. The fluorescein test is useful.

Replantation. In the replantation of amputated digits the key to success is anastomosis of at least two veins and one artery of the affected digit. A specialty team using appropriate magnification and instruments can usually achieve a 90% or better survival rate (Fig. 39-22). Currently accepted indications for replantation include multiple digit amputations, thumb amputations, hand and palm amputations, and amputations in children. Single digits are replanted on a case-by-case basis especially if distal to the flexor digitorum superficialis tendon insertion.

Fractures and dislocations

Fractures of the phalanges and metacarpals are the most common of all fractures. If accompanied

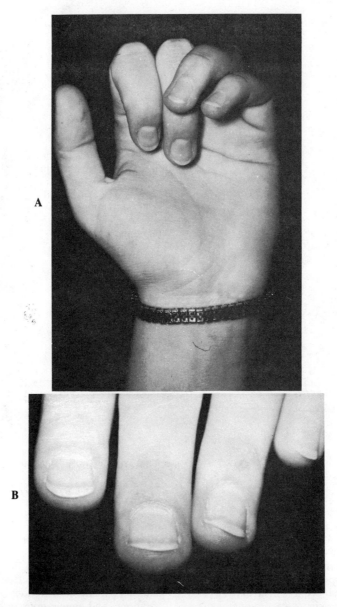

Fig. 39-23. "Scissoring" of fingers. **A,** Fingers overlap when flexed because of poor alignment and rotational malunion from fractures of index and ring proximal phalanges. **B,** Clue to malalignment is nonparallel fingernails.

by no deformity or displacement, they heal quickly with simple immobilization.

Deformity occurs when the fracture creates a disruption in the normal linkage system of the hand. The long bones of the hand constitute a delicate system of levers linked by mobile joints and controlled in space by the balanced pull of the flexor and extensor tendons. With disruption of a long bone a new "joint" is introduced into the system. Since no further controls have been added, the system buckles.

Deformity is tolerated very poorly in the hand, particularly in the proximal and middle phalanges and least of all in the joints. One must always look for rotational deformity, which is confirmed if the nail beds are not parallel or if the fingers tend to overlap in flexion (Fig. 39-23).

In treating deformity caused by fresh fractures one must be sure that reduction is obtained and maintained. If any uncertainty exists, open reduction and internal fixation are warranted.

Immobilization should be continued until there is clinical and roentgenological evidence of union. For simple fractures 3 weeks often suffices; however, transverse fractures of phalangeal or metacarpal shafts often require 5 or 6 weeks. There is no justification for including the arm and shoulder in the immobilization. The patient must faithfully exercise the remainder of the upper limb to prevent disuse atrophy.

Carpus. The most common carpal fracture is of the scaphoid. Classically a fall on the outstretched hand with tenderness in the anatomical snuffbox alerts the examiner to this injury. Even if roentgenographic findings are negative (including scaphoid views), immobilization is mandatory for at least 2 weeks and may be discontinued only if repeat roentgenological and clinical examinations are negative at that time. It is essential to look very closely for evidence of displacement of scaphoid fractures, which may indicate concomitant soft tissue injury and the necessity for open reduction and internal fixation. Furthermore, the possibility of avascular necrosis of the proximal pole of the scaphoid should be considered. It is wise to forewarn the patient of this possibility at the commencement of treatment. At times the scaphoid can be very slow in healing and occasionally many months of immobilization are required to gain satisfactory union and function.

The lunate is the most commonly dislocated carpal bone. It usually dislocates in a volar direction and may compress the median nerve in that position. Reduction can usually be accomplished by closed means but there is a risk of subsequent avascular necrosis. Follow-up roentgenograms are necessary to rule out this complication.

Metacarpus. Bennett's fracture-dislocation is a dislocation of the thumb carpometacarpal joint associated with a fracture of the metacarpal base extending into the joint, with resultant subluxation or dislocation. Skeletal fixation is generally required to maintain reduction.

The most common fracture of the remaining metacarpals is the "boxer's fracture" of the fifth metacarpal, commonly resulting from a fistfight. Fractures of the shaft of the long and ring metacarpals tend to be more stable than those of the border digits.

As a rule, dislocations of the metacarpophalangeal joints are easily reduced and maintained unless a phalangeal or metacarpal head is trapped in a "buttonhole" rent in the joint capsule. In the latter circumstance open reduction of the dislocation is required.

Phalanges. Displaced fractures of the proximal and middle phalanges of an articular surface often require open reduction and internal fixation. Displaced fractures of the distal phalanx are usually caused by crushing injury and are adequately managed by simple immobilization after appropriate soft-tissue management. The fingernail should not be thoughtlessly discarded in these crush injuries, for it often serves as an excellent biological splint.

In a patient with a history of trauma and a swollen, tender digit but without any fracture on roentgenograms, exclusion of significant soft-tissue injury is essential. The extensor apparatus and the collateral ligaments of either the interphalangeal or the metacarpophalangeal joints of the thumb are particularly prone to traumatic disruption.

Burns

Burns of the exposed and vulnerable dorsum of the hand most commonly result from open flames in adults or scalds in children. Suppleness and extensibility of the dorsal skin are destroyed by edema and inflammation and result in troublesome scar tissue formation in deep second-degree and third-degree burns. The resultant claw deformity (Fig. 39-6) is extremely disabling. Therefore in burns of this depth assiduous physical therapy should begin as soon as possible. The joints should move through a full range of motion many times daily. Between exercise periods, plaster or dynamic splints will prevent clawing (Fig. 39-24). If these methods fail or are likely to, internal splinting with Kirschner wires immobilizing the proximal interphalangeal joints in slight flexion may be necessary.

Burns of the palmar surface are most often seen in children who have grasped hot objects. For deep

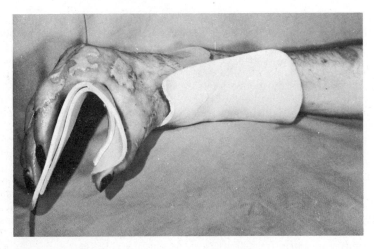

Fig. 39-24. "Anti-claw" splint placed on burned hand when at rest, to prevent claw deformity (see Fig. 39-6). (From Furnas, D.W.: A bedside outline for the treatment of burns, Springfield, Ill., 1969, Charles C Thomas, Publisher.)

second- and third-degree burns skin grafts may be required to prevent flexion deformities.

Electrical burns of the hand usually result from contact of the hand with a high-voltage conductor. Ongoing deep coagulation necrosis imposes an onerous and frustrating therapeutic burden and frequently necessitates amputation. Arterial hemorrhage and gas gangrene are occasional complications.

Inflammatory conditions
Septic (Fig. 39-25)

The dorsum of the hand with hair follicles and sweat and sebaceous glands acquires the same staphylococcal infections seen in the skin elsewhere on the body (folliculitis, carbuncles, furuncles, and subcutaneous abscesses). Simple streptococcal infections of either the dorsal or volar aspect of the hand may lead to lymphangitis or lymphadenitis, which respond promptly to appropriate antibiotics and local wound care. Mixed infections with anaerobic streptococcus, bacteroides, or spirochetes (see Chapter 6) may be very destructive and demand aggressive systemic therapy (I.V. antibiotics) with complete and thorough débridement of the wound. A common source of these dangerous infections is the human bite, resulting from the collision of a closed fist with an open mouth.

Infections originating on the palmar surface or around the nail have distinct characteristics, which are listed in Table 39-3. When these infections are seen quite early in their course, they may be aborted by antibiotics, bed rest, elevation, and warm moist dressings to the hand. If the infection is not aborted, pus will collect and drainage is required.

In recent years the most common cause of hematogenous septic arthritis in the hand in patients under 40 is *Neisseria gonorrhoeae*. Culture of this organism is extremely difficult, and swabs should be taken routinely from the oropharynx, cervix or urethral meatus, anus, blood, and, if possible, the local site.

Nonseptic

Aseptic tenosynovitis is relatively common in the hand and wrist. De Quervain's disorder (Fig. 39-26) is caused by compression of the long abductor and short extensor tendons of the thumb in the fibrous sheath near the radial styloid process. It causes severe pain, particularly if adduction of the thumb is carried out while the wrist is held in ulnar deviation. Trigger finger or thumb results from stenosing tenosynovitis in the proximal portion of the fibrous flexor sheath and from nodule formation in the flexor tendon because of injury or rheumatoid disease. The tendon is trapped momentarily as it passes through the mouth of the sheath and then suddenly releases. Either flexion or extension may be blocked.

Treatment of these entrapment syndromes that fail to settle conservatively is surgical decompression by incision of the roof of the offending fibrous sheath.

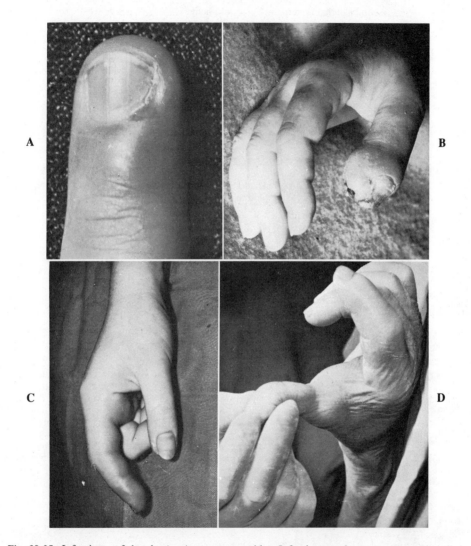

Fig. 39-25. Infections of hand. **A,** Acute paronychia. Infection tends to run around nail in surrounding subcuticular tissue; it may also tunnel beneath nail, forming subungual abscess. **B,** Felon. Pus is localized and tightly compressed within flexor pad or pulp space of tip of thumb. **C,** Tenosynovitis. Finger is (1) uniformly swollen, (2) slightly flexed, and (3) tender along tendon sheath, and (4) passive extension causes exquisite tenderness. **D,** Palmar space infection. Thenar space is swollen, tender, and distended with pus. (See Fig. 39-17.)

Table 39-3. Infections originating on the volar surface or around the nail

Entity	Findings	Cause	Site for incision for drainage of pus	Complications
Paronychia (Fig. 39-24, *A*)	Inflammation of soft tissues around nail that tend to "run around" nail margin	Infection of torn hangnail or cuticle	Directly into pus collection	Subungual abscess
Subungual abscess	Pus collection under nail	Extension from other infections	Excision of proximal portion of nail	
Felon (Fig. 39-24, *B*)	Red, tensely swollen, extremely painful throbbing pulp space of distal phalanx; keeps patient awake	Minor puncture wound of fingertip	Lateral aspect of distal phalanx, cutting through fibrous septa	Necrosis and osteomyelitis of phalangeal bone caused by compression of arteries
Tendon sheath infection (Fig. 39-24, *C*)	Uniform swelling of finger; position of slight flexion of finger; exquisite pain on passive extension; maximum tenderness over tendon sheath area	Puncture wound or extension from other sites	Midlateral line of finger	Necrosis of flexor tendon; spread to palmar spaces or other bursae
Palmar space infections (Fig. 39-24, *D*; Fig. 39-17)	Tenderness and swelling of central and ulnar aspect of palm (*midpalmar space*) or of radial and thenar aspect of palm (*thenar space*)	Extension from tendon sheath infection; direct puncture wound	Skin crease incisions over most prominent area of swelling	Extensive damage to soft tissue of hand; extension to other spaces

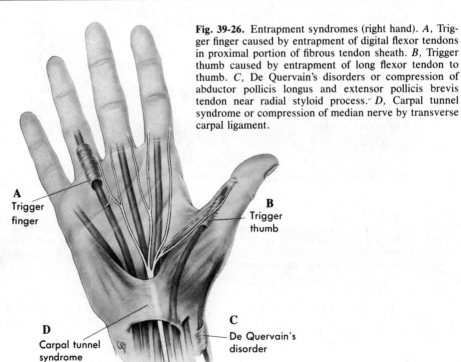

Fig. 39-26. Entrapment syndromes (right hand). *A,* Trigger finger caused by entrapment of digital flexor tendons in proximal portion of fibrous tendon sheath. *B,* Trigger thumb caused by entrapment of long flexor tendon to thumb. *C,* De Quervain's disorders or compression of abductor pollicis longus and extensor pollicis brevis tendon near radial styloid process. *D,* Carpal tunnel syndrome or compression of median nerve by transverse carpal ligament.

A Trigger finger

B Trigger thumb

D Carpal tunnel syndrome

C De Quervain's disorder

Rheumatoid arthritis commonly occurs as an acute arthritis in the wrist or fingers. Multiple symmetrical small joint involvement, fluctuating clinical course, and appropriate laboratory studies serve to differentiate it from other forms of arthritis.

Degenerative changes

Heberden's nodes are the most common form of degenerative change in the hand. These are present at the distal interphalangeal joint and reflect a local process of degenerative arthritis.

The carpometacarpal joint of the thumb is also commonly involved by degenerative processes and, as with Heberden's nodes, may reflect a systemic proclivity for osteoarthritis.

Carpal tunnel syndrome

The carpal tunnel syndrome, caused by compression of the median nerve in the flexor compartment of the wrist by the transverse carpal ligament, may occur as the result of diminution in the size of the canal (as with Colles' fracture) or of increase in the size of the contents (as with rheumatoid synovitis). Characteristically it results in pain in the hand and forearm, hyperesthesia and paresthesia of the three radial digits, and weakness and atrophy of the thenar muscles. Quite commonly the pain is experienced as far proximally as the shoulder. It is most common in middle-aged women and is frequently bilateral. Surgical decompression of the transverse metacarpal ligament

(Fig. 39-26) usually gives results that are gratifying to the surgeon and patient alike.

Tumors and tumorlike conditions
Dupuytren's contracture

Dupuytren's contracture (Fig. 39-27) is a fibrous metaplasia (often bilateral) of the superficial palmar fascia that causes a characteristic flexion contracture in the subcutaneous layer of the palm. A hypertrophic fibrous nodule appears in the palm or finger (most commonly the ring finger) and is followed by the formation of thick, fibrous bands that may extend distally. These bands slowly shorten until extension of the metacarpophalangeal and proximal interphalangeal joints is prevented. The contracture is corrected by excision of the offending metaplastic tissue.

Benign

Ganglia, epidermal cysts, mucous cysts, xanthomas, lipomas, enchondromas, glomus tumors, and neurilemomas are benign tumors characteristically found in the hand (Fig. 39-28, *A* to *E*). These are described in Table 39-4.

Malignant

Squamous cell or epidermoid carcinoma (Fig. 39-29) is the most common malignant tumor of the hand. It usually develops from premalignant keratoses on the dorsum of the hand decades after chronic exposure to sunlight, ionizing radiation, or organic hydrocarbons or after long-standing

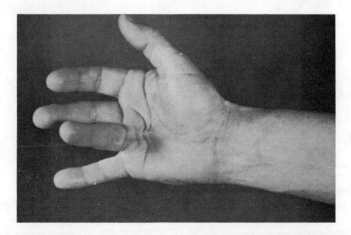

Fig. 39-27. Dupuytren's contracture. Band of hypertrophied and contracted superficial palmar fascia projects distally from nodule in palm; proximal interphalangeal joint of ring finger is forced into permanent flexion.

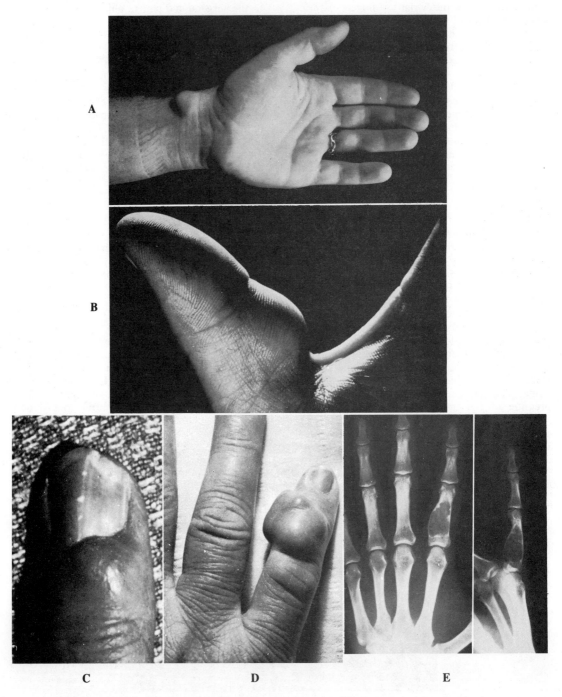

Fig. 39-28. Tumors of hand. **A,** Ganglia. **B,** Epidermal cyst. **C,** Mucus-retention cyst. **D,** Xanthoma. **E,** Enchondroma.

Table 39-4. Benign tumors of the hand

Entity	Description	Comment	Treatment
Ganglia (Fig. 39-28, *A*)	Multilocular cyst growing from capsule of carpal joint (dorsum of wrist, snuffbox, or just proximal to thenar eminence) or volar aspect of metacarpophalangeal joint	Most common (approximately one third of tumors of the hand)	Excision using equipment for major hand surgery (aspiration of cyst, injection of cortisone occasionally effective); recurrences are seen after any type of treatment
Epidermal cyst or implantation cyst, inclusion cyst (Fig. 39-28, *B*)	Subcutaneous cyst filled with epithelial debris located on flexor surface of proximal phalanges or distal palm	Caused by bits of epidermis, stabbed into subcutaneous site by tools or sharp objects	Excision
Mucous cyst (myxomatous cyst, myxoid cyst, or synovial cyst) (Fig. 39-28, *C*)	Translucent cyst embedded in thick, reddish skin just proximal to nail fold; frequently *groove of nail* in direct line with cyst	Filled with synovial fluid; usually communicates with distal interphalangeal joint	Excision of cyst and communication using magnification; avoid injury to extensor tendon
Xanthoma (benign giant cell tumor of tendon sheath; benign synovioma) (Fig. 39-28, *D*)	Firm, irregular, yellowish tumor growing from fibrous flexor tendon sheath	Multinucleated giant cells, synovial clefts, hemosiderin, foam cells seen on microscopic examination	Excision with equipment for major hand surgery
Lipoma	Soft, multinodular fatty mass	Frequently grow forward from middle palmar or thenar space displacing tendons and presenting as mass in palm	Excision with equipment for major hand surgery
Enchondroma (Fig. 39-28, *E*)	Cartilaginous pocket within bone or proximal phalanx (or other phalanges or metacarpal heads)	Usually asymptomatic, incidental finding on x-ray examination	None, unless symptoms of pathological fracture; then curettage and packing with bone chips
Glomus tumors (glomangioma or angioneuromyoma)	Tiny, very painful, reddish purple nodules frequently visible under fingernail, also seen in other sites	Growth of neuromyoarterial glomus, a heat-regulating arterial shunt	Excision
Neurilemoma and neuroma	Painful, tender nodule along course of previously injured nerve; Tinel's sign (distal paresthesias elicited by percussion at site of neurilemoma)	Most common in a digital nerve of thumb or index finger	If nerve is not functioning, excise neuroma and anastomose the nerve, or excise neuroma and bury stump of nerve in a recess where it will not be stimulated

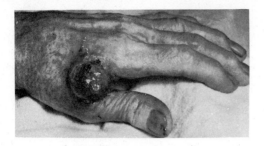

Fig. 39-29. Squamous carcinoma.

chronic dermatological disorders. Ingestion of arsenicals is associated with keratoses and carcinomas of the palmar surface of the hand. Growth is slow, malignancy is low grade, lymph node metastases occur in only about 5% to 15% of cases, and mortality is proportionately low. Wide excision of the lesion and repair of the defect by skin grafts or pedicles is the usual treatment. In far-advanced cases, amputation, axillary lymphadenectomy, and perfusion of the limb with chemotherapeutic agents must be considered. *Basal cell carcinoma* is rare in the hand.

Malignant melanoma of the hand behaves essentially as malignant melanoma elsewhere on the body surface. Wide excision or amputation with or without regional lymphadenectomy or perfusion of chemotherapeutic agents is performed.

40
Neurological Surgery

Hiro Nishioka

Neurological surgery and other surgical specialties constitute areas of limited but essential fields of knowledge for the student. Although details of operative techniques and the complications of surgery are of concern principally to the practitioners of the specialties, the ability to recognize the need for surgical intervention, especially under emergency conditions, remains an indispensable part of every physician's armamentarium.

In considering neurosurgical problems, some basic working principles should be borne in mind. The specialized neurons of the central nervous system, once destroyed, are incapable of replacement. Furthermore, the pathways by which neurons are interconnected cannot be reestablished once severed or interrupted. A cell or its connections may be damaged by pressure, penetration by foreign objects, inflammation, invasion by neoplasm, or biochemical processes. Of these, pressure is the only factor that can be relieved surgically. Reparative surgery in the central nervous system is prophylactic only and is utilized to prevent any additional damage by infection, hemorrhage, or trauma.

The degree of cellular or tract damage by pressure is proportional to the amount of pressure, the rapidity of pressure rise, and its duration. The most severe and permanent damage is produced by the sudden application of pressure, e.g., in acute trauma. Pressure of lesser degrees can be tolerated without permanent damage if its rate of increase is slow, e.g., neoplasm. If surgical decompression is to be worthwhile, it must be performed before irreversible damage has occurred and it must be sufficiently extensive. The surgeon must occasionally sacrifice nervous tissue that appears grossly nonviable or even normal in the interest of preserving useful functioning tissue that appears capable of recovery.

In contrast to the foregoing, the neurosurgical armamentarium contains procedures for the planned focal destruction of tracts and nuclear elements. These operations are utilized for the relief of intractable pain, involuntary movements, and abnormal states of muscle tonus.

The emphasis of this chapter will be directed toward the management of pressure-producing lesions. Descriptions of infrequently used or highly specialized techniques are omitted, so that the reader may concentrate on the commonly encountered neurosurgical problems.

SPECIAL DIAGNOSTIC STUDIES

Neurological examination alone is not sufficiently accurate in localizing intraspinal or intracranial lesions to proceed with operative treatment. Accurate delineation of the extent and location of the lesion prior to operation is desirable and requires the use of special investigative procedures.

Table 40-1 lists the common diagnostic studies utilized. Whenever possible, the specific tests that give the best chances of demonstrating a lesion should be chosen, based on the clinical impression of the location and type of pathosis expected. Although several tests might discover a tumor

Table 40-1. Diagnostic studies utilized most frequently

Diagnostic test	Procedure	Information obtained	Possible complications	Lesions best demonstrated
Noninvasive studies				
Electroencephalography	Application of electrodes to scalp and recording of cortical electrical activity	Abnormal wave forms and seizure discharges from areas irritated or compressed	None	Brain abscess, seizure focus
Echoencephalography	Transmission of ultrasonic waves coronally through the brain and recording echo at brain-fluid or brain-tumor interfaces (requires opening in bone, e.g., open fontanelle)	Ventricular size, neoplasms, or hematomas close to bony opening	None	Hydrocephalus, acute hematomas
Computerized tomography (CT scanning) (Figs. 40-1 and 40-2)	Tomograms of head or spine with computer-derived images of structures of different densities	Outlines of ventricular system and subarachnoid spaces, complete cross-sectional image of brain and spinal cord and of any lesion having densities different from central nervous system structures	None	Cysts, infarcts, hydrocephalus, degenerative lesions, acute and chronic hematomas
Invasive studies				
Lumbar puncture	Insertion of needle into lumbar and subarachnoid space and withdrawal of fluid	Presence of abnormal amounts of cells and alterations in chemical contents of cerebrospinal fluid	Herniation of temporal uncus or cerebellar tonsils with compression of brainstem	Meningitis, subarachnoid hemorrhage
Radioisotope canning (Fig. 40-3)	Parenteral injection of radioactive isotope and observation of its flow through carotid and cerebral arteries, noting its tendency to localize in abnormal areas as determined by radioactive counts over neck and head	Relative rate and volume of flow through carotid and middle cerebral arteries; presence of neoplasms, vascular malformations, and abnormal brain tissues that take up more than normal amounts of isotope	Allergic reaction to isotope or its carrier	Unilateral carotid stenosis or occlusion, middle cerebral thrombosis, arteriovenous malformation, vascular neoplasms, e.g., meningiomas, metastases
Contrast-enhanced computerized tomography (Fig. 40-4)	Tomograms as above after parenteral injection of iodinated contrast media	Circle of Willis and major cerebral arteries, vascular patterns in and around mass lesions in addition to information from unenhanced CT	Allergic reactions to enhancing contrast material	Vascular neoplasms, arteriovenous malformations

Table 40-1. Diagnostic studies utilized most frequently—cont'd

Diagnostic test	Procedure	Information obtained	Possible complications	Lesions best demonstrated
Invasive studies—cont'd				
Angiography (Fig. 40-5)	1. Injection of contrast into superior vena cava and visualization of cervical and intracranial vasculature by computed digital subtraction 2. Injection of contrast directly into carotid or vertebral arteries with rapid serial radiographic examinations	Opacification of cervical and cerebral blood vessels to show vascular abnormalities, or neovascularity and displacement by mass lesions	Thromboembolism with cerebral infarction, local hemorrhage, allergic reaction to contrast medium	Vascular anomalies (aneurysm, arteriovenous malformation) subdural and epidural hematomas, vascular neoplasms, especially meningiomas
Myelography (Fig. 40-6)	Lumbar, cervical, or cisternal puncture and injection of positive contrast medium or air	Outline of spinal subarachnoid space that may be distorted or blocked bv mass lesions in the spinal canal	Spinal arachnoiditis, inflammatory reaction to contrast medium or contaminant	Tumors in the spinal canal, herniated intervertebral disk, avulsion of nerve roots

mass, one of them may provide information that is particularly useful to the operating surgeon, e.g., isotope or computerized tomography (CT) scans may outline a tumor, but an angiogram will show both the internal vascularity and the position of important vascular structures in the immediate vicinity of the tumor (Fig. 40-5). The routine use of a "battery" of tests is to be deplored. All such tests are costly, and some carry significant risks of complications and even death. Therefore careful neurological evaluation is essential to the efficient and safe investigation of the patient. General screening tests are, of course, never to be overlooked. Blood count, urinalysis, chest roentgenogram, and any other appropriate tests should be completed before special investigations.

Electroencephalography, echoencephalography, radioisotope scans, and *computerized tomography* are useful as screening tests, since they can be performed without significant risk or discomfort to the patient. The information thus obtained may be sufficient to proceed directly with surgical treatment. However, in many instances additional preoperative studies, e.g., angiograms or contrast-enhanced tomography (Fig. 40-4), may be utilized to obtain more precise information about a lesion. Two additional methods of obtaining images of intracranial and intraspinal contents are nuclear

magnetic resonance (NMR) scanning and positron-emission tomography (PET). The former provides images somewhat similar to CT scanning by magnetic resonance rather than by radiation, whereas the latter provides information regarding the metabolic activity within the lesion.

Considerable confusion exists in the minds of most students regarding the indications for *lumbar puncture.* Whenever intraspinal pathosis is suspected, lumbar puncture with the Queckenstedt test (compression of the jugular veins) is indicated. The complete lack of any change in pressure with the Queckenstedt maneuver indicates the presence of advanced compression within the spinal canal above the site of the needle. In such circumstances, whenever feasible, radiopaque material for myelographic screening, e.g., Pantopaque, should be instilled immediately, for it may be difficult to repeat the spinal puncture at a later time. Lesser degrees of compression are manifested by abnormally slow rates of rise or fall of fluid pressure during jugular compression and release. These abnormal pressure changes along with the characteristics of the fluid (xanthochromia, increased protein) serve to differentiate surgical from medical neurological problems. It is therefore most important to *measure and record* them accurately.

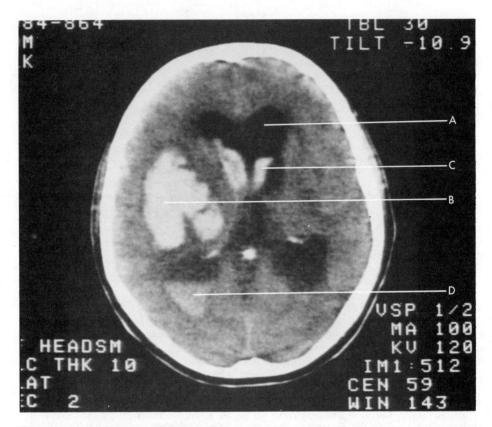

Fig. 40-1. Unenhanced CT scan of head at level of lateral ventricles. Skull appears as dense opaque outline; semisolid brain tissue as intermediate density; fluid in lateral ventricles, *A*, is least dense. Hemorrhage has occurred, *B*, into brain substance and into ventricles, *C*. With patient lying supine, some blood has settled into posterior horn of ventricle, *D*. These differentiations are made without injection of any radiopaque substances.

Fig. 40-2. Unenhanced CT scan of lumbar spine at level of L4-L5 disk. The spinal canal is bordered by ligamentum flavum, *A*, and the intervertebral disk, *B*. Roots of cauda equina, *C*, are greatly compressed by large fragment of herniated disk, *D*, occupying much of the canal. Differentiation of tissues can be accentuated by density-computed highlighting, *E*, without the need for injection of contrast media.

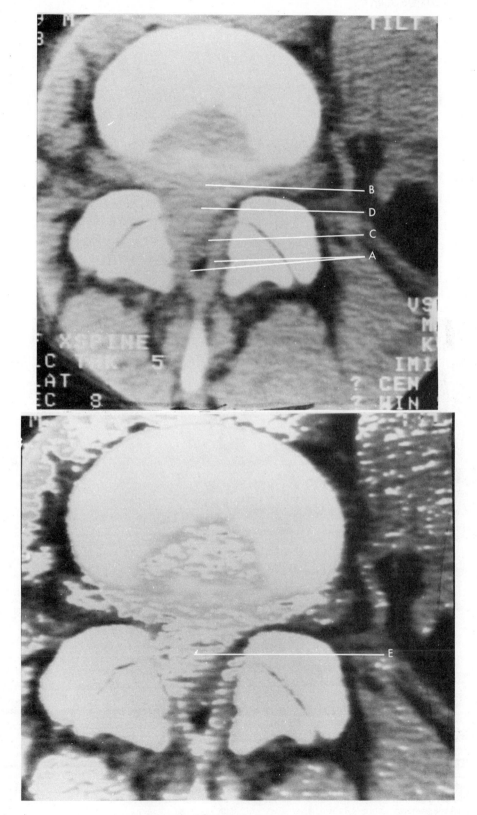

Fig. 40-2. For legend see opposite page.

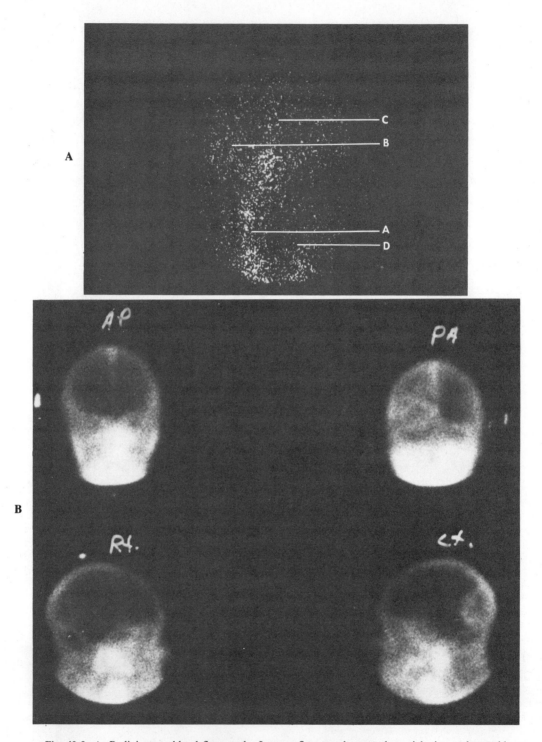

Fig. 40-3. A, Radioisotope blood flow study. Isotope flow can be traced up right internal carotid artery, *A,* and into middle cerebral, *B,* and anterior cerebral arteries, *C.* Severe stenosis or occlusion of left internal carotid artery, *D,* is demonstrated here by lack of isotope flow through cervical region on left side. **B,** Radioisotopic brain scan. Venous sinuses take up relatively heavy concentrations of isotope, whereas normal brain tissue does not. Ringlike area of increased uptake is seen in left occipital region. "Hollow center" indicates necrosis or liquefaction, e.g., abscess, breakdown in rapidly growing neoplasm.

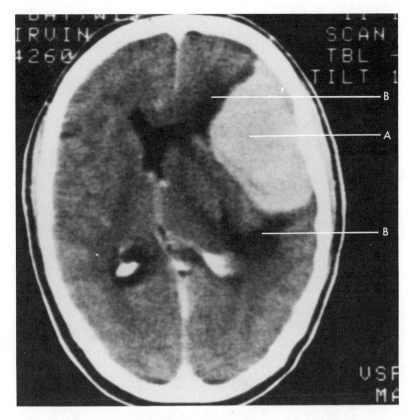

Fig. 40-4. CT scan after intravenous meglumine diatrizoate. Large tumor, *A,* is enhanced by contrast; tumor mass and associated edema, *B,* shift adjacent structures to opposite side. Size and homogeneity of tumor are typical of meningioma.

In the presence of a pressure-producing intracranial pathological condition, lumbar puncture is potentially hazardous to the life of the patient. The withdrawal of spinal fluid from below, and particularly the leakage of fluid into the spinal epidural space after the needle has been removed, encourage herniation of the cerebellar tonsils and temporal lobe uncus, with resultant brainstem compression. Therefore lumbar puncture should be performed for specific indications only. Increased intracranial pressure is usually associated with clinically recognizable symptoms and signs such as vomiting and papilledema. There is no advantage in measuring the exact degree of abnormal pressure in the presence of such signs. The diagnosis of infections (meningitis, encephalitis) and of subarachnoid hemorrhage depends on the finding of the appropriate cells in the cerebrospinal fluid. Lumbar puncture is therefore indicated in all patients suspected of harboring the preceding, based on the clinical finding of *nuchal rigidity.* That these

same conditions are likely to be associated with increased intracranial pressure is apparent, but the possible risks of the procedure are outweighed by the necessity for deriving information that may be vital to the selection of proper treatment. In brain tumors the information obtained from lumbar puncture is usually not worth the hazards; in subdural hematoma the fluid may be entirely normal, misleading the clinician into a false sense of security. The Queckenstedt test, for all practical purposes, should *never* be performed when an intracranial pathosis is suspected, for the potential hazards of uncal or tonsillar herniation are acutely increased by compression of the jugular veins.

INCREASED INTRACRANIAL PRESSURE
Clinicopathological correlations

The addition of fluid, blood, or neoplastic tissue to the normal contents of any body cavity may result in (1) increase in the volume of that cavity, (2) increase in the pressure within the cavity, or (3)

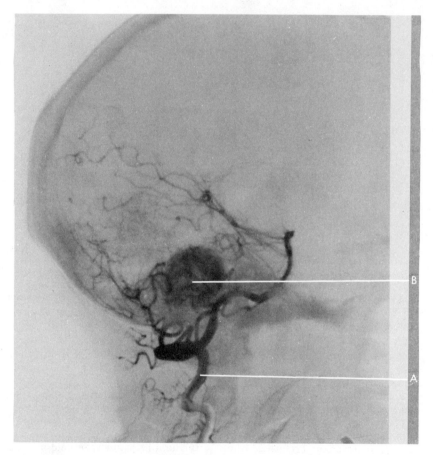

Fig. 40-5. Angiogram performed by injection of meglumine diatrizoate into vertebral artery, *A*. A highly vascularized tumor mass, *B,* lies in fourth ventricle. Lesion was a choroid plexus papilloma.

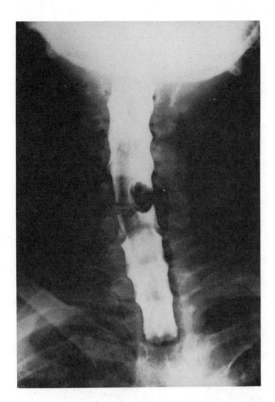

Fig. 40-6. Myelogram showing intradural extramedullary tumor. Sharp outline of tumor mass is diagnostic of lesion inside dura but extrinsic to spinal cord. Neurofibroma and meningioma are usual lesions.

both. Adding to the contents of the cranial cavity results in an increase in the size of the head only in infants when the cranial sutures are still open, but even then the increase can occur only slowly.

For practical purposes the cranial cavity may be regarded as a rigid box divided into two compartments, one above and one below the tentorium. Each has one principal outlet, the tentorial hiatus and the foramen magnum, respectively. Every increase in volume within these compartments is accompanied by a tendency for brain tissue to herniate through their outlets. The herniating tissue directly compresses and distorts the brainstem and is the primary cause of death from increased intracranial pressure.

Institution of treatment before irreversible damage has occurred depends on the recognition of danger signs indicating beginning or advancing herniation. The patient's responses to common environmental stimuli are the most reliable indicators of his intracranial pressure. As pressure increases, the responses are progressively impaired in speed, accuracy, and propriety. Pupillary dilatation is always late in onset, occurring only in the presence of dangerous herniations. The "classical" alterations of vital signs (increasing blood pressure with slowing of the heart rate) may not occur until it is too late for effective treatment, if they occur at all.

Table 40-2 lists the progression of observable responses as intracranial pressure increases. Notice that the categorized responses for each stage are not absolute; these are general guidelines and are subject to some variation. Fig. 40-7 shows how a subdural hematoma distorts the brain and produces the neurological signs of herniation. Dilatation of a pupil signifies herniation of the temporal uncus with compression of the oculomotor nerve. The nerve adjacent to the herniated uncus is usually affected first, resulting in dilatation of the pupil on the side of the lesion. Occasionally, however, the midbrain is shifted to the extent that the opposite oculomotor nerve is compressed against the edge of the tentorium resulting in pupillary dilatation on the side opposite the lesion.

Compression of the cerebral peduncle either directly by the herniating uncus or indirectly by shifting against the opposite tentorial edge results first in a *paresis* on the side opposite the primary lesion (since these fibers cross in the medulla at the decussation of the pyramids), commonly followed by a change in response to *extensor thrust* (decerebration). At this stage vasomotor and respiratory centers are easily compromised, so that cessation of respirations may occur at any moment.

The stage-by-stage progression to total decerebration and finally to complete flaccidity with no response to any stimulus may occur gradually over a period of hours or suddenly within a few seconds. Thus there is no margin of safety after the onset of signs indicating midbrain compression.

CONGENITAL MALFORMATIONS

Three congenital conditions merit the attention of the student. These are meningomyelocele, hydrocephalus, and craniosynostosis.

Meningomyelocele (Fig. 40-8) occurs most frequently in the lumbar region but can occur at any point in the midline of the neuraxis, including the vault of the skull. Lumbar meningomyeloceles are variable in the content of neural tissue; they almost always contain some nervous elements and are frequently associated with varying degrees of paraparesis. If no neural elements are present, the lesion is called a meningocele. Surgical repair of the sac is performed to prevent rupture with its attendant danger of meningitis, but little can be done to improve the neurological deficit.

Table 40-2. Clinical changes with progressive brainstem compression

Stage	Response to:			Pupils	
	Addressing patient by name	*Patting or shaking patient's shoulder*	*Pinching tendon of pectoralis major*	*Relative size*	*Reaction to light*
Normal	Looks at examiner, remains attentive	Looks at examiner, remains attentive	Removes pinching hand quickly and effectively, moves body away	Equal	Reactive
I	Opens eyes but tends to fall asleep while being spoken to	Opens eyes and remains awake as long as stimulus is applied	Removes stimulus and moves away, but not as quickly as in "normal" stage	Equal	Reactive
II	No response	Little or no response	Sluggish and ineffectual attempts to remove stimulus, shrugs shoulders	Dilated on side of lesion*	Sluggish or no reaction
III	No response	No response	Extensor thrust (decerebrate posture) on side opposite the lesion*	Widely dilated on side of lesion	No reaction
IV	No response	No response or bilateral extensor thrusts	Bilateral extensor thrusts	Widely dilated bilaterally	No reaction
V	No response	No response	No response	Moderately dilated	No reaction

*Dilatation of the pupil and the appearance of extensor posturing occasionally occur first on the side opposite that listed in this table. For the anatomical explanation for this phenomenon, refer to text and to Fig. 40-7.

Meningomyeloceles, regardless of location, are very often associated with the *Arnold-Chiari malformation,* a caudal displacement of the medulla and cerebrellar tissue through the foramen magnum into the cervical canal. For reasons that have never been explained adequately, repair of the meningomyelocele is frequently followed by rapid enlargement of the head from *obstructive hydrocephalus.* Numerous methods of shunting the accumulated fluid out of the ventricular system have met with limited success and many complications. At present, the most satisfactory shunting procedures are the ventriculovenous shunt (Fig. 40-9, *A*) and the ventriculoperitoneal shunt (Fig. 40-9, *B*), both incorporating calibrated one-way valve systems that allow fluid to leave the ventricles under controlled pressure and prevent reflux of fluid or blood back into the ventricles. The successful long-term control of pressure usually results in useful survivals—children at least capable of being educated. On the other hand, inadequate control of pressure results in a child with very limited potential for mental development and with a monstrously large head.

Craniosynostosis, or premature closure of the cranial sutures, is a curious condition that affects males six times more frequently than females. The abnormal shape of the head depends on the suture or sutures prematurely fused. In most cases early treatment, within the first 3 months of life, is indicated to prevent mental retardation, blindness, and permanent disfigurement. Operation consists in cutting out an artificial suture (linear craniectomy) and preventing early reclosure.

CRANIOCEREBRAL TRAUMA

The high incidence of head injuries in the general civilian population makes an adequate working knowledge of the problem essential to every physician. The pathological condition that may result from trauma is dependent on the mechanism of injury, so that this must be considered carefully in each patient. In this section the pathogenesis is considered along with the diagnosis and management of the various types of patients.

The management of the patient may be divided into four phases, which are discussed in the following paragraphs.

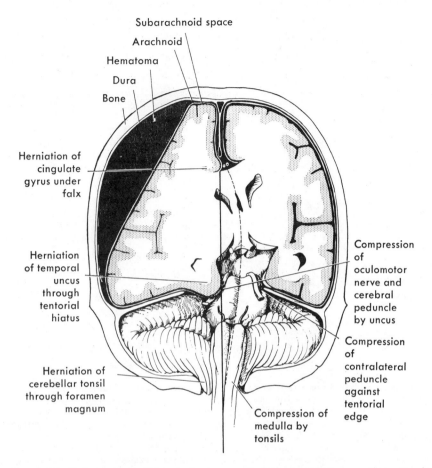

Subarachnoid space

Arachnoid

Hematoma

Dura

Bone

Herniation of cingulate gyrus under falx

Herniation of temporal uncus through tentorial hiatus

Herniation of cerebellar tonsil through foramen magnum

Compression of oculomotor nerve and cerebral peduncle by uncus

Compression of contralateral peduncle against tentorial edge

Compression of medulla by tonsils

Fig. 40-7. Subdural hematoma. Although hematoma displaces and distorts surface of cerebral hemisphere, more serious and life-threatening changes are occurring in deeper structures at some distance from hematoma itself. These changes result in displacement and compression of vital centers within brainstem.

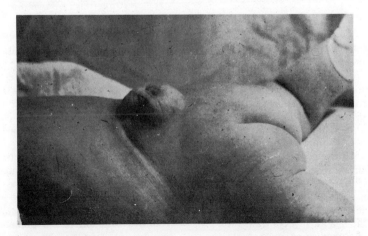

Fig. 40-8. Lumbar meningomyelocele. Lesion usually has wide base, so that closure of skin after excision of sac often requires extensive undermining and rotation of flaps.

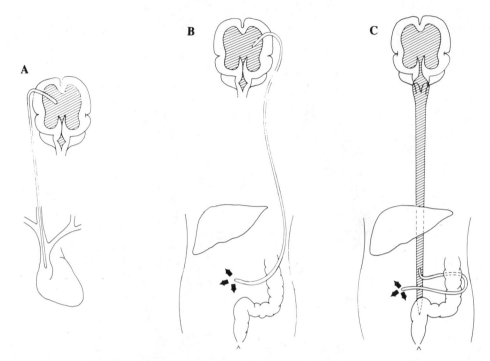

Fig. 40-9. Shunt procedures used most commonly for hydrocephalus. **A,** Ventriculocaval shunt. Fluid is shunted directly back into bloodstream through catheter inserted into jugular vein and threaded downward so that its tip lies in superior vena cava; one-way valve within system prevents reflux of blood upward from vena cava and controls pressure under which fluid drains out of ventricles. **B,** Ventriculoperitoneal shunt. Fluid is shunted into peritoneal cavity to be absorbed back into bloodstream. Catheter is threaded through subcutaneous tunnel over chest and upper abdominal wall to enter peritoneal cavity in lower quadrant. **C,** Lumbar peritoneal shunt. Fluid is shunted from lumbar subarachnoid space through subcutaneous tunnel around patient's flank. This procedure can be utilized only in a communicating hydrocephalus, i.e., when ventricular system communicates freely with spinal subarachnoid space. Any peritoneal shunt can be performed on patient's right or left side.

Phase 1
Assessment of the type and severity of injury

The history of the traumatic event may provide valuable clues to the nature and areas injured. Unfortunately, patients are usually unable to provide this history because they are unconscious or because of amnesia generally associated with the injury. Therefore fragments of information from relatives, spectators, and police officers may have to be pieced together. Since head injury occurs frequently with injuries to other parts of the body, the physician must learn to evaluate quickly the relative severity of each and to determine which deserves priority in the order of treatment. The force of a blow to the head is always transmitted in some degree to the cervical spine, so that one must be aware constantly of the possibility of a fracture

or dislocation of the cervical spine in association with every head injury. Respiratory and cardiovascular distress always take precedence over neurological injury, for they are immediately life threatening, and the resultant hypoxia enhances any damage to other tissues including those of the nervous system. (See Chapter 35.)

The type of injury may be classified according to the mechanism of trauma. It may be kinetic or static, nonpenetrating or penetrating. The kinetic injury results from the differential rates of motion between skull and brain tissues. Nonpenetrating kinetic injuries are by far the most common in civilian life. The stationary head may be struck, resulting in sudden movement of the cranium (acceleration), or the head in motion may strike a stationary object in such a way that motion of the

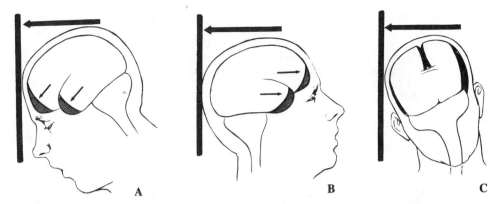

Fig. 40-10. Cortical contusion with relation to direction of head movement. **A,** Head moving forward and striking stationary surface—major injury found at tips of frontal and temporal poles. **B,** Head moving backward and striking stationary surface—major injury found in frontal and temporal lobes (contrecoup). **C,** Head moving laterally and striking stationary surface—major injury found on side opposite that which strikes surface (contrecoup); medial surfaces of hemispheres are also injured by impingement on relatively rigid falx.

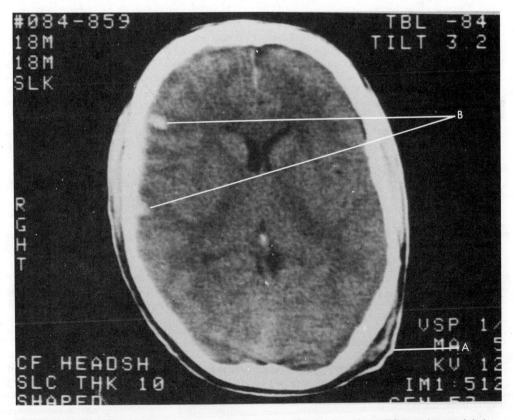

Fig. 40-11. CT scan showing contrecoup injury. Patient fell backwards, striking parieto-occipital region as indicated by swelling of scalp, *A*. Small intracerebral hemorrhages, *B*, are seen farthest from the point of impact on skull.

cranium is suddenly arrested (deceleration). The latter is more common and produces a more severe lesion. When movement is in a forward direction (Fig. 40-10, *A*), the major lesion is usually directly under the point of impact; when movement is in the lateral plane (Fig. 40-10, *C*), there is greater tendency for the maximal damage to occur on the side of the brain opposite the point of impact (contrecoup) (Fig. 40-11). Penetrating injuries are primarily static. In civilian life they are not uncommonly seen after a kick by a horse or after direct blows with small objects such as balls or hammers.

The *key* to the initial and subsequent neurological evaluation of the head-injured patient is the assessment of the *level of responsiveness, or "consciousness."* This point cannot be overemphasized. Instability of the vital signs is common immediately after head trauma, whereas localizing neurological deficits may not become manifest until complications are far advanced. The rapidity, propriety, and accuracy of a patient's responses to verbal commands or to noxious stimulation wherever necessary must be observed carefully and recorded. The Glasgow coma scale (Fig. 40-12) offers a uniform assessment of basic cerebral functions after a head injury and is used widely by medical and paramedical personnel. The patient's cerebral functioning level can be equated to a numerical value and plotted on a chart, so that significant changes in that value may be cause for specific treatment. Because alcoholic intoxication is associated so frequently with head injuries especially from vehicular accidents, the serum ethanol content must be taken into consideration in any assessment of cerebral responses.

The patient should be evaluated according to the *brain* injury as diagnosed by neurological examination and the *bony* injury as diagnosed by physical and radiological examinations.

Brain
  Concussion ⎫
  Contusion ⎬ Hemispheres, brainstem or both
  Laceration ⎭
Bone
  Closed fracture ⎫ Linear
  Open fracture   ⎬ Comminuted with or without depression of fragments

The severity of the brain injury does not correlate with the degree of skull damage. Therefore each component should be described, e.g., cerebral concussion with closed linear fracture, or cerebral laceration from open comminuted fracture with depression of fragments.

Concussion implies that the trauma has been sufficient to impair cerebral function temporarily, that there is no immediate structural damage, and hence that recovery may be expected. *Contusion* denotes a more severe injury, producing bruises or petechial hemorrhages in brain substance. Complete neurological recovery can occur, but severe contusion may progress to infarction with permanent deficits or even death of the patient. *Laceration* denotes a break in the anatomical continuity of brain substance. It is usually associated with penetrating wounds, e.g., depressed fracture and bullet wounds, but it can occur in nonpenetrating injuries.

By far the most common type of head injury seen in practice is concussion with or without skull fracture. A blow to the head sends the victim into a state of unresponsiveness from which he cannot be aroused. Within seconds or minutes, he begins to move his extremities and then to open his eyes. He may be confused and disorientated for minutes or hours. During the first 6 to 12 hours, there may be lethargy, nausea, and vomiting. Within 24 to 48 hours, he is lucid and orientated, with no neurological deficit except for amnesia for the events just before or after the injury, or at both times. Headache and giddiness are common when ambulation is begun, except in young children, who complain very little of symptoms after 24 hours.

Since skull fractures without gross displacement will heal without specific treatment, they are not of therapeutic importance except in two instances. Fractures of the base of the skull with dural and arachnoid tearing resulting in *leakage of cerebrospinal fluid* (mixed with blood) from the ear or nostril may call for prophylaxis against meningitis. Ampicillin is most satisfactory for this purpose. Fractures of the petrous temporal bone frequently cannot be seen in skull roentgenograms, so that *diagnosis is based entirely on the finding of bloody spinal fluid otorrhea.* Fortunately this leakage from the ear will almost invariably cease spontaneously. Cerebrospinal fluid rhinorrhea, however, often persists, with its attendant threat of meningitis. In such cases intracranial repair of the meningeal laceration is necessary. *Depression of bone fragments* of such magnitude or in an area where functional cortex is compressed calls for immediate surgical elevation. In most instances the blow that produces such depression of bone also lacerates the scalp, so that there is danger of infection in sequestrated bone fragments.

Performance of ancillary emergency procedures

Establishment and maintenance of an unobstructed airway are the first and most important considerations. In the unconscious patient *endotracheal intubation* through the mouth or nostril provides an immediate and satisfactory route both for unobstructed breathing and for tracheal suc-

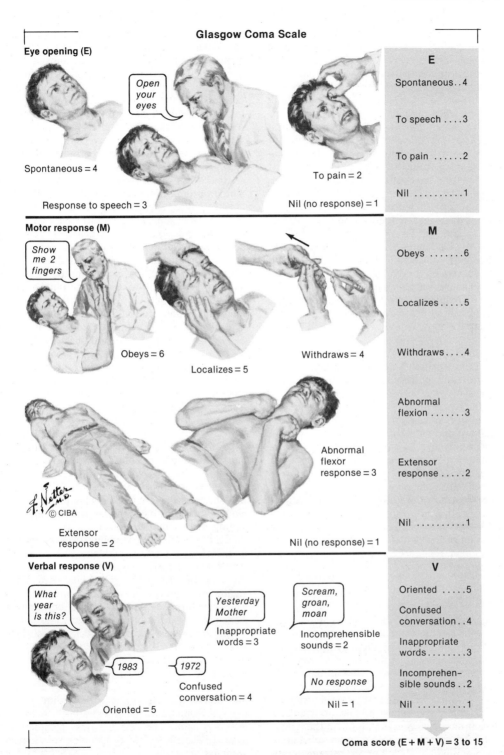

Fig. 40-12. Glasgow coma scale. (© 1983, CIBA Pharmaceutical Company, Division of CIBA-Geigy Corp., Ardsley, N.Y. Reprinted with permission from Clinical Symposia; illustrated by Dr. Frank H. Netter; all rights reserved.)

tion. Where intubation is impossible because of local injuries or deformities, tracheostomy should be performed. These procedures are essential to the safe transport of the patient to a neurosurgical facility. *Replacement of blood loss* from scalp lacerations is not often necessary except in infants and children where the blood loss may become sufficient to result in shock. Bleeding from the scalp edges can be controlled for short periods by tamponing, but if there is an extensive underlying fracture, bleeding from the *bone edges* may continue despite the application of pressure to the scalp. *Débridement* and *suture* of lacerations should be performed with adequate shaving and cleansing of the lacerated area and under good operating conditions. Too often, scalp lacerations are roughly sutured under the premise that the scar will be hidden by hair. Patients who may be expected to remain unresponsive for prolonged periods should have an *indwelling catheter* in the bladder. This will not only facilitate nursing care but will also allow accurate measurement of the urinary output.

Summary of phase I

1. General examination—define areas and extent of injuries and perform necessary emergency measures
2. Record cerebral functional status
   a. Level of responsiveness
   b. Memory and mentation
   c. Motor power in face and extremities
   d. Pupillary size and reactions
   e. Vital signs
3. Examine skull roentgenograms
   a. Type and location of fractures, especially with relation to sinuses and middle meningeal grooves
   b. Position of the pineal gland if calcified
   c. Any other related or unrelated skull abnormality

Phase II
Observation of clinical progress

The clinical course is observed to detect the development of complications. What are these complications, and what are their symptoms and signs? Four types should be under consideration at all times: *increased intracranial pressure, hemorrhage, infection,* and *convulsive seizures.* Increased intracranial pressure after head injury may result from reactive cerebral edema or from the development of a localized hematoma in the epidural or subdural spaces, or within brain substance. Lethargy, vomiting, and dulling of responses are common to all cases regardless of the underlying

pathosis, and localizing neurological deficits are inconstant except in patients with intracerebral hematoma.

Cerebral edema begins immediately after injury and may continue to increase for 48 to 72 hours before beginning to subside. In relatively minor injuries it diminishes after 6 to 12 hours and requires no treatment. After severe cerebral contusions, edema and generalized infarction may convert the white matter into a pulpy mass.

Subdural hematoma is the most common of the complicating hematomas. The acute hematoma, which produces signs within 48 hours of injury, is usually caused by bleeding from a vein bridging between the superficial middle cerebral vein and the sphenoparietal sinus. Hence these hematomas are maximal in the *temporal region.* The clot may become organized and liquefy so that it becomes converted into a cystic cavity limited by a capsule and containing fluid having a much higher osmotic pressure than that of the adjacent cerebrospinal fluid. By osmosis through this semipermeable capsule or membrane, cerebrospinal fluid is imbibed, resulting in gradual expansion of the cavity. Symptoms may then appear after a delay of several weeks or months after injury (chronic subdural hematoma). There may occur small subdural collections that cause no symptoms and require no treatment; they may resolve into thin scars and sometimes become calcified. An intermediate entity, the subacute hematoma, is recognized. Its definition is arbitrary, but generally it applies to hematomas that become clinically manifest between the third and fourteenth day after injury. An alternative explanation for the formation of chronic hematoma is that there is tearing of the pacchionian granulations from their dural attachment, resulting in the immediate leakage of cerebrospinal fluid and blood into the subdural space. This lesion is therefore maximal over the *convexity of the hemisphere.* After a lapse of about 3 months from the time of injury, the possibility of a clinically significant subdural hematoma is so small that for practical purposes it need not be entertained seriously in the differential diagnosis.

Epidural hematoma (Figs. 40-13 and 40-14) usually results from laceration of branches of the middle meningeal artery. Often a fracture line can be seen roentgenologically in the temporal region, crossing the grooves formed in the inner table of the skull by the artery. Because bleeding is arterial, the symptoms are usually rapid both in onset and in progression. This lesion is less common in the elderly because the dura becomes so adherent to the inner table with advancing age that the artery is tamponed effectively.

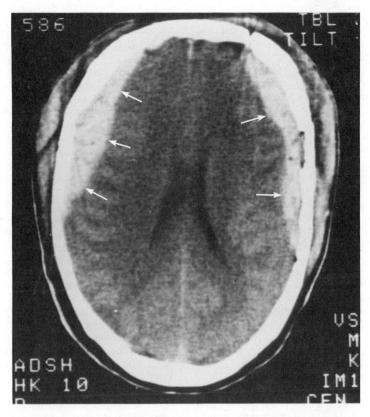

Fig. 40-13. CT scan showing bilateral extracerebral compressing hematomas, *arrows*. Acute hematomas are always of high density and are easily demonstrable by rapid scanning techniques.

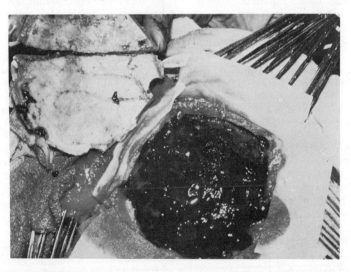

Fig. 40-14. Epidural hematoma. Reflected skull flap shows linear fracture crossing grooves formed by middle meningeal artery. Underlying hematoma is entirely solid clot, so that it could not have been drained through burr holes only.

Intracerebral and intracerebellar hematomas are formed when bleeding occurs into bruised and edematous brain tissue. These "hematomas" are frequently a mixture of blood and necrotic white matter. Most are subclinical and detected only by CT scanning, but occasionally they are large enough to warrant surgical evacuation with concomitant débridement of nonviable adjacent brain tissue.

The appearance of signs of increased intracranial pressure varies with the lesion producing the pressure. Signs develop within the first 24 to 48 hours from cerebral contusion and edema and from epidural hematoma, whereas they tend to appear slightly later with intracerebral hematomas. Evidence of subdural hematoma may appear early or up to 3 months later, by which time the causative traumatic episode may have been forgotten. Since every head injury of any consequence is followed by some degree of increased pressure from reactive edema, one must establish a critical level at which point specific investigation and treatment are indicated. This level is generally reached *when the patient is no longer able to respond appropriately to verbal or nonnoxious tactile stimuli*. If the patient has been incapable of such a response from the time of injury, it is appropriate, in the absence of localizing neurological deficits, to await signs of progression.

The presence of hemiparesis is inconstant and unpredictable in patients with traumatic hematoma. Hemiparesis present immediately after injury is likely caused by cerebral contusion rather than by a compressing hematoma. The slow development of a mild hemiparesis is consistent with the presence of an extracerebral hematoma (epidural or subdural), whereas a dense hemiplegia, especially in an alert patient, is rarely produced by such a lesion. Subdural hematoma may arise with no paresis or with hemiparesis contralateral or ipsilateral to the hematoma. Hence the *neurological picture of subdural hematoma is often confusing and nonspecific.*

Frequent recording of the vital signs—pulse, respirations, blood pressure, and temperature—is an integral part of the observation routine. Unfortunately the so-called classical alterations in the vital signs described under the section on increased intracranial pressure are so *frequently absent* in patients with proved intracranial hematomas that they cannot be relied on to occur. Intracranial pressure may not be assumed to be normal because the vital signs are stable. Shock is never produced by increased intracranial pressure, except in the terminal stages. The development of shock demands a search for an extracranial source of blood loss. (See Chapter 35.)

Hemorrhage from the gastrointestinal tract not uncommonly accompanies severe head injuries, particularly with brainstem damage. The pathophysiology of this phenomenon is presumably the same as stress ulcers associated with burns and other major traumatic incidents. Bleeding may occur from a single acute ulcer or from multiple superficial erosions, and it may cause death by exsanguination. Whenever shock occurs during the clinical course of an unresponsive patient, gastrointestinal hemorrhage should be suspected. Subgaleal bleeding (cephalohematoma) in infants can be of sufficient magnitude to produce shock. In adults it is impossible to lose a sufficient quantity of blood intracranially or into the subgaleal space to produce shock from volume loss alone.

Infections involving the pulmonary and urinary tracts are frequently encountered in patients who remain unresponsive for prolonged periods of time. Tracheostomy is often indicated for adequate removal of tracheobronchial secretions. Prophylactic antibiotic therapy should be given in certain circumstances, particularly in the elderly. *Meningitis* is a threat when an open fracture allows the leakage of cerebrospinal fluid outside the cranial cavity. Whenever there is bleeding from the ears, nose, mouth, or scalp, the blood should be examined for spinal fluid content. Blood containing cerebrospinal fluid is usually watery, forms a pale outer ring when dripped onto a gauze sponge, and does not clot. High fever and nuchal rigidity call for diagnostic lumbar puncture. Abscess formation produces pressure symptoms similar to that of hematoma, except that seizures and localizing paresis are much more common.

Convulsive seizures occur infrequently after head injury. They are much more likely to occur in infants and children under 10 years of age. The seizures may be focal or generalized (grand mal) and usually denote cerebral contusion. Except in infants, subdural hematoma is rarely associated with seizures before treatment.

Progressive facial nerve paralysis occasionally follows basal skull fracture, and so it should be watched for in every patient with cerebrospinal fluid drainage from the ear. It begins 1 to 3 days after injury and may be partial and self-limited, or may progress to total loss of facial nerve function.

Supportive medical care

Vomiting is common during the first 8 hours after head injury, so that oral intake should be withheld during that period. Clear fluids may be given thereafter if the patient desires it, and solid food after 24 to 48 hours depending on the severity of the injury. If parenteral fluids are required, the volume administered during the first 48 hours should be somewhat less than the normal daily requirements—1,500 to 2,000 ml. for an average adult. Overhydration enhances cerebral edema. Feeding by nasogastric tube should be instituted if the patient is unable to swallow after 3 days.

Seizures must be vigorously treated with anticonvulsant drugs. Respiratory embarrassment accompanying convulsive seizures adds the insult of hypoxia to an already injured brain. Phenytoin (Dilantin) should be given intravenously in doses sufficient to establish and maintain a therapeutic serum level (1 to 2 mg.) rapidly. Meanwhile, individual seizures can be stopped by repeated intravenous injections of diazepam (Valium). Sedation should be avoided whenever possible, but the extremely restless, struggling, and vociferous patient should be quieted with small doses of chlorpromazine or other tranquilizing drugs rather than by the simple application of restraining bonds. Progressive facial nerve paralysis usually can be arrested by adrenal corticosteroids, but a complete paralysis may require surgical decompression of the nerve within its canal.

Attention to the care of the eyes, oropharynx, and respiratory and urinary tracts is essential to the prevention of ulcerative and infectious complications. The program for such supportive care is the same as that required after any major operation or trauma.

Phase III
Performance of special diagnostic tests

Traumatic intracranial hematomas are detected and delineated best by computerized tomography (CT scan). The scan may also indicate the degree of cerebral swelling. Therefore optimum evaluation and management planning for any patient who does not regain consciousness fully and rapidly after a head injury should include immediate unenhanced CT scanning. A CT scan may occasionally fail to detect a subdural hematoma that is the same density (isopycnic) as the adjacent brain. In those cases, a cerebral angiogram (Fig. 40-15) may be necessary to reveal the lesion. Certainly any patient whose level of responsiveness is reduced to or is near the critical level discussed previously or who develops a neurological deficit or fails to show satisfactory neurological improvement should have a CT scan or angiogram, or both.

Lumbar puncture is of no value except in the diagnosis of meningitis or gross subarachnoid hemorrhage. Subdural taps can be performed on infants, but only liquefied (chronic) hematomas can be aspirated through the small-bore needles used for such taps.

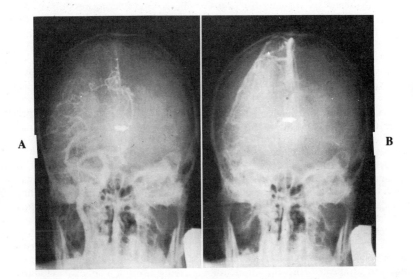

Fig. 40-15. Carotid angiogram demonstrating extracerebral hematoma. Arterial phase, **A,** shows surface arterioles to be displaced inward from inner surface of skull, leaving large avascular area. Anterior cerebral artery *(arrow)* is shifted to left of midline. Venous phase, **B,** shows same avascular area and shift to left of internal cerebral vein *(arrow).* If middle meningeal artery is visualized, subdural hematoma can be differentiated from epidural hematoma; in the former, artery lies in its normal position, whereas in the latter, it is displaced inward along with vessels on surface of brain. Artery is not visible in these photographs.

Phase IV
Nonsurgical treatment

The goal of definitive treatment is to alleviate increased intracranial pressure. Although the removal of a significant hematoma is mandatory, that alone may be insufficient to accomplish this goal if there is severe cerebral swelling. Nonsurgical decompressive aids may then be necessary if the patient is to derive practical benefit from the removal of the primary lesion. These aids are to be used only if a CT scan or angiogram has ruled out the presence of a major hematoma; their indiscriminate use before definitive diagnostic testing not only may mask the signs of a lesion that demands surgical removal but also, by reducing the tamponing effect of the brain adjacent to the hematoma, may *promote* further bleeding and expansion of the hematoma.

Two nonsurgical adjuvants are commonly utilized: the infusion of dehydrating agents and the administration of barbiturates in coma-inducing doses. Intravenously administered mannitol or urea usually produces considerable reductions of intracranial pressure. The degree and duration of this effect depends on the dosage and agent administered. When the effect has been exhausted, intracranial pressure tends to rise to a level even higher than that before the agent was given (rebound phenomenon). Hence the dose of mannitol or urea should be governed by intracranial pressure measurements monitored continuously by implanted sensors. Intravenous thiopental sodium given in high doses to induce and maintain the patient in a comatose state can also reduce intracranial pressure significantly; this technique is reserved for patients with prolonged, dangerous elevations of pressure that cannot be controlled by dehydrating agents. In patients whose respirations are inadequate to maintain at least a normal Pa_{CO_2} (Chapter 3), the intracranial pressure can be lowered when one paralyzes spontaneous respiration with curariform drugs (pancuronium bromide) and then ventilates the patient into a hypocapnic state with a mechanical respirator. High-potency adrenal corticosteroids (e.g., dexamethasone) may reduce the degree of cerebral edema, but their effectiveness in reducing the morbidity and mortality of head injuries has not been proved statistically. Their primary ability to reduce intracranial pressure is too delayed to be worthwhile in acute situations, but they do prolong the beneficial effects of dehydrating agents, and therefore their use as adjuvants to these agents is indicated. Because of the frequency of gastrointestinal hemorrhage in severe head injuries and the possible potentiation of this problem by adrenal corticosteroids, the prophylactic use of cimetidine is advisable. Furosemide also increases the effect of mannitol but, used alone, has minimal effect upon acutely elevated intracranial pressure.

Surgical treatment

Surgical management comprises the evacuation of hematomas, débridement of necrotic nonfunctional brain tissue, and extracerebral decompressive procedures. Chronic liquid hematomas can be drained through simple burr holes, whereas acute solid clots and necrotic brain require larger openings for effective removal. One can provide these by rongeuring the bone (craniectomy) or by removing a full bone flap. Additional decompression may be accomplished by the complete removal of large bone flaps and by sectioning of the tentorium to relieve direct pressure of the brainstem. The use of the latter procedures has largely been supplanted by the application of the nonsurgical adjuvants discussed previously.

In order for surgical treatment to be effective, one must choose an appropriate and adequate operation based upon the history, clinical findings, and the characteristics of the lesion as delineated by a CT scan or angiogram. Hence the patient should be treated in a neurosurgical facility. Although in very rare circumstances, a simple burr hole placed in the emergency room might provide a life-saving decompression of an acute intracranial hematoma, it is much more likely that such an undertaking will be futile and result in delay of transporting the patient to a proper facility for more definitive treatment.

Of special interest in the postoperative care of patients with subacute and chronic subdural hematomas is the high incidence of convulsive seizures. The risk is sufficiently great to warrant routine use of anticonvulsant medications for 3 to 6 months after operation.

Prognosis after head injury

Although the threat of serious or fatal complications attends every head injury, no matter how trivial, some general prognostications may be applied to the majority of patients, depending on their neurological findings immediately after injury. The capacity for neurological recovery is profoundly influenced by the age of the patient. An infant or child suffering a concussion with loss of consciousness for not more than a few minutes will usually be asymptomatic within 48 hours. The young and middle-aged adult often complains of postural headache and giddiness for perhaps a week or more, whereas the elderly patient is often mentally confused for days and complains of symptoms for weeks. Severe brainstem injury with decerebrate responses may be completely reversible in the child and young adult, though several months are required for recovery. With such an injury, chances of fatality are quite high in the middle-aged and even higher in the elderly.

If epidural hematoma is diagnosed and treated in time, complete recovery usually occurs. However, the younger age group sustaining this complication contributes to the low mortality and morbidity. Acute subdural hematoma is fatal in the majority of cases, even with immediate operation. Gross cerebral contusion that accompanies most of these hematomas contributes to high mortality. Chronic subdural hematomas can usually be satisfactorily treated, but the incidence of postoperative complications remains high.

Symptoms that cause varying degrees of prolonged or permanent disability may persist in many forms. The most obvious of these are motor deficits, e.g., hemiparesis and speech disturbances. However, there may be more subtle symptoms noticed by the patient and immediate family that are not easily recognized by the clinician. They include changes in affect and difficulties with cognition and concentration that can be attributed mistakenly to a posttraumatic neurosis. Psychometric testing may be necessary to prove organic brain dysfunction resulting from a head injury,

particularly if the injury appeared to have been mild.

SPINAL TRAUMA

Management of the spine-injured patient may be considered in the same four phases as described for craniocerebral injuries. It is directed toward achieving the following goals:

1. Relief of compression on the spinal cord and nerve roots
2. Prevention of additional trauma to neural elements until bony healing has taken place
3. Provision of conditions such that bony healing will result in permanent stability and satisfactory alignment

Phase I
Assessment of the type and severity of injury

The mechanism of injury, resultant neurological disability, and prognosis differ greatly depending on the level of injury. Table 40-3 lists the types of deficits with relation to the vertebral segments injured. Fracture-dislocations of the cervical spine (Figs. 40-16 and 40-17) usually result from acute hyperextension, e.g., a blow to the forehead or chin driving the head backward. Thus there may be significant craniocerebral injury associated with any cervical spine injury, and, in addition, *any injury to the head may be accompanied by damage*

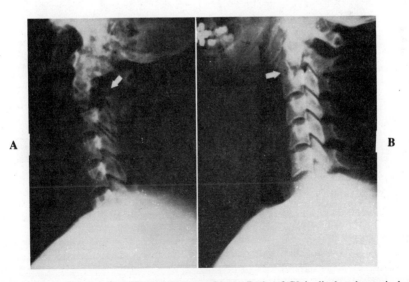

Fig. 40-16. Fracture-dislocation of C2 anteriorly on C3. **A,** Body of C2 is displaced anteriorly, and pedicles are fractured *(arrow)*. **B,** Dislocation has been reduced by traction and anterior interbody fusion performed with insertion of bone graft *(arrow)*.

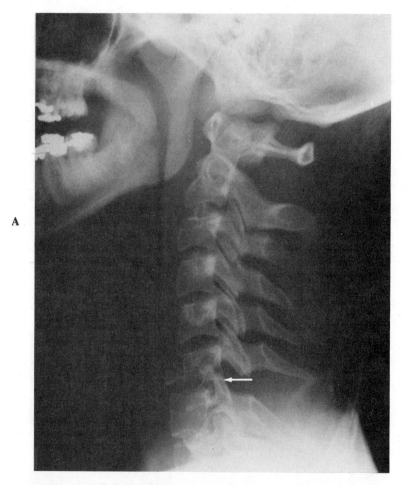

Fig. 40-17. A, Severe fracture-dislocation C6-C7. Body of C6 has sheared, leaving inferior portion aligned with C7 while superior portion is dislocated and its posterior edge, *arrow,* projects dangerously into spinal canal.

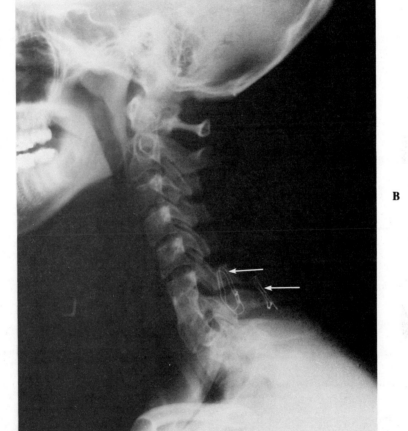

B

Fig. 40-17, cont'd. B, Open reduction was required; spinous processes and laminae of C6 and C7 were wired together, *arrows,* and disrupted vertebral body was replaced with iliac crest graft. This picture 1 year after injury shows solid C6-C7 fusion with no vertebral bone encroaching on spinal canal. Despite severity of dislocation this patient was neurologically intact.

Table 40-3. Clinical picture after injury to the spinal cord and cauda equina

Vertebral segment	Neurological segment	Paralysis resulting from physiological transection	
		Partial transection	*Complete transection*
C1-C4	Spinal cord, cervical plexus level	Quadriparesis, becoming spastic*; Brown-Séquard syndrome	Instant or early death from respiratory failure
C5-T1	Spinal cord, brachial plexus level	Quadriparesis, becoming spastic; Brown-Séquard syndrome	Quadriplegia, becoming spastic
T2-T10	Dorsal spinal cord	Paraparesis, becoming spastic; Brown-Séquard syndrome	Paraplegia, becoming spastic
T11-L1	Conus medullaris	Flaccid or spastic paraparesis	Flaccid or spastic paraplegia
L2-S1	Cauda equina	Flaccid paraparesis	Flaccid paraplegia
Sacrococcygeal	Filum terminale	No deficit	No deficit

*Paresis or paralysis is always flaccid in the acute phase.

to the cervical spine. The thoracic and lumbar spines are more often damaged by hyperflexion (Fig. 40-18).

As in craniocerebral trauma, the spinal injury is considered from two aspects, the neurological and the vertebral:

```
Neurological
   Concussion        ⎫
   Contusion         ⎬  Spinal cord, nerve roots
   Compression       ⎪
   Hematomyelia      ⎭
Vertebral
   Compression          Vertebral body
                     ⎧ Laminal arch (with or
                     ⎪    without dislocation)
   Linear fracture   ⎨ Spinous process (with or
                     ⎪    without dislocation)
                     ⎪ Pedicle (with or without
                     ⎩    dislocation)
Dislocation
   without fracture
```

Description of the injury should include the level of the injury, assessment of major motor and sensory functions, and the bony lesion, e.g., complete paraplegia with motor and sensory loss to the T6 dermatome, fracture of pedicles of T5, with anterior dislocation of T5 on T6.

Concussion and contusion denote the same gross pathological changes as in the brain. Hemorrhage into the substance of the cord may be petechial or localized into a hematoma (hematomyelia). Subdural and epidural hematomas sufficient to produce significant compression are so rare in the spinal canal that they are not of practical importance.

Unfortunately, the neurological picture is frequently that of complete bilateral cord transection.

Table 40-4. Clinical syndromes of partial spinal cord damage

Portion of cord involved	Neurological picture
Central core	Severe paresis at level of injury only, with relatively intact motor and sensory functions below that level
Anterior half	Bilateral paresis and loss of pain and temperature sensation, with relative preservation of touch, position, vibration senses below level of injury
Lateral half	Ipsilateral paresis with contralateral loss of pain and temperature sensations below level of injury (Brown-Séquard syndrome)
Whole cord	Partial loss of all motor and sensory functions to approximately equal degree below level of injury

There is usually a band of hyperesthesia at the dermatomal level of injury, with complete loss of all motor power and sensation, autonomic function (anhydrosis and paralytic ileus), and reflexes below this level. This is the picture of *spinal shock*. Autonomic activity returns in 48 to 72 hours and reflexes in 1 to 5 weeks. Paralysis of voluntary movement is permanent, but hyperactivity of reflexes often leads to severe spasms in paralyzed muscles. Lesser degrees of functional deficits are shown in Table 40-4.

Compression fractures of the vertebral body and linear fractures of laminae and spinous processes are generally not associated with neurological deficit. Fractures of the pedicle are usually accom-

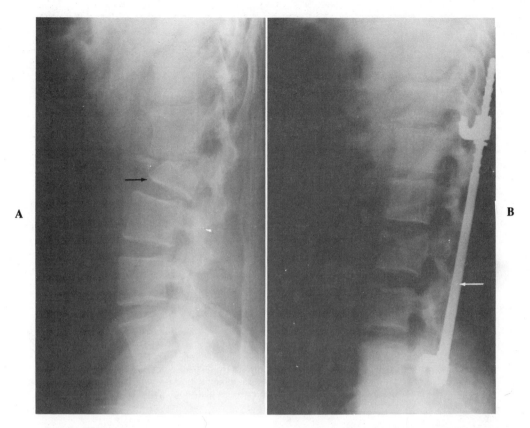

Fig. 40-18. Compression fracture of L2. **A,** Body of L2 has been severely compressed anteriorly *(arrow)* angulating spine forward at L1-L2 junction, stretching and compressing cauda equina. **B,** Normal alignment and vertebral height have been restored surgically by distraction and levering of vertebrae with implanted Harrington rods *(arrow)*.

panied by dislocation and frequently result in neural damage, depending on the extent to which the spinal canal is narrowed. Gross dislocations of the vertebral bodies are still compatible with cord function if fractured laminal arches separate from the bodies so that the spinal cord is not acutely squeezed. Occasionally, severe deficits are present in the absence of any visible bony abnormality. In such cases acute herniation of the intervertebral disk may cause compression of the cord.

In assessing the bony damage radiologically, the patient should be moved as little as possible. In cervical spine injuries the *neck must be protected* against movement at all times until the vertebral alignment has been defined. This is accomplished best by placement of heavy sandbags on each side of the head. If the patient must be moved from the transporting stretcher, his head should be *supported in a neutral position,* preferably with slight *traction.*

Performance of emergency procedures

Any dislocation of cervical vertebrae, with or without associated neurological deficit, requires the immediate application of skull tongs (Gardner-Wells, Crutchfield, or similar type) or wires for skeletal traction (Fig. 40-19). *Halter traction is unsatisfactory and dangerous to life in any patient with upper limb paresis.* The halter may asphyxiate, and the patient with paresis may not have sufficient strength to adjust or remove it. In most instances proper alignment can be restored with traction alone. Traction is begun with 10 to 15 pounds, and weight is added successively as indicated by progress roentgenograms or fluoroscopic monitoring until reduction has been accomplished. Realignment usually occurs with 25 to 35 pounds of traction and can be maintained with 10 to 15 pounds during the period required for bone healing.

Cervical dislocations above C6 associated with

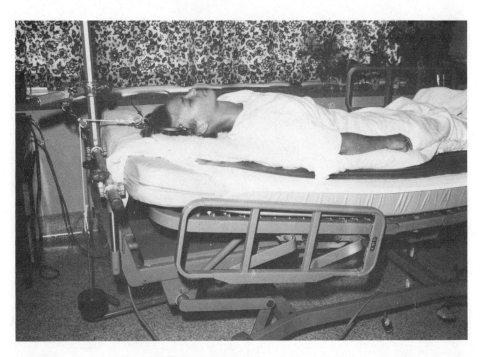

Fig. 40-19. Skeletal traction for dislocation of cervical spine. Gardner-Wells tongs *(arrow)* have been inserted into patient's skull, and traction has been applied by suspension of weights on pulley at head of bed. Position of head required to maintain vertebral alignment varies with individual features of dislocation. Patient is lying on automatic alternating pressure mattress, controlled by motor located at foot of bed.

gross neurological deficit may produce respiratory insufficiency from paresis of intercostal muscles and diaphragm. Tracheostomy plus the assistance of a mechanical respirator may be necessary.

Little can be done initially to restore the alignment after fracture dislocation in the thoracic and lumbar vertebrae except by open operation. Since most of these fractures are the result of hyperflexion, the patient should be placed in bed on soft supports so that the spine is slightly extended. Pelvic traction is of no value.

If the patient is unable to urinate without leaving a significant residual, an indwelling catheter should be placed and drainage established.

Phase II
Observation of progress and supportive medical care

The development of secondary compressive hematomas is so rare after spinal trauma that it is not the major consideration that it is after head injury. However, lack of neurological improvement and certainly any progressive deterioration of function may be indications for surgical exploration and decompression.

Paralytic ileus constantly accompanies paralysis of the limbs, so that oral intake should be withheld until there is evidence of return of good bowel activity. The normal daily requirement of fluids should be given parenterally.

Care of the skin is a major nursing problem in patients who are unable to change position in bed. Decubiti rapidly develop over the sacrum and heels. Use of revolving frame beds, e.g., oscillator, Foster, Stryker, etc., and of the alternating pressure mattress aid in the frequent redistribution of pressure on different areas of skin.

Phase III
Special diagnostic procedures

Evaluation of the degree of pressure on the spinal cord or nerve roots is accomplished best by high-resolution CT scanning through the levels of vertebral injury or the clinical levels of cord injury. Vertebral bodies are frequently comminuted, a fact that cannot be detected by normal roentgenographic techniques, and fracture fragments may project posteriorly, impinging upon neural elements. Soft-tissue projections such as acutely herniated disks can be demonstrated by intrathecal

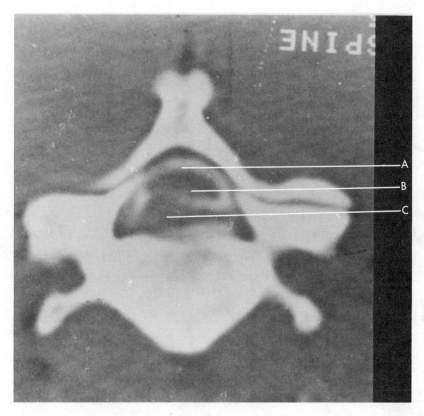

Fig. 40-20. High-resolution computerized tomogram showing compression of cervical cord by herniated disk. Subarachnoid space, *A,* is enhanced by intrathecal instillation of metrizamide. Spinal cord, *B,* is distorted and displaced posteriorly by large fragment of disk extruded into spinal canal, *C.*

contrast enhancement (Fig. 40-20). It should be emphasized that the pathological states revealed by these imaging techniques *do not always require surgical treatment.* The indications for surgical intervention must be determined by the clinician based upon the history, clinical findings, and the roentgenological findings.

Phase IV

Nonsurgical treatment

Contusion and laceration of the spinal cord are accompanied by reactive edema as in brain injuries. Therefore adrenal corticosteroids (dexamethasone) and dehydrating agents (mannitol) may be administered immediately to patients having neurological evidence of spinal cord damage. Because the occurrence of clinically significant hematomas is rare, these nonsurgical adjuncts can be given by the first treating physician before transfer to a neurosurgical facility.

A fractured spine, like any fractured bone, re-
quires approximately 6 weeks of immobilization to heal strongly. Unstable cervical fractures can be immobilized by skeletal traction (Fig. 40-19) or in the ambulatory patient by means of a portable halo traction. After the initial period of healing, a less restrictive support such as a plastic collar can be fitted. Periodic roentgenological checks should be made to detect any subsequent dislocation. Lateral roentgenograms taken with the neck in flexion and then in extension are used to determine the degree of stability or instability. Prolonged immobilization is hazardous to the elderly because of the rapid development of pulmonary complications. Thoracic and lumbar injuries may be mobilized in a body cast or braces. These protective devices are worn for an additional 6 weeks to 3 months.

Surgical treatment

Internal decompression of neural elements is accomplished initially by realignment of dislocated vertebrae. Posterior decompression by removal of

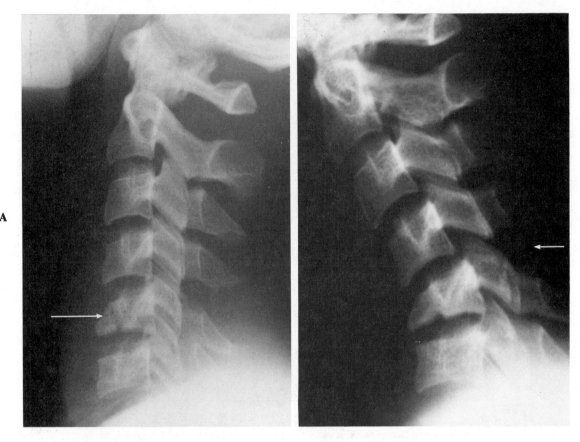

Fig. 40-21. Compression fracture with progressive angulation. **A,** Body of C5, *arrow,* was crushed in diving accident. Alignment was restored by traction and patient immobilized in a halo cast. **B,** Six weeks later, roentgenogram shows anterior angulation has developed because of weakness of C5 vertebral body and rupture of posterior interspinous ligaments, *arrow.*

the laminar arches may also be necessary, particularly when a dislocation is not correctable, e.g., thoracic and lumbar regions. Therefore injuries below T1 associated with neurological deficits and a manometric block on Queckenstedt maneuver are usually treated by decompression and stabilization, even though the chances for functional recovery may be small. Local hypothermia applied directly to the injured segment of spinal cord was shown to be greatly beneficial in the experimental animal, but its efficacy in humans has not been proved.

Operative interbody fusion in cervical fracture-dislocations accomplishes (1) the removal of a possibly herniated and compressing intervertebral disk, (2) much earlier mobilization and discharge from the hospital, and (3) a guarantee, barring complications, of achieving a permanently stable spine. The procedure may be undertaken as soon as the patient has recovered from the immediate constitutional effects of trauma, and ambulation may be begun within 2 weeks of operation. Anterior interbody fusion is applicable to all dislocations between C2 and T1. It is frequently necessary when there has been pronounced subluxation without major fracturing, for while a fracture reunites with strong new bone formation, interspinous ligamentous tears heal poorly and chronic instability is a common result. Simple compression fractures of the cervical vertebrae may heal satisfactorily in 6 to 8 weeks with an external supportive brace, but if the vertebral body has lost too much of its interior structure by shattering and compression, a late progressive gibbus (anterior angulation) may form (Fig. 40-21) and it can result in myelopathy. In such cases, replacement of the damaged body with an iliac crest or rib strut graft bridging to normal bone

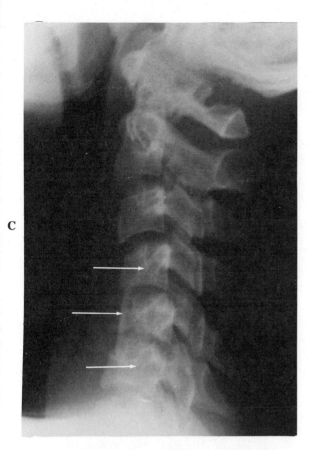

C

Fig. 40-21, cont'd. C, Central portion of C5 was resected and a strut graft used to bridge C4 to C6, *arrows,* and restore good alignment. Once healed, C4, C5, and C6 become one solid block of bone.

will restore and maintain satisfactory alignment until a strong bony fusion has taken place. Odontoid fractures and chronically unstable thoracic and lumbar fracture-dislocations can be fused by use of interlaminar or interpedicular struts. Operative interlaminar fusions in thoracic and lumbar fracture-dislocations carry the same advantages as cervical fusions, plus more accurate restoration of alignment and the prevention of a gibbus, which can progress years after the injury.

Prognosis for recovery after spinal injuries

The prognosis for neurological recovery varies with the neurological segment injured and the severity of the initial deficit. If there is immediate loss of all motor and sensory function below the level of injury, the chances for functional recovery are extremely small regardless of the promptness and type of treatment. Unfortunately, a high percentage of spinal injuries result in immediate functional cord transection with permanent loss of cord function. Any preservation of neurological function alters the prognosis from one of almost complete hopelessness to one of possible, if partial, recovery. Complete recovery is rare with spinal cord injuries but occurs not infrequently when the cauda equina is the only area damaged. Death may ensue early or late as the result of pulmonary or urinary tract infection, especially after cervical cord transection.

The permanently paraplegic patient can usually be rehabilitated to an economically useful life. For some, crutch walking can be accomplished with external bracing of the legs, but for most the wheelchair is the only method of locomotion. The complete quadriplegic is usually a permanent invalid, incapable of gainful employment despite the availability of prosthetic aids.

PERIPHERAL NERVE INJURIES

In contrast to the central nervous system pathways, the peripheral nerves are always capable of regrowth and reestablishment of neural connections after they have been traumatized or severed. The goal of surgical treatment is to provide the best possible conditions for the transected nerve to reestablish its connections with muscles and skin. Without the most optimum conditions, neuronal regrowth may be blocked, retarded, or disorganized and may result in incomplete or ineffective reinnervation.

Pathological changes after injury

Trauma to a peripheral nerve sufficient to produce clinically recognizable denervation may be accompanied by pathological changes both proximal and distal to the site of injury. *Proximally* there is central chromatolysis *(axonal reaction)* in the cells of origin in the central nervous system; this is a temporary change and is reversible. *Distally* there is *wallerian degeneration,* which once begun, is irreversible and continues until all axonal debris is removed. Within 4 to 6 days after the onset of wallerian degeneration, the nerve can no longer be made to conduct an electrical stimulus, so that direct stimulation of the nerve trunk through a needle electrode results in no contraction of the muscles that nerve normally innervates.

Axonal regrowth begins within 48 hours. If a proper pathway is available, regrowth proceeds at a rate of 1 to 1.5 mm. per day until the target (muscle or skin) has been reached. If such a pathway is blocked, the axons curl back upon themselves, forming a heaped-up tangle of fibers called a *neuroma.* Although no recognizable degenerative changes occur in denervated skin, loss of tonus and fiber size occurs in denervatd muscle. The latter is most noticeable in the first 6 weeks after injury. If denervation is prolonged, the muscle becomes progressively replaced with fibrous tissue until it can no longer contract effectively even when stimulated directly. Thus, if effective reinnervation is to occur, the nerve must make contact with its muscle before too much fibrosis has occurred.

Using the foregoing principles, one can calculate the potential for effective treatment of most nerve injuries. Given a minimum neuronal regrowth of *1 mm. per day* or *1 inch per month,* and considering that a muscle remaining denervated for more than 1 year may be extensively fibrosed, then if a nerve is severed more than 1 foot proximal to its muscles, the potential for good functional motor recovery is poor. Furthermore, if, for example, a nerve is severed 9 inches proximal to its muscles but the lesion is neglected or goes undiagnosed for 6 months, a late anastomosis may not restore good function. Thus, although it may be prudent to delay exploration in cases in which the anatomical continuity of a nerve is believed to be preserved, *too long a delay may result in missing the opportunity for functional reinnervation.* There are, of course, exceptions to these mathematical calculations, and so they may not be used as absolute criteria to determine whether surgery is indicated.

Management

The management of peripheral nerve injuries will be considered according to the three types of lesions encountered: stretching, compression and contusion, and laceration.

Stretch injuries affect principally the brachial plexus and, to a lesser extent, the sciatic nerve. A downward blow on the shoulder or falling and landing on the shoulder in such a way that it is forced downward put sudden tension on the roots and trunks of the brachial plexus. Axis cylinders may be ruptured, and the roots may be avulsed from the spinal cord. the result almost invariably is permanent loss of function. Management consists only in placing the limb in such a position that there will be minimal tension on the plexus, i.e., arm abducted 90 degrees and supported by an airplane splint. Myelography may be performed as soon as the patient can tolerate the maneuvers required without undue discomfort; extravasation of contrast medium at the site of an avulsed root is diagnostic. The lesion (Fig. 40-22) is untreatable. Posterior *dislocation of the hip* may result in stretching of the sciatic nerve over the head of the femur; other nerves may occasionally be stretched over the fractured ends of long bones. Surgical treatment of the stretch injury is most unsatisfactory because it is impossible to determine by gross inspection how long a segment of nerve has been damaged. Furthermore, such injuries in the brachial plexus and sciatic nerve at the hip are located so far proximal to denervated muscles that even if regeneration occurs, it cannot reinnervate muscles before extensive fibrosis has occurred.

Compression and contusion most commonly affect nerves that are relatively superficial and not protected by thick layers of muscle. The ulnar nerve at the elbow and the superficial peroneal nerve at the neck of the fibula are such examples. Severe crushing trauma may injure any nerve trunk. There are three possible pathological courses after peripheral nerve compression and contusion:

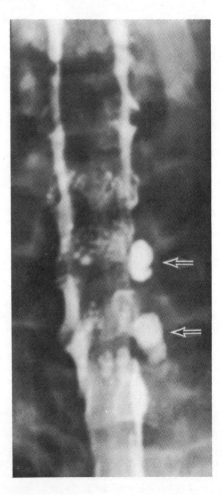

Fig. 40-22. Cervical myelogram showing extravasation of contrast media at site of avulsed C7 and C8 nerve roots *(arrows).*

1. No wallerian degeneration—functional recovery within 2 to 6 weeks regardless of the distance from site of injury to denervated muscle or skin
2. Wallerian degeneration without significant internal fibrosis—regeneration and functional recovery after a delay consistent with the distance as calculated by distance from injury to muscle or skin ÷ rate of regrowth
3. Wallerian degeneration followed by significant internal fibrosis—formation of a neuroma-in-continuity (Fig. 40-23); partial reinnervation only, regardless of length of time elapsed

When there is no reason to suspect that a nerve has been severed (no penetrating wound, no fractured bone ends that might lacerate a nerve), management entails following the patient's course with frequent neurological examination to determine whether regeneration is occurring. Paresthesias referred to the peripheral distribution of a nerve when the nerve is lightly percussed *(Tinel's sign)* indicate the most distal end of the regenerating nerve. If the sign can be elicited more than 2 inches beyond the point of injury, recovery will be likely to occur without surgical intervention. Electromyography is useful in detecting early reinnervation. If after 6 weeks there is no evidence of reinnervation or regeneration, exploration is indicated. If a significant neuroma is present with no electrical conduction distal to it, resection and anastomosis should be performed.

Laceration or transection of a peripheral nerve may be produced by penetrating foreign bodies or internally by the jagged ends of fractured long bones. Whenever such an injury occurs, neurological function must be evaluated accurately and any deficit pointed out to the patient. The importance of the latter lies in the fact that surgical treatment of some kind is usually necessary in the treatment of associated injuries to bones, muscles, and tendons, so that a neurological deficit that is not pointed out before such surgery may be blamed on the surgical procedure rather than on the injury. A clean field free of potential infection is a strict requirement for the anastomosis of a transected nerve. Most open wounds do not fulfill this requirement, and therefore emergency nerve repair is seldom indicated. Apposition of the lacerated ends with one or two sutures prevents their retraction and also facilitates identification at the time of definitive anastomosis. Such wounds should be debrided thoroughly and closed, and anastomosis should be delayed until clean healing has occurred. However, although it is prudent to wait whenever the sterility of a wound is in doubt, there is *equal disadvantage in waiting too long,* particularly when the site of transection is nearly a foot proximal to denervated muscles, for reasons stated previously. Anastomosis can be performed by use of suture or various adhesives. Fresh cuts are made until healthy nerve ends are bared; the nerve trunk proximally and distally may be mobilized with its mesoneurium or transplanted in order to bring the

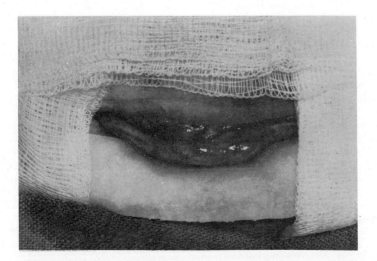

Fig. 40-23. Neuroma-in-continuity. Ulnar nerve in patient who fell on her elbow 6 months before operation and developed partial paralysis of interossei with preservation of all other ulnar nerve functions. Nerve is expanded to double its normal diameter by neuroma.

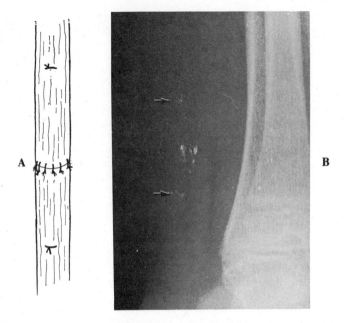

Fig. 40-24. Peripheral nerve anastomosis. **A,** Radiopaque suture is placed through the epineurium on each side of line of anastomosis. Postoperative roentgenogram, **B,** reveals these marking sutures to be approximately equidistant from anastomosis. Separation of nerve ends is diagnosed if marking sutures become separated.

ends together without tension. Marking the ends with radiopaque sutures through the epineurium provides a useful method of checking to see that they have not separated postoperatively (Fig. 40-24).

INTRACRANIAL NEOPLASMS

The morbidity and mortality potentials of an intracranial neoplasm differ from those of tumors elsewhere in the body. Local compression and invasion are as important to the prognosis as the histological picture. Therefore the anatomical localization of a tumor is all-important in the clinical diagnosis. A histologically benign tumor may inevitably be fatal if it is so located that surgical removal cannot be undertaken without undue risk of operative death or the production of an incapacitating neurological deficit. The histologically malignant neoplasms spread infrequently within the subarachnoid space and very rarely outside the central nervous system. They cause death by invading or compressing vital centers.

The symptoms of intracranial neoplasms are of three types:

1. Increased intracranial pressure—headache, lethargy, vomiting

2. Local or neighboring compression and invasion—paralysis and sensory loss

3. Local irritation—convulsive seizures

Persistent headache, often accompanied by subtle changes in mental behavior and by vomiting, indictes abnormal pressure rather than common migraine or nervous tension headaches. The progressive onset of neurological deficit distinguishes neoplasm from cerebrovascular accident with its sudden ictus. Convulsions, especially focal or jacksonian, beginning in adult life are suggestive of neoplasm rather than idiopathic epilepsy.

Objective neurological findings depend on the size, location, and rapidity of growth of the tumor. A slowly growing neoplasm, located at some distance from the sensorimotor cortex, may attain great size before producing recognizable neurological signs other than those of generalized increased intracranial pressure. On the other hand, a small irritative lesion growing within the sensorimotor cortex may produce localized seizures and paresis long before there are any symptoms or signs of increased intracranial pressure.

Any of the foregoing symptoms coupled with any objective neurological abnormality is sufficient to warrant investigation for brain tumor. In certain

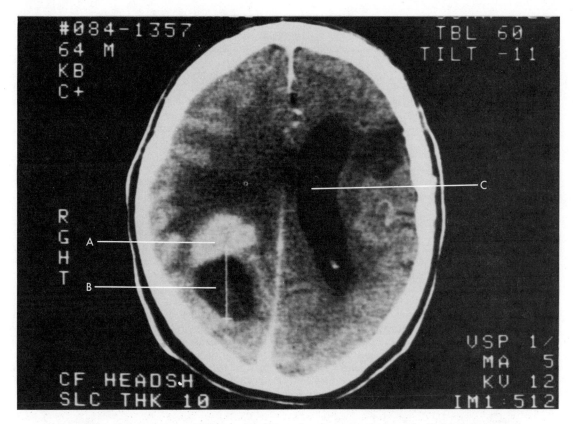

Fig. 40-25. Contrast-enhanced CT scan showing cystic astrocytoma in the parietal lobe. Solid portion of neoplasm, *A*, enhances densely with meglumine diatrizoate. Fluid within cyst, *B*, is slightly more dense than ventricular fluid, *C*.

situations such investigations may be called for in the absence of any recognizable deficit. When it is reasonable to suspect the presence of a brain tumor, the most expeditious and definitive method is by contrast-enhanced CT scanning (Figs. 40-4 and 40-25). If that diagnostic mode is not available in the community, a radioisotope scan (Fig. 40-3, *B*) may disclose the tumor, but the test frequently can miss small or avascular neoplasms. If there is a known history of allergy to iodinated contrast media, a noninvasive study such as a nuclear magnetic resonance scan may be necessary to supplement the unenhanced computerized tomogram.

A classification of more commonly encountered neoplasms is given on the right. For a detailed classification and description of all tumors, refer to textbooks of neuropathology. Only the clinical aspects of the common tumor are discussed here. Those tumors listed in the *plural* occur with varying histological types and grades of differentiation.

Neuroepithelial
  Astrocytoma, grades I, II, III, and IV
  Ependymomas
  Oligodendrogliomas
  Medulloblastoma
  Pinealoma
  Papilloma of choroid plexus
  Paraphyseal (colloid) cyst
  Neurilemoma
Mesodermal
  Meningiomas
  Hemangioblastoma
  Chordoma
Ectodermal
  Craniopharyngioma
  Pituitary adenomas
Congenital
  Epidermoid
  Dermoid

The age of the patient and the anatomical location of the lesion are of considerable importance in allowing prediction of the type of neoplasm. Infants and children under the age of 2 years rarely develop intracranial neoplasms. Up to the age of 15 years, tumors most often arise in the *cerebellum*. Of these, medulloblastoma and cystic astrocytoma comprise the majority. The highly malignant *medulloblastoma* occurs in the cerebellar vermis (disequilibrium) and blocks the outlets of the fourth ventricle (headache, vomiting from obstructive hydrocephalus). Removal of sufficient tissue to unblock the ventricular system followed by radiation therapy is the usual method of treatment. Total surgical removal is impossible because of the infiltrative propensity of the tumor, and although the neoplasm is highly radiosensitive, complete eradication cannot be achieved. It frequently spreads in the subarachnoid space, producing secondary implants along the spinal neuraxis. Survival ranges from 1 to 15 years. The *cystic astrocytoma* occurs in the cerebellar hemisphere (limb ataxia) and later obstructs the fourth ventricle (headache, vomiting). The tumor consists of a large cyst containing xanthochromic fluid (Fig. 40-26) and a small nubbin of solid neoplasm. If this nubbin is resected completely, as it frequently can be, permanent cure results. Tumors of the cerebral hemisphere are less frequent in children, but when they occur, they are likely to be *ependymomas*. These tumors are moderately radiosensitive; therefore as much of the mass as possible is resected, followed by radiation therapy. Recurrence and death within 2 to 3 years are to be expected.

Of the remaining supratentorial tumors of children, *craniopharyngioma* deserves mention. This tumor, rising above the optic chiasm, is very often partially calcified, so that the combination of visual field defect, optic atrophy, and suprasellar calcium deposits provides an almost definitive diagnosis. Complete resection and cures have been reported, but temporary relief by decompression and radiation is frequently all that can be accomplished.

The 30- to 60-year age group produces the largest group of primary neoplasms, most of which are cerebral hemisphere malignancies with survival prognoses of less than 5 years. The *astrocytomas*, particularly the most malignant *glioblastoma* (Fig. 40-27), are the most frequently found lesions. They occur anywhere in the hemispheres, so that the signs and symptoms are dependent on the anatomical location. If the neoplasm is located at the pole of a hemisphere, radical resection with lobectomy may be accomplished, whereas if it is located close to or in the sensorimotor cortex, only a limited excision and external decompression are possible. The neoplasms may infiltrate extensively (Fig. 40-28) and, when located near the midline, tend to cross to the opposite hemisphere via the corpus callosum; therefore recurrence and eventual death of the patient are invariable, even with the most

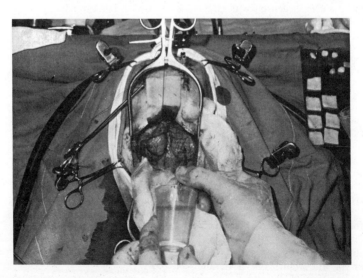

Fig. 40-26. Suboccipital craniectomy for cystic tumor of right cerebellar hemisphere. Cerebellar hemispheres are exposed, and their tonsils are seen herniated downward into cervical canal, right tonsil being larger than left. Cannula has been introduced into right hemisphere and about 25 ml. of fluid is drained off, resulting in collapse of hemisphere. Fluid is usually xanthochromic and often will clot on standing.

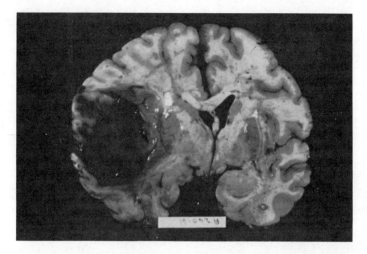

Fig. 40-27. Astrocytoma grade IV (glioblastoma multiforme). Tumor is often hemorrhagic. Its gross demarcation from surrounding brain tissue may appear fairly distinct at times, but microscopic examination will show invasion. Therefore, curative resection is not possible.

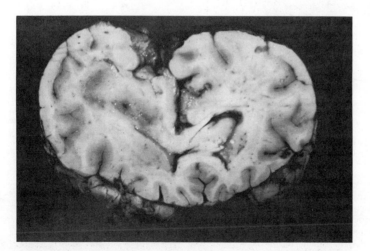

Fig. 40-28. Diffusely infiltrating frontal astrocytoma. Tumor blends imperceptibly with surrounding brain tissue and microscopically infiltrates brain. At operation, it is impossible to determine extent of tumor by gross inspection.

radical resections. The effects of radiotherapy are, at best, moderately palliative; noticeable clinical improvement directly attributable to radiation is seen only infrequently. Chemotherapy with cytotoxic agents has resulted in some increases in postoperative survival, but like radiotherapy the effect in most cases is moderate and not curative.

The most common benign tumor in adulthood is the *meningioma* (Figs. 40-29 and 40-30). A majority of meningiomas occur close to the midline, over the vault, or along the sphenoid wing. In the former position they are closely related to the superior longitudinal sinus and the falx cerebri, and they may invade the sinus or produce hyperostosis of the overlying bone. Focal or jacksonian seizures of months' or years' duration with a slowly developing paresis are typical of this tumor. Total removal can usually be accomplished, but because many of these slow-growing neoplasms reach a large size before they produce symptoms (Fig. 40-4), extensive and permanent structural changes, which may result in significant postoperative morbidity, can occur preoperatively.

Neoplasms of the pituitary gland are common. They may be hormonally active, secreting prolactin (galactorrhea, infertility), ACTH (Cushing's syndrome), or growth hormone (gigantism, acromegaly). These neoplasms are usually small and

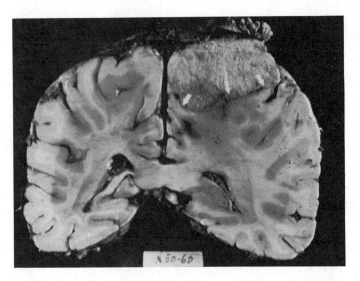

Fig. 40-29. Parasagittal meningioma. Tumor may arise from falx or from convexity and may invade superior longitudinal sinus. It does not invade brain tissue but slowly compresses it inferolaterally.

Fig. 40-30. Convexity meningioma. When tumor arises from convexity and has wide base, it can be removed from its bed in one piece, with it attached to dural flap. Since dura is invaded, flap to which tumor is attached is excised widely. Brain may then be covered with graft of tissue such as pericranium, or bone may simply be replaced over cortex.

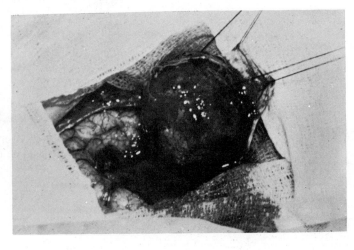

contained within the sella turcica; they can be resected microsurgically by a nasal approach through the sphenoid sinus, or radiated as a primary or postoperative treatment, if necessary. Prolactin-secreting lesions can also be treated medically by use of bromocriptine mesylate. The hormonally inactive pituitary adenoma commonly grows upward out of the sella (Fig. 40-31), compressing the optic nerves and chiasm to produce a characteristic visual field defect (bitemporal hemianopsia) that is the hallmark of this neoplasm. When the tumor is small, it can be resected by the transsphenoidal route or treated by radiation; large tumors may require intracranial resection for ad-

equate and precise decompression of the optic nerves.

The *acoustic neurilemoma* arises from the intracranial portion of the eight cranial nerve and produces tinnitus, loss of hearing, and ataxia of the limbs. This symptom complex, called the *cerebellopontine angle* syndrome, may include impairment of adjacent cranial nerves (fifth and seventh). Complete removal is difficult, except in small tumors, and may result in paralysis of the facial nerve that is intimately associated with the tumor capsule.

Above 50 years of age, the possibility of *metastatic carcinoma* must always be considered in the

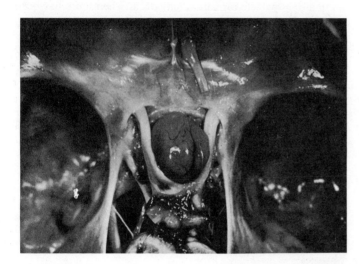

Fig. 40-31. Pituitary adenoma. Having ruptured through diaphragma sellae, tumor balloons upward between optic nerves, stretching them as well as optic chiasm to produce characteristic bitemporal hemianopsia.

Fig. 40-32. Bilateral metastatic neoplasms. Multiplicity of metastases is unfortunate common characteristic. Lesions are grossly quite well demarcated in most instances. They often produce pronounced swelling of white matter. This patient had bronchogenic carcinoma.

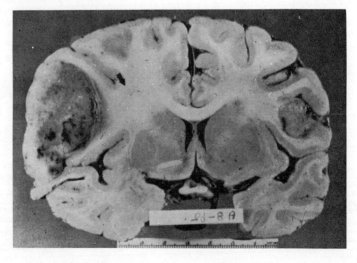

differential diagnosis of any intracranial expanding lesion. The metastases are frequently multiple (Fig. 40-32). In the male the most common source is the lung; in the female the breast is the usual source. A metastasis may become evident months or even years after the primary lesion has been removed; it may be solitary, particularly with hypernephroma, and surgical removal may extend the life expectancy and has even resulted in apparent cures. Despite the ominous prognosis of metastatic carcinoma in the brain, one should not abandon hopes for worthwhile palliation. Surgical removal of any solitary intracranial metastasis may be worthwhile in selected cases, provided, of course, that there are no other known secondaries elsewhere in the body. In most instances a metastatic lesion excites considerable edema in the surrounding white matter. This edema can be overcome with high doses of dexamethasone and may result in dramatic symptomatic improvement. Hormone-dependent carcinomas of the breast and bowel carcinomas that have previously responded to chemotherapy may produce metastases that are sensitive to a combination of hormonal agents and cytotoxic chemicals. With a proper selection of modes of treatment, these unfortunate patients can be offered several months or even years of additional comfortable life. Therefore they should not be abandoned to die untreated simply because of the known presence of metastatic or recurrent malignant disease.

INTRASPINAL NEOPLASMS

Neoplasms within the spinal canal produce symptoms and signs by compression of the adjacent spinal cord or nerve roots and by obstruction of the blood supply to the cord. The patient complains of progressive weakness, clumsiness, or numbness of the extremities below the lesion. If a nerve root is involved, there may be pain radiating out into the dermatomal distribution of that root. In these respects the set of symptoms mimics that of vertebral spondylosis and herniated intervertebral disk. Spinal cord compression per se produces no pain, and loss of specific sensations is often not noticed by the patient.

Tumors involving the spinal cord almost invariably produce recognizable neurological signs *bilaterally* by the time the patient is aware of any deficit. The small diameter of the cord makes it practically impossible for any mass lesion to produce compressive damage to one side only. Therefore, when the findings on examination are strictly unilateral, cord tumor is an unlikely diagnosis. The exact level of compression cannot be established reliably by clinical examination, for paresis and sensory loss do not necessarily extend up to the level of tumor; e.g., a tumor at C5 may produce paresis and sensory loss only to the T4 dermatomal segment. Only in the later stages, when function has been greatly impaired, does the neurological level correlate with the anatomical site of the lesion.

Lumbar puncture with the Queckenstedt maneuver is indicated in all cases, preferably with facilities for immediate myelographic study. Whenever possible, puncture should be performed below and as far away from the lesion as possible. When the needle is inserted below the lesion, varying degrees of block may be shown on jugular compression, and the spinal fluid protein is usually elevated. The color of the spinal fluid should be noted carefully; slight xanthochromia is frequently present, and pellicle formation may occur when there has been long-standing obstruction.

Definitive diagnosis is established by myelography (Figs. 40-6 and 40-33), computerized tomography, and nuclear magnetic resonance scanning. Clinical differentiation between the various types of tumors is difficult and not of practical value to the student. Early recognition of the presence of an intraspinal mass is important, for the sooner the mass is removed, the more rapid and complete will be the neurological recovery. Operation performed after the patient has lost all cord function below the lesion stands little chance of producing worthwhile, if any, neurological recovery.

The common types of tumors are classified as follows:

Intradural
  Intramedullary
    Ependymoma
    Astrocytoma
  Extramedullary
    Primary
      Meningioma
      Neurofibroma
    Secondary
      Medulloblastoma (seeding from cerebellar tumor)
Extradural
  Primary
    Bone tumors
  Secondary
    Carcinomas (from prostate, lung, breast, gastrointestinal tract)
    Lymphoma
    Myeloma

Neoplasms within the cord substance (intramedullary) can be removed microsurgically. However, decompressive laminectomy followed by radiation may be the only treatment possible in some cases. The meningioma and neurofibroma can almost always be totally excised, with excellent neurological results. Metastatic extradural

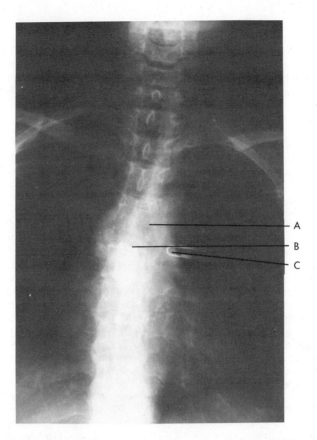

Fig. 40-33. Myelogram showing typical extradural compressive mass. Body of T5 is compressed, and pedicles have been eroded away, *A.* Pantopaque introduced from below passes up to T5 and stops abruptly with irregular cut-off, *B,* indicating extradural block. Paper clip, *C,* has been taped to patient's skin to mark lower level of obstruction.

neoplasms are seen more commonly than the aforementioned primary neoplasms. The history is usually short, with progression from apparently normal neurological status to complete loss of all cord function within a few days. Such rapid progression indicates impairment of blood supply to the cord rather than compression as the principal feature and explains the overall lack of success of emergency decompressions. Laminectomy with partial removal of tumor followed by radiation is offered in the hope of at least delaying progression to total paralysis.

INTRACRANIAL INFECTIONS

Infections within the central nervous system are generally chemotherapeutic rather than surgical problems. Two possibilities for surgical treatment exist, namely, the evacuation of an abscess and the prevention of reinfection. The abscesses are most frequently intracerebral, arising within the white matter by hematogenous spread from the lung, or by contiguous spread through a tract from a paranasal sinus or the middle ear. The symptoms may be acute or chronic, characterized by headache, lethargy, vomiting, and paresis depending on the location of the lesion. Fever is often absent. Abscesses are a common complication of *cyanotic heart disease.* Subdural abscess or empyema is next in frequency, arising almost invariably from a paranasal sinus or middle ear. Symptoms are acute and dramatic, with severe headache, convulsive seizures, and dense neurological deficits. Epidural abscess also arises by direct extension from sinus or bone but is demonstrated less dramatically with pressure signs.

The presence of a focus of infection raises the possibility of abscess in the differential diagnosis of any mass intracranial lesion. It is obviously to the surgeon's advantage to be prepared for the finding of an abscess before intracranial surgery is undertaken. Subdural and epidural abscesses can usually be drained effectively through burr holes. Intracerebral abscesses, whenever encapsulated, are preferably resected completely. Postoperatively, the patient is treated with the same dosages of antibiotics as are used for active meningitis.

After management of the abscess problem, any possible primary source for reinfection should be investigated. Meningitis without abscess formation also deserves such consideration if the responsible organism is other than *Meningococcus* or *Haemophilus influenzae*.

SPONTANEOUS INTRACRANIAL HEMORRHAGE

Intracranial bleeding in the absence of trauma may occur primarily into the brain substance (cerebral hemisphere, brainstem, or cerebellum) or into the subarachnoid space.

Intracerebral and intrapontine hemorrhages are most commonly seen in *hypertensive* patients in the 50- and 70-year age group. They are catastrophic in onset, with initial loss of consciousness and a severe lateralized neurological deficit, e.g., hemiplegia. The hemorrhage usually occurs deep in the cerebral hemisphere near or in the internal capsule in the distribution of the lenticulostriate branches of the middle cerebral artery and frequently ruptures into the ventricular system (Fig. 40-1). The immediate mortality is very high. Surgical treatment is directed toward preservation of

viable functioning tissue by evacuation of hematomas and débridement of swollen and necrotic brain. However, because of the deep location of the hemorrhage and the extensive destruction of tissue, operation is not worthwhile in the majority of cases.

Subarachnoid hemorrhage is most often caused by a ruptured aneurysm of the circle of Willis (Figs. 40-34 and 40-35) and occurs maximally in the 40- to 60-year age group. In over 20%, more than one aneurysm is present, but rarely does more than one aneurysm rupture at any given time. A hemorrhage can cause abrupt apnea and death; thus many victims never reach hospital. Of those who do, 12% to 15% die as a direct result of the initial hemorrhage and an additional 20% within 6 months die of rebleeding from the aneurysm. After 6 months, risk of rebleeding continues at an average rate of 2.2% per year for the next decade. This high risk of aneurysmal rebleeding and death is the indication for surgical treatment. Occlusion of the neck of the aneurysm sac by a spring clip (Fig. 40-35) is the most satisfactory and definitive operation; it is technically feasible in most aneurysms. Surgical mortality may be as low as 3% in patients in good neurological condition, but when the patients are very ill from the effects of the subarachnoid hemorrhage, the operative mobidity and mortality may be very high. Aneurysms that, by their anatomical characteristics, do not lend themselves to clipping are sometimes treated by ligation of the carotid artery in the neck (if the aneurysm arises from the internal carotid artery in the cavernous

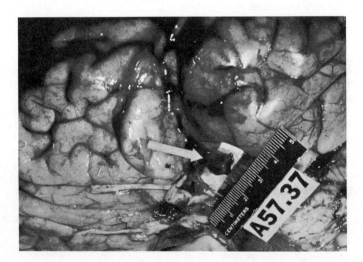

Fig. 40-34. Ruptured aneurysm, internal carotid artery. Aneurysm has ruptured at its neck *(arrow)*, producing fatal subarachnoid hemorrhage. Majority of aneurysmal ruptures occur at dome rather than at neck of sac.

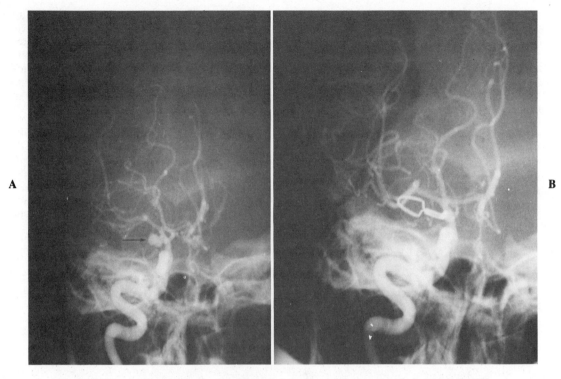

Fig. 40-35. Pre- and postoperative angiograms in patient with aneurysm of circle of Willis. **A,** Aneurysm *(arrow)* arises from right internal carotid artery at origin of posterior communicating artery. **B,** Postoperative angiogram shows neck of aneurysm occluded by metallic clip.

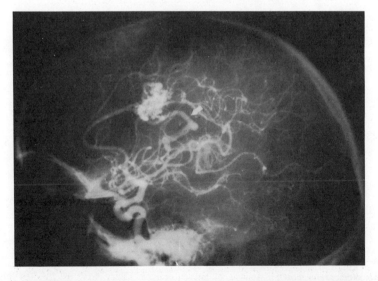

Fig. 40-36. Angiogram showing arteriovenous malformation. Lesion is fed principally by pericallosal artery. Rapid passage of contrast medium through malformation into venous system *(arrow)* is characteristic. Principal feeding and draining vessels depend on location of malformation.

sinus), by the external investment of the sac with gauze or plastics, or by filling of the sac with fine wire to promote intraluminal thrombosis.

Subarachnoid and intraparenchymal hemorrhages occurring in the young (under 30) normotensive patient may result from an *arteriovenous malformation* (Fig. 40-36). The mortality from hemorrhage from this lesion is low, but recurrent hemorrhages are likely to occur over many years or decades. Total extirpation of all abnormal vessels is the goal of surgical treatment but is feasible only in those malformations that are so located that operation does not carry a great risk of producing a disabling neurological deficit.

In approximately 19% of patients with proved subarachnoid hemorrhage, no cause can be estab-

lished by all available diagnostic tests including repeated angiography. The prognosis for recovery and long-term survival for these patients is excellent and bears no relationship to the prognosis after bleeding from an aneurysm or arteriovenous malformation. No surgical treatment is necessary unless there is a localized hematoma of sufficient size to exert a dangerous mass effect.

CEREBROVASCULAR OCCLUSIVE DISEASE

The most common cause of cerebrovascular accident (stroke) is atheromatous occlusive disease. The internal carotid artery in the neck is the most common site of the stroke-producing atheromatous disease, whereas the vertebral artery in the neck and the intracranial vessels are less frequent

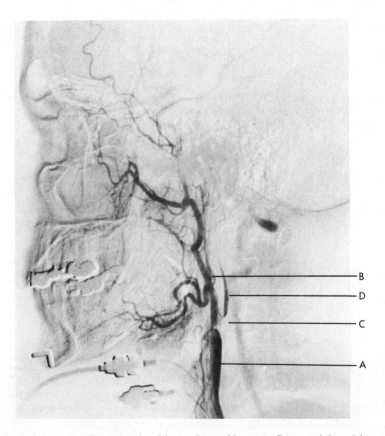

Fig. 40-37. Angiogram showing stenosis of internal carotid artery. Contrast injected into common carotid artery, *A,* passes readily up to external carotid artery, *B,* and its branches. Internal carotid artery, however, is so severely narrowed at its origin, *C,* that only wisp of contrast medium, *D,* has entered lumen.

sites. The age distribution of cerebrovascular disease closely parallels that of coronary artery disease, and the conditions often coexist in the same patient. Ischemia and infarction of the dependent cerebral hemisphere result in varying degrees of neurological deficit that may be transient, temporary, or permanent.

The management of cerebral ischemia consists of angiography of the cervical and intracranial vessels for accurate diagnosis of the location and extent of arterial obstruction, followed by the restoration of vascular pathways by direct or indirect routes whenever feasible. However, if surgical treatment is to be effective, the diagnosis must be established and treatment completed before irreversible major cerebral damage has occurred. It is therefore im-

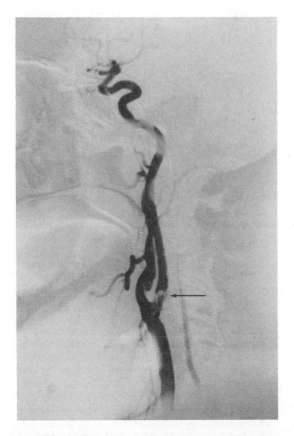

Fig. 40-38. Angiogram showing irregular, ulcerative atheromatous plaque at origin of internal carotid artery *(arrow)*. Such plaques are prone to fragmentation, with resultant embolization of intracranial vessels.

portant to recognize the signs and symptoms of an impending stroke. Clinically recognizable transient cerebral ischemia may precede a major infarction by several weeks or months. In cervical carotid artery disease, the cerebral hemisphere may suffer (with contralateral paresis, numbness, or clumsiness), or the retina may suffer (with ipsilateral loss of vision). In vertebrobasilar disease (brainstem disease) brainstem symptoms occur (vertigo, incoordination, imbalance, or syncope). Such symptoms may be attributable to severe stenosis with inadequate blood flow through proximal vessels (Fig. 40-37) or to embolization of distal vessels from friable ulcerative atheromatous plaques occurring commonly at the origin of the internal carotid artery in the neck (Fig. 40-38). Approximately 85% of patients with significantly stenotic or ulcerative carotid lesions have an audible bruit on auscultation over the neck vessels. Doppler evaluation and oculoplethysmography can provide an indication of the degree of stenosis, but angiography by either direct arterial injection or indirect venous injection with digital subtraction offer the only reliable assessment of the extent of arterial disease.

Carotid endarterectomy in patients with reversible neurological symptoms caused by severe cervical carotid stenosis or ulceration produces excellent results in most cases, with a risk of surgical morbidity of 2% or less. However, not all patients are candidates for the procedure. A completely occluded internal carotid artery can rarely be recanalized satisfactorily. In such cases a bypass anastomosis from the superficial temporal artery or occipital artery to the distal middle cerebral artery may provide useful additional arterial blood to the sensorimotor cortex. The optimum surgical procedure or procedures for a given patient can be determined only after careful physical, neurological, and angiographic evaluations.

PROTRUSION OF INTERVERTEBRAL DISKS AND VERTEBRAL SPONDYLOSIS

Herniation of an intervertebral disk into the spinal canal and degenerative changes in the disk and vertebral bodies resulting in spur formation (spondylosis) may result in compression and irritation of nerve roots and spinal cord. The former is a common condition affecting principally the 30- to 60-year age group, whereas symptomatic spondylosis is seen somewhat later in life (45 to 70 years). Although any vertebral segment may be involved, there are definite sites of predilection. The third, fourth, and fifth lumbar and the fifth and sixth cervical disks are the most frequently herniated; herniation of disks at other levels is distinctly rare. Spondylosis sufficient to produce *neu-*

rological symptoms occurs most commonly in the lower three cervical vertebrae (Fig. 40-39). Spondylotic spurs on the lumbar vertebrae may produce the symptoms and signs of nerve root compression; in the thoracic segments neurological involvement is rare.

The symptoms of the two types of pathosis are clinically indistinguishable from each other. When nerve roots are involved, pain is the principal symptom, accompanied by variable degrees of sensory and motor impairment. The characteristics of the pain are the following:

1. It is referred to the dermatomal distribution of the compressed nerve.
2. It is aggravated by any maneuver that increases intraspinal cerebrospinal fluid pressure such as (a) coughing or sneezing, (b) straining at stool, and (c) compression of jugular veins (Naffziger's test).
3. Cervical root pain is usually aggravated by extension of the neck.
4. Lumbar and sacral root pain is aggravated by straight leg raising, which may be accentuated by forced dorsiflexion of the foot; occasionally, raising the contralateral leg may produce pain referred to the ipsilateral side.

Spinal cord symptoms may be produced either by direct compression of the cord or compression of the incoming radicular arterial supply. The clinical picture is one of progressive spastic quadriparesis (or paraparesis in rare thoracic disk herniations).

Distribution of symptoms and signs depends on the nerve roots compressed, as shown in Table 40-5. Because of individual variations in segmental innervation, the sensory pattern is much less reliable in the upper extremity than in the lower. In contrast, the motor pattern is less reliable in the lower extremity than in the upper.

Management depends on the severity of symptoms and signs. Conservative measures, consisting of bed rest, traction (for cervical root pain), or immobilization, can be tried in all cases in which there is no disabling neurological deficit. If symptoms are relieved satisfactorily, continued support of the involved area with a collar or brace may be the only treatment required. The presence of a definite neurological deficit, particularly muscle weakness and atrophy, usually indicates surgical removal of the compressing lesion. Interference with bladder function by acute disk herniations requires immediate surgical treatment.

The diagnosis of lumbar disk herniation usually can be confirmed by unenhanced computerized tomography (Fig. 40-2), but in some cases myelography is also indicated (Figs. 40-40 and 40-41). Cervical disk herniations are much smaller lesions, averaging 2 to 4 mm. in diameter so that myelogra-

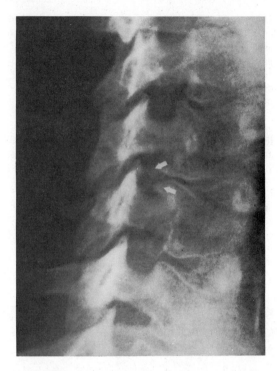

Fig. 40-39. Cervical spondylosis. Oblique view of cervical spine shows presence of osteophytic spurs *(arrows)* encroaching on an intervertebral foramen. Remainder of foramina are normal.

phy or contrast-enhanced CT scanning is necessary to confirm the diagnosis.

Two modes of surgical treatment are available for the treatment of lumbar disk herniation. If the spinal canal is of adequate size and the disk protrusion is relatively small and still contained under the posterior longitudinal ligament, the intradiskal injection of the enzyme chymopapain may provide adequate root decompression and relief of symptoms. However, injection of this substance can produce anaphylactic reactions that can be fatal if not treated appropriately. Hence the procedure is performed under strictly controlled conditions. If the spinal canal is narrow or has become relatively stenotic by arthritic changes, or the herniated disk fragment is very large or extruded into the epidural space, open surgical discectomy through a laminotomy is the treatment of choice. This operation provides immediate relief of root pain in most cases. Cervical root compression by herniated disk or spondylosis can be alleviated by removal of the herniated fragment through a hemilaminotomy and decompression of the root

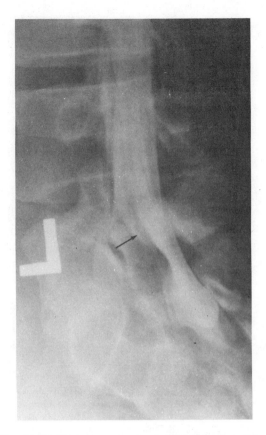

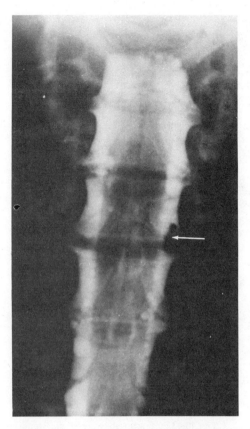

Fig. 40-40. Myelogram showing herniated lumbar disk. Nerve roots are outlined by contrast medium (water-soluble metrizamide). At lumbosacral joint, localized mass indents dye column, and left S1 nerve root *(arrow)* can be seen stretched over mass.

Fig. 40-41. Myelogram showing herniated cervical disk. Cervical canal is outlined by dye column, and nerve roots are seen exiting at each interspace. At C6-C7 interspace, dye column is indented from left *(arrow)* and root shadow is obliterated. At times differentiation between disk and tumor is difficult to make myelographically.

Table 40-5. Neurological manifestations of vertebral spondylosis and herniated intervertebral disk

Intervertebral level	Nerve root involved	Distribution of pain and sensory loss	Principal motor deficit	Reflex diminution
C5-C6	C6	Neck, shoulder, arm, radial side of hand, thumb, index finger	Biceps	Biceps
C6-C7	C7	Neck, shoulder, arm, middle of hand, index and middle fingers	Triceps	Triceps
L4-L5	L5	Lower back, posterior thigh and calf, medial side of foot, medial two or three toes	Anterior tibial group	None
L5-S1	S1	Lower back, posterior thigh and calf, lateral side of foot, lateral two or three toes	Gastrosoleus group	Achilles

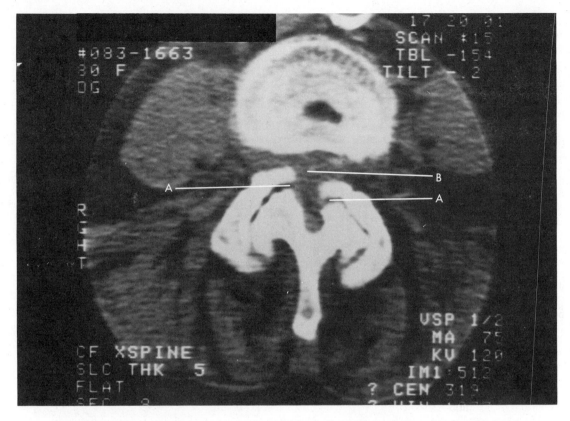

Fig. 40-42. CT scan showing spinal stenosis at L4 level. Facet joints, *A*, have hypertrophied and encroach medially, narrowing spinal canal, *B*, to a slit-like aperture through which roots of cauda equina must pass.

around a bony spur. However, when there is significant spur formation, the decompression can be accomplished better through an anterior interbody approach and the interspace fused with an iliac bone graft to prevent further spondylosis.

Stenosis of the entire spinal canal by bony thickening and overgrowth most commonly affects the lower lumbar segments. The clinical symptoms are numbness, heaviness, cramping, and weakness of the legs consistently brought on by exercise and can mimic *peripheral vascular insufficiency.* Therefore spinal canal stenosis should be considered in the differential diagnosis of claudicatory symptoms in the lower extremities. CT scanning (Fig. 40-42) and myelography confirm the diagnosis, and a *generous* decompressive laminectomy provides excellent relief of symptoms.

PERIPHERAL AND CRANIAL NERVE COMPRESSION SYNDROMES

A variety of sensorimontor disturbances attributable to peripheral nerve compression, entrapment,

or stretching have been identified. The more common anatomical sites of compression are listed as follows:

Median nerve at the carpal tunnel
Median nerve at the bicipital tendon
Ulnar nerve in the hypothenar eminence
Ulnar nerve at the elbow
Radial nerve in the forearm
Radial nerve in the spinal groove
Suprascapular nerve at the suprascapular foramen
Lateral femoral cutaneous nerve at the inguinal ligament
Common peroneal nerve at the fibular neck

The most common of these, the carpal tunnel syndrome, is described in the preceding chapter. The ulnar nerve suffers with almost equal frequency, occasionally as a late complication of a deforming fracture at the elbow joint but more often because of entrapment of the nerve at its entrance to the fibromuscular septum just distal to the medial epicondyle of the humerus. Treatment consists in releasing the nerve from the compressing fascia and transposing it anterior to the epicondyle so that it is not stretched each time the elbow is flexed.

Less common but equally distressing nerve entrapment syndromes respond well to surgical decompression. Their possibility should always be borne in mind in the differential diagnosis of pain, numbness, paresthesias, and weakness in the extremities. *Electromyography* and *nerve conduction studies* are usually essential to confirm the diagnosis.

Trigeminal neuralgia (tic douloureux) is a relatively common condition characterized by lightning-like stabs of pain in the distribution of one or more branches of the trigeminal nerve. Occasionally the pain may follow the distribution of the *glossopharyngeal nerve (glossopharyngeal neuralgia)*. The condition occurs predominantly in the elderly and affects females more frequently than males. Attacks of pain can often be precipitated when one touches or rubs the area of skin involved ("trigger point"). In most instances the causative pathological condition appears to be an abnormal arterial loop or a venous anomaly that presses on the nerve rootlets at their entry into the brainstem. Analgesics are of no value, for the pain is transitory. Carbamazepine is a very effective drug for tic pain, but untoward reactions occur frequently so that drug must be discontinued in a significant proportion of patients. Alcohol injection of peripheral branches usually provides satisfactory relief, but the sensory loss obtained is not permanent so that the pain returns as the nerve regenerates. Intracranial sectioning of preganglionic fibers subserving the area of pain affords permanent relief of pain but leaves an area of permanent numbness that can be distressing. Percutaneous radiofrequency coagulation of the trigeminal ganglion is also effective, with varying degrees of sensory loss, but the pain may recur. Decompression of either trigeminal or glossopharyngeal nerve at the root entry zone by rerouting or padding the compressing arterial loop or vein from the compressed nerve with an interposed sponge or muscle is usually effective and the most satisfactory, but there may be failures or recurrences because of irreversible demyelination of the chronically compressed nerves.

Hemifacial spasm (facial tic) is a motor nerve counterpart of trigeminal neuralgia, in which repetitive, involuntary twitching occurs in the muscles of one side of the face. The condition is frequently blamed on a nervous habit, but in reality it can be attributable to compression of the facial nerve intracranially by a redundant vessel loop just as in the case of the trigeminal and glossopharyngeal nerves. Surgical treatment is similar, i.e., moving the offending vessel away from the nerve or placing a muscle pad between the blood vessel and nerve, or doing both.

SURGICAL RELIEF OF PAIN AND DYSKINESIAS

Intractable pain for which the causative lesion cannot be treated directly may be satisfactorily alleviated only by interruption of the pathways by which painful sensations are perceived. Carcinomas of the cervix, bladder, prostate, and lower bowel frequently produce sever and continuous pain, both in the abdomen from local invasion and in the leg from involvement of the lumbosacral plexus. Advanced carcinomas of the breast and lung may similarly produce pain in the chest and arm, the latter from nodal or rib involvement in the region of the brachial plexus. Analgesics provide only partial and short-lived relief, and the prolonged use of narcotics may result in addiction. Therefore, although every attempt should be made to obtain relief of symptoms by treatment of the causative lesion, the use of neurosurgical procedures should not be withheld unduly in patients with malignant disease.

Table 40-6 shows the two most common procedures in use: *cordotomy* and *rhizotomy*. Spinal rhizotomy is of limited value in the trunk and extremities for two reasons: (1) the extensive overlapping of dermatomal segments necessitates the sectioning of many more roots adjacent to the area of pain, and (2) extensive deafferentation of an extremity renders it *functionally useless* from loss of proprioception, regardless of the integrity of motor innervation. Cerebral destructive procedures, e.g., *prefrontal lobotomy* and *cingulotomy,* designed to alter the patient's interpretation of pain, are useful only in certain specific situations. Malignancies of the oropharynx and paranasal sinuses frequently produce extreme pain and suffering that cannot be satisfactorily alleviated by sensory denervation, unless that denervation is very extensive.

Section of anterior spinal roots (*anterior rhizotomy*) is a procedure reserved for the permanently paraplegic or quadriplegic in whom mass flexor reflexes result in painful spasms of the paralyzed extremities.

From the foregoing descriptions of various techniques, it is apparent that practically any painful area in the body can be rendered analgesic by neurosurgical deafferentation. These procedures are intended primarily for clearly defined painful syndromes such as those occurring with incurable malignancies. They are not generally recommended for the variety of common pain problems that have no provable cause. Once nerve pathways have been purposely destroyed, they can never be reestablished; the resulting sensory loss is per-

Table 40-6. Surgical procedures for the relief of intractable pain

	*Ventrolateral cordotomy**	*Posterior rhizotomy*
Pathway interrupted	Lateral spinothalamic tract	Posterior root proximal to its ganglion
Sensations lost	Pain and temperature	All sensory modalities
Distribution of sensory loss	Up to a level of one to two segments below operation, on the side of the body opposite cordotomy	In the dermatomal distribution of the sectioned root(s) only
Level of operation*	C2	Fifth and ninth cranial nerves
	T2	Any spinal nerve root
Indications	C2—chest and arm pain, e.g., carcinoma of lung	Fifth cranial—trigeminal neuralgia
	T2—abdomen and leg pain, e.g., carcinoma of cervix, prostate	Ninth cranial—glossopharyngeal neuralgia
		Fifth, ninth, C2, C3—oropharyngeal pain, e.g., carcinoma of tongue
Complications	Paralysis from trauma to adjacent lateral corticospinal tract	Same complications as any intracranial operations when fifth and ninth nerves are sectioned

*Cordotomy may be performed percutaneously rather than by open operation; the lesion is produced by a radio-frequency generator through a percutaneously inserted needle.

manent. Trigeminal root section performed for nonmalignant facial pain that is not typically trigeminal neuralgia will leave the patient with a permanently anesthetic face the original pain for which the operation was performed may persist or recur despite the sensory loss. Rhizotomies, cordotomies, or other procedures performed for postherpetic neuralgia or for phantom limb pain fail too frequently to provide lasting relief of symptoms. Denervation should be resorted to only after all reasonable attempts to control the cause of pain have failed. If the patient remains disabled by pain, an operation having permanent consequences may be justified.

Stereotactically placed destructive lesions in the ventrolateral nucleus of the thalamus have, in selected cases, been effective in abolishing or reducing the tremor of Parkinson's disease. Patients under 60 years of age with unilateral tremor and without bradykinesia or pseudobulbar manifestations are the best candidates for the operation. The physiological mechanism by which the tremor is stopped is unknown. The procedure has been tried with little success in the treatment of other disorders characterized by abnormal states of muscle tone and movement (dyskinesias).

41
Urology

Joseph D. Schmidt

Urology is that branch of medicine and surgery devoted to the study, diagnosis, and treatment of diseases and abnormalities of the urogenital tract of the male and the urinary tract of the female.

Urologists must work in close association with members of all other branches of medicine but particularly with internists and surgeons in the study and care of diseases of the adrenal gland, medical diseases of the kidney, and abdominal masses of all types.

The kidney is the most important organ of excretion. A clear understanding of the status of the urinary tract of every patient is essential to a complete evaluation of the patient's condition. Only by a complete history and general examination of the patient, analysis of the urine, estimation of renal function, and radiological visualization of the urinary tract can the physician obtain an accurate knowledge of his patient's urological status. Cystoscopy is often necessary to complete the urinary tract evaluation.

ANATOMY AND PHYSIOLOGY

The kidney has some endocrine functions that are related to the maintenance of blood pressure, hematopoiesis and calcium metabolism, but the kidney's main function is to form urine. This is the main pathway by which water, salts, nitrogenous wastes, and other products are excreted from the body, thereby helping to maintain the internal balance of these substances. The urine that is formed then travels down through the calyces, renal pelves, and ureters to the bladder. In the adult, when about 400 ml. have collected, the desire to urinate triggers contraction of bladder muscle, emptying the urine through the urethra. The kidneys, calyces, pelves, and ureters are normally duplicated, but there is normally only one bladder and urethra.

PATHOLOGY AND SYMPTOMATOLOGY

Diseases of the genitourinary tract conveniently fall into the following general classes: congenital anomalies, injuries, inflammations, neoplasms, and certain miscellaneous diseases. Since its excretory function links the genitourinary tract anatomically and physiologically to other organ systems, lesions involving the urinary tract may give rise to symptoms suggestive of lesions in organs and tissues outside the urinary tract. Moreover, since there is a direct communication and interrelationship between the functions of the various portions of the urinary tract, lesions in one portion may in turn produce disturbances of function in another portion of the urinary tract. These two facts are extremely important to the understanding of urinary tract disease.

Thus disorders of this system may not only be multiple in distribution in the tract itself, but they may also be associated with or influenced or mimicked by lesions arising primarily in other organ systems. This is particularly true in *children* with congenital anomalies of the genitourinary tract. If an early diagnosis is to be made, a complete urological survey must be made of all children with any unexplained symptoms or signs.

One should not infer from the preceding remarks that every person with a genitourinary disease should be subjected at the first visit to all the procedures necessary to evaluate the entire genitourinary system. This is not only unnecessary but in many instances may also be distinctly harmful; e.g., in the presence of an acute inflammation of the urethra, prostrate, or bladder, the instrumentation necessary to examine the urinary tract may be contraindicated. Only those examinations that accurately establish the location and nature of the disease needing immediate treatment are necessary. The more complicated diagnostic manipulations are deferred until the acute inflammatory findings subside or until the progress of the disease makes these examinations imperative.

Since *obstruction* and *infection* are complications common to most urinary tract lesions, the physician must determine whether they are primary or secondary.

THERAPY

Therapy, in general, consists of two phases after an accurate diagnosis has been established. The first phase is designed to relieve pain, dysuria, and increased frequency or signs of infection. The *sine qua non* is the *relief of obstruction* anywhere in the urinary tract, performed in the simplest way possible. In addition, antibiotics are given to control infection. With even this temporary relief of obstructive signs and symptoms, the patient's general condition will improve rapidly, and then one may proceed with the definitive phase of therapy.

The definitive phase is designed to cure, correct, or eradicate the causative lesion. This is done in such a way as not to disturb function but rather to restore it to as near physiological normalcy as possible. Here again, adequate urine drainage is of paramount concern. All therapeutic efforts are aimed at restoring or maintaining normal renal function and urinary transport.

CLINICAL EXAMINATION
Approach

Urological patients may be shy with regard to their complaints because of taboos connected with the genitourinary tract, and it is especially important for the physician and nurse to assume a correct professional attitude toward them. Sympathy must be expressed and embarrassment avoided. They must be made to feel at ease. Deep human understanding and an intense feeling of responsibility on the part of the physician and nurse are mandatory qualities.

Remarks

The patient's history and chief complaint are important because (1) they may point directly to some portion of the genitourinary tract, or (2) they may indicate lesions elsewhere, but these extra–urinary tract disturbances of function may be caused by impaired renal function occurring after primary disease of the genitourinary tract. There may be no symptoms, and only a complete examination of the urinary tract will show the asymptomatic abnormalities.

History

Patients usually relate a history of one or more of the following situations:

1. Trauma with urinary extravasation.
2. Abnormalities of urine.
   a. Pyuria.
   b. Hematuria.
   c. Chyluria.
   d. Pneumaturia.
3. Abnormality in voiding.
   a. Incontinence.
      (1) Ordinary.
      (2) Paradoxic.
      (3) Dribbling between normal urination.
   b. Frequency.
   c. Dysuria.
   d. Oliguria.
   e. Polyuria.
   f. Small stream.
   g. Difficulty or retention.
   h. Dribbling. Is it incontinence or is it associated with apparently normal voiding? The latter is pathognomonic of an ectopic ureteral orifice.
4. Tumors or swellings in urogenital area.
   a. Scrotum.
      (1) Painful.
      (2) Tender.
      (3) Associated redness.
   b. Abdominal masses.
      (1) In the flank.
      (2) Suprapubically.
      (3) In the groin.
5. Pain and tenderness in region of genitourinary tract.
   a. Infection.
   b. Stone.
   c. Trauma.
   d. Congenital or acquired obstruction.
6. Uremia—a blanket term used to designate the syndrome that results from renal insufficiency of any type—may be characterized by nausea, vomiting, stupor, coma, azotemia, oliguria, etc. The signs and symptoms vary with the myriad of variations in pathophysiology associated with renal insufficiency.
7. Azotemia may be part of the picture of renal insufficiency (uremia) but may be present

with no underlying renal disease (dehydration, severe gastrointestinal tract hemorrhage).

8. Chills or fever may mean infection of the urinary tract.
9. Loss of weight may indicate urogenital malignant neoplasm, uremia, or chronic infection.
10. Evidence of metastases to the bones
    a. Osteoblastic lesions usually are metastases from carcinoma of the prostrate in the male.
    b. Hypernephroma frequently metastasizes to the lungs, as does tumor of the testis.
    c. Pulsating bone tumors, osteolytic in nature, usually are metastases from hypernephroma.
11. Poor growth in children may be an indication of renal insufficiency, related to congenital urinary tract obstruction.
12. Sexual dysfunction: Impotence, total or partial, is a common symptom and is based on organic problems in over half the cases. Premature ejaculation is unrelated to organic disease, whereas retrograde ejaculation usually results from anatomic disturbances of either the lumbar sympathetic ganglia or bladder neck (internal sphincter).

Physical examination
General appearance

The general appearance of the patient frequently suggests urinary tract disease. However, many serious diseases of the urinary tract produce no external changes, even in their late stages. In children abnormalities of growth, particularly dwarfism, suggest disease of the urinary tract with associated renal insufficiency. In all ages edema, sallow complexion, shortness of breath, and anemia or dehydration may herald serious genitourinary tract disease.

General findings

General findings often justify careful diagnostic evaluation of the urinary tract.

Fever. Fever may be an indication of primary or secondary urinary tract infection; it is usually high, erratic, and frequently associated with chills.

Hypertension. Hypertension is frequently associated with glomerular disease of the kidneys, late stages of chronic pyelonephritis, congenital polycystic disease of the kidney, decreased perfusion of one or both kidneys or even a segment of one kidney, and acute ureteral obstruction.

Edema. Edema associated with urinary tract disease is of two types. It may be peripheral to venous or lymphatic obstruction caused by primary or metastatic urinary tract neoplasm, or it may be generalized and associated with renal insufficiency or hypoproteinemia.

Abnormalities of growth. Abnormalities of growth in children may be associated with changes in adrenal function or severe renal insufficiency.

Secondary anemia. Secondary anemia is frequently seen with renal insufficiency and urinary tract neoplasm from bleeding and bone marrow involvement.

Evidence of metastasis. Neoplasms of the prostate, kidney, and testis frequently metastasize to the lungs, the brain, and the bones of the torso.

Neurological findings. Diseases of the spinal cord frequently produce abnormalities in function of the bladder and the upper urinary tract, especially infection, stone formation, and residual urine in the bladder and kidney pelves. Early urological work-up is particularly important, since damage to the urinary tract caused by spinal cord disease may be so insidious that a very great change may occur before symptoms arise.

Loss of weight, dehydration. Loss of weight and dehydration are hallmarks of renal insufficiency and other chronic urinary tract diseases.

Abnormal breathing. Abnormal breathing may herald acidosis accompanying renal insufficiency.

Abdominal masses. Abdominal masses require complete urinary tract investigation, including x-ray examination. A suprapubic mass may simply be a full bladder caused by obstruction of the bladder neck. A pelvic or abdominal mass may be an ectopic kidney that should not be removed.

Local examination and findings

Careful examination in the region of the kidneys and ureters should be a part of every physical examination. The skin should be inspected for enlarged, dilated veins that indicate collateral circulation. Palpation of the costovertebral angle for muscle spasm and tenderness should be carefully carried out.

Suprapubic dullness and masses should be noted.

The inguinal canals should be palpated in the standing position for an undescended testis or hernia.

The scrotum should be carefully studied. The vas deferens, the epididymis, and the testis should be examined separately and abnormalities should be noted in their size, consistency, and form. Any mass in the scrotum should be transilluminated. A varicocele on the left side is not of great significance, but a varicocele on the right side may signal a mass in the retroperitoneal area. The patient should be examined in the standing position to allow filling of a varicocele.

The perineum, urethra, and penis should be palpated carefully and inspected for swelling, tenderness, and urethral discharge.

The rectal examination includes the following:

1. The anal sphincter tone should be noted; if lax, it may be an indication of neurological cord disease.
2. Hemorrhoids may be caused by urinary or genital tract neoplasm producing vascular obstruction.
3. The prostate should be palpated carefully. The prostate normally is triangular with its apex caudad, each side measuring 1 inch, and its consistency is firm and rubbery. Hard areas should be noted; they may be caused by chronic inflammation (such as tuberculosis) but are more likely composed of prostatic neoplasms or calculi. The seminal vesicles are not normally palpable; if they are palpable, this may be evidence of inflammation (tuberculosis) or neoplastic invasion.
4. Prostatic secretion should be examined microscopically; one obtains it by digitally milking the prostate after the patient has urinated, so that as the prostatic secretion is discharged through the urethra it will not be contaminated with urethral secretion. Normally five to ten pus cells or fewer are visible in each high-power field. Tumor cells or large numbers of pus cells indicate prostatic neoplasm or infection, respectively. If bacterial prostatitis is suspected, the secretions should be cultured.

Instrumental examination of the urethra

Besides examining the urethra by palpation, one may examine it by means of a catheter, a bougie, a urethroscope, or urethrography. Urethral obstruction will prevent passage of a catheter; its precise cause (stricture, foreign body, or tumor) requires further work-up with urethroscopy and cystourethrography. Spasm of the external urethral sphincter must be differentiated carefully from organic obstruction.

Residual urine in the bladder may be determined as follows: The patient is asked to void, and the character of the stream is observed. A good strong stream resulting in 100 to 300 ml. of urine usually eliminates the possibility of residual urine in the bladder. The patient then lies on his back on the examining table. Suprapubic percussion and palpation are carried out. Any lower abdominal mass, even if it is not in the midline, should be suspected of being a full bladder or an undrained diverticulum of the bladder. Aseptic catheterization should then be performed; more than 30 to 75 ml. of urine in the bladder indicates significant residual urine. The cause of this should be ascertained.

Catheterization in the male. The patient to be catheterized should lie on his back with the thighs slightly separated and moderately flexed. The penis, scrotum, and pubic area are cleaned thoroughly with antiseptic. In the average adult a No. 14 French catheter is used. A sterile tube of lubricant jelly is removed from the antiseptic solution in which it is stored, and the first teaspoonful or so is discarded. Then the nozzle of the tube is inserted into the urethral meatus, and with steady pressure the entire urethra is filled with jelly. Lubrication of the catheter tip alone is inadequate.

The operator stands at the right side of the patient, grasps the shaft of the penis betwen the third and fourth fingers and the glans penis at each side of the meatus with the thumb and index finger of the left hand, so as to open the meatal lips widely enough to admit the tip of the catheter. The penis is drawn gently forward and upward from the body so as to stretch it slightly and thus straighten the anterior urethra. When using soft rubber catheters, the penis is kept in the midline and the catheter is advanced to the bladder; the penile shaft is lowered as the catheter tip passes the external sphincter and enters the bladder. If the catheter does not enter the bladder easily, the tip is probably caught in the urethral bulb or is held by the contracted external sphincter. In the former instance the catheter is withdrawn a little and advanced again drawing the penis over it with the left hand, much as a glove is drawn over a finger, at the same time depressing the penile shaft between the thighs. In case the external sphincter is in spasm, the tip of the catheter is held against it with gentle but continuous pressure for several seconds. The contraction generally relaxes partially, and the catheter enters the bladder. Larger instruments overcome the spasm of the sphincter more easily than small ones. Irrigation is then carried out, since the lubricating jelly may have plugged the lumen of the catheter.

Catheterization in the female. Follow the same general principles in the female as in the male. Since the urethra is short, once the meatus is located, the catherization is easily carried out.

Cystourethroscopic examination. The modern cystoscope is used to visualize the urinary bladder and urethra for diagnostic purposes. It allows operative procedures to be carried out under vision, without an incision being made into the bladder or urethra.

Cystoscopy and urethroscopy may be carried out with ease in patients of all ages, including infants. Ordinarily in the adult female patient, no anesthesia is necessary. In children and adult males, however, or with severe inflammatory lesions, it may be necessary to carry out the procedure under either general or regional anesthesia.

When operative procedures are to be performed, anesthesia is, practically speaking, always necessary.

Asepsis is observed and then the instrument is introduced in much the same manner as a stiff catheter is introduced. After careful observation of the bladder neck, trigone, ureteral orifices, fundus, anterior and lateral walls of the bladder, and the urethra, any indicated operative procedure is carried out.

LABORATORY EXAMINATION—URINE

Urinalysis is an integral part of the examination of any patient. However, important urinary tract abnormalities may occur with relatively normal urine.

Under normal conditions the urine is formed by a process of filtration of the blood plasma through the glomeruli, followed by selective or active reabsorption of a large part of the filtrate by the renal tubules. What is left, plus a few substances that are excreted by the tubules, is the urine.

Abnormalities of the urine may be classified in three separate categories: (1) physical changes, (2) chemical changes, and (3) microscopic changes.

Physical changes
Volume

The amount of urine excreted is of great importance, particularly in relation to the intake. One of the most important single duties of the person in charge of a patient who has a urological condition is to measure accurately the intake and output, especially the urinary output. Normally, the adult excretes anywhere between 1 and 2.5 L. of urine in 24 hours, depending on intake. Children excrete about three times as much as adults per kilogram of body weight. About two thirds of the urine is excreted during the daytime.

Anuria. *Anuria* is the failure to excrete urine. Anuria from renal failure must be differentiated from acute *retention* of urine in which the kidneys secrete a normal amount of urine that cannot be voided because of obstruction somewhere in the drainage system. Bladder outlet obstruction is most common and may readily be determined by urethral catheterization. Occasionally, anuria is caused by bilateral obstruction of the ureters. This is *not* relieved by bladder catheterization and instead mandates supravesical diversion.

Oliguria. When the adult secretes less than 400 to 500 ml. of urine in a 24-hour period, the condition is called *oliguira*. It is definitely pathological; the physician must ascertain its cause. It is *rarely* caused by an obstructive lesion in the urinary passageway.

Polyuria. Polyuria is a condition in which an excess amount of urine is excreted. Diabetes melli-

tus and insipidus and simply a large intake of fluids are the most common causes. Frequency of urination may occur, which must be distinguished from the much more common frequency of urination secondary to bladder outlet obstruction with overflow. Accurate measurement of the total amount of urine excreted in 24 hours will distinguish these two causes for frequency of urination. True polyuria is characterized by urine of a low specific gravity.

Turbidity

Normally the urine is clear. The clarity of the urine may be disturbed by phosphates, fat, chyle, and pus. Most urine becomes cloudy on standing because of the action of bacteria, and therefore turbidity must be studied on the fresh specimen. Phosphaturia will clear when the urine is acidified.

Color

Urine is normally light amber in color. Occasionally it changes because of the administration of drugs, such as methylene blue. With hematuria, it may be smoky, red, or brown, depending on the amount, duration, and age of the blood in the urine. When the urine is brown and turns black on standing after alkalinization, the color may be caused by alkaptonuria (homogentisic acid), or it may be caused by melanin.

Odor

Urine has a characteristic odor. Urea-splitting organisms in the urine give it a distinct ammoniacal smell. These organisms produce severe urinary tract infections and predispose to struvite stones; therefore an ammoniacal odor to the urine requires investigation of the urinary tract. Some commonly prescribed drugs such as ampicillin impart a characteristic odor to the urine.

Reaction

Normally urine has a pH range from 5.0 to 8.0. Renal tuberculosis produces an acid urine, but most other types of urinary tract infections are associated with an alkaline urine. Urine pH is important in the work-up of patients with urolithiasis, since certain types of stones (e.g., cystine, uric acid) tend to occur when the urine is acid, and others (e.g., calcium phosphate, calcium ammonium magnesium phosphate) when the urine is alkaline. Testing a fresh specimen with Nitrazine paper is the most practical way to study the urine pH. Urine pH often reflects the acid-base balance status of the patient. Many of the newer paper-strip indicators (Combistix, Hema-Combistix, and Labstix) afford the patient and the physician an opportunity to detect rather accurately glycosuria, proteinuria, pH, and other urinary changes simultaneously. Similarly, frequent pH testing can monitor a patient's response to therapy for infection or urolithiasis.

Specific gravity

The specific gravity of the urine varies from 1.001 to 1.030, according to the percentage of solutes in the urine. It is usually reduced in chronic renal disease, with a tendency to fixation at 1.010. Inability to concentrate after dehydration is a valuable clinical test indicating poor renal function.

Chemical changes

The following chemical changes in the urine are important: albuminuria, glycosuria, hemoglobinuria, and abnormalities in the excretion of chloride, phosphates, and calcium (Tables 41-1 and 41-2). Albuminuria may be orthostatic in type and transitory because of changes in position that interfere with the circulation through the kidney. It

may be renal in origin because of chronic disease of the kidney, or even extrarenal.

Microscopic changes
Examination

Careful microscopic examination of the urine for casts, red blood cells, leukocytes, epithelial cells, and other formed elements is of great value. Special stains allow study of urinary tract cytology; transitional cell tumors may be diagnosed by this means.

The microscopic examination should always include a thorough search for organisms. Grossly, this is possible in the freshly voided, unstained specimen, but if more positive information is desired, the sediment should be studied with Gram stain. *Staphylococcus, Streptococcus, Gonococcus,* or gram-negative bacilli may be distinguished in this manner. Cultures of the urine are confirmatory and help one select the proper antibiotic. In cases of "sterile pyuria," particularly in an acid urine, cultures for tubercle bacilli should be done (Table 41-3).

ESTIMATION OF RENAL FUNCTION

Evaluation of renal function is an extremely important part of examination of any patient but particularly so in the patient with urological disease. Moreover, the renal function is variable from one time to another, justifying serial evaluations in many patients.

The most common ways by which renal function is estimated are (1) history of loss of appetite or nausea and vomiting, (2) edema or severe dehydra-

Table 41-1. Diagnostic measures in hematuria*

Test	What it detects
General examination (including eye grounds, blood pressure, cuff test, studies of bleeding and clotting mechanisms, etc.)	Nephritis, hemorrhagic diathesis, anticoagulant therapy
Urinalysis†	Verifies presence of blood
Plain roentgenogram (K.U.B.)	Stone, enlarged kidney
Execretory urogram	Tumor, tuberculosis, stone
Cystoscopy (preferably during bleeding)	Source of blood (vesical tumor, stone, renal origin)
Retrograde pyeloureterogram	On side of bleeding; on both sides if not localized to side
Abdominal aortogram and renal arteriogram	Renal neoplasm, vascular malformation
Renal biopsy (open, percutaneous)	Glomerular, interstitial disease
Repeated studies at intervals	To discover lesion at first undetected

*Hematuria must be regarded as serious until unquestionably proved otherwise.
†Red urine does not necessarily contain red blood cells; so this point must be settled by microscopic examination unless clots are present. Other causes of red urine include hemoglobin (March's and cold hemoglobinuria), porphyria, and ingestion of certain azo dyes or large quantities of beets. Malingerers may add blood to the urine; this practice may be difficult to prove if the patient is clever.

Table 41-2. Origin of hematuria in 2,400 cases

Cause	
Neoplasm	800
Inflammation	500
Miscellaneous (systemic, indeterminate, etc.)	400
Stone	425
Tuberculosis	275
TOTAL	2,400
Site	
Vesical	860
Renal	840
Prostatic	300
Ureteral	250
Urethral	60
Systemic	20
Unidentified	70
TOTAL	2,400

tion—"uremic snow," (3) urinary output—quantity, specific gravity, (4) specific renal function tests—the most important of these are the following.

Mosenthal specific gravity test

In progressive renal damage, one of the earliest changes is impairment of the concentrating power of the kidney. In the Mosenthal test fluids are omitted after 6 P.M., and the first urinary specimen passed in the morning is tested for specific gravity. Normally the urine will be concentrated to 1.028. This test may be unreliable during diuresis.

Phenolsulfonphthalein (PSP) test

The PSP test is one primarily of the renal tubular excretion capacity. It shows change relatively early in the course of progressive renal damage and is reduced to zero before much change is found in the blood urea or creatinine.

Procedure. The patient, who should be in bed, drinks two glasses of water. Then, 6 mg. of PSP in 1 ml. of sterile water is injected intravenously. The patient voids every 30 minutes, and four specimens are collected during the next 2 hours. Each specimen is compared colorimetrically with standards to estimate the patient's excretion of the dye.

In a normal person the dye appears in about 3 minutes. About 60% is excreted in the first hour and about 20% in the second hour. The amounts are decreased and sometimes reversed in patients with renal disease. Residual urine in the bladder

Table 41-3. Diagnostic measures in chronic pyuria

Test	What it measures
Two-glass test	Exclusion of urethritis
Culture, Gram stain	Selection of antiseptic or antibiotic
Acid-fast stain, culture	Tuberculosis (skin test, chest roentgenogram)
Residual urine	Prostatism, neurogenic dysfunction, stricture of urethra
Plain roentgenogram (K.U.B.)	Stones, perinephric abscess
Excretory urogram	Stasis, anomalies, tuberculosis, impaired function
Cystourethroscopy	Dilated prostatic ducts, diverticula, etc.
Ureteral catheterization	Source of pyuria, divided cultures
Retrograde pyelogram	When excretory urogram fails or is not possible
Foci of infection	Prostate, cervix, Skene's glands

will make the test less accurate; catheterization prior to the test is required.

Blood urea nitrogen and creatinine

Normally, the blood urea nitrogen is 10 to 20 mg./dl. and the creatinine 0.6 to 1.5 mg./dl. Both values are elevated with considerable renal damage or obstructive disease causing impairment of function.

Urea clearance test

The term *clearance* is defined as the volume of blood in milliliters "cleared" by the kidneys in 1 minute. To carry out the test, one must collect the urine for a 2-hour period and obtain a blood urea determination at the end of the first hour.

Procedure. In the morning after breakfast the patient drinks at least 1 L. of water to ensure maximum diuresis; the bladder is emptied and the specimen is discarded. The next 2-hour urine is the one that is studied. Normally about 75 ml. of blood is cleared of urea per minute.

Excretory urography

Excretory urography is the *most important single test of renal function* available today. It not only gives an estimation of total renal function, but it also differentiates each kidney and gives information about the urinary passageways. With renal impairment, the time of the appearance is delayed, excretion is prolonged, and there is less dense shadow cast on the roentgenogram. On the contrary, with incomplete obstruction, the shadow may be more dense then normal. Known sensitivity to iodinated contrast media is the main contraindication.

Differential renal function tests during cystoscopy

The urine emerging from the ureters at the time of cystoscopic examination may be observed after the intravenous injection of 5 ml. of indigo carmine. Normally, the dye appears in 3 minutes and concentrates to a deep blue.

Another method is to insert ureteral catheters up to each kidney and collect the urines separately; 6 mg. of PSP are injected intravenously, and the appearance time and the total excretion of the dye in 15 minutes are studied.

Endogenous creatinine clearance

The endogenous creatinine clearance test measures a patient's ability to clear the plasma of circulating creatinine. A 24-hour urine collection is made, and a serum creatinine concentration is drawn midway during the collection. The clearance is calculated using the formula $Cl_{cr} = \dfrac{U \times V}{P}$

where *U* represents the urine creatinine concentration, *P* the serum creatinine concentration, and *V* the 24-hour urine volume expressed in milliliters per 1,440 minutes. Correction for body surface area variation should be made for children and large or small adults. The normal range of creatinine clearance is 70 to 130 ml. per minute.

X-RAY EXAMINATION OF THE URINARY TRACT

X-ray examination of the urinary tract is just as important as a chest roentgenogram in a general evaluation of a patient. No other single technique so clearly evaluates renal function or detects urinary tract disease. Early diagnosis is essential to avoid severe and irreparable damage to the urinary tract.

Examination of the urinary tract is carried out by a plain film, by cystograms, urethrograms, excretory urography, and retrograde pyelography. Retrograde pyelography is carried out after cystoscopic examination and the passage of ureteral catheters to the kidney pelvis.

In interpreting the films, it is wise to establish a definite routine for each type of examination and follow that pattern. This may seem tedious, but it produces the best results. The routine that I recommend is presented in the outline that follows:

I. The plain or scout film (kidneys-ureter-bladder, or K.U.B.)
   A. Procedure: The patient lies supine, and the film is taken to include the area from the lower ribs to the pubis.
   B. Bone survey
     1. Look for changes in the ribs, spine, sacrum, pelvis, and femurs (Fig. 41-1).
     2. Metastatic lesions of carcinoma are particularly important
       a. Osteoblastic bone lesions: carcinoma of the prostate
       b. Osteolytic bone lesions: carcinoma of the kidney, thyroid, lung, and urinary bladder
       c. Bone tumors such as multiple myeloma, sarcoma, etc.
     3. Other bone changes such as arthritis, Paget's disease, bone cysts, and fractures

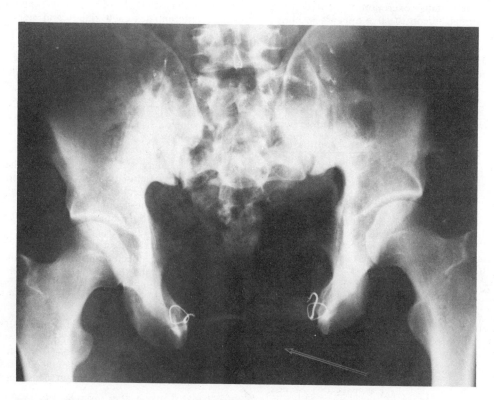

Fig. 41-1. Pelvic roentgenogram of young male with congenital bladder exstrophy and epispadias. *Arrow,* Typical associated defect in pubic symphysis. Metal sutures are seen in pubic arches.

C. Soft-tissue survey
  1. Kidney outline
     a. Size, shape, and position
     b. Frequently not seen because of gas or poor detail
  2. Psoas shadow outline
     a. Are the outlines bilaterally the same?
     b. Notice if the outline is sharp and distinct.
     c. Frequently is not seen because of gas or poor detail
  3. Other soft-tissue shadows
     a. Liver, spleen, tumors
D. Foreign bodies, stones
  1. Show up as opaque or radiodense shadows (Fig. 41-2)
  2. A phlebolith can be differentiated from a stone by its typical lucent center and location with respect to the ureter or kidney pelvis or bladder.

E. Intestinal gas pattern
II. Excretory urography (I.V.P.)
  A. Procedure: Check for sensitivity to iodine. If possible, the patient is prepared previously by being dehydrated—no fluid or food for 12 to 18 hours before the films. (An important exception to the dehydration preparation is the patient with multiple myeloma. These patients should not be dehydrated so that renal failure may be avoided.) First, a plain film (K.U.B.) is taken. Then, 100 to 150 ml. of radiopaque contrast material (Hypaque, Renografin, Renovist, Conray) are injected slowly intravenously. If injected too rapidly, it may cause flushing, abdominal distress, nausea, and vomiting. Exposures, covering the same area as the K.U.B. are usually made at 5, 10, and 25 minutes. A fifth film, the excretory cystogram, is taken over the bladder region alone.

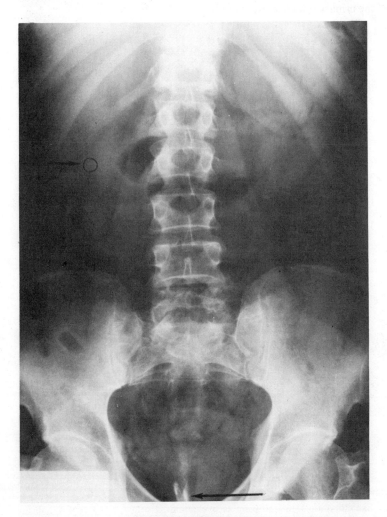

Fig. 41-2. Plain film of abdomen (kidneys-ureter-bladder) reveals extensive prostatic calcifications above pubic symphysis *(large arrow)* and small right renal calculus *(small arrow).*

Visualization of the urinary tract is improved by the technique of infusion urography. Here, the patient need not be dehydrated in advance. An infusion consisting of 1 ml. of contrast per pound of body weight added to an equal volume of 5% dextrose in water is administered intravenously over 15 or 20 minutes. Appropriate films are taken after the infusion is completed. This study is more expensive but results in improved filling of the collecting systems. Oblique and compression films are included.

B. Value of the excretory urogram
1. It is useful when retrograde pyelograms would be difficult or dangerous to do, as with children, urethral or ureteral strictures, impassable stones, suspected rupture of the kidney, suspected anomalies, and poor-risk patients.

2. It is a quick, simple, safe screening test to help rule out pathological conditions of the urinary tract.
3. It is a good indicator of kidney function. A normal kidney is visualized well; a nonfunctioning kidney will not be visualized.
C. The size, shape, and position of the drainage pathways of the tract are established (Fig. 41-3).
D. Iodinated contrast medium may be given intramuscularly or subcutaneously if a vein cannot be entered, as in children. The amount of contrast medium varies from 5 to 20 ml., depending on the age of the child. An infant should take about 5 to 8 ml. and a child over 10 years of age, 15 ml. The contrast medium can be mixed with an equal volume of saline, divided in half, and each portion injected intra-

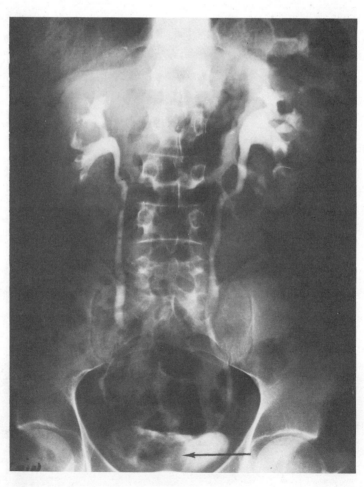

Fig. 41-3. Excretory urogram (intravenous pyelogram). Normal study; arrow indicates rectal gas superimposed on bladder.

muscularly into one buttock. The addition of 1 ml. of hyaluronidase (Wydase) improves absorption of the contrast medium. The first film is exposed in about 10 minutes. The next film taken about 5 minutes later and the third in another 5 to 10 minutes. If the contrast medium is injected intravenously into children, three x-ray exposures are taken 5 minutes apart. This technique has been used in newborns as young as 1 day of age.

III. Cystography: The patient's bladder is entirely emptied by means of a urethral catheter. Any iodinated contrast medium can be used, depending on the effect desired, and there are times when air is used as the contrast medium. The cystogram may be taken in many different positions, depending on the nature of the lesion to be studied. One makes a voiding cystogram by having the patient void while the film is exposed.

IV. Opaque cystogram
   A. Procedure: The patient lies supine and an iodinated contrast solution is instilled into the bladder through a catheter until the patient complains of a feeling of fullness. This amount is usually less than 400 ml. of solution. Anteroposterior and oblique exposures are taken.
   B. Size, shape, and location of the bladder
      1. The normal bladder configuration is a rounded shadow, centrally placed, about the size of a grapefruit.
      2. Chronic cystitis is characterized by an extremely small, spastic bladder; atony by an extremely large, flaccid bladder.
      3. Pelvic tumors displace the bladder from the midline.
   C. Character of the bladder wall
      1. Normally it is smooth.
      2. Long-standing obstruction causes a hypertrophied and greatly roughened bladder wall with many coarse trabeculations.
   D. Diverticula
      1. A diverticulum is a herniation of mucosa through the hypertrophied muscle fibers. This outpouching most commonly results from long-standing obstruction. The normal bladder has no diverticulum.
      2. Sometimes the diverticulum may be larger than the bladder itself, or there may be many diverticula, creating a problem of identifying the true bladder. Distinguishing features of the diverticulum are the following:
         a. It has smooth outline, whereas the obstructed bladder is slightly roughened.
         b. It is usually eccentrically located.
         c. The urethral catheter usually does not enter it.
      3. Emptying: Does the diverticulum empty, or does urine stagnate? This may be distinguished by the position of the diverticulum or by a postevacuation film.
   E. Vesicoureteral reflux
      1. It is not normal to have the contrast solution pass up the ureters.

      2. Ureteral reflux is attributable to incompetence of the ureterovesical valve, caused by infection, long-standing obstruction, congenital anomalies, surgery, or neurogenic disease (Fig. 41-2).
   F. Rupture of the bladder: The contrast extravasates from the bladder.
   G. Bladder contents: The contrast cystogram may outline tumors or foreign bodies within the bladder, but this is better done with the air cystogram.

V. Air cystogram
   A. Procedure: The bladder is emptied of the contrast and washed out. The patient is placed in the right oblique (semilateral) position. The bladder is filled with air, by catheter, until the patient complains of a feeling of fullness.
   B. The air acts as a lucent contrast medium and will help to visualize:
      1. Intravesical position of the prostate
      2. Bladder tumors
      3. Foreign bodies, especially radiolucent stones

VI. Retrograde urethrography
   A. Procedure: Urethrography is of great value in the study of trauma, strictures, contractures, congenital deformities at the bladder neck, and deformities of the prostatic urethra associated with prostatism. A urethrogram is made after the Flocks technique by emptying the bladder of fluid, filling it with air with the patient in the oblique position, and then filling the urethra with a mixture of iodinated contrast and sterile lubricating jelly. During the exposure of the film, 50 ml. of this mixture is injected into the urethra. This gives a simultaneous air cystogram and opaque urethrogram and is particularly valuable for outlining the posterior urethra to evaluate the adequacy of prostatectomy. At times a voiding urethrogram is helpful. This is usually done by filling the bladder with contrast medium and exposing the film during micturition.
   B. The following landmarks should be observed
      1. The pendulous urethra
      2. The bulbous urethra—the usual seat of inflammatory strictures
      3. The external sphincter and the internal sphincter
      4. The prostatic urethra: elongation, widening, and anterior angulation are indicative of benign prostatic enlargement.
         a. Are there prostatic calculi?
         b. Are there periurethral abscesses?

VII. Retrograde pyelography
   A. Retrograde pyelography is a more exact method of visualizing the upper urinary tract. Its purpose is fourfold.
      1. Accurate visualization of the anatomical structure of the upper urinary tract
      2. Procurement of segregated specimens of urine from each kidney for culture, cytology, and microscopy

3. When the ureteral catheters are in place, the differential function of each kidney is determined accurately by the intravenous injection of phenolsulfonphthalein or indigo carmine
4. Relief of ureteral obstruction

B. Procedure: A cystoscope is introduced into the bladder: A cystoscope is introduced into the bladder, and after cystoscopy has been completed, the ureteral orifices are catheterized with catheters that are advanced gently into each renal pelvis. Specimens of urine are then obtained from each renal pelvis for the examinations mentioned previously.

After this, plain films are taken to mark the course of the ureters and to locate any radiopaque density, such as stones. Either air or an iodinated contrast is injected into the kidney pelvis, and roentgenograms are made to visualize the pelvis and calyces accurately. Alternatively the procedure may be performed with fluoroscopic guidance.

If visualization of the ureters is desirable, the catheters are withdrawn to the lower portion of the ureter and contrast is injected for a ureteropyelogram. Air is used instead of contrast to show nonopaque calculi or other relatively nondense filling defects of the ureter. Retrograde pyelography is not an innocuous procedure. Reflex anurias and pyelonephritis are rare complications of retrograde pyelography.

Most cystoscopies and retrograde pyelograms are done without any anesthesia whatsoever, and the patients experience no undue discomfort. All in all, retrograde pyelograms are probably one of the most accurate and definitive diagnostic procedures in medicine.

VIII. Special x-ray studies
There are may special types of studies that have limited use:

A. Perirenal air and gas injections: These are used to outline the kidneys and possible adrenal tumors. This is not an innocuous procedure but does, at times, give sufficient additional information to justify its risk. Ultrasound and computerized tomography have eliminated the need for these studies.

B. Gastric air injections: Air introduced into the stomach may aid in demonstrating a renal mass, especially in children.

C. Nephrotomography: Very valuable particularly to outline masses in the renal area; most uroradiologists now include nephrotomography routinely in excretory urography.

D. Abdominal aortography: Contrast medium injected into the aorta outlines the renal arterial system. Uses:

1. The main advantage of aortography is to differentiate malignant lesions of the kidney from benign cysts. Contrast fills the vascular spaces within a neoplasm but outlines only the periphery of a cyst.

2. The nephrogram demonstrates certain parenchymal lesions before they are large enough to encroach on the calyces or pelvis or to produce detectable reduction of renal function. This is particularly true in early tuberculous and neoplastic renal lesions.

3. Visualization of the renal artery may help diagnose renovascular hypertension (some obstructive mechanism of the arterial supply to the kidney). Massive arterial renal infarct may also be detected by this procedure.

4. The question of renal ptosis versus ectopia is clearly settled, but these usually can be distinguished by retrograde pyelograms.

5. Ectopic vessels that obstruct the ureteropelvic junction in congenital hydronephrosis may be documented by aortography. This may be demonstrated better if one does a retrograde pyelogram immediately preceding the arteriogram, superimposing one on the other.

E. Selective renal angiography: Very useful for visualizing renal artery lesions and renal tumors and has in many instances supplemented aortography. Angiographic infarction of renal tumors is now used instead of, or as a preoperative adjunct to, surgery.

OTHER SPECIAL DIAGNOSTIC STUDIES

Other special diagnostic studies include the following:

1. Radioactive renography
2. Renal scanning
3. Needle biopsy
4. Cinefluorography
5. Urodynamic studies: ureters, kidney pelvis, bladder, and urethra
6. Endocrine function studies
7. Chromatin test for somatic sex and chromosomal analysis (karyotype)
8. Skeletal scanning
9. Ultrasound scanning
10. Computerized tomography (CT) and scanning
11. Nuclear magnetic resonance

KIDNEY
Renal anomalies

The congenital anomalies of the renal parenchyma may be classified as follows: abnormalities of number, position, form, structure, and vascularization.

Number

The most common anomaly is that of number and usually is asymptomatic. Obviously, if both kidneys are absent, life is impossible. Congenital *solitary kidney* does occur. This means that whenever nephrectomy is to be considered, the possibility that the other kidney may be absent or hypoplastic makes preoperative study mandatory. Occasionally a true *supernumerary kidney* may be present. The most common type of abnormality of number is *duplication* of the pelvis and ureter. Many of them are associated with ectopic ureteral openings, usually of the ureter draining the upper kidney pelvis, which are the source of the symptoms. (See discussion of congenital anomalies of the ureter, p. 599.) Many are also associated with anomalies of vascularization that produce partial urinary obstruction.

Position

Anomaly of position occurs when the embryological process of ascent and rotation of the kidney is interfered with at any point. Usually failure of rotation is associated with compression of the pelvis or ureter, or both, by renal vessels, producing obstruction. The *ectopic kidney* can easily be recognized by its short ureter and anterior position of its pelvis. Sometimes *crossed ectopia* with fusion occurs, resembling a large tumor mass. This may actually be all the renal parenchyma the patient has, and removal of such a fused kidney would be lethal.

Form

Anomalies of form occur during upward embryological migration of the kidneys. Their lower poles may fuse to form a *horseshoe kidney*. After fusion one kidney may ascend and pull the other to the opposite side (*crossed ectopia with fusion*). The anterior surface of one may be fused to the posterior surface of the other, and they remain in the pelvis (so-called disk kidney). These anomalies frequently are confused with other masses or are associated with obstruction to the outflow of urine from their pelves from ectopic renal arteries. Treatment is tailored to the exact difficulties each produces.

Structure

Anomalies of structure may be unilateral or bilateral and are characterized by *hypoplasia* or *cystic formation*. If hypoplasia is unilateral, no symptoms may occur. If hypoplasia is bilateral, renal insufficiency will result. Cystic formation may be asymptomatic, but massive replacement of remaining renal tissue will produce renal insufficiency (Fig. 41-4). Multicystic kidney is usually associated with an atretic ureter.

Congenital polycystic disease. Congenital polycystic disease is one of the important anomalies of the kidney. It is usually *bilateral* and *familial* and seems to be caused by a lack of fusion of most of the renal elements with the excretory elements of the tubules. This produces a large number of

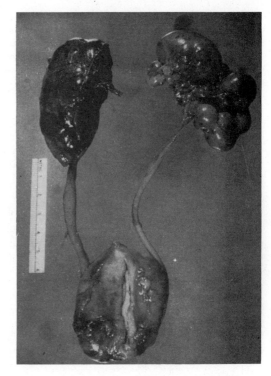

Fig. 41-4. Multicystic kidney, on left.

varying-sized cysts in each kidney that grow slowly, destroy renal substance, and produce gradual renal insufficiency. Bilateral palpable masses usually result. The cysts distort the kidney outlines and the kidney pelves, to produce a characteristic roentgenographic appearance.

If polycystic disease is unilateral, it cannot be readily differentiated from hypernephroma.

When bilateral, the diagnosis is usually easily made. Hypertension with red and white cells and casts in the urine heralds the gradual onset of renal insufficiency. The treatment is symptomatic and operative. *Symptomatic treatment* consists essentially in avoiding trauma and infection to the kidneys, since massive hemorrhage may result. *Surgical treatment* consists in aspirating as many of the cysts as possible to reduce the pressure on the normal-functioning renal substance. This, of course, is purely palliative. The prognosis varies with the rapidity with which renal insufficiency and hypertension develop, which in turn probably depends on the extent of the renal involvement. Some patients live only a few years, most die in middle age, and a few live out their normal span. A small percentage of cases are associated with cystic disease of the liver and lungs and cerebral artery aneurysms. Hemodialysis and renal transplantation have been effective in the treatment of the chronic renal insufficiency related to polycystic kidney disease. Bilateral nephrectomy is indicated to make room for the renal graft or for relief of hypertension.

Vascularization

Anomalies of vascularization may occur in otherwise normal kidneys. They are hazards during operative procedures on the kidney, or they may produce obstruction at the ureteropelvic junction that requires correction.

• • •

Abdominal masses, renal insufficiency, abdominal pain, or urinary symptoms may indicate a congenital anomaly of the kidney. This is true no matter what the age of the patient.

Congenital anomalies of the renal pelvis are essentially *obstructive* from bands, high insertion of the ureter, or stricture at the ureteropelvic junction (Fig. 41-5). They may produce enormous hydronephrotic sacs with renal atrophy. They are bilateral in over 50% of the cases and should be differentiated from renal cysts, renal neoplasms,

and obstructive uropathy originating lower in the urinary tract. They may be silent or produce an ache or pain in the side or evidence of severe infection. They may produce a large abdominal mass. The treatment is surgical—removal or repair—with the surgeon always keeping in mind that the condition is frequently bilateral. The pathognomonic findings are demonstrated readily with intravenous and retrograde pyelography.

Urolithiasis

Stones in the urinary tract are common disorders with distinct geographical variations in incidence (Fig. 41-6). So-called stone belts occur in various parts of the world, in which certain types of stone predominate; e.g., in the southern part of the United States, calcium oxalate stones are common. In the United States as a whole, about 75% to 80% are calcium oxalate, calcium phosphate, or magnesium ammonium phosphate stones. Of the remaining, four fifths are uric acid stones, and the others are cystine stones. Magnesium ammonium phosphate stones commonly occur after infection in the urinary tract with urea-splitting organisms (Fig. 41-7).

Stones in the urinary tract are the result of a

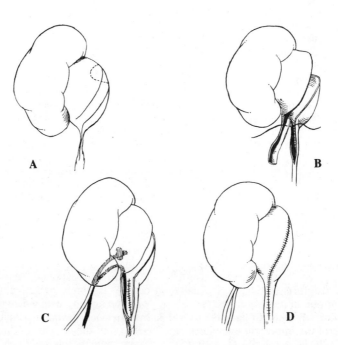

Fig. 41-5. Congenital stricture of ureteropelvic junction and its surgical correction. **A,** Outlined is incision that crosses stricture and raises flap from kidney pelvis. **B,** Flap swung down to widen strictured area. **C,** Nephrostomy tube and ureteral catheter splint inserted. **D,** Result.

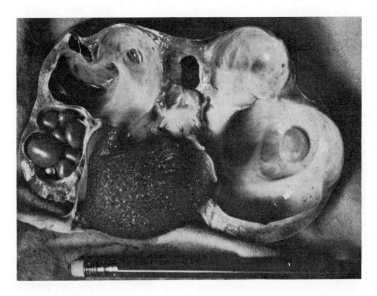

Fig. 41-6. Urolithiasis. Multiple large stones (cystine) have obstructed and totally destroyed kidney.

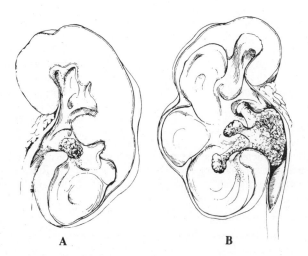

Fig. 41-7. A, Single calculus obstructing and dilating lower renal calyx. **B,** "Staghorn" calculus obstructing and dilating all renal calyces.

series of predisposing factors. Elucidation of these factors is necessary for correct therapy. Renal calculi are a result of one or more of the following: a foreign body in the urinary tract, vitamin A deficiency, urinary tract infection, urinary tract stasis, metabolic disturbances causing increased crystalloid excretion (cystinuria, hyperparathyroidism, etc.), and changes in the urine that lessen the solubility of the crystalloids in the urine. In some instances a matrix, or nucleus, acts as a template for further precipitation of crystalloids. However, in certain types of recumbency calculi, such a matrix is obviously not necessary. Some factors are important in the formation of a nucleus, and others facilitate precipitation of the various stone-forming crystalloids. Some factors that are precursors of certain types of stone should be emphasized.

Foreign body

Any *foreign body* in the urinary tract favors the formation of calcium phosphate and ammonium magnesium phosphate stones. Nonabsorbable suture material used in operations on the bladder or renal pelvis will act as a nucleus around which precipitation of the supersaturated calcium salts occurs. Ulcerating lesions and papillary tumors in the urinary tract act similarly.

Vitamin A deficiency

In man the relationship of *vitamin A deficiency* to urinary calculi is debatable, but in animals it may produce urinary stones in several ways: (1) by producing ulceration of the epithelium of the urinary tract, (2) by causing desquamation of the epithelium (the desquamated epithelium acts as a nucleus), and (3) by predisposing the urinary tract to infection that may change the precipitability of the stone-forming crystalloids.

Urinary tract infection

Urinary tract infection is believed to be the most important single cause of urolithiasis. It may produce a stone by creating a nucleus in a manner similar to vitamin A deficiency, by changing the pH of the urine, or by altering the protective colloids of the urine.

Urinary stasis

Urinary stasis from acquired or congenital obstruction of the urinary passageway is an important predisposing cause of urolithiasis. In a series of 60 patients with obstruction at the ureteropelvic junction without infection who were studied at the University of Iowa Hospitals, the incidence of urolithiasis was 10 times higher than it was in a series of patients without such obstruction. If other

cases for urolithiasis exist and a tiny stone forms, it may pass without becoming clinically manifest if obstruction is not present. If recurrent urolithiasis is to be prevented, urinary stasis must be corrected.

Metabolic disturbances

Certain metabolic disturbances produce qualitative and quantitative changes in the urinary crystalloids that predispose to the formation of calculi, particularly if a nucleus has formed, if urinary stasis and infection occur, or if changes in the urine aid in the precipitation of such crystalloids. The most frequent of these metabolic changes are cystinuria and alterations of calcium and uric acid metabolism.

Cystinuria is a familial abnormality of renal tubular absorption of the amino acid cystine characterized by the excretion of a large amount of cystine in the urine. Normally, 10 to 100 mg. of cystine are excreted in the urine in 24 hours. With abnormal cystine reabsorption, 300 to 1,500 mg. may be excreted in 24 hours. At present, no method for altering this abnormality is known. The following measures are helpful: forced administration of fluids, correction and avoidance of all factors that lead to the formation of a nucleus, correction of urinary stasis if present, and alteration of the hydrogen-ion concentration of the urine so that it will be continuously alkaline (cystine is insoluble in acid urine and highly soluble in akaline urine). The urine usually is made alkaline by administration of sodium bicarbonate, or sodium citrate and potassium citrate. The chelating agent D-penicillamine (Cuprimine) is also indicated in cystinuria. The drug forms a complex with cystine that is more soluble than the cystine alone. Large cystine calculi have been dissolved by such therapy.

Metabolic conditions that predispose to an increased excretion of *calcium phosphate* are very common. The most important of these is recumbency. If other factors that predispose to the formation of urinary calculi can be avoided by a proper regimen, the precipitated calcium salts can be washed out readily before irreparable renal damage occurs. Tiny stones can be demonstrated on x-ray studies of the kidneys even in the first few months of a period recumbency.

Hyperparathyroidism from adenoma or hyperplasia of the parathyroid glands may be the underlying cause of urolithiasis. Up to 50% of patients with hyperparathyroidism will have renal stones. Hyperparathyroidism is characterized by localized or generalized osteoporosis, urinary calculi, and a high serum calcium and low serum phosphorus in the early stage of the disease before renal insufficiency develops. The serum alkaline phosphatase usually is increased. In most cases treatment of the hyperparathyroidism should precede treatment of the urinary calculi. Exceptions to this are cases in which acute urinary obstruction or infection is present.

Other metabolic diseases may be important in the formation of urinary calculi. *Uric acid stones* are seen with hypersecretion of uric acid associated with a disturbance of purine metabolism. The medical management and prevention of these calculi are very similar to those utilized in cases of cystinuria, i.e., an alkaline reaction of the urine and a low purine diet. The xanthine oxidase inhibitor allopurinol (Zyloprim) is useful in that it decreases both serum and urine uric acid concentrations. With improved chemotherapy for various malignancies, more cancer patients are at risk for the hyperuricemia and subsequent hyperuricosuria related to increased cell destruction and release of nucleic acids.

Changes in the urine predisposing to crystalloid precipitation

At the time a urinary stone is formed, the hydrogen-ion concentration of the urine is the final factor that determines the chemical composition of the stone. Infection of the urinary tract plays an important role, since urea-splitting organisms alkalinize the urine to favor the precipitation of calcium phosphate. Treatment includes control of urinary infection and acidification of the urine by the administration of sodium acid phosphate. In addition, this drug decreases the urinary excretion of calcium by as much as 50%. Ascorbic acid (vitamin C) is also useful to acidify the urine.

Other etiological factors

In some cases a primary renal defect may be associated with hyperexcretion of oxalates and calcium phosphate. In such cases diets relatively low in oxalates and phosphorus may be useful.

Stress influences the formation of stones in animals, though its role in humans is obscure. It is believed to be a factor in the production of uric acid and oxalate calculi. Avoidance of stress should be a part of the treatment of patients with these calculi.

The prolonged administration of ACTH and corticosteroids produces osteoporosis and an accompanying hypercalciuria. Hypercalciuria should be considered in any case in which either of these drugs is administered for a long time.

Many patients, particularly young males with recurrent calcium oxalate calculi, have only hypercalciuria (daily excretion of more than 250 mg. of calcium). Newer methods of testing have allowed the subdivision of this category into at least two types: hypercalciuria caused by (1) *gastrointestinal hyperabsorption* and (2) *renal tubular hyperexcretion*. The latter form is best treated by thiazide diuretics, which reduce renal tubular loss of calcium; patients with hyperabsorption should be treated with low calcium diets and the newer phosphate binders.

Ureteral stones

Ureteral stones essentially are renal stones that have passed down into the ureter. They rarely arise in the ureter itself, except when a foreign body, such as a ureteral suture, acts as a nucleus for precipitation of calcium and magnesium ammonium phosphate salts.

In general, stones under 5 to 6 mm. pass spontaneously. Those over that diameter usually must be removed, whether they are causing symptoms or not. Uric acid calculi are nonopaque on roentgenographic examination and show up as filling defects in the pyeloureterogram; they must be differentiated from blood clots and tumors of the ureter (Fig. 41-8).

Vesical stones

Vesical stones are becoming less common. They are associated with infection and obstruction at the bladder neck, or with ulcerating lesions or foreign bodies in the bladder itself. Vesical calculi therefore are found in the bladder itself, though some of them are actually stones that have passed down from the kidney and have been retained in the bladder because of bladder neck obstruction. They may be removed suprapubically or transurethrally by cystolitholapaxy or cystolithotripsy, depending on their size, consistency, and the condition of the bladder itself. Calculi may form in bladder diverticula because of increased stasis. Here treatment must be directed against the underlying cause of the diverticulum and removal of the stone as well.

Nonopaque uric acid stones require differentiation from bladder tumors, large subcervical prostatic lobes, or blood clots. Opaque calculi are readily recognized on the roentgenogram. Since many of them are associated with ulcerative lesions of the bladder or bladder neck obstruction, these accessory or predisposing conditions must be treated simultaneously.

Surgical treatment of renal calculi is shown in Figs. 41-9 and 41-10. Two new methods for removal of renal calculi short of major open surgery are worthy of mention: percutaneous ultrasonic lithotripsy and extracorporeal shock-wave disintegration. In the former method, after a percutaneous nephrostomy tract is obtained and dilated, renal calculi can be either directly removed or shattered

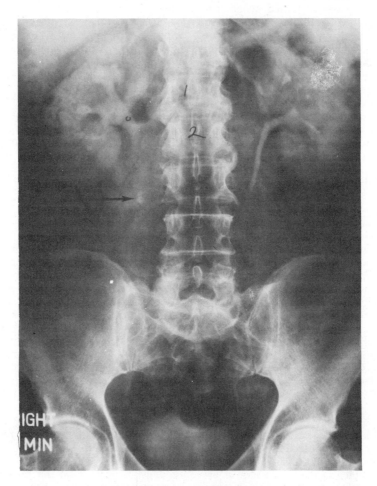

Fig. 41-8. Excretory urogram (I.V.P.) demonstrates right hydroureteronephrosis associated with two opaque calculi in proximal ureter *(arrow);* left upper urinary tract and bladder are normal.

by a special ultrasonic probe. In the latter method, with the patient placed in a waterbath to allow passage of the energy beam, finely focused shock waves are pulsed at the stones. The calculi are fragmented into many tiny particles, which are passed spontaneously down the ureter.

Renal neoplasms

Neoplasms of the kidney are common and are generally malignant. Benign tumors are clinical curiosities. The best clinical classification is related to age. Most tumors in children under 8 years of age are Wilms' tumors, or nephroblastomas. Generally, few malignant tumors occur between 8 years and about 25 or 30 years of age. About 95% of renal tumors in adults are highly malignant neoplasms of the renal parenchyma, the hypernephroma (renal cell carcinoma). The other 5% are tumors of the renal pelvis: transitional cell, squamous cell, or adenocarcinoma.

The general trend in the treatment of malignant renal neoplasms favors more radical surgery. Preoperative or postoperative x-ray therapy is not helpful for hypernephroma, though the current consensus strongly endorses irradiations as part of the therapy for Wilms' tumor.

Childhood neoplasms

Renal neoplasms of childhood are mixed mesenchymal tumors (Wilms' tumors, or nephroblas-

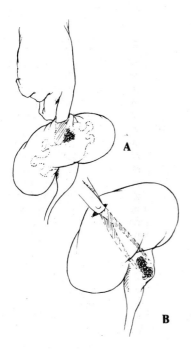

Fig. 41-9. A, Transrenal digital removal of stone from calyx. **B,** Transrenal removal of stone from kidney pelvis by instrument.

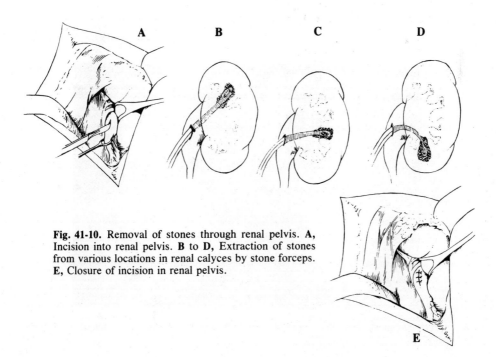

Fig. 41-10. Removal of stones through renal pelvis. **A,** Incision into renal pelvis. **B to D,** Extraction of stones from various locations in renal calyces by stone forceps. **E,** Closure of incision in renal pelvis.

toma). They appear very early in life and constitute one of the most frequent malignant tumors of childhood, rivaled in incidence by neuroblastoma, which frequently invades the kidney and resembles Wilms' tumor. Wilms' tumors grow rapidly and metastasize early through the bloodstream and lymphatics, with the lungs being frequently involved. Over 30% of patients have metastases when first seen: the most common sign is a large abdominal mass. The urine is often normal, and there are generally no urinary symptoms. Gastrointestinal disturbances and pain are frequent because of the weight and bulk of the tumor. Metastatic lesions produce a variety of symptoms and signs. The diagnosis is usually readily made by means of urography; intravenous pyelograms show a mass deformity or no function from the involved kidney, and retrograde pyelograms show a distorted and deformed pelvis. Wilms' tumors must always be differentiated from congenital hydronephrosis and cystic disease of the kidney, which are frequently bilateral and in which removal of a kidney might be contraindicated. A differential diagnosis between neuroblastoma and Wilms' tumor should also be made, since therapy is different: a very fine stippled calcification is seen in the neuroblastoma, which involves the kidney only indirectly (by pushing it down and involving the cortex or a portion of the cortex so that the intravenous pyelogram shows good function in a portion of the kidney) (Fig. 41-11). On the other hand, Wilms' tumor usually involves the entire kidney and usually has no calcification.

In addition Wilms' tumor must be distinguished from a fetal hamartoma (mesoblastic nephroma), a benign developmental renal mass presenting in the first year of life and generally in the newborn period. Fetal hamartoma requires only simple nephrectomy as therapy.

Treatment. The treatment of Wilms' tumor consists of three modalities: (1) surgical removal of the primary tumor, (2) irradiation therapy, and (3) chemotherapy. For Wilms' tumors, actinomycin D seems to be almost specific. Treatment must be carried out over a long period of time so that metastatic lesions are destroyed. Results have been steadily improving, so that in patients who do not have obvious metastases an 80% 5-year survival can be expected. Vincristine sulfate and doxorubicin (Adriamycin) are also useful in chemotherapy for Wilms' tumor.

Adult neoplasms (Fig. 41-12)

A. General
   1. All neoplasms are malignant, with rare exceptions.
   2. There is no definite agreement on the pathological classification of these tumors, but for practical purposes they are all hypernephromas (renal cell carcinoma, clear cell carcinoma, adenocarcinoma).
   3. Treatment is the same—surgery
B. Metastases
   1. Most frequent to the lung and x-ray evidence is characteristic (snowball lesion)
   2. Almost as frequent to bone (pulsating osteolytic lesion)
   3. 30% have metastases when first seen

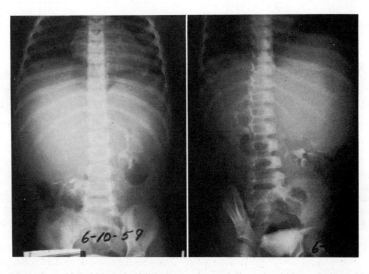

Fig. 41-11. Mass above right kidney in child, depressing and distorting kidney. Oblique view on right. Neuroblastoma.

C. Cardinal signs and symptoms
1. Pain
2. Mass—unilateral
3. Hematuria
D. Diagnosis
1. Suspicion is aroused by
   a. Any of the preceding cardinal signs or symptoms
   b. Unexplained fever
   c. Unexplained weight loss
   d. Unexplained anemia
2. However, diagnosis at the stage when these signs and symptoms appear is usually too late for curative therapy.
3. Cytological studies of the urine show promise of aiding early diagnosis in those tumors developing close to the urothelium.
4. Endocrinopathies (paraneoplastic syndromes): erythrocytosis, hypercalcemia, hyperreninemia
5. X-ray diagnosis
   a. Characteristic urogram (Fig. 41-13)
      (1) Characteristic splaying or spiderlike deformity of calyces
      (2) Asymmetrical enlargement of kidney substance on film
      (3) Obscuring of the renal outline
      (4) Irregular calcifications
   b. Renal ultrasound
      (1) Echogenic mass lesion
      (2) Any mass that is not clearly echolucent (cystic)

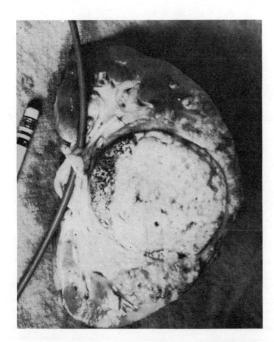

Fig. 41-12. Carcinoma of kidney parenchyma.

c. Computerized axial tomography (CAT or CT scan)
   (1) Mass lesion or lesions more dense than normal renal parenchyma
   (2) Obliteration of perinephric spaces
   (3) Retroperitoneal lymphadenopathy
   (4) Renal vein or inferior vena cava involvement
   (5) Identification of hepatic masses as possible metastases
d. Aortography (renal arteriography) (Fig. 41-13)
   (1) Hypervascular or neovascular pattern in mass
   (2) Parasitic (collateral) vessels
   (3) Arteriovenous fistula
   (4) Nodal or hepatic metastases may be visualized
e. Chest roentgenogram
   (1) Pulmonary metastasis
   (2) Mediastinal lymphadenopathy
f. Bone films
   (1) Osteolytic metastatic lesions
   (2) Pathological fractures
E. Differential diagnosis
1. Congenital lesions
   a. Cysts
      (1) Polycystic—usually bilateral
      (2) Solitary—cannot tell by roentgenographic examination, calcification less frequent, radiolucent center, smooth wall
      (3) Multiple solitary—same as for solitary
2. Trauma: hematoma—history, blood clot is not smooth in outline, clot is generally mobile in the pelvis and will gradually disappear.
3. Infection
   a. Renal carbuncle—tenderness, renal mass, chills and fever, W.B.C. count elevated, history of diabetes mellitus
   b. Tuberculosis—history of contact and above
   c. Parasites, e.g., hydatid disease
4. Stone—smooth, movable, does not disappear, x-ray evidence, blood chemistry studies

Treatment. Surgical removal (nephrectomy) has improved results. A 40% to 70% 5-year survival is expected if there are no metastases when the diagnosis is made. Radical nephrectomy with regional lymphadenectomy is the procedure of choice.

Neoplasms of the urothelium

Tumors arising from the urothelium are relatively uncommon but present a serious diagnostic problem (Fig. 41-14). The most common symptoms are gross hematuria and pain that simulates a renal calculus. Retrograde pyelography shows filling defects or distortions of the calyces that are quite characteristic but need to be distinguished from nonopaque stone and blood clot. They frequently metastasize along the ureter or into the bladder. Sometimes this causes a problem in differential

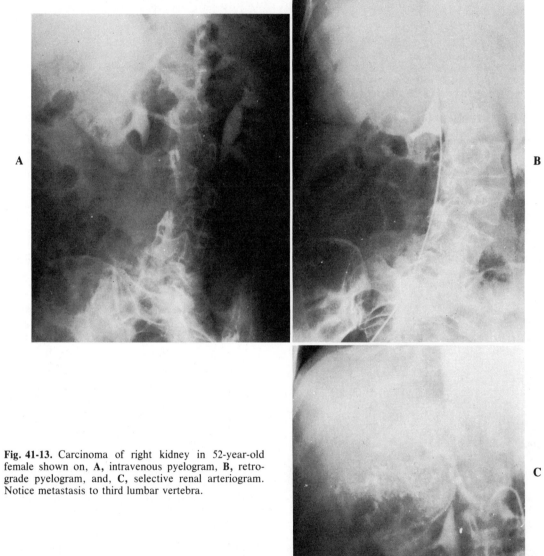

Fig. 41-13. Carcinoma of right kidney in 52-year-old female shown on, **A,** intravenous pyelogram, **B,** retrograde pyelogram, and, **C,** selective renal arteriogram. Notice metastasis to third lumbar vertebra.

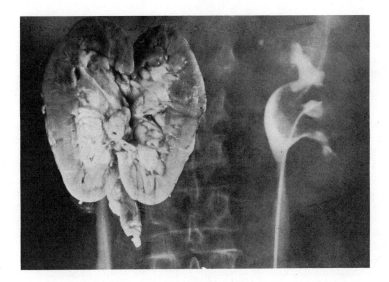

Fig. 41-14. Carcinoma of renal pelvis; pyelogram and specimen.

diagnosis in that the tumor blocks the ureter, presents itself in the bladder that is blocking off the outflow of urine from the kidney. Separate bladder tumors are seen in about half the patients with renal pelvic or ureteral tumors.

The treatment is surgical (nephroureterectomy). Cytology of the urine from the ureters is helpful in differential diagnosis.

Renal injuries

Renal injuries may be divided into two types: *penetrating* and *blunt*. The former are caused by bullet or knife wounds, and the latter are caused by indirect injury. With regard to the latter type, a kidney that is already the seat of a pathological lesion is more easily injured because (1) inflamed or tumor tissue is more friable and (2) the increased size of the diseased kidney makes it more accessible to the forces producing the injury. Renal injuries may also be classified according to the extent of the injury: (1) a slight tear or *contusion,* (2) a large tear of the renal substance, (3) a tear of the kidney substance involving the renal pelvis, (4) a hematoma about the kidney, and (5) injuries (including avulsion) to the vascular pedicle or ureter.

The ensuing symptoms, signs, and pathological changes depend on the nature and extent of the lesion. Extravasation of urine into the kidney substance may occur, producing necrosis and subsequent infection. Massive hemorrhage or massive renal infarction may result. Serious late sequelae to kidney trauma can occur, including scarring and caliectasis with poor drainage from portions of the kidney, leading to hypertension, stone formation, and renal infection.

Symptoms and diagnosis. After the history of injury, pain, hematuria, a mass on the injured side, strong muscle spasm, and tenderness with shock may appear. Physical, urine, blood, and roentgenographic examinations should be done immediately. The findings are varying degrees of shock, hemorrhage, a mass with tenderness in the area of the renal injury, and abdominal distension. Hematuria is variable, depending on whether the blood has access to the ureter. Intravenous and retrograde pyelograms confirm the diagnosis, though intravenous pyelograms are useless if the patient is in shock. Abdominal aortography plus renal arteriography and even celiac axis injection are most helpful in the identification of the site and character of vascular injuries. Pyelography may be required in the operating room. Careful consideration of both kidneys and all the renal substance involved is necessary. The best surgical approach is transabdominal to allow evaluation of all other intraabdominal organs as well as both renal arteries and both kidneys. The surgical procedure is tailored to the precise injury, from simple suture to nephrectomy (Fig. 41-15).

Postinjury examinations should be done every 3 months for at least a year (with intravenous pyelography) to evaluate possible permanent damage to the kidney. Ultrasound examinations are helpful in monitoring blood or urine accumulation resulting from trauma.

One other form of injury associated with trauma,

called *crush syndrome,* must be considered. Massive amounts of crushed tissue can cause severe oliguria and acute tubular necrosis. Fluids must be managed carefully. (See Chapter 3.) In severe cases peritoneal or hemodialysis may be required.

Renal tuberculosis

Renal tuberculosis is decreasing in incidence with more effective general control of the disease by public health measures and antituberculous drugs, since it is part and parcel of hematogenous dissemination from a primary focus in the lung or gastrointestinal tract. The primary focus produces a temporary bacteremia of tubercle bacilli, which are filtered out in the cortex of both kidneys and produce lesions that usually go on to repair themselves. Occasionally, however, they progress and involve the collecting system to produce an open renal tuberculosis. Before the advent of specific chemotherapy, this condition became bilateral in nearly 100% of the cases and required prolonged sanatorium care. With gross unilateral involvement, nephrectomy was the treatment of choice. At the present time, with the use of isoniazid (INH), ethambutol, and rifampin, most of these cases can be controlled if massive lesions can be removed surgically.

Hematuria or pyuria is present with no evidence of pyogenic organisms, but with tubercle bacilli in the urine detected by acid-fast stains and cultures. Any patient with severe pyuria, with no obvious organisms on smear or ordinary culture, should be suspected of having renal tuberculosis. This is particularly true if there is a history of pulmonary tuberculosis, even though inactive and completely healed. Urography usually shows the typical lesion: scarring and obliteration of some of the infundibula of the calyces and distortion and irregularity of several of the calyces in a kidney (Fig. 41-16). Tuberculous lesions frequently calcify. In fact, renal tuberculosis can be first seen in so many different ways that it might be called "the great masquerader" and is similar to generalized syphilis in this regard. If there is no substantial destruction of renal tissue or abscess formation, the treatment should be conservative and medical. If surgery is contemplated, chemotherapy before and after the surgical procedure for 6 months to 2 years is indicated.

Nontuberculous infections of the urinary tract

Renal infections are common and may arise as primary lesions, with entrance of the organisms into the kidney from a *hematogenous* source,

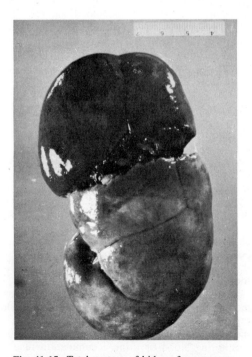

Fig. 41-15. Total rupture of kidney from trauma.

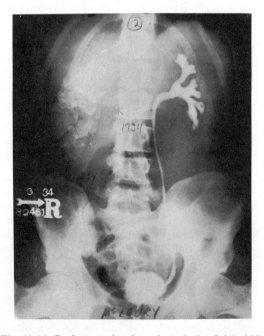

Fig. 41-16. Pyelogram showing tuberculosis of right kidney ("putty kidney").

much as described in renal tuberculosis. On the other hand, they may be associated with *ascending infection,* starting with lesions primarily in the urethra and prostate in the male, the urethra in the female, and the bladder in both. They may also arise from *infections outside the urinary tract,* producing lesions that allow the entrance of organisms into the perirenal and periureteral lymphatics. If the ureterovesical junctions are incompetent because of bladder infection, congenital anomaly, or neurogenic involvement of the bladder, renal infection is almost sure to ensue because of reflux of the infected urine into the renal pelvis.

Symptoms and signs. Urinary tract infection may manifest itself in many different ways. It may be discovered in an asymptomatic patient whose urinalysis shows bacteriuria or pyuria. It may produce disturbances of urination or pain over the region of the bladder or kidney. It may be associated with chills, fever, and leukocytosis, indicative of a general reaction. The history is important to rule out previous infections elsewhere in the body that might have acted as a primary source or some other pathological lesion in the urinary transport system. Thus excretory urography, cystography (to evaluate ureteral reflux), careful examination and culture of the urine, and cystourethroscopy may all be necessary for complete evaluation.

General supportive therapy, specific antibiotics for the organism that is cultured, and correction of urinary tract obstruction or other lesions that predispose to infection are keystones of treatment. An ulcerated bladder tumor, stones, bladder neck obstruction, benign prostatic hypertrophy in the adult male, and urethral stenosis in the elderly female produce obstruction that sustains the infection. These lesions *must* be corrected if the infection is to be eliminated. Pyuria or bacteriuria does not mean pyelonephritis. It means simply that an infection exists somewhere in the urinary passageway or the kidney. Newer methods detecting presence of antibody-coating may better localize the source of urinary infections. Intelligent management demands a thorough quest for contributory anatomical deformities. The eventual sequelae of uncontrolled urinary tract infection are loss of renal function (renal failure) and destruction of the urinary transport system.

URETER
Congenital anomalies

Anomalies of the ureter are frequently associated with anomalies of the kidney, which have been discussed previously. They include duplications, fused ureters, and aberrant course.

Ureterocele

Ureterocele is a cystic dilatation of the vesical end of the ureter caused by a congenital narrowing of the ureteral orifice (Fig. 41-17). It is asymptomatic until obstruction leads to hydronephrosis, stone formation, and infection. Diagnosis is made by cystoscopic examination and urography. Cystoscopy reveals a thin-walled cystic body that intermittently fills and balloons with urine and then collapses as the urine is discharged from the tiny orifice. Urograms may show the cystic radiolucent mass in the bladder and the secondary damage to ureter and kidneys. Treatment consists of removal of the ureterocele with ureteral reimplantation.

Megaloureter

Megaloureter is a tremendously atonic and dilated ureter (Fig. 41-18). The cause is obscure, though a functional disturbance of the neuromuscular mechanism of the ureter is the most likely. The condition is asymptomatic until hydronephrosis, infection, and stone formation occur.

Diagnosis is made by cystoscopy and urography. On cystoscopy the ureteral orifice may be normal. Urograms reveal a dilated and tortuous ureter. The essence of treatment is to secure good drainage and relieve stasis, which may require ureterovesical reimplantation or cutaneous ureterostomy.

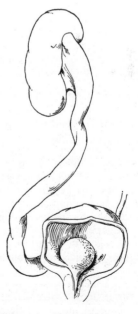

Fig. 41-17. Right ureterocele.

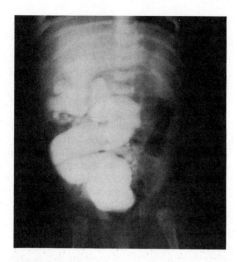

Fig. 41-18. Pyelogram showing right-sided megaloureter and hydronephrosis.

Ectopic ureteral orifices

Ectopic ureteral orifices are often associated with other congenital anomalies of the genitourinary passageways. In the female the aberrant opening of the ureteric orifice may be found in the vesical trigone, urethra, vagina, or even uterus. In the male the ectopic ureter opens proximally to the external sphincter. The symptoms affecting micturition vary greatly. In the female, sphincter control of the ectopic ureter is absent, and urinary incontinence is always present.

Diagnosis is made by history, urography, and cystoscopy. If the abnormality is discovered before renal damage is serious, the ureter may be implanted into the bladder, but if it is discovered after hydronephrotic atrophy and infection have occurred, nephrectomy is indicated if adequate renal function remains on the other side.

Other relatively rare congenital anomalies of the ureter include valves, diverticulum, postcaval ureter, and stricture. Postcaval ureter is actually an anomaly of the vascular system, for the vena cava forms in front of, instead of behind, the ureter. The ureter is compressed by this overlying vena cava, causing a hydronephrosis that may later become infected. True congenital strictures are rare; they result in hydroureter and hydronephrosis.

Injuries

Injuries from external violence are relatively infrequent because of musculoskeletal protection and relative mobility of the ureter. When injury does occur, it is accompanied by other injuries of great severity, such as shattered pelvis, and generally involves complete division of the lower ureter. In addition a fracture of one or more lumbar vertebral transverse processes must raise the possibility of trauma to the ureter.

Injuries from instrumentation are most frequently perforations made while one is attempting to extract a stone or to pass a catheter.

Injuries from surgery, particularly gynecological pelvic surgery, are the most common cause of ureteral injury. Normally the uterine artery and ureter are only 2.5 cm. apart, but neoplastic or inflammatory disease distorts this relationship and makes identification difficult. Injuries include incision, complete transection, occlusion, and necrosis from interference with blood supply.

Symptoms with unilateral injury include urinary fistula, progressive silent hydronephrosis, or pyonephrosis after infection. Symptoms with bilateral injury include anuria, uremia, and death.

Diagnosis. Indications of ureteral injury are the following:

1. Urinary fistula exists without bladder injury.
2. If methylene blue solution is introduced into the bladder and no dye appears through the fistula but dye does appear through the fistula when methylene blue is given intravenously, ureteral fistula must be suspected.
3. Further confirmation is obtained by cystoscopy and pyelographic studies.

Treatment. Treatment varies with the extent of injury to the ureter and the location of the lesion. Small incisions or minor damage to the ureteral wall may require no repair. Large incisions or transections should be repaired over a ureteral catheter, if possible, and the catheter left in place for 8 to 10 days. Other procedures include ureterovesical anastomosis, ureterointestinal anastomosis, cutaneous ureterostomy, transureteroureterostomy, autotransplantation, or even nephrectomy.

Calculus

Etiology. A ureteral calculus is usually a small stone that has passed down from the kidney pelvis. It rarely starts in the ureter, though an impacted fragment may grow larger there. The majority are composed of uric acid or calcium oxalate, since the phosphatic and cystine stones rapidly grow too large to pass down the ureter. The etiological factors responsible for stones in the kidney pelvis are also responsible for ureteral stones, particularly those of stasis associated with strictures and congenital hydroureter.

Symptoms. The types of symptoms produced by ureteral calculi are the same as those produced by a stone in the kidney. However, pain, hematuria, evidences of obstruction, infection, and renal insufficiency are more common with ureteral stones than they are with renal stones. Rarely ureteral calculi may be present for long periods of time without producing symptoms. They may produce gradual destruction of the urinary tract above because of obstruction.

Diagnosis. History, particularly of the known predisposing factors, chemical examination of the blood and urine, and dramatic relief of pain when a ureteral catheter is passed beyond the obstruction are important in diagnosis. Roentgenographic examination is important, particularly oblique films that will show the relationship of the stone to the course of the ureter (Fig. 41-8).

Differential diagnosis. Calcified lymph nodes, phleboliths, pills, gas in the bowel, and skin moles must be distinguished roentgenographically from ureteral calculi. Of course, all other causes of acute abdominal disease must be ruled out.

Treatment. Generally all stones over 1 cm. in diameter anywhere in the ureter, whether they are causing symptoms, should be removed.

Stones under 6 mm. in diameter may pass spontaneously. Antispasmodics and narcotics are given as needed, and fluids are forced. If the stone does not pass, a ureteral catheter is inserted above the stone for 48 hours. The catheter is then removed for another trial at passing the stone. If the stone is already down in the lower one third of the ureter, an extractor is used to attempt to remove it under general or spinal anesthesia after having dilated the ureter with an indwelling ureteral catheter for 2 to 3 days. Attempted basket extraction of calculi in the upper or middle third of the ureter is associated with a significantly increased complication rate. Ureterolithotomy is usually a safer procedure.

Carcinoma

Carcinoma of the ureter may be either primary, arising from the urothelium, or secondary, arising from such organs as the ovary or the gastrointestinal tract. The reported age incidence varies from 22 to 89 years. There seems to be no sex difference or preference for either side. The lower third of the ureter is the most common site of primary carcinoma.

Pathology. The most striking characteristic of ureteral tumors is their ability to seed elsewhere on the urothelium (Fig. 41-19). The primary growth may be in the renal pelvis, and the secondary "seedlings" may appear in the ureter, the bladder, or even the urethra. Some investigators believe that carcinogens are the cause of these new growths, or there may exist a multifocal instability of the urothelium. Ureteral tumors characteristically are slow growing and confined to the urinary

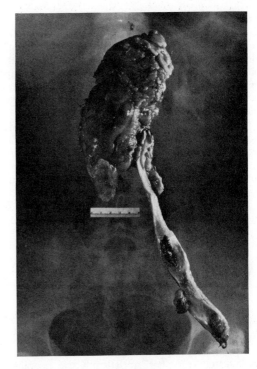

Fig. 41-19. Pyelogram and specimen of multiple tumors of ureter.

tract. Two general types of tumor are recognized: *papillary transitional cell carcinoma,* which may either be pedunculated or have a base as large as the tumor mass itself, and the *squamous cell* type, which is nonpapillary, more solid, less cellular, and tends to be invasive. Metastases occur in the areas drained by the lymphatics of the ureter.

Symptoms. Hematuria is the initial symptom in 70% of patients with ureteral neoplasms; renal colic or a mass in the flank area are less common heralding complaints. The hematuria is usually painless and may be accompanied by "fishworm" or "shoestring" clots. Pain may be colicky because of obstruction of the ureter but is more commonly dull and aching in character. The mass usually is a hydronephrotic kidney and not the tumor itself. Weight loss, easy fatigue, and a general rundown feeling are late symptoms of ureteral tumors.

Diagnosis. The urine consistently contains red blood cells, either grossly or microscopically. The significance of hematuria is that it tells you *where* the pathological condition is, not *what* the pathological condition is. Cystoscopy is indicated to locate the source of the bleeding: bleeding from a ureteral tumor is usually continuous, not episodic, and the tumor may protrude from the meatus at each efflux of the urine. The drip from the ureteral catheter may be bloody initially and then suddenly clear as the catheter rises above the source of the bleeding. On the other hand, vigorous hemorrhage may be provoked by the passage of a ureteral catheter. All of these signs point toward a tumor of the ureter.

The intravenous urograms may show nonfunction or hydronephrosis on the involved side. The retrograde pyelograms may indicate hydronephrosis and hydroureter, but the most reliable sign of ureteral tumor is a constant filling defect in the ureter.

Nonopaque stones or a blood clot must be distinguished from ureteral tumors. The nonopaque stone is usually sharp in outline, its position may move from time to time as progressive x-ray studies are made, and it may scratch a waxed catheter bulb. A blood clot may also change position or disappear, indicating that the lesion is not constant.

One of the more recent and reliable methods of differentiating a ureteral tumor from a nonopaque stone or blood clot is the examination of the urinary sediment for abnormal cells, i.e., "cytology studies." Characteristically, the neoplastic cells have an increased nuclear: cystoplasmic ratio, a thickened nuclear membrane, and prominent and bizarre nucleoles, and often the cells are tadpolelike, indicating their origin from transitional cell epithelium. Cytological detection of abnormal cells in the urine is a useful adjunct but does not replace any standard diagnostic procedures.

Treatment. The classic treatment of ureteral neoplasia is early nephroureterectomy, with extirpation of the entire upper urinary tract, including a cuff of the bladder at the ureterovesical junction. (Remember that these tumors tend to seed themselves on the urothelium.) A single-stage procedure is usually employed.

An attractive alternative treatment is local resection of the neoplasm and adjacent ureter with end-to-end ureteroureterostomy. This therapy obviously conserves renal function in a disease that tends to be bilateral and recurrent. Follow-up includes interval urine cytology, excretory urography, and cystoscopy.

Prognosis. The prognosis of ureteral tumor is good in the papillary type, especially if the tumor is small, if the pathological sections show noninvasive characteristics, and if the involved ureter is completely removed with the accompanying kidney. The squamous cell type has a poor prognosis; invasion and metastases occur early.

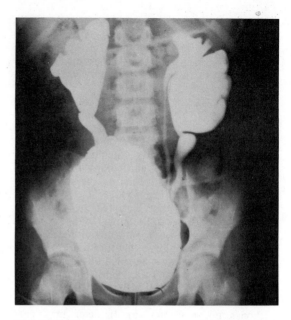

Fig. 41-20. Cystogram showing congenital bladder neck stricture with dilated bladder, bilateral ureteral reflux, and hydronephrosis.

Reflux

Ureteral reflux (Figs. 41-20 and 41-21) has captured the interest of urologists. Although the relationship of ureteral reflux to chronic bladder infection has been known for many years, the common occurrence of ureteral reflux in many other conditions was not generally recognized until the past two decades. Ureteral reflux plays a major role in renal infection and gradual renal deterioration in patients with neurogenic bladder and in children with bladder infections from undetected causes. Renal failure may result from neglected bilateral reflux.

In some instances ureteral reflux is associated with a congenital patulous state of the ureteral orifice with failure of the ureterovesical valvelike mechanism to prevent ureteral reflux. Urinary tract obstruction or infection may well predispose to ureteral reflux. Many operative procedures have been devised for its correction, the most common being the submucosal "tunneling procedure." This is usually successful in patients who do not have greatly dilated ureters and in whom infection can be controlled satisfactorily. Ureteral reflux is usually readily demonstrated by cystography or by voiding cystourethrography.

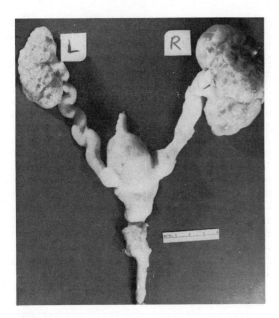

Fig. 41-21. Specimen of congenital bladder neck stricture.

URINARY BLADDER

The function of the bladder is twofold: to store urine and to remove it from the body. Any pathological condition changing these functions will usually be accompanied by frequent, difficult, and painful urination, nocturia, hematuria, and pyuria. These symptoms are discussed thoroughly under the primary pathological conditions responsible for producing them.

A greatly or moderately distended bladder is percussible or palpable on abdominal examination. A midline suprapubic tumor should always make one consider the possibility of a distended bladder, which may also be palpated rectally as a fullness above the prostate. Evaluation of the size of the prostate by rectal examination is hindered by a distended bladder.

Bladder function may be accurately assessed by simple tests. Catheterization will yield a great deal of information. *Residual urine,* the amount of urine remaining in the bladder after voiding, is diagnostically important. Residual urine in the bladder in any amount is significant of abnormal bladder function.

X-ray examination of the bladder may reveal valuable information. Stones and radiopaque foreign bodies will be seen on the plain film. The injection of radiopaque medium through a catheter into the bladder (cystography) outlines the size and shape of the bladder, trabeculation, diverticula, and ureteral reflux. Extravasation of radiopaque medium indicates bladder rupture. Micturition cystograms (roentgenograms of the bladder taken after the patient voids after instillation of radiopaque media into the bladder) pinpoint the presence and location of residual urine (which may reside in a diverticulum). Air cystograms best demonstrate filling defects from tumors, nonradiopaque stones, and foreign bodies.

Examination of the interior of the bladder by cystoscopy allows precise evaluation of the mucosa for inflammation, trabeculation, stones, ulcers, tumors, scars, and fistulous tracts. Cystoscopy is also valuable in determining the source of hematuria, i.e., whether it is coming from the bladder or the right or left ureteral orifice.

Cystometry is useful in determining the neuromuscular function of the bladder.

Congenital anomalies

Complete aplasia of the bladder is rare and is usually diagnosed at autopsy. *Double bladder* is also rare; it may be complete or incomplete, transverse or sagittal. An hourglass bladder with a constricting fibrous band in the midportion has also been described. *Exstrophy of the bladder* occurs about once in every 50,000 births. Complete exstrophy of the bladder is characterized by a lack of the anterior bladder wall with a fasciomuscular defect in the anterior abdominal wall. The posterior wall of the bladder and the trigone occupy this defect. Exstrophy in the male is usually accompanied by complete epispadias, undescended testes, and a bifid scrotum. In the female the clitoris is bifid, the labia are separated, and the urethra is epispadic. In both sexes the symphysis is absent, with a wide separation of the pubic bones (Fig. 41-1). This creates the characteristic waddling gait of these children. Incomplete exstrophy of the bladder presents only a defect in the upper or lower portion of the anterior bladder wall. About 90% of exstrophies occur in males. The bladder wall is basically defective and often is associated with hydroureteronephrosis or even reflux.

Clinical picture. The diagnosis of exstrophy of the bladder is easy. The exstrophied bladder is seen as a red outpouching of mucous membrane on the anterior abdominal wall in which the ureteral orifices and the interureteric ridge are clearly visible. The patient is constantly urine soaked and is physically and socially miserable.

The anomaly is not compatible with long life because of upper urinary tract damage leading to renal failure. Another complication of exstrophy of the bladder is malignant change of the epithelium of the exstrophied bladder, which occurs in about 5% of the cases. An adenocarcinoma is the most common malignancy developing in an exstrophied bladder.

The management of bladder exstrophy consists of diversion of the urinary stream and resection of the exstrophied bladder. Attempts to close and reconstruct the bladder have been generally unsatisfactory. Diversion of the urinary stream is carried out either into the sigmoid colon (ureterosigmoidostomy), or into a rectal bladder from which feces have been diverted. This is a very successful operation if the anal sphincters are functioning. Otherwise an ileal conduit urinary diversion is indicated.

Results of treatment by this method are uniformly good and offer the patient comfort, social acceptability, and a good prognosis. At a later time the associated epispadias and undescended testes are surgically corrected. In all female patients and in some male patients, adequate sexual relationships and procreation can be achieved.

The *urachus* may give rise to anomalies that create definite clinical entities. Patent urachus is characterized by a fistula draining urine at the umbilicus, or in the midline between the symphysis and the umbilicus. The urachus may obliterate at the upper end only, forming a pouch off the bladder that may harbor stones and infection. Both ends of the urachus may obliterate, leaving a blind pouch in which calculi may also form. Adenocarcinoma and sarcoma in these urachal cysts have also been reported. Diagnosis of these lesions is confirmed by (1) cystography and (2) cystoscopy and endoscopic examination of the lower urinary tract. The treatment consists of surgical removal of such lesions.

Hernias of the bladder are uncommon. They are usually found in "sliding" direct inguinal or femoral hernias.

Injuries

Traumatic perforations of the urinary bladder result in two different pathological entities: intraperitoneal or extraperitoneal urinary extravasation. Rupture of the bladder is caused by a variety of agents: instrumentation, penetrating wounds, and direct or indirect blows. The most common causes of ruptured bladder are comminuted fracture of the bony pelvis and operative damage incurred during transurethral manipulation or open pelvic operations. Penetrating wounds of the blad-der are commonly associated with damage to other abdominal viscera. Sudden changes in directional force when the bladder is full may cause rupture of the urethra at the junction of the prostatic and membranous portion.

Diagnosis. The diagnosis of bladder or urethral rupture is not always simple. A history of trauma followed by hematuria and pain suprapubically with voiding abnormalities is suggestive of a ruptured bladder. Extraperitoneal extravasation of urine may produce only moderate tenderness and rigidity of the lower abdomen, though later a mass becomes apparent on the anterior abdominal wall that may extend upward to the umbilicus and laterally to the inguinal ligament, or may be felt as a mass above the prostate on rectal examination. By this time the patient is extremely ill with fever, chills, nausea, and vomiting. Urinalysis reveals gross or microscopic hematuria. Leukocytosis is also present.

If the rupture is intraperitoneal, the patient will have generalized abdominal tenderness and rigidity, paralytic ileus, shock, and the other well-known signs of generalized peritonitis.

Final diagnosis rests on visualization of the bladder extravasation by cystography with radiopaque media. Differentiation between rupture of the bladder and the prostatic urethra is important; if a catheter passes easily into the bladder, it is presumptive evidence that the urethra is intact.

Treatment. The treatment of a ruptured bladder is prompt surgical closure of the rent with perivesical drainage. The bladder itself is drained with an indwelling urethral or suprapubic catheter. Supportive treatment and antibiotic therapy are vitally important. To temporize by catheter drainage alone in a suspected rupture of the bladder invites disaster.

Foreign bodies

Foreign bodies arrive in the bladder in a number of different ways. They may come through the bladder wall, through the urethra, or through fistulous openings into the bladder from some other viscera. The variety and number of foreign bodies introduced into the bladder through the urethra by children and adults are amazing: e.g., paraffin, chewing gum, hairpins, matches, insects, worms, snakes, rubber tubing, and balloons.

The clinical features are those of pronounced bladder irritation: frequency, dysuria, tenesmus, hematuria, and pyuria are prominent. The diagnosis of foreign bodies rests on demonstration by roentgenographic and cystoscopic studies.

Treatment is removal either transurethrally with an instrument or through a suprapubic cystotomy.

Inflammatory disease

Inflammatory disease of the bladder is very common. This is true in women of all ages but particularly in young girls and elderly women. It is associated with frequency, dysuria, aching in the suprapubic area, and bacteria and pus cells in the urine in abnormal quantities.

Extravesical sources for the infection must be ruled out, as well as vesical tumor, vesical stones, and obstructions.

Ureteral reflux is evaluated by cystography. Cystoscopy will distinguish a vesical infection from some other underlying lesion such as a diverticulum, neurogenic bladder, stone or tumor, or bladder-neck contracture. The urethra must be calibrated to rule out urethral stenosis. Careful study of the bladder neck is indicated to rule out congenital bladder-neck contracture, valves at the bladder-neck, or some other bladder-neck obstruction. Prostatitis in the male is a common cause. When these conditions are eliminated, the diagnosis of primary bladder infection is made. The treatment is straightforward. Culture and sensitivity tests indicate the proper antibiotic to be used, generally one with a broad spectrum of effect because colon bacilli of various kinds are almost invariably responsible. Vaginal infections and cervical infections must be treated because the short female urethra allows reinfection from these adjacent areas. Topical application of 1:1,000 or 1:750 silver nitrate solution helps in the treatment of the local infection.

Interstitial cystitis or *Hunner's ulcer* is a peculiar type of cystitis, found much more frequently in women than in men. It is characterized by sterile, clear urine, without inflammatory cells but with painful and frequent urination. Cystoscopic examination reveals areas of hemorrhage and cracking of the vesical mucosa, usually in the fundus, when the bladder is distended. This lesion responds to increasing strength of silver nitrate solution instilled into the bladder, starting with 1:1,000 and going up to about 1:500. The cause of this lesion is unknown, though current research points to either a quantitative or qualitative difference in the normal protective layer of mucopolysaccharides (glycosaminoglycans) lining the urothelium.

Other treatments include anticholinergic drugs and hydraulic dilatation performed under anesthesia. The anti-inflammatory agent dimethylsulfoxide (DMSO), when instilled intravesically as a topical treatment, relieves symptoms of interstitial cystitis at least temporarily in about half the patients. An unfortunate sequela of interstitial cystitis is the small-capacity, contracted fibrotic bladder. In situ carcinoma may masquerade as interstitial cystitis.

Enuresis

All patients 5 years of age or older with enuresis should be studied roentgenologically and often endoscopically to rule out an underlying lesion. Ectopic ureteral orifices, urethral diverticulum, foreign body in the bladder, congenital obstructions to the outflow of urine, and other bladder lesions are often the cause of enuresis. If a search for anatomical abnormality is unrewarding, therapy consists of anticholinergic agents and general psychological support for both child and parents. Many children with enuresis have delayed maturation of their central nervous systems, resulting in persistent infantile, small-capacity bladders.

Neurogenic bladder

In the adult, function of the normal bladder is controlled by conditioned reflexes, the highest center of which is in the cortex; any break in the pathway or derangement affecting the cortical center produces some type of neurogenic vesical dysfunction.

In infancy the bladder is controlled by a simple reflex arc synapsing in the sacral cord (S2 to S4). Sensory stimulation from distension of the bladder is carried to this sacral center, triggering motor impulses over the efferent limb that cause the detrusor muscle to undergo a series of contractions of increasing amplitude until a massive contraction occurs and the bladder evacuates its contents. This pattern is influenced by training and environment until, in a normal child, the bladder is completely controlled by the conditioned reflex mechanism arising in the cortex. The contractions occurring in an infant bladder may be termed uninhibited contractions and do not occur in the normal adult bladder.

The bladder may be evaluated neurologically much as any other portion of the nervous system, for perception of temperature, pain, touch, contraction, and filling. The motor function of the bladder is examined by cystometry. Table 41-4 lists the types of neurogenic bladders and summarizes the features.

Diverticulum

Diverticulum and trabeculation of the bladder are produced by obstruction to the outflow of urine from the bladder itself. Urethral stricture, bladder neck contracture, benign prostatic hypertrophy, urethral stenosis, and congenital valves are the most common causes. Diverticula of the bladder may occur at any age, and the large ones should be

Table 41-4. The neurogenic bladder

Type	Voluntary control	Condition of bladder; muscle tone	Bladder capacity	Micturition
Sensory paralytic	Present early	Flaccid and distended; myogenic tone decreased	Considerably increased	Early stage—incomplete emptying Late stage—overflow incontinence; dribbling
Motor paralytic	Absent	Flaccid and distended; myogenic tone decreased	Considerably increased	Early stage—incomplete emptying; sense of distension Late stage—overflow incontinence; dribbling
Autonomous	Absent	Myogenic tone preserved	Variable—may be increased or somewhat reduced	Early stage—inability to void; distended bladder Late stage—dribbling and straining
Reflex (automatic)	Absent	Variable—may be below normal, normal, or above normal	Variable—may be reduced or increases	Early stage—inability to void Late stage—reflex and precipitous urination
Uninhibited	Maintained by external sphincter but often insufficient to preserve continence	Normal to increased	Decreased	Precipitous and frequent

Residual urine	Infection	Etiology	Responsible conditions	Comment
Large volume	Common	Loss of sensory supply to bladder, as in lesions of posterior roots and columns	Acute (shock) stage of spinal injury; tabes dorsalis; diabetic radiculitis; subacute combined sclerosis	With the subsidence of spinal shock this type will merge into the reflex bladder unless severe myogenic disturbance has occurred through overdistension
Large volume	Common	Loss of motor supply to bladder, as in lesions of anterior horns and roots of sacral segments 3 and 4	May be part of the picture of spinal shock or occur in acute poliomyelitis	This type of bladder disturbance is also susceptible to myogenic disturbance, as above, but usually not to such severe degree
Present, usually in small or moderate amounts	Generally present	Complete interruption of reflex arc when both the sensory and motor components are destroyed	Trauma of sacral cord or conus; spina bifida manifesta; trauma of nervi erigentes	Patient may be able to express some urine by straining or manual compression
Present in variable amounts, depending on muscle tone of bladder	Often present	Complete interruption of upper motor neuron control; spinal arc present	Trauma of spinal cord above sacral level (after period of shock); spinal cord tumor; multiple sclerosis	Patient may discover "trigger areas" for induction of micturition
None in absence of infravesical obstruction	Absent	Loss of cerebral inhibitory control	Cerebral arteriosclerosis; brain tumor; brain injury, incomplete lesions of spinal cord; delayed development of cerebral inhibitory mechanism	This type shows least variance from normal bladder activity

removed surgically and their cause eliminated. They occur in at least 10% of the patients with benign prostatic hypertrophy.

Carcinoma

Carcinoma of the bladder is the second most common genitourinary neoplasm. The fact that most of these cancers occur near the trigone and ureteral orifices, is suggestive of the action of a carcinogenic agent in the urine acting on the bladder mucous membrane. No proof of this hypothesis exists, except in patients who are exposed to hydrocarbons, as in the dye industry. One carcinogenic agent is beta-naphthylamine. Chronic irritation, vesical calculi, and chronic cystitis are not present in any sizable portion of the cases. Studies are being carried out to see if tryptophan derivatives may be related to vesical cancer.

Fig. 41-22 shows the four classifications (degree of invasion) of bladder tumors. Cure and survival rates are directly related to the stage and grade of lesions.

Signs and symptoms. Although painless hematuria is the cardinal sign of carcinoma of the bladder, some patients do not manifest hematuria at all or only in the latter stages. Any disturbance of micturition or change in the urine may be a manifestation of carcinoma of the bladder. In many instances patients have been referred to the hospital with a mistaken diagnosis of chronic prostatitis or cystitis. Therefore any patient over 40 years of age who has any disturbance of micturition should have a cystoscopic examination to rule out carcinoma of the bladder. Early diagnosis makes a tremendous difference in the type of therapy recommended and the result of treatment. In one series of 540 patients the average time interval between the occurrence of the first symptom and the diagnosis was 1½ years.

Diagnosis. Absolute diagnosis is based on cystoscopic examination with biopsy of suspicious tissue. The lateral air cystogram and the intravenous pyelogram may visualize a bladder tumor, particularly if it is large and papillary or if it obstructs a ureter (Figs. 41-23 and 41-24).

Cytology studies of the bladder urine may reveal suspicious cells; bladder washings increase the yield of positive cytological tests.

The differential diagnosis between transitional cell carcinoma of the bladder (urachal rest tumor), carcinoma of an adjacent organ invading the bladder (sigmoid colon, prostate, cervix, uterus), and intense chronic cystitis may be difficult even after microscopic study of sections of the tumor. All these lesions require thorough investigation.

Treatment. The treatment of carcinoma of the bladder is summarized as follows:
1. Destruction by means of electrocoagulation, either through the resectoscope transurethrally or through an open cystostomy
2. Removal by open surgical procedure (partial cystectomy or total cystectomy with diversion of the urinary stream) to include the removal of the regional lymph nodes
3. Palliative treatment: transurethral resection, high-energy x-ray therapy, or diversion of the urinary stream

Transurethral resection or fulguration is well-

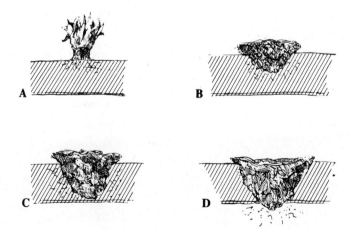

Fig. 41-22. Bladder tumors. **A**, Papillary, noninvasive. **B**, Partially invading bladder wall. **C**, Invading bladder wall completely. **D**, Invading perivesical tissue, generally with metastases.

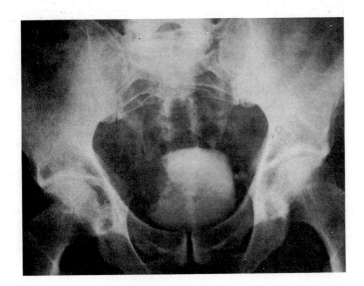

Cystogram of tumor producing
'ect" in right side of bladder.

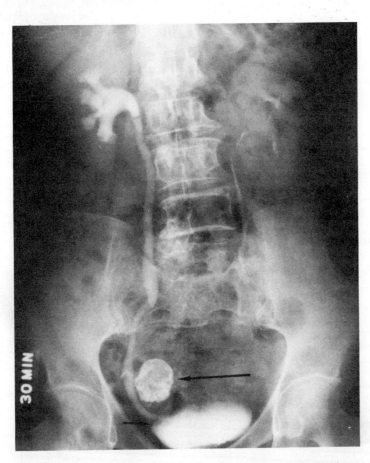

Fig. 41-24. Excretory urogram (I.V.P.) demonstrates right hydroureteronephrosis associated with infiltrating bladder tumor seen as filling defect *(small arrow)*. Calcified uterine fibroid is also present *(large arrow)*.

suited for low-grade, low-stage papillary tumors. Although 40% to 70% will recur given enough time, the treatment can be repeated successfully because most of the new tumors continue to have a similar histological appearance. On the other hand, the high-grade, high-stage (invasive, solid) tumors require aggressive treatment. Even so, only about 50% of patients with tumors invading the bladder muscular wall will live 5 years free of disease. Most treatment failures are attributable to distant metastases previously undetectable.

In recent years surgical treatment has been greatly aided by the ileal conduit (ureteroileal cutaneous anastomosis) and colon conduit for supravesical diversion. They have proved to be superior to ureterosigmoid anastomosis, particularly in patients treated with irradiation. External beam irradiation is a valuable therapeutic aid. Systemic chemotherapy continues to be studied. Local application of thio-TEPA for recurrent superficial tumors has been of proved value.

PROSTATE
Congenital anomalies

Congenital anomalies of the prostate are extremely rare and are found only in association with other anomalies of the genitourinary tract, such as hypospadias. Congenital cysts of müllerian duct remnants arise between the lobes of a normal prostate. They may be felt on bimanual (rectal and abdominal) examination and are treated by complete excision.

Inflammatory lesions

Inflammatory lesions of the prostate are quite common, particularly during middle life. They are caused by enteric bacteria, gonorrhea, or tuberculosis. They may be acute or chronic and can produce abscesses. The signs and symptoms vary, depending on the organism, the stage of the infection, and whether an abscess has formed. Acute prostatitis is characterized by dysuria (frequency, burning, smarting) and retention of urine if a large abscess or an acutely swollen gland compresses the urethra. On the other hand, a dull, aching sensation in the perineum may be the only symptom of chronic prostatitis.

Treatment consists of general supportive care, prostatic massage, drainage (if an abscess is present), and appropriate antimicrobial therapy after the organisms have been cultured. Tuberculous prostatitis justifies a search for a primary tuberculous focus elsewhere in the body, and appropriate antituberculous therapy.

Prostatic calculi may be an underlying cause for chronic prostatitis and may need to be removed, either transurethrally or by open prostatectomy.

Frequently prostatitis is associated with impotence and with infertility. Both of these problems improve once the infection has been cleared.

Benign prostatic hypertrophy
Etiology

Benign prostatic hypertrophy is a common disease, probably the second most common disease of the aged male (Fig. 41-25) (generalized arteriosclerosis is first). It is of tremendous importance in geriatric practice; 75% of all males over 60 years of age have benign prostatic hypertrophy, which causes complete bladder outlet obstruction in 50% of these (i.e., 38% of the total).

The prostate is a compound racemose structure composed of 100 or more outer (paraurethral) glands and 100 or more inner (periurethral) glands. A true capsule surrounds the entire gland, known as Denonvilliers' fascia. In benign prostatic hypertrophy the inner glands hypertrophy as nodules of fibroadenomatous tissue. These nodules push inward to distort the prostatic urethra and outward to compress the tissue between the inner and outer glands. Thus the outer (paraurethral) glands are not involved in benign prostatic hypertrophy. The hyperplasia so distorts the urethra as to cause a ball-valve effect leading to urinary retention. The disease first manifests itself as small spheroids of hypertrophy beneath the mucosa of the prostatic urethra that interfere with urination, not by constricting the urethra but by acting as a valve.

With long-standing obstruction in the prostatic urethra, the bladder muscle hypertrophies and the bladder wall becomes trabeculated. Later, small herniations of vesical mucosa are pushed outward between these hypertrophied muscle bundles,

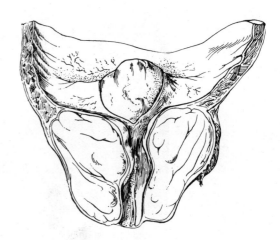

Fig. 41-25. Benign prostatic hypertrophy (trilobar).

forming diverticula. Stagnation of urine, infection, and sometimes stone formation occur in these diverticula.

Eventually, the bladder can no longer compensate by hypertrophy, and the bladder wall becomes stretched and atonic. The ureterovesical valve becomes impaired by constant back pressure; reflux, hydroureter, hydronephrosis, destruction of kidney tissue, uremia, and death result. *The most common cause of a lower abdominal mass in males over 50 years of age is a full bladder obstructed by benign prostatic hypertrophy.*

Symptoms and signs

Urinary obstruction from prostatic hypertrophy has many clinical manifestations, including frequency, nocturia, hesitancy, urgency, inability to empty the bladder completely, episodes of complete retention, hematuria, pyuria, dysuria, episodes of chills and fever, back pain, renal colic, and a progressive history of slowing of the stream and diminution in its caliber. Oddly enough, hematuria is more common in benign prostatic hypertrophy than in carcinoma of the prostate, with about 25% of patients complaining of initial or terminal hematuria.

Long-standing bladder obstruction with renal damage also produces nonspecific complaints of poor appetite, anemia, general weakness, and at times excessive thirst and spells of disorientation.

The residual urine that remains after the patient attempts to empty his bladder is the most conspicuous sign of urinary obstruction. True, rectal examination can estimate the size of the prostate, but it cannot determine the degree of obstruction. Frequently, a huge gland will cause no destruction, whereas a tiny nodule, strategically located, can cause complete retention.

Differential diagnosis of obstructive uropathy of the bladder

Many conditions, outlined as follows, produce obstruction to the outflow of urine from the bladder. In adult males benign hypertrophy of the prostate is the most common.

A. Conditions of the prostate that cause obstruction
 1. Acute prostatitis
 2. Prostatic abscess
 3. Tuberculous prostatitis
 4. Prostatic cyst
 5. Prostatic calculi
 6. Benign hypertrophy
 7. Carcinoma of the prostate
 8. Sarcoma of the prostate
B. Conditions about the prostatic urethra that cause obstruction
 1. Perirectal abscess
 2. Carcinoma or sarcoma adjacent to the urethra
C. Conditions of the prostatic urethra that cause obstruction
 1. Congenital conditions
  a. Enlargement of the verumontanum
  b. Urethral valve
  c. Congenital stricture
 2. Urethral stone
 3. Traumatic stricture of the prostatic urethra
D. Conditions in the bladder that cause obstruction
 1. Vesical stone
 2. Ureterocele
 3. Bladder-neck contracture
E. Conditions of the bladder that cause obstruction
 1. Disturbances of position—prolapse
 2. Diverticulum
 3. Neurogenic
  a. Upper motor neuron
  b. Lower motor neuron
 4. Spasm of the sphincters
 5. Myogenic atony
 6. Carcinoma of the bladder
F. Conditions outside the bladder that cause obstruction
 1. Abscess in the pelvis
 2. Carcinoma of the cervix
 3. Diverticulitis of the sigmoid colon
 4. Carcinoma of the sigmoid colon

Disturbances of urination are the chief symptoms of diseases that involve any portion of the urinary tract and not just those originating in the bladder or prostate. Thus the characteristic symptoms of obstructive uropathy must be regarded merely as evidence of nonspecific urogenital disease, until definite abnormality of the bladder or prostate is proved. Only complete urological investigation will differentiate among the many conditions that produce obstruction to the outflow of urine from those conditions that give symptoms of bladder dysfunction without obstruction.

Diagnosis

The following procedures are necessary for diagnosis.

Rectal examination. The prostate is smooth, usually symmetrical, elastic, and mobile. On rectal examination it is usually graded from 1+ to 4+, 1+ being a gland of small size and 4+ being one so large that the examining finger cannot go over it.

Residual urine. After voiding, the patient is catheterized and the amount of urine remaining in the bladder is measured. The normal bladder is able to empty itself to less than 1 ml. of urine. But on practical clinical grounds residual urine volumes of less than 50 to 75 ml. are not considered "significant" unless complications such as infection, calculi, or severe voiding difficulty supervene. The urine obtained in this manner should be examined for pH, specific gravity, blood, pus, sugar, and microscopic elements.

Cystourethrograms, cystoscopy, pyelography, renal function tests. Use cystourethrograms, cystoscopy, pyelography, and renal function tests as indicated (Fig. 41-26).

Urinary flow rate. A fairly recent yet simple test to study the balance between bladder detrusor activity and the resistance of the outflow tract (the bladder neck and all structures distal to it) is uroflowmetry (uroflow test, urinary flow rate measurements). The total urine volume voided and the time required for this voiding are measured by devices as simple as a stopwatch and calibrated beaker or by pressure-transducer equipment. The minimal information gained is the average or mean urinary flow rate (milliliters per second); the pressure-transducer equipment also records on graph paper the peak or maximum urinary flow rate and the pattern of voiding. Abnormally low peak and average flow rates are compatible with both obstructive and neurogenic diseases and are helpful in monitoring response to any therapy utilized.

General physical examination, particularly car-

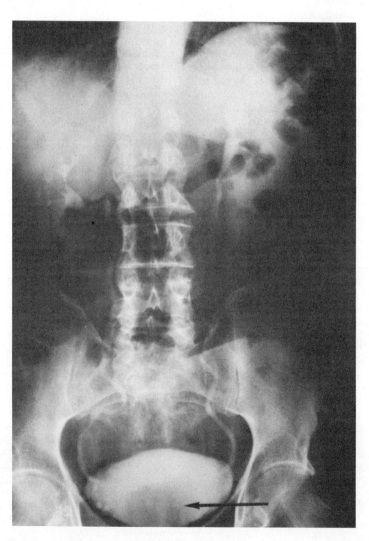

Fig. 41-26. Excretory urogram (I.V.P.) in older male with prostatism. Study is normal except for large filling defect in bladder base *(arrow)* consistent with intravesical prostatic enlargement.

diac status. The patient must be evaluated as a whole to determine whether he will benefit from surgical relief of his bladder-neck obstruction.

Treatment

Treatment includes nonsurgical treatment, treatment of acute retention, and surgical treatment.

Nonsurgical. In mild cases with an acute episode of retention, conservative measures are often successful for a time. Prostatic massage, hot sitz baths, urinary antiseptics, antibiotics, bed rest, and catheter drainage may take the patient through an acute episode and avoid surgery. Hormonal agents to "shrink" the prostate are still being investigated.

Acute retention. The essence of treatment of acute retention is to drain the bladder slowly enough to prevent hemorrhage and bladder spasm, yet rapidly enough to draw off more urine than is being formed. Should the patient develop bladder spasms or hemorrhage, fluid is immediately replaced into the bladder and the patient is watched carefully. Once equilibrium has been achieved, surgical treatment is carried out.

Surgical. The four surgical approaches to the prostate for the treatment of benign prostatic hypertrophy are (1) *transurethral,* (2) *suprapubic,* (3) *perineal,* and (4) *retropubic* prostatectomy. Although called "prostatectomy," they are truly only an adenectomy, or a partial prostatectomy. The end result of each approach is identical—removal of the adenoma to the plane of cleavage at the surgical capsule, with the outer prostatic glands left undisturbed. In none of these methods is the entire prostate removed. The operation called the radical (total) prostatectomy is not performed for benign prostatic hypertrophy; see discussion of cancer on p. 614.

Transurethral resection (TUR). In transurethral resection the resectoscope is introduced into the urethra, and under direct vision the adenomatous tissue is cut away with a high-frequency current until the plane of the surgical capsule is reached (Fig. 41-27). *Advantages* are (1) low mortality and morbidity with short and mild convalescence, (2) average postoperative hospital stay is 3 to 5 days, (3) the disadvantages of open surgery are avoided, and (4) damage to the rectum or external sphincter is avoided. *Disadvantages* are that (1) the procedure is technically difficult and hard to learn and (2) hemolytic reactions, urethral trauma, and stricture sometimes occur.

Suprapubic (transvesical) prostatectomy. In suprapubic prostatectomy the bladder is opened extraperitoneally through an incision above the pubis, and the adenoma is enucleated with the finger. *Advantages* are that (1) this is an easy operative technique, best suited for the surgeon who infrequently does prostatic surgery and (2) it avoids the rectum and external sphincter. *Disadvantages* are (1) relatively high mortality and morbidity and (2) delayed healing with urinary fistula and long hospitalization (up to 2 weeks).

Perineal prostatectomy. The approach in perineal prostatectomy is through the perineum (Fig. 41-28). The prostate is detached from the rectum when the rectourethralis muscle is cut. The plane of cleavage is established, and the adenoma is enucleated. *Advantages* are (1) low mortality and

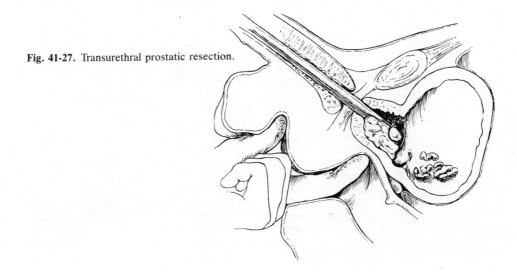

Fig. 41-27. Transurethral prostatic resection.

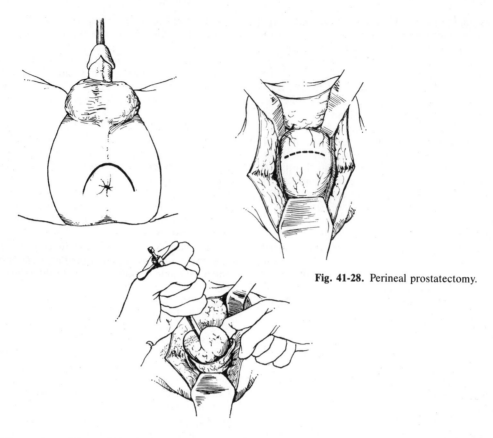

Fig. 41-28. Perineal prostatectomy.

morbidity and a mild convalescence second only to transurethral resection and (2) dependent drainage. The *disadvantage* is that the operation is technically difficult and occasionally damages the rectum and external sphincter.

Retropubic prostatectomy. In retropubic prostatectomy an incision is made just above the symphysis. The prostate is exposed in the prevesical space beneath the pubic arch. The plane of cleavage is established below the level of the internal sphincter, and the adenoma is enucleated through an incision in the anterior prostatic capsule. *Advantages* are (1) relatively low mortality and morbidity and a relatively short hospital stay and (2) a simple anatomical approach that avoids the rectum and external sphincter. *Disadvantages* are the hemorrhage from the prostatic venous plexus is not infrequent, and osteitis pubis may (rarely) complicate the convalescence.

Vasectomy. Many clinics precede a prostatectomy by vasectomy in hopes of preventing epididymitis. I have found approximately the same incidence of epididymitis with or without vasectomy. Probably bilateral vasectomy has its greatest place in preventing postprostatectomy epididymitis when

it is performed *prior* to any urethral instrumentation. The scrotal route is most often employed, but an intrapelvic vasectomy can be achieved at the time of open prostatectomy.

Prognosis and results. The overall mortality in recent years for all types of prostatic resection in this country is less than 1%. Patients void well after resection, and only a small percentage suffer from incontinence or sufficient regrowth to cause prostatic obstruction to recur.

Cancer

Cancer of the prostate is the most common malignant growth in aged males, and next to carcinoma of the lung it is the most frequent cause of death from cancer in the male in the United States. It is relatively rare below 40 years of age but occurs in 20% of all white males over the age of 50. About 40% of all elderly males suffer from urinary obstruction, and one fifth of these cases are attributed to carcinoma of the prostate. There is no causal relationship between prostatic carcinoma and other lesions of the gland such as benign prostatic hypertrophy or chronic inflammatory disease. The cause is unknown.

Unlike benign prostatic hypertrophy, carcinoma arises in the periphery of the prostate (in the outer glands). Thus rectal examination may detect a carcinomatous nodule before it gives symptoms of obstruction and frequently before metastases have occurred, if rectal examination is carried out routinely. The neoplasm may remain limited to the gland itself for a relatively long period of time; then by direct invasion it involves the inner glands, the seminal vesical area, and the vas deferens. Later it breaks through the capsule to involve the urethra and bladder, rectum, periurethral tissues and the lymph nodes along the internal and external iliac vessels. Blood-borne metastases carry the malignancy to the bones, primarily the spine and pelvis, and to the lung. In advanced cases metastases occur to any other portion of the body.

Grossly, carcinoma of the prostate is a firm, white-yellow, irregular mass. Histologically, it is an adenocarcinoma, which characteristically produces an increase in the serum acid phosphatase when it has disseminated. Bony metastases are usually osteoblastic and associated with an elevation of the serum alkaline phosphatase as well.

Signs, symptoms, and diagnosis. Carcinoma of the prostate produces no symptoms until there is a spread to the urethra or until the bones are involved, causing pain. Urethral involvement produces dysuria, hematuria, and difficulty in urination. Detection of a hard prostatic nodule palpable on rectal examination requires confirmatory biopsy of the nodule. Chronic inflammatory disease of the prostate and prostatic calculi may mimic prostatic carcinoma. Once the biopsy findings confirm prostatic cancer, the following studies are performed for staging: radionuclide bone scan, excretory urogram (IVP), serum acid and alkaline phosphatases, and in some patients a computerized axial tomogram (CAT scan) of the abdomen and pelvis or pedal lymphangiogram.

Clinical staging is as follows: Stage A is defined as prostatic cancer discovered coincidentally to surgery performed for clinically benign disease; Stage B, nodular areas confined to the substance of the prostate gland on rectal examination; Stage C, evidence of periprostatic infiltration (rectum, seminal vesicles, bladder) on rectal examination; Stage D, distant metastatic disease, most commonly skeletal.

Treatment. The treatment for prostatic carcinoma depends on the stage. Stage A lesions, when low grade and focal, need no further treatment but only observation. The high-grade or diffuse stage A lesion, on the other hand, requires aggressive treatment, either radical surgery or definitive radiotherapy. If the lesion is localized completely to the prostatic area, a total (radical) prostatectomy can be carried out with a high incidence of cure (80% to +90% 5-year survival free of disease). On the other hand, once the lesion has invaded the capsule, the base of the bladder, or the area around the seminal vesicles, there is a 50% chance that the regional lymph nodes are involved and a 10% to 15% chance of vascular metastases. External irradiation (linear accelerator) has also been used as therapy for this type of patient. If dissemination has occurred, local therapy to relieve obstructive symptoms must be supplemented by systemic treatment. The local therapy usually is by transurethral prostatic resection.

Palliative systemic therapy of disseminated prostatic cancer consists essentially in altering the hormonal environment of the lesion by orchiectomy or the administration of estrogens. Progesterone-like agents and alkylating agents have some effect on disseminated prostatic carcinoma. Controlled clinical trials to evaluate the efficacy of chemotherapeutic agents in this disease are now being conducted at several institutions. Recently open cryosurgical destruction of the malignant prostate has been utilized to destroy the large local lesion and alleviate pain from bony metastases. As yet there is no good objective evidence of regression of metastases or of an enhanced immunological defense mechanism.

URETHRA
Congenital anomalies
Male urethra

Congenital valves of the posterior urethra may obstruct the passage of urine and, if not detected early, will produce strong back pressure with hydroureter, hydronephrosis, and ultimately renal insufficiency. Treatment consists of destruction of the valve leaflets by the resectoscope, to relieve the obstruction. Plastic procedures on the bladder, ureters, and kidney pelvis may be required to correct the effects of long-standing back pressure on the urinary transport system.

Hypospadias. The urethra opens on the ventral surface of the penis in hypospadias, the distal urethra not having been formed. In addition, there is pronounced ventral curvature, or *chordee,* of the penis. The corrective operations must first straighten the penis by removal of the fibrous band causing the chordee; then, a tube is fashioned of skin leading from the intact urethra to the glans penis. The untreated patient must urinate in the sitting position and is sterile, even if the chordee is mild enough to permit coitus, since ejaculation occurs outside the vagina.

Epispadias. In epispadias the urethra opens dorsally on the penis, appearing as a flat strip of mucous membrane on the upper surface of the penis between the separated corpora cavernosa. The severe forms involve the sphincters, causing incontinence of urine, and often are associated with exstrophy of the bladder. Treatment consists of closure of the urethral groove by plastic operation.

Diverticulum of the urethra. Urethral diverticulum is rare; treatment is surgical excision.

Female urethra

The female urethra is homologous with the posterior urethra in the male. Congenital anomalies are associated with defective development of the bladder, as in exstrophy and epispadias. In epispadias the urethra appears as a trough in the mons veneris.

Urethral stenosis. Congenital urethral stenosis is a possible cause of urinary obstruction in the female. It may be associated with urethral valves. The obstruction must be corrected, usually by dilatation.

Infections

Infections of the urethra are common. They may produce prostatitis in the male and stricture formation in both the male and the female, with backpressure effects on the urinary transport system. They are the result of various types of organisms (pyogenic, *Trichomonas vaginalis,* pleuropneumonia-like organisms) and tuberculosis.

Treatment centers around identification of the specific organism and administration of appropriate antibiotics. Obstruction to urine drainage must be relieved.

Gonococcal urethritis, caused by venereally transmitted *Neisseria gonorrhoeae,* continues to be the most common specific urethral infection. Symptoms in the male are an intense dysuria and a yellow-green purulent urethral discharge, whereas the female is usually asymptomatic. Diagnosis can be made in addition by identification of gramnegative intracellular diplococci on a Gram-stained urethral discharge or by new culture techniques. Treatment in nonallergic persons consists of high-dose parenteral penicillin G (4.8 to 9.6 million units) plus probenecid, given orally, to increase further tissue drug levels. A combination of oral ampicillin and probenecid is an alternative: Patients allergic to penicillin can be given either spectinomycin, administered intramuscularly, or tetracycline, administered orally. Treatment of sexual contacts as well will reduce the reinfection rate.

Stricture

Stricture of the urethra narrows the urethral channel and is generally caused by cicatrix from old inflammation. It is seen in both sexes but is more common in the male. It develops gradually, months or years after the initial episode of urethritis.

The urethral stricture is evaluated by roentgenograms or cystourethroscopy, with its length noted and the size of the lumen calibrated. Minor strictures may respond to dilatations, but severe ones require surgical therapy to restore the natural size of the lumen. Unless this is done, there is gradual persistent damage to the proximal portion of the urinary transport system. Periurethral abscess, urinary fistulas, and infertility are other complications of urethral stricture.

Urethral strictures that are not easily managed by simple dilatation and yet are symptomatic can now be treated by two new methods. The simpler of the two is that of *direct visual internal urethrotomy,* an endoscopic procedure that allows the operator to incise the stricture under visual control. Failures of this and other more conservative measures can be handled by *patch graft urethroplasty,* in which the stricture is incised through an open approach and a free graft of preputial or penile skin is sutured into the resulting urethral defect.

Injuries

Simple contusion may be caused by forcible instrumentation, false passage, or acts of sexual violence. There is slight to moderate bleeding. Treatment generally is by splinting the area of injury with an indwelling catheter, or suture of the area if accessible.

If *severe trauma* occurs, one must differentiate among ruptures of the anterior urethra, posterior urethra, and bladder.

Rupture of the anterior urethra is most frequently caused by forcible use of urethral instruments or lacerating wounds (Fig. 41-29). Injuries to the bulbous urethra are generally caused by straddle injuries or direct blows to the perineum. In both of these injuries there is a continuous drip of blood from the urethral meatus. A hematoma may form under Buck's fascia. The patient has no desire to urinate and later develops lower abdominal pain. He may have difficulty in urinating, and urine may extravasate into the scrotum. Treatment is by antibiotic administration, immediate drainage of the area of extravasation, and splinting of the urethra with an indwelling catheter.

Rupture of the posterior prostatic urethra is usually associated with fractures of the pelvis, severe physical trauma, and occasionally instrument perforations during transurethral resection. The patient becomes just as ill and "toxic" as in rupture of the anterior urethra, but there is no dripping of blood from the urethra, no hematoma

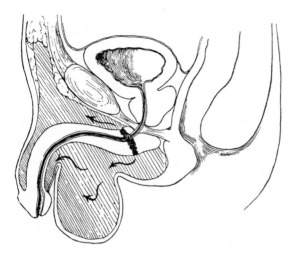

Fig. 41-29. Traumatic rupture of anterior urethra; *shaded areas,* routes of extravasation. Treatment consists in catheter splinting and drainage.

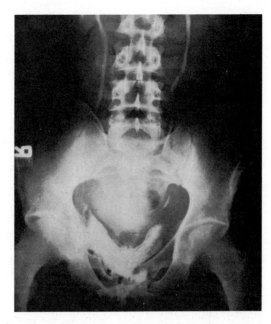

Fig. 41-30. Cystourethrogram with intravenous pyelogram showing rupture of posterior (prostatic) urethra with fractured pelvis. Notice extravasation of contrast medium about base of bladder, which has been displaced upward.

under Buck's fascia, and no scrotal swelling; instead the urine extravasates posteriorly into the ischiorectal fossa or anteriorly into the suprapubic area. The urethral catheter passes easily but may go through the false passageway rather than into the bladder (Fig. 41-30). Injection of contrast through the catheter determines if the catheter is really in the bladder. The patient will not void spontaneously even though the bladder is distended with urine because of spasm. Many of these patients die of shock or sepsis, if treatment is neglected.

Treatment of rupture of the posterior urethra is by a suprapubic cystostomy, with drainage of the prevesical space. Later, plastic procedures may be necessary if fibrosis and scarring produce urethral stricture leading to chronic infection and calculi formation (Fig. 41-31). Long-term complications of posterior urethral injuries include impotence, urinary incontinence, and stricture.

Rupture of the bladder occurs from severe external trauma, usually with associated fracture of the pelvis, or from operative trauma. There is no immediate suprapubic extravasation or scrotal swelling, and frequently the patient is able to void. Diagnosis is suspected when saline solution injected into the bladder by catheter is not returned, and it is readily confirmed by cystography. Treatment is by immediate suprapubic drainage with surgical repair of the wound.

Neoplasms
Benign

Benign neoplasms of the urethra occur rarely in both sexes. They are usually caruncles, papillomas, or adenomatous polyps. Initial hematuria is the most frequent initial complaint. Treatment is by electrocoagulation through the panendoscope or direct excision.

Malignant

Etiology. Primary carcinoma of the urethra is a very rare disease that, unlike carcinoma of the penis, occurs in both circumcised and uncircumcised men. A history of chronic urethral stricture is common.

Pathology. This neoplasm is usually an epidermoid carcinoma but may be an adenocarcinoma; it is a relatively slow-growing neoplasm that arises with equal frequency in the anterior and posterior urethra. Urethral carcinoma spreads to the inguinal, external iliac, hypogastric, and common iliac nodes. One should suspect spread to the pelvic nodes if there is pronounced local extension into the corpora or metastases to the inguinal nodes.

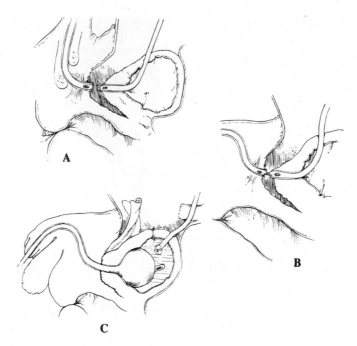

Fig. 41-31. Diagram showing traumatic rupture of posterior (prostatic) urethra and its repair. **A,** Catheter passed from urethra and bladder to meet at point of rupture. **B,** Catheter ends joined, and urethral catheter pulled on into bladder. **C,** Urethral catheter bag inflated and pulled down to splint urethra; perivesical space drained, suprapubic catheter placed.

Symptoms. The symptoms result from progressive narrowing of the urethra and associated infection: diminution in size and caliber of the stream, dysuria, pyuria, and hematuria.

Diagnosis. Diagnosis is made by palpation of an indurated urethral mass and confirmed by panendoscopy.

Treatment. If there are no pelvic node metastases, I advocate preoperative radiotherapy and wide surgical excision. Palliative treatment consists in providing a free passageway for urine and amputation of the penis for cosmetic purposes in neglected cases.

PENIS
Anomalies

The most common anomalies of the penis are associated with hypospadias and epispadias (discussed on p. 615). Anomalies of absence or multiplicity are extremely rare, as are micropenis and macropenis.

Phimosis may be either congenital or acquired and consists of a long, narrow prepuce with a minute orifice that limits the urinary flow and causes local irritation and inflammation. Treatment is by circumcision with or without a preliminary dorsal slit.

Paraphimosis results from the retraction of the prepuce behind the glans. The prepuce becomes so edematous that replacement becomes difficult, and local ulceration or gangrene may result. Again the treatment is by reduction and circumcision. A dorsal slit may be required if manual reduction is unsuccessful.

Inflammatory lesions

Inflammatory lesions of the penis are relatively common. They consist essentially of balanitis, chancre, granuloma inguinale, chancroidal infection, and lymphogranuloma venereum. These are all venereal in nature and yield to cleanliness, accurate diagnosis, and proper antimicrobial therapy. Serological testing may be necessary to rule out syphilis. Yeast or fungal infections may not respond completely to anti-infective agents until circumcision is performed. Condylomata acuminata can be eradicated by topical podophyllin or by excision. Herpes progenitalis, caused by the herpes simplex virus, is usually self-limited with proper hygiene and prevention of secondary bacterial infection. Recent clinical studies have demonstrated the efficacy of the antiviral agent acyclovir in initial cases of herpes progenitalis.

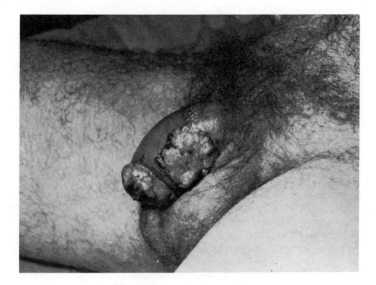

Fig. 41-32. Carcinoma of penis.

However the drug has yet to be proved useful for the vexing problem of recurrent herpetic infection.

Neoplasms

Neoplasms of the penis are not uncommon. Venereal warts are probably caused by a viral infection and are associated with poor hygiene and a redundant foreskin. They are readily treated by circumcision, coagulation of the papillomatous areas, or topical podophyllin. They may be precursors to carcinoma and should be cleared up at all costs.

Carcinoma of the penis is very rare in patients who have been circumcised in childhood or adolescence, Uncircumcised people who live in a hot, humid climate and have poor genital hygiene are predisposed to carcinoma of the penis. It is a slow-growing, painless, fungating epidermoid carcinoma that usually begins as a small pimple or wart on the glans, prepuce, or shaft of the penis (Fig. 41-32). Diagnosis is readily made by biopsy; certain types of chronic inflammatory lesions (chancre and chancroid) need to be differentiated. The treatment is by penectomy (partial or total), sometimes with inguinal lymphadenectomy. The prognosis is good if the regional lymph nodes are not involved.

Small premalignant and malignant lesions, e.g., erythroplasia of Queyrat, carcinoma in situ, can be successfully treated by wide local excision and circumcision. Alternative therapies include topical 5-fluorouracil and external beam irradiation using special penile molds.

Idiopathic

A fairly common lesion identifiable in middle-aged and older males is that of Peyronie's disease or idiopathic penile fibrosis. Symptoms include penile curvature with erection (sometimes to the extent that vaginal penetration is impossible), localized pain or the presence of subcutaneous penile nodules. Characteristically, variable areas of induration are palpable in the corpora cavernosa. Histologically, these penile plaques develop deep to the tunica albuginea covering each of the paired corpora but do not involve the corpus spongiosum or urethra. Treatment is exasperating, with vitamin E being used for its antifibrotic activity in mild to moderate cases. Severely symptomatic men may require plaque incision or excision with the placement of a penile prosthesis, since impotence is a long-term result of the disease.

SCROTUM AND SCROTAL CONTENTS
Anomalies

Anomalies of the scrotum are rare and have little significance. A bifid scrotum usually is seen with congenital anomalies of the urethra such as epispadias, severe hypospadias, and intersex conditions. Congenital deformities of the scrotum are of importance only for cosmetic reasons.

Diseases

Carcinoma of the scrotum is seen occasionally as a soft, warty growth that soon becomes ulcerated. *Sebaceous cysts* of the scrotum are common; they are yellowish, rounded, firm and may grow to the size of a marble. The cysts are asymptomatic unless secondarily infected; then they should be treated by excision rather than by incision.

TESTIS
Anomalies

Anomalies of position of the testis are common, but anomalies of number are very rare. There are two types of anomalies of position: failure of descent (cryptorchidism) and abnormal location (ectopia).

Cryptorchidism is usually unilateral but may be bilateral; it occurs in approximately 1 out of every 25 boys and is commonly associated with an inguinal hernia. The cause of undescended testis is not completely understood, but it is probably related to maldevelopment of the structural route along which the testis must descend, to an abnormal testis, or to atrophy of the gubernaculum testis. Cryptorchidism is frequently associated with atrophy and alteration in the composition of the testis itself; degenerative changes of the seminiferous tubules are progressive with sterility resulting unless the testis is surgically brought into the scrotum (orchidopexy) early in childhood.

Failure of the testis to enter the scrotum is not abnormal until after the first year of life; after this, orchidopexy should be seriously considered and in all cases should be carried out before 5 years of age. The use of gonadotropic hormones from the anterior lobe of the pituitary gland has many advocates, particularly in bilateral cryptorchidism. However, I believe it is better to bring the testis down surgically rather than depend on hormones or wait until the onset of puberty.

Inflammation of the testis and epididymis
Orchitis

Orchitis may be either acute or chronic. Chronic orchitis is usually associated with tuberculous epididymitis and is discussed later. Acute orchitis, too, may be associated with infection of the epididymis, vas deferens, and seminal vesicles, or it may be primary and not involve the cord structures. Primary orchitis is seen most commonly in adults who develop mumps and other contagious diseases more characteristic of childhood. The diagnosis is made by palpation of an acutely tender, swollen testicle with or without involvement of the epididymis and vas deferens.

Mild cases of orchitis are treated conservatively and symptomatically with bed rest, analgesics, elevation of the scrotum, and application of heat. However, severe orchitis is treated surgically by incision and drainage of the tunica vaginalis and albuginea; this will prevent the severe testicular atrophy that otherwise might occur. Corticosteroid therapy is indicated in postpubertal mumps orchitis to prevent postinflammatory fibrosis and subsequent sterility.

Acute epididymitis

Etiology. Acute epididymitis may be gonorrheal or nonspecific in origin. In either case the pathogenesis and treatment are generally the same. Usually epididymitis is associated with infection of the lower urinary tract from prostatitis, urethral manipulation, or too vigorous prostatic massage. The infection travels by a direct route from these structures up the seminal vesicles, through the vas deferens, and to the tail of the epididymis.

Diagnosis. The diagnosis is made by palpation of a greatly inflamed, hot, tender, and swollen epididymis, with or without involvement of the testis. Usually, the epididymis can be palpated separately from the testis. Accompanying these findings are systematic reactions with chills, fever, and leukocytosis.

Treatment. The treatment of acute epididymitis is medical, be it gonorrheal or nonspecific. The use of large doses of antibiotics, elevation of the part, bed rest, and local heat will usually arrest the process within a few days. However, it may be a matter of months before the swelling and induration have completely subsided. One should eradicate the focus of infection in the lower urinary tract to prevent the opposite epididymis from subsequently becoming involved.

Complications. The principal complication of acute epididymitis is sterility, caused by obliteration of the epididymal canals and lumen of the vas deferens. Complete aspermia is commonly found after bilateral epididymitis even though testicular biopsy reveals entirely normal testicular tissue.

Chronic epididymitis—tuberculosis

Etiology. Chronic epididymitis is often tuberculous in origin and should be considered such until proved otherwise. Whether epididymal tuberculosis is primary or secondary is in dispute. Many believe that it arises from the prostate and seminal vesicles just as acute epididymitis does, traveling to the epididymis through the vas deferens. Others believe that it arrives in the epididymis by embolic metastases and spreads down along the genital tract into the testis.

Signs and symptoms. Tuberculous epididymitis begins in the globus minor as a painless mass and may reach an advanced stage before the patient is aware of its presence. Palpation reveals a hard, irregular, and commonly fixed mass involving a part or all of the epididymis; the vas deferens is often irregular and beaded, and there may be a secondary hydrocele. Chronic epididymitis may be bilateral and associated with one or many draining scrotal sinuses.

Diagnosis. The diagnosis is often difficult. A history of pulmonary tuberculosis (usually arrested) is helpful. Careful palpation of the vas deferens and rectal examination may disclose tuberculous involvement of other genital organs. One must rule out testicular tumor. A spermatocele will frequently cause confusion, but spermatoceles usually can be transilluminated. Tumors of the epididymis are rare and seldom confusing.

Treatment. The treatment of tuberculous epididymis continues to be surgical. Prompt removal as soon as the diagnosis is made frequently prevents testicular involvement by direct extension. It may also prevent involvement of the other side. Simple epididymectomy usually suffices.

Chemotherapy has not yet proved itself capable of curing any but the superficial tuberculous lesions, but it is helpful as an adjunct in the treatment of genitourinary tuberculosis. Treatment for up to 2 years is indicated.

Torsion

Etiology. Torsion of the testis is caused by a sudden twisting of the spermatic cord producing an acute partial or total obliteration of the vascular supply to the part. Torsion may occur in a normal testis, but it is more frequently seen in the cryptorchid. It frequently follows minor trauma and may be confused with an acute epididymitis. The immediate and mechanical cause of the torsion is believed to be a spastic contraction of the cremasteric muscle. The combination of an abnormal attachment of the testis, a deficiency in the gubernaculum, or an unusually large tunica vaginalis more frequently leads to a partial or complete rotation with subsequent vascular obstruction.

Diagnosis. Sudden pain usually occurs, followed by swelling, induration, and tenderness. It may be extremely difficult to differentiate from an acute epididymitis, but usually careful history will assist in clinching the diagnosis. Elevation of the testis relieves the pain of acute epididymitis but does not help in testicular torsion. The testis undergoing torsion may assume a more horizontal axis and superior position because of shortening of the spermatic cord. Newer diagnostic modalities used for identifying torsion include radionuclide testis scanning and evaluation of the vascular supply utilizing the Doppler principle.

Treatment. The treatment of torsion of the testis is a serious, distinct emergency, and, if relief is not prompt, sterility and subsequent atrophy will occur. The scrotum should be explored as soon as the diagnosis is even suspected. If, after straightening

of the cord, the testis regains its normal color, it should be fixed securely in the scrotum. Unfortunately, by the time the diagnosis is made the testis is often infarcted, and the only recourse is surgical extirpation. In either event the contralateral scrotum should be explored and orchiopexy carried out, since the tendency to testicular torsion is often bilateral.

Neoplasm

Incidence. In general, most tumors of the testis are malignant and should be removed if the diagnosis is suspected. Tumors of the testis constitute about 1% of all malignant tumors in the male. Although uncommon, the significance of these tumors lies in the age group affected, which is 20 to 40 years.

In descending order of frequency, malignant tumors of the testis are as follows: seminoma, embryonal carcinoma, teratocarcinoma, adult teratoma, and, the least common, chorioepithelioma or choriocarcinoma.

Etiology. Although the cause of testicular tumors is unknown, the undescended testis is distinctly a predisposing factor. All cryptorchid testes should be either removed or brought down into the scrotum in early childhood as prophylaxis against testicular tumor development.

Pathology. There is no unanimity in the pathological classification of testicular tumors. From a practical viewpoint, they are probably best understood when they are classified according to cells. They may develop from any cell type found in the testicular tissue but usually from the germ cells.

The seminoma closely resembles the cells of the seminiferous tubules. Seminomas are believed to be derived from the primordial and primitive sex cells. They usually are unicellular tumors and are the most common of the testicular tumors. They are definitely malignant. Their hormone production is usually nil.

The embryonal carcinoma is a more highly malignant tumor and elaborates gonadotropic hormone in the urine but to a lesser degree than chorioepitheliomas. Embryonal carcinomas grow rapidly and metastasize readily. Grossly they are soft, often necrotic appearing, and hemorrhagic in the cut specimen. They may be unicellular, in which case they are difficult to differentiate from the seminomas. Usually they are multicellular and may appear either papillary or adenomatous. These tumors are therefore often spoken of as either embryonal *adenocarcinoma* or embryonal *papillary adenocarcinoma*.

The teratocarcinoma is a mixture of fairly well-differentiated teratoid structures. This tumor is definitely malignant, unlike the adult teratoma. The teratoid structures are seen intermingling with masses of malignant cells recognized as embryonal carcinoma, seminoma, or chorioepithelioma. Grossly, they are solid and contain many cystic areas. The solid areas contain the malignant tissue.

The adult *teratomas* are believed to arise from isolated blastomeres. They are a mixed cell type, relatively benign, and uncommon. They cause no gonadotropic hormone to be excreted in the urine; grossly they may be solid or cystic. They are encapsulated. The cysts contain sebaceous and mucoid material. Microscopically they are characterized by a variety of well-differentiated and often unrecognizable structures.

The most malignant and fortunately the rarest of the testicular tumors is the *chorioepithelioma*. These tumors elaborate large quantities of gonadotropic hormone. Grossly, the primary lesion may be small and often hidden until postmortem examination, at which time there may be metastases throughout the body. The tumors are soft, extremely hemorrhagic, and necrotic, because of the tumor's propensity to outgrow its own blood supply. Microscopically it is distinguished by cytotrophoblasts and syncytiotrophoblast cells.

Metastases. The mode of metastases is primarily lymphatic, passing up along the cord to the regional nodes: the para-aortic, mediastinal, and supraclavicular nodes. These tumors may, in addition, metastasize through the bloodstream; lung metastases have occasionally been excised with apparent cure and no systemic treatment.

Signs and symptoms. Testicular tumors arise insidiously. The initial symptoms are usually a painless swelling of the testis and a sensation of increased weight. Because of the tumor's insidious onset, minor trauma to the part frequently directs attention to the mass. The mass slowly enlarges and continues to be painless. However, all too frequently the testicular mass goes unnoticed until widespread metastases have developed with weight loss, abdominal mass, abdominal or back pain, edema of the lower extremities, or pulmonary complaints. Lastly, gynecomastia is suggestive of chorioepithelioma.

Diagnosis. Testicular tumors must be differentiated from hydroceles. Differentiation is often very difficult since a hydrocele frequently accompanies the tumor. Usually the mass cannot be transilluminated, but if any doubt remains, the scrotum should be explored from an inguinal approach. Hematocele may be rules out by palpation. Chronic or acute epididymitis is frequently confused with testicular tumors.

Biological markers. It is now well established that many nonseminomatous testicular tumors secrete substances that can be fairly easily measured in serum. The two most promising of these tumor markers are alpha-fetoprotein (AFP) and the beta subunit of human chorionic gonadotropic hormone (β-HCG). The presence of either or both of these markers in abnormal concentrations, along with the presence of a scrotal mass, generally indicates an embryonal cell carcinoma, teratocarcinoma, choriocarcinoma, or some combination of these with or without seminoma. The return of these markers to normal levels after therapy (e.g., high inguinal orchiectomy and retroperitoneal lymphadenectomy) is helpful in assessment of the adequacy of treatment. Follow-up serum measurements of such markers are indicated to detect recurrences that otherwise would remain silent for many weeks to months.

Prognosis. The prognosis of testicular tumors largely depends on the type of tumor and the time elapsing between its onset and adequate treatment. The cure rate for seminoma should approach 100%.

Treatment. The treatment of seminoma of the testis is high inguinal orchiectomy followed by irradiation therapy over the common routes of metastasis. In all other types of malignant testicular neoplasms, high inguinal orchiectomy plus complete node dissection of the iliac and para-aortic nodes up to the renal arteries is indicated. Irradiation therapy is not so helpful for lesions other than seminoma. Chemotherapy is the treatment of choice in disseminated testicular tumors, and the effective agents are the combination of vinblastine sulfate, bleomycin, and *cis*-platinum (Einhorn regimen).

VARICOCELE

Etiology. Varicocele is the name given to varicosities of the pampiniform venous plexus. The veins become distended, elongated, and tortuous; 97% of varicoceles are found on the left side, and 5% are bilateral. Although the cause is unknown, the high incidence of left-sided varicoceles indicates that the 90-degree angle by which the left spermatic vein enters the renal vein may be, in some way, causative. On the right side the spermatic vein empties into the inferior vena cava at an oblique angle. Since obstruction of the inferior vena cava may produce a varicocele on the right side, all right-sided varicoceles must be thoroughly investigated to rule out this cause. Defective valves in the spermatic venous system may also cause varicocele.

Varicoceles are usually seen between 15 and 30 years of age. Frequently they are asymptomatic. Some patients complain of a dragging sensation or neuralgia of the testis. Each male evaluated for infertility needs to be examined for the presence of an asymptomatic varicocele, since this lesion is often implicated in the "stress-pattern" seminogram: poor motility, increased numbers of abnormal spermatozoa, and a sperm concentration that may be normal to decreased. The pathogenesis of this form of infertility is yet unknown; because of cross circulation of the scrotal contents, the unilateral varicocele results in bilateral spermatogenic changes.

Diagnosis. The diagnosis of a varicocele is simple. The involved testis hangs distinctly lower than its mate, and its cord has a "bag of worms" sensation to palpation. The distended veins empty when the scrotum is elevated, and the "bag of worms" sensation disappears, only to return when the patient stands. If the varicocele does not disappear with scrotal elevation, an intra-abdominal tumor or vena cava obstruction must be suspected. The Doppler stethoscope can detect varicoceles that are otherwise not obvious.

Treatment. The treatment of varicocele is controversial. In most instances varicoceles tend to disappear spontaneously with time. Furthermore, surgical ligation of the involved veins rarely relieves the neuralgia and may be followed by atrophy of the testicle, hydrocele, hemorrhage, thrombosis, and epididymitis, leaving the patient worse off than before surgery. Therefore I recommend a scrotal support as the only treatment of simple varicocele. However, infertility associated with varicocele may respond to ligation of the spermatic veins. Improvement in sperm count, motility, and morphology with subsequent pregnancy has been reported in up to 50% of men so treated. Although this surgery can be performed at the scrotal or inguinal levels, I prefer the retroperitoneal route to expose the internal spermatic veins superior to the internal inguinal ring.

SPERMATOCELE

Etiology. Spermatoceles are retention cysts of the vasa efferentia or epididymis, and they contain spermatozoa. Most spermatoceles are believed to arise from scarring and deformity of the epididymis because of inflammatory obliteration of the lumen of the vasa efferentia, though some are traumatic in origin.

Signs and symptoms. Spermatoceles are manifest as slowly enlarging cystic masses of the scrotum in young and old men, and generally they produce only mild local discomfort.

Diagnosis. A spermatocele is palpable as a cystic mass separate and distinct from the testis, usually arising from the globus major. It can be transilluminated as well as a hydrocele, the fluid contents being gray-white and containing inactive spermatozoa.

Treatment. Spermatoceles usually require no treatment. When they become large, they may be excised.

HYDROCELE

Etiology. A hydrocele is an accumulation of fluid within the serous sac of the scrotum lying between the tunica vaginalis and the tunica albuginea. Hydroceles are classified as idiopathic or congenital, acute or chronic, and may involve the testis or the cord.

By far the most common hydrocele is the idiopathic variety, which may occur at any age. Congenital hydrocele occurs in the infant with an imperfect closure of the processus vaginalis; it may be associated with a congenital type of inguinal hernia, depending on the size of the opening into the peritoneal cavity.

Hydrocele of the cord may also be congenital. In this case there is obliteration of the funicular process proximally and distally, leaving an intervening lumen in which fluid accumulates. Hydrocele of the cord presents as a cystic mass along the cord, which transilluminates and is separate from both the testis and the epididymis.

Diagnosis. Diagnosis of hydrocele is established by palpation and transillumination, which will usually rule out a hernia and hematocele. It must then be differentiated from spermatocele. In a hydrocele the testis is either not felt or is palpated within the hydrocele sac. The spermatocele is felt as a mass distinct from the testis.

Treatment. The treatment of hydrocele may be either medical or surgical. The hydrocele may be aspirated from time to time, with infection being the most likely complication of this conservative form of treatment. Surgical treatment is by excision of the redundant portion of the hydrocele sac or a plication procedure that enhances reabsorption of fluid produced by the tunica vaginalis testis.

DISEASES OF THE VAS DEFERENS

The vas deferens is afflicted by the same diseases as the epididymis. Vasitis may be of gonorrheal or nonspecific origin, as well as tuberculous. The acute pyogenic infections cause pain, swelling, and tenderness on deep palpation over the vas deferens and the lower quadrants of the abdomen. Systemic manifestations are nausea, vomiting, fever, and leukocytosis.

The treatment of vasitis is the same as for epididymitis: bed rest, heat applications, and antibiotics. The prognosis is usually good, with infection subsiding in approximately a week to 10 days. However, obliteration of the lumen is a distinct possibility, leading to sterility.

Chronic infection of the vas is usually tuberculous in origin and has been discussed in the section on tuberculous epididymitis.

DISEASES OF THE SEMINAL VESICLES

Seminal vesiculitis may be of gonorrheal, non-specific, or tuberculous origin. Gonorrheal and non-specific vesiculitis is often associated with prostatitis and epididymitis and is simply a part of a general infection of the genital tract. The posterior urethra is the most frequent source of infection, which involve the vesicles by direct extension.

The acute phase of seminal vesiculitis begins with pronounced engorgement of the vesicles, which may progress to suppuration and abscess formation if the process fails to resolve. Later, a chronic stage develops with thickening and induration of the vesicles. This accounts for the ease with which they are palpated on rectal examination in the chronic stage of seminal vesiculitis.

Acute seminal vesiculitis may begin with systemic manifestations of chills and fever with or without urinary disturbances. Pain is variable; when present, it is referred to the suprapubic and inguinal regions but rarely as high as the kidney. In nongonorrheal seminal vesiculitis the onset is more insidious, with few systemic manifestations and little discomfort. Chronic vesiculitis is frequently asymptomatic except for pain in the perineum, hip, and low back area. Because it is frequently associated with prostatitis, there may be increased urinary frequency, dysuria, and the symptoms of prostatitis.

On examination one finds tenderness, induration, and thickening of the vesicles, in addition to epididymitis and vasitis. Seminal vesiculitis will frequently be followed by aspermia, oligospermia, or even a complete lack of ejaculate.

Treatment of acute seminal vesiculitis is by massive doses of antibiotics, bed rest, and sedation. Chronic vesiculitis is treated with antibiotics and massage or stripping of the vesicles. No treatment is needed if the patient is asymptomatic. Hematospermia is a common symptom.

STERILITY IN THE MALE

Etiology. Fertility in the male requires (1) normal, actively motile spermatozoa formed within the testis, (2) free transport of the spermatozoa through the epididymis, vas deferens, and ultimately out the urethra, and (3) deposition of the sperm into the vaginal fornix.

There is a multitude of causes for sterility. *Impotence* may produce a relative state of sterility because of the inability to deliver spermatozoa into the vaginal vault. Impotence may be either neurological or psychogenic in origin. If the lesion is psychogenic, the prognosis is good with proper psychiatric care, but if it is neurological, the prognosis is usually poor.

Hypospadias frequently results in sterility on the same basis as impotence, the chordee and foreshortened urethra precluding delivery of the ejaculated specimen into the vaginal vault.

Stricture of the urethra will produce aspermia or oligospermia if the lumen is so narrow as to prohibit the extremely viscid semen from passing.

Prostatitis and *seminal vesiculitis* are believed by many to cause sterility by altering the pH of the prostatic secretions to decrease seriously the motility and longevity of otherwise healthy spermatozoa.

The most common cause of sterility in the male is bilateral *epididymitis*. It may be acute, gonorrheal, or nonspecific, perhaps resulting from a prostatitis. In any case, after the acute inflammatory reaction, scarring of the tubules results with either total or partial obliteration of their lumen.

Orchitis is another common cause of sterility. Mumps orchitis usually occurs during or after puberty and may result in extreme atrophy of the seminiferous tubules. Since the Leydig cells are much more resistant to injury, impotence usually does not occur.

Patients with cryptorchidism after the age of puberty are sterile on the involved side, and complete aspermia is the usual finding if the disease is bilateral. Secondary sex characteristics will develop normally, since the testicular atrophy does not involve the interstitial cells of Leydig.

Diagnosis. The examination for sterility should include a careful history of past or present prostatitis, seminal vesiculitis, epididymitis, or orchitis.

The testes, epididymides, vasa deferentia, seminal vesicles, prostate, and urethra are examined carefully because a pathological condition anywhere along the genital tract may eventuate in either partial or complete sterility.

Examination of the semen. After a complete history and physical examination, the semen is examined. It must be obtained after at least 3 days of sexual abstinence, so that the sperm count can return to its optimal level. Most clinics obtain the semen specimen by masturbation, and it is extremely rare that the patient complains of this method. There are other less satisfactory methods of obtaining semen specimens. Coitus interruptus may result in a partial loss of the fluid, making the count unreliable. The semen may be obtained from the vaginal vault of the female partner, but this, too is an unsatisfactory method, since it is impossible to obtain the total volume of ejaculate. The use of a condom to collect the ejaculate is wholeheartedly condemned since the latex rubber is impregnated with solutions and powders designed to act as spermicides.

The semen is first checked grossly. Normal semen is milky in appearance, of a thick consistency, and has a high viscosity. The volume averages 3 to 4 ml.; the pH varies from 7.7 to 8.5. Any appreciable alteration from these norms should be noted; a low pH will result in decreased motility and longevity of the spermatozoa. A positive fructose test indicates the presence of seminal vesicle fluid; this function is extremely sensitive to even low concentrations of plasma testosterone.

The specimen is studied best microscopically about 30 minutes after delivery. By this time it has lost its high viscosity and can be diluted easily for an accurate count; little change in the motility of the sperm occurs during this interval of time. Normally, 80% or more of the sperm are actively motile; any decrease of the motility percentage lowers fertility.

A cell count of the semen, which normally averages 40 to 150 million spermatozoa per mililiter, is next done. The specimen is diluted in a white blood cell pipette in the same manner as for a white blood cell count, using a diluent composed of 1% formalin and 5% sodium bicarbonate in water. This immediately kills the sperm cells. Two large squares are counted, as for a white blood cell count, and the result is multiplied by 100,000 (i.e., add 5 zeros to the total count). This will give the spermatozoa count per milliliter.

Although great reliance is placed on the total sperm count, it has little practical significance inasmuch as only the actively motile spermatozoa can impregnate the ovum. Many clinics classify their degree of fertility on the actively motile count, obtained by this formula: % motility × sperm count per mililiter × volume of specimen in milliliters. At least three seminograms are required for a base-line value in any patient.

Medical treatment. Thyroid extract, vitamin E, steroids, and gonadotropins have been found on careful experimentation to produce no significant increase in sperm count. Parenteral testosterone therapy predictably results in a decreased sperm count. Some authors have described a subsequent "rebound" phenomenon to justify the treatment, but most studies do not bear this out. Furthermore, and more importantly, since the entire process of spermatogenesis requires 75 to 90 days, any attempt to assess the efficacy of a treatment modality on the seminogram should be postponed until about 3 months after the initiation of the therapy.

Men with infertility and oligospermia should have measurements made of their plasma levels of both luteinizing hormone (LH) and follicle-stimulating hormone (FSH). Men demonstrating significant elevations of FSH and LH probably have primary testicular failure with expected increased pituitary hormone levels. On the other hand, men with normal LH and FSH levels may have hypothalamic or anterior pituitary dysfunction with secondary testicular impairment. This latter group of subfertile men may benefit from long-term cyclic administration of the drug clomiphene citrate, which in turn stimulates the hypothalamus-pituitary-testis axis.

Surgical treatment. The surgical treatment of male sterility is disappointing. The surgery may be divided into prophylactic and therapeutic. Prophylactic surgery is of vital importance: undescended testes should be brought into the scrotum in early childhood, and patients with severe orchitis associated with mumps may be saved from sterility by prompt opening and draining of the tunica vaginalis and tunica albuginea or by corticosteroid therapy. Urethral strictures should be dilated, and hypospadias with chordee should be corrected by appropriate plastic surgery.

Surgery has little to offer aspermic patients. Epididymis–vas deferens anastomosis has been attempted in patients with sterility associated with old epididymitis with little success. Catheterization of the ejaculatory duct and injection of the vas deferens are mentioned only in condemnation. Vasovasostomy is successful in 50% to 80% of patients previously rendered sterile by bilateral vasectomy.

Bilateral testicular biopsy is recommended for patients with oligospermia or aspermia. This procedure may be done under local anesthesia. The biopsy specimen is fixed in Bouin's solution, stained, and studied microscopically to determine the degree of spermatogenesis and to lend some insight into the cause of the sterility. Biopsy allows a more accurate prognosis of fertility.

Treatment of low-fertility patients. Discouraging as the medical and surgical approaches to male sterility are, definite progress is being made in the management of low-fertility males. The date of ovulation must be determined accurately to allow the maximum number of spermatozoa to be ejaculated at the most opportune time. Spermatozoa are rarely viable fore more than 48 hours in the uterus. The date of ovulation may be estimated by a sharp drop in the daily basal temperatures, taken just after awakening. This method will usually localize the time of ovulation to within 48 hours. It has proved a definite boon to the subfertile males, even though its accuracy is limited. Recent tests may be accurate to within 6 to 12 hours of ovulation.

Instructions to the low-fertility groups. After determining the exact time of ovulation, I am able to suggest the following course: sexual abstinence for a week before the date of ovulation; then coitus the day before, twice during the 8-hour period of ovulation, and daily for the next 3 days. By this method the husband will be able to concentrate the maximum number of spermatozoa at the most crucial period. Strict adherence to this routine has produced encouraging results in subfertile couples.

Men with documented high-volume ejaculates (6 to 10 ml.) usually have their spermatozoa concentrated in the first portion of the ejaculate, whereas the overall sperm count may be normal or low. Instruction about the technique of coitus interruptus at the time of expected ovulation to deliver the undiluted active spermatozoa has resulted in pregnancies in this select group of subfertile couples.

Artificial insemination. The initial successes with artificial insemination occurred at the University of Iowa. Two general types are now practiced: artificial insemination by husband (A.I.H.) and artificial insemination by donor (A.I.D.). The former is indicated when physical abnormalities make normal sexual intercourse impossible or in the use of split ejaculates when coitus interruptus is unsuccessful. Unidentified donor insemination (A.I.D.) has many medicolegal ramifications, and the exact status of this technique may vary from state to state. Presumably its use would benefit those couples in which the husband is sterile, the wife is fertile, and adoption is considered less attractive.

The newer techniques of in vitro fertilization and embryo transference are under the aegis of the obstetrician-gynecologist specializing in infertility. However, the close cooperation of a urologist in evaluation of the potential father's fertility status must be emphasized.

42
Head and Neck Surgery

Charles J. Krause
Brian F. McCabe

A clear understanding of otolaryngological and head and neck diseases is important for the general physician, since somewhere between 20% and 40% of all the illnesses he treats will center above the clavicles. Upper respiratory tract infections (nasal, sinal, aural, and pharyngeal) are by far the most common sources of infection. A knowledge of these diseases is important for the specialist as well, because even the specialist must occasionally practice some general medicine. Furthermore, the specialist must not neglect disease in another organ system while treating that disease for which he is primarily trained. We must continuously dedicate ourselves to the welfare of the whole patient.

This chapter deals primarily with identification of otolaryngological disease by pointing out the *nature* of the process. Principles of diagnosis are stressed, and treatment methods are described only so far as they are pertinent. The student is cautioned that treatment methods in this field change very rapidly.

CONGENITAL ANOMALIES
Congenital anomalies with respiratory obstruction

Congenital abnormalities of the head and neck are important because they may affect vital processes such as respiration, deglutition, and nourishment. Some anomalies in this region impair the important modalities of communication. Of no small import are the cosmetic defects imposed by congenital abnormalities of the head and neck. Function is the most important consideration, but appearance is also of concern. Here we do not speak of the gross abnormalities, such as anen-

cephaly or cyclops deformity, and the other monstrous deformities that are for the most part incompatible with life. The minor abnormalities, such as prominent nose, outstanding ears, cleft lip, and hypognathia, though not necessarily compromising function, are major concerns to the patient as a person. The good physician bears in mind that in one's physiognomy dwells the entity that a person calls "himself."

In this section we will consider chiefly those entities that alter function and therefore demand early recognition and treatment.

Respiratory obstruction in the newborn is a problem of prime importance, and a thorough knowledge of its differential diagnosis is essential. The following is a list of some of the important causes:

1. Secretory obstruction (mucus or amniotic fluid)
2. Choanal atresia
3. Tracheoesophageal fistulas
4. Congenital vascular ring
5. Laryngeal cysts and webs
6. Congenital laryngeal stridor
7. Pierre-Robin syndrome
8. Treacher-Collins syndrome
9. Rhinomeningoceles or encephaloceles
10. Laryngomalacia and tracheomalacia
11. Laryngeal paralysis
12. Diaphragmatic hernia
13. Bronchial or pulmonary agenesis
14. Brain damage or agenesis, or both

Secretory obstruction of the nasal airways may result from the retention of thick mucus or amniotic fluid during the perinatal period. The treatment consists of removal of the thick secretions using a flexible nasal suction. This results in an immediate improvement in the nasal airway, differentiating secretory obstruction from the other more serious causes discussed below.

Choanal atresia is obstruction of the posterior nares attributed to retention of the embryonic plate that separates the nasal chambers from the nasopharynx. The atresia may be unilateral or bilateral. Neonates afflicted with this abnormality do not breathe normally because *mouth breathing is not normal to the infant within the first 2 weeks of life.* Careful observation of the infant with bilateral choanal atresia reveals the following sequence of events: cyclical episodes of upper airway obstruction when the mouth is closed, associated with cyanosis and labored respiratory efforts that are dramatically relieved when he cries. Air is freely exchanged when the infant cries, he becomes pink and quiet, closes his mouth, and the cycle is then repeated. The infant cannot rest, and feedings are often aspirated because of the airway obstruction that this provokes. There exists a true respiratory emergency. The diagnosis is made by inability to pass a catheter through the nasal chamber into the oropharynx. Radiocontrast studies confirm the diagnosis: lateral skull films show complete retention of dye instilled into the nasal chambers while the infant is supine. Treatment consists in tiding the infant over the 2-week period required for mouth breathing to be learned. Feedings are given by orogastric tube. A patent airway is obtained by whatever means proves most satisfactory: decubi-

tus positioning, frequent suctioning, placement of an oropharyngeal airway, and occasionally a tracheostomy is required. The nasopharyngeal plate may be perforated with a blunt instrument, or with a mastoid drill and operative microscope, but extreme care must be taken to avoid passing the instrument through the fragile and largely cartilaginous cervical vertebrae into the brainstem. Definitive operation for removal of the atresia plate transpalatally can be carried out as early as 1 year of age.

Tracheoesophageal fistulas are discussed in Chapter 28.

Congenital vascular ring is discussed in Chapter 31.

Laryngeal cysts and webs produce respiratory obstruction of the larynx and usually result in hoarseness. In the infant this is manifested as a husky or nonclear cry. Cysts arise anywhere within the endolarynx or hypopharynx and are caused by malformations of mucous glands. Web formation occurs through incomplete separation of the true vocal cords. The cords are joined at the anterior commissure, much as fingers are connected in syndactylism. The laryngeal web is of minor consequence if it involves only the anterior commissure but is serious if it is nearly total with only a small airway at the posterior commissure. *Subglottic stenosis* is a less common condition of congenital narrowing of the airway at the level of the cricoid cartilage. Diagnosis is made by direct laryngoscopy. The treatment includes tracheotomy with excision of the stenotic area or expansion of the

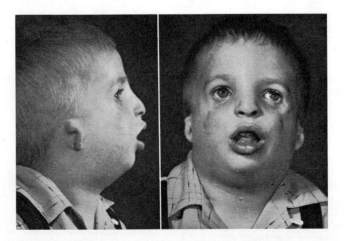

Fig. 42-1. Treacher-Collins syndrome, one of the congenital craniofacial dysplasias. "Bird shape" to face and eye and ear anomalies are striking. It is extremely important to place bone-conduction hearing aid on such patient by age 1 or 2, so that normal speech and intellectual development may occur.

cricoid lumen through splitting it and interposing a cartilage graft. An indwelling stent for a period of several weeks is frequently necessary.

Congenital laryngeal stridor produces a clear, sharp inspiratory stridor on crying or straining. When the infant is breathing normally and quietly, the stridor is not present. Mild cyanosis is seen occasionally, but unconsciousness attributable to hypoxia does not occur. The lesion is caused by immaturity of the epiglottis ("infantile" or omega-shaped epiglottis), so that on sharp inspiration the aryepiglottic folds are drawn down into the glottic aperture, with consequent stridor. The stridor occurs *only on inspiration*. The condition is self-limiting. The child usually outgrows his symptoms during the second year of life, as the epiglottis gains maturity.

Pierre-Robin syndrome is one of the family of mandibulofacial dysplasias produced by anomalies of the first and second branchial arches. Respiratory obstruction of the oropharynx is immediate and alarming with the baby supine but is relieved in the prone position. The syndrome is recognizable at birth by simple observation of hypognathia, glossoptosis, cleft palate, and usually a cleft lip. The descriptive term *micrognathia* is used if there is no cleft palate. There is not room for the relatively large tongue in the patient's oropharynx because of the failure of anterior growth of the mandible. This must be differentiated from cretinism, in which the tongue is abnormally large and cannot be accommodated by the oral cavity of normal size. On inspection, the bulging floor of the mouth may resemble the tongue, but when this is pushed down, the tip of the tongue can be seen

pointing up toward the hard palate, well back in the mouth. Although feeding may be difficult, airway obstruction is the most acute threat to life. Careful positioning is necessary for gravity to prolapse the dependent tongue away from the posterior pharyngeal wall to disobstruct the airway. An anterior tongue-tie with a base of tongue suture to the mandible may also hold the tongue forward to keep the airway clear. Tracheotomy may be necessary. Tube feedings are often required. Curiously, the airway problems improve with time. Other congenital anomalies are frequently present. The mortality is high, exceeding 20% in most series.

Treacher-Collins syndrome, another of the mandibulofacial dysplasias, is a striking developmental defect of the first and second branchial arches and the first branchial groove (Fig. 42-1). Hypognathia and glossoptosis are present, as in the Pierre-Robin syndrome. In addition, there is an underformed maxilla producing the appearance of an abnormally prominent nose, outward and downward slanted eyes (sometimes called "antimongoloid"), a notched lower lid, bony atresia of both external auditory canals with severe conductive hearing loss, and small, low-set, and deformed ears. The palate and the lip are usually intact. Early in life, the respiratory problem requires attention, but past infancy the mandible grows enough for adequate respiratory exchange without obstruction or stridor. In the second and third years of life, deafness is the greatest problem; the child needs a bone conduction hearing aid to develop speech and learn at an adequate rate. The external auditory canal atresia is corrected surgically to improve hearing at about the time the child enters school; this should

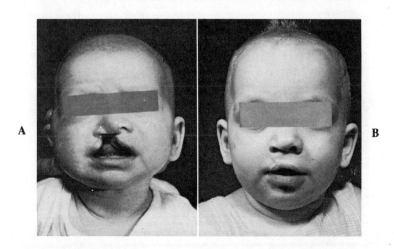

Fig. 42-2. Cleft palate and lip. **A,** Preoperative. **B,** Postoperative.

take precedence over cosmetic improvement of the external ears. These patients have such a characteristic appearance that they are sometimes called "bird people" (Fig. 42-1).

In *rhinomeningoceles* or *encephaloceles* cerebral contents herniate through an unformed cribriform plate or other portions of the floor of the anterior cranial fossa to produce masses in the nasal chamber of the newborn that may obstruct the airway. The appearance externally may be normal, or paranasal masses may pulsate. Rhinomeningoceles or encephaloceles are smooth, pale, and pulsate on close inspection. Roentgenograms reveal a bony defect in the floor of the anterior cranial fossa. Biopsy may be disastrous, of course, and must be avoided by awareness of this diagnostic possibility. Rhinomeningoceles are approached by anterior craniotomy, and the mass is retracted back into the cranial cavity with repair of the defect.

Laryngomalacia and *tracheomalacia* are congenital defects in the ground substance of the airway cartilage, which cannot retain its shape on inspiration. The walls of the airway collapse proportionate to the degree of negative pressure created during inspiration. The only treatment is tracheotomy when airway obstruction is severe. Congenital laryngeal stridor may be misdiagnosed as laryngomalacia and wrongly treated by tracheotomy.

Laryngeal paralysis may be unilateral or bilateral. If unilateral, the condition is asymptomatic, but if bilateral, severe inspiratory stridor is present at birth, and tracheotomy is mandatory. Bilateral laryngeal paralysis seldom occurs without associated neurological disturbances, such as cerebral palsy. The diagnosis is made by direct laryngoscopy; the cords stay at or near the midline and do not abduct on inspiration.

Diaphragmatic hernia is discussed in Chapter 27, *pulmonary agenesis* in Chapter 30, and *central nervous system disturbances* in Chapter 40.

Congenital anomalies not associated with respiratory obstruction

Branchial and *thyroglossal remnants* are discussed in Chapter 28.

A *cleft lip* or *cleft palate* (Fig. 42-2, *A*) is always alarming to the parents of the afflicted newborn, and they need reassurance that the child can develop almost normally in function and appearance with medical care that is properly timed and carried out. The appearance of the cleft lip or cleft palate is so varied as to defy description. It ranges all the way from a minor notch or slight alteration of the vermilion portion of the upper lip to complete clefts of both sides of the upper lip that extend into the floor of the nostrils and nasal chambers, completely back through the hard and soft palate. Restoration of the intact palate is as important for function as repair of the lip is for cosmetic appearance (Fig. 42-2, *B*). Multiple operations, properly timed, are needed to avoid inter-

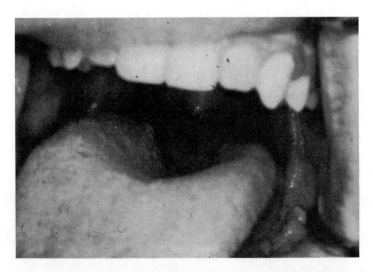

Fig. 42-3. Lingual thyroid, occurring at foramen cecum of tongue. Notice intact, unulcerated covering. Such lesions may be biopsied for diagnosis but should not be removed as a tumor, for this may be the only thyroid tissue patient has. [131]I scintiscan is simpler method of diagnosis.

ference with proper growth of the middle third of the face. Dental anomalies, sometimes gross and bizarre, are invariably present. Speech and nourishment are difficult and require special help; cleft palate adds vexing ear problems, such as repeated acute infections and chronic serous otitis media. Thus the modern care of cleft palate patients is a multidisciplinary effort of a highly specialized team. The cleft palate team includes an otolaryngologist, a plastic surgeon, an orthodontist, a prosthodontist, a speech therapist, a pediatrician, a pedodontist, an audiologist, a social worker, and a psychologist.

Lingual thyroid, a prominent mass overlain by normal mucosa (Fig. 42-3), is located at the junction of the middle and posterior thirds of the tongue. It is diagnosed by biopsy or scintiscan. Lingual thyroid should not be removed until it is proved that other thyroid tissue is present, unless thyroid replacement is given.

Outstanding ears (lop-ears) result from failure of development of the anthelix of the auricle, so that

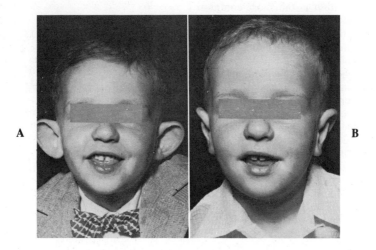

Fig. 42-4. Lop ears. **A,** Preoperative. **B,** Postoperative.

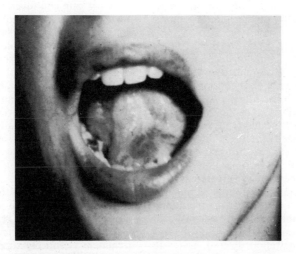

Fig. 42-5. Ranula, with intact epithelium over it. It is soft and cystic. Such lesions may be superficial in floor of mouth ("pseudoranula") or have deep extensions into diaphragm of floor of mouth and genioglossus muscles ("true" ranula).

the rim of the ear stands outward from the skull (Fig. 42-4, *A*). The ear is often cup shaped. Otoplasty will restore good contour if the patient is sensitive about the cosmetic deformity (Fig. 42-4, *B*).

Pretragal cysts or granulomas appear just anterior to the tragus of the ear and are caused by entrapped skin below the surface, from the developing hillocks of cartilage that form the outer ear. Incision and drainage are inadequate treatment; the entire skin-lined tract must be removed to effect a cure.

Floor-of-the-mouth cysts and tumors may be of many varieties. The *ranula* is the most common (Fig. 42-5). The *pseudoranula* is merely a blocked minor salivary gland in the floor of the mouth and is submucosal. The *true ranula* is an embryological deformity of the sublingual glands and perhaps other glands, with fingerlike ramifications into the substance of the genioglossus muscles. Simple intraoral excision of the pseudoranula suffices. The true ranula generally requires an external approach for complete excision, though it may be managed satisfactorily by creation of a fistula of the ranula into the mouth. *Dermoid* and *epidermoid cysts* cannot be distinguished clinically. They are fusion-fault cysts, in which epithelial tissue is trapped between the joining mandibular arches. Differential diagnosis includes *minor salivary gland tumors, salivary gland calculi,* and *desmoid* or *desmoplastic tumors.*

INFECTIONS

Certain principles in the diagnosis and treatment of head and neck infections are important. Infections in this region are very common and may constitute as much as 20% of the family doctor's office practice.

Despite their frequency, head and neck infections should not be taken lightly or dismissed with a superficial evaluation. The complications may be serious and life threatening, e.g., extension to bone or metastatic spread to other organ systems such as the kidney, heart, or joints. On the other hand, they hold no mystery to the alert physician who understands the specialized structures involved.

In the treatment of acute infections, full-dosage antibiotic therapy must be instituted early and maintained for several days after symptoms have subsided. Whenever possible, cultures should be obtained before antibiotic therapy is instituted. Selection of a specific antibiotic will rest on what organism is suspected, a history of drug allergy, and the route of administration desired. Later it may be necessary to change the antibiotic when culture and sensitivity results are available. Acute abscesses, whether in the middle ear, neck, or

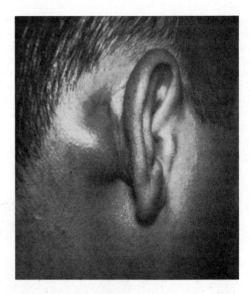

Fig. 42-6. Acute mastoiditis. Swelling with pain and fluctuant mass in this region is most unlikely to be misdiagnosed. Incidence of acute mastoiditis has been very low in antibiotic era, but that of chronic mastoiditis is steadily rising. This patient has acute exacerbation of chronic mastoiditis. Disease chose to perforate mastoid cortex. If it had chosen rather the middle fossa plate (roof of mastoid) or inner ear, results could have been disastrous.

another part of the body, must be afforded the time-honored principle of incision and drainage. Supportive measures are necessary, including aspirin for pain and fever, local wet or dry heat, bed rest, and increased fluid intake.

Chronic infections in this region, especially chronic sinusitis, mastoiditis (Fig. 42-6), and tonsillitis, are seldom amenable to antibiotic therapy alone. The treatment of chronic infections in this region is surgical. When bone is infected acutely, it is usually amenable to antibiotic therapy, but when chronic infection is present, the bone must be removed. This can usually be done without significant alteration of function or cosmetic deformity.

Viral

The *viral nose cold* is the most common infection of man. Little need be said about it except that antibiotics of any kind render the patient a disservice. The symptoms are well known, and the treatment is entirely supportive. The nose cold is generally said to be 3 days coming, 3 days present, and 3 days going. Any nose cold lasting longer than this is probably becoming complicated by suppura-

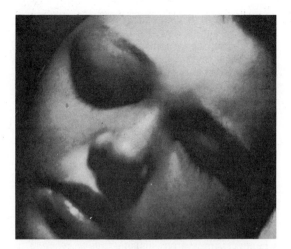

Fig. 42-7. Acute right frontal sinusitis that has perforated floor of sinus and produced an orbital abscess. Disease is now surgical. Differential diagnosis includes orbital cellulitis, cavernous sinus thrombosis or fistula, frontal or ethmoid neoplasm, and osteomyelitis.

tive infections of the nose, sinuses, or lower respiratory tract. *APC fever* (adenopharyngoconjunctival fever) is a mildly epidemic viral infection of the nasopharynx that, after several days of sore throat, produces a nonsuppurative conjunctivitis of first one and then the other eye. *Infectious mononucleosis* is also a mildly epidemic disease of young people, often heralded by petechiae of the palate or buccal mucosa. The tonsils are usually involved in the nonsuppurative process. The tonsillitis may on occasion be extreme, with severe sore throat and necrotic slough of the surface of each tonsil. The diagnosis is made when two of the following are present: (1) posterior cervical adenopathy, (2) a significant rise in the number of atypical "foamy" lymphocytes in peripheral blood, and (3) a positive heterophile agglutinin test in rising titer. The treatment is nonspecific but should include prolonged bed rest because of the possible complications of the disease, which include hepatitis and a prolonged postinfectious fatigue state.

Bacterial
Acute suppurative oropharyngitis, nasopharyngitis, laryngitis, and tonsillitis

As with acute suppurative infections anywhere, acute infections of the oropharynx, nasopharynx, larynx, and tonsils result in fever, general malaise, pain in the affected organ, and altered function. The diagnosis is made when pus is observed over the greatly inflamed tissue. Antibiotic and support-

ive therapy is the treatment. A mirror is necessary in the diagnosis of all head and neck infections, or one may be led astray; e.g., the oropharynx of a patient with acute suppurative nasopharyngitis may be profusely inflamed but without pus visible on tongueblade examination, suggestive of a viral oropharyngitis. These infections are not communicable, though there are infections of this region that are communicable (diphtheria and Vincent's infection). When the suppuration involves the larynx or trachea, modified voice rest must be a part of therapy to avoid the complication of speaker's nodule, vocal cord granuloma, or vocal polyp.

Paranasal sinusitis

Clinically, the important forms of sinusitis are acute and chronic suppurative. Other forms of sinusitis exist, e.g., atrophic sinusitis, rhinoscleromatous sinusitis, and tuberculous sinusitis, but they are rare.

Acute suppurative sinusitis is accompanied by the usual signs of acute infection together with facial pain, usually over the involved sinus, and a purulent rhinorrhea (Fig. 42-7). The pain of sphenoiditis is either fronto-occipital or bitemporal. The history is that of change of the watery nasal discharge to a suppurative one at the end of a viral nose cold. The diagnosis is not difficult to make on examination: pus at one of the sinus ostia within the nasal chamber. The edematous nasal mucosa is easily shrunk with a drop or spray of 1% to 3% ephedrine in normal saline solution, or with any of the commercial nose drops. The treatment is similar to that for any acute febrile infection, as described previously. Codeine may be necessary for relief of pain, and some benefit is afforded by antihistamines or similar agents to produce mucosal shrinkage, aid drainage, and diminish the mucoid element of the discharge. Most acute suppurative sinus infections are never seen by the physician, resolving spontaneously after a course of several weeks—but the *complications* of acute sinusitis always bring the patient to the physician. The most common complication is that of chronicity, and this is discussed later. Perhaps the second most common complication is *acute serous otitis media*, producing a stuffy ear, deafness, tinnitus, and autophony, of which the patient may complain bitterly without mention of the nasal complaint. The sinusitis is then discovered as the cause during routine examination. More serious complications are *acute osteomyelitis, orbital abscess* (Fig. 42-7), *epidural, subdural, and brain abscess, cavernous sinus thrombosis*, and *acute empyema* of the sinus. All these complications are of major consequence, and each is accompanied by a specific set of symptoms that requires treatment by an appropriate specialist. They all produce external swelling and a rapid worsening of the general condition of the patient, which should immediately alert the physician.

Chronic suppurative sinusitis, however, is unaccompanied by facial pain, headache, or any signs of systemic infection, unless complicated. Let us dispel the widely prevalent notion that frontal (or frontal and occipital) headache plus a stuffy nose is equatable with chronic sinus disease. This set of symptoms generally signals tension headaches plus chronic vasomotor rhinitis. The diagnosis of chronic suppurative sinusitis is untenable if pus is not visible at one of the sinal ostia. This is true almost regardless of the x-ray findings, especially report of a "cloudy sinus." Perhaps the only diagnostic x-ray sign is that of an air-fluid level. The "cloudy sinus" frequently means nothing more than thickening of the lining—testimony of an old healed infection and scarification (Fig. 42-8, *A*).

The treatment of chronic suppurative sinusitis is surgical (the nasoantral window operation, or sinusectomy). Sinusectomy is accomplished transorally (antral region), intranasally (ethmoid or sphenoid sinus), or externally (for the frontal or frontoethmoid sinus). The *complications* of chronic sinusitis are of major importance, including those listed under acute sinusitis, plus one other, mucocele. *Mucocele* arises as a slowly enlarging cyst filled with mucus, or mucopus (*mucopyocele*), from the frontal sinus or a frontal ethmoid cell; it invades the surrounding sinuses and the orbit, often taking several years to produce proptosis and a down-and-outward displacement of the eye (Fig. 42-8, *B*). A cystic mass is felt above the inner canthus of the eye. The treatment is always surgical removal.

The *role of allergy* in suppurative sinus disease deserves mention. There is no question that patients with allergic rhinitis are more predisposed to acute and chronic suppurative sinusitis than nonallergic patients. Identification of the underlying allergy directs treatment beyond that of the infection alone, which will not produce resolution of the basic disease. Allergic hyposensitization is then in order. An allergic component should be suspected whenever suppurative sinusitis fails to respond to the usual measures. Generally there is a family history of extrinsic allergy or a positive history of drug or food allergy in the patient, asthma in childhood, a labile nasal airway, perennial hay fever, or merely prolonged repetitive bouts of sneezing and epiphora. Pale, boggy, or violaceous nasal mucosa is often a clue, and the presence of allergic polyps (which resemble peeled grapes) is usually diagnostic. The treatment of allergic polyps is always surgical, but prior hyposensitization is carried out if allergies are found.

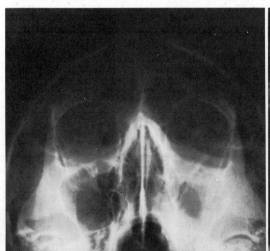
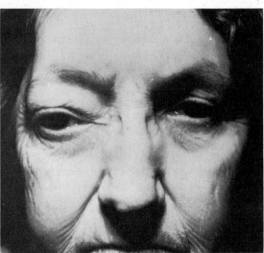

Fig. 42-8. A, Thickened lining of right maxillary antrum; this is not diagnostic of chronic sinusitis but may represent old healed disease. Only diagnostic radiographic sign of active sinusitis is air-fluid level. View roentgenograms you order; the good physician realizes that if roentgenogram is worth ordering, it is worth going to look at. **B,** Frontal mucocele; right eye is pushed down, out, and forward; cystic mass is palpable and easily visible above inner canthus of eye. This is one of complications of chronic suppurative sinusitis. Surgical intervention is indicated.

Infections of the ear

External otitis, frequently mistermed otomycosis or "fungus of the ear canal," is a suppurative infection of the skin of the ear canal. In the *acute form* it is extremely painful and produces considerable edema of the skin. It does not produce deafness unless the canal is occluded by the edematous skin or exudate. Over half the reported cases are caused by *Pseudomonas aeruginosa*, and the remainder are caused by streptococci, staphylococci or *Haemophilus influenzae*. Since it is an acute pyoderm, the treatment is the administration of topical antibiotics (not systemic antibiotics). A cotton wick is placed deeply into the ear canal and kept soaked with Burow's solution or antibiotic-cortisone eardrops. The pain is relieved in 24 to 48 hours if the cotton wick extends the entire length of the ear canal. The wick is left in place for 1 to 3 days, after which drops are continued along with meticulous periodic cleaning of the ear canal until the infection has subsided.

The *chronic form of external otitis* may have a number of causes. The most frequent is atrophy of the cerumen glands resulting in a chronically dry, pruritic canal. Other causes are seborrheic dermatitis, eczematoid dermatitis, and the end result of an untreated acute external otitis. Repeated trauma to the canal is the usual result of the pruritus. Such trauma from a finger, cotton-tipped applicator, or pin propagates the infection. The treatment is by avoidance of all trauma, careful cleaning by a physician, and long-term use of cortisone cream or ointment.

Acute suppurative otitis media is second in incidence to the nose cold. Few children escape it. It is also called *acute otitis media, middle ear abscess, acute ear, red ear,* and *bulging drum.* Signs and symptoms are those of an acute febrile infection with ear pain, which may be severe and protracted. Relief of the pain comes with either spontaneous drainage or the myringotomy knife. In the infant irritability and diarrhea may be the only symptoms; this has been termed "cholera infantum." The cause is the ascension of suppurative organisms from the nasopharynx (streptococci, pneumococci, *Haemophilus influenzae*, staphylococci, sometimes other organisms) through the eustachian tube or more probably through the peritubal lymphatics. It should be stressed here that not all "red ears" are acute suppurative middle ear infections. Distinction must be made from mere hyperemia of the membrane or tympanum, which can be caused by holding a struggling, crying child for otoscopy. Diagnosis is made by observation of a bulging, inflamed tympanic membrane, or pus in the ear canal that has recently perforated the tympanic membrane. Bulging is recognized by a diminished or absent prominence of the short process of the malleus. The eardrum changes may be obscured by the thickening and desquamation that occur in the tympanic membrane in the medial portion of the canal with acute middle ear infection, requiring cleaning of the canal.

The treatment is by myringotomy (if the drum is bulging) and appropriate antibiotic therapy for at least 10 days. The following complications of an acute suppurative otitis media are probably more important than the disease itself.

Acute mastoiditis
Acute osteomyelitis of the temporal bone
Acute petrositis
Facial nerve paralysis
Chronic nonsuppurative otitis media
Chronic suppurative otitis media
Subperiosteal abscess
Acute suppurative labyrinthitis
Acute meningitis
Sigmoid sinus thrombus
Epidural abscess
Subdural abscess
Brain abscess (cerebellar or temporal lobe)

Each of these complications poses its own diagnostic and treatment problems. The most common complication of acute suppurative otitis media, *chronic nonsuppurative otitis media*, is considered in the following paragraphs.

Chronic nonsuppurative otitis media is the most common cause of deafness in children and is conductive in type. It is of the magnitude of about 30 decibels (dB). The precise cause is not completely understood, though it follows eustachian tube obstruction and antibiotic-treated acute suppurative otitis media. Mucus-secreting glands migrate from the eustachian tube epithelium into the middle ear mucosa and produce a thick, viscid, gluelike substance. The eardrum is gray, lusterless, retracted, and immobile. A synonym for the disease is *glue ear.* Treatment includes adenoidectomy, resolution of any suppurative disease of the upper respiratory tract, eustachian tube inflations by Valsalva maneuver or politzerization (forcible insufflation of the ear into the nasal chambers), elimination of inhalant allergies, antihistaminics, and, in recalcitrant cases, temporary intubation of the tympanic membrane to give the middle ear a rest. In each case, myringotomy and aspiration of the gluelike material should accompany any other treatment.

Chronic nonsuppurative otitis media, with true secretion of mucus into the middle ear, should be differentiated from acute nonsuppurative otitis media, which is a transudation of thin amber fluid into the middle ear after acute eustachian tube obstruction. This is most commonly caused by a viral upper respiratory infection, with edema about the nasopharyngeal end of the tube. However, the physician must be aware that neoplasms of the nasopharynx usually result in a middle ear effusion, and he must carefully examine the nasopharynx of each patient with middle ear effusion.

Chronic suppurative otitis media is another sequela of acute middle ear infection. It is essentially a nonresolution of the acute infection. This is always accompanied by a perforation of the tympanic membrane and chronic, usually fetid, otorrhea. It is incumbent on the physician to distinguish a *safe* from a *dangerous* chronic suppurating ear. A "safe ear" seldom shortens anyone's life by one day; a "dangerous ear" produces the same complications that may occur after acute suppurative otitis media. The following criteria for this distinction demand careful consideration:

1. Character of the discharge
2. Site of the perforation
3. Presence of a cholesteatoma
4. Progressive unexplained hearing loss
5. Presence of bone destruction on inspection or roentgenographic examination
6. Presence of vascular pyogenic granulation tissue growing on bone
7. Positive reservoir sign
8. Positive fistula test

The *discharge* is suggestive of dangerous chronic osteomyelitis if it is highly fetid, the result of bone digestion by bacterial enzymes. Simple mucosal infection produces predominantly a mucoid discharge with no odor, or merely a musty odor from stasis and the action of saprophytic organisms.

Marginal perforation, including "attic" perforations or those in the pars flaccida, generally indicate a dangerous ear condition. Central perforations, or those in the pars tensa away from the annular region, generally indicate a nondangerous ear condition.

A *cholesteatoma (skin in the middle ear, where skin does not belong)*, is virtually diagnostic of a dangerous ear condition. Once skin enters the middle ear space, it casts off layer upon layer of desquamated epithelium, which is surrounded by the thinned-out matrix. The matrix is the surrounding layer of living skin. The cholesteatoma invades and destroys bone by two processes: enzymatic digestion in the presence of vascular pyogenic granulation tissue, and pressure necrosis by a solid ball of cholesteatoma whose center is filled with desquamated keratin debris or "squame." The cholesteatoma may enlarge slowly over many years with no symptoms except the chronic otorrhea and perhaps *increasing deafness*. Then the cholesteatoma invades one of the many vital struc-

tures surrounding the middle ear, and catastrophe follows. These vital structures are the cochlea, the vestibular labyrinth, the sigmoid sinus, the jugular bulb, the dura of the cerebellum, the dura of the temporal lobe, and the subarachnoid space. Septic retrograde thrombosis of vessels may also be induced by chronic osteomyelitic bone. The cholesteatoma is recognized by its characteristic cheesy-white, flaky content. *The presence of bone destruction on either visual inspection or x-ray examination* indicates either a destructive osteomyelitic process or an expanding cholesteatoma. *Vascular pyogenic granulation tissue growing on bone* is diagnostic of chronic osteomyelitis. The *positive reservoir sign* is the re-formation of pus a few minutes after it has been thoroughly wiped away. A *positive fistula test* is conjugate deviation of the eyes to the opposite side on compression of the air in the external auditory canal, diagnostic of a fistula through the bone over a semicircular canal, without actual suppurative invasion of the inner ear. It is then only a matter of a few days to a few weeks before suppurative invasion takes place. When this occurs, sudden irrevocable total deafness follows, together with severe and prolonged vertigo and nystagmus. A labyrinthectomy is then necessary.

Only a few of these criteria may be present in a given patient, and no single test (except the positive fistula test in a chronic draining ear) is absolutely diagnostic of a dangerous ear. Thus it becomes a matter of meticulous observation, careful interpretation, and judgment to establish this. Recognition of the dangerous state is crucial *because the impending complication may be diagnosed in advance and prevented by surgical intervention.* Recognition is the physician's responsibility.

Fascial space abscesses

Peritonsillar abscess (quinsy) is the most common fascial space abscess. The organism is usually *Streptococcus* or *Staphylococcus* and the cause is an acute or chronic tonsillitis. Pronounced edema of the tonsillar bed with fanning out of the anterior pillar over the swollen mass occurs. The uvula may be pushed across the midline. It is severely painful, causing sharp odynophagia and pain on opening the mouth. True trismus may be present. Incision and drainage is the treatment, along with antibiotic therapy. Distinction between peritonsillar abscess and peritonsillar cellulitis may be difficult. The cellulitis precedes the abscess, which takes at least 48 hours to form.

Retropharyngeal space abscesses are uncommon. They are generally seen in children, in whom an infected retropharyngeal lymph node gives rise to the infection. These nodes are usually absent in the adult. The diagnosis is made by a characteristic spongy or cystic feel to the posterior pharyngeal wall and widening of the retropharyngeal space on the lateral soft-tissue roentgenogram of the neck. The collection of pus exists between the superior constrictor muscle and the prevertebral fascia. The treatment is incision and drainage.

Pharyngomaxillary space abscess (lateral or parapharyngeal space) is an abscess in the potential space between the fascia of the parotid gland and the internal pterygoid muscle laterally, and the fascia of the superior constrictor muscle medially. In it are the carotid sheath structures and the styloid process with its muscle group. The abscess is recognized by medial displacement of the tonsil *and* lateral angle of the pharynx and brawny induration of the upper neck just below the angle of the mandible. However, bulging may be present in only one of these places. Trismus is pronounced. The treatment is external incision and drainage with antibiotic therapy.

A *masticator space abscess*, usually of dental origin, is an abscess under the periosteum of the mandible. Trismus is usually present. Ludwig's angina is a floor-of-the-mouth phlegmon and is also usually of dental origin. The patient frequently is a diabetic. The floor of the mouth is greatly swollen, and the tongue is pushed up and back, endangering the airway. Tracheotomy must be contemplated. Later, all the potential spaces of the floor of the mouth are involved, and the infection may spread down to the clavicular level. Wide incision and drainage is frequently necessary, though intensive antibiotic therapy early in the infection may suffice.

TRAUMA

Automobile accidents account for most severe maxillofacial trauma today. Although reduction and fixation of facial bone fractures may be delayed for as much as 14 days, a very careful evaluation of the patient must be carried out at the time of the injury. Other emergency conditions that require immediate attention may be developing such as airway obstruction, cervical vertebra fracture, long bone fracture, progressive intracranial or intra-abdominal injury, or soft-tissue lacerations.

Nose

The *nasal bone* is the most commonly *fractured* bone in the body. Even relatively minor nasal trauma may result in a fracture. When the patient is evaluated immediately after the trauma has occurred, the diagnosis may be obvious. Mobility of the nasal bones on palpation is diagnostic. X-ray studies may be misleading when old fractures have healed with scar tissue or when recent fractures are not demonstrated. Within a few hours after trauma the swelling about the nose may be extensive,

making a clinical evaluation extremely difficult. In such a case, treatment may be delayed for as much as 7 days to allow the swelling to subside. Because of their intimacy, both nasal bones are usually fractured. After the nose is anesthetized, a blunt instrument may be placed beneath the nasal bone on the concave side and elevated outward. The other nasal bone is then moved medially into its proper position. This position is maintained with external splinting. When the nasal fracture is allowed to heal in a deviated position, a rhinoplasty is required later to restore normal nasal contour (Fig. 42-9).

Fracture of the nasal septum sometimes occurs without nasal bone fracture. If the fractured septum is displaced significantly, it produces permanent airway obstruction. Fractures of the nasal septum are often difficult to reduce because the septum becomes dislocated off the maxillary crest. If the septum does not go easily back to the midline, nasal septal reconstruction (discussed on this page) may be required at the time of the acute fracture.

Another late sequela of untreated septal fracture is a *saddle deformity of the nose*. The middle third of the dorsum of the nose is supported by the nasal septum and not by the nasal bones. The support is lost by an inward fracture of the septum that may not be apparent immediately on external examination because a hematoma forms in its place, so that the nose retains roughly its former appearance. The "saddle" deformity then becomes apparent after resolution of the hematoma and contraction of the resulting scar tissue. Correction of this deformity requires a bone graft and rhinoplasty, a complicated procedure.

Deviation of the nasal septum may also be acquired by a differential growth pattern. Nasal septal spurs and bending of the nasal septum with encroachment of one nasal chamber are usually the result of unequal growth of the two sides of the septum. Deflection of the caudal (anteroinferior) edge of the septum into one nasal vestibule is usually traumatic. Septal deflections are important to the degree they produce airway obstruction. Significant obstructions should be treated by nasal septal reconstruction. In this operation the mucoperiosteum and mucoperichondrium of each side of the septum are elevated, and the deviated part of the cartilaginous septum is scored to allow it to straighten. Deviated bone is removed. These operations are relatively minor and often produce gratifying results. Deviated septa do not cause headaches, sinus disease, nervousness, weight loss, or the like.

Digital trauma to the nasal septum may eventually cause a septal perforation and today is its most common cause. Years ago, the most common cause was *syphilis*. A perforated nasal septum is not significant unless it produces annoying crusting and bleeding from perichondritis or chondritis at the edge of the perforation. This is treated when the cartilage and bone are cut back well beneath the mucosal covering when the perforation is covered with a silicone rubber prosthesis. Occasionally a septal perforation causes whistling in the airstream, when the perforation is of a critical size relative to the speed of the airstream. This may be resolved or the septal perforation is closed with a special surgical procedure.

Epistaxis (nosebleed)

Epistaxis is an almost invariably benign disease but frequently a trying one because it is frightening to the patient and difficult for the physician to treat.

The single most common cause of epistaxis in the adult is *hypertension*. The most common season is the late fall, when the home heating plant is turned on and the humidity drops precipitously. This dries out the inspired air, cracking or splitting the delicate respiratory mucosa. In children *digital trauma* to the anterior area of the nose promotes this cracking, as crusts build up inside the nares. The usual location of the bleeding vessel is at the anteroinferior portion of the nasal septum, where a plexus of submucosal vessels is located (Kiesselbach's plexus) in *Little's area*. The plexus is formed by the confluence of the septal branch of the sphenopalatine artery, the anterior ethmoid artery, and the perforating branch of the anterior palatine artery. Such epistaxes are termed *anterior bleeders;* they account for nine out of ten nosebleeds.

The management of *posterior epistaxis* is sometimes difficult. In addition, the patients deserve a complete work-up in search of specific causes, such as hypertension, leukemia, neoplasms of the nasal chambers and paranasal sinuses, and hemorrhagic disorders.

The first step in the management of a patient with epistaxis is to locate the bleeding vessel. The important principles are threefold: *spot lighting, spot suction,* and *spot hemostasis.* Spot lighting requires a head mirror or a head light, because overhead operating room lighting or a flashlight is totally inadequate to the task. Spot suctioning apparatus (which will reach 25 mm. Hg negative pressure with a high flow) is available in every hospital emergency room. To this should be added a (Frazier type) suction tip, which has a finger cutoff valve. All clots are aspirated from the nasal chamber with the patient in a sitting or semi-Fowler's position, and the free-flowing source of blood is located.

Anterior septal bleeders may be managed as a rule by silver nitrate bead cautery. The silver nitrate bead must be placed directly over the opening in the bleeding vessel and held in position for 10 to 15 seconds. The patient is cautioned

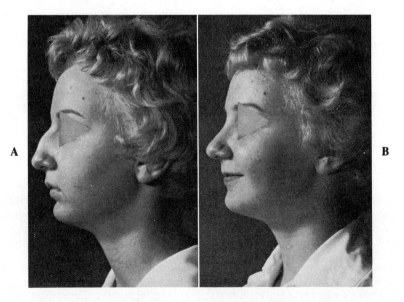

Fig. 42-9. Old nasal fracture. **A,** Unreduced. **B,** After rhinoplasty.

against straining and noseblowing for several days. Occasionally petroleum jelly gauze packing is necessary. The use of topical vasoconstrictor agents such as epinephrine on a cotton tampon must be looked on as a temporary measure in the treatment of epistaxis.

Posterior epistaxis arises from either the ethmoid arteries (a part of the internal carotid system) or from the sphenopalatine arteries (a part of the external carotid system). In the former the bleeding will be from above the level of the middle turbinate and in the latter from below the level of the middle turbinate. This distinction is of vital importance should all local methods fail and vascular ligation be necessary.

Control of posterior epistaxis is usually possible by careful packing of ½-inch strip gauze impregnated with antibiotic ointment against the bleeding site. This packing is left in place for 4 or 5 days while the patient is hospitalized for observation. When the bleeding site is too far posterior to be controlled in this manner, a posterior pack of lamb's wool or Foley catheter balloon is added to the anterior pack. Recurrent or persistent severe epistaxis usually requires ligation of the internal maxillary artery or ethmoid artery, or both. Ligation of the internal maxillary artery is usually carried out following a transantral route, with removal of the anterior and posterior walls of the maxillary sinus to gain access to the artery.

Facial bones

Fractures of the middle third of the face involving the maxilla have been conveniently classified by LeFort (Fig. 42-10). Type I is a fracture involving the alveolar ridges or palate, and the bodies of the maxillary bones are intact. Type II involves the medial portion of the middle third of the face, with the fracture line crossing the zygomaticomaxillary suture lines, so that grasping the incisor teeth allows motion of the entire middle third of the face and not just the palatal portion. Type III is termed a craniofacial separation, with the fracture line on almost a horizontal plane, separating the maxillary and zygomatic bones from the rest of the skull. *Proper treatment is very important because occlusion of the teeth is involved as well as cosmetic appearance.* Improper treatment results in malocclusion of varying types and degrees. If the molar teeth come together before the incisor teeth, biting through food with the front teeth is impossible. Arch bars are wired to the maxillary and mandib-

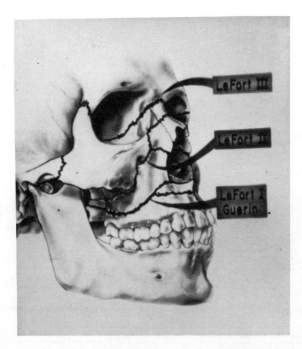

Fig. 42-10. Mid-third (maxillary) fractures of face tend to occur along certain lines and may be classified. LeFort classification is pictured here. LeFort III is craniofacial separation, LeFort II is pyramid-shaped fracture, and LeFort I is palatal separation.

ular teeth and then joined together with intermaxillary wires, so that the teeth are locked together in the natural occlusal relationship. The middle third of the face is stabilized when the arch bars are snugged up to the base of the skull with suspension wires circling the arches of the zygoma or passed subcutaneously through drill holes in the lateral orbital rims.

The supraorbital ridge, being very thick, is fractured only by a heavy blow. The infraorbital rim, however, is formed by thin bone and may be fractured by a relatively minor blow. A blow to the orbit may generate tremendous elevations of intraorbital pressure and result in a "blowing out" of the thin, bony orbital floor with herniation of orbital contents into the maxillary sinus below. Such an injury may result in enophthalmos, a depressed interpupillary line, and limitation of upward gaze in the affected eye (Fig. 42-11). Failure to recognize this fracture may result in permanent enophthalmos and diplopia. Treatment consists in retrieving the herniated tissue and restoring the integrity of the orbital floor.

Fractures of the zygoma occur from a direct blow high over the cheek. A crushing blow may fracture the arch of the zygoma to produce cos-metic deformity. The *tripodal fracture* involves the zygomaticofrontal suture, the zygomaticomaxillary suture, and the arch, resulting in a depression of the malar eminence. This fracture usually requires open reduction and fixation to assure a good cosmetic result.

Mandibular fractures are important for the same reason that maxillary fractures are important: faulty treatment will produce nutritionally crippling malocclusion. The most common types are *subcondylar,* which results in trismus; *ramus,* with displacement of the fracture ends produced by different muscle pulls exerted on the fragments; *body,* usually across the mental foramen; and *symphyseal.* Treatment is usually accomplished with simple closed reduction and stabilization with intermaxillary fixation. Occasionally, open reduction with fixation of the fragments is necessary.

Fractures of the frontal sinus are important to recognize in order to avoid the late sequelae of *cosmetic deformity, obstruction of the nasofrontal duct* (with ultimate production of a mucocele of the frontal sinus), and *cerebrospinal fluid leak* from a fracture tear of the posterior wall to which dura is firmly attached. An unrecognized cerebrospinal fluid leak may result in repeated meningitis,

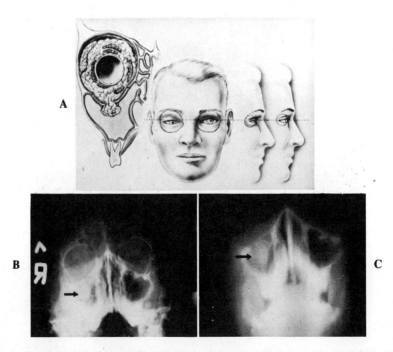

Fig. 42-11. Blowout fracture of orbit. Sharp blow to soft tissues of eye may fracture thin floor of orbit and allow orbital contents to drop into antrum, **A,** Eye is thus dropped, becomes enophthalmic, and upward-following gaze is lost. This is permanent unless recognized and treated. Water's view of sinuses can be very helpful, **B,** but sometimes laminagram, **C,** is necessary.

months or years apart. Open reduction is usually necessary.

Temporal bone

Temporal bone fractures are the result of severe head injury, with the fracture line extending through the base of the skull, of which the temporal bone is a part. Hemorrhage from the ear canal or cerebrospinal fluid otorrhea is frequent, though not invariable. If there has not been a direct blow to the soft tissue over the mastoid, a bruise in this area is diagnostic (Battle's sign).

Temporal bone fractures are of two types. *Transverse temporal bone fractures* occur across the internal auditory canal and inner ear, producing immediate total deafness, labyrinthine vertigo and nystagmus, and frequently a facial nerve paralysis. *Longitudinal temporal bone fractures* cross the posterosuperior canal wall, middle ear, and eustachian tube, producing conductive deafness. A facial paralysis in this type is less common. Immediate facial nerve paralysis indicates severance of the nerve, which should be repaired as soon as the patient's general condition permits. A delayed facial nerve paralysis usually will resolve spontaneously.

Larynx

Laryngeal fractures are extremely important to recognize and treat early to avoid loss of the important faculties of speech and normal breathing. *In any patient with a neck injury, particularly an anterior blow to the neck, the symptoms of hoarseness or dyspnea demand immediate laryngoscopy.* Because progressive swelling continues for several hours after injury, airway symptoms that are very mild on admission to an emergency room may suddenly become severe and life threatening. Therefore, any patient with even mild airway symptoms must be carefully monitored for evidence of progression and treated with endotracheal intubation or tracheostomy should progression occur.

Within a week or 10 days of injury the diameters of the larynx can be reconstituted to restore normal speech and breathing. After this time, consequent scarring may require repeated operations on the larynx before the tracheotomy tube can be removed or may even sentence the patient to a permanent tracheostoma. The preceding points are of extreme importance and should be firmly in the mind of every physician attending an emergency room or treating acutely traumatized patients.

Frostbite

Cold injuries to the head and neck most frequently involve the external ear and the tip of the nose. The old maxim that a frozen member should be rubbed with snow is false. This results only in needless trauma to already damaged tissue. Cold, or frostbite, produces its injury by infarction and through cellular rupture by large ice crystals that form when tissue is slowly cooled below the crystallization point. Some tissue loss is then inevitable, but frequently this need be only the outer layers of the skin.

There is no uniformly successful method of treating frostbite, but it is generally agreed that the frozen tissue should be thawed reasonably rapidly. Further injury to the tissue should be avoided by immobility. Anticoagulation is not widely accepted. The skin should be protected against drying, fissuring, and the development of superficial infection by the application first of petrolatum jelly, and later antibiotic ointments if necessary.

NEOPLASMS
Face

Basal cell carcinoma (rodent ulcer) is the most common neoplasm of the skin of the face. The lesion begins as a roughened area that ulcerates and fails to heal, classically above a line drawn from the tragus of the ear to the nasal ala. Farmers, because of their high exposure to actinic radiation, are prone to develop this lesion, as well as other skin neoplasms in exposed areas. Basal cell carcinomas rarely metastasize but continue to enlarge and destroy anything in their path until properly treated. The treatment is adequate excision, with closure of the excision site within skin lines to obtain optimal cosmetic results, especially for small lesions. When large basal cell carcinomas are excised, some type of skin flap is required for coverage. Excellent results are also obtainable by radiation therapy given in cancericidal doses, which usually means at least several weeks of daily treatments. Dermatologists frequently prefer to treat by electrodesiccation and curettage, or chemosurgery.

Epidermoid (squamous cell) carcinoma occurs anywhere on the face, including the lips, nose, lids, and external ear. Classically, the ulcerated lesion has a rolled, pearly border. The indurated border represents infiltration of adjacent normal tissue. In contrast to basal cell carcinoma, epidermoid carcinoma can metastasize. The nodes first involved are the submaxillary or submental nodes and then the deep cervical nodes, or the deep cervical nodes alone. Treatment is by adequate excision of the primary lesion, which must include 1 cm. of normal tissue around its borders. Radiation therapy is also effective, but higher doses are necessary than in the basal cell carcinoma. When lymph nodes are involved, a radical neck dissection is necessary.

Carcinomas of the lids, lips, or external ear pose special problems in treatment and are best treated by a specialist. Where cartilage is immediately subjacent, as in the ear or nasal ala, special handling is required to prevent chondritis, whether treated surgically or by irradiation. Immediate reconstruction is necessary if the ear, eye, or nose is removed or is grossly deformed. Eyelid lesions must be managed with special care to avoid entropion, ectropion, and exposed cornea, which may lead to corneal damage and blindness. Lip lesions are treated by wedge resection or vermilionectomy. If the wedge is large, a plastic reconstructive procedure must be performed to supplant the tissue sacrificed so that a tight lip that limits speech and feeding does not ensue.

The *differential diagnosis* of facial skin cancer includes senile keratoses, seborrheic keratoses, nevi, and the keratoacanthoma. The last is an ulcerating reactive lesion of the skin that closely resembles cancer but is a self-limiting disease.

Mouth and oropharynx

Epidermoid (squamous cell) carcinoma is by far the most common neoplasm of the mouth and oropharynx. This lesion occurs most commonly in the tongue, floor of the mouth (Fig. 42-12), buccal mucosa, and tonsil but may involve the palate, alveolar ridges, mucosa of the jaws, uvula, and oropharyngeal walls. Treatment is simple excision to include an area 1 cm. around the periphery or radiation therapy if the lesion is 2 cm. or smaller in size. A wedge resection is performed if the primary lesion involves the tongue. Tonsillar lesions are treated differently because of their propensity for

early metastasis; small lesions are treated by irradiation, but those larger than 2 cm. have usually metastasized and require neck dissection for cure. The involved cervical lymph nodes may be impalpable (subclinical metastases). Epidermoid carcinomas of the mouth and oropharynx that are larger than 2 cm. in diameter require a large operation. Combination therapy is frequently used, including radiation therapy in a submaximal dose and surgical resection of the primary lesion with in-continuity radical neck dissection. Resection of the primary lesion frequently requires partial mandibulectomy, partial glossectomy, or pharyngectomy. Reconstruction of the surgical defect is begun immediately to provide early functional and cosmetic rehabilitation. Five-year survival may approach 75% in small lesions located anteriorly in the mouth, whereas large lesions posteriorly with regional lymph node metastasis represent 25% or less 5-year survival.

Adenocarcinomas also occur in the mouth and oropharynx that are identical to those of the major salivary glands, because they arise in one of the many minor salivary glands in the region. They may be of many types. (See the discussion of salivary glands on p. 646.) Thus mixed salivary gland tumors may occur on the palate, tonsillar pillars, or lateral angle of the pharynx. Treatment is always surgical because adenocarcinomas generally are not radiosensitive. The prognosis for these lesions is less favorable than for epidermoid carcinomas.

Connective tissue tumors are not unusual in this

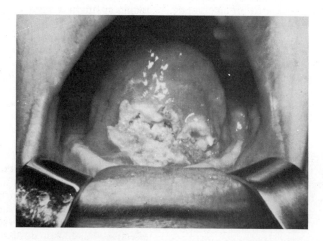

Fig. 42-12. Epidermoid carcinoma of floor of mouth. Notice its exophytic character and purulent membrane over entire ulcerated surface. Indurated lesions with ulceration anywhere in mouth demand biopsy.

area. The most common are lymphomas that occur in tonsillar tissue. There may be connective tissue tumors of the bones of the jaws, such as osteogenic sarcoma, fibrosarcoma, and giant cell tumor of bone. Muscle tumors such as rhabdomyosarcoma occur here, as well as neoplasms of other connective tissue elements, e.g., myxomas, fibromas, lipomas, and hemangiomas (Fig. 42-13).

Tumors of dental origin appear as expansile lesions widening the alveolar ridge or the body of the mandible, or, less commonly, the upper jaw. The only common neoplasm of this type is the adamantoma (ameloblastoma), a neoplasm of the enamel organ of the developing tooth. This is a benign tumor, cured by adequate simple excision. A dentigerous cyst is not a neoplasm, but it requires simple excision because it can be distinguished from an adamantoma only by histological examination.

Leukoplakia (white plaque) occurs wherever there is moist, stratified squamous, nonkeratinizing or respiratory epithelium. It appears as a thin, whitish plaque, most commonly in areas subject to chronic irritation, and can be identified in almost any denture-wearing patient. It is also very common on the buccal mucosa, lips, mucosa over the ascending ramus of the mandible, floor of the mouth, tongue and palate. It occasionally takes on a lacy pattern and may resemble lichen planus. Histologically, there may be any degree of abnormality from hyperkeratosis to invasive carcinoma.

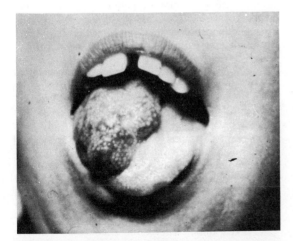

Fig. 42-13. Hemangioma of tongue. This lesion is common in upper digestive tract. Lesion is characteristically deep blue and empties and refills slowly on application and release of pressure. Varices on undersurface of tongue should be readily distinguishable from them and do not require treatment.

Not all leukoplakia requires treatment, but it must be observed periodically. If the lesion becomes thickened and palpable, this condition may indicate premalignant change, or if punctate ulceration occurs, excision must be carried out. If the area of leukoplakia is large, it may be excised in stages, or cryotherapy may be considered. Ordinarily, radiation therapy is not utilized unless there is evidence of malignant change.

The *differential diagnosis* of oral cancer includes the *epulides, chronic specific granulomas,* and *trauma* from ill-fitting dentures or jagged teeth. Giant cells epulis is not a neoplasm but a reactive phenomenon, found most frequently on the alveolar ridges. It is caused by trauma or great alterations in hormonal levels, as in pregnancy. Chronic specific granulomas masquerading as neoplasms include *tuberculosis* (rare), *Vincent's angina, histoplasmosis* (Fig. 42-14), *actinomycosis, syphilis,* and *lethal midline granuloma* perforating the hard palate. The *brown hairy tongue* (Fig. 42-15), a peculiar biological phenomenon that is poorly understood, should not be mistaken for a neoplasm. It is common in the chronically ill patient but also is seen in a healthy person. Brown hairy tongue is essentially hypertrophy of filiform papillae, with proliferating chromogen bacteria deeply embedded between the papillae. The treatment consists in repeatedly trimming the hypertrophied material with sharp dissection.

Early biopsy of lesions of the mouth and oropharynx is essential to cure. Once the lesion becomes larger than 1 cm., the cure rates drop precipitously. The prudent physician biopsies any suspicious lesion in this area. Practically no harm can be done, as functional or cosmetic losses from mouth or oropharyngeal biopsy are virtually negligible, but a positive biopsy of a small lesion will yield high dividends for the patient. Retain a high index of suspicion. The physician should never feel chagrined at a negative biopsy.

Nasopharynx

Cancer of the nasopharynx is common, especially in people of Oriental extraction. *Epidermoid carcinoma* and *lymphoepithelioma* of the nasopharynx are most insidious neoplasms, for in the majority of patients the first symptom is hearing loss from a middle ear effusion. Symptoms that may follow are presence of a firm mass in the neck, odynophagia, epistaxis, or blood-streaked oral secretions. Any patient with a middle ear effusion or a hard mass in the neck must have a thorough examination of the nasopharynx before treatment is instituted. The treatment of the primary nasopharyngeal carcinoma is radiation therapy. Once the primary tumor is controlled, neck dissection is

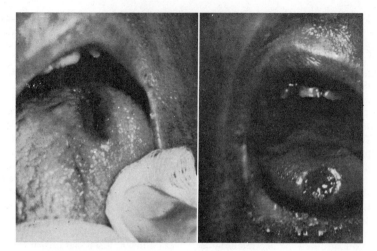

Fig. 42-14. Histoplasmosis of tongue. Notice sharp margination of ulceration and lack of exophytic response. This probably occurs by primary inoculation from chronic weed chewing. It is easy to confuse this or any other chronic specific granuloma with malignancy.

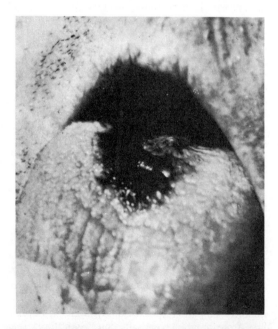

Fig. 42-15. Brown hairy tongue. This is not a disease per se but is often a great concern to patient. It is a frequent accompaniment of chronic disease state. Chromogen bacteria growing between greatly elongated filiform papillae produce picture. Treatment is by "tongue shave."

performed if the cervical nodes are involved.

Connective tissue neoplasms of the malignant variety, including reticulum cell sarcoma, lymphosarcoma, and giant follicular lymphoma, may also occur in this area. Liposarcoma and fibrosarcoma are rare neoplasms of the nasopharynx.

Benign tumors of the nasopharynx include the juvenile nasopharyngeal angiofibroma. This is a highly vascular tumor of young boys that is believed to arise in cartilaginous rests of sphenoid ossification centers. Its symptoms are nasal obstruction and epistaxis. The tumor can be diagnosed by mirror examination of the nasopharynx. The tumor contains a great many dilated blood spaces unlined with smooth muscle, and even biopsy may provoke profuse bleeding. Although it does not metastasize, it erodes the base of the skull. The treatment is by excision, usually with preoperative vascular embolization. The operation is extremely difficult and attended with much blood loss. *Craniopharyngioma* is a tumor arising from the embryonic Rathke's pouch. Most of these neoplasms are intracranial, but if the stalk of Rathke's pouch is persistent and becomes entrapped in the sphenoid bone, a sphenoid or nasopharyngeal tumor will result. This is also a benign tumor that is dangerous because of its position; an aid to diagnosis is calcification of the embryonic notochord. Chordomas occur most frequently in the body of the sphenoid bone and in the sacrum. Contents of the tumors are usually gelatinous; thus the tumor may be thought to be merely a cyst.

However, unless excision of the entire capsule is accomplished, it will recur.

Differential diagnosis. The differential diagnosis of tumors in this area includes *chronic sphenoiditis, sphenoid mucocele, mucus-retention cyst of nasopharyngeal mucosa, Tornwaldt's bursa,* and *chronic adenoiditis.*

Larynx and hypopharynx

Epidermoid carcinoma of the larynx afflicts men more commonly than women, in a ratio of about 10:1. One classification of neoplasms of the larynx is by location and divides into (1) glottic, including the entire true cord, (2) supraglottic, including the false vocal cord, aryepiglottic folds, epiglottis, and valleculae, and (3) subglottic, involving the conus elasticus and upper trachea. Cancer of the true cord has a good prognosis, ranking second only to epidermoid carcinoma of the skin in curability. The overall cure rate of carcinoma of the larynx is about 80%.

Carcinomas of the true cord are highly curable for two reasons: (1) symptoms (hoarseness, excessive throat clearing) annoy the patient enough to prompt an early visit to the physician, and (2) there is a paucity of lymphatics in the true cord so that metastases are rare. The 5-year cure rate of carcinomas of the true cord is between 80% and 90%. Treatment is by radiation therapy if cord mobility is unimpaired and the lesion extends to neither end of the cord; hemilaryngectomy is preferred if the lesion does extend to either end of the true cord. Because lesions of this area are so amenable to cure and so readily visible, *any patient with hoarseness of 2 weeks' duration or longer must have examination of his larynx.*

Larger glottic or supraglottic lesions without vocal cord fixation may be treated with a partial laryngectomy. These patients retain a serviceable voice with survival rates equal to those with total laryngectomy. Even larger lesions require total laryngectomy and radical neck dissection. The patient must learn esophageal speech to gain full speech rehabilitation. Five-year survival is approximately 70%.

Epidermoid carcinoma of the laryngopharynx involves the lateral pharyngeal wall, posterior pharyngeal wall, or piriform sinus. Carcinomas that arise in the introitus of the esophagus are referred to as postcricoid lesions. These lesions are more common in women than in men. Dysphagia is the first symptom, and loss of laryngeal crepitus is the most outstanding finding on examination. Laryngeal crepitus is that crackling sensation obtained when one pushes the larynx side to side over the cervical vertebrae. Barium swallow is indicated, and esophagoscopy confirms the diagnosis.

The treatment is by partial or total laryngopharyngectomy and radical neck dissection followed by irradiation to 6000 rads. Five-year survival is approximately 50%.

Differential diagnosis. *Leukoplakia* occurs on the true vocal cords and may be indistinguishable from carcinoma in situ or early invasive carcinoma. *Speaker's nodules* occur at the junction of the anterior and middle thirds of the vocal cords in patients who use their voices excessively. The nodules may be pinhead in size, or polypoid and ulcerated, resembling a neoplasm. *Laryngocele* is a progressive enlargement of a noncommunicating portion of the laryngeal ventricle, producing a laryngeal cyst. Initially the laryngocele is internal, encroaching on the airway, and then it dissects up over the thyroid cartilage and externalizes as a neck mass. Laminagrams of the larynx are helpful in diagnosis of laryngocele. *Retention cysts* ordinarily present no problems in diagnosis because of their typical smooth, yellow-domed appearance. They are most common in the valleculae and on the aryepiglottic folds. The *chronic specific granulomas (syphilis, tuberculosis, actinomycosis,* and *lethal midline granuloma)* may present an identical appearance to cancer and require biopsy for distinction.

Nose and paranasal sinuses

Epidermal carcinoma is relatively rare in the nasal chamber but is common in the antrum and the ethmoid sinus. Unfortunately, the cure rate of this lesion is low because it does not produce significant symptoms until it has reached a large size. Ordinarily an antral carcinoma is not diagnosed or even suspected until it has eroded through one of its bony walls. Any of its walls may be eroded, with the symptoms depending on which wall is involved. When the anterior wall is involved, the symptoms are a fullness in the cheek, a mass, and a numbness of the infraorbital region caused by infiltration of that nerve. Involvement of the inferior wall produces loosening or extrusion of teeth, widening of the alveolar ridge producing a poorly fitting denture, and a mass on the palate. Erosion of the medial wall produces blood-tinged nasal secretions and nasal airway obstruction. Erosion of the superior wall produces infraorbital nerve paresthesias and paralysis, proptosis, and interference with extraocular muscles. Bone destruction is present on appropriate x-ray examination. The treatment is a combination of radiation therapy and maxillectomy, which usually means sacrifice of that side of the hard palate. The patient can be rehabilitated in speech and chewing by the placement of an oral prosthesis that contains teeth.

Adenocystic carcinoma (adenoid cystic carcinoma, pseudoadenomatous basal cell carcinoma, cylindroma) is the most common adenocarcinoma of the region. This may involve any of the paranasal sinuses or the nasal chamber. It is an extremely lethal neoplasm, somewhat sensitive to radiation therapy but generally treated by surgical means. Other adenocarcinomas may occur here, arising in minor salivary glands, and the types are as listed in the discussion of salivary glands on this page.

Solitary myeloma of the respiratory tract (extramedullary myeloma) occurs in the ethmoid sinus or nasal chamber and produces symptoms of epistaxis and airway obstruction. It may exist as a solitary myeloma for many years, but frequently evidence of disseminated myeloma follows shortly. The treatment is by excision or radiation therapy. Fibrosarcoma is another malignant connective tissue neoplasm occasionally arising in this general area.

Olfactory neuroepithelioma (esthesioneuroblastoma) has been described only relatively recently. It is believed to arise from the neural elements of the olfactory epithelium. It is of relatively low-grade malignancy in most patients, though it may metastasize, and it is certainly malignant by position. There appears to be some radiosensitivity to this lesion. The treatment consists of wide surgical excision.

Osteoma is the most common benign tumor of connective tissue origin that arises in the nasal and paranasal cavities. Osteoma usually involves the frontal sinus; it tends to grow slowly but may become very large. Excision must be carried out, especially if it arises adjacent to the nasofrontal duct or threatens to erode the inner wall of the sinus and the dura. *Ossifying fibroma* is one of the bony dysplasias that is not a true neoplasm but tends to act like one. The ethmoid sinus is the most common location, roentgenographic examination is diagnostic, and treatment is excision by external approach. *Giant cell tumor of bone* may affect any age group, is of generally low-grade malignancy, and may be treated either by surgical excision or by irradiation.

Differential diagnosis. *Chronic vestibulitis* of the eczematoid variety is distinguished with difficulty from skin cancer of the nasal vestibule. When seen in a localized area of the nasal vestibule, or particularly when a brief trial of treatment fails, biopsy is mandatory. *Nasal polyposis* of the hyperplastic or allergic types should present no difficulty in distinction from cancer, since a nasal polyp has a striking resemblance to a peeled grape, and the surface epithelium is always intact. Beefy red polyps associated with chronic sinusitis are a different matter, demanding prompt biopsy to rule out neoplasm. The presence of pus with inflammatory polyps does not exclude polypoid nasal malignancy because neoplasms of the nose alter nasal physiology, and infection is the rule. *Nasal glioma*, representing heterotopic glial tissue, may be present anywhere in the nasal chamber and is overlain by normal skin or mucosa. *Meningocele* or *meningoencephalocele* should always be considered when a smooth nonulcerated mass is present in a nasal chamber. Pulsation of the mass is suggestive of meningocele and precludes biopsy. The chronic specific granulomas include *lethal midline granuloma, sarcoidosis, actinomycosis,* and *syphilis. Rhinoscleroma* and *rhinosporidiosis* are rare in this country.

Salivary glands

Classification
1. Benign
   a. Mixed salivary gland tumor
   b. Benign mucoepidermoid tumor
   c. Adenoma
      (1) Papillary cystadenoma lymphomatosum (Warthin's tumor)
      (2) Serous cell adenoma
      (3) Acidophilic cell adenoma
2. Malignant
   a. Epidermoid carcinoma (well and poorly differentiated, including lymphoepithelioma)
   b. Mucoepidermoid carcinoma
   c. Adenocarcinoma
      (1) Adenocystic carcinoma
      (2) Acinic (serous) carcinoma
      (3) Acidophilic (oxyphilic) cell carcinoma
   d. Unclassified salivary gland carcinoma

Connective tissue tumors also occur in salivary glands, though they are relatively rare. They include neurofibromas, fibromas, and neurofibrosarcomas. Salivary glands may also be the site of infiltration by lymphomas.

The physician should be aware of the relative frequency of malignant tumors found in various salivary glands. In the parotid gland approximately 25% of neoplasms are malignant; in the submandibular gland approximately 50% are malignant; and in the minor salivary glands approximately 70% are malignant.

About 60% of all salivary gland tumors are the so-called *mixed salivary gland tumor (pleomorphic adenoma),* which is almost always benign (Fig. 42-16). It acquired its name by virtue of an apparent mixture of two germ cell layers in its histological pattern: nests, cords, and sheets of epithelial cells interspersed by a myxomatous stroma that sometimes condenses into pseudocartilage. It is characteristically a slowly growing, firm, freely mobile mass most commonly found in the tail of the parotid gland. When it is less than 2 cm. in diameter, it may feel so mobile and superficial that the physician is tempted to remove it in the office. *This is always a mistake.* Adequate treatment for a mixed salivary gland tumor is lateral lobectomy. In our experience nothing short of this carries any assurance against recurrence. The mixed salivary gland tumor is notorious for its ability to produce seedling recurrences. This fre-

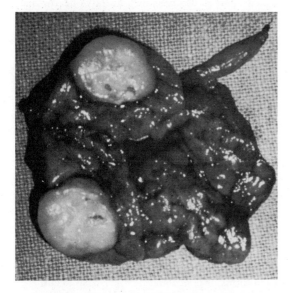

Fig. 42-16. Mixed salivary gland tumor involving submaxillary salivary gland. This particular neoplasm is much more common in parotid gland and may also occur in minor salivary glands of mouth and throat, particularly around palatine tonsil.

quently happens when the tumor capsule is broken at the time of removal, or the tumor is simply shelled out.

Warthin's tumor is characteristically soft and almost cystic and occurs in the tail of the parotid gland, usually in old men. It may be bilateral. Simple excision effects a cure.

The distinction between a benign and a malignant salivary gland tumor is frequently a very difficult one. The surgeon is caught between Scylla and Charybdis: he does not want to biopsy a mass lest it be a mixed tumor, and yet he wants to go to the operating room prepared for whatever radical operation is necessary. Therefore it is wise to perform total parotidectomy for any parotid tumor. The only characteristic clinical feature of a malignant parotid tumor is a branch paralysis or total paralysis of the facial nerve. Benign tumors reach tremendous size without producing any paralysis of the facial nerve. Other characteristics of malignant tumors are fixation, pain, and tenderness (Fig. 42-17). However, benign tumors may be tender or painful as well, if recent hemorrhage into the tumor produces capsular stretch. If either one of these features is present, the surgeon should assume malignancy and make appropriate preparations. The facial nerve is not sacrificed at operation unless it is involved by tumor, in which event it is immediately grafted, using a sensory nerve as donor (Fig. 42-18).

Epidermoid carcinoma is the single most common malignant tumor of salivary glands, but the adenocarcinomas as a group are more common than the epidermoid carcinoma. *Adenocystic carcinoma* is highly lethal, tending to metastasize early in regional lymphatics and to lung. *Mucoepi-*

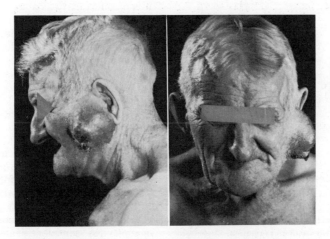

Fig. 42-17. Large, ulcerating adenocarcinoma of parotid gland.

dermoid carcinoma is rare. Rarer still is *acidophilic cell adenocarcinoma,* which is believed to arise from ductal epithelium and is a tumor of old men. *Acinic cell adenocarcinoma* is the second most common of the adenocarcinoma group, occurring in females predominantly, and it tends to act more like a sarcoma than a carcinoma in that it metastasizes through the bloodstream.

Differential diagnosis. *Salivary gland calculi* may mimic neoplasm by obstruction of salivary flow, but usually there is a clear history of fluctuation in the size of the gland. *Mikulicz's disease* and *Sjögren's syndrome* may resemble neoplasms, but they are diffuse diseases of the gland rather than localized; biopsy may be necessary to rule out cancer, and this is permissible in diffuse diseases of the salivary glands. A *high cervical lymph node* may be mistaken for a tumor in the tail of the parotid gland. If the mass can be brought out over the body or ramus of the mandible, it is a parotid gland mass rather than a cervical chain lymph node. A *hypertrophied masseter* or a *wing mandible* may be confused with a diseased parotid gland.

HEARING LOSSES AND MICROSURGERY OF THE EAR
Sensorineural hearing loss

Sensorineural deafness (sensory—hair cells of the organ of Corti; neural—eighth nerve or above this level in the central nervous system) is often called "nerve" deafness or perceptive deafness. It is the most common form of deafness. Here are some causes:

1. Congenital
2. Traumatic
3. Toxic
4. Vascular
5. Infection
6. Neoplasm
7. Ménière's disease
8. Degenerative

Congenital sensorineural deafness is usually very severe. As a rule it is bilateral, and so serious that the patient can hear only the loudest of sounds and, of these, only low tones. Such a person will never develop normal speech and needs training in special schools all during his early years. Congenital deafness may be attributable to Rh incompatibilities, birth trauma, in utero virus infection, malformation of the inner ears, or other causes. Mild forms of congenital deafness also occur.

Traumatic sensorineural deafnesses are of three kinds: noise-induced deafness, otic concussion, and transverse temporal bone fracture. The most commin is *noise-induced deafness,* often called acoustic trauma, which results from an accumulation of the effects of intense sound over months or years. This is becoming more and more prevalent. It is manifest early as a selective 4,906 hertz (Hz.) dip on the audiogram, not impairing speech reception. *Otic concussion* produces a high-tone deafness and is the result of either cerebral concussion or the convergence of lines of force through the skull, which center on the temporal bone. *Transverse temporal bone fracture* (see p. 641) causes a total inner ear deafness.

Toxic deafness in the United States is generally caused by drugs, the most common of which are aspirin, streptomycin, and kanamycin. This is a direct effect of the drug on the hair cell.

Vascular deafness is the result of occlusion of the end artery to the labyrinth and produces total deafness together with loss of vestibular function. It is sometimes called "otic apoplexy."

Viral infection, the most common of which is the mumps virus, can cause deafness. Fortunately, this almost always spares one ear. It is quite common in

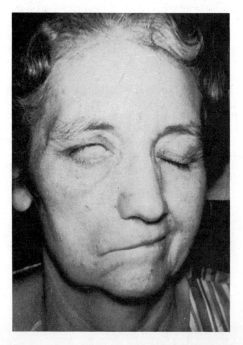

Fig. 42-18. Right complete peripheral facial paralysis with pronounced "Bell's phenomenon." This may be attributable to lesion anywhere along course of facial nerve trunk: internal auditory canal, middle ear, mastoid, or parotid gland. If cause is not determinable on complete work-up, diagnosis is Bell's palsy. This patient has just had parotid malignancy removed and facial nerve grafted. Facial motion will return in 9 to 12 months.

children and may not be discovered until adult life or on a routine school audiometric program. Loss of hearing in one ear produces the inability to localize sound and the loss of stereo effect of hearing, preventing the person from separating one voice from another when there are multiple conversations in the room; this is sometimes called the "cocktail party effect" of binaural hearing. Bacterial infection from meningitis or from chronic mastoiditis can invade the inner ear and produce immediate total deafness and loss of vestibular function.

Neoplasms that begin in the middle ear, the mastoid, or the auditory nerve produce deafness by growth and infiltration. Of these, the most common are acoustic neuroma, glomus jugulare tumor, and epidermoid carcinoma.

Ménière's disease is listed separately because we do not know whether it is caused by vascular, toxic, or metabolic factors. It is a pure hair cell deafness and as such is accompanied by a severe discrimination loss and *recruitment* (the abnormal growth of loudness in a deafened ear). The deafness fluctuates. The disease is characterized by tinnitus and vertigo, the spells lasting 20 minutes to many hours. The treatment is diuretics, vasodilators, and a low-sodium diet. Generally only one ear is affected. If treatment fails, destruction labyrinthotomy may be necessary.

Degenerative sensorineural deafness is called *presbycusis.* It is the result of gradual loss of hair cells or first-order neurons, or both, because of the aging process. This strikes virtually all people and begins in the very high tones. It goes on all through life, but only in the middle-aged or older patient does it produce noticeable deafness by finally involving the upper and then the middle speech frequencies. Even a person 20 years of age does not have as extensive high tone hearing as a younger person. There is no treatment for presbycusis. All the preceding causes of deafness tend to be additive to degenerative deafness, so that presbycusis may occur in such patients at an earlier age than otherwise.

Conductive hearing loss

A *conductive deafness* is any form of deafness that tends to impede sound from reaching the sensorineural apparatus. There are many causes, the most common of which are the following:

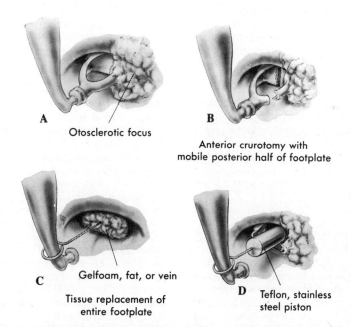

A Otosclerotic focus

B Anterior crurotomy with mobile posterior half of footplate

C Gelfoam, fat, or vein
Tissue replacement of entire footplate

D Teflon, stainless steel piston

Fig. 42-19. Various methods of handling otosclerotic deafness. **A,** Focus of spongiotic bone is visible at anterior portion of footplate binding stapes in oval window. **B,** Anterior crurotomy has been done. Footplate is fractured behind otosclerotic focus, and posterior assembly is mobile. **C,** Entire stapes has been removed; footplate is replaced with tissue graft or Gelfoam and crura with stainless steel wire; knot holding tissue graft is buried in it. **D,** Teflon piston secured by wire around incus replaces central portion of footplate.

1. Chronic nonsuppurative otitis media
2. Chronic suppurative otitis media
3. Canal problems, including congenital atresia and stenosis
4. Perforation of the tympanic membrane
5. Ossicular destruction or fixation, including otosclerosis
6. Trauma

Chronic nonsuppurative otitis media and *chronic suppurative otitis media* have been discussed on pp. 635 and 636. *Canal problems* that produce deafness do so by complete blockage of the canal. If even a very small passageway remains for air to reach the tympanic membrane, hearing is unaffected. Wax impactions and acute external otitis are the most common in this category. Other causes are osteomas of the canal, neoplasms of the skin of the canal, neoplasms about the ear such as neurofibromatosis, and congenital atresia, either occurring singly or as a part of a more general anomaly such as Treacher-Collins syndrome. A *perforation* of the tympanic membrane from unresolved middle ear infection or trauma produces a conductive deafness by virtue of loss of the sound-gathering ability of the tympanic membrane. *Clinical otosclerosis* is a disease of young adults caused by ankylosis of the stapes by an overgrowth of spongiotic bone from the enchondral layer of the otic capsule. It is slowly progressive, and a history of repeated earaches or otorrhea is absent. There is usually a positive family history. It is slightly more common in females than in males. A normal tympanic membrane is compatible with this diagnosis. The deafness is frequently purely conductive, though there may be a mild to moderate sensorineural deafness superimposed. This form of deafness can usually be helped by an operation (Fig. 42-19). *Traumatic deafness* can be caused by a bursting of the tympanic membrane that has failed to heal, a dislocation of the ossicles in the middle ear, or a temporal bone fracture of a longitudinal nature.

Hearing testing

The *decibel* (dB.) is the measure used to describe degrees of hearing loss. It is important to note that the decibel is not a unit of measurement but a ratio. Hearing loss is expressed logarithmically, because the ear is able to work over a great expanse of energy input. The decibel is a logarithmic ratio between an observed sound pressure level and a reference level. For every increase in sound of 6 dB., there is a doubling of sound pressure.

The *audiogram* indicates hearing levels at thresholds over a frequency range of 125 to 8,000 hertz (Hz.). Across the ordinate of the audiogram, the threshold of hearing from 0 to 100 dB. loss is indicated at that frequency. One also measures hearing thresholds at each of the speech frequencies (250, 500, 1,000, 2,000 Hz.) by bone conduction, placing a transducer over the mastoid bone and stimulating the sensorineural receptor apparatus directly rather than through the ossicular chain and tympanic membrane.

With use of the audiometer, *discrimination testing* can be performed. This is a test of how clearly words are understood by the ear. The volume is raised 40 dB. above the threshold of hearing, and the number of phonetically balanced words the patient can understand is recorded. The normal ear can understand at least 80% of these words. When discrimination ability is definitely impaired, it indicates a sensory or a neural deafness. Conductive deafnesses do not impair word discrimination ability.

Tuning fork tests are important in the identification of hearing loss. The tuning forks most useful are the 512 and 1,024 Hz. and frequently the 256 and 2,048 Hz. The *Rinne test* is performed when one places the stem of the fork sounded above threshold first over the mastoid bone just behind and above the external canal and then over the external canal an inch away from the ear. If bone conduction is louder than air conduction, the Rinne test is said to be negative, and if air conduction is louder than bone conduction, it is positive. A negative Rinne test is characteristic of a conductive deafness. A positive Rinne test is compatible with normal hearing or a sensorineural deafness. It is important to mask the opposite ear when there is a significant difference of hearing between the two ears, so that during bone conduction testing the sound is not perceived in the opposite or better ear. The *Weber test* is performed when one places the stem of the fork somewhere in the midline: the vertex, the forehead, or the upper incisor teeth. The fork will lateralize to the better ear in a sensorineural deafness or to the deaf ear in a conductive deafness. It is a rather sensitive test.

Tuning fork tests are supplemented by *whisper and speech tests* to determine the approximate level of the deafness. The normal or very slightly deaf ear can perceive the lightest "residual air" whispered voice. Perception of a light whispered voice audible a few inches from the ear indicates hearing with 20 dB, a medium whispered voice tests at a 30 to 40 dB level, a low spoken voice at a 50 to 60 dB level, and a medium spoken voice at the 70 to 80 dB level. If the ear cannot hear a loud-spoken voice or a shout with the other ear properly masked, it is said to be profoundly deaf.

A number of *special auditory tests* provide a

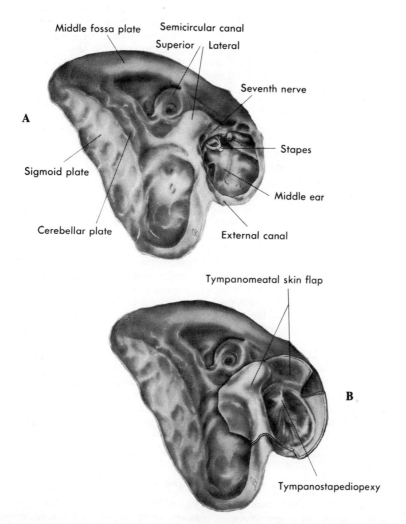

Fig. 42-20. A, Radical mastoidectomy; here, one large common chamber is created, including mastoid bowl, middle ear, and external auditory canal; ossicles are removed except for stapes; this is essentially sculpturing of bony plates surrounding temporal bone and is reserved for advanced tympanomastoid disease. **B,** Modified radical mastoidectomy; if mesotympanum can be preserved, tympanic membrane is tilted inward to contact stapes and is held in this new position by reflection of tympanomeatal canal skin flap onto facial ridge and roof of cavity; this preserves hearing.

relatively high degree of localization of the lesion; i.e., these special tests may tell us whether the deafness is hair cell, neural, or cortical in origin. Some of them are the short increment sensitivity index (SISI test), tone fatigue testing, Bekesy audiometry, and recruitment. There is also a wide variety of tests available for malingered deafness. There are even special tests available for objective evaluation of auditory acuity, not involving a judgment on the part of the patient. These include psychogalvanic skin response and evoked cortical potential recording using an analog computer.

Tinnitus aurium

Tinnitus aurium means nothing more than ringing in the ears. This is a symptom and not a disease. Tinnitus of varying degrees is almost invariably associated with deafness, and it is present to the degree that the ear is deaf. Usually, the tinnitus will be at about the same frequency as the deafness, such that presbycusis or high-tone deafness produces a high-pitched ringing and conductive deafness produces a panfrequency or "white noise" ringing. Tinnitus may be subdivided into *subjective* and *objective*. Subjective tinnitus is that which the patient alone can hear, and the physician is unable to detect any sound using his stethoscope over the external canal or over the temporal region. Objective tinnitus is that which the physician can hear as well. Objective tinnitus always means that there is a physical basis for the tinnitus instead of a sensory or neural lesion. Examples of objective tinnitus are that produced by a cavernous sinus fistula, eddy currents of blood in the carotid system from an arteriosclerotic plaque, eustachian tube clicks, and tympanic muscle clicks from spasm of the tensor tympani muscle or stapedius

muscle. The only treatment for tinnitus is detection of the underlying cause and its correction if possible.

Mastoidectomy

Mastoidectomy is performed for acute or chronic suppurative bone infection of the mastoid portion of the temporal bone (Fig. 42-6). The incidence of mastoidectomy for acute disease has dropped precipitously since antibiotics have become available, but at the same time, mastoidectomy done for chronic bone infection has risen.

A *simple mastoidectomy* is performed for acute osteomyelitis of the mastoid bone. The mastoid cortex and all air cells and diseased bone are removed. This usually means removal of the mastoid tip. The ossicles, tympanic membrane, and posterior bony canal wall are left intact. If the middle ear recovers, hearing is unaffected.

A *modified radical mastoidectomy* is performed for chronic suppurative mastoiditis and otitis media. The mastoid cortex is removed, and a meticulous removal of all mastoid air cells is done as the first step. The posterior canal wall is then removed, with the skin of the posterior and superior canal wall being preserved. The epitympanum is then exenterated of disease, and the incus and the head and neck of the malleus are removed. The tympanic membrane is reflected medially until it comes into contact with the head of the stapes, and the skin of the canal is used to line the mastoid cavity, sealing the middle ear from the remaining cavity. This operation joins the external canal and the mastoid cavity, making one large chamber. The cavity then heals by secondary intention, becoming lined with skin in a matter of weeks. Wax and skin debris must be removed from this cavity at twice

---

Fig. 42-21. A, Tympanoplasty type I. Notice that all structures are normal in the middle ear and mastoid, except for the perforation of tympanic membrane in its lower portion. Vein or fascia graft may be placed over perforation after careful removal of surrounding skin. More commonly, graft material is placed inside tympanic membrane. **B,** Tympanoplasty type II. Ossicular chain is preserved because it is free of disease. External auditory canal and mastoid bowl are one common chamber, from which middle ear is sealed. Normal hearing is obtainable with this operation. **C,** Tympanoplasty type III. Because of disease, malleus and incus were sacrificed, and tympanic membrane rests against head of stapes; otherwise it is same as tympanoplasty type II. Excellent hearing is attainable, because only lever ratio of ossicular chain is sacrificed and areal ratio (tympanic membrane to footplate) is maintained. This operation is same as modified radical mastoidectomy. **D,** Tympanoplasty type IV. Stapedial arch required sacrifice or was absent through disease. Footplate is left exposed to outside, and tympanic membrane is sealed against promontory. Round window (shaded area in center of hypotympanum) is thus joined with eustachian tube orifice as closed air-containing chamber. Because areal ratio is sacrificed as well as lever ratio, normal hearing is not obtainable; the best level that is theoretically obtainable is 26 dB. below normal.

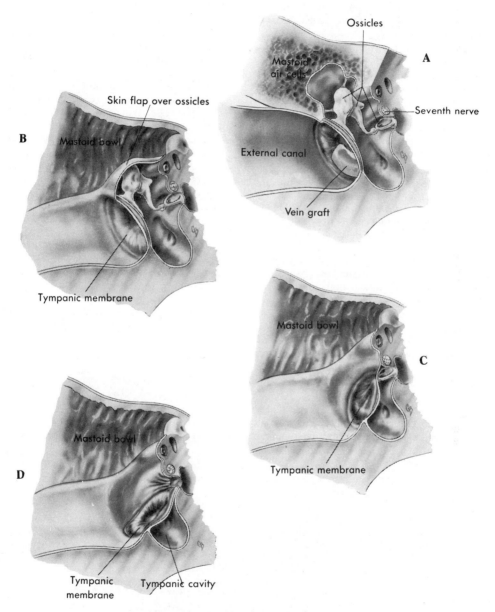

Fig. 42-21. For legend see opposite page.

yearly intervals, because it does not have the normal debris-removing characteristics of the normal ear canal. Excellent hearing may possibly occur after this operation. Theoretically only the lever ratio of the ossicular chain is sacrificed, and thus it is possible to have as little as a 2 dB. hearing loss (Fig. 42-20, *B*).

A *radical mastoidectomy* is the same as the modified operation except that portions of the middle ear and tympanic membrane are removed. The contents of the middle ear are exenterated, except for the stapes. Thus one large chamber is created, comprising the external canal, mastoid cavity, and middle ear, open for inspection the rest of the patient's life. The consequent hearing loss is, of course, severe: between 45 and 60 dB. (Fig. 42-20, *A*).

Microsurgery of the ear

Deafness is still man's most common physical impairment, despite the myriad ways modern man has found to maim and injure himself. Fortunately, a significant number of deafnesses are surgically correctable, especially those caused by defects in the tympanic membrane, ossicular chain, and stapedovestibular joint. Since that part of the tympanum containing the hearing mechanism is quite small (Fig. 42-21), these operations are done under magnification and are termed microsurgical operations. Some diseases causing deafness that may be helped by microsurgery are (1) tympanic perforation, (2) ossicular chain disruption with or without an intact tympanic membrane, (3) chronic suppurative otitis media (after mastoid disease is controlled), (4) certain varieties of chronic adhesive otitis media, (5) tympanosclerosis, and (6) otosclerosis.

These operations may be performed transmeatally or across the mastoid after mastoidectomy has been performed. The binocular operating microscope is used, which provides a coaxially lighted image of brilliant intensity, magnified from 6 to 40 times. Operations are done under general or local anesthesia. Where the tympanic membrane is intact, as in otosclerosis or tympanosclerosis, a skin flap is elevated from the posterior canal wall hinged on the posterior half of the tympanic membrane. Access to the tympanum is gained between the fibrocartilaginous annular ligament and the bony annulus of the tympanum. This renders the posterior half of the tympanum visible and, with it, almost all the conductive apparatus. A wide variety of special instruments is necessary for these operations. They are electrical and air turbine drills, chisels, needles, picks, hooks, knives, elevators, scissors, saws, suction tips, and various forceps. They are unique primarily in their diminutive size. Since these instruments are all hand-held and not moved by micromanipulators, the surgeon's touch must be developed to an uncommon deftness. This usually takes several years of practice.

43
Gynecology

John T. Soper
Daniel L. Clarke-Pearson

Gynecology is the medical and surgical specialty that is concerned with the study of the female genital tract. Although this specialty may appear to be restricted, the gynecologist participates in the evaluation and therapy of normal reproductive function and a variety of benign and malignant diseases of pelvic structure and function. Diseases of the pelvic organs may affect other organ systems. In addition, the gynecologist deals with gynecological symptoms arising from localized or systemic diseases. The gynecologist must also screen women for nongynecological diseases, since many women seek primary medical care from gynecologists. Finally, many gynecological disorders may directly affect the patient's psychological self-image or, conversely, genital symptoms may reflect psychopathological problems.

GYNECOLOGICAL HISTORY

Similar to all medical histories, the gynecological history is developed from the women's chief complaint to her total history, emphasizing menstrual, obstetrical and sexual function. Key gynecological symptoms include abnormal vaginal bleeding or discharge, pelvic relaxation, coital dysfunction, abdominopelvic pain, and urinary and gastrointestinal tract symptoms. Previous pelvic examinations, genital cytology, past obstetrical and contraceptive histories, and abdominopelvic operations also provide important data for constructing a thorough gynecological history.

GYNECOLOGICAL EXAMINATION

The gynecological examination is an integral part of the complete physical examination of a woman.

Ultrasonic or computerized tomography scans are poor substitutes for a physical examination of the pelvis. The gynecological examination most conveniently follows the general examination after the patient has emptied her bladder and rectum. This allows optimal palpation of the pelvic organs and improves rapport with the patient.

Basic equipment consists of a table with foot stirrups, an adequate light source, a bivalve speculum, gloves, lubricating jelly, and equipment necessary for obtaining a Papanicolaou smear. Additional useful items include ring forceps with cotton balls, tenaculum, cervical and endometrial biopsy instruments, material for endometrial cytology, cotton swabs with normal saline for vaginal smears, Thayer-Martin culture plates, local anesthetics, instruments for vulvar biopsies, and silver nitrate sticks or Monsell's solution for hemostasis. Lugol's solution and acetic acid are useful for staining the cervix for directed biopsies. A colposcope is invaluable for directing the examination of patients with abnormal cytological or gross pathological disorders of the cervix, vagina, or vulva.

The external genitalia are examined and carefully palpated for abnormalities of the mons, labia, clitoris, perianal region, and Bartholin's and vestibular glands. The urethra, perineum, and hymenal ring are carefully palpated. A warm speculum is inserted into the introitus, and the entire vaginal canal and cervix are visualized (Fig. 43-1, *A*). Findings are recorded in relation to the patient's right and left or anterior and posterior. A convenient method of recording cervical lesions is in reference to the face of the clock (e.g., 12 o'clock

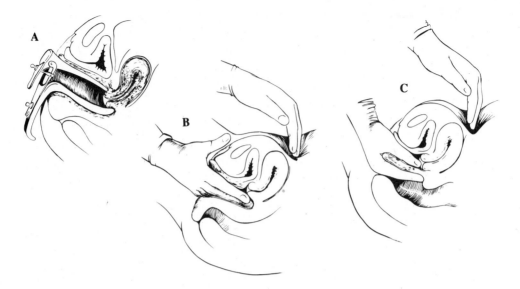

Fig. 43-1. Pelvic examination. **A,** Insertion of vaginal speculum. **B,** Bimanual abdominovaginal palpation of uterus and adnexa. **C,** Bidigital rectovaginal exam (forefinger in vagina and middle finger in rectum).

corresponds to the anterior position and 6 o'clock to the posterior). Papanicolaou smears are obtained from the cervix; both direct smear from the cervical portio and endocervical swab or aspirate are utilized. Any abnormal discharge is sampled for microscopic evaluation. Grossly visible lesions of the vulva or cervix are biopsied. The bimanual examination (Fig. 43-1, *B*) is utilized to assess systematically the pelvic structures. Cervical consistency, mobility, and tenderness with motion are noted first. The uterine position, size, shape, and contour are determined. Each adnexal region is palpated to determine the size and shape of the ovaries and to search for tenderness, masses, or nodularity. Normal fallopian tubes are usually not palpable. Finally, a bidigital rectovaginal examination (Fig. 43-1, *C*) is performed to palpate the posterior aspect of the uterus, adnexal structures, cul-de-sac, and the cardinal and uterosacral ligaments. Stool is tested for occult blood.

Pelvic findings are described in terms of anatomic (patient's) right or left and size expressed in conventional units of measurement (centimeters). The shape, consistency, mobility, and tenderness of the structures are described. Uterine size is usually expressed in terms of gestational size (weeks). Experience in performing the pelvic examination increases the ability to appreciate subtle variations in normal pelvic anatomy and detect pelvic pathological disorders.

BENIGN GYNECOLOGICAL CONDITIONS: GENERAL DIAGNOSTIC PROCEDURES AND TESTS

Papanicolaou (Pap) test. The Papanicolaou test utilizes smears of scrapings from the external cervical os and the cervical canal for cytological evaluation (Fig. 43-2). Smears can also be obtained from the posterior vaginal fornix, directly from lesions of the vagina and vulva, or aspirates or brushings from the endometrial cavity. In general usage, Pap smear refers to endocervical and cervical samples. After microscopic examination, the smear is reported as negative, containing cells suggestive of inflammation, containing atypical cells suggestive of dysplasia, or containing cells consistent with carcinoma. We believe that sexually active women should have an annual pelvic examination including Pap smear, regardless of age. The optimal accuracy rate for detection of invasive cervical carcinoma probably exceeds 90%, but it is less efficient for the detection of endometrial or ovarian carcinoma or other endometrial lesions. A major purpose for obtaining the Pap smear is to screen for premalignant cervical lesions, which can be treated conservatively. The management of the patient with an abnormal cervical Pap test is considered in detail later.

Wet vaginal smears. Direct microscopic evaluation of a wet-smear vaginal discharge (leukorrhea) often will be diagnostic in determining the cause of vaginitis, as in the following.

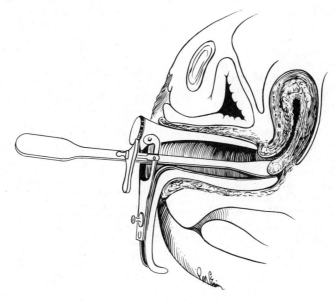

Fig. 43-2. Papanicolaou test—cervical scraping smear.

Trichomonas vaginitis. A mixture of vaginal discharge and normal saline solution examined immediately under the microscope may reveal motile, flagellated, pear-shaped parasites. The *Trichomonas* is intermediate in size between a white blood cell and an epithelial cell.

Candidal vaginitis. One drop of 10% potassium hydroxide (KOH) solution dissolves squamous epithelium but not yeast forms. Long thin septate hyphae and oval yeast buds are present. The vaginal aspirate may be incubated on Nickerson's medium and will produce dark brown colonies in a few days.

Gardnerella vaginitis. A normal saline smear reveals multiple white blood cells and bacteria with white blood cells containing intracellular bacteria (clue cells).

Atrophic vaginitis. Few quantified superficial cells and many basal epithelial cells are seen in the wet prep, a feature of estrogen deficiency. Superimposed vaginitis of a different cause may also produce many white blood cells, bacteria, trichomonads, or fungal forms.

Schiller's test. The normal squamous epithelium of the vagina and cervix contains a large amount of glycogen and stains a dark brown when exposed to concentrated iodine solution. Areas that do not stain are abnormal, and the test is considered "positive." The Schiller-positive areas may be caused by epithelial abnormalities and should be biopsied for histological analysis. Cervical biopsies usually require no anesthesia, and vaginal biopsies may be performed with a small amount of local anesthetic. In the past, this test was utilized to evaluate abnormal Pap smears but has been largely replaced by colposcopy.

Colposcopy. (See discussion of evaluation of abnormal Pap smear on p. 669.)

Pregnancy tests. Pregnancy tests are biological, immunological and radioimmunological assays that detect portions of human chorionic gonadotropin (hCG). Biological assays have been replaced by immunological and radioimmunological assays. Radioimmunological assays for hCG may become positive 6 or 7 days after ovulation at the time of implantation of the fertilized ovum. Less sensitive latex agglutination inhibition tests of urine are reliable approximately 2 weeks after the first missed menstrual period.

Dilatation and curettage (D&C) and endometrial biopsy. Cervical dilatation with separate endocervical and endometrial curettage is both a diagnostic and therapeutic procedure. It is utilized in the evaluation of abnormal, most frequently postmenopausal or perimenopausal, vaginal bleeding. The D&C is most adequately performed under general anesthesia. After examination under anesthesia the endocervical canal is curetted, the uterine cavity is sounded and endocervical canal serially dilated. The endometrial cavity is explored for polyps with forceps, and endometrial curettage is performed. Specimens are submitted separately for histological evaluation.

Endometrial biopsy or aspirate is a simple outpatient procedure that can be utilized as the initial diagnostic test for evaluation of women with abnormal uterine bleeding. It is 75% to 90% accurate in the diagnosis of endometrial carcinoma when compared to D&C. However, negative endometrial biopsy results must be confirmed by D&C in women with perimenopausal or postmenopausal bleeding who have persistent symptoms.

Laparoscopy. The laparoscope is utilized to visualize pelvic organs and perform simple operative procedures. General anesthesia is usually utilized. The peritoneal cavity is insufflated with carbon dioxide through a Verre needle, and the laparoscopic trochar is introduced through a small periumbilical incision. A fiberoptic light source is passed through the trochar sheath, and pelvic and abdominal contents are visualized (Fig. 43-3). Often a second probe or instrument is introduced through a second suprapubic incision. Simple surgical procedures such as tubal sterilization may be performed through the laparoscope. The incidence of complications decreases with operator experience, but many severe complications from this seemingly minor surgical procedure have been reported. Some indications, operative procedures, complications, and contraindications of laparoscopy are listed as follows:

1. Indications
   a. Pelvic pain
   b. Infertility
   c. Pelvic mass
   d. Selected genital anomalies and amenorrhea
2. Operative procedures
   a. Tubal coagulation
   b. Lysis of adhesions
   c. Fulguration of endometriosis
   d. Evaluation for residual carcinoma after primary therapy of ovarian carcinoma
3. Complications
   a. Hemorrhage, hematoma
   b. Bowel perforation
   c. Electrical burns
   d. Gas embolism
   e. Cardiorespiratory problems
   f. Infection
   g. Anesthetic complications
4. Contraindications
   a. Peritonitis
   b. Ileus
   c. Abdominopelvic mass or ascites
   d. Aortic aneurysm
   e. Failed pneumoperitoneum
   f. Ventral hernia
   g. Previous abdominal surgery (relative)

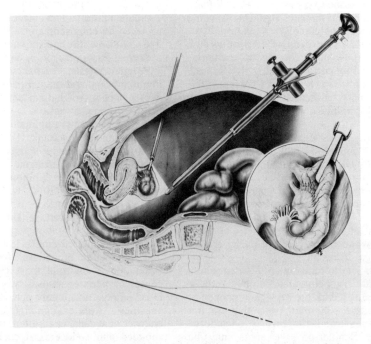

Fig. 43-3. Laparoscopy showing laparoscope and grasping forceps. Inset shows placement for tubal sterilization by coagulation.

INFECTIONS AND BENIGN DISORDERS OF THE LOWER GENITAL TRACT AND VULVA

Vulva

Chronic vulvar dystrophy. White lesions of the vulva have been described by a variety of confusing terms in the past. This classification has been simplified to take into account both atrophic and hypertrophic changes resulting from disordered epithelial growth as follows:

1. Vulvar dystrophies
   a. Hyperplastic dystrophy
      (1) Without atypia
      (2) With atypia
   b. Atrophic dystrophy (lichen sclerosis)
   c. Mixed dystrophy
      (1) Without atypia
      (2) With atypia
2. Vulvar atypia (with or without dystrophy)
   a. Mild
   b. Moderate
   c. Severe

These vulvar lesions may be elevated or flat, white, hyperpigmented or erythematous and are associated with changes caused by chronic irritation such as fissures, weeping, lichenification, ulceration, and excoriation. Pruritus and discomfort are the main symptoms. Since gross appearances are rarely diagnostic, all abnormalities should be biopsied with local anesthesia to exclude in situ or invasive carcinoma. Colposcopic examination of the vulva or evaluation of the vulva with toluidine blue staining may help to direct biopsies.

Benign vulvar dystrophy may be treated conservatively with improved local hygiene, treatment of coexistent vaginitis, and topical medications. Hyperplastic dystrophies are best treated with topical corticosteroids. Topical 2% testosterone proprionate in a petroleum base is effective treatment of lichen sclerosis. Mixed lesions may require both topical agents. Treatment with testosterone preparations may result in clitoral growth, hirsutism, and increased libido as a result of systemic absorption. Atypical and carcinomatous lesions require special therapy as discussed later.

Bartholin's cyst. Bartholin's cyst results from inflammation of the Bartholin's gland and occluded Bartholin's duct. When the cyst is infected, a Bartholin's abscess is extremely painful and tender and should require incision and drainage. After treatment of acute inflammation, the cyst may be totally excised or marsupialized to form a new duct opening. Any Bartholin's cyst in a menopausal woman should be biopsied to exclude a rare adenocarcinoma arising in Bartholin's gland.

Vagina

Trichomonas vaginitis. The trichomonad is a venereally transmitted parasite. The diagnosis of *Trichomonas* vaginitis is confirmed by visualization of the organism on wet smear. Patients complain of a thin, irritating vaginal discharge. Metronidazole is the treatment of choice. Both the patient and sexual partner need stimultaneous treatment, since the male is often an asymptomatic carrier. Metronidazole is contraindicated in pregnancy because of the risk of congenital malformation. Topical vaginal medications such as furazolidone or diiodohydroxyquin may be used during pregnancy.

Candidal vaginitis. Candidal (formerly monilial) vaginitis is seen frequently in patients who are pregnant, diabetic, immunosuppressed, or taking oral contraceptives or broad-spectrum antibiotics. The vaginal discharge resembles cottage cheese and may cause a severe erythematous vulvovaginitis. Topical antifungal agents such as nystatin or miconazole nitrate are the treatment of choice. Occasionally, patients may require treatment with topical gentian violet painting of the entire vaginal wall.

Atrophic vaginitis. Estrogen deficiency in postmenopausal or surgically castrate women results in thinning of the vaginal mucosa. This predisposes to infection, synechial formation, and symptoms of pruritus without significant discharge. The atrophic epithelium is susceptible to coital injury. Associated atrophy of the bladder epithelium may produce symptoms of cystitis. Systemic or local estrogen therapy is the treatment of choice and will alleviate systemic symptoms of estrogen deficiency simultaneously. Topical estrogen cream is absorbed systemically across the vaginal mucosa and should not be considered "topical" treatment only.

Nonspecific vaginitis. "Nonspecific" vaginitis is caused by *Gardnerella* bacteria. The symptoms are leukorrhea and vaginal odor. Topical therapy with sulfonamide-containing cream is ineffective. Metronidizole systemic therapy is the treatment of choice; however nonspecific vaginitis will frequently be recurrent unless the sexual partner is treated.

Vulvovaginitis in children. The most common cause of a purulent or bloody vaginal discharge in children is a vaginal foreign body. Often, a vaginal foreign object can be palpated on rectal examination or detected on plain film of the abdomen. Urethroscopic examination of the vagina is valuable and manual extration of the foreign object can frequently be performed without anesthesia. Pinworm infestation may also cause vulvovaginal discharge and pruritus. Rarely, a gonococcal infection of the vagina can cause a purulent vaginal discharge. When a gonococcal infection is diagnosed, the child should be evaluated for sexual abuse.

Gartner's duct cyst. Gartner's duct cysts arise in the lateral vaginal wall from wolffian duct remnants. These are frequently asymptomatic. Total excision for histological assessment is recommended.

Vaginal changes from diethylstilbestrol. Several gross and microscopic changes of the upper vagina and cervix have been noticed in female offspring of mothers who received diethylstilbestrol (trade name DES) or other estrogen during early pregnancy. These changes include vaginal adenosis, cervical erosion, and malformations of the vaginal fornices and cervical shape. These changes are not necessarily related to clear cell carcinoma of the vagina and cervix, which may also develop in children exposed in utero to diethylstilbestrol. Initial evaluation of women with a history of exposure to diethylstilbestrol should include complete physical evaluation with colposcopy and cytological smears from the cervix and upper vagina. The vaginal tube should be carefully palpated to detect any abnormal masses. Women exposed in utero to diethylstilbestrol have an increased incidence of abnormalities of the uterine cavity, which may predispose to infertility or pregnancy loss.

Fistulas. Rectovaginal, vesicovaginal, and urethrovaginal fistulas may result from obstetrical and surgical trauma, carcinoma, and pelvic radiation. Enterovaginal fistulas generally occur after radiation therapy. Traumatically induced fistulas are surgically repaired several months after fistula formation to allow resolution of inflammation. A temporary colostomy may be required for rectovaginal fistulas. Fistulas resulting from radiation therapy often require repair with a vascularized pedicle transposed into the defect to allow healing. Larger postradiation fistulas or enterovaginal fistulas require diversion of the urinary or gastrointestinal tract.

Cervix

Chronic cervicitis. The majority of sexually active women develop some degree of infection involving the columnar epithelium of the endocervical canal. This may become prominent if the squamocolumnar junction is located on the ectocervix with an eversion of the columnar epithelium. Most often, cervical eversions are asymptomatic but occasionally may produce a malodorous, mucopurulent discharge. Cytological screening should be utilized. Symptomatic cervicitis may be treated with systemic or topical antibiotics. Cryotherapy may be required for chronic symptomatic cervicitis after proper screening for cervical neoplasias.

BENIGN DISEASES OF THE UTERUS

Leiomyomas (fibroids). Leiomyomas are benign tumors of smooth muscle origin arising from the myometrium. Leiomyomas are, to a certain extent, hormonally responsive. The highest incidence of leiomyomas are found in blacks and nulligravidas and during the later years of reproductive life. The majority of leiomyomas regress after menopause. Leiomyomas may remain confined to the uterine wall (intramural) or may bulge into the endometrial cavity (submucosal) or peritoneal cavity (subserosal). Subserosal fibroids may extend into the broad ligament (intraligamentous) or become pedunculated. Rarely, they may draw blood supply from adjacent tissues with regression of the uterine blood supply (parasitic). Less than 10% arise from the cervix. Benign degenerative changes of hemorrhage, calcification, or liquefaction are frequently seen. Leiomyosarcomas develop in less than 1% of uterine leiomyomas.

Clinical manifestations of leiomyomas include crampy menstrual pain, excessive menstrual or intermenstrual bleeding, and symptoms of pelvic pressure. Occasionally degenerative changes may cause enlargement or acute pelvic pain. Rarely, a fibroid may impede labor and delivery during pregnancy. Uterine leiomyomas are usually diagnosed by pelvic examination. A pedunculated subserosal fibroid may mimic an adnexal mass.

The majority of uterine fibroids are small and asymptomatic and require no therapy. Most gynecologists recommend that a fibroid uterus larger than a gestational size of 12 weeks should be removed to exclude the possibility of uterine sarcoma or ovarian neoplasia. Total abdominal hysterectomy is indicated if the patient has significant symptoms of pelvic pain, develops significant anemia from menorrhagia, or has ureteral obstruction. Occasionally, leiomyomas can be "shelled out" (myomectomy) if they appear to cause infertility.

Adenomyosis. Adenomyosis is occasionally referred to as endometriosis interna and is caused by projections of endometrial tissue deep into the myometrium. Microscopically, this appears as diffuse or localized areas of endometrial glands and stroma interdigitated between normal myometrium. The symptoms and signs are menorrhagia, progressive dysmenorrhea, and an enlarged uterus. Adenomyosis is associated with advanced age and multiparity. The diagnosis is usually made after hysterectomy is performed to relieve symptoms.

Endometriosis. Endometriosis is characterized by hormonally responsive endometrial tissue implants in extrauterine sites. Most common sites for endometriosis are the ovaries, peritoneal surfaces of the pelvis, uterosacral ligaments, cul-de-sac, posterior part of the uterus, and Fallopian tubes (Fig. 43-4). Less common sites are the bowel, umbilicus, cervix, external genitalia, abdominal and episiotomy scars, and rarely distant sites such as the lungs. Probably several mechanisms are

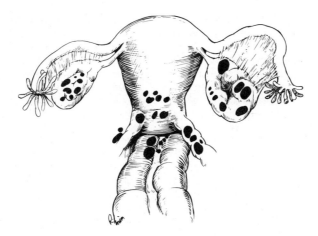

Fig. 43-4. Common sites of pelvic endometriosis.

responsible for the development of endometriosis, including retrograde menstruation through the tubes, lymphatic or hematogenous dissemination, and coelomic epithelial metaplasia.

Endometriosis is usually not detected in teen-age women. It may be progressive throughout reproductive years but usually disappears after menopause. The typical patient has complaints of progressive dysmenorrhea, dyspareunia, or cyclic bowel and bladder pain. The patient is frequently in her late twenties or early thirties and infertile.

Physical examination may reveal tenderness and nodularity of the cul-de-sac and uterosacral ligaments, retroflexion and fixation of the uterus, ovarian enlargement, or pelvic tenderness.

Although the diagnosis is suggested by history and physical examination, laparoscopy is generally performed for diagnosis. Typical endometriosis implants have a "powder-burn" appearance though hemorrhagic cysts of the ovaries can result from hemorrhage into larger implants. Differential diagnoses include pelvic inflammatory disease, uterine leiomyomas, and other causes of adnexal mass.

Regression of endometriosis often occurs during pregnancy. Hormonal manipulation such as combination oral contraceptives may be appropriate for mild endometriosis. A pseudopregnancy regimen consists in increasing doses of combination progestin-estrogen contraceptive pills or progestin alone to cause amenorrhea for 6 to 9 months. Side effects may include weight gain, fluid retention, nausea, and breakthrough bleeding. Hormonal manipulation is generally not curative but may result in sufficient atrophy of endometriosis to provide relief of symptoms and fertility. Danazol is also employed as an androgen with antiestrogen activity.

Danazol produces regression of endometrial tissue by suppressing gonadotropins and ovarian steroid output. Side effects are related to androgen activity. Danazol is very expensive but can produce a pregnancy rate of approximately 50% in previously infertile patients with endometriosis.

Conservative surgical therapy is utilized for moderate to severe endometriosis when fertility is desired or medical therapy has failed. This includes excision or fulguration of peritoneal implants, resection of ovarian endometriomas, lysis of adhesions, suspension of the uterus, and occasionally presacral neurectomy for relief of pain. Often conservative surgery is followed by danazol or hormonal therapy. When symptomatic endometriosis exists and fertility is no longer desirable, appropriate treatment is total abdominal hysterectomy with bilateral salpingo-oophorectomy. Retention of an ovary will result in a 25% to 30% recurrence of endometriosis, but residual endometriosis is rarely stimulated by exogenous hormonal replacement.

PELVIC INFLAMMATORY DISEASE AND VENEREAL DISEASES

Gonorrhea. Gonorrhea is one of the most common communicable bacterial diseases, with an estimated 1 to 3 million cases per year. It is epidemic among young men and women in the 16- to 24-year age group.

Although most males develop symptoms of urethritis, approximately 80% of women are clinically asymptomatic. Most of these asymptomatic carriers will have complaints of vaginal discharge or mild urethritis. The gonoccoccus invades columnar and transitional epithelium. The most common sites of infection in females are endocervical canal, urethra, Bartholin's and Skene's glands, and the rectum. Gonococcal pharyngitis is also a form of uncomplicated gonococcal infection. Approximately 15% to 25% of patients with untreated gonorrhea will develop complications, including pelvic inflammatory disease and disseminated gonococcemia with septic arthritis and meningitis.

Culture of the endocervical canal is most effective for screening asymptomatic persons. Ideally, cultures should be obtained from the endocervix, urethra, oral pharynx, and rectum in symptomatic patients or patients with a history of exposure. The gonococcus is a fastidious organism requiring a high carbon dioxide content and special culture medium (Thayer-Martin medium). Despite the emergence of relative penicillin-resistant strains and penicillinase-producing strains of gonorrhea, aqueous procaine penicillin G remains the treatment of choice for uncomplicated gonorrhea. One half hour before treatment, 1 gram of probenecid is given orally to decrease renal excretion of penicillin. Aqueous procaine penicillin G, 4.8 million units, is then given intramuscularly (this will also treat incubating syphilis). Alternatively, a large dose of ampicillin or amoxicillin may be given as a one-time oral treatment. Tetracycline, spectinomycin, or erythromycin are used in patients who are allergic to penicillin. After treatment of uncomplicated gonorrhea, cultures are repeated. Antibiotic sensitivity testing is done to rule out penicillinase-producing gonorrhea or reinfection if cultures are positive. Resistant gonorrhea can be treated with spectinomycin, cefoxitin, or cefotaxime.

Pelvic inflammatory disease (PID). Pelvic inflammatory disease (PID) is a spectrum of infections involving the uterus, tubes, and ovaries along with the pelvic peritoneum. In the United States, approximately 30% to 80% are associated with gonococcal infections. *Chlamydia trachomatis* may be isolated from 30% to 50% cases of salpingitis. Pelvic tuberculosis is rarely a cause of PID. The majority of cases of PID will have several pathogenic aerobic and anaerobic bacteria isolated from the fallopian tubes.

Frequently PID is caused by an ascending infection occurring at the time of menses when the cervical mucus barrier is breeched. Patients usually present with pelvic pain and fever. The clinical diagnosis of PID is made in a patient with symptoms, signs, and laboratory findings of acute pelvic peritonitis. The uterus and cervix are exquisitely tender to motion. Bilateral adnexal tenderness is present and tubal enlargement or bilateral adnexal masses may be palpated. Differential diagnosis includes other acute abdominal infections such as appendicitis, diverticulitis, pyelonephritis, and cys-

titis. Laparoscopy will aid in the early diagnosis of pelvic inflammatory disease.

Treatment is by broad-spectrum antibiotics. Patients should be treated with regimens that will be curative for gonococcus. Clinical response usually occurs in 1 to 3 days, but antibiotics are continued for 7 to 10 days beyond the disappearance of fever. Frequent evaluation including pelvic examination during therapy is necessary to detect pelvic abscesses. Aggressive management of acute PID is mandatory to preserve patient fertility.

Before the advent of broad-spectrum antibiotics, pelvic abscesses were frequently drained vaginally through the posterior cul-de-sac. The development of a tubo-ovarian or cul-de-sac abscess refractory to antibiotic therapy will require surgical removal and drainage. Traditionally, this has entailed total abdominal hysterectomy with bilateral salpingo-oophorectomy. However, some patients may be selected for more conservative resection of unilateral abscesses in an attempt to preserve fertility.

Repeated episodes of acute PID lead to chronic PID (Fig. 43-5), characterized by tubal destruction and formation of hydrosalpinx or pyosalpinx tubo-ovarian abscess, and chronic tubal adhesions. Patients with chronic PID may develop chronic pelvic pain, recurrent fever, and infertility. Although conservative tuboplasty may be employed to preserve fertility, the majority of patients with chronic PID and pelvic pain require total abdominal hysterectomy with bilateral salpingo-oophorectomy for definitive treatment.

Occasionally, patients with gonococcal or chlamydial PID will develop an acute perihepatic peritoneal inflammation (Fitz-Hugh and Curtis syndrome). Rarely, this syndrome may be mistaken for acute cholecystitis. Occasionally, such patients require lysis of "violin-string" adhesions between the diaphragm and liver for treatment of chronic right upper quadrant pain.

Other venereal diseases and toxic shock syndrome (TSS). Other venereal diseases include syphilis, herpes progenitalis, chlamydial infections, and the less common diseases of chancroid, lymphogranuloma venereum, and granuloma inguinale. Toxic shock syndrome (TSS) is a multisystemic disease associated with various staphylococcal toxins and antigenic proteins.

Syphilis is much less common than gonorrhea. The causative organism, *Treponema pallidum,* is a spirochete that can be demonstrated by dark-field microscopy of luetic lesions. The primary stage is characterized by an infectious hard chancre and secondary stage by generalized rash, systemic symptoms, and mucocutaneous patches. Tertiary lues may involve the central nervous system, cardiovascular system, and soft tissues. History,

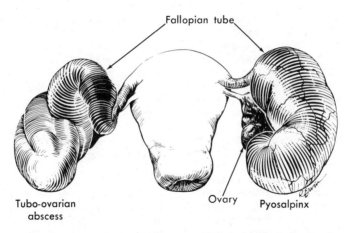

Fig. 43-5. Chronic pelvic inflammatory disease. On biological right, tubo-ovarian abscess. On biological left, pyosalpinx.

dark-field microscopy, serological tests (RPR, VDRL), and clinical manifestations of tertiary lues establish the diagnosis. Penicillin remains the antibiotic of choice.

Herpes progenitalis is caused by the herpes simplex virus types I and II. Approximately 3 to 5 million new cases occur each year in the United States. Manifestations of primary herpes include painful vesicles on an erythematous base that involve the lower genital tract. Other symptoms include fever, inguinal lymphadenopathy, and urinary retention. Disseminated herpes virus infection or aseptic meningitis are rare manifestations. After a primary herpes infection, the virus enters into a latent phase of infection where viral particles can be demonstrated in the lumbosacral dorsal nerve root ganglia. Secondary recurrences are frequently observed, though the manifestations are generally not so severe as during the primary infection. Topical or systemic acyclovir is effective in reducing the duration and severity of the symptoms of primary herpes, but its effectiveness in preventing recurrence is unknown. Otherwise, therapy is by use of analgesics, sitz baths, and other symptomatic measures.

The exact incidence of significant chlamydial infections of the genital tract is unknown because of insufficient culture techniques. *Chlamydia* species may cause symptomatic infections of the cervix, endometrium, fallopian tubes, urethra, and bladder. Previously, chlamydial urethritis was recognized as sterile "nonspecific" urethritis after successful eradication of gonorrhea. Treatment of choice is tetracycline.

Toxic shock syndrome (TSS) is a spectrum of multisystemic diseases mainly affecting menstruat-ing women and is associated with vaginal infection with *Staphylococcus aureus*. The majority of affected women are tampon users. Clinical manifestations include fever, orthostatic hypotension, and rash in association with multisystemic signs and symptoms. Patients may develop nausea and vomiting, diarrhea, myalgias, mucous membrane ulceration, renal or hepatic failure, thrombocytopenia, or neurological symptoms. Treatment is by aggressive intravenous fluid hydration and beta lactamase–resistant antibiotics. Vasopressors, steroids, dialysis, and artificial ventilation may be required in selected patients. A range of mortality from 2% to 13% has been reported. Patients are at a 20% to 30% risk for a later recurrence. It is recommended that patients who develop TSS have follow-up cultures to ensure that vaginal colonization of staphylococcus has been eradicated. They should discontinue the use of tampons indefinitely.

DISORDERS OF PELVIC SUPPORT AND URINARY STRESS INCONTINENCE

Pelvic relaxation commonly results from obstetrical trauma with resultant stretching and thinning of the pelvic supporting tissues. The postmenopausal atrophy of hormone-sensitive tissues caused by estrogen deficiency may accentuate pelvic relaxation. A cystocele or urethrocele is caused by weakening of the anterior vesicovaginal fascia so that the bladder and urethra bulge into the vagina. Relaxation of the posterior rectovaginal fascia results in a rectocele. A true hernia of the posterior cul-de-sac may occur through the apex of the vagina or along the rectovaginal septum. This peritoneum-lined sac generally contains loops of small intestine and is termed an enterocele. Relaxation of pelvic supporting tissues is often accompanied by uterine descensus. In its extreme form, the uterus may prolapse through the vaginal introitus. Abnormalities of pelvic support usually coexist.

The descent of the bladder neck and distortion of the normal posterior urethrovesical angle produced by cystocele and urethrocele causes urinary stress incontinence. This is involuntary loss of urine accompanying increased intra-abdominal pressure from Valsalva maneuvers such as laughing, coughing, or straining. Stress incontinence must be differentiated from other types of incontinence that cannot be cured by surgical therapy including unstable bladder (detrusor dyssynergia), urgency incontinence produced by cystitis, overflow incontinence from neurogenic bladder, and continuous incontinence from a vesicoovaginal fistula. A careful history and physical examination will often allow the physician to distinguish these entities. Not infrequently, patients have a combination of anatomic urinary stress incontinence and detrusor dyssynergia. Cystometric and cystoscopic evaluation may help distinguish these entities. Before surgical correction of urinary stress incontinence, patients with mixed disorders should be treated with anticholinergic drugs to determine the true extent of stress incontinence.

Other components of pelvic relaxation may produce symptoms of pelvic pressure. Rectoceles are usually asymptomatic but may cause constipation. Incarcerated enteroceles may rarely produce bowel obstruction and infarction.

The key to surgical management of pelvic relaxation is to identify and correct all components of pelvic relaxation. Frequently, this is best accomplished by the vaginal route: vaginal hysterectomy, cul-de-sac plication, and posterior colporrhaphy correct uterine descensus, enterocele, and rectocele. Restoration of the normal posterior urethrovesical angle can be accomplished vaginally by Kelly plication of the urethrovesical angle and anterior colporrhaphy.

An alternative to the vaginal surgical correction of stress incontinence is retropubic urethropexy, which can be combined with abdominal hysterectomy and vaginal repair of a rectocele. Colpocleisis, obliteration of the vaginal canal, can be used in a small number of patients who are no longer sexually active and who are not candidates for a more definitive operative procedure because of medical complications.

Frequently, patients develop vaginal prolapse with or without associated cystocele or rectocele after a vaginal or abdominal hysterectomy. In the majority of these patients, a small enterocele was not corrected at the time of the primary procedure. Surgical repair includes obliteration of the entero-

cele and suspension to the sacrospinous ligament as a transvaginal procedure, or transabdominal suspension of the vaginal vault to the sacral periosteum using Marlex mesh.

Some patients will develop recurrent urinary stress incontinence after one or more surgical procedures. These patients may require a combined vaginal and abdominal approach to correct the incontinence. Ofter a sling of synthetic material or fascia is utilized to support the posterior vesicourethral angle.

ABORTION

Abortion (AB) is the spontaneous or induced termination of pregnancy during the first 24 weeks of gestation. Spontaneous abortion usually occurs in the first 12 to 14 weeks of gestation and is frequently caused by a blighted or chromosomally abnormal ovum. Spontaneous abortion is clinically recognized in approximately 15% of gestations, whereas the actual incidence is probably higher. *Threatened abortion* refers to spotting, cramping, or bleeding in early pregnancy without cervical dilatation. This may progress to cervical dilatation (*inevitable abortion*) or passage of products of conception (*incomplete abortion*). The dilated cervical os predisposes to uterine infection, and bleeding associated with abortion may be sufficient to cause hypovolemic shock. Treatment is by suction D&C to prevent further hemorrhage or infection. Only rarely is complete expulsion of the products of conception (*complete abortion*) observed.

Habitual abortion refers to three consecutive spontaneous abortions, usually occurring in the first trimester. Metabolic disorders such as diabetes and thyroid disease, chronic infection, uterine anomalies, and parental chromosomal anomalies should be excluded in the evaluation of habitual abortion. The majority of causes for habitual abortion are never determined, but a treatable disorder must be ruled out.

Second trimester abortions may result from uterine anatomic anomalies or incompetent cervix. The classical history for incompetent cervix is of repetitive painless second-trimester cervical dilatation and premature rupture of the amniotic sac or second trimester delivery of an immature fetus after a relatively short labor. Frequently, the pregnancy terminates at an earlier gestational age with each successive pregnancy. Placement of a nonabsorbable encircling suture at the level of the internal cervical os before significant cervical dilatation corrects an incompetent cervix. The cerclage should not be placed after labor has begun or after significant cervical dilatation or rupture of membranes has occurred, since under these circumstances the chance of success is low and the chance of inducing an infection of the intrauterine contents is high. After attainment of term gestation, the cerclage suture may be removed to allow vaginal delivery or may be left in place and delivery effected by cesarean section.

Elective abortion has become more common since liberalization of abortion laws in the early 1970s. Elective abortion is performed by suction D&C in the first trimester or in the second trimester by intra-amniotic installation of saline solution or prostaglandin. Dilatation and evacuation of the uterine contents (D&E) is also performed in some centers for the elective termination of second trimester gestations. Although the risk of complications such as uterine perforation increases with gestational age, second trimester D&E is a safe procedure when employed by skilled practitioners.

The legalization of elective abortion has resulted in a lower incidence of septic abortion caused by unsterile termination of pregnancy either by self-manipulation of instrumentation by nonmedical personnel. Septic abortion is a fulminant mixed gram-negative and anaerobic infection of the products of conception, endometrium, and myometrium. Septic abortion is a life-threatening emergency, requiring aggressive management with broad-spectrum antibiotics, fluid resuscitation, and often vasoactive agents. Uterine evacuation by D&C is necessary after stabilization and initiation of antibiotics. Occasionally hysterectomy may be required to remove infected or necrotic tissues.

ECTOPIC PREGNANCY

Ectopic pregnancy results when a fertilized ovum fails to migrate and implant normally in the endometrial cavity. Most ectopic pregnancies involve the ampullary region of the fallopian tube (95%), but implantation may occur in the isthmic or cornual regions of the tube, on or in the ovary, in the abdominal cavity, or in the endocervical canal. Combined intrauterine and extrauterine pregnancies may rarely coexist. The most common predisposing factor for ectopic pregnancy is salpingitis with resultant tubal agglutination and adhesions. Other factors mechanically interfering with normal tubal transport of fertilized ovum may cause ectopic implantation such as endometriosis, adhesions from previous gynecological or infertility surgery, or tubal ligation. The ectopic implantation site lacks the stroma necessary for normal placental development. Usually, the pregnancy undergoes abortion or the trophoblastic tissue invades into adjacent vessels resulting in hemorrhage. The incidence of ectopic pregnancy has increased alarmingly in the last 10 years, paralleling an increase in the incidence of gonococcal and nongonococcal salpingitis.

Signs of hemorrhagic shock indicate tubal rupture. Aspiration of the cul-de-sac may yield non-clotting blood indicating intraperitoneal hemorrhage. After stabilization of the patient the ectopic pregnancy must be removed, most frequently by salpingectomy. The entire fallopian tube is removed to the uterine cornual region. The ipsilateral ovary is not removed. Elective reconstructive surgery of the contralateral adnexal structures is deferred until hemorrhage and inflammation from the ectopic pregnancy have resolved.

With the employment of serum hCG testing and laparoscopy, unruptured tubal pregnancies are being more frequently diagnosed. Conservative surgical management of unruptured tubal pregnancies includes linear salpingostomy and segmental resection of the involved tube. These procedures may preserve the potential for normal pregnancies in patients with a damaged or absent contralateral tube and do not seem to increase the incidence of repeat ectopic pregnancies. In any event, future prospects for normal pregnancy are limited. Approximately 15% of patients will have a second ectopic pregnancy, and only one third will have a subsequent normal viable intrauterine pregnancy.

Most often the classical historical and physical findings are absent. The patient may relate episodes of vaginal bleeding interpreted as normal menses and may not have distinct physical findings. Often, routine urinary pregnancy tests are negative because of low-level hCG secretion from the abnormally implanted placenta, but more sensitive serum beta-hCG assays will usually be positive. Other conditions that must be differentiated from ectopic pregnancy include early threatened abortion, bleeding or pain associated with a functional ovarian cyst, and pelvic inflammatory disease. The laparoscope may be useful in evaluating patients with atypical findings and, coupled with serum hCG assays, may detect unruptured ectopic pregnancies.

BENIGN OVARIAN TUMORS AND ADNEXAL MASSES

The ovary contains many components that can give rise to both benign and malignant neoplasms, functional cysts, and other lesions simulating ovarian neoplasms (Table 43-1). Additionally, the adnexal regions may contain masses related to uterine, tubal, or bowel pathoses. Therefore the management of an adnexal mass is aimed at exclusion of ovarian or tubal malignancy, prevention of acute complications of benign neoplasms (torsion or rupture), and avoidance of surgical intervention for benign functional events associated with the menstrual cycle. Functional cysts of the follicle or corpus luteum are frequently found in menstruating women. They rarely exceed 5 cm. in diameter or persist for more than one menstrual cycle. Benign

Table 43-1. Histogenic classification of ovarian tumors

Epithelial	Serous
	Mucinous
	Endometrioid
	Brenner
Sex cord–stromal	Granulosa
	Theca
	Sertoli-Leydig
Germ cell	Dysgerminoma
	Teratoma
	Immature
	Mature
	Endodermal sinus
	Embryonal carcinoma
	Choriocarcinoma
	Mixed forms
Miscellaneous	Lymphoma
	Sarcoma
	Metastatic tumors

epithelial neoplasms occur during or after reproductive years. Cystic mature teratomas (dermoid cysts) are the most common ovarian germ cell tumor. They may contain tissue from all germinal cell layers: endoderm, mesoderm, and ectoderm. Teeth, hair, and a thick, greasy sebaceous material are frequently present in the cyst. Occasionally, calcifications resembling teeth may be detected on a plain film of the pelvis, which is a finding indicative of a benign dermoid cyst. Ovarian stromal neoplasms may produce either estrogen or androgen and systemic symptoms related to hormonal excess. Other conditions may produce an adnexal mass indistinguishable from an ovarian mass and include endometriosis, hydrosalpinx, peduculated leiomyomas or paraovarian cysts. Nongynecological conditions such as chronic appendicitis or diverticulitis may also give rise to adnexal masses.

Often benign causes of adnexal mass cannot be distinguished clinically from malignancy. The management of an adnexal mass depends on the patient's age and findings on pelvic examination. Asymptomatic, smooth, cystic adnexal masses less than 7 or 8 cm. in a woman of reproductive age may be safely followed with serial pelvic examination for one or two menstrual cycles. Persistent masses, masses greater than 8 cm. in diameter, or masses associated with ascites must be further evaluated and require surgical exploration with extirpation. Any ovarian enlargement in premenarcheal or postmenopausal women is abnormal and should result in surgical intervention.

Preoperative evaluation includes routine laboratory blood studies, intravenous pyelography to evaluate the location of the ureters, and chest roentgenogram. Data from barium enema and upper gastrointestinal series should be obtained if the patient has significant gastrointestinal symptoms. A pelvic ultrasound scan may be helpful if the patient is obese and examination unsatisfactory, or if intrauterine pregnancy is suspected. In general, ultrasound is not more accurate than a careful pelvic examination in determining the size, location, or consistency of adnexal masses and does *not* yield a histological diagnosis. A few patients may be evaluated with laparoscopy to determine whether surgical extirpation is required, but most patients should undergo exploratory laparotomy through a midline incision to allow surgical removal and staging of a possible ovarian malignancy.

CONGENITAL ANOMALIES

Vaginal anomalies. An imperforate hymen or a transverse vaginal septum may result from failure of the urogenital sinus to fuse with the müllerian duct systems. These anomalies are usually detected after menarche when accumulation of menstrual flow collects above the obstruction causing pain and an abdominopelvic mass. Patients with these anomalies must be distinguished from those with primary amenorrhea because surgical removal of the septum is curative.

Congenital absence of the upper two thirds of the vagina often coexists with an absent or anomalous uterus and normal ovaries. Infrequently a normal uterus, cervix, and small segment of upper vagina are present. Since the prospect for normal fertility is limited if the cervix is absent, the major therapeutic goal usually is creation of a functional vagina. At the time of sexual maturity, a space is created surgically between the bladder and rectum and lined with a split-thickness skin graft sutured around a vaginal mold. The vaginal mold is removed postoperatively, and the vaginal canal is kept patent through sexual activity and mechanical dilatation. An alternative to surgical creation of a neovagina is the Frank method of progressive elongation of the rudimentary vaginal dimple using pressure with silicone rubber dilators. If a relatively normal cervix or uterus is lacking, the uterus and tubal structures should be removed to prevent reflux menstruation and development of endometriosis.

Total absence of the ovaries, tubes, uterus, and vagina is rare. Testicular feminization (androgen-insensitive syndrome) should be suspected and gonads removed if the patient has a male karotype (46,XY).

Uterine anomalies. The fallopian tubes, uterus, cervix, and most of the vaginal tube are created by fusion of the paired müllerian ducts. Failure of fusion can result in a wide spectrum of anomalies ranging from a uterus with a small intrauterine septum in the upper fundus to complete duplication with separate uterine horns, cervices, and vaginas. An isolated vaginal septum may exist. These anomalies may cause no problems or may result in repeated abortions, premature labor, or infertility. If a uterine septum or duplication is the cause of repeated pregnancy wastage or infertility, the uterus may be reunified surgically by excision of the septum. A vaginal septum should be removed to prevent difficulties with delivery. In all anomalies of the female reproductive tract, except for an imperforate hymen, a preoperative intravenous pyelogram should be performed to rule out frequently associated urinary tract malformations.

PREMENSTRUAL SYNDROME

Although clinically recognized for many years, premenstrual syndrome (PMS) remains an inadequately defined and poorly understood spectrum of symptoms associated with the luteal phase of the menstrual cycle. A large segment of the female population is affected by this syndrome in one form or another. Clinical manifestations of premenstrual syndrome include cyclic headache, breast swelling and tenderness, abdominal bloating, fluid retention, mood alterations, skin eruptions, and gastrointestinal symptoms. Symptoms usually worsen during the second half of the menstrual cycle and abate after menstruation begins. Symptoms vary greatly in severity ranging from mild to incapacitating. Many causes have been proposed for premenstrual syndrome, including estrogen excess, progesterone deficiency, vitamin deficiency, and neuroendocrine abnormalities. Since the cause is poorly understood and the spectrum of illness encompasses many symptoms, it is understandable that a variety of different therapies are employed in the management of this syndrome. Oral contraceptives, vaginal progestin, diuretics, and analgesics may provide relief of some of the symptoms of premenstrual syndrome for selected women.

DYSMENORRHEA

Primary dysmenorrhea is defined as pain with menstruation in the absence of a definite cause (e.g., endometriosis). Symptoms are cramping pelvic pain beginning immediately before or at the onset of menses and gradually decreasing over several days after the onset of menstruation. Primary dysmenorrhea is most commonly observed in younger women and may improve after pregnancy or with the use of oral contraceptives. Since the syndrome is caused by production of local prostaglandins, prostaglandin synthetase inhibitors (e.g., indomethacin) have been successfully used in treating primary dysmenorrhea. Persistent dysmenorrhea despite an adequate trial of prostaglan-

din synthetase inhibitors or abnormalities detected on serial pelvic examinations warrant further investigation to rule out other causes of pelvic pain and dysmenorrhea.

PELVIC PAIN

The symptom of pelvic pain may result from many organic and functional causes. Initial evaluation of the patient with pelvic pain of short duration should be directed toward ruling out acute organic disease. Managing the patient with chronic pelvic pain requires patience and diligence to determine the cause. Frequently psychiatric counseling is helpful in determining psychological causes for pelvic pain. Often, laparoscopy is required to exclude organic pelvic disease and to reassure the patient who requires long-term psychiatric therapy. Without clear organic cause, surgical removal of the uterus and ovaries rarely resolves these chronic pelvic symptoms.

GYNECOLOGICAL ONCOLOGY
Vulvar intraepithelial neoplasia

Vulvar in situ carcinoma and Paget's disease of the vulva are preinvasive intraepithelial vulvar malignancies. These lesions may appear 10 years earlier than invasive vulvar carcinoma and may coexist with invasive carcinoma. In situ carcinoma frequently occurs in dystrophic areas of the vulva. Recent evidence indicates a possible association with human papovavirus and herpesvirus infections, though these have not been proved as causal agents.

The lesions of carcinoma in situ are raised and may be white or hyperpigmented. They are usually asymptomatic but may be associated with pain and pruritus. Paget's disease has a similar appearance to Paget's disease of the breast and presents as an erythematous, pruritic plaque. Histologically Paget's disease of the vulva is characterized by large, polygonal clear cells infiltrating the basal epithelium. Normal-appearing skin is frequently involved beyond the visible margins of the gross lesion. Occasionally, it may be difficult to distinguish melanoma from Paget's disease without special stains being used. Unlike Paget's disease of the breast, the vulvar lesion is infrequently associated with an underlying carcinoma of the apocrine glands.

Since many lesions of the vulva have similar gross appearances and in situ carcinoma is frequently associated with invasive carcinoma, biopsy should be used liberally to establish the diagnosis and exclude invasion. Toluidine blue staining or colposcopy may aid in directing biopsies. Wide local excision is the therapy of choice. In multifocal disease, a skinning vulvectomy with split-thickness skin grafting of the operative bed maintains normal vulvar appearance and clitoral function. Topical 5-fluorouracil cream and laser vaporization of lesions are alternative modes of therapy. Despite operative therapy, these lesions have a high recurrence rate and the patient should be closely followed for life.

Invasive vulvar carcinoma

Invasive vulvar carcinomas account for 4% of all female genital malignancies. A rising incidence of vulvar carcinoma has been observed recently and parallels increased life expectancy. The average age of patients with invasive vulvar carcinoma is in the midsixties, with the majority being over 60 years of age.

Although this disease occurs on the body surface and is amenable to early diagnosis, many patients delay seeking treatment because of false modesty or a reluctance to undergo pelvic examination. Physician delay caused by treatment of vulvar lesions without biopsy is unfortunately also common. Because of the advanced age of the patient with vulvar cancer, many patients have associated medical diseases such as diabetes, hypertension, and cardiovascular disease. Approximately 25% of patients will have second primaries, most frequently carcinoma of the cervix.

Symptoms and diagnosis. The initial lesion is usually a small nodule that eventually enlarges and ulcerates. Occasionally the carcinoma may mimic a condyloma in appearance. Pruritus and discomfort are frequent symptoms. The majority of lesions arise on the labia majora (Fig. 43-6). The diagnosis is established by either incisional or excisional biopsy. Small lesions may be completely excised under local anesthesia for assessment of the depth of invasion. Biopsy shold be obtained from the worst-appearing portion of any vulvar lesion.

Approximately 85% to 90% of vulvar malignancies are well-differentiated squamous cell carcinoma, with melanoma, sarcoma, and adenocarcinoma being less common.

Pattern of spread and treatment. Vulvar carcinoma is usually indolent, locally invasive, and metastasizes primarily through the lymphatics. Lymphatic drainage begins with interconnecting subepithelial and subdermal plexuses that form larger subcutaneous channels that drain to the superficial inguinal and femoral lymph nodes. The channels run anterolaterally, medial to the labio-

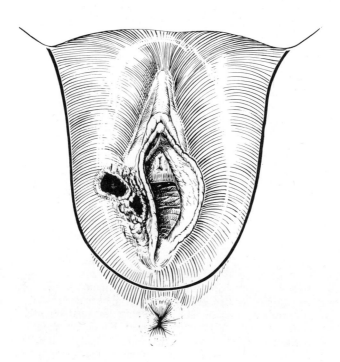

Fig. 43-6. Gross appearance of vulvar carcinoma. *Solid line*, Perineal resection margin of radical vulvectomy.

crural fold, and do not extend into the thigh. Lymph node involvement is usually orderly, with initial involvement of the superficial inguinal nodes located above the cribriform fascia before involvement of the femoral and finally external iliac nodes (Fig. 43-7). Cloquet's node is the last node of the deep femoral group: pelvic nodal involvement is rarely seen without involvement of Cloquet's node. Although lymphatics from the clitoris may drain directly to the deep pelvic lymph nodes, the clinical significance of this route of drainage appears to be minimal.

Surgical management of invasive vulvar carcinoma is based upon the lymphatic drainage of the vulva. Historically the treatment of choice has been the en bloc dissection or radical vulvectomy with inguinal and femoral lymphadenectomies (Fig. 43-8). This removes the mons, clitoris, labia, and underlying tissues to the periosteum of the symphysis, the efferent lymphatics, and both primary and secondary lymph nodes. With this therapy, 5-year survival rate for early vulvar carcinoma is approximately 90%. If femoral lymph nodes are involved, the operation can be extended to include a deep pelvic lymphadenectomy or the patient may be treated with whole pelvic radiation therapy. As expected, the morbidity from this procedure is significant: wound breakdowns are frequent and removal of the deep femoral lymph nodes often results in significant chronic lymphedema of the extremity.

An alternative approach to the surgical therapy of small (less than 2 cm.) early invasive vulvar carcinoma is the combination of bilateral superficial inguinal lymphadenectomy with wide local excision of the vulvar lesion. The superficial inguinal nodes are submitted for immediate frozen-section analysis, and a radical vulvectomy with complete inguinal and femoral lymphadenectomies is performed if metastases are present. For properly selected patients, this procedure would appear to reduce the morbidity without significantly compromising survival. Occasionally, patients will have extensive disease involving the vagina or rectum, and exenterative surgery or radiation therapy may be required.

The survival of patients with vulvar carcinoma mirrors lymphatic involvement. Early vulvar carcinoma without regional metastases has a 5-year survival of approximately 90%, which is reduced to approximately 40% when regional lymph nodes are involved. Only 20% of patients with positive pelvic nodes will survive 5 years or more.

Evaluation of abnormal Pap smear

The cervix and lower genital tract of the female are uniquely accessible for direct observation and cytological screening. Data from several studies indicate that premalignant lesions of the cervix (cervical intraepithelial neoplasia, CIN) are detected reliably by cytological means. Although many patients with early CIN will have spon-

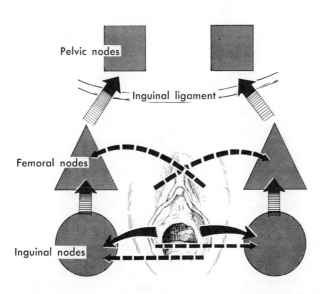

Fig. 43-7. Lymphatic dissemination of vulvar carcinoma. *Solid arrows*, Most common routes; *broken arrows*, less common routes.

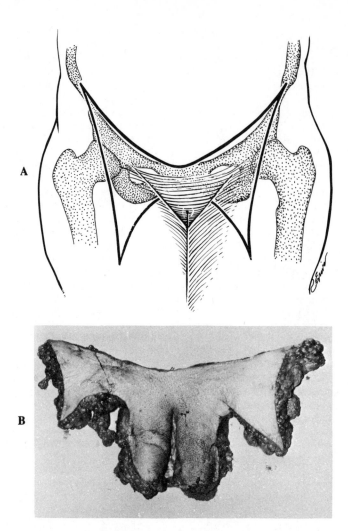

Fig. 43-8. A, Marshall incision for radical vulvectomy and bilateral groin dissection. **B,** Radical vulvectomy specimen with en bloc dissection of vulva, efferent lymphatics, and groin.

Table 43-2. Classification of cervical intraepithelial neoplasia

Type	Degree	Extent of atypia
CIN I	Mild dysplasia	Basal third
CIN II	Moderate dysplasia	Lower two thirds
CIN III	Severe dysplasia	Full epithelial
	Carcinoma in situ	thickness

taneous regression of the abnormal cytological condition to a normal pattern, a significant proportion of patients with CIN will develop invasive squamous cell carcinoma of the cervix if left untreated. Once CIN has been identified, progression can usually be prevented by simple outpatient therapy and continuing surveillance. "Cervical intraepithelial neoplasia (CIN)" has generally replaced the terms "dysplasia" and "carcinoma in situ" as terms referring to the histological characterization of premalignant cervical epithelial changes (Table 43-2). In lesions of CIN I and CIN II, the basal cell layer of the cervical squamous epithelium undergoes proliferation with nuclear

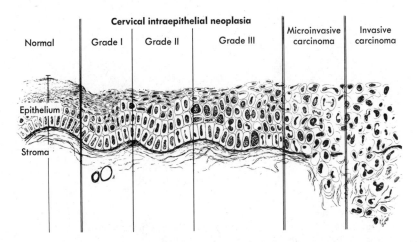

Fig. 43-9. Progression of histological changes from normal cervical epithelium through cervical intraepithelial neoplasia to invasive squamous cell carcinoma.

atypia, changes in the nuclear: cytoplasmic ratio, and loss of polarity (Fig. 43-9). The upper layers of the epithelium undergo maturation, and often a few layers of stratified epithelium are present on the surface. When the architecture of the epithelium is completely disrupted and loss of polarity through all cell layers has occurred without invasion of underlying cervical stroma, the lesion is referred to as CIN III (Fig. 43-9). Exfoliated cells from the surface of the epithelium are detected cytologically and form the basis for the Papanicolaou smear.

Many epidemiological studies have inferred associations of CIN and cancer of the cervix with multiple interdependent social factors. These disorders are more common in multiparous women with an early age of first coitus and multiple sexual partners. Cervical carcinoma is rare in celibate groups. A male factor has been hypothesized. A viral cause has also been proposed, with both herpesvirus type II and human papovavirus having been associated with CIN and invasive carcinoma of the cervix.

Lesions of cervical intraepithelial neoplasia are asymptomatic and frequently not observed on routine examination. The natural history of early CIN is extremely variable. Frequently, lesions of CIN I or CIN II will spontaneously revert to normal. Lesions of CIN III less frequently regress but frequently progress to invasive carcinoma over a variable length of time.

Screening for CIN and carcinoma of the cervix is by means of the cervical Pap smear. This test should be performed annually on all women who are sexually active. The Pap test is a screening mechanism only and is valid only in screening for cervical neoplasia. The cervix must be sampled at the squamocolumnar junction where most lesions originate. The Pap smear should evaluate both the endocervix and the ectocervix.

The interpretation of an abnormal Pap smear should take into account all possible explanations for the abnormal cytological pattern. In the past, evaluation of a patient with an abnormal Pap smear included repeat cytology tests, random cervical biopsies, directed biopsies in areas that did not stain with Lugol's solution, and conization of the cervix (Fig. 43-10) to rule out invasive cancer. Recently colposcopy has led to a more conservative evaluation and therapy scheme for the patient with an abnormal Pap smear (Fig. 43-11). The colposcope is a binocular stereoscopic microscope with low magnification. The cervix is stained with 3% acetic acid, and the colposcope is utilized to visualize the entire portion of the cervix and the squamocolumnar junction. Acetic acid accentuates the difference between normal and abnormal culposcopic patterns. In most instances, the entire lesion can be visualized, and the most atypical area can be selected for biopsy. If the lesion extends into the endocervical canal or endocervical curettage reveals atypical cells, diagnostic conization will be necessary to define disease. The major advantage of colposcopy is that a skilled colposcopist can establish the definitive diagnosis by directed biopsy and avoid surgical conization. This is most important in the younger patient desirous of childbearing in whom cone biopsy may result in impaired fertility. Additionally, conization is a pro-

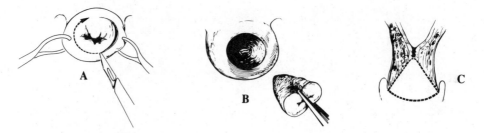

Fig. 43-10. Cone biopsy of cervix. **A,** Line of incision. **B,** Specimen removed. **C,** Frontal section of cervix and lower corpus demonstrating extent of conization.

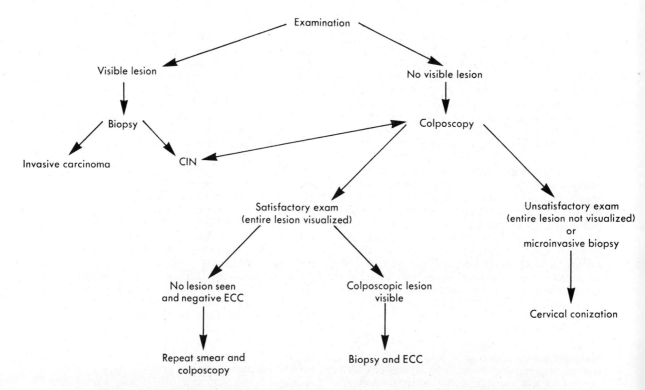

Fig. 43-11. Evaluation of abnormal cervical smear. *CIN*, cervical intraepithelial neoplasia; *ECC*, endocervical curettage.

cedure that requires anesthesia and hospitalization. The majority of patients with CIN can thus receive appropriate outpatient treatment.

Patients selected for outpatient therapy are those in whom satisfactory colposcopy yields evaluation of the entire squamocolumnar junction, the entire lesion is visualized and biopsy is confirmatory of an abnormal cytological pattern, and in whom the endocervical curettage is negative for dysplasia. Outpatient therapy for CIN includes cryotherapy, electrocautery, and laser destruction. All therapeutic modalities are successful in eradicating CIN in more than 90% of patients.

If colposcopy does not allow visualization of the entire lesion or the entire squamocolumnar junction, if the directive biopsy reveals questionable stromal invasion, or if the endocervical curettage is positive, cone biopsy is necessary for definitive diagnosis. The limits of the ectocervical incision can be delineated by use of the culposcope and the smallest possible cone obtained to excise all atypical epithelium. The depth of the incision as it tapers toward the endocervical canal is determined by the length of the cervical canal and suspected depth of involvement. Bleeding from the operative bed is controlled by hemostatic sutures. Cervical stenosis, cervical incompetence, infertility, and hemorrhage are possible but rare complications of cone biopsy. Cone biopsy may be therapeutic in patients whose lesion is contained in the cone biopsy specimen. Definitive therapy of CIN may also be attained with hysterectomy in patients who do not desire further childbearing.

Regardless of the therapeutic modality employed, patients with CIN are at a higher risk for recurrence of genital tract lesions and should be followed with genital cytology tests for the remainder of their lives.

Invasive cervical carcinoma

The incidence of invasive cervical carcinoma has decreased with the availability of routine cytological screening in the United States. At the same time, the number of advanced cervical carcinomas has decreased, along with the mortality from invasive cervical carcinoma. Approximately 16,000 new cases of cervical carcinoma occur annually in the United States, with approximately 7,000 deaths being attributable to cervical carcinoma. Of cervical carcinoma, 95% are of the squamous cell variety and the remaining 5% are primarily adenocarcinomas arising from the endocervical mucus-producing glands. The epidemiology of cervical squamous carcinoma is similar to the epidemiology of CIN, in that squamous carcinoma is more frequently seen among patients with early onset of coital activity and frequent sexual partners.

The typical patient with invasive cervical carcinoma is between 45 and 55 years of age. The most common early symptom of cervical carcinoma, a thin bloody vaginal discharge, is frequently unrecognized. The classical symptom is abnormal intermenstrual bleeding, often occurring as postcoital spotting. Late symptoms of disease include flank or leg pain that is usually secondary to the involvement of ureters, pelvic wall, and sciatic nerve roots. Some patients develop urinary and bowel symptoms because of local invasion. Distant metastases and persistent edema of the lower extremities are late manifestations of primary or recurrent disease. Occasionally patients will present with profound genital hemorrhage or uremia from advanced pelvic disease.

Staging. Cervical carcinoma is clinically staged, preferably confirmed with examination under anesthesia. The international staging for cervical carcinoma allows limited diagnostic aids for determining the stage including physical examination, routine chest roentgenograms, intravenous pyelogram, barium enema, colposcopy, cystoscopy, and proctoscopy. Clinical staging allows a rough assessment of prognosis, and communication of treatment results between one institution and another. Staging does not limit the therapeutic plan, and therapy is tailored to the extent of disease in each patient. The clinical stages of cervical cancer are as follows:

Allowed studies for determining stage
  1. History, physical exam, routine blood studies
  2. Chest roentgenogram, intravenous pyelogram, barium enema
  3. Colposcopy, cystoscopy, sigmoidoscopy
Stage 0: Carcinoma in situ
Stage I: Carcinoma confined to the cervix
  Stage Ia: Microinvasion
  Stage Ib (occult): Not recognized visually
  Stage Ib: All other cancers limited to cervix
Stage II: Involvement of upper vagina or infiltration of parametria, not involving pelvic sidewall
  Stage IIa: Upper two thirds of vagina but not parametria
  Stage IIb: Infiltration of parametria, not involving pelvic sidewall
Stage III: Involvement of lower vagina or parametria with extension to pelvic sidewall
  Stage IIIa: Lower third of vagina but not to pelvic sidewall if parametria are involved
  Stage IIIb: Infiltration of one or both parametria to the pelvic sidewall; obstruction of one or both ureters by intravenous pyelogram
Stage IV: Extension outside of reproductive tract
  Stage IVa: Involvement of bladder or rectal mucosa
  Stage IVb: Distant metastases

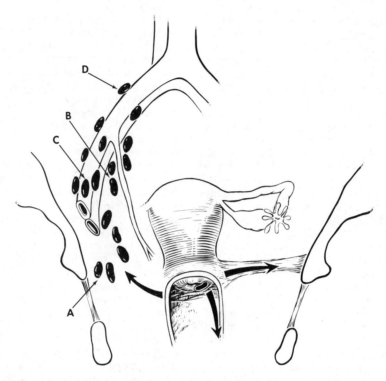

Fig. 43-12. Routes of spread of cervical carcinoma. Left side shows spread by extension along cardinal ligaments to lateral pelvic wall and into vagina. Right side demonstrates commonly involved pelvic lymph nodes. *A*, Obturator; *B*, hypogastric; *C*, external iliac; *D*, common iliac.

The major routes of spread for cervical carcinoma (Fig. 43-12) are: (1) into the vaginal mucosa, (2) into the lower uterine segment, (3) direct extension into the paracervical and parametrial tissues, (4) into the paracervical lymphatics and pelvic lymph nodes, and (5) directly into the bladder or rectum. Pelvic lymph node metastases are well correlated with the stage of disease, and they increase from 10% to 20% in stage I disease to greater than 50% in stage III disease. The primary lymphatic drainage of the cervix is along the cardinal and uterosacral ligaments to the pelvic lymph nodes with secondary involvement of the common iliac, para-aortic, and inguinal lymph nodes. Systemic dissemination is frequently present when the para-aortic nodes are involved.

Treatment. Therapy of cervical carcinoma is tailored to the extent of disease (Table 43-3). In many institutions, the primary modality of therapy is radiation; however surgery is appropriate for early lesions. Since the incidence of nodal metastases is extremely low in microinvasive lesions

confined to a depth of 3 mm. or less without lymphatic or vascular space involvement, patients with these lesions may be appropriately treated with simple vaginal or abdominal hysterectomy. Younger patients who are acceptable surgical risks may have radical surgical therapy of selected stage Ib and IIa cervical carcinomas. The radical hysterectomy involves en block removal of the uterus, lateral paracervical and uterosacral ligaments to the pelvic sidewalls, cervix, and a portion of the upper vagina. The pelvic lymph nodes are removed completely from the external iliac and obturator nodes. Presacral, common iliac and para-aortic lymphadenectomies are also performed. The ovaries are retained in younger patients to permit normal ovarian function until menopause. With modern surgical techniques and antibiotics, the operative mortality and morbidity of radical surgery are extremely low; long-term survival for patients with stage Ib cervical carcinoma after radical hysterectomy is approximately 90%.

Otherwise, the therapy of cervical carcinoma at

Table 43-3. Therapy of cervical carcinoma

Stage	Whole pelvis (rad)	Brachytherapy applications	Optional surgery
Ia	—	—	Simple extrafascial hysterectomy
Ib	2000-4000	2	Radical hysterectomy with pelvic lymphadenectomy
IIa	4000	2	
IIb	4000-5000	2	
IIIa	5000-6000	1 or interstitial implant	
IVa	6000	2	
IVb	1000 pulse for central palliation		

Recurrent cervical carcinoma:
1. Central—consider pelvic exenteration
2. Distant metastases—chemotherapy

stages Ib, IIa, IIb, IIIa, and IIIb is based on external radiation combined with intracavitary radium or cesium brachytherapy. The normal pelvic tissues are able to tolerate an extremely high dose of radiation therapy, particularly the cervix and upper vagina. Intracavitary brachytherapy is ideally suited to the treatment of cervical carcinoma because it is possible to place a radiation source in proximity to the lesion and thus deliver high central doses approaching 15,000 to 20,000 rad. This is combined with external radiation therapy to increase the dose to the pelvic sidewall for treatment of parametrial and retroperitoneal disease. The addition of radiation sensitizers such as hydroxyurea increases the effects of radiation on malignant cells.

Acute treatment complications occurring during radiation therapy included irritation of the rectum, small bowel, bladder, skin, and mild bone marrow suppression. Late radiation complications include fibrostenotic changes of the intestinal and bladder walls with atrophic gastrointestinal and genitourinary mucosa. Radiation produces an obliterative endarteritis. Chronic complications can be progressive and manifest several months or years after completion of radiation therapy. Occasionally, such complications may require small bowel bypass, colostomy, or urinary diversion. In general, serious morbidity of pelvic radiation is low if external radiation is below 5,000 rad.

Approximately 35% of patients with invasive cervical carcinoma will have recurrent or persistent disease after therapy. The triad of weight loss accompanied by leg edema and back or pelvic pain is ominous and indicative of pelvic sidewall recurrence. Vaginal bleeding or discharge is strongly suggestive of central recurrence. Patients with central recurrence after radiation therapy are occasionally candidates for ultraradical exenterative surgical therapy. Reirradiation for recurrent disease inside previously radiated fields is generally not possible because of the radiation tolerance of normal tissues. *cis*-Platinum (*cis*-diaminodichloroplatinum) is the most active single agent in the chemotherapy of metastatic or recurrent cervical carcinoma.

Endometrial carcinoma

Endometrial carcinoma is the most common malignancy of the female reproductive organs. Approximately 40,000 new cases occur in the United States annually, with approximately 3,500 patients dying from endometrial carcinoma. The majority of patients are postmenopausal, and the average age at diagnosis is 60 years. Adenocarcinoma of the endometrium accounts for 95% of uterine corpus malignancies, with the balance being sarcomas.

Estrogen has been implicated as an etiological factor in endometrial carcinoma. Endometrial carcinoma occurs more frequently in women with unopposed estrogen as in polycystic ovary disease, hormone-secreting ovarian tumors, and exogenous estrogen. In general, women who develop endometrial carcinoma have low parity, menstrual irregularity, and late menopause. Patients are frequently obese with associated hypertension and diabetes mellitus. Obese patients have a high rate of peripheral conversion of adrenal and ovarian androstenedione to estrone. This results in unopposed endogenous estrogen exposure.

Diagnosis. Early symptoms of endometrial carcinoma include a thin, serosanguineous vaginal discharge, but postmenopausal or intermenstrual vaginal bleeding generally brings the patient to the physician's attention. Any episode of postmenopausal bleeding requires investigation with endometrial biopsy or D&C. The routine Pap smear is ineffective in detecting endometrial carcinoma. Although cytological studies of the endometrial cavity may prove useful in some patients, a histological technique such as endometrial biopsy or D&C is preferred for the diagnosis of endometrial carcinoma. Staging of endometrial carcinoma requires sounding of the uterus and endocervical curettage in addition to routine pelvic examination and histological diagnosis of endometrial carcinoma.

Pathology. Adenocarcinomas of the endometrium may produce a varied pattern including mixed adenosquamous, papillary, clear cell, and adenoacanthoma patterns. A well-differentiated tumor retains glandular differentiation (grade 1). A moderately differentiated tumor has a mixture of solid and glandular areas (grade 2), and a poorly differentiated tumor (grade 3) loses glandular differentiation.

The premalignant precursors of endometrial carcinoma are less well characterized than for cervical carcinoma. Adenomatous hyperplasia can progress under estrogen stimulation; approximately 20% will develop endometrial carcinoma if untreated. Adenomatous hyperplasia will frequently respond to progestin therapy. Adenomatous hyperplasia with cellular atypia is less likely to respond to hormonal therapy and requires hysterectomy both for treatment and to rule out a coexistent endometrial carcinoma. Cystic hyperplasia of the endometrium has an extremely low malignant potential.

Staging. Initially, endometrial carcinoma spreads along the surface of the uterine cavity and locally invades the myometrium. Deeply invasive and poorly differentiated lesions can metastasize through hematogenous or lymphatic routes to adnexal structures and the pelvic or para-aortic lymph nodes. Involvement of the endocervical canal results in more frequent extension into the lateral parametria and pelvic lymph node metastases. Intraperitoneal metastases may occur through seeding of peritoneal surfaces by freefloating malignant cells, which can be detected by peritoneal cytology tests. Hematogenous spread to lungs, liver, and brain are late manifestations. Survival is roughly correlated with clinical stage of endometrial carcinoma. The stages of endometrial carcinoma follow:

> Stage I: Carcinoma confined to the corpus
> > Stage Ia: Length of uterine cavity 8 cm. or less
> > Stage Ib: Length of uterine cavity more than 8 cm.
> Stage I carcinomas are subgrouped according to histological grade:
> > Group 1: Highly differentiated adenocarcinoma
> > Group 2: Differentiated adenocarcinoma with partly solid areas
> > Group 3: Predominantly solid or undifferentiated carcinomas
> Stage II: Carcinoma involving the corpus and cervix
> Stage III: Carcinoma extending outside of the uterus but not outside the true pelvis
> Stage IV: Carcinoma extending outside of the true pelvis or involving the bladder or rectal mucosa

The most significant prognostic factors in early endometrial carcinoma are histological differentiation, depth of myometrial invasion, and the presence or absence of malignant cells in peritoneal washings. Pelvic and para-aortic lymph node metastases are associated with lack of histological differentiation, deep myometrial invasion, and adnexal metastases.

Treatment. The majority of endometrial carcinomas are treated by total abdominal hysterectomy with bilateral salpingo-oophorectomy and examination of peritoneal cells. Sampling of pelvic and para-aortic lymph nodes are performed in cases with deeply invasive grade 1 lesions and all grade 2 or grade 3 lesions. The surgical findings dictate the necessity for adjuvant radiation therapy. Intraperitoneal instillation of radioactive chromic ^{32}phosphate is effective therapy for patients with malignant peritoneal cells as the only poor prognostic factor. Adjuvant whole pelvic radiation therapy of 4,500 to 5,000 rads is usually given to patients with cervical involvement, pelvic metastases, or pelvic lymph node metastases. Radiation fields may be extended to include involved para-aortic lymph nodes.

Using individualized therapy selected on the basis of surgical staging, 5-year survival rates are approximately 90% to 95% for stage I lesions. Stage II endometrial cancers have a much poorer prognosis if true invasion of cervical stroma is present, with a 50% to 60% survival. Survival for patients with stage III and stage IV cancers is dependent on the sites of metastatic involvement and response to progestin therapy. *cis*-Platinum and doxorubicin (formerly called adriamycin) are active chemotherapeutic agents against endometrial carcinoma, but overall survival in advanced endometrial cancer is less than a range of 10% to 15%.

Ovarian carcinoma

Ovarian carcinoma is the third most common gynecological malignancy with approximately 17,000 new cases annually, but it is the leading cause of death among gynecological malignancies with approximately 12,000 deaths. The incidence of ovarian carcinoma is increasing in industrialized nations for unknown reasons. The risk of developing ovarian carcinoma approaches 1%, with the peak incidence in the fifth and sixth decades. From 85% to 90% of all ovarian carcinomas are derived from celomic epithelium. Germ cell tumors are the second most frequent type of ovarian malignancy and are more frequently found in patients under 25 years of age.

Unfortunately, the majority of ovarian carcinomas are detected at a late stage because of insidious, nonspecific symptoms of early ovarian carcinoma. No effective techniques are available to detect ovarian carcinoma early. Immunological techniques aimed at detection of tumor-specific antigens are at present too nonspecific to serve in this capacity.

Diagnosis and therapy. Most symptoms caused by ovarian carcinoma are related to intestinal involvement, ascites, or pleural effusion when the malignancy is far advanced. Therefore even asymptomatic adnexal masses must not be ignored. Frequently patients will have nonspecific complaints of early satiety, bloating, or constipation. Increasing abdominal girth may be attributable to ascites. Abdominal pain and nausea or vomiting may reflect intestinal obstruction.

A woman with ascites in the 40- to 70-year age group, without other evidence of liver or cardiac disease, should be considered to have ovarian carcinoma until proved otherwise. Diagnostic paracentesis is not recommended, since a peritoneal cytological examination may not establish the diagnosis and malignant cells may seed the needle tract. Occasionally, a large contained cyst may be mistaken for ascites and rupture during attempted paracentesis.

Preoperative evaluation of a patient suspected of having ovarian carcinoma should include a chest roentgenogram to screen for pulmonary metastases, and an intravenous pyelogram and small bowel series or barium enema if bowel involvement is suspected. Abdominal CT scan and ultrasound scan do not yield a histological diagnosis and are rarely valuable in staging these patients.

Ovarian carcinoma is surgically staged as follows:

Stage I	Growth limited to the ovaries
Stage Ia	Growth limited to *one* ovary; no ascites
	(i) No tumor on the external surface; capsule intact
	(ii) Tumor present on the external surface or capsules ruptured, or both features
Stage Ib	Growth limited to *both* ovaries; no ascites
	(i) No tumor on the external surface; capsule intact
	(ii) Tumor present on the external surface or capsule(s) ruptured, or both features
Stage Ic	Tumor either stage Ia or stage Ib, but with ascites* present or positive peritoneal washings
Stage II	Growth involving one or both ovaries with pelvic extension
Stage IIa	Extension or metastases to the uterus or tubes
Stage IIb	Extension to other pelvic tissues
Stage IIc	Tumor either stage IIa or stage IIb, but with ascites* present or positive peritoneal washings
Stage III	Growth involving one or both ovaries with intraperitoneal metastases outside the pelvis or positive retroperitoneal nodes
	Tumor limited to the true pelvis with histologically proved malignant extension to small bowel or omentum
Stage IV	Growth involving one or both ovaries with distant metastases
	If pleural effusion is present, there must be positive cytology tests to allot a case to stage IV
	Parenchymal liver metastases equals stage IV
Special category	Unexplored cases which are believed to be ovarian carcinoma

Therefore laparotomy establishes the diagnosis and determines the extent of disease. Two thirds of patients have stage III or stage IV disease at the time of diagnosis. Exploration for ovarian carcinoma includes sampling ascites or peritoneal washings for cytological examination, examination and biopsy of the right hemidiaphragm, and visual or palpatory examination of all serosal and peritoneal surfaces with biopsies of suspicious areas. Even in the absence of gross involvement, partial omentectomy should be performed to detect occult metastases.

In early disease, total abdominal hysterectomy

---

*Ascites is peritoneal effusion that in the opinion of the surgeon is pathological or clearly exceeds normal amounts.

with bilateral salpingo-oophorectomy and omentectomy should be performed with sampling of pelvic and para-aortic lymph nodes. Young patients who desire to retain fertility may have more conservative extirpation of disease if the tumor is of borderline malignant potential or is well differentiated and there is no extraovarian spread. In the presence of more advanced disease, every attempt is made to reduce the tumor burden by surgical resection. "Debulking" appears to enhance a response to chemotherapy.

Early-stage ovarian carcinoma is usually treated with adjuvant single-agent alkylating chemotherapy, since overall survival is approximately 60% in patients treated with surgery alone. Intraperitoneal radioactive isotopes (e.g., chromic ^{32}phosphate) may also be used. This has the advantage of requiring only a single application with fewer side effects than with chemotherapy.

Recently, advanced stage ovarian carcinoma has been treated with combination chemotherapy, usually based around *cis*-platinum in combination with alkylating agents and doxorubicin. Multiple-agent chemotherapy improves the response when compared to single-agent alkylating therapy, and the duration of survival appears to be longer. However, the ultimate cure rate for advanced-stage ovarian carcinoma is less than 15%.

External-beam radiation therapy to the whole abdomen is limited by the radiosensitivity of the liver, kidneys, and bowel. Ovarian carcinoma has a propensity to spread over all peritoneal surfaces; therefore radiation therapy directed at the pelvis alone is rarely successful.

Prognosis of ovarian epithelial carcinoma is most closely related to stage of disease (p. 677). The histological grade of the tumor affects the prognosis within each stage. The estimated 5-year survival rates range from 90% in stage Ia (i) borderline or well-differentiated lesions, to less than 15% for disease at stages III and IV.

Carcinoma metastatic to ovary. Endometrial adenocarcinoma frequently metastasizes to the ovary. The most common extragenital carcinomas that metastasize to the ovary are from gastrointestinal and breast primaries. Bilateral ovarian enlargement from metastatic mucinous carcinoma (generally of gastric origin) are frequently called "Krukenberg tumors," an imprecise term.

Gestational trophoblastic neoplasia

Gestational trophoblastic neoplasia (GTN) is a term applied to the rare placental neoplasms called hydatidiform mole, chorioadenoma destruens, and choriocarcinoma. In contrast to primary choriocarcinoma of the gonad, these neoplasms are essentially disorders of pregnancy and contain paternal genetic material. Normal trophoblast is locally invasive and also has the ability to metastasize. Normal villi are found in maternal lungs during many normal pregnancies, particularly in the third trimester of pregnancy. The viability of normal

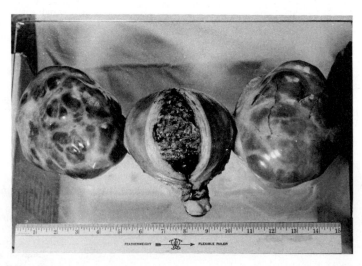

Fig. 43-13. Hydatidiform mole. Surgical specimen showing molar tissue in uterine cavity and bilateral theca-lutein cysts.

trophoblastic tissue is self-limited, probably under the influence of hormonal or immunological controls.

Hydatidiform mole. The incidence of hydatidiform mole in the United States is approximately 1 in 1,500 to 2,000 pregnancies. "Complete" moles are usually of karyotype 46,XX and contain paternal chromosomal material. "Partial" moles have a less frequent incidence of malignant sequelae and are generally triploid. Vaginal bleeding in the first half of pregnancy is the most frequent sign, with passage of molar tissue in the second trimester. Molar tissue is composed of multiple translucent vesicles ranging in size up to 1 cm. Approximately

half the patients will have a uterus that is large for gestational age, but one fourth will have a small-for-dates uterine size. Unilateral or bilateral theca lutein cysts (Fig. 43-13) are present in approximately 20% of cases, resulting from ovarian hyperstimulation by high levels of circulating human chorionic gonadotropin (hCG). Fetal heart tones are absent. Approximately 20% to 25% of patients have hyperemesis. Toxemia of pregnancy before 24 weeks of gestation is highly suspicious for mole.

Slightly more than 50% of molar pregnancies are diagnosed before the expulsion of vesicles. The diagnostic method of choice is ultrasound (Fig. 43-14), which demonstrates a mixed echogenic

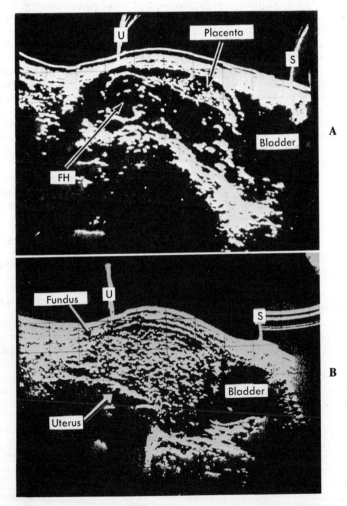

Fig. 43-14. Longitudinal midline ultrasound scans of abdomen. **A,** Normal 22-week gestation showing fetal head, *FH,* and placenta. *U,* Umbilicus; *S,* symphysis. **B,** Hydatidiform mole showing diffuse homogeneous echo pattern in uterus enlarged to 22-week size with absence of fetal parts.

diffuse pattern in the uterus without fetal parts. This is preferred to arteriography, amniography, or roentgenography, since ultrasound is noninvasive and poses no threat to mother or fetus. After the diagnosis of hydatidiform mole, the patient is screened for systemic metastases with a chest roentgenogram and a base-line serum hCG titer is obtained. The uterus is evacuated by suction curettage. If the patient desires sterilization, hysterectomy is employed. The lutein cysts require no therapy and regress spontaneously when hCG stimulation is removed. Prophylactic chemotherapy is not recommended, since it does not eliminate the need for postmolar surveillance and may result in serious toxicity.

After evacuation, the patient is followed with serial hCG titers at 1- or 2-week intervals. Serum radioimmunoassays for the beta chain of hCG are preferred, since they do not cross-react with serum luteinizing hormone and are sufficiently sensitive to detect small amounts of viable trophoblastic tissue. After remission, titers are followed for 12 months at 1- to 2-month intervals. During this time, contraception is employed. After remission of 1 year, the patient may become pregnant. If the hCG titer rises or plateaus for more than three successive hCG titers, the patient is considered to have malignant gestational trophoblastic neoplasia and appropriate therapy is warranted.

Malignant gestational trophoblastic neoplasia. Malignant gestational trophoblastic neoplasia (GTN) was previously a devastating, rapidly progressive malignancy of young women with an almost uniformly fatal outcome when metastases were present. However, the advent of effective chemotherapy and hCG titer surveillance have made malignant GTN one of the most curable of human malignancies.

Approximately 20% of molar pregnancies will develop malignant sequelae. On the other hand, one third to one half of malignant GTN cases are preceded by nonmolar gestations. Histologically, malignant GTN can be divided into chorioadenoma destruens (invasive mole) and choriocarcinoma. Chorioadenoma destruens demonstrates maintenance of villous architecture with pronounced trophoblastic proliferation and direct invasion of the myometrium and may metastasize. Choriocarcinoma is histologically characterized by sheets of malignant trophoblastic cells without villous architecture. The prognosis and treatment of both entities are similar depending on the presence or absence of metastases and clinical features suggestive of poor response to single-agent chemotherapy. Before the advent of chemotherapy, the cure rate for nonmetastatic malignant GTN was less than 50% in patients treated by hysterectomy

alone. Several chemotherapeutic regimens are effective for the treatment of malignant GTN, and therapy is monitored through the use of serum hCG titers as a tumor marker.

After the diagnosis of malignant GTN, the patient should be staged with a base-line (pretherapy) serum hCG titer, chest roentgenogram, brain scan or CT scan of the brain, and liver-spleen scan or CT scan of the liver to screen for high-risk metastases. The most common sites of metastases are lungs, vagina, brain, and liver. Brain and liver metastases have a poorer prognosis than metastases in other sites.

Nonmetastatic gestational trophoblastic neoplasia. Patients with nonmetastatic GTN are managed with single agent chemotherapy utilizing methotrexate or actinomycin D. Cycles of chemotherapy are repeated until hCG titers become negative. The reported cure rates for nonmetastatic GTN utilizing this approach are excellent, with cure of virtually all patients. The majority of patients can be treated without hysterectomy, though hysterectomy may be combined with chemotherapy to shorten the duration of chemotherapy.

Metastatic gestational trophoblastic neoplasia. Patients with metastatic GTN are divided into good-prognosis and poor-prognosis groups on the basis of whether or not one or more high-risk clinical feature is present, which would predict failure of single-agent chemotherapy. If a patient has none of the following, she has good-prognosis metastatic GTN, if one or more, she has poor-prognosis metastatic GTN:

1. Pretherapy hCG titer greater than 40,000 mIU/ml. serum beta hCG titer
2. Duration of disease greater than 4 months
3. Brain or liver metastases
4. Antecedent term pregnancy
5. Previous unsuccessful single agent chemotherapy

Patients with good-prognosis metastatic GTN are treated with repetitive cycles of single-agent methotrexate or actinomycin D, and cure rates in excess of 90% have been reported (Fig. 43-15). Patients with poor prognosis metastatic GTN should be initially treated with multiagent chemotherapy, since the expectations for cure with single-agent chemotherapy are low and the risk of severe toxicity when secondarily treated with combination chemotherapy is high. Adjuvant radiation therapy to cerebral or hepatic metastases is given to control hemorrhage, since metastases are highly vascular.

Chemotherapy is individualized according to the hCG titer response and is recycled on a frequent basis. Patients are monitored closely for toxicity including bone marrow depression, stomatitis, nau-

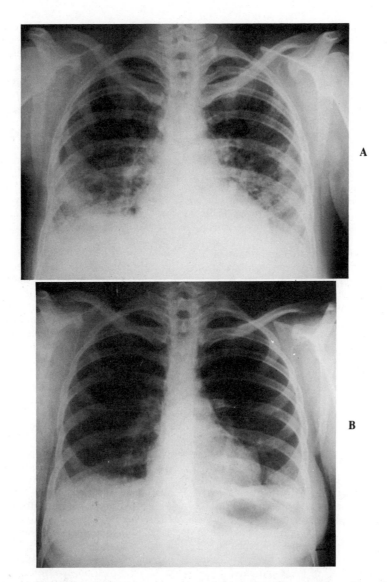

Fig. 43-15. Regression of pulmonary metastases of choriocarcinoma after treatment with methotrexate. **A,** Chest roentgenogram before chemotherapy. **B,** Appearance after three courses of methotrexate.

sea and vomiting, and alopecia. When hCG titer remission is achieved, patients are followed with hCG titers at 2-week intervals for 3 months followed by 1-month intervals for 3 months, followed by 2-month intervals for the remainder of 1 year of hCG titer surveillance. If the patient remains in prolonged hCG titer remission, titer surveillance is then performed at 6-month intervals indefinitely. Fertility is excellent after successful therapy of malignant GTN. There has not been an increase in congenital anomalies among the offspring of women who have been successfully treated.

ENDOCRINOLOGY, CONTRACEPTION, AND INFERTILITY
Amenorrhea

Amenorrhea is defined as the absence of menses by 14 years of age in the absence of secondary sexual development, absence of menstruation by 16 years of age, or the absence of menses for a length of time equivalent to three previous menstrual cycles in a woman who has been menstruating. Amenorrhea may be caused by disorders of any of the components of the hypothalamic-pituitary-ovarian-gonadal-genital system.

Primary amenorrhea

Patients with primary amenorrhea will have one of the following general causes.

Congenital anomalies. Patients with congenital anomalies of the müllerian tract have normal secondary sexual characteristics and normal karyotype. Pelvic examination should show the abnormality (i.e., transverse vaginal septum) that prevents normal menses, as discussed previously.

Gonadal dysgenesis. Gonadal dysgenesis ranges from the classic "Turner's" (45,XO) karyotype with short stature and other somatic abnormalities to mosaic variants with normal physical appearance but with secondary amenorrhea and early ovarian failure. Patients with elevated gonadotropins (FSH greater than 40 mIU/ml.) should have a chromosome karyotype to identify XY mosaicism. Gonadectomy is indicated in patients with a Y chromosome to prevent potential neoplasm formation. These patients are infertile and require estrogen replacement.

Intersex. Intersex patients have divergent phenotypes. Patients with testicular feminization have an XY karyotype but appear as normal females lacking pubic and axillary hair. The gonads are testicles, but androgen-sensitive tissues in these patients lack intracellular androgen receptors or are unable to convert testosterone to dihydrotestosterone. These patients lack a uterus and upper vagina because they do respond to müllerian duct–inhibiting substance secreted by the testes. The gonads are either intra-abdominal or located in the inguinal canal. They should be removed because of potential tumor formation. Estrogen replacement and formation of a neovagina are indicated to fulfill the female sexual identity of these patients.

Overproduction of androgens from adrenal or ovarian sources can cause hirsutism, acne, deep voice, and clitoral hypertrophy along with primary amenorrhea. Polycystic ovarian syndrome can occasionally develop similar manifestations. Adrenogenital syndrome with cliteromegaly may rarely not be diagnosed until adolescence.

Hypothalamic amenorrhea. Patients with normal female karyotype, low gonadotropin, and hypoestrogenism usually have suppression of hypothalamic releasing factors. Psychogenic stress and certain drugs can alter the synthesis and metabolism of monoamine neurotransmitters and produce functional alterations of the hypothalamic gonadotropin regulating centers. Pituitary or peripituitary tumors are rare but can also produce hypothalamic amenorrhea. Constitutional delayed onset of menarche with delayed maturation of the hypothalamic regulatory centers is another cause. Bone growth should be assessed and low doses of estrogen may be employed to facilitate development of secondary sexual characteristics.

Secondary amenorrhea

Secondary amenorrhea is defined as absence of menses for three menstrual cycles in a previously menstruating woman. The causes are as follows:

Pregnancy. Pregnancy should be considered and excluded by examination and hCG testing.

Hyperprolactinemia. Many women with secondary amenorrhea have elevated prolactin levels. Many of these patients have galactorrhea. Pituitary prolactinomas should be ruled out by CT scan or tomography of the pituitary sella in women who have prolactin levels elevated about 20 ng./ml. Low-level elevations of prolactin may be caused by psychotropic medications (e.g., narcotics, major and minor tranquilizers) and hypothyroidism with elevated TSH. If a prolactinoma is present, transsphenoidal microsurgery is generally utilized to remove the tumor. Bromocriptine, a dopamine agonist, is also utilized for the conservative therapy of prolactinomas.

Excess androgen syndrome. Polycystic ovarian syndrome with chronic anovulation and mild androgen excess is a common cause of anovulation. Signs of virilization such as clitoral hypertrophy, temporal balding, and deepening of the voice is indicative of an androgen-producing tumor and is confirmed by testosterone levels elevated to normal male levels. Laboratory findings of polycystic ovarian syndrome include withdrawal bleeding with progesterone administration, elevated serum LH, slightly elevated testosterone, elevated urinary 17-ketosteroid or blood dehydroepiandrosterone sulfate levels. Management varies, depending on the goal as discussed in the section on polycystic ovarian syndrome, and includes ovulation induction, cycling with combination estrogen-progestin contraceptive pills, or monthly administration of progestin.

Hypothalamic amenorrhea. Patients with disruption of normal hypothalamic-pituitary-ovarian function may secrete enough gonadotropin to stimulate the ovary, resulting in low levels of estrogen but without a midcycle estradiol peak and LH surge. Some patients have extremely low levels of FSH and LH resulting in no follicular development and minimal estrogen output. These patients are hypoestrogenic and do not respond to a progesterone challenge test. Many causes for hypothalamic amenorrhea have been documented including acute and chronic stress, weight loss, and psychogenic causes. Since nonfunctioning pituitary tumors can cause hypothalamic amenorrhea, these must be ruled out. Management depends on the cause and desires of the patient. Treatment may include estrogen supplementation, weight gain, removal of stress, and psychotherapy.

Ovarian failure. Cessation of menses associated with an FSH level over 40 mIU/ml. is diagnostic of ovarian failure. Causes include chromosomal mosaicism, autoimmune disorders, gonadotropin-resistant ovaries, and premature menopause. Patients with ovarian failure are sterile and require estrogen replacement.

MISCELLANEOUS GYNECOLOGICAL ENDOCRINE DISORDERS
Polycystic ovarian disease

Patients with polycystic ovarian disease (PCOD) may present with a wide range of symptoms suggestive of chronic anovulation and production of androgens by ovarian stromal cells. The classical Stein-Leventhal syndrome includes amenorrhea, hirsutism, and obesity, but these patients comprise only a relatively small number of patients with PCOD. Frequently, patients will have an elevated LH and normal FSH. A small percentage will have elevated prolactin. Continuous ovarian stromal production of androstenedione with peripheral conversion to estrone may result in anovulatory bleeding or amenorrhea. Patients are infertile and do not demonstrate a normal basal body temperature rise indicative of ovulation if they are having regular menses. Ovarian stromal production of testosterone and androstenedione may result in hyperandrogenism with hirsutism or acne. Rarely do patients with PCOD have true virilism.

Management depends on the therapeutic goal. If fertility is desired, clomiphene citrate, an antiestrogen ovulation-inducing agent, may be used. The unopposed endogenous estrogenic stimulation of the endometrium will predispose to endometrial hyperplasia and possibly endometrial carcinoma. Therefore patients not desiring fertility should be cycled with either combination estrogen-progestin contraceptives or monthly progestin. Cosmetic improvement of acne and hirsutism may be obtained with combination oral contraceptives that increase hepatic production of sex hormone–binding globulin, decrease free testosterone, and interfere with androgen action on target tissues. Spironolactone is also effective in ameliorating hirsutism. Medical management does not cause the hirsutism to regress, but rather ceases progression. Electrolysis may be employed to remove unwanted facial hair. After failure of medical management for induction of fertility or control of hirsutism, bilateral wedge resection of the ovaries may be considered. This decreases circulating levels of androgens and may result in ovulation.

Dysfunctional uterine bleeding (DUB)

Irregular and occasionally excessive anovulatory uterine bleeding is caused by uninterrupted estrogen effect. Prolonged exposure to estrogen may lead to endometrial hyperplasia. DUB is frequently seen at the extremes of reproductive life: in the adolescent before she develops consistent ovulation and in the perimenopausal woman as ovarian function declines. Excessive bleeding can be managed by cyclic estrogen-progestin hormonal therapy, but older patients require endometrial sampling to rule out endometrial carcinoma.

Estrogen replacement therapy

Perimenopausal and postmenopausal estrogen replacement relieves vasomotor symptoms (hot flashes), improves atrophic genital tissue, retards osteoporosis, and may possibly have cardiovascular benefits. The most widely publicized risk of estrogen replacement therapy is the increased risk for developing endometrial carcinoma in patients who have received exogenous estrogens. Estrogen replacement does not appear to increase the risk of breast carcinoma but should not be used in a patient with a prior history of an estrogen-dependent tumor. Estrogen replacement should be administered at the lowest effective dose in a cyclical manner (21 to 25 days each month). The addition of progestin during the last 10 days of each cycle appears to protect against endometrial hyperplasia and endometrial carcinoma. Endometrial biopsies should be employed liberally in these patients if they develop vaginal bleeding.

CONTRACEPTION AND STERILIZATION

Currently the most effective method of contraception is the oral combination estrogen-progestin pill. The oral combination pill results in continuous therapeutic levels of estrogen and progestin, causing hypothalamic suppression of releasing factors with decreased gonadotropin secretion leading to inhibition of ovulation. The therapeutic levels of estrogen and progestin affect many physiological and metabolic processes. Common side effects include nausea, spotting, minor psychological disturbances, and weight gain. More serious side effects include thromboembolism, increased serum lipids, hypertension, and altered liver function. Rare liver neoplasms have been caused by oral contraceptives. The majority of these serious metabolic effects are associated with estrogen; therefore it is recommended that pills containing less than 50 µg. of estrogen initially be prescribed. Older patients should employ some other form of contraception, since there is an increased incidence of coronary artery disease associated with oral contraceptives. This risk is further increased among smokers. The theoretical effectiveness of the combination oral contraceptive approaches 99%. The "minipill" consists of a low dose of progestin, which is taken daily. A higher failure rate and frequent breakthrough bleeding is observed with its use.

The intrauterine device (IUD) is another effective mode of contraception. Devices include inert plastic IUD's, IUD's wound with copper wire, and progestin-saturated IUDs. The effects are generally limited to the female genital tract and appear as chronic endometritis and alteration of cervical mucus. The IUD does not usually prevent fertilization but prevents implantation of the fertilized ovum. Problems associated with the IUD include uterine perforation, dysmenorrhea, menorrhagia, uterine expulsion, and pelvic inflammatory disease. Attached to the end of the IUD generally is a string, which is placed through the cervical canal and is visualized in the vagina. If the string of an IUD is not visualized, the patient should be evaluated with ultrasound or abdominal plain film to confirm intrauterine placement of the IUD and exclude the possibility of a late perforation or IUD expulsion. Since the IUD protects against uterine implantation, there is a higher incidence of ectopic pregnancy in women who become pregnant with an IUD in place.

Barrier methods of contraception include the diaphragm combined with spermacidal jelly, cervical cap, vaginal contraceptive foam, and condom. These are less effective contraceptive techniques but have no systemic side effects.

Permanent contraception may be achieved by surgical sterilization. Although tubal ligation may be performed by either the abdominal or the vaginal route with low morbidity or mortality, vasectomy in the male is a less morbid procedure and should be seriously considered for a couple desiring permanent sterilization. Tubal sterilization by laparoscopy has become the most frequent sterilization procedure. It can often be performed as an outpatient but should be considered a major surgical procedure.

INFERTILITY

Infertility is defined as 1 year of unprotected intercourse without pregnancy and affects approximately 15% of couples. Approximately one third involve a male factor. The most common causes of female infertility are anovulation and tubal obstruction. Cervical factors are occasionally found. No cause will be found in 15% to 20% of infertile couples.

Infertility evaluation

After a complete medical and sexual history and physical examination with pelvic examination, a "factor analysis" should be performed (Table 43-4).

Therapy

Male. The infertile male should consult a urologist. Artificial insemination may be required for an unfavorable seminogram.

Cervical factor. Thick, "hostile" cervical mucus at the time of ovulation can be improved with preovulatory estrogen. Many white blood cells in cervical mucus are suggestive of cervicitis and should be treated with antibiotics. The presence of

Table 43-4. Factor analysis

Factor	Test	Normal findings
Male	Seminogram	20 million sperm with 75% motility and normal forms/ml.
Cervical	Sims-Huhner (obtain endocervical mucus at ovulation time, 2 to 6 hours after coitus)	Clear elastic mucus containing 2 to 20 motile sperm/hpf*; minimal cells; few nonmotile sperm
Tubal	Rubin's (CO_2 uterotubal insufflation)	Shoulder pain; normal tracing on machine
	Hysterosalpingogram (water-soluble radiopaque medium instilled under fluoroscopy)	Normal uterine cavity, tubes, and intraperitoneal spill
Ovulatory	Basal body temperature	Biphasic pattern with 14-day rise
	Endometrial biopsy	Dated secretory changes
	Plasma progesterone	5 to 20 ng./ml. on day 22
	Urinary pregnanediol	Over 3 mg./24 hr.
Miscellaneous	Laparoscopy	No evidence of endometriosis, adhesions, or ovarian pathosis

hpf, High-powered field.

antisperm antibodies in the cervical mucus are suggested when the sperm are nonmotile. There is a wide variety of techniques for measuring antisperm antibodies, but unfortunately none has proved to be clinically reliable. Condoms can be utilized for 6 months along with corticosteroids in an attempt to reduce antisperm antibodies.

Tubal factor. Tuboplasty is utilized in patients who have abnormalities of the tube identified on hysterosalpingography or laparoscopy. Patients who do not have bilateral tubal occlusion should have a complete evaluation of the patient and her partner for other factors before employing surgery. Tuboplasty procedures include salpingolysis, fimbrioplasty, salpingostomy, tubal anastomosis, and cornual implantation. Intraperitoneal high molecular weight dextran is employed to reduce postoperative adhesions. Postoperative tubal hydrotubation also appears helpful. Microsurgical techniques with meticulous attention to hemostasis and minimizing tissue trauma improve pregnancy rates.

Ovulatory factor. Clomiphene citrate is the most commonly used agent for inducing ovulation. Clomiphene has an antiestrogenic effect on the hypothalamus resulting in increased gonadotropin-releasing factors and gonadotropins. An intact hypothalamic-pituitary-ovarian axis with endogenous estrogen production is necessary for ovulation induction with clomiphene. The dose of clomiphene is escalated during succeeding cycles until ovulation is achieved. Ovulation can be achieved in approximately 80% of patients, but only half of these will become pregnant. The incidence of spontaneous abortion and twin gestation is increased. Ovarian hyperstimulation may result in ovarian cysts, which are treated conservatively.

Menopausal gonadotropins (Pergonal) and human chorionic gonadotropin (hCG) acting as an LH substitute may be used in patients who are resistant to clomiphene or who lack an intact hypothalmic-pituitary-ovarian axis. Pergonal requires daily injections with frequent monitoring of estrogen levels to avoid hyperstimulation of the ovaries. Multiple pregnancies are often observed. Gonadotropin-releasing factors are not yet available for routine ovulation induction.

Miscellaneous. If no causative factor for infertility is determined, laparoscopy should be performed to exclude tubal or peritoneal causes of infertility. Positive findings approach 20%.

Previously, options for infertile couples unable to achieve pregnancy by any of the aforementioned treatments have been limited to adoption. Currently, the application of techniques utilized in animal husbandry for in vitro fertilization and embryo transfer offer new options to these couples. In vitro fertilization is achieved by producing ovarian hyperstimulation using menopausal gonadotropins. Ova are harvested by laparoscopy and selected ova are fertilized with sperm. After appropriate maturation, the embryo is implanted into the endometrial cavity. Currently, the cost and success rate for in vitro fertilization make it prohibitive for routine use. Embryo transfer techniques may have a higher success rate but, as with surrogate motherhood, ethical and legal issues have yet to be resolved for this controversial procedure.

Bibliography

CHAPTER 1
Origin of Surgical Disease

Anson, B.J., and McVay, C.P.: Surgical anatomy, Philadelphia, 1984, W.B. Saunders Co.

Cuschieri, A., Giles, G.R., and Moosa, A.R.: Essential surgical practice, London, 1983, John Wright & Sons, Ltd.

Dunphy, J.E., and Botsford, T.W.: Physical examination of the surgical patient, Philadelphia, 1975, W.B. Saunders Co.

Greenfield, L.: Complications in surgery and trauma, Philadelphia, 1984, J.B. Lippincott.

Hardy, J.: Textbook of surgery, Philadelphia, 1983, J.B. Lippincott Co.

Maingot, R.: Abdominal operations, ed. 7, New York, 1980, Appleton-Century-Crofts.

Nora, P.F.: Operative surgery, ed. 2, Philadelphia, 1980, Lea & Febiger.

Rosai, J.: Ackerman's surgical pathology, ed. 6, St. Louis, 1981, The C.V. Mosby Co.

Sabiston, D.C.: Christopher's textbook of surgery, ed. 12, Philadelphia, 1983, W.B. Saunders Co.

Schwartz, S.I., Shires, T.C., et al., editors: Principles of surgery, ed. 4, New York, 1984, McGraw-Hill Book Co.

Shackelford, R.T., and Zuidema, G.: Surgery of the alimentary tract, ed. 3, Philadelphia, 1982, W.B. Saunders Co.

Zollinger, R.M., and Zollinger, R.M., Jr.: Atlas of surgical operations, ed. 5, New York, 1983, The Macmillan Co.

CHAPTER 2
Wounds, Wound Healing, and Drains

Dineen, P., and Hildick Smith, G.: The surgical wound, Philadelphia, 1981, Lea & Febiger.

Gabbiani, G., et al.: Granulation tissue as a contractile organ, J. Exp. Med. **135:**719, 1972.

Morton, D., Madden, J.W., and Peacock, E.E.: Effect of a local smooth muscle antagonist on wound contraction, Surg. Forum **23:**511, 1972.

Mujino, G., Gabbiani, G., et al.: Contraction of granulation tissue in vitro: similarity to smooth muscle, Science **173:**548, 1971.

Peacock. E.E., and Van Winkle, W.: Wound repair, ed. 3, Philadelphia, 1984, W.B. Saunders Co.

Rudolph, R.: Contraction and the control of contraction, World J. Surg. **4:**275, 1980.

CHAPTER 3
Fluids and Electrolytes

Cohen, J.J., and Jassirer, J.P.: Acid-base, Boston, 1982, Little, Brown & Co.

Davenport, H.W.: The ABC of acid-base chemistry, ed. 6, Chicago, 1974, The University of Chicago Press.

Kinney, J.M., Lister, J., and Moore, F.D.: Relationship of energy expenditure to total exchangeable potassium, Ann. N.Y. Acad. Sci. **110:**711, 1963.

Kwun, K.B., Boucherit, T., Wong, J., Richards, Y., and Bryan-Brown, C.W.: Treatment of metabolic alkalosis with intravenous infusion of concentrated hydrochloric acid, Am. J. Surg. **146:**328, 1983.

Leaf, A.: The clinical and physiological significance of the serum sodium concentration, N. Engl. J. Med. **267:**24, 77, 1962.

Mason, E.E.: Fluid, electrolyte and nutrient therapy in surgery, Philadelphia, 1974, Lea & Febiger.

Mason, E.E., and Dryer, R.L.: The implications of abnormal sodium concentration, Surg. Gynecol. Obstet. **105:**273, 1957.

Mundy, G.R., and Martin, T.J.: The hypercalcemia of malignancy: pathogenesis and management, Metabolism **31:**1247-1277, 1982.

Shapiro, B.A., Harrison, R.A., and Walton, J.R.: Clinical application of blood gases, ed. 2, Chicago, 1977, Year Book Medical Publishers, Inc.

Winters, R.W.: Principles of pediatric fluid therapy, ed. 2, Boston, 1982, Little, Brown & Co.

CHAPTER 4
Disorders of Hemostasis: Diagnosis and Treatment

Colman, R.W., Hirsh, J., Marder, V.J., and Salzman, E.W.: Hemostasis and thrombosis: basic principles and clinical practice, Philadelphia, 1982, J.B. Lippincott Co.

Colman, R.W., Robboy, S.J., and Minna, J.D.: Disseminated intravascular coagulation: a reappraisal, Annu. Rev. Med. **30:**359, 1979.

Goldsmith, J.C.: Medical management of dental patients with bleeding disorders, J. Iowa Med. Soc. **71:**291, 1981.

Goldsmith, J.C., Chung, K.S., Blatt, P.M., and Roberts, H.R.: The role of the normal and diseased liver in blood coagulation. In Seligson, D., and Schmidt, R.M., editors: CRC handbook of hematology, sect. 1, vol. 3, Boca Raton, 1980, CRC Press.

Goldsmith, J.C., Unger, H.A., and Fried, F.A.: Successful prostatectomy in patients with inherited abnormalities of the factor VIII molecule, J. Urol. **124:**570, 1980.

Mannucci, P.M., Canciani, M.T., Rota, L., and Donovan, B.S.: Response of factor VIII/von Willebrand factor to DDAVP in healthy subjects and patients with haemophilia A and von Willebrand's disease, Br. J. Haematol. **47:**283, 1981.

Rapaport, S.I.: Preoperative hemostatic evaluation: which tests, if any? Blood **61:**229, 1983.

Thompson, A.R., and Harker, L.A.: Manual of hemostasis and thrombosis, Philadelphia, 1983, F.A. Davis Co.

Triplett, D.A.: Laboratory evaluation of coagulation, Chicago, 1982, American Society of Clinical Pathologists Press.

CHAPTER 5
Shock

Altemeier, W.A., Todd, J.C., and Wellford, W.I.: Gram-negative septicemia: a growing threat, Ann. Surg. **116:**530, 1967.

Collins, J.A.: The pathophysiology of hemorrhagic shock, Prog. Clin. Biol. Res. **108:**5, 1982.

Hardaway, R.M., et al.: Intensive study and treatment of shock in man, J.A.M.A. **199:**779, 1967.

Holcraft, J.W., and Trunkey, D.D.: Pathophysiology of shock and adult respiratory distress syndrome, Surg. Ann. **15:**1, 1983.

Lillehei, R.C., et al.: The nature of irreversible shock: experimental and clinical observations, Ann. Surg. **160:**682, 1964.

MacLean, L.D.: Shock: causes and management of circulatory collapse. In Sabiston, D.C., Jr.: Davis-Christopher textbook of surgery, ed. 12, Philadelphia, 1981, W.B. Saunders Co.

MacLean, L.D., et al.: Patterns of septic shock in man: a detailed study of 56 patients, Ann. Surg. **166:**543, 1967.

Parker, M.M., and Parrillo, J.E.: Septic shock: hemodynamics and pathogenesis, J.A.M.A. **250:**3324, 1983.

Rackow, E.C., Fein, I.A., and Siegel, J.: The relationship of the colloid osmotic: pulmonary artery wedge pressure gradient to pulmonary edema and mortality in critically ill patients, Chest **82:**433, 1982.

Rackow, E.C., et al.: fluid resuscitation in circulatory shock: a comparison of the cardiorespiratory effects of albumin, hetastarch, and saline solution in patients with hypovolemic and septic shock, Crit. Care Med. **11:**839, 1983.

Reingold, A.L., et al.: Nonmenstrual toxic shock syndrome, Ann. Intern. Med. **96:**871, 1982.

Resnekov, L.: Cardiogenic shock, Chest **83:**893, 1983.

Shoemaker, W.C.: Shock, Springfield, Ill., 1967, Charles C Thomas, Publisher.

Shubin, H., and Weil, M.H.: Bacterial shock, J.A.M.A. **235:**421, 1976.

Swan, H.J.C., et al.: Catheterization of the heart in man with use of a flow-directed balloon-tipped catheter, N. Engl. J. Med. **283:**447, 1970.

Vargish, T.: The role of endogenous opiates in the pathophysiology of hypovolemic shock and their interrelationship with the pituitary-adrenal axis, Adv. Shock Res. **10:**57, 1983.

Wagner, G.P.: Toxic shock syndrome: a review, Am. J. Obstet. Gynecol. **146:**93, 1983.

Wilson, J.N., et al.: Central venous pressure in optimal blood volume maintenance, Arch. Surg. **85:**563, 1962.

Wilson, R.F.: Shock: the principles and techniques of critical care, Kalamazoo, Mich., 1976, Upjohn Co., Inc.

CHAPTER 6
Surgical Infection

Alexander, J.W.: Host defense mechanisms against infection, Surg. Clin. North Am. **52**(6):1367-1378, 1972.

Altemeier, W.A., and Fallen, W.D.: Prevention and treatment of gas gangrene, J.A.M.A. **217**(6):806-813, 1971.

Baxter, C.R.: Surgical management of soft tissue infection, Surg. Clin. North Am. **52**(6):1483-1499, 1972.

Bessman, A.N., and Wagner, W.: Nonclostridial gas gangrene, J.A.M.A. **233**(9):958-963, 1975.

Edwards, L.D.: The epidemiology of 2,056 remote site infections and 1,966 surgical wound infections occurring in 1,865 patients, Ann. Surg. **184**(6):758-766, 1976.

Flynn, N.M.: Antimicrobial prophylaxis for surgery, Hosp. Physician, pp. 110-119, Feb. 1984.

Kalisman, M., Millendorf, J.B., and Schiffman, E.: Clinical tetanus: prevention and management of an uncommon disease, Infection in Surg. **3**(4):291-302, 1984.

Kerstein, M.D.: Introduction. In Kerstein, M.D., editor: Management of surgical infections, Mt. Kisco, N.Y., 1980, Futura Publishing Co., Inc.

Maki, D.G.: The epidemiology of surgical wound infection. In Condon, R.E., and Gorbach, S.L., editors: Surgical infections, Baltimore, 1981, The Williams & Wilkins Co.

Polk, H.C., Fry, D., and Flint, L.M.: Dissemination and causes of infection, Surg. Clin. North Am. **56**(4):817-829, 1976.

Rothstein, R.J., and Baker, F.J.: Tetanus: prevention and treatment, J.A.M.A. **240**(7):675-676, 1978.

Weinstein, L., and Barza, M.A.: Gas gangrene, N. Engl. J. Med. **289**(21):1129-1131, 1973.

Young, L.S.: Advances in managing gram-negative septicemia, Drug Therapy, pp. 24-30, Feb. 1984.

CHAPTER 7
Surgical Nutrition

American College of Surgeons Committee on Pre- and Postoperative Care, Dudrick, S.J., et al.: Manual of preoperative and postoperative care, ed. 3, Philadelphia, 1983, W.B. Saunders Co.

Baker, J.P., et al.: Nutritional assessment: a comparison of clinical judgment and objective measurements, N. Engl. J. Med. **306:**960, 1982.

Cerra, F.B., et al.: Septic autocannibalism: a failure of exogenous nutritional support, Ann. Surg. **192:**570, 1980.

Delany, H.M., et al.: Postoperative nutritional support using needle catheter feeding jejunostomy, Ann. Surg. **186:**165, 1977.

Fischer, J.E.: Nutritional support in the serious ill patient, Curr. Probl. Surg. **17:**1 (entire issue), Sept. 1980.

Freeman, J.B.: Peripheral parenteral nutrition, Can. J. Surg. **21:**489, 1978.

Goodgame, J.T., Jr.: A critical assessment of the indications for total parenteral nutrition, Surg. Gynecol. Obstet. **151:**433, 1980.

Heymsfield, S.B., et al.: Enteral hyperalimentation: an alternative to central venous hyperalimentation, Am. Intern. Med. **90:**63, 1979.

Johnson, D.G.: Total intravenous nutrition in newborn surgical patients: a three-year perspective, J. Pediatr. Surg. **5:**601, 1970.

Mullen, J.L., et al.: Reduction of operative morbidity and mortality by combined preoperative and postoperative nutritional support, Ann. Surg. **192:**604, 1980.

Mullen, J.L., editor: Surgical nutrition, Surg. Clin. North Am. (June) **61:**427 (entire issue), 1981.

Sheldon, G.F., and Baker, C.: Complications of nutritional support, Crit. Care Med. **8:**35, 1980.

CHAPTER 8
Preoperative Care

American College of Surgeons Committee on Pre- and Postoperative Care, Dudrick, S.J., et al.: Manual of preoperative and postoperative care, ed. 3, Philadelphia, 1983, W.B. Saunders Co.

Brenowitz, J.B., Williams, C.D., and Edwards, W.S.: Major surgery in patients with chronic renal failure, Am. J. Surg. **134:**765, 1977.

Bunker, J.P., and Wennberg, J.E.: Operation rates, mortality statistics and the quality of life, N. Engl. J. Med. **289:**1249, 1973.

Gaensler, E.A., and Weisel, R.D.: The risks in abdominal and thoracic surgery in COPD, Postgrad. Med. **54:**183, 1973.

Goldman, D.R.: Medical care of the surgical patient, Philadelphia, 1982, J.B. Lippincott Co.

Goldman, L., Caldera, D.L., Nussbaum, S.R., et al.: Multifactorial index of cardiac risk in noncardiac surgical procedures, N. Engl. J. Med. **297:**845, 1977.

Kyle, J., and Hardy, J.D.: Scientific foundations of surgery, London, 1981, William Heinemann, Ltd.

Lee, Y.N.: Effect of anesthesia and surgery on immunity, J. Surg. Oncol. **9:**425, 1977.

Strunin, L.: Preoperative assessment of the patient with liver dysfunction, Br. J. Anaesth. **50:**25, 1978.

CHAPTER 9
Anesthesia

Caplan, J.A.: Cardiac anesthesia, vol. 1, New York, 1979, Grune & Stratton, Inc.

Caplan, J.A.: Cardiac anesthesia, vol. 2, New York, 1983, Grune & Stratton, Inc.

Churchill-Davidson, H.C.: A practice of anaesthesia, Philadelphia, 1979, W.B. Saunders Co.

Gray, T.C., Nunn, J.F., and Utting, J.E.: General anaesthesia, Woburn, Mass., 1980, Butterworth Publishers.

Miller, R.D.: Anesthesia, Edinburgh, Scotland, 1981, Churchill Livingstone.

Tinker, J.H., and Rapin, M.: Care of the critically ill patient, Berlin, 1983, Springer-Verlag.

CHAPTER 10
Postoperative Care

American College of Surgeons Committee on Pre- and Postoperative Care, Dudrick, S.J., et al.: Manual of preoperative and postoperative care, ed. 3, Philadelphia, 1983, W.B. Saunders Co.

Fariello, R.G., and Mutani, R.: Treatment of hiccup, Lancet **2:**1201, 1974.

Freischlag, J., and Busuttil R.W.: The value of postoperative fever evaluation, Surgery **94:**358, 1983.

Greenfield, L.J.: Complications in surgery and trauma, Philadelphia, 1984, J.B. Lippincott Co.

Shapiro, B.A., Harrison, R.A., and Trout, C.A.: Clinical application of respiratory care, ed. 2, Chicago, 1979, Year Book Medical Publishers.

CHAPTER 11
Malignant Neoplasms

Carter, S.K., Bakowski, M.T. and Hellmann, K.: Chemotherapy of cancer, New York, 1977, John Wiley & Sons.

del Regato, J.A., and Spjut, H.J.: Ackerman and del Regato's Cancer: diagnosis, treatment, and prognosis, ed. 5, St. Louis, 1977, The C.V. Mosby Co.

Holland, J.F., and Frei, E.: Cancer medicine, ed. 2, Philadelphia, 1978, Lea & Febiger.

Proceedings of the American Cancer Society–National Cancer Institute National Conference on Advances in Cancer Management, Part II: Detection and diagnosis, Cancer **37**(suppl.):1, 1976.

Proceedings of the 1977 Workshop on Large Bowel Cancer, National Large Bowel Cancer, National Large Bowel Cancer Project, Cancer **40**(suppl.):5, 1977.

Proceedings of the National Cancer Institute Division of Cancer Research Resources and Centers, Clinical Investigations Branch, and the Cancer Clinical Investigation Review Committee Conference on Cancer Epidemiology and the Clinician, Cancer **39**(suppl.):4, 1977.

Raven, R.W., editor: Outlook on cancer, New York, 1979, Plenum Publishing Co.

Mikol, Y.B., and Lipkin, M.: Methionine dependence in skin fibroblasts of humans: affects with familial colon cancer or Gardner's syndrome, National Cancer Institute Monogr. **72:**19-22, 1984.

Proceedings of the American Cancer Society On Breast Cancer 1983, Cancer **54**(suppl.):589-828, Feb. 1984.

Gyres, J.W., et al.: A totally implanted infection port system for blood drawing and chemotherapy administration, J.A.M.A. **251**:2538-2541, 1984.

CHAPTER 12
The Skin

Apfelberg, D.B., Maser, M.R., and Lash, H.: Argon laser treatment of cutaneous vascular abnormalities, Ann. Plast. Surg. **1**:14, 1978.

Breslow, A.: Thickness, cross-sectional areas and depth of invasion in the prognosis of cutaneous melanomas, Ann. Surg. **172**:902, 1970.

Clark, N.H., Fromm, L., Bernardino, E.A., et al.: The histogenesis and biologic behavior of primary human malignant melanomas of the skin, Cancer Res. **29**:705, 1969.

Cosman, B.: Experience in the argon laser therapy of port wine stains, Plast. Reconstr. Surg. **65**:119, 1980.

Edgerton, M.T.: The treatment of hemangiomas with special reference to the role of steroid therapy, Ann. Surg. **183**:517, 1976.

Fergin, P.E., Chu, A.C., and McDonald, D.M.: Basal cell carcinomas complicating nevus sebaceus, Clin. Exp. Dermatol. **6**:111, 1981.

Fitzpatrick, T.B., Eisen, A.C., Wolff, K., et al., editors: Dermatology in general medicine, New York, 1979, McGraw Hill Book Co.

Lever, W.F., and Schaumberg-Lever, G.: Histopatology of the skin, ed. 6, Philadelphia, 1983, J.B. Lippincott Co.

McGovern, V.J. Mihm, M.C., et al.: The classification of malignant melanoma and its histologic reporting, Cancer **32**:1446, 1973.

Pathak, M.A.: Sunscreens: topical and systemic approaches for protection of human skin against harmful effects of solar radiation, J. Am. Acad. Dermatol. **7**:285, 1982.

Williams, H.B.: The use of dermabrasion in giant pigmented nevi, Chapter 32 in Williams, H.B., editor: Symposium on Vascular Malformations in Melanotic Lesions, Vol. 22, St. Louis, 1983, The C.V. Mosby Co.

Wisnicki, J.L.: Hemangiomas and vascular malformations, Ann. Plast. Surg. **12**:41, 1984.

CHAPTER 13
The Thyroid Gland

Block, M.A.: Management of carcinoma of the thyroid, Ann. Surg. **185**:133, 1977.

Bradley, E.L., and Liechty, R.D.: Modified subtotal thyroidectomy for Graves' disease: a two institution study, Surgery **94**:955, 1983.

Cady, B.: Surgery of thyroid cancer, World J. Surg. **5**:3, 1981.

Degroot, L.J., and Larsen, P.R.: Thyroid and its diseases, New York, 1984, John Wiley & Sons, Inc.

Hubert, J.P., Kiernan, P.D., Beahrs, O.H., et al.: Occult papillary carcinoma of the thyroid, Arch. Surg. **115**:394, 1980.

Liechty, R.D., and Zimmerman, D.: Solitary thyroid nodules, Arch. Surg. **112**:59, 1977.

Lowhagen, T., Willem, J.S., and Lundell, G.: Aspiration biopsy cytology in diagnosis of thyroid cancer, World J. Surg. **5**:61, 1981.

Johnston, I.D.A., and Thompson, N.W.: Endocrine surgery, London, 1983, Butterworth & Co.

Kaplan, E.L.: Surgery of the thyroid and parathyroid glands, Edinburgh, 1983, Churchhill Livingstone.

Werner, S.C., and Ingbar, S.H.: The thyroid, ed. 4, Philadelphia, 1978, J.B. Lippincott Co.

CHAPTER 14
Parathyroid Glands

Haussler, M.R., and McCain, T.A.: Basic and clinical concepts related to vitamin D metabolism and action, N. Engl. J. Med. **297**:974, 1041, 1977.

Johnston, I.D.A., and Thompson, N.W.: Endocrine surgery, London, 1983, Butterworth & Co.

Kaplan, E.L.: Surgery of the thyroid and parathyroid glands, Edinburgh, 1983, Churchhill Livingston.

Liechty, R.D. and Weil, R.: The anatomy of parathyroid hyperplasia, Surgery **96**:1099, 1984.

Paloyan, E., Lawrence, A.M., and Straus, F.H.: Hyperparathyroidism, New York, 1973, Grune & Stratton Inc.

Purnell, D.C., Scholz, D.A., and Beahrs, O.H.: Hyperparathyroidism due to single gland enlargement, Arch. Surg. **112**:369, 1977.

Saxe, A.W., and Brennan, M.F.: Strategy and technique of reoperative parathyroid surgery, Surgery **89**:417, 1981.

Wells, S.A., Gunnells, C.J., Shelburne, J.D., et al.: Transplantation of the parathyroid glands in man: clinical indications and results, Surgery **78**:34, 1975.

CHAPTER 15
The Adrenal Glands

Bigos, S.T., Somma, M., Rasio, E., et al.: Cushing's disease: management by transsphenoidal microsurgery, J. Clin. Endocrinol. Metab. **50**:348, 1980.

Friesen, S.R.: Surgical endocrinology: clinical syndromes, Philadelphia, 1978, J.B. Lippincott Co.

Johnston, I.D.A., and Thompson, N.W.: Endocrine surgery, London, 1983, Butterworth & Co.

Prinz, R.A., Brooks, M.H., Lawrence, A.M., et al.: Cushing's disease: the role of adrenalectomy and autotransplantation, Surg. Clin. North Am. **59**:159, 1979.

Sisson, J.C., Frager, M.S., Yalk, T.W., et al.: Scintigraphic localization of pheochromocytoma, N. Engl. J. Med. **305**:12, 1981.

Thompson, N.W., and Vinik, A.I.: Endocrine surgery update, New York, 1983, Grune & Stratton.

Welbourn, R.B.: Some aspects of adrenal surgery, Br. J. Surg. **67**:723, 1980.

Grant, C.S., Carpenter, P., van Heerden, J.A., et al.: Primary aldosteronism, Arch. Surg. **119**:585, 1984.

CHAPTER 16
The Breast

Bonadonna, G., Rossi, A., Valagussa, P. et al.: The CMF program for operable breast cancer with positive axillary nodes, Cancer **39**:2904, 1977.

Bonadonna, G., Valagussa, P.: Dose-response effect of adjuvant chemotherapy in breast cancer, N. Engl. J. Med. **304**:10, 1981.

Donegan, W.L., and Spratt, J.S.: Cancer of the breast, Philadelphia, 1979, W.B. Saunders Co.

Fisher, B., Montague, E., Redmond, C., et al. Comparison of radical mastectomy with alternative treatments for primary breast cancer, Cancer, **39**:2827, 1977.

Fisher B., Glass, A., Redmond, C., and Fisher, E.R., et al.: L-Phenylalanine mustard (L-PAM) in the management of primary breast cancer, Cancer **39**:2883, 1977.

Haagensen, C.D.: Diseases of the breast, ed. 2, Philadelphia, 1971, W.B. Saunders Co.

Henderson, I.C., and Canellos, G.P.: Cancer of the breast: the past decade, N. Engl. J. Med. **302**:17, 78, 1980.

Macdonald, I.: The natural history of breast cancer, Am. J. Surg. **3**:435, 1966.

McDivitt, R.W., Urban, J.A., and Farrow, J.H.: Cystosarcoma phyllodes, Johns Hopkins Med. J. **120**:33, 1967.

Moxley, J.H., Allegra, J.C., Henney, J., and Muggia, F.: Treatment of primary breast cancer: summary of the National Institutes of Health Consensus Development Conference, J.A.M.A. **244**:797, 1980.

Peters, M.V.: The effect of pregnancy in breast cancer. In Forrest, A.P.M., and Kunkler, P.B., editors: Prognostic factors in breast cancer, Edinburgh, 1968, E. & S. Livingstone, Ltd.

Rosemond, G.P., Maier, W.P., and Brobyn, T.J.: Needle aspiration of breast cysts, Surg. Gynecol. Obstet. **128**:351, Feb. 1969.

Rhoads, J.E., editor: Proceedings of an NIH Consensus Conference on Steroid Receptors, Cancer **46**:2759, 1980.

Rhoads, J.E., editor: Proceedings of the 1979 Conference on Breast Cancer, Cancer **46**:859, 1980.

Shapiro, S.: Evidence on screening for breast cancer from a randomized trial, Cancer **39**:2772, 1977.

CHAPTER 17
Liver and Biliary Tract

Barone, R.M., et al.: Intra-arterial chemotherapy using an implantable infusion pump and liver irradiation for the treatment of hepatic metastases, Cancer **50**:850, 1982.

Bennion, L.J., and Grundy, S.M.: Risk factors for the development of cholelithiasis in man (2 parts), N. Engl. J. Med. **299**:1161 and 1221, 1978.

Bismuth, H.: Surgical anatomy and anatomical surgery of the liver, World J. Surg. **6**:3, 1982.

Bodvall, B.: The postcholecystectomy syndromes, Clin. Gastroenterol. **2**:103, 1973.

Burnstein, M.J., Vassal, K.P., and Strasberg, S.M.: Results of combined biliary drainage and cholecystokinin cholangiography in 81 patients with normal oral cholecystograms, Ann. Surg. **196**:627, 1982.

Fischer, J.E.: Amino acids in hepatic coma, Dig. Dis. Sci. **27**:97, 1982.

Gracie, W.A., and Ransohoff, D.F.: The natural history of silent gallstones: the innocent gallstone is not a myth, N. Engl. J. Med. **307**:798, 1982 (also the delightful accompanying editorial).

Lees, C.D., et al.: Carcinoma of the bile ducts, Surg. Gynecol. Obstet. **151**:193, 1980.

LeVeen, H.H., et al.: Ascites: its correction by peritoneovenous shunting, Curr. Probl. Surg. **16**:1, Feb. 1979.

Lewis, J.W., Chung, R.S., and Allison, J.G.: Injection sclerotherapy for control of acute variceal hemorrhage, Am. J. Surg. **142**:592, 1981.

Lindner, H.H., and Green, R.B.: Embryology and surgical anatomy of the extrahepatic biliary tract, Surg. Clin. North Am. **44**:1273, 1964.

McSherry, C.K., and Glenn, F.: The incidence and causes of death following surgery for nonmalignant biliary tract disease, Ann. Surg. **191**:271, 1980.

Pitt, H.A., et al.: Factors influencing outcome in patients with postoperative biliary strictures, Am. J. Surg. **144**:14, 1982.

Rattner, D.W., and Warshaw, A.L.: Impact of choledochoscopy on the management of choledocholithiasis: experience with 499 common duct explorations at the Massachusetts General Hospital, Ann. Surg. **194**:76, 1981.

Rikkers, L.F.: Operations for management of esophageal variceal hemorrhage, West. J. Med. **136**:107, 1982.

Scharschmidt, B.F., Goldberg, H.I., and Schmid, R.: Current concepts in diagnosis: approach to the patient with cholestatic jaundice, N. Engl. J. Med. **308**:1515, 1983.

Sherlock, S.: Diseases of the liver and biliary system, ed. 6, Oxford, England, 1981, Basil Blackwell Publisher.

Sherlock, S.: Patterns of hepatocyte injury in man, Lancet **1**:782, 1982.

Sugiura, M., and Futagawa, S.: Further evaluation of the Sugiura procedure in the treatment of esophageal varices, Arch. Surg. **112**:1317, 1977.

Thompson, J.E., Tompkins, R. K., and Longmire, W.P.: Factors in management of acute cholangitis, Ann. Surg. **195**:137, 1982.

Van der Linden, W., and Edlund, G.: Early versus delayed cholecystectomy: the effect of a change in management, Br. J. Surg. **68**:783, 1981.

Verlenden, W.L., III, and Frey, C.F.: Management of liver abscess, Am. J. Surg. **140**:53, 1980.

Walt, A.J.: The mythology of hepatic trauma or Babel revisited, Am. J. Surg. **135**:12, 1978.

CHAPTER 18
Pancreas

Bradley, E.L., Clements, J.L., and Gonzalez, A.C.: The natural history of pancreatic pseudocysts: a unified concept of management, Am. J. Surg. **137**:135, 1979.

Deveney, C.W., Deveney, K.E., Stark, D., Moss, A., Stein, S., and Way, L.W.: Resection of gastrinomas, Ann. Surg. **198**:546, 1983.

Ebid, A.M., Murray, P.D., and Fischer, J.E.: Vasoactive intestinal peptide and the watery diarrhea syndrome, Ann. Surg. **187**:411, 1978.

Frey, C.F., Child, C.G., and Fry, W.: Pancreatectomy for chronic pancreatitis, Ann. Surg. **184**:403, 1976.

Friesen, S.R.: Tumors of the endocrine pancreas, N. Engl. J. Med. **306**:580, 1982.

Friesen, S.R.: Treatment of the Zollinger-Ellison syndrome, Am. J. Surg. **143**:331, 1982.

Graham, J.M., Mattox, K.L., and Jordan, G.L.: Traumatic injuries of the pancreas, Am. J. Surg. **136**:744, 1978.

Harrison, T.S., Child, C.G., Fry, W.J., Floyd, J.C., and Fajans, S.S.: Current surgical management of functioning islet cell tumors of the pancreas, Ann. Surg. **178**:485, 1973.

Jones, R.C.: Management of pancreatic trauma, Ann. Surg. **187**:555, 1978.

Kelly, T.R.: Gallstone pancreatitis: pathophysiology, Surgery **80**:488, 1976.

McCarthy, D.M.: The place of surgery in the Zollinger-Ellison syndrome, N. Engl. J. Med. **302**:1344, 1980.

Meinke, W.B., Twomey, P.L., Guernsey, J.M., Frey, C.F., Higgins, G., and Keehn, R.: Gastric outlet obstruction after palliative surgery for cancer of head of pancreas, Arch. Surg. **118**:550, 1983.

Miller, T.A., Lindenauer, S.M., Frey, C.F., and Stanley, J.C.: Pancreatic abscess, Arch. Surg. **108**:545, 1974.

Prinz, R.A., Badrinath, K., Banerji, M. et al.: Operative and chemotherapeutic management glucagon producing tumors, Surgery **90**:713, 1981.

Prinz, R.A., and Greenlee, H.B.: Pancreatic duct drainage in 100 patients with chronic pancreatitis, Ann. Surg. **194**:313, 1981.

Ranson, J.H.C.: Conservative surgical treatment of acute pancreatitis, World J. Surg. **5**:351, 1981.

Ranson, J.H.C., and Spencer, F.C.: The role of peritoneal lavage in severe acute pancreatitis, Ann. Surg. **187**:565, 1978.

Ranson, J.H.C., Rifkind, K.M., Roses, D.F., et al.: Prognostic signs and the role of operative management in acute pancreatitis, Surg. Gynecol. Obstet. **139**:69, 1974.

Ranson, J.H.C., and Spencer, F.C.: Prevention, diagnosis, and treatment of pancreatic abscess, Surgery **82**:99, 1977.

Ranson, J.H.C.: The timing of biliary surgery in acute pancreatitis, Ann. Surg. **189**:654, 1979.

Safrany, L., and Cotton, P.B.: A preliminary report: urgent duodenoscopic sphincterotomy for acute gallstone pancreatitis, Surgery **89**:424, 1981.

Sankaran, S., and Walt, A.J.: The natural and unnatural history of pancreatic pseudocysts, Br. J. Surg. **62**:37, 1975.

Semel, L., Schrieber, D., and Fromm, D.: Gallstone pancreatitis, Arch. Surg. **118**:901, 1983.

Thompson, J.C., Lewis, B.G., Wiener, I., and Townsend C.M.: The role of surgery in the Zollinger-Ellison syndrome, Ann. Surg. **197**:594, 1983.

van Heerden, J.A., Edis, A.J., and Service, F.J.: The surgical aspects of insulinomas, Ann. Surg. **189**:677, 1979.

Warren, K.W., Christophi, C., Armendariz, R., and Basu, S.: Current trends in the diagnosis and treatment of carcinoma of the pancreas, Am. J. Surg. **145**:813, 1983.

Weaver, D.W., Walt, A.J., Sugawa, C., and Bouwman, D.L.: A continuing appraisal of pancreatic ascites, Surg. Gynecol. Obstet. **154**:845, 1982.

CHAPTER 19
Spleen

Block, G.E., and Exelby, P.R.: Chapter 30 in Nora, P.F., editor: Operative surgery, ed. 2, Philadelphia, 1980, Lea & Febiger.

Burrington, J.D.: Surgical repair of a ruptured spleen in children: report of eight cases, Arch. Surg. **112**:417, 1977.

Claret, I., Morales, L., and Montaner, A.: Immunological studies in the post splenectomy syndrome, J. Pediatr. Surg. **10**:59, 1975.

Ein, S.H., Shandling, B., Simpson, J.S., and Stephens, C.A.: Nonoperative management of traumatized spleen in children: how and why, J. Pediatr. Surg. **13**:117, 1978.

Erkalis, A.J., and Filler, R.M.: Splenectomy in childhood: a review of 1413 cases, J. Pediatr. Surg. **7**:382, 1972.

Hebeler, R.F., Ward, R.E., Miller, P.W., and Ben-Menachem, Y.: The management of splenic injury, J. Trauma **22**:492, 1982.

Keisewetter, W.B., and Patrick, D.B.: Childhood splenectomy: indications for and results from, Ann. Surg. **37**:135, 1971.

McClure, P.D.: Idiopathic thrombocytopenic purpura in children: diagnosis and management, Pediatrics, **54**:68, 1975.

Pearson, H.A.: Splenectomy: its risks and its roles, Hosp. Pract., p. 85, Aug. 1980.

Pearson, H.A., et al.: The born-again spleen, N. Engl. J. Med. **298**:1389, 1978.

Ratner, M.H., Garrow, E., Valda, V., Shashikumar, V.L., and Somers, L.A.: Surgical repair of the injured spleen, J. Pediatr. Surg. **12**:1019, 1977.

Scheele, J., Gentsch, H.H., and Matteson, E.: Splenic repair by fibrin tissue adhesive and collagen fleece, Surgery **95**:6, 1984.

Schwartz, P.E., et al.: Postsplenectomy sepsis and mortality in adults, J.A.M.A. **248**:2279, 1982.

Sherman, R.T., et al.: Panel: splenic injuries, J. Trauma **22**:507, 1982.

Soper, R.T.: Splenic salvage, Hosp. Physician **19**:73, 1983.

Traub, A.C., and Perry, J.F.: Splenic preservation following splenic trauma, J. Trauma **22**:496, 1982.

Velcek, F.T., et al.: Posttraumatic splenic replantation in children, J. Pediatr. Surg. **17**:879, 1982.

CHAPTER 20
Peritoneum and Acute Abdominal Conditions

Botsford, T.W., and Wilson, R.E.: The acute abdomen, vol. X, Major problems in clinical surgery, ed. 2, Philadelphia, 1977, W.B. Saunders Co.

Cope, Z. (revised by Silen, W.): The early diagnoses of the acute abdomen, ed. 15, New York, 1979, Oxford University Press.

Jones, P.F., and Dudley, H.A.: Emergency abdominal surgery in infancy, childhood and adult life, Philadelphia, 1974, J.B. Lippincott Co.

Requarth, W.: Indication for operation for abdominal trauma, Surgery **46**:461, 1959.

Simmons, R.L., and Howard, R.J.: Surgical infectious diseases, New York, 1982, Appleton-Century-Crofts.

Thomford, N.R.: Appendicitis, Cont. Ed. Family Phys., pp. 49-54, Dec. 1979.

Warren, K.W.: Acute surgical conditions of the abdomen in the aged and the poor risk patient, Surg. Clin. North Am. **34**:745, 1954.

CHAPTER 21
Intestinal Obstruction

Davis, S., and Sperling, L.: Obstruction of the small intestine, Arch. Surg. **99**:424, 1969.

Quan, S.H.Q., and Stearns, M.W., Jr.: Early postoperative intestinal obstruction and postoperative intestinal ileus, Dis. Colon Rectum **4**:307, 1961.

Wangensteen, O.H.: Intestinal obstruction, ed. 3, Springfield, Ill., 1955, Charles C Thomas, Publisher.

Wangensteen, O.H.: Great ideas in surgery—understanding the bowel obstruction problem, Am. J. Surg. **135**:131, 1978.

Welch, C.E.: Intestinal obstruction, Chicago, 1958, Year Book Medical Publishers, Inc.

CHAPTER 22
Gastrointestinal Hemorrhage

Adams, J.T.: Therapeutic barium enema for massive diverticular bleeding, Arch. Surg. **101**:457, 1970.

Albo, R.J., Grimes, O.F., and Dunphy, J.E.: Management of massive lower gastrointestinal hemorrhage, Am. J. Surg. **112**:264, 1966.

Alavi, A., Dann, R.W., Baum, S., et al.: Scintigraphic detection of acute gastrointestinal bleeding, Radiology **124**:753, 1977.

Athanasoulis, C.A.: Angiographic methods for control of gastric hemorrhage, Am. J. Dig. Dis. **21**(2):174, 1976.

Baum, S., and Nusbaum, M.: The control of gastrointestinal hemorrhage by selective mesenteric arterial infusion of vasopressin, Radiology **98**:497, 1971.

Boley, S.J., Sammartano, R., Adams, A., et al.: On the nature and etiology of vascular ectasias of the colon, Gastroenterology **72**:650, 1977.

Corry, R.J., Mundth, E.D., and Bartlett, M.K.: Massive upper gastrointestinal tract hemorrhage, Arch. Surg. **97**:531, 1968.

Corry, R.J., Bartlett, M.K., and Cohen, R.B.: Erosions of the cecum: a cause of massive hemorrhage, Am. J. Surg. **119**:106, 1970.

Eckstein, M.R., and Athanasoulis, C.A.: Gastrointestinal bleeding, an angiographic perspective, Surg. Clin. North Am. **64**:37, 1984.

Freeark, R.J., Norcross, W.J., Baker, R.J., and Strohl, E.H.: The Mallory-Weiss syndrome, Arch. Surg. **88**:882, 1964.

Hastings, P.R., Skillman, J.J., Bushnell, L.S., and Silen, W.: Antacid titration in the prevention of acute gastrointestinal bleeding: a controlled, randomized trial of 100 critically ill patients, N. Engl. J. Med. **298**(19):1041, 1978.

Hedberg, S.E.: Early endoscopic diagnosis in upper gastrointestinal hemorrhage: an analysis of 323 cases, Surg. Clin. North Am. **46**:499, 1966.

Johnson, W.C., Widrich, W.C., Ansell, J.E., et al.: Control of bleeding varices by vasopressin: a prospective randomized study, Ann. Surg. **186**:369, 1977.

Lewis, J., Chung, R.S., and Allison, J.: Sclerotherapy of esophageal varices, Arch. Surg. **115**:476, 1980.

Malt, R.A.: Portasystemic shunts, N. Engl. J. Med. **295**:24, 80, 1976.

Malt, R.A.: Medical intelligence—current concepts: control of massive upper gastrointestinal hemorrhage, N. Engl. J. Med. **286**:1043, 1972.

Orloff, M.J., Bell, Jr., J.R., Hyde, P.V., and Skivolecki, W.P.: Long term results of emergency portacaval shunt for bleeding esophageal varices in unselected patients with alcoholic cirrhosis, Ann. Surg. **192**:325, 1980.

Papp, J.P.: Endoscopic electrocoagulation in the management of upper gastrointestinal tract bleeding, Surg. Clin. North Am. **62**:797, 1982.

Sugiura, M., and Futagawa, S.: Further evaluation of the Sugiura procedure in the treatment of esophageal varices, Arch. Surg. **112**:1317, 1977.

Welch, C.E., Athanasoulis, C.A., and Galdabini, J.J.: Hemorrhage from the large bowel with special reference to angiodysplasia and diverticular disease, World J. Surg. **2**:73, 1978.

CHAPTER 23
Stomach and Duodenum

Bushkin, F.L., and Woodward, E.R.: Postgastrectomy syndromes, Philadelphia, 1976, W.B. Saunders Co.

Diehl, J.T., Hermann, R.E., Cooperman, A.M., and Hoerr, S.O.: Gastric carcinoma—a ten-year review, Ann. Surg. **198**:9, 1983.

Dragstedt, L.R.: Gastrin and peptic ulcer, Arch. Surg. **91**:1005, 1965.

Eiseman, B., and Heyman, R.L.: Stress ulcer—a continuing challenge, N. Engl. J. Med. **282**:372, 1970.

Goligher, J.C.: A technique for highly selective (parietal cell or proximal gastric) vagotomy for duodenal ulcer, Br. J. Surg. **61**:337, 1974.

Hardy, J.D., and Doolittle, P.D.: Zollinger-Ellison syndrome: special considerations, Ann. Surg. **185**:661, 1977.

Howard, R.J., Murphy, W.R., and Humphrey, E.W.: A prospective randomized study of the elective surgical treatment for duodenal ulcer: two to ten-year follow-up study, Surgery **73**:256, 1973.

Hoerr, S.O.: A review and evaluation of operative procedures used for chronic duodenal ulcer, Surg. Clin. North Am. **56**:1289, 1976.

Johnson, A.G.: Peptic ulcer and the pylorus, Lancet **1**:710, 1979.

Johnston, D., and Goligher, J.C.: Selective, highly selective, or truncal vagotomy? In 1976—a clinical appraisal, Surg. Clin. North Am. **56**:1313, 1976.

Jordan, P.H., Jr.: A follow-up report of a prospective evaluation of vagotomy-pyloroplasty and vagotomy-antrectomy for treatment of duodenal ulcer, Ann. Surg. **180**:259, 1974.

Kennedy, F., Mackay, C., Bedi, B.S., and Kay, A.W.: Truncal vagotomy and drainage for chronic duodenal ulcer disease: a controlled trial, Br. Med. J. **1**:71, 1973.

Knight, C.D., Jr., van Heerden, J.A., and Kelly, K.A.: Proximal gastric vagotomy: update, Ann. Surg. **197**:22, 1983.

Maclean, L.D., Rhode, B.M., and Shizgal, H.M.: Nutrition following gastric operations for morbid obesity, Ann. Surg. **198:**347, 1983.

Mason, E.E.: Evolution of gastric reduction for obesity, Contemp. Surg. **20:**1982.

Menguy, R.: Gastric ulcerations. In Hardy, J.D., editor: Advances in surgery, vol. 6, Chicago, 1972, Year Book Medical Publishers, Inc. pp. 103-139.

Moody, F.G., and McGreevy, J.M.: Stomach. In Schwartz, S.I., Shires, G.T., Spencer, F.C., and Storer, E.H., editors: Principles of surgery, ed. 4, New York, 1983, McGraw-Hill Book Co.

Moore, F.D.: Surgery in search of a rationale: eighty years of ulcerogenic surgery, Am. J. Surg. **105:**304, 1963.

Nyhus, L.M., and Wastell, C.: Surgery of the stomach and duodenum, ed. 3, Boston, 1977, Little, Brown & Co.

Nyhus, L.M., Donohue, P.E., Krystosek, R.J., Pearl, R.K., and Bombeck, C.T.: Complete vagotomy: the evolution of an effective technique, Arch. Surg. **115:**264, 1980.

Penn, I.: Management of the perforated duodenal ulcer, Heart Lung **7:**111, 1978.

Penn, I.: Surgical and medical treatment of peptic ulcer disease, Contin. Educa. for the Fam. Physician **11:**39, 1979.

Rosato, F.E., and Noto, J.A.: Gastric polyps, Am. J. Surg. **111:**647, 1966.

Schein, P.S., Smith, F.P., Woolley, P.V., and Ahlgren, J.D.: Current management of advanced and locally unresectable gastric carcinoma, Cancer **50:**2590, 1982.

Skillman, J.J.: Pathogenesis of peptic ulcer: a selective review, Surgery **76:**515, 1974.

Spiro, H.M.: Clinical gastroenterology, ed. 2, New York, 1977, The Macmillan Co.

Wara, P., Kristensen, E.S., Sørensen, F.H., Boné, J., Skovgaard, S., and Amdrup, E.: The value of parietal cell vagotomy compared to simple closure in a selective approach to perforated duodenal ulcer: operative morbidity and recurrence rate, Acta Chir. Scand. **194:**585, 1983.

Zollinger, R.M., and Ellison, E.H.: Primary peptic ulcerations of the jejunum associated with islet cell tumors of the pancreas, Ann. Surg. **142:**709, 1955.

CHAPTER 24
Small Intestine

Colcock, B.P., and Fortin, C.: Surgical treatment of regional enteritis: review of 85 cases, Ann. Surg. **161:**812, 1965.

Colcock, B.P., and Braasch, J.W.: Surgery of the small intestine in the adult, Philadelphia, 1968, W.B. Saunders Co.

Kutscher, A.H., Zegardli, E.V., Rankow, R.M., and Mercandante, J.L.: Peutz-Jeghers syndrome: follow-ups on patients reported on in the literature, Am. J. Med. Sci. **238:**180, 1959.

McPeak, C.J.: Malignant tumors of the small intestine, Am. J. Surg. **114:**402, 1967.

Rankin, G.B., and Turnbull, R.B., Jr.: Transmural colitis: medical and surgical management, Hosp. Practice, p. 65, Jan. 1971.

Read, J.D.: Intestinal carcinoma in the Peutz-Jeghers syndrome, J.A.M.A. **229:**833, 1974.

Sherman, N.J., et al.: Regional enteritis in childhood, J. Pediatr. Surg. **7:**585, 1972.

Skinner, D.B., et al.: Mesenteric vascular disease, Am. J. Surg. **128:**835, Dec. 1974.

CHAPTER 25
Large Intestine

Bacon, H.E., and Pezzutti, J.E.: Granulomatous ileocolitis, J.A.M.A. **198:**1330, 1966.

Burkitt, D.P.: Epidemiology of cancer of the colon and rectum, Cancer **28:**3, 1971.

Coller, F.A., Ransom, H.K., and Regan, W.J.: Cancer of the colon and rectum, Monograph, New York, 1956, American Cancer Society.

Crespi, M., Weissman, G.S., and Gilbertsen, V.A., et al.: The role of proctosigmoidoscopy in screening for colorectal neoplasia, CA **34:**158, 1984.

Goligher, J.C.: Surgery of the anus, rectum, and colon, ed. 4, New York, 1980, The Macmillan Co.

Goligher, J.D., De Dombal, F.T. and Watts, F.M.: Ulcerative colitus, Baltimore, 1968, The Williams & Wilkins Co.

Hawk, W.A., Turnbull, R.B., and Farmer, R.G.: Regional enteritis of the colon, J.A.M.A. **201:**738, Sept. 1967.

Miller, F.E., and Liechty, R.D.: Adenocarcinoma of the colon and rectum in persons under thirty years of age. Am. J. Surg. **113:**507, 1967.

Spratt, J.S., Ackerman, L.V., and Moyer, C.A.: Relationship of polyps of the colon to colonic cancer, Ann. Surg. **148:**682, 1958.

Thomson, J.P.S., Nicholls, R.J., and Williams, C.B.: Colorectal diseases, New York, 1981, Appleton-Century-Crofts.

Turnbull, R.B., Jr., et al.: Cancer of the colon: the influence of the no-touch isolation technique on survival rates, Ann. Surg. **166:**420, 1967.

Welch, C.E., and Hedberg, S.: Polypoid lesions of the gastrointestinal tract, Philadelphia, 1975, W.B. Saunders Co.

Wilson, S.M., and Beahrs, O.H.: The curative treatment of colonic carcinoma of the sigmoid, rectosigmoid and rectum, Ann. Surg. **183:**556, 1976.

Winawer, S.J., and Sherlock, P.: Surveillance for colorectal cancer in average-risk patients, familial high-risk groups, and patients with adenomas, Cancer, **50:**2609, 1982.

CHAPTER 26
Anorectum

Beahrs, O.H.: Complete rectal prolapse: an evaluation of surgical treatment, Ann. Surg. **161:**221, 1965.

Buckwalter, J.A., and Jurayj, M.D.: Relationship of chronic rectal disease to carcinoma, Arch. Surg. **75:**352, 1957.

Dunphy, J.E.: Surgical anatomy of the anal canal, Arch. Surg. **57:**791, 1948.

Dunphy, J.E., and Pikula, J.: Fact and fancy about fistula-in-ano, Surg. Clin. North Am. **35:**1469, 1955.

Goligher, J.C.: Surgery of the anus, rectum, and colon, ed. 4, New York, 1980, The Macmillan Co.

Goligher, J.C., Leacock, A.G., and Brossy, J.J.: The surgical anatomy of the anal canal, Br. J. Surg. **43**:51, 1955.

Harkins, H.N.: Correlation of the newer knowledge of surgical anatomy of the anorectum, Dis. Colon Rectum **8**:154, 1965.

Nesselrod, J.P.: Clinical proctology, ed. 3, Philadelphia, 1964 W.B. Saunders Co.

Page, B.H.: The entry of hair into a pilonidal sinus, Br. J. Surg. **56**:32, 1969.

Parks, A.G.: Haemorrhoidectomy, Surg. Clin. North Am. **45**:1305, 1965.

Patey, D.H.: A reappraisal of the acquired theory of sacrococcygeal pilonidal sinus, Br. J. Surg. **56**:462, 1969.

Sawyers, J.L.: Epidermoid cancer of the perianus and the anal canal, Surg. Clin. North Am. **45**:1173, 1965.

Thomson, J.P.S., Nicholls, R.J., and Williams, C.B.: Colorectal disease, New York, 1981, Appleton-Century-Crofts.

CHAPTER 27
Abdominal Hernias

Adelman, S., Benson, C.D.: Bochdalek hernias in infants: factors determining mortality, J. Pediatr. Surg. **11**:569, 1976.

Anson, B.J., Morgan, E.H., and McVay, C.B.: Surgical anatomy of the inguinal region based upon a study of 500 body halves, Surg. Gynecol. Obstet. **111**:707, 1960.

Bettex, M.: Surgical treatment of hiatus hernia and cardioesophageal chalasia in infants and children, Paediatrician **3**:161, 1974.

Bombeck, G.T., and Nyhus, L.M.: Chapter 32 in Nora, P.F., editor: Operative surgery, ed. 2, Philadelphia, 1980, Lea & Febiger.

McGregor, D.B., Halverson, K., and McVay, C.B.: The unilateral pediatric inguinal hernia: should the contralateral side be explored? J. Pediatr. Surg. **15**:313, 1980.

McVay, C.B.: Inguinal and femoral hernioplasty, Surgery **57**:615, 1965.

Nyhus, L.M., and Condon, R.E.: Hernia, ed. 2, Philadelphia, 1978, J.B. Lippincott Co.

Nyhus, L.M., and Harkins, H.N.: Hernia, ed. 2, Philadelphia, 1979, J.B. Lippincott Co.

Osebold, W.R., and Soper, R.T.: Congenital posterolateral diaphragmatic hernia past infancy, Am. J. Surg. **131**:748, 1976.

Ponka, J.L.: Hernias of the abdominal wall, Philadelphia, 1980, W.B. Saunders Co.

Ravitch, M.M.: Repair of hernias, Chicago, 1969, Year Book Medical Publishers, Inc.

Ruff, S.J., et al.: Pediatric diaphragmatic hernias, Am. J. Surg. **139**:641, 1980.

Safaie-Shirazi, S., Zike, W.L., Anuras, S., Condon, R.E., and DenBesten, L.: Proceedings: Nissen fundoplication without crural repair: a cure for reflux esophagitis, Arch. Surg. **108**:424, 1974.

Shirazi, S.S.: Hernias of the diaphragm and abdominal wall, Garden City, N.Y., 1981, Medical Examination Publishing Co., Inc.

Smith, L.A., et al.: Treatment of defects of the anterior abdominal wall in newborns, Mayo Clinic Proc. **58**:797, 1983.

Soper, R.T.: Hernia in infants and children, Postgrad. Med. **40**:523, 1966.

Talbert, J.L.: Surgical management of massive ventral hernias in children, J. Pediatr. Surg. **12**:63, 1977.

Zimmerman, L.M., and Anson, B.J.: The anatomy and surgery of hernia, ed. 2, Baltimore, 1967, The Williams & Wilkins Co.

CHAPTER 28
Pediatric Surgery

Bain, K.: The physically abused child, Pediatrics **31**:895, 1963.

Ehrenpreis, T.: Hirschsprung's disease, Chicago, 1970, Year Book Medical Publishers, Inc.

Froehlich, L.A., and Fujikura, T.: Significance of a single umbilical artery, Am. J. Obstet. Gynecol. **92**:274, 1966.

Gross, R.E.: The surgery of infancy and childhood, Philadelphia, 1953, W.B. Saunders Co.

Holder, T.M., and Ashcraft, K.W.: Pediatric surgery, Philadelphia, 1980, W.B. Saunders Co.

Izant, R.J., and Hubey, C.A.: Annual injury of 15,000,000 children, J. Trauma **6**:65, 1966.

Nadler, H.L.: Prenatal diagnosis of inborn defects: a status report, Hosp. Practice, p. 41, June 1975.

Randolph, J.G., Ravitch, M.M., Welch, K.J., Benson, C.D., and Aberdeen, E.: The injured child, Chicago, 1979, Year Book Medical Publishers, Inc.

Raffensperger, J.G.: Swenson's pediatric surgery, ed. 4, New York, 1980, Appleton-Century-Crofts.

Rickman, P.P., Soper, R.T., and Stauffer, U.: Synopsis of pediatric surgery, Stuttgart, 1975, Georg Thieme Verlag.

Rickham, P.P., Lister, J., and Irving, I.M.: Neonatal surgery, ed. 2, Sevenoaks, Kent, 1978, Butterworth & Co., Ltd.

Spits, L., Steiner, G. M., and Zachary, R.B.: Color atlas of pediatric surgical diagnosis, Chicago, 1981, Year Book Medical Publishers, Inc.

Stephens, F.D., and Smith, E.D.: Ano-rectal malformations in children, Chicago, 1971, Year Book Medical Publishers, Inc.

Touloukian, R.J.: Pediatric trauma, New York, 1978, John Wiley & Sons, Inc.

Velcek, F.T., Weiss, A., DiMaio, D., Klotz, D.H., Jr., and Kottmeier, P.K.: Traumatic death in urban children, J. Pediatr. Surg. **12**:375, 1977.

Young, D.G.: Fluid balance in pediatric surgery, Br. J. Anaesth. **45**:953, 1973.

CHAPTER 29
Intensive care

Beal, J.M., Critical care for surgical patients, New York, 1982, Macmillan Publishing Co.

Berk, J.L., and Sampliner, J.E.: Handbook of critical care, Boston, 1982, Little, Brown & Co.

Condon, R.,E., and Nyhus, L.M.: Manual of surgical therapeutics, Boston, 1981, Little, Brown & Co.

Costrini, N.V., and Thomson, W.M.: Manual of medical therapeutics, Boston, 1977, Little, Brown & Co.

Greenfield, L.: Complications in surgery and trauma, Philadelphia, 1984, J.B. Lippincott Co.

Hill, D.W., and Dolan, A.M.: Intensive care instrumentation, New York, 1982, Grune & Stratton.

Kinney, J.M., Bendixen, H.H., and Powers, S.R.: Manual of surgical intensive care, Philadelphia, 1977, W.B. Saunders Co.

Swan, J.H.C., Ganz, W., and Forrester, J.: Catheterization of the heart in man with the use of a flow-directed balloon-tipped catheter, N. Engl. J. Med. **283**:447-451, 1970.

Walker, W.F., and Taylor. D.E.M.: Intensive care, Edinburgh, 1975, Churchill Livingstone.

CHAPTER 30
Thoracic and Pulmonary Surgery

Bates, D.V., Macklem, P.T., and Christie, R.V.: Respiratory function in disease, ed. 2, Philadelphia, 1971, W.B. Saunders Co.

Comroe, J.L., Jr., Foster, R.E., II, DuBois, A.B., Brisco, W.A., and Carlson, E.: The lung, ed. 3, Chicago, 1965, Year Book Medical Publishers, Inc.

Doty, D.B., Anderson, A.E., Rose, E.F., Go, R.T., Chiu, C.L., and Ehrenhaft, J.L.: Cardiac trauma: clinical and experimental correlations of myocardial contusion, Ann. Surg. **180**:452, 1974.

Edwards, F.R.: Foundations of thoracic surgery, Baltimore, 1966, The Williams & Wilkins Co.

Effler, D.B., editor: Blades' surgical diseases of the chest, ed. 4, St. Louis, 1978, The C.V. Mosby Co.

Flavell, G.: An introduction to chest surgery, New York, 1957, Oxford University Press.

Glenn, W., editor: Thoracic and cardiovascular surgery, ed. 4, East Norwalk, Conn., 1983, Appleton-Century-Crofts.

Johnson, J., and Kirby, C.K.: Surgery of the chest, ed. 4, Chicago, 1970, Year Book Medical Publishers, Inc.

Nelson, A.R.: The surgical treatment of pulmonary coccidioidomycosis, Curr. Probl. Surg., pp. 1-48, 1974.

Robin, E.D.: A clinical approach to the diagnostic management of pulmonary embolism. In Bang, N.U., Glover, J.L., Holden, R.W., and Triplett, D.A., editors: Thrombosis and atherosclerosis, Chicago, 1982, Year Book Medical Publishers, Inc.

Slonim, N.B., and Hamilton, L.H.: Respiratory physiology, ed. 3, St. Louis, 1976, The C.V. Mosby Co.

West, J.B.: Ventilation/blood flow and gas exchange, ed. 2, Philadelphia, 1970, F.A. Davis Co.

Zavala, D.C., and Rossi, N.P.: Nonthoracotomy diagnostic techniques for pulmonary disease, Arch. Surg. **107**:152, 1973.

CHAPTER 31
Cardiac Surgery

National Academy of Sciences–National Research Council Ad Hoc Committee: Cardiopulmonary resuscitation, J.A.M.A. **198**:372, 1966.

Berne, R.M., and Levy, M.N.: Cardiovascular physiology, ed. 3, St. Louis, 1977, The C.V. Mosby Co.

Blalock, A., and Taussig, H.B.: Surgical treatment of malformation of the heart in which there is pulmonic stenosis or pulmonic atresia, J.A.M.A. **128**:189, 1945.

Cohn, L.H.: The long-term results of aortic valve replacement, Chest **85**:387, 1984.

DeWall, R.A., Grage, T.V., McFee, A.S., and Chiechi, M.A.: Theme and variations on blood oxygenators. I, Bubble oxygenators, Surgery **50**:931, 1961.

Gentsch, T.O., Bopp, R.K., Siegel, J.H., Cev, M., and Glenn, W.W.L.: Experimental and clinical use of a membrane oxygenator, Surgery **45**:301, 1960.

Glenn, W.L., Baue, A.E., Geha, A.S., Hammond, G.L., and Laks, H.: Thoracic and cardiovascular surgery, ed. 4, East Norwalk, Conn., 1983, Appleton-Century-Crofts.

Hill, J.D.: I, The development of the first successful heart-lung machine, Ann. Thorac. Surg. **34**:337, 1982.

Kirklin, J.K., and Kirklin, J.W.: Management of the cardiovascular subsystem after cardiac surgery, Ann. Thorac. Surg. **32**:311, 1981.

Kirklin, J.W., and Karp, R.B.: The tetralogy of Fallot from a surgical viewpoint, Philadelphia, 1970, W.B. Saunders Co.

Loop, F.D.: Progress in surgical treatment of coronary atherosclerosis (part 1), Chest **84**:611, 1983.

Loop, F.D.: Progress in surgical treatment of coronary atherosclerosis (part 2), Chest **84**:740, 1983.

McGoon, D.C.: Cardiac surgery, Philadelphia, 1982, F.A. Davis Co.

Parsonnet, V., Candice, C.C., Crawford, M.A., and Bernstein, A.D.: The 1981 United States survey of cardiac pacing practices, J. Am. Coll. Cardiol. **3**:1321, 1984.

Potts, W.J., Smith, S., and Gibson, S.: Anastomosis of aorta to pulmonary artery, J.A.M.A. **132**:627, 1946.

Sabiston, D.C., Jr., and Spencer, F.C.: Gibbon's surgery of the chest, ed. 4, Philadelphia, 1983, W.B. Saunders Co.

Utley, J.R.: Pathophysiology and techniques of cardiopulmonary bypass, vol. II, Baltimore, 1983, The Williams & Wilkins Co.

Weber, K.T., and Janicki, M.S.: Intra-aortic balloon counter pulsation: a collective review, Ann. Thorac. Surg. **17**:602, 1974.

CHAPTER 32
Peripheral Arteries

Baker, W.H., String, S.T., Hayes, A.C., and Turner, D.: Diagnosis of peripheral occlusive disease, Arch. Surg. **113**(11):1308, 1978.

Barker, W.F.: Peripheral arterial disease, ed. 2, Philadelphia, 1975, W.B. Saunders Co.

Barnes, R.W.: Hemodynamics for the vascular surgeon, Arch. Surg. **115**:216, 1980.

Bergan, J.J., and Yao, J.S.T.: Gangrene and severe ischemia of the lower extremities, New York, 1978, Grune & Stratton, Inc.

Blaisdell, F.W., and Hall, A.D.: Axillary-femoral artery bypass for lower extremity ischemia, Surgery **54**:563, 1963.

Boley, S.J., Sprayregan, S., Siegelman, S.S., and Veith, F.J.: Initial results from an aggressive roentgenological and surgical approach to acute mesenteric ischemia, Surgery **82**:848, 1977.

Brewster, D.C., and Darling, R.C.: Optimal methods of aortoiliac reconstruction, Surgery **84**:739, 1978.

Burgess, E.M., Romano, R.L., and Zettl, J.H.: The management of lower extremity amputations, TR 10-6, Washington, D.C., 1969, U.S. Government Printing Office.

Council on Scientific Affairs (AMA): Percutaneous transluminal angioplasty, J.A.M.A. **251:**764, 1984.

Dale, W.A., and Lewis, M.R.: Management of ischemia of the hand and fingers, Surgery **67:**63, 1970.

Dent, T.L., Lindenauer, S.M., Ernst, C.B., and Fry, W.J.: Multiple arteriosclerotic arterial aneurysms, Arch. Surg. **105:**338, 1972.

DePalma, R.G., and Clowes, A.W.: Interventions in atherosclerosis: a review for surgeons, Surgery **84:**175, 1978.

Eastcott, H.H.G.: Arterial surgery, Philadelphia, 1969, J.B. Lippincott Co.

Eastcott, H.H.G., Pickering, G.W., and Rob, C.G.: Reconstruction of internal carotid artery in a patient with intermittent attacks of hemiplegia, Lancet **2:**994, 1954.

Fairburn, J.F., et al., editors: Allen-Barker-Hines peripheral vascular disease, ed. 4, Philadelphia, 1972, W.B. Saunders Co.

Fogarty, T.J., Cranley, J.J., Krause, R.J., Strasser, E.S., and Hafner, C.D.: A method for extraction of arterial emboli and thrombi, Surg. Gynecol. Obstet. **116:**241, 1963.

Leather, R.P., Powers, S.R., and Karmody, A.M.: A reappraisal of the in situ saphenous vein arterial bypass, Surgery **86:**453, 1979.

Linton, R.R.: Atlas of vascular surgery, Philadelphia, 1973, W.B. Saunders Co.

Linton, R.R., and Wilde, W.L.: Modifications in the technique for femoral popliteal saphenous vein bypass autografts, Surgery **67:**234, 1970.

Mannick, J.A.: Femoro-popliteal and femoro-tibial reconstruction, Surg. Clin. North Am. **59:**581, 1979.

Nath, R.L., Menzoian, J.O., Kaplan, K.H., McMillian, T.N., Siroky, M.B., and Krane, R.J.: The multidisciplinary approach to vasculogenic impotence, Surgery **89:**124, 1981.

O'Donnell, T.F., Darling, R.C., and Linton, R.R.: Is 80 years too old for aneurysmectomy?, Arch. Surg. **111:**1250, 1976.

Pilcher, D.B., Barker, W.F., and Cannon, J.A.: An aortoiliac endarterectomy case series followed 10 years or more, Surgery **67:**5, 1970.

Russell, J.B., Watson, T.M., Modi, J.R., Lambeth, A., and Sumner, D.S.: Digital subtraction angiography for evaluation of extracranial carotid occlusive disease: comparison with conventional arteriography, Surgery **94:**604, 1983.

Stanley, J.C., and Fry, W.J.: Surgical treatment of renovascular hypertension, Arch. Surg. **112:**1291, 1977.

Stoney, R.J., and Wylie, E.J.: Surgical treatment of ruptured abdominal aneurysms, Calif. Med. **111:**1, 1969.

Strandness, D.E.: Peripheral arterial disease, London, 1969, J. & A. Churchill Ltd.

Szilagyi, D.E., Smith, R.F., DeRusso, F.J., Elliott, J.P., and Sherrin, F.W.: Contribution of abdominal aortic aneurysmectomy to prolongation of life, Ann. Surg. **164:**678, 1966.

Weale, F.E.: An introduction to surgical haemodynamics, Chicago, 1967, Year Book Medical Publishers, Inc.

Wylie, E.J., and Ehrenfeld, W.K.: Entracranial occlusive cerebrovascular disease: diagnosis and management, Philadelphia, 1970, W.B. Saunders Co.

CHAPTER 33
Peripheral Veins

Bell, W.R., and Meek, A.G.: Guidelines for the use of thrombolytic agents, N. Engl. J. Med. **201**(23):1266, 1979.

Bernstein, E.F., editor: Noninvasive diagnostic techniques in vascular disease, St. Louis, 1978, The C.V. Mosby Co.

Borrow, M., and Goldson, H.: Postoperative venous thrombosis: evaluation of five methods of treatment, Am. J. Surg. **141:**245, 1981.

Coon, W.W.: Epidemiology of venous thromboembolism, Ann. Surg. **186**(2):149, 1977.

Coon, W.W., and Willis, P.W., III: Recurrence of venous thromboembolism, Surgery **73:**823, 1973.

Cranley, J.J., Canos, A.J., and Sull, W.J.: The diagnosis of deep vein thrombosis: fallibility of clinical symptoms and signs, Arch. Surg. **111:**34, 1976.

Dale, W.A., and Allen, T.R.: Unusual problems of venous thrombosis, Surgery **78:**707, 1975.

Dodd, H., and Cockett, F.B.: Pathology and surgery of veins of the lower limb, ed. 2, Baltimore, 1970, The Williams & Wilkins Co.

Donaldson, G.A., Linton, R.R., and Rodkey, G.V.: A twenty-year survey of thromboembolism at the Massachusetts General Hospital, 1932-1959, N. Engl. J. Med. **265:**208, 1961.

Donaldson, M.C., Wirthlin, L.S., and Donaldson, G.A.: Thirty-year experience with surgical interruption of the inferior vena cava for prevention of pulmonary embolism, Ann. Surg. **191:**363, 1980.

Fairbairn, J.F., et al., editors: Allen-Barker-Hines peripheral vascular disease, ed. 4, Philadelphia, 1972, W.B. Saunders Co.

Goldsmith, H.W., de los Santos, R., and Beattie, E.J., Jr.: Relief of chronic lymphedema by omental transposition, Ann. Surg. **166:**573, 1967.

Greenfield, L.J., Peyton, R., Crute, S., and Barnes, R.W.: Greenfield vena cava filter experience: late results in 156 patients, Arch. Surg. **116:**1451, 1981.

Gurewich, V., Thomas, D.P., and Stuart, R.K.: Some guidelines for heparin therapy of venous thromboembolic disease, J.A.M.A. **199:**116, 1967.

Hobbs, J.J., editor: The treatment of venous disorders, Philadelphia, 1977, J.B. Lippincott Co.

Kakkar, V.V., Corrigan, T.P., and Fossard, P.P.: An international multicentre trial: prevention of fatal postoperative pulmonary embolism by low doses of heparin, Lancet **2:**34, 1975.

Lansing, A.M., and Davis, W.M.: Five-year follow-up study of ileofemoral venous thrombectomy, Ann. Surg. **168:**620, 1968.

Lofgren, K.A.: Pitfalls in vein surgery, J.A.M.A. **188:**17, 1964.

Madden, J.L., and Hume, M., editors: Venous thromboembolism, New York, 1976, Appleton-Century-Crofts.

Sabiston, D.C.: Pathophysiology, diagnosis and management of pulmonary embolism, Am. J. Surg. **128**:384, 1979.

Salzman, E.W., and Davies, G.C.: Prophylaxis of venous thromboembolism: analysis of cost effectiveness, Ann. Surg. **191**:207, 1980.

Salzman, E.W., Deykin, D., Shapero, R.M., and Rosenberg, R.: Management of heparin therapy, N. Engl. J. Med. **292**:1046, 1975.

Shepard, J.T., and Vanhoutte, P.M.: Role of the venous system in circulatory control, Mayo Clin. Proc. **53**:246, 1978.

Stallworth, J.M., Bradham, G.B., Kletke, R.R., and Price, R.G.: Phlegmasia cerulea dolens: a ten year review, Ann. Surg. **161**:802, 1965.

CHAPTER 34
Plastic and Reconstructive Surgery

Achauer, B.M., et al.: Cyclosporine and the treatment of burns. Presented to American Burn Association annual meeting, San Francisco, 1984 (American Burn Association, Durham, N.C.).

Daniel, R.R., and Kerrigan, C.L.: Skin flaps: an anatomical and hemodynamic approach, Clin. Plast. Surg. **6**:181, 1979.

Flowers, R.W.: Unexpected postoperative problems in skin grafting, Surg. Clin. North Am. **50**:439, 1970.

Furnas, D.W., Black, K.S., Hewitt, C.W., Fraser, C.A., and Achauer, B.M.: Cyclosporine and long-term survival of composite tissue allografts (limb transplants) in rats, Transplant. Proc. **15**:3063, 1983.

Grabb, W.C., and Smith, J.W., editors: Plastic surgery, ed. 3, Boston, 1979, Little, Brown & Co.

Harii, K.: Microvascular tissue transfer: fundamental techniques and clinical applications, Tokyo, 1983, Igaku Shoin.

Hoopes, J.E.: Pedicle flaps: an overview. Chapter 28 in Krizek, T.J., and Hoopes, J.E., editors: Symposium on Basic Science in Plastic Surgery, St. Louis, 1976, The C.V. Mosby Co.

Smahel, J.: The healing of skin grafts, Clin. Plast. Surg. **4**:409, 1977.

CHAPTER 35
Care of the Acutely Injured Patient

Ballinger, W.F., Zuidema, G.D., and Rutherford, R.B.: The management of trauma, ed. 4, Philadelphia, 1984, W.B. Saunders Co.

Shires, G.T.: Care of the trauma patient, ed. 3, New York, 1984, Blakiston Division, McGraw-Hill Book Co.

Walt, A.J., editor: Early care of the injured patient, American College of Surgeons, Committee on Trauma, ed. 3, Philadelphia, 1982, W.B. Saunders Co.

CHAPTER 36
Transplantation

Borel, J.F., and Lafferty, K.J.: Basic science summation (cyclosporine), Transplant. Proc. **15**:3097, 1983.

Calne, R.Y., editor: Liver transplantation, New York, 1983, Grune & Stratton, Inc.

Jamieson, S.W., Baldwin, J., Stinson, E.B., et al.: Clinical heart-lung transplantation, Transplantation **37**:81, 1984.

Lafferty, K.J., Prowse, S.J., and Simeonovic, C.J.: Immunobiology of tissue transplantation: A return to the passenger leukocyte concept. Annu. Rev. Immunol. **1**:143, 1983.

Morris, P.J. editor: Kidney transplantation: principles and practice, New York, 1984, Grune & Stratton, Inc.

Najarian, J.S., and Simmons, R.L.: Transplantation, Philadelphia, 1972, Lea & Febiger.

Penn, I.: The price of immunotherapy, Curr. Probl. Surg. **18**(11):681, 1981.

Shumway, N.E.: Recent advances in cardiac transplantation, Transplant. Proc. **15**:1221, 1983.

Starzl, T.E., Iwatsuki, S., Van Thiel, D.H., et al.: Evolution of liver transplantation, Hepatology **2**(5):614, 1982.

Starzl, T.E., Hakala, T.R., Shaw, B.W., et al: A flexible procedure for multiple cadaveric organ procurement, Surg. Gynecol. Obstet. **158**:223, 1984.

Sutherland, D.E.R.: Pancreas transplantation: overview and current status of cases reported to the registry through 1982, Transplant. Proc. **15**:2597, 1983.

Veith, F.J., Kamholz, S.L., Mollenkopf, F.P., and Montefusco, C.M.: Lung transplantation 1983, Transplantation **35**:271, 1983.

Washer, G.F., Schröter, G.P.J., Starzl, T.E., and Weil, R., III: Causes of death after kidney transplantation, J.A.M.A. **250**:49, 1983.

CHAPTER 37
Thermal Injuries

Achauer, B.M., Allyn, P.A., Furnas, D.W., and Bartlett, R.H.: Pulmonary complications of burns: the major threat to the burn patient, Ann. Surg. **177**:311, 1973.

Andreasen, N.J.C., Noyes, R., Jr., Hartford, C.E., Brodland, G., and Proctor, S.: Management of emotional reactions in seriously burned adults, N. Engl. J. Med. **286**:65, 1972.

Artz, C.P., Moncrief, J.A., and Pruitt, B.A., Jr.: Burns: a team approach, Philadelphia, 1979, W.B. Saunders Co.

Bromberg, B.E., and Song, I.C.: Homografts and heterografts as skin substitutes, Am. J. Surg. **112**:28, 1966.

Burke, J.F., Bondoc, C.C., and Quinby, W.C.: Primary burn excision and immediate grafting: a method shortening illness, J. Trauma **14**:389, 1974.

Collentine, G.E., Waisbren, B.A., and Mellender, J.W.: Treatment of burns with intensive antibiotic therapy and exposure, J.A.M.A. **200**:939, 1967.

Colocho, G., Graham, W.P., III, Greene, A. E., Matheson, D.W., and Lynch, D.: Human amniotic membrane as a physiologic wound dressing, Arch. Surg. **109**:370, 1974.

Curreri, P.W., Asch, M.J., and Pruitt, B.A.: The treatment of chemical burns: specialized diagnostic, therapeutic, and prognostic considerations, J. Trauma **10**:634, 1970.

Evans, E.B., Larson, D.L., Abston, S., and Willis, B.: Prevention and correction of deformity after severe burns, Surg. Clin. North Am. **50**:1361, 1970.

Foley, F.D.: Pathology of cutaneous burns, Surg. Clin. North Am. **50**:1201, 1970.

Hartford, C.E.: Fluid resuscitation of the burned patient. In Mason, E.E., editor: Fluid, electrolyte and nutrient therapy in surgery, Philadelphia, 1974, Lea & Febiger, p. 286.

Hartford, C.E., and Ziffren, S.E.: Electrical injury, J. Trauma **11**:331, 1971.

Jelenko, C., III: Chemicals that "burn," J. Trauma **14**:65, 1974.

Law, E.J., Kim, O.J., Stieritz, D.D., and MacMillan, B.G.: Experience with systemic candidiasis in the burned patient, J. Trauma **12**:543, 1972.

Mason, A.D., Jr., Pruitt, B.A., Jr., Lindberg, R.B., Moncrief, J.A., and Foley, F.D.: Topical Sulfamylon chemotherapy in the treatment of patients with extensive thermal burns. In Matter, P., Barclay, T.L., and Konickova, Z., editors: Research in burns, Berne, 1971, Hans Huber Medical Publisher, p. 120.

Polk, H.C., Jr., and Stone, H.H., editors: Contemporary burn management, Boston, 1971, Little, Brown & Co.

Price, P.B., Brown, C.R., King, T.C., et al.: Bacterial invasion in experimental burns, Surg. Forum **6**:64, 1955.

Pruitt, B.A., Jr., Foley, F.D., and Moncrief, J.A.: Curling's ulcer: a clinical-pathological study of 323 cases, Ann. Surg. **172**:523, 1970.

Sevitt, S.: Burn pathology and therapeutic applications, Sevenoaks, Kent, 1957, Butterworth & Co., Ltd.

Stone, H.H., and Humphrey, C.P.: Burn septicemia—a clinical and bacteriological study. In Matter, P., Barclay, T.L., and Konickova, Z., editors: Research in burns, Berne, 1971, Hans Huber Medical Publisher, p. 201.

Teplitz, C.: Pathogenesis of pseudomonas vasculitis and septic lesions, Arch. Pathol. **80**:297, 1965.

Whitesides, T.E., Jr., Haney, T.C., Harada, H., Holmes, H.E., and Morimoto, K.: A simple method for tissue pressure determination, Arch. Surg. **110**:1311, 1975.

Wilmore, D.W.: Nutrition and metabolism following thermal injury, Clin. Plast. Surg. **1**:603, 1974.

CHAPTER 38
Orthopedics

American Orthopaedic Association: Manual of orthopaedic surgery, Chicago, 1966, the Association.

Blount, W.P.: Fractures in children, Baltimore, 1955, The Williams & Wilkins Co.

Brashear, H.R., and Raney, R.B.: Shand's handbook of orthopaedic surgery, ed. 9, St. Louis, 1978, The C.V. Mosby Co.

Cooper, R.: Fractures in children: fundamentals of management, J. Iowa Med. Soc. **54**:472, 1964.

Cooper, R.: Management of common forearm fractures in children, J. Iowa Med. Soc. **54**:689, 1964.

Edmondson, A.S., and Crenshaw, A.H.: Campbell's operative orthopaedics, ed. 6, St. Louis, 1980, The C.V. Mosby Co.

Hart, V.L.: Acute osteomyelitis in children, J.A.M.A. **108**:524, 1937.

Jaffe, H.L.: Metabolic, degenerative and inflammatory diseases of bones and joints, Philadelphia, 1972, Lea & Febiger.

Larson, C.B.: Low back pain, Disease a Month, Chicago, 1957, Year Book Medical Publishers, Inc.

Lovell, W., and Winder, R.: Pediatric orthopaedics, Philadelphia, 1978, J.B. Lippincott Co.

Mercer, W., and Duthie, R.B.: Orthopedic surgery, Baltimore, 1964, The Williams & Wilkins Co.

Ponseti, I.V.: Congenital dislocation of the hip in the infant. In American Academy of Orthopaedic Surgeons: Instructional course lectures, vol. 10, Ann Arbor, 1953, J.W. Edwards.

Ponseti, I.V.: Legg-Perthes disease. Observations on the pathological changes in two cases, J. Bone Joint Surg. **38A**:739, 1956.

Ponseti, I.V., and Friedman, B.: Prognosis in idiopathic scoliosis, J. Bone Joint Surg. **32A**:381, 1950.

Ponseti, I.V., and Smoley, E.N.: Congenital club foot: the results of treatment, J. Bone Joint Surg. **45A**:261, 1963.

Rockwood, C.A., and Green, D.P.: Fractures, ed. 2, Philadelphia, 1983, J.B. Lippincott Co.

Stone, D.B., and Bonfiglio, M.: Pyogenic vertebral osteomyelitis: a diagnostic pitfall for the internist, Arch. Intern. Med. **112**:491, 1963.

Turek, S.L.: Orthopaedics: principles and their application, ed. 2, Philadelphia, 1967, J.B. Lippincott Co.

CHAPTER 39
The Hand

Beasley, R.W.: Hand injuries, Philadelphia, 1981, W.B. Saunders Co.

Boswick, J.A., Jr., editor: Current concepts in hand surgery, Philadelphia, 1983, Lea & Febiger.

Flatt, A.E.: The care of minor hand injuries, ed. 4, St. Louis, 1979, The C.V. Mosby Co.

Flynn, J.E., editor: Hand surgery, ed. 3, Baltimore, 1982, The Williams & Wilkins Co.

Kilgore, E.S., and Graham, W.P., editors: The hand: surgical and nonsurgical management, Philadelphia, 1977, Lea & Febiger.

Weeks, P.M.: Acute bone and joint injuries of the hand and wrist, St. Louis, 1981, The C.V. Mosby Co.

Weeks, P.M., and Wray, R.C.: Management of acute hand injuries: a biological approach, ed. 2, St. Louis, 1978, The C.V. Mosby Co.

CHAPTER 40
Neurological Surgery

Friedman, W.A.: Head injuries, Clin. Symp. **35**:4, 1983.

Jennet, B., and Teasdale, G.: Management of head injuries, Philadelphia, 1981, F.A. Davis Co.

Milhorat, T.H.: Pediatric neurosurgery, Philadelphia, 1978, F.A. Davis Co.

Omer, G.E., and Spinner, M.: Management of peripheral nerve problems, Philadelphia, 1980, W.B. Saunders Co.

Schneider, R.C., Kahn, E.A., Crosby, E.A., and Taren, J.A.: Correlative neurosurgery, ed. 3, Springfield, Ill., 1982, Charles C Thomas, Publisher.

Shillito, J., and Matson, D.D.: An atlas of pediatric neurosurgical operations, Philadelphia, 1982, W.B. Saunders Co.

Youmans, J.R.: Neurological surgery, ed. 2, Philadelphia, 1982, W.B. Saunders Co.

CHAPTER 41
Urology

Banner, M.P., and Pollack, H.M.: Evaluation of renal function by excretory urography, J. Urol. **124:**437, 1980.

Buchsbaum, H.J., and Schmidt, J.D.: Gynecologic and obstetric urology, ed. 2, Philadelphia, 1982, W.B. Saunders Co.

Cinman, A.C.: Genitourinary tuberculosis, Urology **20:**353, 1982.

Duckett, J.W.: Hypospadias, Urol. Clin. North Am. **8:**371, 1981.

Flocks, R.H., and Culp, D.A.: Surgical urology, ed. 4, Chicago, 1975, Year Book Medical Publishers, Inc.

Flocks, R.H., and Kadesky, M.C.: Malignant neoplasms of the kidney: an analysis of 353 patients followed five years or more, Trans. Am. Assoc. Genitourin. Surg. **49:**105, 1957.

Fonkalsrud, E.W., and Mengel, W.: The undescended testis, Chicago, 1981, Year Book Medical Publishers, Inc.

Glenn, J.F.: Urologic surgery, ed. 3, Philadelphia, 1983, Harper & Row, Publishers, Inc.

Harrison, J.H., Gittes, R.F., Perlmutter, A.D., Stamey, T.A., and Walsh, P.D.: Campbell's urology, ed. 4, Philadelphia, 1978, W.B. Saunders Co.

Javadpour, N.: The role of biologic tumor markers in testicular cancer, Cancer **45:**1775, 1980.

Johnson, D.E., and Boileau, M.A.: Genitourinary tumors: fundamental principles and surgical techniques, New York, 1982, Grune & Stratton.

Marshall, V.F.: Symposium on bladder tumors, Cancer **9:**543, 1956.

McDonald, M.W.: Current therapy for renal cell carcinoma, J. Urol. **127:**211, 1982.

Pak, C.Y.C.: Medical management of nephrolithiasis, J. Urol. **128:**1157, 1982.

Ransley, P.G.: Vesicoureteric reflux: continuing surgical dilemma, Urology **12:**246, 1978.

Ross, L.S.: Diagnosis and treatment of infertile men: a clinical perspective, J. Urol. **130:**847, 1983.

Scott, W.D., Menon, M., and Walsh, P.C.: Hormonal therapy of prostatic cancer, Cancer **45:**1929, 1980.

Walsh, P.C., and Jewett, H.J.: Radical surgery for prostatic cancer, Cancer **45:**1906, 1980.

Wein, A.J.: Classification of neurogenic voiding dysfunction, J. Urol. **125:**605, 1981.

Williams, D.I., and Johnston, J.H.: Paediatric urology, ed. 2, Sevenoaks, Kent, 1982, Butterworth & Co.

Witten, D.M., Myers, G.H., Jr., and Utz, D.C.: Emmett's clinical urography, Philadelphia, 1977, W.B. Saunders Co.

CHAPTER 42
Head and Neck Surgery

Anson, B.J., and Donaldson, J.A.: Surgical anatomy of the temporal bone and ear, Philadelphia, 1973, W.B. Saunders Co.

DeWeese, D.D., and Saunders, W.H.: Textbook of otolaryngology, ed. 5, St. Louis, 1977, The C.V. Mosby Co.

Jesse, R.H., and Fletcher, G.H.: Treatment of the neck in patients with squamous cell carcinoma of the head and neck, Cancer **39**(2 suppl.):868-872, Feb. 1977.

Jesse, R.H., and Lindberg, R.D.: The efficacy of combining radiotherapy with a surgical procedure in patients with cervical metastasis from squamous cancer of the oropharynx and hypopharynx, Cancer **35:**1163-1166, April 1975.

Paparella, M.M., and Shumrick, D.A., editors: Otolaryngology, Philadelphia, 1973, W.B. Saunders Co.

Schuller, D.E., McGuirt, W.F., Krause, C.J., et al.: Increased survival with surgery alone versus combined therapy, Laryngoscope **89**(4):582-594, April 1979.

Sessions, D.G.: Surgical pathology of cancer of the larynx and hypopharynx, Laryngoscope **86**(6):814-839, June 1976.

Shambaugh, G.D., Jr., and Glasscock, M.E., III: Surgery of the ear, ed. 3, Philadelphia, 1980, W.B. Saunders Co.

Suen, J.Y., and Myers, E.N., editors: Cancer of the head and neck, Edinburgh, 1981. Churchill Livingstone.

The Centennial Conference on Laryngeal Cancer, Toronto, Canada, May 24-31, 1974, papers presented, published in the Laryngoscope, Feb.-Nov. 1975.

CHAPTER 43
Gynecology

Creasman, W.T., Clarke-Pearson, D.L., Ashe, C., et al.: The abnormal pap smear—what to do next? Cancer **48:**515, 1981.

Cunningham, F.G., Hauth, J.C., Gilstrap, L., et al.: The bacterial pathogenesis of acute pelvic inflammatory disease, Obstet. Gynecol. **52:**161, 1978.

Danforth, D.N., Dignam, W.J., Hendricks, C.H., and Mack, J.V.S., editors: Obstetrics and gynecology, ed. 4, Philadelphia, 1982, Harper & Row Pubs, Inc.

DiSaia, P.J., and Creasman, W.T.: Clinical gynecologic Oncology, St. Louis, 1984, The C.V. Mosby Co.

DiSaia, P.J., Creasman, W.T., and Rich, W.M.: An alternative approach to early cancer of the vulva, Am. J. Obstet. Gynecol. **133:**825, 1979.

Jones, H.: Treatment of adenocarcinoma of the endometrium, Obstet. Gynecol. Surv. **30:**147, 1975.

Judd, H.L., Cleary, R.E., Creasman, W.T., et al.: Estrogen replacement therapy, Obstet. Gynecol. **58:**267, 1981.

Kolstad, P., and Stafl, A.: Atlas of colposcopy, Baltimore, 1977, University Park Press.

Mattingly, R.F.: Te Linde's operative gynecology, ed. 5, Philadelphia, 1977, J.B. Lippincott Co.

Osser, S., and Persson, K.: Epidemiologic and serodiagnostic aspects of chlamydial salpingitis, Obstet. Gynecol. **59:**206, 1982.

Reid, R.C., and Yen, S.S.C.: Premenstrual syndrome, Am. J. Obstet. Gynecol. **139:**85, 1981.

Schwarz, R.H., editor: Sexually transmitted diseases, Clin. Obstet. Gynecol. **26:**109, 1983.

Speroff, L., Glass, R.H., and Kase, N.G.: Clinical gynecologic endocrinology and infertility, ed. 3, Baltimore, 1983, The Williams & Wilkins Co.

Townsend, D.E., and Morrow, C.P.: Synopsis of gynecologic oncology, New York, 1981, John Wiley & Sons, Inc.

Wager, G.P.: Toxic shock syndrome: a review, Am. J. Obstet. Gynecol. **146:**93, 1983.

Index